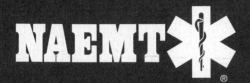

NAEMT®

In Cooperation With

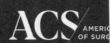ACS AMERIC... OF SURG...

M000200370

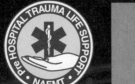

PHTLS

Prehospital Trauma Life Support

TENTH EDITION

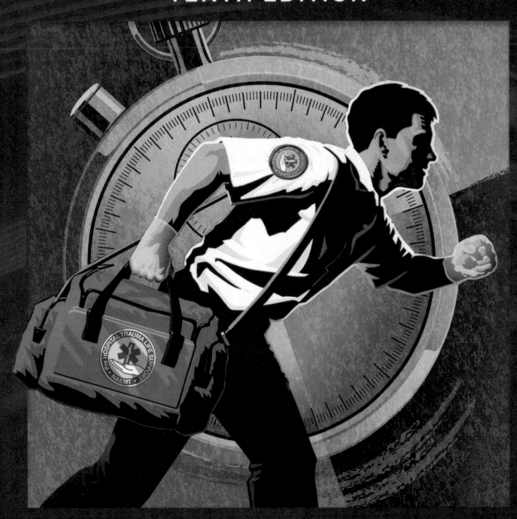

Endorsed By

east
Eastern Association for the
Surgery of Trauma

Special Operations
Medical Association

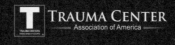
T TRAUMA CENTER
Association of America

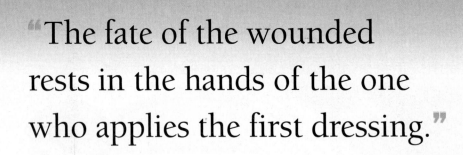

"The fate of the wounded rests in the hands of the one who applies the first dressing."

~ Nicholas Senn, MD (1844–1908)
American Surgeon (Chicago, Illinois)
Founder, Association of Military Surgeons of the United States

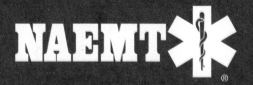

In Cooperation With

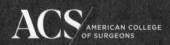

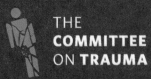

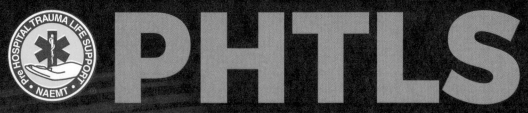

PHTLS
Prehospital Trauma Life Support

TENTH EDITION

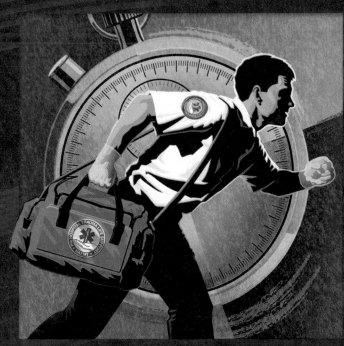

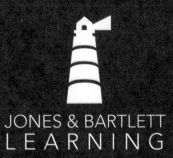

JONES & BARTLETT
LEARNING

Endorsed By

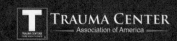

east
Eastern Association for the
Surgery of Trauma

Special Operations
Medical Association

TRAUMA CENTER
Association of America

World Headquarters
Jones & Bartlett Learning
25 Mall Road
Burlington, MA 01803
978-443-5000
info@jblearning.com
www.jblearning.com
www.psglearning.com

Jones & Bartlett Learning books and products are available through most bookstores and online booksellers. To contact the Jones & Bartlett Learning Public Safety Group directly, call 800-832-0034, fax 978-443-8000, or visit our website, www.psglearning.com.

Production Credits

Vice President, Product Management: Marisa R. Urbano
Vice President, Product Operations: Christine Emerton
Director, Product Management: Laura Carney
Director, Content Management: Donna Gridley
Manager, Content Strategy: Tiffany Sliter
Content Strategist: Ashley Procum
Content Coordinator: Mark Restuccia
Development Editor: Heather Ehlers
Director, Project Management and Content Services: Karen Scott
Manager, Project Management: Jackie Reynen
Project Manager: Madelene Nieman
Senior Digital Project Specialist: Angela Dooley
Director, Marketing: Brian Rooney

VP, International Sales, Public Safety Group: Matthew Maniscalco
Director, Sales, Public Safety Group: Brian Hendrickson
Content Services Manager: Colleen Lamy
VP, Manufacturing and Inventory Control: Therese Connell
Composition: S4Carlisle Publishing Services
Cover and Text Design: Scott Moden
Senior Media Development Editor: Troy Liston
Rights & Permissions Manager: John Rusk
Rights Specialist: Liz Kincaid
Cover Image (Title Page, Part Opener, Chapter Opener): © Ralf Hiemisch/Getty Images; © National Association of Emergency Medical Technicians (NAEMT)
Printing and Binding: LSC Communications

Library of Congress Cataloging-in-Publication Data

Names: National Association of Emergency Medical Technicians (U.S.), issuing body.
Title: PHTLS: prehospital trauma life support / National Association of Emergency Medical Technicians (NAEMT).
Other titles: PHTLS (1986) | Prehospital trauma life support
Description: Tenth edition. | Burlington, Massachusetts : Jones & Bartlett Learning, [2023] | Includes bibliographical references and index.
Identifiers: LCCN 2022007832 | ISBN 9781284264746 (paperback)
Subjects: MESH: Wounds and Injuries--therapy | Advanced Trauma Life Support Care | First Aid--methods | Emergency Medical Services | Emergencies | Traumatology
Classification: LCC RC86.7 | NLM WO 700 | DDC 616.02/5--dc23/eng/20220613
LC record available at https://lccn.loc.gov/2022007832

6048

Printed in the United States of America
26 25 24 23 22   10 9 8 7 6 5 4 3 2 1

Brief Contents

Table of Contents

Division 2 Assessment and Management 47

Chapter 3 Shock: Pathophysiology of Life and Death 49

Chapter 4 The Physics of Trauma 103

Chapter 5 Scene Management 149

Chapter 13 Burn Injuries   431

Chapter 14 Pediatric Trauma   461

Chapter 15 Geriatric Trauma   493

Division 4 Prevention   513

Chapter 16 Injury Prevention   515

Division 5 Mass Casualties and Terrorism   537

Chapter 17 Disaster Management   539

Chapter 18 Explosions and Weapons of Mass Destruction   565

Division 6 Special Considerations   603

Chapter 19 Environmental Trauma I: Heat and Cold   605

Chapter 20 Environmental Trauma II: Lightning, Drowning, Diving, and Altitude   653

Chapter 21 Wilderness Trauma Care   697

Chapter 22 Civilian Tactical Emergency Medical Support (TEMS)   735

Specific Skills Table of Contents

Acknowledgments

Contributors

Medical Editor–Tenth Edition

Andrew N. Pollak, MD, FAAOS
The James Lawrence Kernan Professor and Chairman
Department of Orthopaedics
University of Maryland School of Medicine
Chief Clinical Officer
University of Maryland Medical System
Medical Director Baltimore County Fire Department
Special Deputy U.S. Marshal
Baltimore, Maryland

Editor–Military Edition

Frank K. Butler Jr., MD
Capt, MC, USN (Retired)
Chairperson
Committee on Tactical Combat Casualty Care
Joint Trauma System
Pensacola, Florida

Chapter Editors

Heidi Abraham, MD, EMT-B, EMT-T, FAEMS
Deputy Medical Director Austin/Travis County Office of the Chief Medical Officer
Austin, Texas
Medical Director New Braunfels Fire Department
New Braunfels, Texas

Faizan H. Arshad, MD
Section Chief, Division of EMS
EMS Medical Director—Vassar EMS part of NuVance Health
Asst Residency Program Director—Dept of Emergency Medicine
USAF-R Flight Commander—Critical Care Air Transport Team
Evaluations Subcommittee Chair, Hudson Valley REMAC, New York
Host and Producer of EMS Nation Podcast
Hudson Valley, New York

Robert D. Barraco, MD, MPH, FACS, FCCP
Chief Academic Officer
Lehigh Valley Health Network
Associate Dean for Educational Affairs
USF Health Morsani College of Medicine–Lehigh Valley
Allentown, Pennsylvania

Thomas Colvin, NREMT-P
Firefighter/Paramedic
Houston Fire Department
Houston, Texas

Alexander L. Eastman, MD, MPH, FACS, FAEMS
Senior Medical Officer—Operations
Medical Operations/Office of the Chief Medical Officer
Countering Weapons of Mass Destruction Office
U.S. Department of Homeland Security
Tactical Medical Director, NAEMT Prehospital Trauma Committee
Washington, D.C.

Emily Esposito, DO
Assistant Professor, Department of Emergency Medicine
University of Maryland School of Medicine
R Adams Cowley Shock Trauma Center
Baltimore, Maryland

Samuel M. Galvagno Jr., DO, PhD, MS, FCCM
Professor and Executive Vice Chair
Department of Anesthesiology
University of Maryland School of Medicine
State Medical Director, Critical Care Coordination Center (C4), Maryland Institute for Emergency Medical Services Systems
Baltimore, Maryland

Mark Gestring, MD, FACS
Medical Director, Kessler Trauma Center
Chief, Acute Care Surgery Division
Professor of Surgery, Emergency Medicine and Pediatrics
University of Rochester School of Medicine
Rochester, New York

Jennifer M. Gurney, MD, FACS
COL, MC, U.S. Army
Surgeon, U.S. Army Institute of Surgical Research
Chief, Defense Committee on Trauma and Chair, Committee on Surgical Combat Casualty Care, Joint Trauma System
San Antonio, Texas

Danielle Hashmi, DO, MS
Trauma/Burn/Surgical Critical Care
Crozer Chester Medical Center
Upland, Pennsylvania

Seth C. Hawkins, MD
Associate Professor of Emergency Medicine, Wake Forest University
Medical Director, Western Piedmont Community College Emergency Services Programs
Medical Director, North Carolina State Parks
Medical Director, National Association for Search & Rescue
Medical Director, Landmark Learning
Chief, Appalachian Mountain Rescue Team
Morganton, North Carolina

Nancy Hoffmann, MSW
Senior Director, Education Publishing
National Association of Emergency Medical Technicians
Hopkinton, New Hampshire

Michael Holtz, MD
Clinical Assistant Professor of Emergency Medicine
UNLV School of Medicine
Las Vegas, Nevada

Jay Johannigman, MD, FACS
Chief Medical Officer
Knight Aerospace's
Trauma Surgeon
Brooke Army Medical Center
San Antonio, Texas

Brandon Kelly, MD
Orthopedic Surgery Resident
University of Minnesota
Minneapolis, Minnesota

Spogmai Komak, MD, FACS
Assistant Professor, Department
of Surgery
McGovern Medical School
University of Texas Health—Houston
Houston, Texas

Matthew J. Levy, DO, MSc
Deputy Director of Special Operations
Associate EMS Fellowship Director
Associate Professor of Emergency
Medicine
Johns Hopkins University School of
Medicine
Baltimore, Maryland

Angel Ramon Lopez, MD
General and Trauma Surgeon
Trauma Medical Director
Yuma Regional Medical Center
Yuma, Arizona

Anthony Loria, MD
Department of Surgery, Emergency
Medicine and Pediatrics
University of Rochester School of
Medicine
Rochester, New York

Steven C. Ludwig, MD
Professor of Orthopaedics
Chief of the Division of Spine Surgery
Spine Surgery Fellowship Director
Department of Orthopaedics
University of Maryland Medical Center
Baltimore, Maryland

Angela Lumba-Brown, MD
Associate Professor and Associate Vice
Chair
Department of Emergency Medicine
Stanford University School of Medicine
Co-Director, Stanford Brain Performance
Center
Palo Alto, California

Faroukh Mehkri, DO
Assistant Professor
Division of Emergency Medical Services
Department of Emergency Medicine
University of Texas at Southwestern
Medical Center at Dallas
Deputy Medical Director, Dallas Fire
Rescue
Police Officer & Tactical Physician, Dallas
SWAT
Dallas Police Department
Dallas, Texas

Vince Mosesso, MD, FACEP, FAEMS
Professor of Emergency Medicine
Associate Chief, Division of EMS
University of Pittsburgh School of Medicine
Medical Director, UPMC Prehospital Care
Medical Director, NAEMT Advanced
Medical Life
Support Committee
Pittsburgh, Pennsylvania

Jessica A. Naiditch, MD, FACS
Trauma Medical Director
Dell Children's Medical Center of
Central Texas
Assistant Professor of Surgery &
Perioperative Care
Dell Medical School
University of Texas—Austin
Austin, Texas

Daniel P. Nogee, MD, MHS
Medical Toxicology Fellow
Department of Emergency Medicine
Emory University School of Medicine
Atlanta, Georgia

Jean-Cyrille Pitteloud, MD
Head of Anesthesiology, HJBE Hospital
Bern County, Switzerland
EMS Medical Director, Jura County
Switzerland
At-Large Member, NAEMT Prehospital
Trauma Committee
Sion, Switzerland

Christine Ramirez, MD, FACS
Acute Care Surgeon
Associate Chief Medical Information
Officer
St. Luke's University Health Network
Clinical Assistant Professor of Surgery
Department of Surgery, Lewis Katz School
of Medicine at Temple University
Philadelphia, Pennsylvania

**Katherine Remick, MD, FAAP,
FACEP, FAEMS**
Medical Director, San Marcos Hays
County EMS System
Executive Lead, National EMS
for Children Innovation and
Improvement Center
Associate Professor, Departments of
Pediatrics and Surgery, Dell Medical
School at the University of Texas at
Austin
EMS Director, Pediatric Emergency
Medicine Fellowship, Dell Medical
School
Medical Director, NAEMT Emergency
Pediatric Care Committee
Austin, Texas

Christopher H. Renninger, MD
Orthopaedic Traumatology
Chief, Orthopaedic Trauma, Tumor and
Foot & Ankle Surgery
Walter Reed National Military Medical
Center
Bethesda, Maryland

Thomas Scalea, MD
Physician in Chief, R Adams Cowley
Shock Trauma Center
Distinguished Francis X Kelly Professor
of Trauma
University of Maryland School of
Medicine
Baltimore, Maryland

Andrew Schmidt, MD
Chair, Department of Orthopaedic Surgery
Hennepin Healthcare
Professor, Department of Orthopaedic
Surgery
University of Minnesota
Minneapolis, Minnesota

Justin R. Sempsrott, MD, FAAEM
Executive Director, Lifeguards Without
Borders
Director, International Drowning
Researchers' Alliance
Kuna, Idaho

Jesse Shriki, DO, MS, FACEP
Department of Critical Care
Vice Chair of Quality and Safety,
Department of Medicine
Assistant Clinical Professor, Creighton
University
Omaha, Nebraska

**R. Bryan Simon, RN, MSc,
DiMM, FAWM**
Co-owner of Vertical Medicine Resources
Owner, Peripatetic Solutions
Director, New River Alliance of Climbers
Associate Editor, Medical Screening for
Outdoor Activities
Fayetteville, West Virginia

Gerard Slobogean, MD, MPH, FRCSC
Associate Professor
Director of Clinical Research
Department of Orthopaedics
University of Maryland School of Medicine
R Adams Cowley Shock Trauma Center
Baltimore, Maryland

Will Smith, MD, Paramedic, FAEMS
Medical Director, Teton County
  Search and Rescue, Grand Teton
  National Park, Jackson Hole Fire/
  EMS, USFS-BTNF
Clinical Assistant Professor, University
  of Washington School of Medicine
Colonel, MC, U.S. Army Reserve—
  62A (EMS and Emergency Medicine)
Emergency Medicine, St. John's Health
Jackson, Wyoming

Deborah M. Stein, MD, MPH
Professor of Surgery
University of Maryland School of
  Medicine
Director for Critical Care Services
University of Maryland Medical Center
Baltimore, Maryland

Alexandra E. Thomson, MD, MPH
Spine Research Fellow
Department of Orthopaedics, Spine
  Division
University of Maryland School of
  Medicine
Baltimore, Maryland

John Trentini, MD, PhD, FAWM
Major, USAF, MC
United States Air Force
Las Vegas, Nevada

David Tuggle, MD, FACS, FAAP
Associate Trauma Medical Director
Dell Children's Medical Center in Texas
Former Vice-Chair of Surgery and Chief
  of Pediatric Surgery, OU Medical Center
Austin, Texas

Brian H. Williams, MD, FACS
Professor of Trauma and Acute Care
  Surgery
University of Chicago Medicine
Robert Wood Johnson Foundation
  Health Policy Fellow
National Academy of Medicine
Chicago, Illinois

Kelsey Wise, MD
Orthopedic Surgery Resident
University of Minnesota
Minneapolis, Minnesota

Ivan B. Ye, MD
Spine Research Fellow
Department of Orthopaedics, Spine
  Division
University of Maryland School of
  Medicine
Baltimore, Maryland

National Association of Emergency Medical Technicians 2022 Board of Directors Officers

President: Bruce Evans, MPA, NRP,
  CFO, SPO
President-elect: Susan Bailey, MSEM,
  NRP
Secretary: Troy Tuke, RN, NRP
Treasurer: Christopher Way, BA,
  Paramedic
Immediate Past President: Matt
  Zavadsky, MS-HSA, NREMT

Directors:
Region I:
Robert Luckritz, NRP, Esq.
Steven Kroll, MHA, EMT
Region II:
Melissa McNally, MMSC, BCEM,
  PA-C, NRP
Juan Cardona, MPA, NRP
Region III:
Garrett Hedeen, MHA, Paramedic
David Edgar, MHA, CCP
Region IV:
Macara Trusty, MS, LP
Karen L. Larsen, DNP, MSN, APRN,
  NP-C, CEN, CFRN, CPEN, FP-C,
  Paramedic
At-Large:
Allison G. S. Knox, MPH, MA, EMT-B
Maria Beermann-Foat, PhD, MBA, NRP
Medical Director:
Douglas F. Kupas, MD, FAEMS, FACEP

PHTLS–Medical Directors

Warren Dorlac, MD, FACS
PHTLS Medical Director
Col (Retired), USAF, MC, FS
Medical Director, Trauma and Acute
  Care Surgery
Medical Center of the Rockies
Loveland, Colorado

Margaret M. Morgan, MD, FACS
PHTLS Associate Medical Director
Medical Director, Perioperative Services
UC Health Memorial
Colorado Springs, Colorado

PHT Committee

Dennis W. Rowe, EMT-P
Chair, PHT Committee
Director of Government and Industry
  Relations
Priority Ambulance
Knoxville, Tennessee

**Alexander L. Eastman, MD, MPH,
  FACS**
Tactical Medical Director
Senior Medical Officer—Operations
Medical Operations/Office of the Chief
  Medical Officer
Countering Weapons of Mass
  Destruction Office
U.S. Department of Homeland Security
Washington, D.C.

Frank K. Butler Jr., MD
Military Medical Advisor, PHT
  Committee
CAPT, MC, USN (Retired)
Tactical Combat Casualty Care
  Consultant to the Joint Trauma
  System
Pensacola, Florida

Jean-Cyrille Pitteloud, MD
At-Large Member, PHT Committee
Head of Anesthesiology, HJBE Hospital
  Bern County, Switzerland
EMS Medical Director, Jura County
  Switzerland
Sion, Switzerland

**Anthony S. Harbour, BSN, MEd,
  RN, NRP**
Member, PHT Committee
Acute Care/EMS Educator, Center for
  Trauma and Critical Care Education
Virginia Commonwealth University,
  School of Medicine
Richmond, Virginia
Paramedic/Quality Assurance &
  Performance Improvement
  Committee
Goochland County Department of Fire-
  Rescue and Emergency Services
Goochland, Virginia

**Jim McKendry, BSc, MEM, ACP
  (Retired)**
Member, PHT Committee
Winnipeg, Manitoba, Canada

Joanne Piccininni, MBA, NRP, MICP
Member, PHT Committee
Program Director, Assistant Professor
Bergen Community College Paramedic
  Science Program
Lyndhurst, New Jersey

Brian Simonson, MBA, NRP, CHEC
Member, PHT Committee
SERAC Trauma Coordinator
Novant New Hanover Regional Medical
  Center
Wilmington, North Carolina

Reviewers

Tenth Edition Reviewers

William Armonaitis, DHPE, MS, NRP, NCEE
University Hospital EMS
Newark, New Jersey

Ryan Batenhorst, MEd, NRP
Creighton University
Omaha, Nebraska

Shawn Bjarnson, AEMT
EMS Instructor
Retired Law Enforcement Officer
Gunnison Valley Hospital
Gunnison, Utah

Mark A. Boisclair MPA, NRP
EMS Education
Chattahoochee Valley Community
   College
Phenix City, Alabama

Dr. Susan Braithwaite
Western Carolina University
Cullowhee, North Carolina

Edward Caballero, MBA, NRP, FP-c, CCP-c
University of Hawai'i at Kapi'olani
   Community College
Honolulu, Hawaii

Bernadette Cekuta
Dutchess Community College
Poughkeepsie, New York

Joshua Chan
Flight Paramedic
Life Link III
Minneapolis, Minnesota
EMS Educator/Paramedic
Glacial Ridge Health System
Glenwood, Minnesota

Claudia Clark, MA, NRP
Anne Arundel Community College
Arnold, Maryland

Kevin Curry, AS, NRP, CCEMTP
United Training Center
Lewiston, Maine

Charles Dixon, NRP, NCEE
Nucor Steel Berkeley
Huger, South Carolina

Joel Ellzie, BS, NRP
University of South Alabama
Mobile, Alabama

Ronald Feller Sr., BSEd, MBA, NRP
Oklahoma EMS Education
Oklahoma City, Oklahoma

John A. Flora, Firefighter/ Paramedic, EMS-I
EMS Coordinator
Urbana Fire Division
Urbana, Ohio

Victoria Gallaher, FP-C, CCP
Nauvoo Fire Protection District
Nauvoo, Illinois

Jeffery D. Gilliard, PMD, NRP, CCEMTP, FPM, MEd
EMETSEEI Institute, Inc.
Rockledge, Florida

David Glendenning
Captain/Education Coordinator
New Hanover Regional EMS
Wilmington, North Carolina

James E. Gretz, MBA, NRP, CCP-C
JeffSTAT – Jefferson Health
Philadelphia, Pennsylvania

Jason D. Haag, CCEMT-P, CIC
Upstate Medical University
Syracuse, New York

Frederick A. Haas Jr., NRP, BS
Sussex County EMS
Georgetown, Delaware

Randy Hardick, MA, NREMT-P
EMS Department Chair, Paramedic
   Program Director
Saddleback College
Mission Viejo, California

Greg P. Henington, Paramedic, FP-C, BBA, MBA
Terlingua Fire & EMS
Terlingua, Texas

Melanie Jorgenson, BLS Education Specialist
Regions Hospital EMS Education
St. Paul, Minnesota

Alan F. Kicks, BSEE
EMT/BLS/PHTLS Instructor
Bergen County EMS Training Center
Paramus, New Jersey

Robert Loiselle, MA, NRP, IC
Patriot Ambulance Service
Flint, Michigan

Josh Lopez, MA, BS-EMS, NRP, I/C
University of New Mexico School of
   Medicine
Department of Emergency Medicine
   EMS Academy
Albuquerque, New Mexico

Michael McDonald, RN, NRP
Loudoun County Combined Fire and
   Rescue System
Leesburg, Virginia

Gregory S. Neiman, MS, NRP, NCEE
VCU Health System
Richmond, Virginia

Keito Ortiz, Paramedic, NYS CIC, NAEMSE Level II
Pre-Hospital Care Training Coordinator
Jamaica Hospital Medical Center
Queens, New York

Kevin Ramdayal
EMS Deputy Chief
FDNY EMS Training Academy
Queens, New York

Josh Steele, MBAHA, NRP, FP-C, CMTE
Hospital Wing
Memphis Medical Center Air
   Ambulance, Inc.
Memphis, Tennessee

Melissa Stoddard, MPH, NRP
Tacoma Community College
Tacoma, Washington

Brian Turner, CCEMT-P, RN
Genesis Medical Center
Davenport, Iowa

Jackilyn E. Williams, RN, MSN, NRP
Portland Community College Paramedic
   Program
Portland, Oregon

Rich Wisniewski, MA, NRP
South Carolina Department of Health
   and Environmental Control
Columbia, South Carolina

Karen "Keri" Wydner Krause RN, CCRN, EMT-P
Lakeshore Technical College
Cleveland, Wisconsin

Ninth Edition Reviewers

Alberto Adduci, MD, ED
Molinette Hospital
Turin, Italy

J. Adam Alford, BS, NRP
Old Dominion EMS Alliance
Bon Air, Virginia

Justin Arnone, BS, NRP, NCEE, TP-C
East Baton Rouge Parish EMS
Baton Rouge, Louisiana

Hector Arroyo
New York City Fire Department Bureau
of Training
Bayside, New York

Ryan Batenhorst, MEd, NRP
Southeast Community College
Lincoln, Nebraska

Nick Bourdeau, RN, Paramedic I/C
Huron Valley Ambulance
Ypsilanti, Michigan

Dr. Susan Smith Braithwaite, EdD, NRP
Western Carolina University
Cullowhee, North Carolina

Lawrence Brewer, MPH, NRP, FP-C
Rogers State University/Tulsa
LifeFlight
Claremore, Oklahoma

Aaron R. Byington, MA, NRP
Davis Technical College
Kaysville, Utah

Bernadette Cekuta
Dutchess Community College
Wappingers Falls, New York

Ted Chialtas
Fire Captain/Paramedic, Paramedic
Program Coordinator
San Diego Fire-Rescue Department
Paramedic Program
San Diego, California

Hiram Colon
New York City Fire Department Bureau
of EMS
New York, New York

Kevin Curry, AS, NRP, CCEMT-P
United Training Center
Lewiston, Maine

Charlie Dixon, NRP, NCEE
Nucor Steel Berkeley
Huger, South Carolina

John A. Flora, FF/Paramedic, EMS-I
Urbana Fire Division
Urbana, Ohio

Fidel O. Garcia, EMT-P
Professional EMS Education
Grand Junction, Colorado

Jeff Gilliard, NRP/CCEMT-P/FPC, BS
President/CEO, Central Florida Office
Emergency Medical Education &
Technology Systems Inc.
Rockledge, Florida

David Glendenning, EMT-P
Education & Outreach Officer
New Hanover Regional EMS
Wilmington, North Carolina

Conrad M. Gonzales, Jr., NREMT-P
San Antonio Fire Department (retired)
San Antonio, Texas

David M. Gray, BS, EMTP-IC
Knoxville Fire Department
Knoxville, Tennessee

Jamie Gray, BS, AAS, FF, NRP (NAEMT/NAEMSE/ATOA)
State of Alabama Office of EMS
Montgomery, Alabama

Kevin M. Gurney, MS, CCEMT-P, I/C
Delta Ambulance
Waterville, Maine

Jason D. Haag, CCEMT-P, CIC, Tactical Medic
Finger Lakes Ambulance
Clifton Springs, New York
Wayne County Advanced Life
Support Services
Marion, New York
Finger Lakes Regional Emergency
Medical Services Council
Geneva, New York

Poul Anders Hansen, MD
Medical Director
EMS North Denmark Region
Chairman PHTLS Denmark

Anthony S. Harbour, BSN, MEd, RN, NRP
Executive Director

Southern Virginia Emergency Medical
Services
Roanoke, Virginia

Brad Haywood, NRP, FP-C, CCP-C
Fairfax County Fire and Rescue
Academy
Fairfax, Virginia

Greg Henington
Terlingua Fire & EMS
Terlingua, Texas

Paul Hitchcock, NRP
Front Royal, Virginia

Sandra Hultz, NREMT-P
Holmes Community College
Ridgeland, Mississippi

Joseph Hurlburt, BS, NREMT-P, EMT-P I/C
Instructor Coordinator/Training Officer
Rapid Response EMS
Romulus, Michigan

Melanie Jorgenson
Regions Hospital EMS
Oakdale, Minnesota

Travis L. Karicofe, NREMT-P
EMS Officer
City of Harrisonburg Fire Department
Harrisonburg, Virginia

Brian Katcher NRP, FP-C
Warrenton, Virginia

Alan F. Kicks, EMT
PHTLS Instructor
Bergen County EMS Training Center
Paramus, New Jersey

Jared Kimball, NRP
Tulane Trauma Education
New Orleans, Louisiana

Timothy M. Kimble, AAS, NRP
Education Coordinator
Carilion Clinic Life Support Training
Center
Craig County Emergency Services
New Castle, Virginia

Don Kimlicka, NRP, CCEMT-P
Executive Director
Clintonville Area Ambulance Service
Clintonville, Wisconsin

Jim Ladle, BS, FP-C, CCP-C
South Jordan City Fire Department
South Jordan, Utah

Frankie S. Lobner
Mountain Lakes Regional EMS Council
Queensbury, New York

Robert Loiselle, MA, NRP, EMSIC
Bay City, Michigan

Joshua Lopez, BS-EMS, NRP
University of New Mexico EMS
    Academy
Albuquerque, New Mexico

Kevin M. Lynch, NREMT, NYS CIC
Greenburgh Police Department: EMS
White Plains, New York

Christopher Maeder, BA, EMT-P
Chief
Fairview Fire District
Fairview, New York

Jeanette S. Mann, BSN, RN, NRP
Director of EMS Programs
Dabney S. Lancaster Community College
Clifton Forge, Virginia

Michael McDonald, RN, NRP
Loudoun County Fire Rescue
Leesburg, Virginia

Jeff McPhearson, NRP
Southside Regional Medical Center
Petersburg, Virginia

David R. Murack, NREMT-P, CCP
EMS Educator
Lakeshore Technical College
Assistant Chief of Emergency Operations
City of Two Rivers Fire/Rescue
Cleveland, Wisconsin

**Stephen Nacy, FP-C, TP-C, CCEMT-P,
    NRP, DMT**
Leesburg, Virginia

**Gregory S. Neiman, MS, NRP, NCEE,
    CEMA(VA)**
VCU Health System
Richmond, Virginia

Norma Pancake, BS, MEP, NREMT-P
Pierce County EMS
Tacoma, Washington

Deb Petty
St. Charles County Ambulance District
St. Peter's, Missouri

Mark Podgwaite, NECEMS I/C
Waterbury Ambulance Service
Waterbury, Vermont

Jonathan R. Powell, BS, NRP
University of South Alabama
Mobile, Alabama

Kevin Ramdayal
New York City Fire Department Bureau
    of EMS
New York, New York

**Christoph Redelsteiner, PhD, MSW,
    MS, EMT-P**
Academic Director Social Work (MA)
Danube University, Krems Austria
Scientific Director
Emergency Health Services Management
    Program
University of Applied Sciences St. Pölten

Les Remington, EMT-P, I/C, FI1
EMS Educator, Trauma Course
    Coordinator Genesys EMS and
    Employee Education
Grand Blanc, Michigan

Ian T.T. Santee, MPA, MICT
City and County of Honolulu
Honolulu, Hawaii

Edward Schauster, NREMT-P
Air Idaho Rescue
Idaho Falls, Idaho

Justin Schindler, BS, NRP
Monroe Ambulance
Rochester, New York

**Kimberly Singleton, APRN, MSN,
    FNP-C**
Gwinnett Medical Center
Lawrenceville, Georgia

Jennifer TeWinkel Smith, BA, AEMT
Regions Hospital Emergency Medical
    Services
Oakdale, Minnesota

**Josh Steele, MBAHA, BS, AAS, NRP,
    FP-C, I/C**
Hospital Wing (Memphis Medical Center
    Air Ambulance, Inc.)
Memphis, Tennessee

Richard Stump, NRP
Central Carolina Community College
Erwin, North Carolina

William Torres, Jr., NRP
Marcus Daly Memorial Hospital
Hamilton, Montana

Brian Turner, CCEMT-P, RN
Genesis Medical Center
Davenport, Iowa

Scott Vanderkooi, BS, NRP
Department of EMS Education
University of South Alabama
Mobile, Alabama

Gary S. Walter, NRP, BA, MS
Union College
International Rescue & Relief
Lincoln, Nebraska

Mitchell R. Warren, NRP
Children's Hospital and Medical
    Center
Omaha, Nebraska

David Watson, NRP, CCEMT-P, FP-C
Pickens County EMS
Pickens, South Carolina

Jackilyn E. Williams, RN, MSN, NRP
Portland Community College Paramedic
    Program
Portland, Oregon

Earl M. Wilson, III, BIS, NREMT-P
Nunez Community College
Chalmette, Louisiana

Rich Wisniewski, BS, NRP
Columbia, South Carolina

**Karen "Keri" Wydner Krause, RN,
    CCRN, EMT-P**
Lakeshore Technical College
Cleveland, Wisconsin

Dawn Young
Bossier Parish School for Technology
    and Innovative Learning
Bossier City, Louisiana

Photoshoot Acknowledgments
We would like to thank the following
    people and institutions for their
    collaboration on the photoshoot for
    this project. Their assistance was
    appreciated greatly.

**Technical Consultants and
    Institutions**
UMass Memorial Paramedics,
    Worcester EMS
Worcester, Massachusetts

Richard A. Nydam, AS, NREMT-P
Training and Education Specialist, EMS
UMass Memorial Paramedics, Worcester
    EMS
Worcester, Massachusetts

Southbridge Fire Department
Southbridge, Massachusetts

Jerry Flanagan
Account Manager
BoundTree Medical
Dublin, Ohio

Foreword

It is an honor to recognize the significant accomplishments of the Prehospital Trauma Life Support (PHTLS) program with the launch of the 10th Edition of the PHTLS textbook. For over 40 years, PHTLS has been the gold standard for training EMS professionals in the latest strategies to minimize death and disability after severe injury. Thanks to the long-standing collaboration between the National Association of Emergency Medical Technicians (NAEMT) and the American College of Surgeons (ACS) Committee on Trauma (COT), the PHTLS course has evolved in parallel to the Advanced Trauma Life Support (ATLS) program, ensuring seamless care of patients from the prehospital to hospital environment.

This year, as the ACS Committee on Trauma celebrates our Centennial, we reflect on the history of the evolution of EMS in the United States. Optimizing the prehospital care of injured patients has been a priority of the ACS since 1922 when Transportation of the Injured was established as one of the first subcommittees of the original ACS Committee on Fractures. In the 1950s and 60s, surgeons of the COT developed standards for ambulance equipment and for the training of ambulance personnel and first responders in basic trauma care. As EMS systems began to develop, Norman E. McSwain Jr., MD, FACS, a founding member of NAEMT and Chair of the ACS COT's Subcommittee on Emergency Services Prehospital (1981–1986), saw the need for a comprehensive education program for prehospital providers comparable to the ATLS course, and so PHTLS was born.

Like ATLS, PHTLS has grown exponentially into a global program taught across the world as a uniform, evidence-based approach to care for the most critically injured. PHTLS has expanded to support both civilian and military prehospital care and has been instrumental in the implementation of the Tactical Combat Casualty Care guidelines developed during the wars in Iraq and Afghanistan. In return, lessons learned in the care of combat casualties have enhanced the care of civilian trauma patients.

This edition of PHTLS also incorporates the recently updated 2021 National Guidelines for the Field Triage of Injured Patients, which recognize the critical importance of the triage decisions of EMS clinicians in ensuring the right patient receives the right level of care in the right amount of time. EMS is the first link in the chain of survival for critically injured patients and the portal of entry into our trauma systems.

Dr. McSwain taught us, *"Trauma is a surgical disease from beginning to end. Trauma begins when the incident occurs. Trauma care begins when the first emergency medical technician or first responder arrives on the scene, not when the patient arrives at the hospital. At least half of the care provided in the golden hour is in the hands of the [paramedics and] EMTs. Trauma is a team effort and EMS is a critical part of that team."* (Scudder Oration on Trauma, 2003)

This 10th Edition of PHTLS ensures a standardized approach to the immediate care of these patients, which will save lives and support optimal outcomes for all those impacted by traumatic injury.

Eileen M. Bulger, MD, FACS
Medical Director of Trauma Programs
American College of Surgeons
Professor of Surgery & Chief of Trauma
Harborview Medical Center, University of Washington

Preface

PHTLS Textbook Development Philosophy

When we began to develop the 10th edition of this textbook, we very purposefully intended it to serve as a resource. However, we did not want it to be merely a resource that just sits on a shelf for when questions arise. We also did not want it to simply serve as the academic medicine that supports the PHTLS course. We wanted this book to be something that prehospital trauma practitioners read and then use to begin or to sustain a lifelong journey through the literature. And we wanted to provide them with a way to prepare.

When taking care of trauma victims, it is necessary to have a plan. That plan can be based on local protocols, jurisdictional algorithms, or even nationally driven standards. But as famous boxer Mike Tyson once said, *"Everyone has a plan until they get punched in the mouth."* Trauma often represents that punch in the mouth. The punch may knock your plan out from under you, but a solid foundation of knowledge and critical thinking prepares you for the unexpected.

Patients present with different challenges in different scenarios, and being prepared for the unexpected requires knowledge and reading. Being prepared requires learning from the mistakes and successes of others and requires understanding the literature written about those mistakes or successes. Whether in architecture, surgery, or prehospital trauma care, understanding the literature begins with thoroughly reading textbooks and continues with using the references in those books to delve further into the journal articles, textbook chapters, and further readings that comprise the supporting evidence.

Preparing for anything involves reading the history of what others have done before in similar situations and what they have learned. Former Marine Corps General and former Secretary of Defense James Mattis has advocated for continual preparation through reading. He argues that every problem warriors are likely to face in battle has likely been faced previously and has likely already been described in the literature. He further argues that preparing for battle by voraciously reading this literature is the solemn obligation of every warrior. You could certainly make an argument that the same is true in trauma care. Whatever constellation of injuries a patient presents with, it is highly likely that trauma victims have presented with similar injuries in the past. It is also highly likely that someone has already written about what worked and what didn't work in the care of such a patient. Gen. Mattis is famously quoted as having said, *"'Winging it' and filling body bags as we sort out what works reminds us of the moral dictates and the cost of incompetence in our profession."* While he intended for that statement to apply to performing the job of leading soldiers into battle, it certainly applies equally well to the task of caring for the injured. We cannot afford to 'wing it' when patients' lives are at stake.

In addition to serving as an important general resource for the trauma practitioner, this book is also intended to help prepare and guide students through the formal PHTLS course. While studying trauma care and the science behind it is critically important, so too is training. Prehospital trauma care practitioners must consistently and frequently practice their skills and be thoroughly prepared to perform those skills under stressful situations.

Ancient Greek poet and mercenary Archilochus wrote, *"We don't rise to the level of our expectations, we fall to the level of our training."* He, too, was referring to performance of warriors in battle, but the quote applies equally to the response of trauma care practitioners in the care of injured patients. Understanding the skills we perform and developing the muscle memory necessary to apply those skills perfectly under duress must also be part of every prehospital care practitioner's regular work of preparation.

It is the combination of planning, learning, and practicing that allows any practitioner to be as prepared as possible to care for trauma patients. This book is intended to be an important resource to allow practitioners to train effectively, to avoid 'winging it,' and to prepare to be punched in the mouth once or twice.

Why PHTLS?

Course Education Philosophy

Prehospital Trauma Life Support (PHTLS) focuses on principles, not preferences. By focusing on the principles of good trauma care, PHTLS promotes critical thinking. The PHT Committee of the National Association of Emergency Medical Technicians (NAEMT) believes that emergency medical services (EMS) practitioners make the best decisions on behalf of their patients when prepared with a sound foundation of key principles and evidence-based knowledge. Rote memorization of mnemonics without understanding their foundation is discouraged. Furthermore, there is no one 'PHTLS way' of performing a specific skill. The principle of the skill is taught, and then one acceptable method of performing the skill that meets the principle is presented. The authors realize that no one method can apply to the myriad unique situations encountered in the prehospital setting.

Up-to-Date Information

Development of the PHTLS program began in 1981, on the heels of the inception of the Advanced Trauma Life Support (ATLS) program for physicians. As the ATLS course is revised every 4 to 5 years, pertinent changes are incorporated into the next edition of PHTLS. This 10th edition of the PHTLS program has been revised based on the forthcoming 2022 ATLS course, the 10th edition of the ATLS textbook, discussions with members of the ACS-COT, and subsequent publications in the medical literature. Although aligned with ATLS principles, PHTLS is specifically designed to prepare learners to address the unique challenges encountered when caring for trauma outside of the hospital. All chapters have been revised and updated to reflect current evidence. Video clips of critical skills and an eBook are available online.

Scientific Base

The authors and editors have adopted an evidence-based approach that includes references from medical literature supporting the key principles, and additional position papers published by national organizations are cited when applicable. References have been added or updated, allowing those prehospital care practitioners with inquisitive minds to read the original scientific papers that form the evidentiary basis for our recommendations.

PHTLS—Commitment and Mission

As we continue to pursue the potential of the PHTLS course and the worldwide community of prehospital care practitioners, we must remember the goals and objectives of the PHTLS program:

- To provide a description of the physiology and kinematics of injury
- To provide an understanding of the need for and techniques of rapid assessment of the trauma patient
- To advance the participant's level of knowledge with regard to examination and diagnostic skills

- To enhance the participant's performance in the assessment and treatment of the trauma patient
- To advance the participant's level of competence in regard to specific prehospital trauma intervention skills
- To provide an overview and establish a management method for the prehospital care of the multisystem trauma patient
- To promote a common approach for the initiation and transition of care beginning with civilian first responders continuing up and through the levels of care until the patient is delivered to the definitive treatment facility

It is also fitting to reprise our mission statement, which was written during a marathon session at the NAEMT conference in 1997:

> *The Prehospital Trauma Life Support (PHTLS) program of the National Association of Emergency Medical Technicians (NAEMT) serves trauma victims through the global education of prehospital care providers of all levels. With medical oversight from the American College of Surgeons Committee on Trauma (ACS-COT), the PHTLS programs develop and disseminate educational materials and scientific information and promote excellence in trauma patient management by all providers involved in the delivery of prehospital care.*

The PHTLS mission also enhances the achievement of the NAEMT mission. The PHTLS program is committed to quality and performance improvement. As such, PHTLS is always attentive to changes in technology and methods of delivering prehospital trauma care that may be used to enhance the value of this program.

Support for NAEMT

NAEMT provides the administrative structure for the PHTLS program. All profits from the PHTLS program are reinvested into NAEMT to support programs that are of prime importance to EMS professionals, such as educational conferences and advocacy efforts on behalf of prehospital care practitioners and their patients.

PHTLS Is a World Leader

Because of the unprecedented success of the prior editions of PHTLS, the program has continued to grow rapidly. PHTLS courses continue to proliferate across civilian and military sectors in the United States. It has also been taught worldwide in more than 80 nations, with more countries expressing interest in PHTLS to improve prehospital trauma care.

Prehospital care practitioners have the responsibility to assimilate this knowledge and these skills in order to use them for the benefit of their patients. The editors and authors of this material and the PHT Committee of NAEMT hope that you will incorporate this information into your practice and that you will rededicate yourself to the care of trauma patients.

National Association of Emergency Medical Technicians

Founded in 1975, NAEMT is the only national organization in the United States that represents and serves the professional interests of EMS practitioners, including paramedics, emergency medical technicians, emergency medical responders, and other professionals providing prehospital and out-of-hospital emergent, urgent, or preventive medical care. NAEMT members work in all sectors of EMS, including government service agencies, fire departments, hospital-based ambulance services, private companies, industrial and special operations settings, and the military.

NAEMT serves its members by advocating on issues that impact their ability to provide quality patient care, providing high-quality education that improves the knowledge and skills of practitioners, and supporting EMS research and innovation.

One of NAEMT's principal activities is EMS education. The mission of NAEMT education programs is to improve patient care through high-quality, cost-effective, evidence-based education that strengthens and enhances the knowledge and skills of EMS practitioners.

NAEMT strives to provide the highest quality education programs. All NAEMT education programs are developed by highly experienced EMS educators, clinicians,

and medical directors. Course content incorporates the latest research, newest techniques, and innovative approaches in EMS learning. All NAEMT education programs promote critical thinking as the foundation for providing quality care. This is based on the belief that EMS practitioners make the best decisions on behalf of their patients when given a sound foundation of evidence-based knowledge and key principles.

Once developed, education programs are tested and refined to ensure that course materials are clear, accurate, and relevant to the needs of EMS practitioners. Finally, all education programs are reviewed and updated every 4 years or as needed to ensure that the content reflects the most up-to-date research and practices.

NAEMT provides ongoing support to its instructors and the EMS training centers that hold its courses. Over 2,500 training centers, including colleges, EMS agencies, fire departments, hospitals, and other medical training facilities located in the United States and more than 80 other countries, offer NAEMT education programs. NAEMT headquarters staff work with the network of education program faculty engaged as committee members; authors; national, regional, and state coordinators; and affiliate faculty to provide administrative and educational support.

Andrew N. Pollak, MD, FAAOS
Medical Editor, PHTLS
The James Lawrence Kernan Professor and Chairman
Department of Orthopaedics
University of Maryland School of Medicine
Chief Clinical Officer
University of Maryland Medical System
Medical Director Baltimore County Fire Department
Special Deputy U.S. Marshal

Dedication

This edition of PHTLS is dedicated to all the prehospital practitioners who are on the front lines of trauma care in Eastern Europe and other regions around the globe.

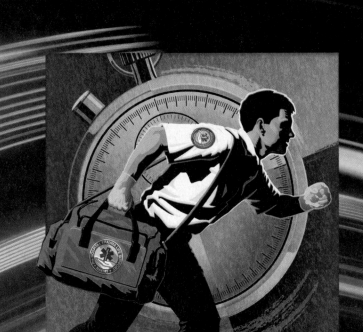

Introduction

© Ralf Hiemisch/Getty Images

CHAPTER 1

PHTLS: Past, Present, and Future

Lead Editors
Andrew N. Pollak, MD, FAAOS
Nancy Hoffmann, MSW

© Ralf Hiemisch/Getty Images

CHAPTER OBJECTIVES

At the completion of this chapter, you will be able to do the following:

- Understand the history and evolution of prehospital trauma care.
- Recognize the magnitude of the human and financial impact of traumatic injury.

- Understand the three phases of trauma care.

INTRODUCTION

Our patients did not choose us. We chose them. We could have chosen another profession, but we did not. We have accepted the responsibility for patient care in some of the worst situations—when we are tired or cold, when it is rainy and dark, when we cannot predict what conditions we will encounter. We must either accept this responsibility or surrender it. We must give to our patients the very best care that we can—not while we are daydreaming, not with unchecked equipment, not with incomplete supplies, and not with yesterday's knowledge. We cannot know what medical information is current, we cannot purport to be ready to care for our patients if we do not read and learn each day. The Prehospital Trauma Life Support (PHTLS) Course provides a part of that knowledge to the working prehospital care practitioner, but, more importantly, it ultimately benefits the person who needs our all—the patient. At the end of each run, we should feel that the patient received nothing short of our very best.

History of Trauma Care in Emergency Medical Services (EMS)

The stages and development of the management of the trauma patient can be divided into several time periods, as described by Norman McSwain, MD, in the Scudder Oration of the American College of Surgeons in 2003.[1] The four time periods described in this chapter are (1) the ancient period, (2) the Larrey period, (3) the Farrington era, and (4) the modern era. This text, the entire PHTLS Course, and care of the trauma patient are based on the principles developed and taught by the early pioneers of prehospital care. The list of these innovators is long; however, a few deserve special recognition.

Ancient Period

All of the medical care that was accomplished in Egypt, Greece, and Rome, by the Israelites, and up to the time of Napoleon is classified as premodern EMS. Most of the medical care was accomplished within some type of rudimentary medical facility; little was performed by prehospital care practitioners in the field. The most significant contribution to our knowledge of this period is the Edwin Smith Papyrus from approximately 4,500 years ago, which describes the medical care in a series of case reports.

Larrey Period (Late 1700s to Approximately 1950)

In the late 1700s, Baron Dominique Jean Larrey, Napoleon's chief military physician, recognized the need for prompt prehospital care. In 1797, he noted that "the remoteness of our ambulances deprive the wounded of the requisite attention. I was authorized to construct a carriage which I call flying ambulances."[2] He developed these horse-drawn "flying ambulances" for timely retrieval of warriors injured on the battlefield and introduced the premise that individuals working in these "flying ambulances" should be trained to provide on-scene and en route medical care for patients.

By the early 1800s, he had established the following elements of the basic theory of prehospital care that we continue to use to this day:

- Rapid transport
- Proper training of medical personnel
- Movement into the field during battle for patient care and retrieval
- Field control of hemorrhage
- Transport to a nearby hospital
- Provision of en route care
- Development of frontline hospitals
- Field triage based on severity of injury

He developed hospitals that were close to the front lines (much like the military of today) and stressed the rapid movement of patients from the field to medical care. Baron Larrey is now recognized by many as the father of EMS in the modern era.

Unfortunately, the type of care developed by Larrey was not used by the Union Army in the United States 60 years later at the beginning of the American Civil War. At the First Battle of Bull Run in August 1861, the wounded lay in the field—3,000 for 3 days, 600 for up to a week.[1] Jonathan Letterman was appointed Surgeon General and created a separate medical corps with better organized medical care (**Figure 1-1**). At the Second Battle of Bull Run 13 months later, there were 300 ambulances, and attendants collected 10,000 wounded in 24 hours.[3]

In August 1864, the International Red Cross was created at the First Geneva Convention. The convention recognized the neutrality of hospitals, of the sick and wounded, of all involved personnel, and of ambulances,

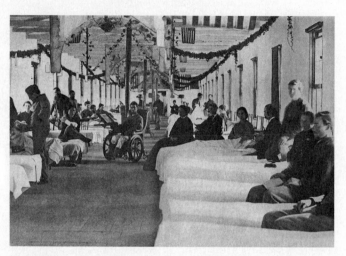

Figure 1-1 During the American Civil War, patient care practices for soldiers developed by Larrey, such as building temporary hospitals near the front lines, were put in place.
© Unknown/Alamy Stock Photo

and it guaranteed safe passage for ambulances and medical personnel to move the wounded. It also stressed the equality of medical care provided, regardless of which side of the conflict the victim was on. This convention marked the first step toward the Code of Conduct used by the U.S. military today. This Code of Conduct is an important component of the Department of Defense's Tactical Combat Casualty Care (TCCC) Course.

Hospitals, Military, and Mortuaries

In 1865, the first private ambulance service in the United States was created in Cincinnati, Ohio, at Cincinnati General Hospital.[3] Soon thereafter, several EMS systems were developed in the United States: Bellevue Hospital Ambulance[3] in New York in 1867; Grady Hospital Ambulance Service (the oldest continuously operating hospital-based ambulance) in Atlanta in the 1880s; Charity Hospital Ambulance Services in New Orleans, created in 1885 by a surgeon, Dr. A. B. Miles; and numerous other facilities in the United States. These ambulance services were run primarily by hospitals, the military, or mortuaries until 1950.[1]

In 1891, Nicholas Senn, MD, the founder of the Association of Military Surgeons, said, "The fate of the wounded rests in the hands of one who applies the first dressing." Although prehospital care was rudimentary when Dr. Senn made his statement, in many ways the words are even more true today. Care rendered and decisions made long before trauma victims reach the hospital often determine whether an injured patient will or will not survive.

Some changes in medical care occurred during the various wars up until the end of World War II, but generally the system and the type of care rendered prior to arrival at the Battalion Aid Station (Echelon II) in the military or at the back door of the civilian hospital were relatively unchanged until the mid-1950s.

During this period, many ambulances in the major cities that had teaching hospitals were staffed by interns during their first year of training. The last ambulance service to require physicians on ambulance runs was Charity Hospital in New Orleans in the 1960s. Despite the fact that physicians were present, most of the trauma care they were able to deliver was primitive. The equipment and supplies had not changed significantly from those used during the American Civil War.[1]

Farrington Era (Approximately 1950 to 1970)

The era of J. D. "Deke" Farrington, MD (1909 to 1982), began in 1950. Dr. Farrington, the father of EMS in the United States, stimulated the development of improved prehospital care with his landmark article, "Death in a Ditch."[4] In the late 1960s, Dr. Farrington and other early leaders, such as Oscar Hampton, MD, and Curtis Artz, MD, brought the United States into the modern era of EMS and prehospital care.[1] Dr. Farrington was actively involved in all aspects of ambulance care. His work as chairman of the committees that produced three of the initial documents establishing the basis of EMS—the *Essential Equipment List for Ambulances* of the American College of Surgeons Committee on Trauma,[4] the ambulance design specifications of the Department of Transportation (DOT),[5] and the first emergency medical technician (EMT) basic training program—also propelled the idea and development of prehospital care. In addition to the efforts of Dr. Farrington, others actively helped to promote the importance of prehospital care for the trauma victim. Robert Kennedy, MD, was the author of *Early Care of the Sick and Injured Patient.*[6] Sam Banks, MD, along with Dr. Farrington, taught the first prehospital training course to the Chicago Fire Department in 1957, initiating the process of educating first responders in the proper care of the trauma patient.

A 1965 text edited and compiled by George J. Curry, MD, a leader of the American College of Surgeons and its Committee on Trauma, stated:

> Injuries sustained in accidents affect every part of the human body. They range from simple abrasions and contusions to multiple complex injuries involving many body tissues. This demands efficient and intelligent primary appraisal and care, on an individual basis, before transport. It is obvious that the services of trained ambulance attendants are essential. If we are to expect maximum efficiency from ambulance attendants, a special training program must be arranged.[7]

The landmark white paper, *Accidental Death and Disability: The Neglected Disease of Modern Society,* further accelerated the process in 1967.[8] The National Academy of Sciences/National Research Council (NAS/NRC) issued this paper just 2 years after Dr. Curry's call to action.

Modern Era of Prehospital Care (Approximately 1970 to Today)

1970s

The modern era of prehospital care began with a Dunlap and Associates report to the DOT in 1968 defining the curriculum for EMT-Ambulance Training. This training later became known as EMT-Basic; it is known simply as EMT today.

The National Registry of EMTs (NREMT) was established in 1970, and it developed the standards for testing and registration of trained EMS personnel as advocated in the NAS/NRC white paper. Rocco Morando was the Executive Director of the NREMT for more than 15 years and was associated with Drs. Farrington, Hampton, and Artz.

Dr. Curry's call for specialized training of ambulance attendants *for trauma* was initially answered by using the educational program developed by Drs. Farrington and Banks in the initial development and publication of *Emergency Care and Transportation of the Sick and Injured* (the "Orange Book") by the American Academy of Orthopaedic Surgeons (AAOS), by the EMT training programs from the National Highway Traffic Safety Administration (NHTSA), and by NAEMT through the PHTLS Course. The first training efforts were primitive; however, they have progressed significantly in a relatively brief time.

The first textbook of this era was *Emergency Care and Transportation of the Sick and Injured.* It was the brainchild of Walter A. Hoyt, Jr., MD, and was published in 1971 by the AAOS.[1] The text is now in its 12th edition.

During this same period, the Glasgow Coma Scale (GCS) was developed in Glasgow, Scotland, by Dr. Graham Teasdale and Dr. Bryan Jennett for research purposes. Dr. Howard Champion brought it to the United States and incorporated it into the care of the trauma patient for assessment of the continued neurologic status of the patient.[3] The GCS is a sensitive but effectively reproducible indicator of improvement or deterioration of such patients.

In 1973, federal EMS legislation was created to promote the development of comprehensive EMS systems. The legislation identified 15 individual components that were needed to have an integrated EMS system. Dr. David Boyd, under the Department of Health and Human Services (DHHS), was placed in charge of implementing this legislation. One of these components was education. This became the basis for the development of training curricula for EMT-Basic, EMT-Intermediate, and

EMT-Paramedic care throughout the United States. Today, these levels of training are called Emergency Medical Technician (EMT), Advanced Emergency Medical Technician (AEMT), and Paramedic. The curriculum was initially defined by the DOT through the NHTSA and became known as the National Standard Curriculum or the DOT curriculum.

Dr. Nancy Caroline, an early pioneer in EMS education, defined the standards and the curriculum for the first paramedic program, and she wrote the initial textbook, *Emergency Care in the Streets*, used in the training of paramedics. This text is now in its ninth edition.

The Blue Star of Life was originally designed by the American Medical Association (AMA) as the symbol for a "Medic Alert"—an indication that a patient had an important medical condition that should be noted by EMS. Later, the AMA gave this symbol to the NREMT to use as their logo. Because the American Red Cross would not allow the "Red Cross" logo to be used on ambulances as an emergency symbol, Lew Schwartz, the chief of NHTSA's EMS branch, asked Dr. Farrington, the chairman of the NREMT board, to allow NHTSA to use the symbol for ambulances. Permission was granted by NREMT, and the Blue Star of Life has since become an international symbol of EMS systems.[1]

The National Association of Emergency Medical Technicians (NAEMT) was established in 1975 with the financial support of NREMT (**Figure 1-2**). NAEMT is the nation's only organization dedicated solely to representing the professional interests of all EMS practitioners, including paramedics, AEMTs, EMTs, emergency medical responders, and other professionals working in prehospital emergency medicine.

1980s

In the mid-1980s it became apparent that trauma patients were different from cardiac patients from the perspective of prehospital care and education. Trauma surgeons such as Frank Lewis, MD, and Donald Trunkey, MD, recognized the key distinction between these two groups: For cardiac patients, all or most of the tools needed for reestablishment of cardiac output (cardiopulmonary resuscitation [CPR], external defibrillation, and supportive medications) were available to properly trained paramedics in the field. For trauma patients, however, the most important tools (surgical control of internal hemorrhage and replacement of blood) were not available in the field. The importance of moving patients rapidly to the correct hospital became apparent to both prehospital care practitioners and EMS medical directors. A well-prepared facility incorporated a well-trained trauma team comprising emergency physicians, surgeons, trained nurses, and operating room (OR) staff; a blood bank; registration and quality assurance processes; and all of the remaining components necessary for the management of trauma patients. All of these resources needed to be ready and waiting for the arrival of the patient, with the surgical team standing by to take the patient directly into the OR if necessary. Over time, these standards were modified to include such concepts as permissive hypotension (Dr. Ken Mattox) and a transfusion ratio close to one part red blood cells for one part plasma (1:1).[9-12] However, the bottom line of rapid availability of a well-equipped OR has not changed.

Rapid treatment of trauma patients depends on a prehospital care system that offers easy access to the system. This access is aided by a single emergency phone number (e.g., 9-1-1 in the United States), a good communication system to dispatch emergency medical units, and well-prepared and well-trained prehospital care practitioners. Many people have been taught that early access and early CPR can save the lives of those experiencing cardiac arrest. Trauma can be approached in the same way. The principles just listed serve as the bases for good patient care; to these basic principles has been added the importance of internal hemorrhage control, which cannot be accomplished outside of the trauma center and OR. Thus, rapid assessment, proper packaging, and rapid delivery of the patient to a facility with OR resources immediately available has become the additional principle that was not as fully understood or embraced until the mid-1980s. These basic principles remain the bedrock of EMS care today.

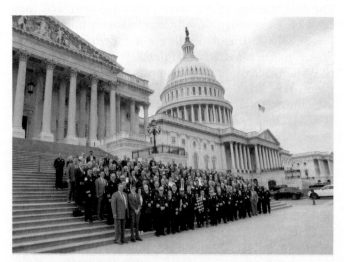

Figure 1-2 Formed in 1975, NAEMT is the only national association representing the professional interests of all emergency and mobile healthcare practitioners, including EMTs, AEMTs, emergency medical responders, paramedics, advanced practice paramedics, critical care paramedics, flight paramedics, community paramedics, and mobile integrated healthcare practitioners.

The accomplishments of these great physicians, prehospital care practitioners, and organizations stand out; however, there are many others, too numerous to mention, who contributed to the development of EMS. To all of them, we owe a great debt of gratitude.

Advances in the New Millennium

Every period of armed conflict gives rise to major advances in trauma care, and the past 20 years have been no exception. The military engagements of the past two decades have seen some of the most substantial changes in battlefield management of wounded military personnel in recent history. Some of the key organizations driving these advancements include the Department of Defense Joint Trauma System and the Committee on Tactical Combat Casualty Care. The Department of Defense established the Joint Trauma System with an aim of providing the optimal chance for survival and maximal chance for functional recovery to every service person wounded in battle. To this end, the Department of Defense established a Trauma Registry (previously known as the Joint Theater Trauma Registry) to collect data and statistics regarding wounded military personnel and the care they receive. The Committee on Tactical Combat Casualty Care uses these data and additional resources as a basis for research that can then lead to the development of clinical practice guidelines. These clinical practice guidelines are deployed to medical personnel in the field for use in the treatment and stabilization of wounded military personnel. Implementing best practices for the care of those wounded in battle has become an agile process that adapts to changing circumstances on the front lines.

The result of this ongoing process has been lives saved. Mortality rates for those wounded in battle have decreased markedly when compared to previous conflicts. The survival rate for those wounded in combat has increased to over 90%.[13,14] In patients where massive transfusion is necessary, typically the most gravely wounded, the implementation of damage control resuscitation (discussed later in this chapter) has reduced mortality from 40% to 20%.[15]

The benefit of these advancements in trauma care is not limited to military health care. The civilian world is rapidly adopting these changes for use in hospitals far away from the front lines. The use of damage control resuscitation in large trauma centers is becoming a standard of care. Tourniquet use, once considered a last resort, has unequivocally become the primary intervention for severe bleeding in the field and during stabilization in the emergency department (ED). The lessons learned from treating wounded military personnel over the past 20 years will have a significant impact on the quality and delivery of civilian trauma care for decades to come.

Philosophy of PHTLS

PHTLS provides the tools for prehospital practitioners to understand anatomy and physiology, the pathophysiology of trauma, the assessment and care of trauma patients using the XABCDE approach, and the skills needed to provide that care—no more and no less. Patients who are bleeding or breathing inadequately have a limited amount of time before their condition results in severe disability or becomes fatal (**Box 1-1**). Prehospital care practitioners must possess and apply critical-thinking skills to rapidly make and carry out decisions that will enhance the survival of trauma patients. PHTLS does not advocate for or train prehospital care practitioners to memorize a "one-size-fits-all" approach. Rather, PHTLS teaches practitioners to develop an understanding of trauma care and critical thinking. Each prehospital care practitioner–patient contact involves a unique set of circumstances. If the prehospital care practitioner understands the basis of medical care and the specific needs of the individual patient given the circumstances at hand, then precise patient care decisions can be made that ensure the greatest chance of survival for that patient.

The overarching tenets of PHTLS are that prehospital care practitioners must have a good foundation of knowledge, must be critical thinkers, and must have appropriate technical skills to deliver excellent patient care, even in less-than-optimal circumstances. PHTLS neither proscribes nor prescribes specific actions for the prehospital care practitioner; instead, it supplies the appropriate knowledge and skills to enable the prehospital care practitioner to use critical thinking to arrive at decisions regarding the best care for each patient.

The opportunity for a prehospital care practitioner to help a patient can be profound. Because trauma impacts people who are often in the most productive years of their lives, the societal impact of survival of a trauma patient who receives excellent trauma care, in both the prehospital and the hospital setting, is compelling. Prehospital care practitioners can lengthen the life span and productive years of trauma patients and benefit society by virtue of the care provided. By delivering effective care to trauma victims, prehospital care practitioners can have a significant positive impact on society.

Epidemiology and Financial Burden

Injury has a profound effect on society. Each day some 14,000 people will die worldwide as a result of injury. Unintentional injury is the leading cause of death in people between the ages of 1 and 45.[16] Each year, approximately 4.4 million people in the world die as a result

Box 1-1 XABCDE

ABCDE is a traditional mnemonic used to remember the steps in the primary survey (Airway, Breathing, Circulation, Disability, Expose/Environment). That approach was modified in the last edition of this text to include immediate focus on exsanguinating extremity or junctional hemorrhage when present, recognizing the immediate and irreversible consequences of such blood loss. The "X" placed before the traditional "ABCDE" describes the need to address eXsanguinating hemorrhage immediately after establishing scene safety and, when personnel resources are limited, before addressing airway. Severe exsanguinating hemorrhage, particularly arterial bleeding, has the potential to lead to loss of total or near total blood volume in a relatively short period of time. Depending on the pace of the bleeding, that time can be just a few minutes. Furthermore, in the prehospital environment, absent the ability to respond with blood transfusion, it will be impossible to correct the problem after the blood volume has been lost because crystalloid resuscitation will not restore the capacity to transport oxygen to the cells. Thus, even prior to airway stabilization, controlling severe bleeding from a limb or other compressible external site takes precedence. Managing airway threats, ensuring adequate breathing, assessing circulatory status and disability, and exposing the body to allow a thorough evaluation follow.

For those who may have taken the American College of Surgeons Advanced Trauma Life Support (ATLS) Course and note a difference in the approach to the primary survey, it is important to understand that this difference does not reflect any disagreement in philosophy between the two courses relative to the importance of early hemorrhage control. Instead, it represents recognition of several distinctions between prehospital and in-hospital care. First, in most Level I or Level II trauma centers, there are sufficient personnel present when the trauma patient arrives that addressing extremity hemorrhage and achieving airway control can be accomplished simultaneously. Second, truly exsanguinating extremity or junctional hemorrhage such as that associated with a femoral artery transection in the groin will no longer be problematic by the time the patient arrives at the hospital if it was not addressed effectively in the field. Finally, if a patient arrives in the trauma bay with blood squirting from an artery in the groin, it must be addressed immediately, but it is also possible to begin massive transfusion protocols to replace the blood already lost, which is just not feasible in most prehospital scenarios.

of injury, accounting for nearly 8% of all deaths.[16] The combined total of deaths caused by diseases such as tuberculosis, malaria, and HIV/AIDS amounts to only a little more than half the number of deaths that result from injury.[16] For further perspective, approximately 3 million people died during the first year of the COVID-19 pandemic.[17] Although it is not difficult to see that trauma is a problem of pandemic proportions that occurs each and every year, understanding the cause of traumatic injury and the most effective means of treating it remains complicated, despite the abundance of data available on the subject.

In the United States, the Centers for Disease Control and Prevention (CDC) reports fatalities resulting from trauma under the umbrella terms "unintentional injury and violence-related injury."[18] When attempting to research trauma as a cause of death, these data are confounded by the fact that not all unintentional injury is traumatic. Unintentional injury encompasses a number of proximate causes, including drowning, poisoning, firearms, falls, and motor vehicle crashes. Consider the fact that poisoning is a cited cause of unintentional injury, and that deaths as a result of opioid overdose are included in this category.[18] This example demonstrates how careful analysis of the available data is necessary to fully understand the problem at hand.

To provide important context, it is helpful to evaluate the trends regarding some of the most common unintentional injury causes of death across the spectrum of age. When this approach is taken, areas of emphasis for prevention, training, and public education can be identified. A few of these areas can be seen in **Figure 1-3** and **Figure 1-4**, which clearly illustrate that drowning and motor vehicle crashes are significant causes of death early in life. As age increases, the number of deaths secondary to drowning begins to fall, and motor vehicle crashes surge to become the leading cause of death until around 25 years of age, when poisoning emerges as the leading cause of unintentional injury leading to death.[19] Poisoning remains the leading cause of death due to unintentional injury until approximately 65 to 70 years of age, when the leading cause becomes falls.[19]

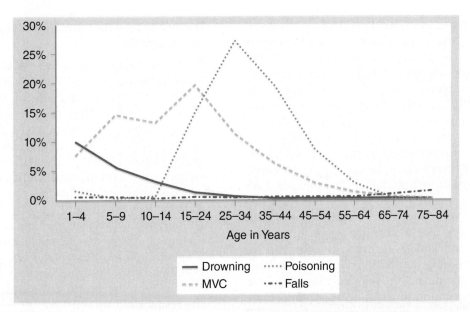

Figure 1-3 Percentage of all deaths by selected cause—ages 1 to 85 years, 2019.

Data from the National Center for Injury Prevention and Control: WISQARS. 10 leading causes of death, United States, 2019, all races, both sexes. Centers for Disease Control and Prevention. https://wisqars.cdc.gov/fatal-leading

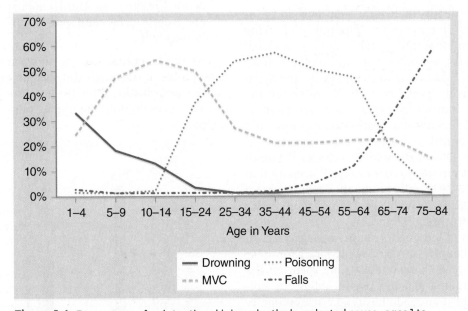

Figure 1-4 Percentage of unintentional injury deaths by selected cause—ages 1 to 85 years, 2019.

Data from the National Center for Injury Prevention and Control: WISQARS. 10 leading causes of death, United States, 2019, all races, both sexes. Centers for Disease Control and Prevention. https://wisqars.cdc.gov/fatal-leading

When the data are broken down in this manner, it becomes clear that across the spectrum of age, motor vehicle crashes persist as a major cause of death, while the most likely cause of death early in life is drowning. While not considered a traumatic cause of death, poisoning is growing as a leading cause of death secondary to unintentional injury, a trend that is likely to continue into the future if the opioid epidemic, seemingly worsened during the COVID-19 pandemic, persists.

These statistics demonstrate alarming trends with regard to the causes of unintentional injury, and while the trends may not be new, the regions in the world that are most affected by these trends are changing. Efforts to reduce fatalities caused by motor vehicle crashes have led to an overall decrease from previous decades in developed countries, yet the overall number of deaths globally due to motor vehicle crashes is increasing.[16] Each day, almost 3,700 people are killed globally in crashes involving motor vehicles, bicycles, or pedestrians.[20] This trend is largely a result of the rapidly rising use of motorized vehicles in developing countries, outpacing the ability of local infrastructure and resources (including EMS) to respond to the demands presented by the increased traffic. A similar pattern is expected in the coming decades with regard to deaths resulting from fall-related injuries. Falls are the second most common cause of death from unintentional injury worldwide. They result in more than 650,000 deaths each year worldwide; again, disproportionately in low- and middle-income countries.[21] In response to the increasing mortality from falls each year, developed countries have initiated fall risk screening, education, and prevention programs. Still, in the United States, 3 million older Americans are treated in an ED for fall-related injuries each year, and over 800,000 of them are eventually hospitalized. In 2015, the estimated total medical cost for these (fatal and nonfatal) injuries exceeded $50 billion.[22]

Analyzing the deaths that result from falls and motor vehicle crashes illuminates the importance of trying to address unintentional injury and trauma on a global scale. A 2014 report identified falls and motor vehicle crashes as the only traumatic causes of death predicted to increase worldwide by the year 2030.[23] Although the burden of these injuries is experienced everywhere, 93% of the world's road traffic deaths occur in low- and middle-income countries despite these countries accounting for only 60% of the world's vehicles.[24] Subsequent to the 2014 report, the UN resolved formally that the decade of 2021–2030 will become the *Second Decade of Action for Road Traffic Safety* with a goal of reducing worldwide road traffic deaths by 50%.[25]

While the loss of life due to trauma is staggering, so too is the financial burden incurred while caring for those victims who survive. Billions of dollars are spent on the management of trauma patients, not including the dollars lost in wages, insurance administration costs, property damage, and employer costs. The National Safety Council estimated that the economic impact in 2019 from both fatal and nonfatal trauma was approximately $1.1 trillion in the United States.[26] Prehospital care practitioners have an opportunity to reduce the societal costs of trauma. For example, proper protection of the fractured cervical spine by a prehospital care practitioner may make the difference between lifelong quadriplegia and a productive, healthy life of unrestricted activity. Saving an individual life by identifying life-threatening hemorrhage, and transporting patients expeditiously to a trauma center for resuscitation and hemorrhage control, can save society $1.2 million per patient in lifetime wage and productivity losses.[26]

The following data come from the World Health Organization (WHO):

- *Road traffic injuries are a huge public health problem.* Road traffic crashes kill 1.3 million people per year worldwide, with an average of more than 3,500 people every day. They are the number one cause of death among persons between the ages of 5 and 29. Road traffic crashes account for nearly 4% of all deaths globally. WHO predicts that without improvements in prevention, road traffic accidents will rise to become the seventh leading cause of death worldwide by the year 2030.[27]
- *The majority of road traffic injuries affect people in low-income and middle-income countries, with three out of four road deaths occurring among men.* While individuals in low- and middle-income countries own only half of the world's vehicles, these countries are responsible for 90% of all road traffic deaths (**Figure 1-5**).[27]
- *Worldwide, 4.4 million people die annually from injury, both unintentional and intentional.* Whereas road traffic incidents are the most common cause of death (roughly one-third), approximately one-sixth are from suicide and one-tenth are secondary to homicide.[16]

As these statistics clearly show, trauma is a worldwide problem. Although the specific events that lead to injuries and deaths differ from country to country, the consequences do not. The impact of preventable injuries is global.

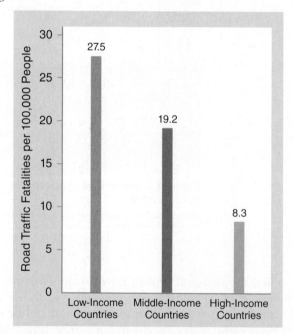

Figure 1-5 Worldwide distribution of road traffic fatalities per 100,000 people.

Data from World Health Organization. Global Status Report on Road Safety 2018. World Health Organization; 2018. https://www.who.int/publications/i/item/9789241565684

We who work in the trauma community have an obligation to our patients to prevent injuries, not just to treat them after the injuries occur. An often-told story about EMS best illustrates this point. On a long, winding mountain road, there was a curve where cars would often slide off the road and plummet 100 feet (30.5 meters) to the ground below. The community decided to station an ambulance at the bottom of the cliff to care for the patients involved in these crashes. The better alternative would have been to place guardrails along the curve to prevent these incidents from occurring in the first place.

The Phases of Trauma Care

Trauma is no accident, even though it is often referred to as such. An accident is often defined as either a chance event or an event caused by carelessness. Most trauma deaths and injuries fit the second definition but not the first and are thus preventable. Prevention has had a great deal of success in developed countries but has a long way to go in developing countries, where poorly developed infrastructures present a major barrier for education and prevention efforts. Traumatic incidents fall into two categories: *intentional* and *unintentional*. Intentional injury results from an act carried out on purpose with the goal of harming, injuring, or killing. Traumatic injury that occurs not as a result of a deliberate action, but rather as an unintended or accidental consequence, is considered unintentional.

Trauma care is divided into three phases: pre-event, event, and post-event. Actions can be taken to minimize the impact of traumatic injury during any of the three phases of trauma care. The prehospital care practitioner has critical responsibilities during each phase.

Pre-event Phase

The **pre-event phase** involves the circumstances leading up to an injury. Efforts in this phase are primarily focused on injury prevention. To achieve maximum effect, strategies to address traumatic death and injury in the pre-event phase should focus on the most significant contributors to mortality and morbidity. According to the most recent data available, unintentional injury is the fourth overall leading cause of death among all ages annually in the United States. Almost half of the deaths caused by injury in the United States are a result of either a motor vehicle crash, a fall, or a firearm (**Figure 1-6**).[28]

Approximately 85% of Americans owned a smartphone in 2021 as compared to 35% in 2011.[29] This growth has been associated with a progressive increase in the number of deaths due to distracted driving. The CDC estimates that distracted driving results in approximately 3,000 deaths per year, with younger drivers at disproportionately higher risk.[30] Prevention efforts involving public awareness campaigns such as "It Can Wait" and "U Drive. U Text. U Pay" have been developed in recent years with the goal of curbing this rising trend (**Figure 1-7**).[30] In some states, these programs have been

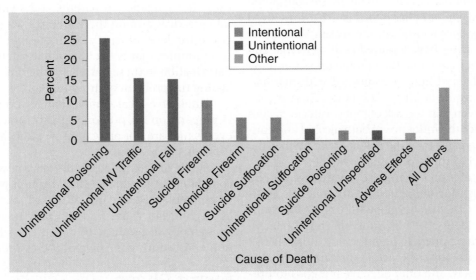

Figure 1-6 Motor vehicle trauma, falls, and firearms account for almost half of the deaths that result from injury.

Data from National Center for Injury Prevention and Control. 10 leading causes of death by age group highlighting violence-related injury deaths, United States - 2018. https://www.cdc.gov/injury/images/lc-charts/leading_causes_of_death_by_age_group_violence_2018_1100w850h.jpg

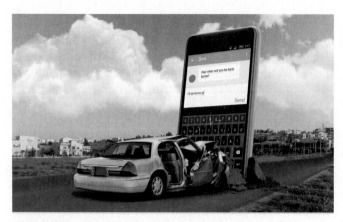

Figure 1-7 Increasingly, public awareness campaigns emphasize the risks of distracted driving.
© Mosab Bilto/Shutterstock

combined with laws targeting the use of cell phones and mobile devices while operating a motor vehicle. According to the Governor's Highway Safety Association, an organization focused on highway safety, 24 states have primary enforcement laws in place banning the use of handheld phones by all individuals while driving.[31] Texting and driving is banned in 48 states. The use of cell phones by novice drivers (drivers younger than 18 years) has been banned entirely in 37 states and the District of Columbia. This type of graded legal enforcement by age and experience is aimed specifically at preventing traffic accidents in these vulnerable groups.[31]

Another preventable cause of motor vehicle crashes is driving while intoxicated.[32] Significant efforts have been aimed at targeting this issue during the pre-event phase. As a result of increased public awareness, education, and pressure to change state laws regarding the minimum blood alcohol content at which individuals are considered legally intoxicated, the number of drunk drivers involved in fatal crashes has been consistently decreasing since 1989. Recently, several states have legalized both medicinal and recreational use of marijuana. Data on the impact of these changes on deaths and injuries associated with marijuana-impaired driving are lacking at this point. There is concern, however, given that the risk of motor vehicle crashes from driving under the influence of both alcohol and cannabis together is greater than the risk of driving under the influence of either of the two substances alone.[33]

Promoting programs that raise awareness among populations at risk for falling is also an area of significant efforts. The CDC has developed the STEADI (Stopping Elderly Accidents, Deaths, and Injuries) initiative for healthcare practitioners to identify individuals at risk for falling, recognize any risk factors that are modifiable for those individuals, and offer effective methods to prevent falls before they occur. Prehospital care practitioners are in a unique position to play a role in fall prevention. With one of the leading risk factors for a fall resulting in

injury or death among older adults being a previous fall incident,[34] it is entirely possible that local EMS personnel are encountering at-risk individuals during calls for lift assistance or minor injury. These calls present an important opportunity for local public safety departments to collaborate with other healthcare practitioners and organizations to develop an evidence-based fall prevention program in the community.[35]

Increasing water safety education, especially in underserved and lower socioeconomic populations, must remain a priority.[36] Worldwide, drowning is the third most common cause of death from unintentional injury.[37] Local code enforcement guidelines that require fencing around swimming pools have been implemented in cities across the United States. Additionally, programs that offer guidance to parents and swimmers regarding safe practices around the water are widely available.[38-41] Given the level of trust and the unique position in local communities that is held by public safety agencies, their participation in these outreach programs is crucial to mitigating the problem of drowning in the pre-event phase.

Another critical component of the pre-event phase is preparation by prehospital care practitioners for the events that are not prevented by public safety awareness programs (**Box 1-2**).

While unintentional injury may never be eliminated completely, it is possible that through programs such as those mentioned, the magnitude of unintentional injury as a significant cause of death may be minimized. EMS personnel will continue to play a crucial role in prevention efforts during the pivotal pre-event phase.

Event Phase

The **event phase** is the moment of the actual trauma. Actions taken during the event phase are aimed at minimizing injury as the result of the trauma. The use of safety equipment has significant influence on the severity of injury caused by the traumatic event. Motor vehicle safety restraint systems, airbags, and motorcycle helmets commonly play a role in injury reduction and avoidance during the event phase. (See Chapter 4, *The Physics of Trauma.*)

The history surrounding motorcycle helmet laws offers a good illustration of the impact that laws mandating the use of certain safety equipment can have on the incidence and severity of traumatic injury. In 1966, the U.S. Congress gave the DOT the authority to penalize states that failed to pass legislation mandating the use of motorcycle helmets.[42] Over the next 10 years, 47 states enacted universal helmet laws. Congress rescinded this authority from the DOT in 1975, and, incrementally, states began repealing their universal helmet laws. Whereas motorcycle deaths had been steadily declining since the early 1980s, by 1998, just over two decades after the threat of penalty for states with no motorcycle helmet law had been lifted, those rates began to rise. As of August 2021, only 18 states plus the District of Columbia have laws in place requiring all riders to wear helmets, 30 states have partial laws in place requiring some riders (generally persons 17 years of age and younger—although specific ages vary from 17–25) to wear helmets, and two states (Illinois and Iowa) have no laws regulating helmet use for any riders, regardless of age or license status.[43,44] This is the lowest number of states having helmet laws since Congress originally granted authority to the DOT to influence states to pass helmet law legislation. According to NHTSA, the number of deaths related to motorcycle accidents was 5,014 in 2019, down slightly from 5,038 the year prior, but increased markedly from 1997 when 2,056 people were killed in motorcycle crashes in the United States.[45] The complex history regarding helmet law legislation over the past 50 years is just one example of how legal statute and enforcement regarding the use of certain safety equipment can dramatically alter patient outcomes during the event phase of trauma care.

Another way to minimize the potential for traumatic injury is through the use of child safety seats. Many trauma centers, law enforcement organizations, and EMS and fire systems conduct programs to educate parents in the correct installation and use of child safety seats. When correctly installed and properly used, child safety seats offer infants and children the best protection during the event phase of trauma care.

Certain steps taken by EMS personnel play a large role in the outcome of the event phase. "Do no further harm" is the admonition for good patient care. Whether driving a personal vehicle or an emergency vehicle, prehospital care practitioners need to protect themselves and teach by example. You are responsible for yourself, your partner, and the patients under your care while in your medic unit. It only makes sense to maintain the same commitment to the safety of yourself and others when operating your personal vehicle; therefore, prevent injury by safe and attentive driving. The same level of attention you give to your patient care should be given to all of your driving. Always use the personal protective devices available, such as vehicle restraints, in the driving compartment and in the passenger or patient care compartment. Avoid distractions while driving. Set your GPS or wayfinding software for your car or smartphone before you start to drive. Avoid using your phone while driving unless absolutely necessary and then only in hands-free mode. Remember, in addition to the risks your own actions lead to, as an EMS professional, you are a role model for others. If people see you texting and driving, not wearing a seat belt, or otherwise engaged in dangerous driving behavior, they may adopt the same habits themselves. Similarly, the good example you set can stimulate others to do the same. Others understand that if your experiences in caring for people who have been involved in MVCs lead you to employ these safety measures, there is potential merit in their doing the same.

Post-event Phase

The **post-event phase** deals with the outcome of the traumatic event. Obviously, the worst possible outcome of a traumatic event is death of the patient. Trauma surgeon Donald Trunkey, MD, has described a trimodal distribution of trauma deaths.[46] The *first phase* of deaths occurs within the first few minutes and up to an hour after an incident. Many of these deaths occur immediately or within seconds after the traumatic injury. Some, however, occur due to massive hemorrhage during the short period of time that elapses while waiting for medical care to arrive. The best way to combat these deaths is through injury prevention strategies and public education programs. In addition, recent public awareness campaigns include education on the use of tourniquets by lay responders and the increased presence of hemorrhage control kits available in public areas and in police cruisers.[47] These efforts can help control the compressible hemorrhage events that often lead to death of the patient during that first phase. The *second phase* of deaths occurs between one and several hours of an incident. These deaths can often be prevented by good prehospital care and hospital care. The *third phase* of deaths occurs several days to several weeks after the incident. These deaths are generally caused by multiple organ failure. Studies suggest that this phase is decreasing as a result of modern trauma and critical care.[48] Damage control resuscitation is an evolving trend in trauma care that addresses third-phase deaths by combining staged surgical intervention with intensive care unit (ICU) stabilization in patients with massive trauma.[49-51] The evidence

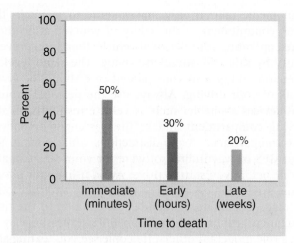

Figure 1-8 Immediate deaths can be prevented by injury-prevention and public emergency response education. Early deaths can be prevented through timely, appropriate prehospital care and transport to an appropriate trauma center. Late deaths can be prevented through modern damage control techniques to control hemorrhage, resuscitation with blood and products, and proceeding with staged reconstruction of injuries after adequate physiologic stabilization of the patient.

© National Association of Emergency Medical Technicians (NAEMT)

indicates that patient outcomes are improved when crystalloid resuscitation is limited and the initial surgical intervention is brief and only addresses major sources of bleeding, allowing the patient to be transferred to the trauma ICU where the patient can be physiologically stabilized to an appropriate metabolic state.[52-54] Once this ICU stabilization is complete, additional surgical interventions can be performed in a staged fashion with intermittent ICU re-stabilization as needed by the patient. Early and aggressive management of shock with blood and blood products as opposed to crystalloid solutions in the prehospital setting also plays a major role in preventing some of these deaths (**Figure 1-8**). In regions of the world where access to combined ICU and trauma care is available, early intervention by EMS with aggressive control of hemorrhage along with rapid transfer to a capable trauma center and damage control resuscitation in the hospital improves outcomes in trauma patients.

R. Adams Cowley, MD, founder of the Maryland Institute of Emergency Medical Services Systems (MIEMSS), one of the first trauma centers in the United States, defined what he called the Golden Hour.[55] Based on his research, Dr. Cowley believed that patients who received definitive care soon after an injury had a much higher survival rate than those whose care was delayed. One reason for this improvement in survival is prompt treatment of hemorrhage and preservation of the body's ability to produce energy to maintain organ function. For the prehospital care practitioner, this translates into maintaining oxygenation and perfusion and providing rapid transport to a facility that is prepared to continue

the process of resuscitation using blood and plasma (damage control resuscitation) and to provide access to the immediate surgical intervention necessary to achieve prompt hemorrhage control.

Because this critical period of time is not literally 1 hour, the Golden Hour is better thought of as the "Golden Period." Some patients have less than an hour in which to receive care, whereas others have more time. In many urban prehospital systems in the United States, the average time between activation of EMS and arrival to the scene is 8 to 9 minutes, not including the time between injury and call to the public safety answering point. A typical transport time to the receiving facility is another 8 to 9 minutes. If the prehospital care practitioners spend only 10 minutes on the scene, over 30 minutes of time will have already passed by the time a patient arrives at the receiving facility. Every additional minute spent on the scene is additional time that the patient is bleeding, and valuable time is ticking away from the Golden Period.

Research data support the concept of rapid transport to definitive care.[56-59] One of these studies showed that critically injured patients had a significantly lower mortality rate (17.9% vs. 28.2%) when transported to the hospital by a private vehicle rather than an ambulance.[56] This unexpected finding was most likely the result of prehospital care practitioners spending too much time on the scene.

In the 1980s and 1990s, a trauma center documented that EMS scene times averaged 20 to 30 minutes for patients injured in motor vehicle crashes and for victims of penetrating trauma. This finding brings to light the questions that all prehospital care practitioners need to ask when caring for trauma victims: "Is what I am doing going to benefit the patient? Does that benefit outweigh the risk of delaying transport?"

One of the most important responsibilities of a prehospital care practitioner is to spend as little time on the scene as possible and instead expedite the field care and transport of a trauma patient. In the first precious minutes after arrival at a scene, a prehospital care practitioner rapidly assesses the patient, performs lifesaving maneuvers, and prepares the patient for transport. An important articulated goal of PHTLS has been to decrease prehospital scene times by allowing all practitioners (fire, police, and EMS) to perform as a cohesive unit in a uniform style and by employing a standard methodology across emergency services. This has hopefully contributed to the increase in patient survival during this time period. A second responsibility is transporting the patient to an appropriate facility. A factor that is extremely critical to a compromised patient's survival is the length of time that elapses between the incident and the provision of definitive care.

With the management of trauma patients, time from injury to arrival at the appropriate trauma center is critical to survival. Definitive care for trauma patients usually involves control of hemorrhage and restoration of adequate

---

Box 1-3 Trauma Centers

The American College of Surgeons (ACS) establishes the requirements for trauma centers in a document entitled *Resources for Optimal Care of the Injured Patient.* State and local jurisdictions utilize these requirements, and the ACS Committee on Trauma (COT) Verification Review Committee's reports from trauma site surveys, to designate trauma centers at varying levels. According to the ACS, there should be no difference in clinical requirements for level I and level II trauma centers. The primary difference between the two levels is that medical education, research, specialty services, and patient volume are higher at level I trauma centers. Level I trauma centers serve as a hub for organizing trauma care in a given region. Level III trauma centers generally have fewer resources and are typically located in suburban or rural areas. Their primary role is immediate treatment

and stabilization, combined with rapid and efficient transport to the higher level of care provided at a level I or II trauma center. Level IV trauma centers have few resources other than a 24-hour staffed ED, and their major role is to serve as a guide for immediate basic care and stabilization with rapid transfer to a higher level trauma center.[60]

It is important to note that the ACS *does not* designate which institutions are considered trauma centers; they simply verify that hospitals have or have not met the recommended criteria for a specific level of trauma service. The decision to designate a particular hospital as a trauma center, and what level trauma center that hospital will be, lies with state and local government, usually after verification from the ACS that certain criteria have been met.

© National Association of Emergency Medical Technicians (NAEMT)

perfusion by replacement of fluids as near to whole blood as possible. Administration of reconstituted whole blood (packed red blood cells and plasma, in a ratio of 1:1) to replace lost blood has produced impressive results by the military in Iraq and Afghanistan and now in the civilian community. These fluids replace the lost oxygen-carrying capacity, the clotting components, and the oncotic pressure to prevent fluid loss from the vascular system. They are not widely available for use in the field and are an important reason for rapid transport to the hospital. En route to the hospital, balanced resuscitation (see Chapter 3, *Shock: Pathophysiology of Life and Death*) has proven to be important. Hemostasis (hemorrhage control) cannot always be achieved in the field or in the ED; often, it can be achieved only in the OR. Therefore, when determining an appropriate facility to which a patient should be transported, it is important that the prehospital care practitioner use the critical-thinking process and consider the transport time to a given facility and the capabilities of that facility.

A trauma center that has a trained and prepared trauma surgeon available either at the time of or shortly after the arrival of the patient, a well-trained and trauma-experienced resuscitation team, and an OR team immediately available can have a trauma patient with life-threatening hemorrhage in the OR rapidly after the patient's arrival, and this can make the difference between life and death (Box 1-3).

On the other hand, a hospital without in-house surgical capabilities must await the arrival of the surgeon and the surgical team before transporting the patient from the ED to the OR. Additional time may then elapse

before the hemorrhage can be controlled, resulting in an associated increase in mortality rate (**Figure 1-9**). There is a significant increase in survival if all severely injured patients are taken directly to a trauma center, bypassing closer nontrauma hospitals if necessary.[61-69]

Experience, in addition to the initial training in surgery and trauma, is important. Studies have demonstrated that more experienced surgeons in a busy trauma center have a better outcome than trauma surgeons with less experience.[69,70]

PHTLS—Past, Present, Future

Advanced Trauma Life Support

As happens so often in life, a personal experience brought about the changes in emergency care that resulted in the birth of the Advanced Trauma Life Support (ATLS) Course, and eventually, the PHTLS Program. ATLS started in 1978, 2 years after a private plane crash in a rural area of Nebraska. The ATLS Course was born out of that mangled mass of metal, the injured, and the dead. An orthopaedic surgeon, his wife, and his four children were flying in their twin-engine airplane when it crashed. His wife was killed instantly. The children were critically injured. They waited for help to arrive, but it never did. After approximately 8 hours, the orthopaedic surgeon walked more than half a mile along a dirt road to a highway. After two trucks passed him by, he flagged down a car. Together, they drove to the

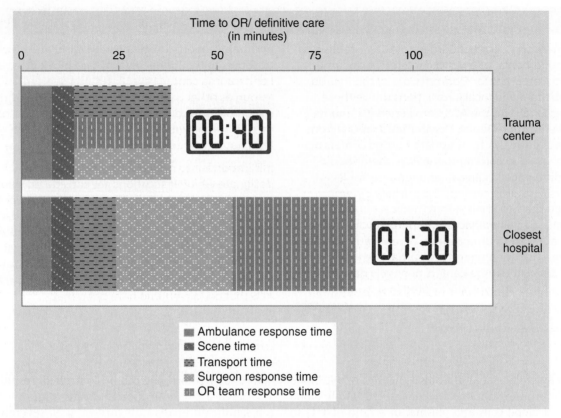

Figure 1-9 In locations in which trauma centers are available, bypassing hospitals not committed to the care of trauma patients can significantly improve patient care. In severely injured trauma patients, definitive patient care often occurs in the OR. An extra 10 to 20 minutes spent en route to a hospital with an in-house surgeon and in-house OR staff can substantially reduce the time to definitive care in the OR.

© National Association of Emergency Medical Technicians (NAEMT)

accident site, loaded the injured children into the car, and drove to the closest hospital, a few miles south of the crash site.

When they arrived at the ED door of the local rural hospital, they found it was locked. The on-duty nurse called the two general practitioners in the small farming community who were on call. After examining the children, one of the doctors carried one of the injured children by the shoulders and the knees to the x-ray room. Later, he returned and announced that the x-rays showed no skull fracture. An injury to the child's cervical spine had not been considered. The doctor then began suturing a laceration the child had sustained. The orthopedic surgeon called his physician partner in Lincoln, Nebraska, and told him what had happened. His partner said that he would arrange to get the surviving family members to Lincoln as soon as possible.

The doctors and staff in this little rural hospital had little or no preparation for assessing and managing multiple patients with traumatic injuries. Unfortunately, there was a lack of training and experience on triage and on assessment and management of traumatic injuries. In the years that followed, the Nebraska orthopaedic surgeon

and his colleagues recognized that something needed to be done about the general lack of a trauma care delivery system to treat acutely injured patients in a rural setting. They decided that rural physicians needed to be trained in a systematic manner on treating trauma patients. They chose to use a format similar to Advanced Cardiovascular Life Support (ACLS) and call it Advanced Trauma Life Support (ATLS).

A syllabus was created and organized into a logical approach to manage trauma. The "treat as you go" methodology was developed as well as the ABCs of trauma (airway, breathing, and circulation) to prioritize the order of assessment and treatment. In 1978, the ATLS prototype was field tested in Auburn, Nebraska, with the help of many surgeons. Next, the course was presented to the University of Nebraska and eventually to the American College of Surgeons Committee on Trauma.

Since that first ATLS Course in Auburn, Nebraska, more than four decades have passed and ATLS keeps spreading and growing. What was originally intended as a course for rural Nebraska has become a course for the whole world and for all types of trauma settings. It is this course that is the basis of PHTLS.

PHTLS

As Dr. Richard H. Carmona, former U.S. Surgeon General, stated in his foreword to the sixth edition of PHTLS:

> It has been said that we stand on the shoulders of giants in many apparent successes, and PHTLS is no different. With great vision and passion, as well as challenges, a small group of leaders persevered and developed PHTLS over a quarter of a century ago.

In 1958, Dr. Farrington convinced the Chicago Fire Department that fire fighters should be trained to manage emergency patients. Working with Dr. Sam Banks, Dr. Farrington started the Trauma Training Program in Chicago. Millions have been trained following the guidelines developed in this landmark program. Dr. Farrington continued to work at every level of EMS, from the field, to education, to legislation, to help expand and improve EMS as a profession. The principles of trauma care set forth by Dr. Farrington's work form an important part of the nucleus of PHTLS.

The first chairman of the ATLS ad hoc committee for the American College of Surgeons and Chairman of the Prehospital Care Subcommittee on Trauma for the American College of Surgeons, Dr. Norman E. McSwain, Jr., FACS, knew that ATLS would have a profound effect on the outcomes of trauma patients. Moreover, he had a strong sense that an even greater effect could come from bringing this type of critical training to prehospital care practitioners.

Dr. McSwain, a founding member of the board of directors of NAEMT, gained the support of the association's president, Gary LaBeau, and began to lay plans for a prehospital version of ATLS.[71] President LaBeau directed Dr. McSwain and Robert Nelson, NREMT-P, to determine the feasibility of an ATLS-type program for prehospital care practitioners.

As a professor of surgery at Tulane University School of Medicine in New Orleans, Louisiana, Dr. McSwain gained the university's support in putting together the draft curriculum of what was to become PHTLS. With this draft in place, a PHTLS committee was established in 1983. This committee continued to refine the curriculum, and later that same year, pilot courses were conducted in Lafayette and New Orleans, Louisiana; the Marian Health Center in Sioux City, Iowa; the Yale University School of Medicine in New Haven, Connecticut; and the Norwalk Hospital in Norwalk, Connecticut.

Richard W. Vomacka (1946 to 2001) was a part of the task force that developed the initial PHTLS Course. PHTLS became his passion as the course came together, and he traveled around the country in the early 1980s conducting pilot courses and regional faculty workshops. He worked with Dr. McSwain and the other original task force members to fine-tune the program. Vomacka was instrumental in forging a relationship between PHTLS and the U.S. military. He also worked on the first international PHTLS Course sites.

National dissemination of PHTLS began with three intensive workshops taught in Denver, Colorado; Bethesda, Maryland; and Orlando, Florida, between September 1984 and February 1985. The graduates of these early PHTLS Courses formed what would be the "barnstormers." These individuals were PHTLS national and regional faculty members who traveled the country training additional faculty members, spreading the word on the core PHTLS principles. Alex Butman, NREMT-P, along with Vomacka worked diligently, frequently using money out of their own pockets, to bring the first two editions of the PHTLS Program to fruition.

Throughout the growth process, medical oversight has been provided through the American College of Surgeons Committee on Trauma. For over 30 years, the partnership between the American College of Surgeons and NAEMT has ensured that PHTLS Course participants receive the opportunity to help give trauma patients their best chance at survival.

Between 1994 and 2001, Dr. Scott B. Frame, FACS, FCCM (1952 to 2001), was the associate medical director for the PHTLS Program. His major emphasis was in the development of the audiovisuals for PHTLS and its promulgation internationally. At the time of his death, he had assumed responsibility for the fifth edition of the PHTLS Course. This included the revision of not only the textbook but also of the instructor's manual and all of the associated teaching materials. He was appointed as medical director of the PHTLS Course when the fifth edition was published. The PHTLS Program grew tremendously under Dr. Frame's leadership, and its continuation into the future owes much to his efforts and the part of his life that he lent to PHTLS and to his patients.

It is on the shoulders of these individuals and other individuals too numerous to mention, that PHTLS stands and continues to grow.

PHTLS in the Military

Beginning in 1988, the U.S. military aggressively set out to train its combat medics in PHTLS. Coordinated by the Defense Medical Readiness Training Institute (DMRTI) at Fort Sam Houston in Texas, PHTLS was taught to combat medics in the United States and to those stationed overseas. In 2001, the Army's 91WB program standardized the training of over 58,000 combat medics to include the PHTLS Course.

In the fourth edition of PHTLS, a military chapter was added to better address the needs of military practitioners treating combat-related injuries. After the fifth edition was published, a strong relationship was forged between the PHTLS committee and the newly established

Committee on Tactical Combat Casualty Care of the Defense Health Board in the Department of Defense. As a result of this relationship, a military version of PHTLS, with an extensively revised military chapter, was published as a revised fifth edition in 2005. This collaboration between the PHTLS committee and the Committee on Tactical Combat Casualty Care led to the creation of multiple military chapters for the military version of the sixth edition of PHTLS. In 2010, NAEMT began to offer the Department of Defense's TCCC Course.

International PHTLS

The sound principles of prehospital trauma management emphasized in the PHTLS Course have led prehospital care practitioners and physicians outside the United States to request the importation of the program to their various countries. Beginning in the early 1990s, PHTLS was launched internationally, first in the United Kingdom and Mexico, and then in other countries.

In 2019, over 25,600 international prehospital practitioners received PHTLS education and, since the publication of this edition, PHTLS has been taught in more than 70 countries across the globe. During the global COVID-19 pandemic, NAEMT training centers around the world taught fewer PHTLS Courses, as prehospital practitioners turned their attention to pandemic patient care and immunization efforts. NAEMT, through its Education and PHT Committees, worked to support those training centers through innovative approaches to virtual teaching. The global network of PHTLS faculty continue to teach this vital trauma program far and wide, both virtually and in the classroom.

Translations

Our growing international family has spawned translations of the PHTLS text, which is currently available in languages including Arabic, Dutch, English, French, German, Greek, Italian, Korean, Norwegian, Polish, Portuguese, Simplified Chinese, Spanish, Swedish, and Traditional Chinese.

Vision for the Future

The PHTLS Program will continue its mission to provide the highest quality prehospital trauma education to all who need and desire this opportunity. PHTLS is always driven by the latest evidence in prehospital trauma, and we are committed to seeking out this evidence from all reputable sources.

As prehospital trauma care evolves and improves, so too must the PHTLS Program. We are dedicated to ongoing evaluation of the program and to identifying and implementing improvements wherever needed. We will pursue new methods and technologies for delivering PHTLS to enhance the clinical and service quality of the program.

We will strive to ensure that our program meets the needs of prehospital patients in all countries. Since 2010, PHTLS faculty in Europe have met to discuss methods for measuring program quality and to identify areas for improvement. This group evolved into the Regional European Education Committee, which was established in 2018. Similar committees have been established in Latin America (2019) and the Middle East (2021). Since 2012, the World Trauma Symposium has been held annually to present the latest evidence, trends, and controversies in prehospital trauma care. These programs bring the work of practitioners and researchers from around the globe together to examine the continuing evolution of trauma care. Their contributions, as well as the contributions of the PHTLS family of instructors, medical directors, coordinators, authors, and reviewers worldwide, all volunteering countless hours of their lives, will ensure that the PHTLS Program continues to thrive and grow.

PHTLS will maintain its unwavering commitment to our patients by ensuring that PHTLS practitioners are able to do the following:

- Assess their patients rapidly and accurately.
- Identify shock and hypoxemia.
- Initiate the right interventions at the right time.
- Transport their patients to the right place, for the right care, at the right time.

SUMMARY

- Prehospital care as we know it today can be traced back to the late 1700s, when Baron Dominique Jean Larrey, Napoleon's chief military physician, recognized the need for prompt prehospital care. Progress in prehospital care was relatively slow until about 1950, when J. D. "Deke" Farrington, MD, stimulated the development of improved prehospital care. Ever since, improving prehospital trauma care has been a steady and ongoing effort.
- The overarching tenets of Prehospital Trauma Life Support (PHTLS) are that prehospital care practitioners must have a good foundation of knowledge, must be critical thinkers, and must have appropriate technical skills to deliver

SUMMARY (CONTINUED)

- excellent patient care, even in less-than-optimal circumstances.
- Worldwide, injury is a leading cause of death and disability, impacting not only the people directly involved, but, given the magnitude of its financial ramifications, society as a whole.
- Improving outcomes from trauma can be considered in three phases: pre-event, event, and post-event. Actions can be taken to minimize the impact of traumatic injury during any of the three phases of trauma care. The prehospital care practitioner has critical responsibilities during each phase.
- The concept of a Golden Hour or Golden Period guides prehospital care. Research has shown that

- prompt transport to definitive care is a key to improving patient outcomes.
- The PHTLS Course is modeled after the Advanced Trauma Life Support (ATLS) Course created in 1978, which emphasized rapid patient transport and treatment en route. As the PHTLS Program has grown, medical oversight has been provided through the American College of Surgeons Committee on Trauma. For over 30 years, the partnership between the American College of Surgeons and the National Association of Emergency Medical Technicians has ensured that PHTLS Course participants receive the opportunity to help give trauma patients their best chance at survival.

References

1. McSwain NE. Prehospital care from Napoleon to Mars: the surgeon's role. *J Am Coll Surg.* 2005;200(44):487-504.

2. Larrey DJ. *Mémoires de Chirurgie Militaire, et Campagnes* [Memoirs of Military Surgery and Campaigns of the French Armies]. Paris, France: J. Smith and F. Buisson; 1812-1817. English translation with notes by R. W. Hall of volumes 1-3 in 2 volumes; 1814. English translation of volume 4 by J. C. Mercer; 1832.

3. Rockwood CA, Mann CM, Farrington JD, et al. History of emergency medical services in the United States. *J Trauma.* 1976;16(4):299-308.

4. Farrington JD. Death in a ditch. *Bull Am Coll Surg.* 1967; 52(3):121-132.

5. Federal Specifications for Ambulance, KKK-A-1822D. United States General Services Administration, Specifications Section, November 1994.

6. Kennedy R. *Early Care of the Sick and Injured Patient.* American College of Surgeons; 1964.

7. Curry G. *Immediate Care and Transport of the Injured.* Charles C. Thomas Publisher; 1965.

8. Committee on Trauma and Committee on Shock, Division of Medical Sciences. *Accidental Death and Disability: The Neglected Disease of Modern Society.* National Academy of Sciences/National Research Council; 1966.

9. Holcomb JB, Jenkins D, Rhee P, et al. Damage control resuscitation: directly addressing the early coagulopathy of trauma. *J Trauma.* 2007;62(2):307-310.

10. Holcomb JB, Tilley BC, Baraniuk S, et al. Transfusion of plasma, platelets, and red blood cells in a 1:1:1 vs a 1:1:2 ratio and mortality in patients with severe trauma: the PROPPR randomized clinical trial. *JAMA.* 2015;313(5): 471-482.

11. Borgman MA, Spinella PC, Perkins JG, et al. The ratio of blood products transfused affects mortality in patients receiving massive transfusions at a combat support hospital. *J Trauma.* 2007;63(4):805-813.

12. Holcomb JB, Wade CE, Michalek JE, et al. Increased plasma and platelet to red blood cell ratios improves outcome in 466 massively transfused civilian trauma patients. *Ann Surg.* 2008;248(3):447-458.

13. Eastridge BJ, Jenkins D, Flaherty S, et al. Trauma system development in a theater of war: experiences from Operation Iraqi Freedom and Operation Enduring Freedom. *J Trauma.* 2006;61(6):1366-1372.

14. Ling GS, Rhee P, Ecklund JM. Surgical innovations arising from the Iraq and Afghanistan wars. *Annu Rev Med.* 2010;61:457-468.

15. Borden Institute. *Emergency War Surgery 2014.* 4th ed. Office of the Surgeon General; 2014.

16. World Health Organization. Injuries and violence. Published March 19, 2021. Accessed November 11, 2021. https://www.who.int/news-room/fact-sheets/detail/injuries-and-violence

17. World Health Organization. The true death toll of COVID-19. Accessed November 11, 2021. https://www.who.int/data/stories/the-true-death-toll-of-covid-19-estimating-global-excess-mortality

18. Centers for Disease Control and Prevention. Accessed November 11, 2021. Fatal injury and violence data. https://www.cdc.gov/injury/wisqars/fatal.html

19. Centers for Disease Control and Prevention. 10 leading causes of death, United States, 2019, all races, both sexes. Accessed November 11, 2021. https://wisqars.cdc.gov/fatal-leading

20. Centers for Disease Control and Prevention. Road traffic injuries and deaths—A global problem. Last reviewed December 14, 2020. Accessed November 11, 2021. https://www.cdc.gov/injury/features/global-road-safety/index.html

21. World Health Organization. Falls. Published April 26, 2021. Accessed November 11, 2021. https://www.who.int/news-room/fact-sheets/detail/falls

22. Centers for Disease Control and Prevention. Important facts about falls. Last reviewed February 10, 2017. Accessed November 11, 2021. https://www.cdc.gov/homeandrecreationalsafety/falls/adultfalls.html

23. World Health Organization. Injuries and violence: the facts, 2014. Published 2014. Accessed November 11, 2021. http://apps.who.int/iris/bitstream/10665/149798/1/9789241508018_eng.pdf

24. World Health Organization. Road traffic injuries. Published June 21, 2021. Accessed November 11, 2021. https://www.who.int/news-room/fact-sheets/detail/road-traffic-injuries

25. United Nations General Assembly. Improving global road safety. Resolution adopted by the General Assembly on 31 August 2020. Published September 2, 2020. Accessed November 11, 2021. https://undocs.org/en/A/RES/74/299

26. National Safety Council. *Injury facts: Societal costs*. Accessed November 11, 2021. https://injuryfacts.nsc.org/all-injuries/costs/societal-costs/

27. World Health Organization. World traffic injuries: the facts. Accessed November 11, 2021. http://www.who.int/violence_injury_prevention/road_safety_status/2015/magnitude_A4_web.pdf?ua=1

28. Centers for Disease Control and Prevention. 10 leading causes of injury deaths by age group highlighting violence-related injury deaths, United States – 2018. Accessed November 11, 2021. https://www.cdc.gov/injury/images/lc-charts/leading_causes_of_death_by_age_group_violence_2018_1100w850h.jpg

29. O'Dea S. Percentage of U.S. adults who own a smartphone from 2011 to 2021. *Statista*. Published May 12, 2021. Accessed November 11, 2021. https://www.statista.com/statistics/219865/percentage-of-us-adults-who-own-a-smartphone/

30. Centers for Disease Control and Prevention. Distracted driving. Last reviewed March 2, 2021. Accessed November 11, 2021. https://www.cdc.gov/transportationsafety/distracted_driving/index.html#problem

31. Governors Highway Safety Association. Distracted driving. Accessed August 18, 2021. https://www.ghsa.org/state-laws/issues/distracted%20driving

32. Mothers Against Drunk Driving. Accessed November 11, 2021. http://www.madd.org/

33. Sewell RA, Poling J, Sofuoglu M. The effect of cannabis compared with alcohol on driving. *Am J Addict*. 2009;18(3)185-193.

34. Centers for Disease Control and Prevention, National Center for Injury Prevention and Control. Fact sheet: risk factors for falls. Published 2017. Accessed November 11, 2021. https://www.cdc.gov/steadi/pdf/Risk_Factors_for_Falls-print.pdf

35. Centers for Disease Control and Prevention, National Center for Injury Prevention and Control. Preventing falls: a guide to implementing effective community-based fall prevention programs. Published 2015. Accessed November 11, 2021. https://www.cdc.gov/homeandrecreationalsafety/pdf/falls/fallpreventionguide-2015-a.pdf

36. American Red Cross. Red Cross launches campaign to cut drowning in half in 50 cities. Published May 20, 2014. Accessed November 11, 2021. https://www.redcross.org/about-us/news-and-events/press-release/red-cross-launches-campaign-to-cut-drowning-in-half-in-50-cities.html

37. World Health Organization. Drowning. Published April 27, 201. Accessed November 11, 2021. https://www.who.int/news-room/fact-sheets/detail/drowning#:~:text=Key%20facts,000%20annual%20drowning%20deaths%20worldwide

38. Ramos W, Beale A, Chambers P, Dalke S, Fielding R. Primary and secondary drowning interventions: The American Red Cross Circle of Drowning Prevention and Chain of Drowning Survival. *Int J Aquatic Res Educ*. 2015;9(1):89-101.

39. American Red Cross. Water safety. Accessed November 11, 2021. http://www.redcross.org/get-help/how-to-prepare-for-emergencies/types-of-emergencies/water-safety

40. Association of Aquatic Professionals. Drowning prevention education. Accessed November 11, 2021. https://aquaticpros.org/drowning-prevention-education

41. YMCA. Water safety and swimming. Accessed November 11, 2021. https://www.ymca.org/what-we-do/healthy-living/water-safety

42. Goodwin A, Kirley B, Sandt L, et al., eds. *Countermeasures That Work: A Highway Safety Countermeasure Guide for State Highway Safety Offices*. 7th ed. National Highway Traffic Safety Administration; 2013:5-7.

43. Insurance Institute of Highway Safety. Motorcycles: motorcycle helmet use. Data updated November 2021. Accessed November 11, 2021. https://www.iihs.org/topics/motorcycles/motorcycle-helmet-laws-table

44. Edgar Synder and Associates. Motorcycle helmet laws—by state. Accessed November 11, 2021. https://www.edgarsnyder.com/motorcycle-accidents/state-helmet-laws

45. Insurance Information Institute. Facts and statistics: Motorcycle crashes. Accessed November 11, 2021. https://www.iii.org/fact-statistic/facts-statistics-motorcycle-crashes

46. Trunkey DD. Trauma. *Sci Am*. 1983;249(2):28-35.

47. U.S. Department of Homeland Security. Stop the bleed. Published June 16, 2017. Accessed November 11, 2021. https://www.dhs.gov/stopthebleed

48. Cuschieri J, Johnson JL, Sperry J, et al. Benchmarking outcomes in the critically injured trauma patient and the effect of implementing standard operating procedures. *Ann Surg*. 2012;255(5):993-999.

49. Rotondo MF, Zonies DH. The damage control sequence and underlying logic. *Surg Clin North Am*. 1997;77(4):761-777.

50. Sugrue M, D'Amours SK, Joshipura M. Damage control surgery and the abdomen. *Injury*. 2004;35(7):642-648.

51. Beldowicz BC. The evolution of damage control in concept and practice. *Clin Colon Rectal Surg*. 2018;31(1):30-35.

52. Rotondo MF, Schwab CW, McGonigal MD, et al. "Damage control": an approach for improved survival in exsanguinating penetrating abdominal injury. *J Trauma*. 1993;35(3):375-382.

53. Schreiber MA. Damage control surgery. *Crit Care Clin*. 2004;20(1):101-118.

54. Parr MJ, Alabdi T. Damage control surgery and intensive care. *Injury*. 2004;35(7):713-722.

55. University of Maryland Medical Center. Tribute to R Adams Cowley, MD. Accessed November 11, 2021. https://www.umms.org/ummc/health-services/shock-trauma/about/history

56. Demetriades D, Chan L, Cornwell EE, et al. Paramedic vs. private transportation of trauma patients: effect on outcome. *Arch Surg.* 1996;131(2):133-138.

57. Cornwell EE, Belzberg H, Hennigan K, et al. Emergency medical services (EMS) vs. non-EMS transport of critically injured patients: a prospective evaluation. *Arch Surg.* 2000;135(3):315-319.

58. Kotwal RS, Howard JT, Oramn JA, et al. The effect of a golden hour policy on the morbidity and mortality of combat casualties. *JAMA Surg.* 2016;151(1):15-24.

59. Alarhayem AQ, Myers JG, Dent D, et al. Time is the enemy: mortality in trauma patients with hemorrhage from torso injury occurs long before the "Golden Hour." *Am J. Surg.* 2016;212(6):1101-1105.

60. American Academy of Surgeons. *Resources for Optimal Care of the Injured Patient.* 6th ed. American College of Surgeons; 2014. Accessed November 11, 2021. https://www.facs.org/quality-programs/trauma/tqp/center-programs/vrc/resources

61. Demetriades D, Martin M, Salim A, Rhee P, Brown C, Chan L. The effect of trauma center designation and trauma volume on outcome in specific severe injuries. *Ann Surg.* 2005;242(4):512-519. doi: 10.1097/01.sla.0000184169.73614.09

62. Peleg K, Aharonson-Daniel L, Stein M, et al. Increased survival among severe trauma patients: the impact of a national trauma system. *Arch Surg.* 2004;139(11):1231-1236.

63. Edwards W. Emergency medical systems significantly increase patient survival rates, Part 2. *Can Doct.* 1982;48(12):20-24.

64. Haas B, Jurkovich GJ, Wang J, et al. Survival advantage in trauma centers: expeditious intervention or experience? *J Am Coll.* 2009;208(1):28-36.

65. Scheetz LJ. Differences in survival, length of stay, and discharge disposition of older trauma patients admitted to trauma centers and nontrauma center hospitals. *J Nurs Scholarsh.* 2005;37(4):361-366.

66. Norwood S, Fernandez L, England J. The early effects of implementing American College of Surgeons level II criteria on transfer and survival rates at a rurally based community hospital. *J Trauma.* 1995;39(2):240-244; discussion 244-245.

67. Kane G, Wheeler NC, Cook S, et al. Impact of the Los Angeles county trauma system on the survival of seriously injured patients. *J Trauma.* 1992;32(5):576-583.

68. Hedges JR, Adams AL, Gunnels MD. ATLS practices and survival at rural level III trauma hospitals, 1995-1999. *Prehosp Emerg Care.* 2002;6(3):299-305.

69. Konvolinka CW, Copes WS, Sacco WJ. Institution and per-surgeon volume vs. survival outcome in Pennsylvania's trauma centers. *Am J Surg.* 1995;170(4):333-340.

70. Margulies DR, Cryer HG, McArthur DL, et al. Patient volume per surgeon does not predict survival in adult level I trauma centers. *J Trauma.* 2001;50(4):597-601; discussion 601-603.

71. McSwain NE. Judgment based on knowledge: a history of Prehospital Trauma Life Support, 1970-2013. *J Trauma Acute Care Surg.* 2013;75:1-7.

Suggested Reading

Callaham M. Quantifying the scanty science of prehospital emergency care. *Ann Emerg Med.* 1997;30:785.

Cone DC, Lewis RJ. Should this study change my practice? *Acad Emerg Med.* 2003;10:417.

Haynes RB, McKibbon KA, Fitzgerald D, et al. How to keep up with the medical literature: II. Deciding which journals to read regularly. *Ann Intern Med.* 1986;105:309.

Keim SM, Spaite DW, Maio RF, et al. Establishing the scope and methodological approach to out-of-hospital outcomes and effectiveness research. *Acad Emerg Med.* 2004;11:1067.

Lewis RJ, Bessen HA. Statistical concepts and methods for the reader of clinical studies in emergency medicine. *J Emerg Med.* 1991;9:221.

MacAvley D. Critical appraisal of medical literature: an aid to rational decision making. *Fam Pract.* 1995;12:98.

Reed JF III, Salen P, Bagher P. Methodological and statistical techniques: what do residents really need to know about statistics? *J Med Syst.* 2003;27:233.

Sackett DL. How to read clinical journals: V. To distinguish useful from useless or even harmful therapy. *Can Med Assoc J.* 1981;124:1156.

CHAPTER 2

Golden Principles, Preferences, and Critical Thinking

Lead Editors
Andrew N. Pollak, MD, FAAOS
Nancy Hoffmann, MSW

CHAPTER OBJECTIVES

At the completion of this chapter, you will be able to do the following:

- Describe the difference between principles and preferences in relation to decision making in the field.
- Given a trauma scenario, discuss the principles of trauma care for the specific situation.
- Given a trauma scenario, use critical-thinking skills to determine the preferred method for accomplishing the principles of emergency trauma care.
- Relate the four principles of ethical decision making to prehospital trauma care.
- Given a trauma scenario, discuss the ethical issues involved and how to address them.
- Relate the importance of the "Golden Hour" or "Golden Period."
- Discuss the 14 "Golden Principles" of prehospital trauma care.
- Identify the components and importance of prehospital research and literature.

SCENARIO

You and your partner (a paramedic and an EMT) arrive at the scene of a two-vehicle T-bone collision. You are currently the only available unit. In a pickup truck, there is a young, unrestrained adult male driver who smells strongly of alcohol and has an obvious forearm deformity. The truck struck the passenger's side front door of a small sedan, with significant intrusion into vehicle. There is an older adult female in the front passenger seat who does not appear to be breathing; the windshield is starred directly in front of her. The female driver of the sedan is also injured but conscious and extremely anxious. In the rear seats, there are two children restrained in car seats. The child on the passenger side appears to be approximately 3 years old and is unconscious and slumped over in the car seat. On the driver's side, a restrained 5-year-old boy is crying hysterically in a booster seat and appears to be uninjured.

The driver of the pickup truck is obviously injured, with an open arm fracture, but he is belligerent and verbally abusive and is refusing treatment. Meanwhile, the driver of the sedan is frantically inquiring about her children and her mother.

(continues)

INTRODUCTION

Medicine has changed a great deal since the painting by Sir Luke Fildes that shows a concerned and frustrated physician sitting at the bedside of a sick child (**Figure 2-1**). At that time, there were no antibiotics, only a superficial understanding of most diseases and illness, and rudimentary surgery. Medication consisted primarily of herbal remedies. For many years, medicine was not an exact science but more of an art form. Now, considerable advancements have been made in our understanding of disease, development of pharmaceuticals, and application of technology. Research has allowed us to provide better patient care through evidence-based medicine. However, even though the practice of medicine has become more science-based and less of an art form, the art remains.

It was not until the 1950s that consideration went into training individuals who encounter patients prior to their arrival in the emergency department (ED). The education of prehospital care practitioners has significantly advanced since that time. Beyond the knowledge gained during the initial training and certification process however, each prehospital care practitioner also has a need to remain proficient, from both cognitive and technical perspectives, with an ever-expanding base of medical knowledge. Proficiency is maintained by reading and attending continuing medical education (CME) classes. Skills improve with experience and critique, like those of a surgeon or an airplane pilot. Just as a pilot does not fly solo after one flight, an emergency medical technician (EMT) or paramedic does not achieve proficiency in a skill after performing it once or in only one type of situation.

As discussed throughout this text, the science of prehospital care involves a working knowledge of the following:

1. Anatomy—the organs, bones, muscles, arteries, nerves, and veins of the human body
2. Physiology—the understanding of how the organs and tissues of the body interact with one another to result in human function

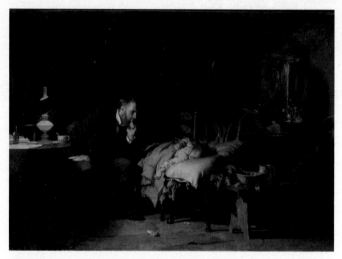

Figure 2-1 "The Doctor" by Sir Luke Fildes shows a concerned physician sitting by the bedside of an ill child. The relatively primitive state of health care offered few options for intervention beyond hopeful waiting and watching.
© Tate, London 2014

3. Pharmacology—the science of medications and how they interact with the body
4. The relationship among these components and how they affect one another

By applying one's understanding of these elements, practitioners can understand the injuries their patients have sustained and the logic behind treatments employed to mitigate the effects of those injuries.

Major improvements in the science of medicine include technological advancements and the evolution of diagnostic tools. The ability to assess, diagnose, and treat a patient has dramatically improved with the imaging techniques of computed tomography (CT) scans, ultrasound, and magnetic resonance imaging (MRI); clinical laboratories can measure almost any electrolyte, hormone, or substance found in the human body. The pharmaceutical industry is continuously developing new medications. Treatments are becoming less invasive and less morbid through endovascular and interventional radiologic techniques. The emergency medical services (EMS) communications system has dramatically improved, and the global positioning system (GPS) helps find patients even in more remote areas. Rural outreach and response times have decreased, and overall patient care has improved secondary to technological advancements.

In order to take advantage of all of these scientific medical advances, emergency first responders must be skilled in the art of linking that knowledge base to the needs of individual patients. Prehospital care practitioners need to be able to determine which patients are seriously injured and require rapid transport to which level of care; they need to be able to balance which interventions may be helpful to the patient's outcome without risking a worsening of the outcome. Being able to choose which adjuncts and techniques to use to accomplish the end goal, which in the case of shock is end-organ perfusion, is critical. This capability describes the art that is the practice of medicine.

Medicine, like all other artistic endeavors, has guiding principles. In particular, this chapter includes an exploration of the Golden Principles of Trauma Care. One foundational principle of the Prehospital Trauma Life Support (PHTLS) Program is that patient care should be *knowledge* driven and not purely *protocol* driven—hence the Golden Principles that assist prehospital care practitioners in improving patient outcomes and include making rapid assessments, rapidly applying key field interventions, and transporting trauma patients to the closest appropriate facilities. Of course, that is not to say that protocols do not have a role in the prehospital care of trauma patients. Rather, it means that the application of protocols must always be guided by; influenced by; and, when appropriate, superseded by a thorough understanding of the anatomy and physiology of a patient's injuries and how to best mitigate the detrimental impact of those injuries.

Principles and Preferences

The science of medicine provides the basis for the **principles** of medical care. Simply stated, principles define what the prehospital care practitioner must accomplish to maximize the chance of patient survival with the best possible outcome. How these principles are implemented by the individual practitioner to most efficiently manage the patient depends on the **preferences**, which describe how a system and its individual practitioners choose to apply scientific principles to the care of patients. This is how the *science* and *art* of medicine come together for the good of patient care.

An example such as airway management can illustrate the difference between principle and preference.

The *principle* is that air, containing oxygen, must be moved through an open airway into the alveoli of the lungs to facilitate oxygen–carbon dioxide exchange with red blood cells (RBCs) so they may deliver oxygen to other tissues. This principle is true for all patients. The *preference* is the method by which airway management is carried out in a particular patient. In most cases, patients will be able to maintain their own airways; in other patients, the prehospital care practitioner will have to decide which adjunct is best to facilitate airway management. In other words, the practitioner will determine the best method to ensure that the air passages are open to get oxygen into the lungs and, secondarily, to get carbon dioxide out. The art, or preference, is how the practitioner makes this determination and carries it out to achieve the principle. Some of this art is directed by information from high-quality randomized clinical trials. This is what is referred to as evidence-based medicine. Much of it, however, is often based on experience and anecdote. Standards of care describe basic minimum performance requirements that practitioners must meet in the process of delivering care to individual patients.

The preferences of how to accomplish the principles depend on several factors: the situation, the patient's condition, the practitioner's knowledge base of the available medical evidence, the practitioner's skills and experience, local protocols, and the equipment available (**Box 2-1**).

The foundation of PHTLS is to teach the prehospital care practitioner to make appropriate decisions for patient care based on knowledge and not purely on protocol. The goal of patient care is to achieve the principle. How this is achieved (i.e., the decision made by the practitioner to manage the patient) is the preference based on the situation, patient condition, medical evidence, and the skill, local protocols, and equipment available at the time—the several components outlined in Box 2-1.

Box 2-1 Principles Versus Preferences

Principle—a fundamental scientific or anatomy-based tenet for patient improvement or survival

Preference—how the specific prehospital care practitioner achieves a particular principle

The preference used to accomplish the principle depends on several factors:

- Situation that exists
- Condition of the patient
- Fund of knowledge, skills, and experience of the prehospital care practitioner
- Local protocols
- Equipment available

The philosophy of the PHTLS Program is that each situation and patient is different. PHTLS teaches the importance of having a strong understanding of the subject matter and the skills necessary to accomplish necessary interventions. The judgments and decisions made on scene should be individualized to the needs of the specific patient being managed at *that* specific time and in *that* specific situation. Protocols are helpful for guidance and direction, but they must be sufficiently flexible when there is variability in an event. Appropriate decisions can be made by understanding the principles involved and using critical-thinking skills to achieve the end goal.

Given that the preference is the way an individual prehospital care practitioner achieves the end goal, the principle will not be accomplished the same way every time. Not all practitioners have skill mastery in every technique. The equipment to carry out these techniques is not available at every emergency. Just because one instructor, lecturer, or physician medical director prefers one technique does not mean it is the best technique for *every* practitioner in *every* situation. The important point is to achieve the principle. How this is done and how the care is provided to the patient depend on the factors listed in Box 2-1. These factors are described in more detail in the following sections.

Situation

The situation involves all of the factors at a scene that can affect what care is provided to a patient. These factors include, but are not limited to, the following:

- Hazards on the scene, including infectious hazards
- Number of patients involved
- Location of the patient
- Position of the vehicle
- Contamination or hazardous materials concerns
- Fire or potential for fire
- Weather
- Scene control and security by law enforcement
- Time/distance to medical care, including the capabilities of the closest hospital versus the nearest trauma center
- Number of prehospital care practitioners and other possible helpers on the scene
- Bystanders
- Transportation available on the scene
- Other transportation available at a distance (i.e., helicopters, additional ambulances)

All of these conditions and circumstances, as well as many others, may be constantly changing and will affect the way a prehospital care practitioner can respond to the needs of the patient.

Take, for example, the following situation: a single-vehicle crash into a tree on a rural road in a wooded area. The weather is clear and dark (time 0200 hours). The transport time by ground to the trauma center is 35 minutes. A medical helicopter can be requested by prehospital care practitioners on the scene with approval of online medical direction. Startup time for the helicopter is 5 minutes, and travel time is 15 minutes; a non–trauma center hospital is 15 minutes away and has a helipad. Do you transport by ground to the trauma center, stop at the non-trauma hospital for initial evaluation, transport to the helipad to meet the helicopter, or stay on scene and wait for the helicopter?

Some examples of how the situation affects a procedure such as spinal stabilization include the following:

Situation 1

- Automobile crash
- Starburst pattern fracture of the windshield
- Warm, sunny day
- No traffic on the road

Management

- Patient examined in the car—significant back pain and lower extremity weakness noted
- Cervical collar applied
- Patient extricated onto backboard
- Removed from the car
- Placed on the stretcher
- Physical assessment completed
- Patient transported to the hospital

Situation 2

- Same as Situation 1, except gasoline is dripping from the gas tank, engine is smoking and no fire suppression units are on scene
- Concern for fire

Management

- Rapid extraction techniques used
- Patient moved significant distance from the vehicle
- Patient examined and need for implementation of spinal motion restriction determined
- Physical assessment completed
- Patient transported to the hospital

Condition of the Patient

The next component of the decision-making process concerns the medical condition of the patient. The major question that will affect decision making is, "How sick is this patient?" Some information points that will facilitate this determination include age of the patient, physiologic factors that affect end-organ perfusion (blood pressure, pulse, ventilatory rate, skin temperature, etc.), mechanism of injury, the patient's medical condition prior to the event, medication that the patient is using, and drug or alcohol intoxication. These factors and more require critical thinking to determine what needs to be done before and during transport, and what method of transportation should be used.

Let us return to the scenario of the single-vehicle crash with a tree: The patient is breathing with difficulty at a rate of 30 breaths/minute, his heart rate is 110 beats/minute, his blood pressure is 90 millimeters of mercury (mm Hg) by palpation, and the patient is not following commands; he is in his mid-20s, he was not wearing a seat belt, and his position is against the dashboard, away from the driver-side airbag; he has a deformed right leg at mid-thigh and an open left ankle fracture with significant hemorrhage. There is approximately 1 liter of blood on the floorboard near the ankle.

Fund of Knowledge of the Prehospital Care Practitioner

The fund of knowledge of the prehospital care practitioner comes from several sources, including initial training, CME courses, ongoing reading and study, local protocols, overall experience, and skill set.

Let us again use airway management as an example. The level of knowledge and experience a prehospital care practitioner possesses significantly impacts decision making with regard to airway management. The comfort level practitioners have with any particular technical skill depends on the frequency with which they have performed it in the past. As the practitioner, you might consider: Can the patient maintain a patent airway without assistance? If not, what devices are available, and of those, which ones do you feel comfortable using? When was the last time you performed an intubation? How comfortable are you with the laryngoscope? How comfortable are you with the anatomy of the oropharynx? How many times have you done a cricothyroidotomy on a live patient or even an animal training model? Without the appropriate skills and experience, the patient would likely be better off and the practitioner would be more comfortable if they were to choose a nasopharyngeal or oropharyngeal airway plus bag-mask device rather than a more advanced intervention such as endotracheal intubation or a surgical airway as the preference for management. Regardless, the option that leads you to the fastest control of the airway with the least associated risk for complications is the one you should choose.

Returning to the example of the patient in the single-vehicle crash, the responding prehospital care practitioners have been working together for 2 years. Both are nationally registered paramedics (NRPs). Their last update training for endotracheal (ET) intubation was 1 year ago. One paramedic last placed an ET tube 2 months ago; his partner placed one a month ago. They are not authorized to use paralytic drugs for ET insertion, but they can use sedation if necessary. They were just trained on hemorrhage control using tourniquets and hemostatic agents. How will their training impact what will be done to manage this patient in the field at this very moment?

Local Protocols

A PHTLS practitioner's scope of practice is defined by what they are trained to do, certified as competent to do, licensed to do, and credentialed by their agency medical director to do. Protocols define under what circumstances the practitioner should apply their scope of practice. While these protocols should not and cannot describe in cookbook fashion how to care for every patient, they are intended to guide the approach to patients in a way that is systematic and consistent with best practices, local resources, and training. In the scenario of the single-vehicle crash, rapid-sequence induction with intubation may be valuable and indicated in some situations, but if the skill set is not included in the local protocols, the paramedics will not have it at their disposal. Local protocols often dictate which procedures and transport destinations the practitioner should select. They may, for example, direct the practitioner to request air medical assets for assistance with transport or to transport the patient to a specific trauma center.

Equipment Available

The experience of prehospital care practitioners does not matter if they do not have the appropriate equipment available. Practitioners must use the equipment or supplies that are available. As an example, blood may be the best resuscitation fluid for trauma victims. However, blood is frequently not available in the field; therefore, crystalloid may be the only resuscitative fluid available. Another consideration is whether permissive hypotension would be a better choice given the nature of the patient's injuries. This particular issue is discussed in more detail in Chapter 3, *Shock: Pathophysiology of Life and Death*.

Once again let us return to the patient in the single-vehicle crash: There is complete paramedic equipment available, and it was checked at the beginning of the shift. It includes ET tubes, laryngoscopes, supraglottic airways, nasopharyngeal airways, oropharyngeal airways, tourniquets, and other equipment and supplies as supported by the 2020 National Association of EMS Physicians (NAEMSP) Joint Position Statement on Recommended Essential Equipment for Basic Life Support and Advanced Life Support Ground Ambulances.[1] The paramedics have hemostatic agents available. The patient is not trapped; therefore, the most expeditious form of transport to the trauma center is by ground. The patient is independently capable of maintaining an airway. However, given his difficulty breathing, the paramedics assist his ventilation using a bag-mask device with supplemental oxygen. Ongoing bleeding is minimal after extrication from the vehicle; therefore, the paramedics apply manual pressure to the open ankle injury and are able to achieve control. They choose a collar plus a long backboard to stabilize the patient's cervical and thoracolumbar spine. They splint the patient's femur to the board to save time and transport him directly to the nearby trauma center.

Another example of principle versus preference is when a nonbreathing patient is encountered, the *principle* is that the airway must be opened and oxygen delivered to the lungs. The *preference* chosen depends on the preference factors (situation, patient condition, fund of knowledge, protocols and experience/skill, equipment available). A bystander on the street with only cardiopulmonary resuscitation (CPR) training may perform mouth-to-mask ventilation; the EMT may choose an oral airway and bag-mask ventilation; the paramedic may choose to place an ET tube or may decide that it is more advantageous to use the bag-mask device with rapid transport; the Corpsman in combat may choose a cricothyroidotomy or nothing at all if the enemy fire is too intense; and the physician in the ED may choose paralytic drugs or fiber-optic–guided ET tube placement. None of the choices is wrong at a specific point in time for a given patient; similarly, none is correct all of the time.

This concept of principle and preference for the care of the trauma patient has its most dramatic application in the combat situation in the military. For this reason, the Committee on Tactical Combat Casualty Care (Co-TCCC) wrote the military component of the PHTLS textbook. For the military medic, the scene situation will include whether there is active combat, the location of the enemy, the tactical situation, the weapons currently being used, and protection available for sheltering the wounded. Although obvious differences relate to patient care in combat situations, similar considerations exist for civilian tactical emergency medical support practitioners and those prehospital care practitioners who work in hazardous environments such as fire scenes. For example, in the middle of a house that is fully involved in fire, a firefighter–paramedic discovers a patient who is down. It is not safe or even rational in such a situation to stop and assess the patient's airway or hemodynamics. The first step is to get the patient out of the burning building and away from the immediate danger of the fire. Only then is it appropriate to assess the patient's airway and pulse.

For the military medic who is potentially involved in combat, the three-step process for casualty management developed by the Co-TCCC is as follows:

1. *Care under fire/threat*—management in the middle of a fire fight
2. *Tactical field care*—management after the shooting is over but danger still exists
3. *Tactical evacuation care*—treatment of the casualty once the situation is considered safe

Courtesy of the Committee on Tactical Combat Casualty Care.

While the principles of patient care never change, the preferences with regard to how patient care is delivered may be dramatically different. For further discussion, details, and clarification, refer to Chapter 22, *Civilian Tactical Emergency Medical Support (TEMS)* or the military version of PHTLS. (These situational differences are described in more detail in Chapter 5, *Scene Management*.)

Critical Thinking

To successfully address the principle that applies to a particular patient's condition and to choose the best preference to implement the principle, critical-thinking skills are crucial. Critical thinking in medicine is a process in which the healthcare practitioner assesses the situation, the patient, and all of the resources that are available (**Box 2-2**). The practitioner then rapidly analyzes this information and determines the optimal means to provide the best care possible to the patient. The critical-thinking process requires that the healthcare practitioner develop a plan of action, initiate this plan, reassess the plan as the process of caring for the patient moves forward, and make adjustments to the plan as the patient's condition changes until that phase of care is completed (**Box 2-3**). Critical thinking is a learned skill that improves with use and experience.[2] If prehospital care practitioners are to function successfully, they must be equipped with the critical-thinking skills necessary to acquire and process information in a rapidly and ever-changing world.[3]

For the prehospital care practitioner, critical thinking begins with processing the initial information provided at the time of dispatch and continues until transfer of care at the hospital. Critical thinking is also involved in the selection of receiving facility level, because resources available and the transport time need to be considered.

All of these critical decisions are based on the situation, the patient condition, the fund of knowledge of the practitioner, and the skills and equipment available.

The critical-thinking process cannot be dogmatic or gullible; instead, it must be open-minded, with skepticism.[4] The prehospital care practitioner must question the scientific accuracy of all approaches. This is the reason why the practitioner must have a strong, well-grounded fund of knowledge that can be used to make appropriate decisions. However, the questioning cannot be taken so far that it would delay care. Aristotle suggested that one should not require more certainty than the subject allows.[5] When a practitioner is assessing and caring for a patient, withholding action in hopes of securing absolute certainty in the patient's diagnosis would be foolish; such certainty is impossible, and seeking it would only delay needed interventions. A practitioner must make the most informed assessment and decision possible given the information available at the time.

The basis of appropriate medical care advocated by PHTLS relies on critical thinking: "judgment based on knowledge." Robert Carroll described critical thinking as concepts and principles, not hard-and-fast rules or step-by-step procedures.[4] The emphasis throughout PHTLS education is that protocols should always leave room for and be accompanied by critical thinking. Guidelines and formal pathways for patient care must be flexible. Critical thinking requires that flexibility. Protocols are put into place to serve as guidelines to assist prehospital care practitioners in aligning their thought process. They also play a crucial role in ensuring that important steps in the delivery of care are not missed. For example, protocols often mandate checking both waveform end-tidal CO_2 ($ETCO_2$) levels and breath sounds after endotracheal intubation to verify proper tube placement. If the situational reality is that you simply cannot hear breath sounds, not because the tube is malpositioned but because you happen to be in the back of a moving helicopter, you may need to rely on $ETCO_2$ alone, recognizing that this does not provide the same level of verification of tube position as does checking for breath sounds or obtaining a chest x-ray, neither of which are possible in the situation.

Using Critical Thinking to Control Biases

All healthcare practitioners have biases that can affect critical-thinking processes and decision making about patients. These biases must be recognized and not allowed to influence the patient care process. Biases usually arise from several sources. A previous experience that resulted in either a significant positive or negative impact could be a source. Two thought processes help protect patients: (1) Assume the worst-case scenario until proven otherwise, and (2) uphold the principle of *primum non nocere*,

---

Box 2-2 Components of Critical Thinking in Emergency Medical Care

1. Assess the situation.
2. Assess the patient.
3. Assess the available resources.
4. Analyze the possible solutions.
5. Weigh the relative risks and benefits of treatment options in determining the best way to manage the situation and patient.
6. Develop the plan of action.
7. Initiate the plan of action.
8. Reassess the response of the patient to the plan of action.
9. Make any needed adjustments or changes to the plan of action.
10. Continue with steps 8 and 9 until this phase of care is completed.

© National Association of Emergency Medical Technicians (NAEMT)

Box 2-3 Steps in Critical-Thinking Assessment

What is going on? What needs to be done? What are the resources to achieve the goal? Analysis will involve:

- Scene assessment
- Identification of any hazards to either the patient or the prehospital care practitioner
- Condition of the patient
- Rapidity required for resolution
- Location of the care (in the field, during transport, and after arrival to the hospital)
- Number of patients on the scene
- Number of transport vehicles required
- Need for more rapid transport
- Destination of the patient for the appropriate care

Analysis

Each of these conditions must be individually and rapidly analyzed, and they must be cross-referenced with the prehospital care practitioner's fund of knowledge and the resources available. Steps must be defined to provide the best care.

Construction of a Plan

The plan to achieve the best outcome for the patient is developed and critically reviewed. Is any step incorrect? Are the planned steps all achievable? Are any steps missing? Are the resources available that will allow the plan to move forward? Will they, more likely than not, lead to a successful outcome? Is there a better plan?

Action

The plan is initiated and put into motion. This is done decisively and with assertiveness so that there is no confusion regarding what needs to be accomplished or who is in command and making the decisions. If the decisions are not effective for the outcome of the patient, the prehospital care practitioner in command must again assess relative risks and benefits and make appropriate changes. Suggestions for change can come from the commander or from other participants.

Reassessment

Has the situation on scene changed? Does anything in the action plan need to be changed? What is the patient's condition and has it changed? Has the treatment plan improved the patient's condition or has it worsened?

Changes Along the Way

Any changes that are identified by the prehospital care practitioner are assessed and analyzed as described here, and alterations are made accordingly to allow the practitioners to continue to deliver the best possible care for the patient. Alterations in decision making that are based on reassessments of the patient should not be viewed as indicative of failures or earlier incorrect patient care, as the patient and situation are ever-changing and may call for a change in plan. Having the ability to think critically and remain dynamic based on the situation is a sign of strength in a leader.

or "first do no harm." The patient's treatment plan is designed regardless of the opinion of the prehospital care practitioner regarding the "apparent" conditions that might have led to the current circumstances. For example, the initial impression that a driver is intoxicated may be correct, but other conditions may exist as well. Patients who are intoxicated may also be seriously injured. Because the patient is impaired from intoxication does not mean that some of the alteration in mental status might not be due to brain injury or decreased cerebral perfusion because of shock.

Frequently, the complete picture cannot be understood based on the initial presentation; therefore, the critical thinking and response of the prehospital care practitioner must be based on worst-case scenario assumptions. Judgments must be made based on the best information available. The critical thinker is constantly looking for "other information" as it becomes available and then acting on it. The critical-thinking process must continue throughout the assessment of the patient, the

situation, and the conditions. The practitioner should always be anticipating and thinking several steps ahead.

Using Critical Thinking in Rapid Decision Making

EMS is a field of quick action and reliance on the innate ability of the prehospital care practitioner to respond decisively to varying presentations and varying diseases in a timely manner. Efficiency and accuracy are important. Combining protocol and preference efficiently is optimal.

Critical thinking at the site of an emergency must be swift, thorough, flexible, and objective. The prehospital care practitioner at the site of an emergency may have only seconds to assess the situation, the condition of the patient(s), and the resources available before needing to make decisions and commence patient care. Sometimes the practitioner may have a downright luxurious amount of time to think through a situation and should take advantage of the luxury of time, but this is often not the case.

Using Critical Thinking in Data Analysis

Information is gathered using four of the five senses: vision, smell, touch, and hearing. (This will be taught in Chapter 6, *Patient Assessment and Management*.) The prehospital care practitioner then analyzes this information or data obtained based on the primary survey and determines the overall plan of care for the patient until care is transferred to a hospital practitioner.

Typically, the evaluation of a trauma patient begins with the primary survey of XABCDE (eXsanguinating hemorrhage, Airway, Breathing, Circulation, Disability, Expose/Environment), but critical thinking guides the prehospital care practitioner to the most critical condition first. If the patient is in shock because of external hemorrhage, then applying direct pressure over the source of hemorrhage is the appropriate initial step after assessment. Critical thinking is the recognition that following the standard ABC priority as would be appropriate for medical patients may lead to a trauma patient who has an airway but who has now exsanguinated; so, instead of attention to the airway, control of obvious severe exsanguinating hemorrhage is the appropriate first step. Critical thinking is the process of recognizing that if direct pressure is not working, then something else needs to be done. Critical thinking is understanding that relatively minor bleeding from an extremity is not the same thing as exsanguinating hemorrhage and should not be addressed until after the remainder of the primary survey has been completed. Critical thinking is about synthesizing the data immediately available and making decisions based on the needs of the patient at the time, the overall situation, the fund of knowledge of the practitioner, the skills of the practitioner, and the equipment available.

> Critical thinking is a pervasive skill that involves scrutinizing, differentiating, and appraising information and reflecting on the information gained in order to make judgments and inform clinical decisions.[6]

Using Critical Thinking Throughout the Phases of Patient Care

The art and science of medicine, the knowledge of principles, and the appropriate application of preferences will lead to the anticipated outcome of the best care possible for the patient in the circumstances in which the care is provided. There are essentially four phases in the process of caring for patients with acute injuries:

1. The prehospital phase
2. The initial (resuscitative) phase in the hospital
3. The stabilization and definitive care phase
4. The long-term resolution and rehabilitation phase to return the patient to a functional status

The same principles of patient care apply in each phase. Each of the healthcare practitioners throughout the phases of the patient's care must use critical thinking. Critical thinking continues from the time of the injury until the time that the patient goes home. EMS personnel are directly involved in the initial prehospital phase of care and use critical-thinking skills to help identify and prioritize treatment decisions. Prehospital care practitioners must often think beyond the current situation to the definitive care needs and the patient's ultimate outcome. The goal is to help treat the patient in a way that will ultimately promote healing and allow the patient to return to the highest level of function possible—ideally just as before injury. For example, critical thinking involves recognizing that even though splinting the fractured forearm of a multisystem trauma patient is not one of the initial priorities of care, when considering the definitive outcome of the patient and the ability to lead a productive life, the preservation of limb function and the prevention of additional injury during transport (and thus splinting of the limb) is an important concern in the patient's prehospital treatment.

Ethics

Prehospital professionals often face ethically challenging scenarios that are both emergent and time sensitive. However, the lack of prehospital-specific ethics education can leave prehospital care practitioners feeling both unprepared and unsupported when confronted with ethical challenges.[7] Critical-thinking skills can provide a sound basis for helping to work through some of the difficult ethical decisions sometimes required of practitioners.

The goal of this section is to use bioethical principles and concepts to begin to develop ethical awareness and ethical reasoning skills and to provide common frameworks and vocabulary to help understand ethically challenging cases. This section will rely on the traditional elements of basic bioethics education, which are familiar to many healthcare practitioners, but will use prehospital examples and cases to provide content that is authentic, practical, and applicable to the field setting. Additionally, by exposing prehospital care practitioners to common bioethics principles and concepts, ethics conversations across healthcare disciplines and settings can be facilitated.

Ethical Principles

Everyone uses some set of values, beliefs, or social rules to make decisions. These rules are generally accepted beliefs about moral behavior and are often referred to as principles. Ethics is the use of a set of moral principles to assist in identifying the right thing to do. In medicine, the set of principles that is often relied on to ensure ethical behavior, to guide clinical practice, and to assist in ethical decision making includes elements of **autonomy**, **nonmaleficence**, **beneficence**, and **justice**. The use of these four principles, often referred to as **principlism**, provides a framework within which one can weigh and balance benefits and burdens, generally within the context of treating a specific patient, in order to act in the patient's best interest.[5]

Autonomy is defined as the patient's right to direct their own health care. The principle of nonmaleficence obligates the medical practitioner not to take actions that are likely to harm the patient. Beneficence means "to do good" and requires prehospital care practitioners to act in a manner that maximizes the benefits and minimizes the risks to the patient. Justice, in the context of trauma care, commonly thought of as that which is fair or just, usually refers to how we distribute medical resources.

In trauma, the concept of justice must be considered when faced with circumstances in which the available resources are overwhelmed by the need for patient care. For example, when triaging an emergency multiple-casualty incident, those with the greatest medical needs are prioritized over those with less critical needs. Thus, the most vulnerable are often given a greater portion of healthcare goods and services based on a shared community value of caring for the sick and marginalized.

In a mass-casualty incident, triage is based partially on probability of survival, and some of the sickest or most vulnerable are moved to an expectant category to allow for resources to be focused on those with more survivable injuries. Therefore, what is most just in a particular situation may depend on the availability of resources and the fairest way of using and distributing those resources in that specific case.[8]

There are some important challenges in the delivery of trauma care that are better understood in the context of considering these ethical principles. For example, a patient's ability to make autonomous decisions may be compromised by brain injury, shock, or chemical intoxication. In trauma, eligible surrogates are often unavailable to help with decision making. The practitioner should make every effort to explain the situation to patients, when possible, in a way that will allow them to make informed decisions autonomously. Not every piece of information will be available at the initial presentation, but those that are available should be shared with patients who are conscious and capable of understanding in order to allow those patients to retain their autonomy. Similarly, the principle of nonmaleficence requires practitioners to limit motion in the thoracolumbar spine of a patient with high-energy trauma and difficulty breathing

due to morbid obesity. The complicated trauma scenario would suggest that one very acceptable and efficient way to limit such motion is to stabilize the patient onto a backboard. The principle of beneficence would suggest that elevating the patient's head to facilitate breathing is in order, but this is in conflict with the goal of nonmaleficence. The solution of elevating the patient's head by tilting the board upward at the head by 30 degrees or moving the stretcher to a reverse Trendelenburg position addresses both principles for the patient.

Informed Consent

Informed consent is a process through which a medical practitioner provides a patient who has decision-making capacity, or a surrogate decision maker (a person who is chosen to make healthcare decisions on the patient's behalf if the patient is not able to make decisions for themself),[5] with the information necessary to provide informed consent for, or refusal of, the medical treatment being offered. Although many people think of informed consent as a legal form, in reality, the form itself is only a record of the consent conversation. There is an ethical obligation on the part of a healthcare practitioner to give patients the appropriate medical information to allow them to make health decisions based on their own values, beliefs, and wishes.

In order for an informed consent to be valid, the following must be true for patients:

- Must have decision-making capacity
- Must have the ability to communicate their understanding of their diagnosis, prognosis, and treatment options
- Must be able to give consent or refusal voluntarily
- Must actively refuse or consent to treatment[5,9,10]

Assessing any one of these elements can be hard enough to accomplish in a controlled clinical setting, but in an emergency trauma situation, it is especially difficult. Although many people use the terms *competence* and *decision-making capacity* interchangeably, **competence** is a legal term referring to a person's general ability to make good decisions for themself, and decision-making capacity refers to a patient's ability to make decisions regarding a specific set of medical treatment options or therapies.

Assessing the capacity of a patient is particularly difficult in the context of trauma. There is rarely knowledge of the patient's baseline on initial presentation, and the assessment is often made when the patient is acutely injured. When assessing the decision-making capacity of an adult patient, it is necessary to attempt to determine their level of understanding. Can the patient understand the medical options and weigh the risks and benefits associated with those options? Patients should also have the capacity to appreciate the anticipated outcomes of their choices, as well as be able to express their wishes to the healthcare practitioner. Although the informed consent process respects the rights of patients to make their own decisions, the informed consent requirement may be overridden in emergency situations under certain conditions:

1. The patient lacks decision-making capacity due to unconsciousness or significant cognitive impairment and there is no surrogate available.
2. The condition is potentially life or health threatening and the patient may suffer irreversible damage in the absence of treatment.
3. A reasonable person would consent to the treatment, in which case a healthcare practitioner may proceed with treatment in the absence of an autonomous consent from the patient or a surrogate.[7]

Privacy and Confidentiality

In the healthcare context, **privacy** refers to the right of patients to control who has access to their personal health information. **Confidentiality** refers to the obligation of healthcare practitioners not to inappropriately share patient information that has been disclosed to them. Within the context of the patient–practitioner relationship, any information a practitioner obtains should be considered confidential. It should not be disclosed to any individuals other than those the patient has authorized, other medical professionals involved in the patient's care, or agencies responsible for processing state and/or federally mandated reporting, such as in cases of child or elder abuse.

Depending on the circumstances, prehospital care practitioners may need to rely on and interact with people other than an incapacitated patient (family, friends, or neighbors) in order to gain the information necessary to care for the patient. However, great effort should be made to protect patient information from those who are not healthcare practitioners, such as observers or news media who may be at the scene of an injury or loss of life, and to limit information given to others until an appropriate surrogate decision maker is identified.

Truth Telling

Truth telling can also present ethical challenges.[10] Truthfulness is both an expectation and a necessary part of building a trusting patient–practitioner relationship. Communicating honestly shows respect for the patient and enables decision making based on truthful information. However, especially in the prehospital setting, there are situations in which telling a patient the truth has the potential to cause great harm, such as in cases of multivictim trauma in which survivors are inquiring about the condition of nonsurviving or critically injured loved ones. At such times, the immediate obligation to tell the truth may sometimes be somewhat mitigated by the obligation to do no harm, depending on the level of injury and the condition of the patient who is asking.[7] It is never acceptable to lie to a patient. But withholding, or more accurately, delaying communication of, certain sensitive information may at times be necessary in the context of prioritizing lifesaving care over communicating distressing information to a patient who may be unprepared to fully process it.

The Golden Period: Time-Sensitive Conditions

In the late 1960s, R. Adams Cowley, MD, conceived the idea of a crucial time period during which it is important to begin definitive patient care for a critically injured trauma patient. In an interview he said:

> There is a "golden hour" between life and death. If you are critically injured, you have less than 60 minutes to survive. You might not die right then—it may be three days or two weeks later—but something has happened in your body that is irreparable.[11]

While occasionally taken literally, Dr. Cowley was actually describing a concept, and as such, it is important to realize that a patient does not always have the luxury of an entire "Golden Hour." The "hour" was intended to be a figurative as opposed to a literal description of a period of time. A patient with a penetrating wound to the heart may have only a few minutes to reach definitive care before the shock caused by the injury becomes irreversible; however, a patient with slow, ongoing internal hemorrhage from an isolated femur fracture may have several hours or longer to reach definitive care and resuscitation.

Because the Golden *Hour* is not a strict 60-minute time frame and varies from patient to patient based on the injuries, it is better thought of as the Golden *Period*. If a critically injured patient can obtain definitive care—that is, hemorrhage control and resuscitation—within that particular patient's Golden Period, the chance of survival is improved greatly.[12] The American College of Surgeons Committee on Trauma has used this concept to emphasize the importance of transporting trauma patients to facilities where expert trauma care is available in a timely manner.

The management of serious prehospital trauma must reflect these contingencies. The following goals, however, do not change:

1. Gain access to the patient.
2. Identify and treat life-threatening injuries.
3. Minimize on-scene time through rapid assessment, rapid patient packaging, and reducing

on-scene treatments to only those to reverse immediately life-threatening conditions.

4. Transport the patient to the closest appropriate facility by the most expeditious mode of transport.

The majority of the techniques and principles discussed are not new, and most are taught in initial training programs. However, PHTLS is different in the following ways:

- It provides current, evidence-based management practices for the trauma patient.
- It provides a systematic approach for establishing priorities of patient care for trauma patients who have sustained injury to multiple body systems.
- It provides an organizational scheme for interventions.

Why Trauma Patients Die

Studies that analyze the causes of death in trauma patients demonstrate some variability depending on place and time. A 1975 study from Russia of more than 700 trauma deaths found that most patients who rapidly succumbed to their injuries fall into one of three categories: massive acute blood loss (36%), severe injury to vital organs such as the brain (30%), and airway obstruction and acute ventilatory failure (25%).[13] A study published in 2010 from Dallas documented that 76% of patients who died rapidly did so from nonsurvivable injuries to the head, aorta, or heart.[14] In 2020, Kalkwarf and colleagues in Houston reported that 17% of trauma deaths were due to hemorrhage and that 45% of those deaths were preventable or potentially preventable with earlier resuscitation and hemorrhage control.[15] A study published in 2013 found a reduction in deaths from multiple organ failure, or the third phase of death (see Chapter 1, *PHTLS: Past, Present, and Future*).[16] This reduction in deaths may be attributed to improvements in modern trauma care both in the field and in the hospital.

Clearly the severity and duration of hypotension affect outcome as well as the speed to surgical hemorrhage control. In 2002, Clarke and colleagues in Philadelphia demonstrated that for hypotensive patients with intra-abdominal trauma, prolonged time in the ED prior to surgical intervention was an independent risk factor for death with mortality increasing by 1% for each additional 3 minutes of delay.[17] In 2016, Meizoso and his co-authors in Miami reported that delays of greater than 10 minutes from arrival in the ED to surgery tripled the risk of death for victims of gunshot wounds who present with hypotension.[18]

But what is happening to these patients on a cellular level? The metabolic processes of the human body are driven by energy, similar to any other machine. This is discussed further in Chapter 3, *Shock: Pathophysiology of Life and Death*. Shock can be viewed as a failure of energy production in the body caused by a failure to deliver oxygen to and retrieve carbon dioxide from body tissues. As with machines, the human body generates its own energy but must have fuel to do so. Fuel for the body is oxygen and glucose. The body can store glucose as complex carbohydrates (glycogen) and fat to use at a later time. However, oxygen cannot be stored. It must be constantly supplied to the cells of the body. Atmospheric air, containing oxygen, is drawn into the lungs by the action of the diaphragm and intercostal muscles. Oxygen diffuses across the alveolar and capillary walls, where it binds to the hemoglobin in the RBCs and is then transported to the body's tissues by the circulatory system. In the presence of oxygen, the cells of the tissues then "burn" glucose through a complex series of metabolic processes (glycolysis, Krebs cycle, and electron transport) to produce the energy needed for all body functions. This energy is stored as adenosine triphosphate (ATP). Without sufficient energy in the form of ATP, essential metabolic activities cannot occur normally, cells begin to die, and organ failure occurs.

Acidosis, hypothermia, and coagulopathy—also known as the lethal triad of trauma—are factors that combine with shock in trauma patients to increase the risk of death. These are not independent variables. Bleeding and shock cause acidosis because of increased anaerobic metabolism. Acidosis impairs clotting. Bleeding leads to shock and to loss of clotting factors from the blood. As a result of the loss of these factors, clotting is impaired and bleeding worsens during the early hours after injury, resulting in worsening of the shock state. Later in the patient's course, platelet and clotting factor activation actually leads to hypercoagulable states that increase risks of clotting-related disorders such as pulmonary embolism and multiple organ dysfunction syndrome. As many as 25% of severely injured civilians and a third of severely injured military personnel who are in shock are also coagulopathic.[19,20] Similarly, while hypothermia may be primarily related to exposure to cold atmospheres, blood loss and shock decrease the body's ability to respond to cold temperatures. Hypothermia is an independent contributor to coagulopathy and thus contributes to ongoing hemorrhage. The trio of acidosis, hypothermia, and coagulopathy is particularly deadly and must be reversed promptly.

The sensitivity of the cells to oxygen deprivation varies from organ to organ (**Box 2-4**). The cells within an organ can be fatally damaged but can continue to function for a period of time. (See Chapter 3, *Shock: Pathophysiology of Life and Death* for complications of prolonged shock.) This delayed death of cells, leading to organ failure, is what Dr. Cowley was referring to in his earlier quote. Shock results in death if a patient is not treated promptly.

Box 2-4 Shock

When the heart is deprived of oxygen, the myocardial cells cannot produce enough energy to pump blood to the other tissues. For example, a patient has lost a significant number of RBCs and blood volume following a gunshot wound to the aorta. The heart continues to beat for several minutes before failing. Refilling the vascular system after the heart has been without oxygen for too long will not restore the function of the injured cells.

Although ischemia, as seen in severe shock, may result in damage to any tissues, the damage to the organs does not become apparent initially. In the lungs, acute respiratory distress syndrome often develops up to 48 hours after an ischemic insult, whereas acute renal failure and hepatic failure typically occur several days later. Although all body tissues are affected by insufficient oxygen, some tissues are more sensitive to ischemia. For example, a patient who has sustained a brain injury due to shock and anoxia may develop permanent brain damage. Although brain cells cease to function and die, the rest of the body can survive for years.

For this reason, Dr. Cowley advocated the rapid transport of the patient to the operating room for control of internal hemorrhage.

The Golden Hour or Period represents a crucial interval during which the cascade of events can worsen the long-term survival and overall outcomes of the patient; if proper care is received rapidly during this period, much of the damage is reversible. Failure to initiate appropriate interventions aimed at improving oxygenation and controlling hemorrhage allows shock to progress, eventually leading to death. In addition, reversal of acidosis, hypothermia, and coagulopathy must occur as soon as possible. For trauma patients to have the best chance of survival, interventions should start with an easily accessible and functional emergency communications system. Trained dispatchers can begin the process of providing care in the field by offering prearrival instructions such as hemorrhage control. Care in the field continues with the arrival of prehospital care practitioners and proceeds to the ED, the operating room, the intensive care unit, and when appropriate, the rehabilitation facility. Trauma is a true "team sport." The patient "wins" when all members of the trauma team—from those in the field to those in the trauma center—work together to care for the individual patient.

The Golden Principles of Prehospital Trauma Care

This text discusses the assessment and management of patients who have sustained injury to specific body systems. Although the body systems are presented individually, many severely injured patients have injury to more than one body system—hence the term *multisystem trauma* patient (also known as *polytrauma*). A prehospital care practitioner needs to recognize and prioritize the treatment of patients with multiple injuries, following the Golden Principles of prehospital trauma care. Note that these principles may not necessarily be performed in the exact order listed, but they must all be accomplished for optimal care of the injured patient. The Golden Principles are reviewed briefly in the following discussion. References are given to specific chapters in which each principle is more directly applied to prehospital trauma care. **Table 2-1** offers a quick reference to these principles.

1. Ensure the Safety of the Prehospital Care Practitioners and the Patient

Scene safety remains the highest priority on arrival to all calls for medical assistance. Trauma calls represent some of the highest risk responses prehospital practitioners face. Situational awareness of all scene types can help practitioners understand how to mitigate the risks (**Figure 2-2**). This awareness includes the safety of all emergency responders as well as the safety of the patient. Based on information provided by dispatch, potential threats can often be anticipated before arrival at the scene. Chapters that discuss this principle include Chapter 16, *Injury Prevention* and Chapter 5, *Scene Management*.

2. Assess the Scene Situation to Determine the Need for Additional Resources

During the response to the scene and immediately upon arrival, prehospital care practitioners should perform a quick assessment to determine the need for additional or specialized resources. Examples include additional EMS units to accommodate the number of patients, fire suppression equipment, special rescue teams, medical helicopters, and EMS physicians where available. The need for these resources should be considered and requests made as soon as possible, and a designated communications channel should be secured. Chapter 5, *Scene Management* discusses this principle in detail.

Table 2-1 Reference Guide for the 14 Golden Principles

Golden Principle	Related Chapter(s)
1. Ensure the safety of the prehospital care practitioners and the patient.	Chapter 5, *Scene Management* Chapter 16, *Injury Prevention*
2. Assess the scene situation to determine the need for additional resources.	Chapter 5, *Scene Management* Chapter 17, *Disaster Management* Chapter 18, *Explosions and Weapons of Mass Destruction*
3. Control any significant external hemorrhage.	Chapter 3, *Shock: Pathophysiology of Life and Death* Chapter 11, *Abdominal Trauma* Chapter 12, *Musculoskeletal Trauma* Chapter 21, *Wilderness Trauma Care* Chapter 22, *Civilian Tactical Emergency Medical Support (TEMS)*
4. Use the primary survey approach to identify life-threatening conditions.	Chapter 6, *Patient Assessment and Management*
5. Recognize the physics of trauma that produced the injuries.	Chapter 4, *The Physics of Trauma*
6. Provide appropriate airway management while maintaining spinal motion restriction as indicated.	Chapter 7, *Airway and Ventilation* Chapter 8, *Head and Neck Trauma* Chapter 9, *Spinal Trauma*
7. Support ventilation and deliver oxygen to maintain an SpO_2 greater than or equal to 94%.	Chapter 7, *Airway and Ventilation* Chapter 8, *Head and Neck Trauma*
8. Provide basic shock therapy, including appropriately splinting musculoskeletal injuries and restoring and maintaining normal body temperature.	Chapter 3, *Shock: Pathophysiology of Life and Death* Chapter 12, *Musculoskeletal Trauma* Chapter 19, *Environmental Trauma I: Heat and Cold* Chapter 21, *Wilderness Trauma Care*
9. Apply appropriate spinal motion restriction principles based on the patient's complaints and mental status and considering the mechanism of injury.	Chapter 9, *Spinal Trauma* Chapter 21, *Wilderness Trauma Care*
10. For critically injured trauma patients, initiate transport to the closest appropriate facility as soon as possible after EMS arrival on scene.	Chapter 6, *Patient Assessment and Management* Chapter 8, *Head and Neck Trauma* Chapter 10, *Thoracic Trauma* Chapter 13, *Burn Injuries*
11. Initiate fluid replacement en route to the receiving facility as necessary to restore basic perfusion.	Chapter 3, *Shock: Pathophysiology of Life and Death* Chapter 13, *Burn Injuries*

Golden Principle	Related Chapter(s)
12. Ascertain the patient's medical history, and perform a secondary survey when life-threatening problems have been satisfactorily managed or have been ruled out.	Chapter 6, *Patient Assessment and Management*
13. Provide adequate pain relief.	Chapter 6, *Patient Assessment and Management* Chapter 10, *Thoracic Trauma* Chapter 11, *Abdominal Trauma* Chapter 12, *Musculoskeletal Trauma* Chapter 13, *Burn Injuries* Chapter 14, *Pediatric Trauma* Chapter 15, *Geriatric Trauma*
14. Provide thorough and accurate communication regarding the patient and the circumstances of the injury to the receiving facility.	Chapter 6, *Patient Assessment and Management*

© National Association of Emergency Medical Technicians (NAEMT)

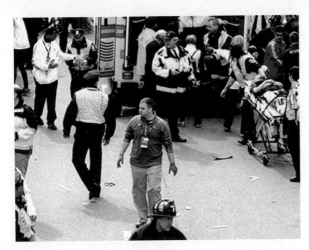

Figure 2-2 Scene safety remains the highest priority on arrival to all calls for medical assistance. Maintaining situational awareness is one way to help practitioners mitigate risk.
© Charles Krupa/AP Images

3. Control Any Significant External Hemorrhage

In the trauma patient, significant external hemorrhage is a finding that requires immediate attention. Although measures aimed at resuscitation are often the immediate priority in patient care, attempted resuscitation will never be successful in the presence of severe ongoing external hemorrhage. Even in the growing number of situations where blood is available for administration in the prehospital setting, hemorrhage control is a paramount concern for prehospital care practitioners in order to maintain a sufficient number of circulating RBCs; *every red blood cell counts*. Bleeding control is a recurring topic throughout this text and is particularly relevant in Chapter 3, *Shock: Pathophysiology of Life and Death*; Chapter 11, *Abdominal Trauma*; Chapter 12, *Musculoskeletal Trauma*; Chapter 21, *Wilderness Trauma Care*; and Chapter 22, *Civilian Tactical Emergency Medical Support (TEMS)*.

4. Use the Primary Survey Approach to Identify Life-Threatening Conditions

This brief survey allows vital functions to be rapidly assessed and life-threatening conditions to be identified through systematic evaluation of the XABCDEs (**Box 2-5**). The primary survey involves a "treat as you go" philosophy. As life-threatening problems are identified, care is initiated at the earliest possible time, with many aspects of the primary survey performed simultaneously when resources allow. This principle is discussed in Chapter 6, *Patient Assessment and Management*.

5. Recognize the Physics of Trauma that Produced the Injuries

Understanding the physics of trauma provides the reader with a foundation of how kinetic energy can translate into injury to the trauma patient. See Chapter 4, *The Physics of Trauma* for a full discussion. As the prehospital care

Box 2-5 Critical or Potentially Critical Trauma Patient: Scene Time of 10 Minutes or Less

Presence of any of the following life-threatening conditions:

1. Inadequate or threatened airway
2. Impaired ventilation, as demonstrated by any of the following:
   - Respiratory rate (RR) < 10 or > 29 breaths/min
   - Respiratory distress or need for respiratory support
   - Hypoxia (oxygen saturation [SpO_2] < 90% on room air)
   - Dyspnea
   - Chest wall instability, deformity, or suspected flail chest
3. Active bleeding requiring a tourniquet or wound packing with continuous pressure
4. Shock, even if compensated
5. Abnormal neurologic status
   - Unable to follow commands (motor GCS < 6)
   - Seizure activity
   - Suspected spinal injury with new motor or sensory loss
6. Penetrating trauma to the head, neck, or torso, or proximal to the elbow and knee in the extremities
7. Amputation or near-amputation proximal to the wrist or ankle

© National Association of Emergency Medical Technicians (NAEMT)

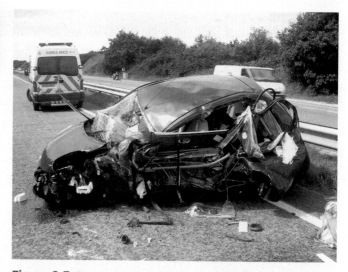

Figure 2-3 Recognize the physics of trauma that produced the injuries.
Courtesy of Dr. Mark Woolcock.

Box 2-6 Mechanism of Injury Criteria for Triage to Trauma Centers

- Falls
  - Greater than 10 feet (3 meters [m]) (one story is equal to 10 feet) (all ages)
- High-risk auto crash (**Figure 2-4**)
  - Intrusion, including roof: Greater than 12 inches (0.3 m) occupant site; greater than 18 inches (0.5 m) any site
  - Need for extrication (i.e., physical entrapment of a body part requiring extrication)
  - Ejection (partial or complete) from automobile
  - Death in same passenger compartment
  - Vehicle telemetry data consistent with a high risk of injury
  - Pedestrian/bicycle rider thrown, run over, or with significant impact
  - Rider separated from transport vehicle with significant impact (e.g., motorcycle, all-terrain vehicle, horse, etc.)

Source: Adapted from *Field Triage Guidelines.* American College of Surgeons—Committee on Trauma. 2021.

Modified from the Field Triage Decision Scheme: The National Trauma Triage Protocol, U.S. Department of Health and Human Services, Centers for Disease Control and Prevention.

practitioner approaches the scene and the patient, they should be considering the physics of trauma of the situation (**Figure 2-3**). Knowledge of specific injury patterns aids in predicting injuries and knowing what to look for. Consideration of the physics of trauma should not delay the initiation of patient assessment and care but can be included in the global scene assessment and in the questions directed to the patient and bystanders. The physics of trauma may also play a key role in determining the destination facility for a given trauma patient (**Box 2-6**).

6. Provide Appropriate Airway Management While Maintaining Spinal Motion Restriction as Indicated

After establishing scene safety and controlling exsanguinating hemorrhage, management of the airway is the highest priority in the treatment of critically injured patients. All prehospital care practitioners must be able to perform the "essential skills" of airway management with ease: head and neck stabilization, manual clearing of the airway, manual maneuvers to open the airway (jaw thrust and chin lift), suctioning, and the use of oropharyngeal and nasopharyngeal airways. This principle is discussed most directly in Chapter 7, *Airway and Ventilation*, but it is also a key consideration in Chapter 8, *Head and Neck Trauma* and Chapter 9, *Spinal Trauma*.

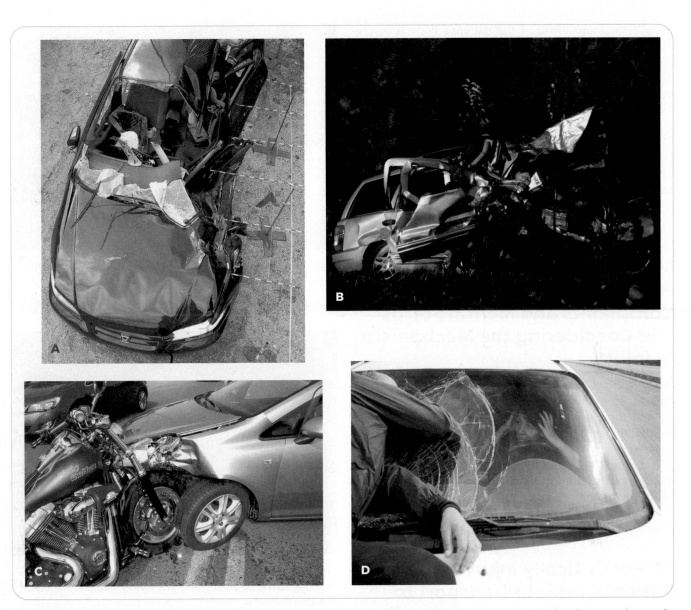

Figure 2-4 High-risk auto crashes. **A.** Significant side impact. **B.** Significant engine compartment crumple. **C.** Axle separation crash. **D.** Pedestrian struck with significant impact.

Courtesy of Stewart C. Wang, MD.

7. Support Ventilation and Deliver Oxygen to Maintain an SpO$_2$ ≥ 94%

Assessment and management of ventilation is another key aspect in the management of the critically injured patient. Prehospital care practitioners must recognize a ventilatory rate that is too slow (bradypnea) or too fast (tachypnea) and assist ventilations with a bag-mask device connected to supplemental oxygen. Trauma patients with obvious or suspected life-threatening conditions also need supplemental oxygen management. This principle is discussed in detail in Chapter 7, *Airway and Ventilation*, and it is put into action in Chapter 8, *Head and Neck Trauma*.

8. Provide Basic Shock Therapy, Including Appropriately Splinting Musculoskeletal Injuries and Restoring and Maintaining Normal Body Temperature

Once significant external blood loss has been controlled, the prehospital care practitioner must consider other causes and complications relating to shock. A fracture, for example, can produce internal bleeding that cannot be observed visually and cannot be stopped through bandaging or pressure; realignment of the fractured limb may reduce this blood loss in the prehospital setting. Severe hypothermia can ensue if the patient's body temperature is not maintained. Hypothermia drastically impairs the ability of the body's blood clotting system to achieve hemostasis. Therefore, it is important to maintain body heat through the use of blankets and a warmed environment inside the ambulance. Chapter 12, *Musculoskeletal Trauma* discusses methods of splinting extremity injuries. Measures for keeping the patient warm and avoiding hypothermia are discussed throughout the text, but particularly relevant discussions can be found in Chapter 19, *Environmental Trauma I: Heat and Cold* and Chapter 21, *Wilderness Trauma Care*.

9. Apply Appropriate Spinal Motion Restriction Principles Based on the Patient's Complaints and Mental Status and Considering the Mechanism of Injury

When contact with the trauma patient is made, manual stabilization and motion restriction of the cervical and thoracolumbar spine should be established and maintained throughout transport or until the patient is deemed not to meet indications for spinal motion restriction (**Figure 2-5**). See Chapter 9, *Spinal Trauma* for a full discussion of the indications for and methods of spinal stabilization; Chapter 21, *Wilderness Trauma Care* includes additional information related to the unique spinal motion restriction challenges associated with this environment.

10. For Critically Injured Trauma Patients, Initiate Transport to the Closest Appropriate Facility as Soon as Possible After EMS Arrival on Scene

Patients who are critically injured (see Box 2-6) should be transported as soon as possible after EMS arrival on scene, ideally within 10 minutes, whenever possible—the "Platinum 10 Minutes" (**Figure 2-6**). Although prehospital care practitioners have become more proficient at airway management, ventilatory support, and administration of IV fluid therapy, most critically injured trauma patients are in hemorrhagic shock and are in need of two things that often cannot be provided in the prehospital setting: (1) blood to carry oxygen and (2) plasma to provide internal clotting and control of internal hemorrhage. Prehospital care practitioners must keep in mind that the *closest* hospital may not be the *most appropriate* facility for many trauma patients; they must carefully consider the patient's needs and the receiving facility's capabilities to determine

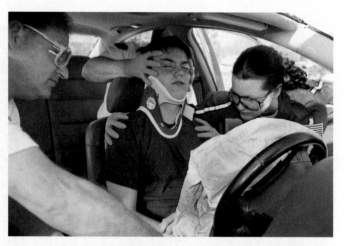

Figure 2-5 Maintain spinal motion restriction in vulnerable patients throughout transport.
Courtesy of Rick Brady.

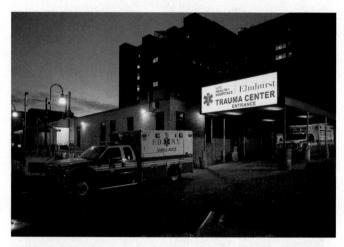

Figure 2-6 For critically injured trauma patients, initiate transport to the closest appropriate facility within 10 minutes of arrival on scene.
© Massimo Giachetti/iStock Editorial/Getty Images Plus/Getty Images

which destination will most promptly manage the patient's condition. Such decisions are discussed in Chapter 6, *Patient Assessment and Management*. This principle applies to all trauma situations and is well illustrated in Chapter 8, *Head and Neck Trauma* and Chapter 13, *Burn Injuries*.

11. Initiate Fluid Replacement en Route to the Receiving Facility as Necessary to Restore Basic Perfusion

Initiation of transport of a critically injured trauma patient should never be delayed simply to insert IV catheters and administer fluid therapy. Although crystalloid solutions do restore lost volume and improve perfusion, they do not transport oxygen. Additionally, restoring normal blood pressure may result in additional hemorrhage from clot disruption in damaged blood vessels that initially clotted off, thereby increasing patient mortality. Thus, the priority, as discussed in the preceding principle, is to deliver the patient to a facility that can meet their needs. Nonetheless, administration of crystalloid solution can be valuable in certain situations. For example, patients with evidence of traumatic brain injury and acute hypotension. While fluid administration can come into play in nearly any trauma scenario, Chapter 3, *Shock: Pathophysiology of Life and Death* and Chapter 13, *Burn Injuries* demonstrate this principle in action.

12. Ascertain the Patient's Medical History and Perform a Secondary Survey When Life-Threatening Problems Have Been Satisfactorily Managed or Have Been Ruled Out

If life-threatening conditions are found in the primary survey, key interventions should be performed and the patient transported within the Platinum 10 Minutes. However, if life-threatening conditions are not identified, a secondary survey is performed. The secondary survey is a systematic, head-to-toe physical examination that serves to identify all injuries. A SAMPLER history (**S**ymptoms, **A**llergies, **M**edications, **P**ast medical history, **L**ast meal, **E**vents preceding the injury, **R**isk factors) is also obtained during the secondary survey.

The patient's airway, respiratory, and circulatory status along with vital signs should be reassessed frequently because patients who initially present without life-threatening injuries may subsequently develop them. This principle is discussed in Chapter 6, *Patient Assessment and Management.*

13. Provide Adequate Pain Relief

Patients who have sustained serious injury typically will experience significant pain. It was once thought that providing pain relief would mask the patient's symptoms and impair the ability of the trauma team to adequately assess the patient after arrival to the hospital. Numerous studies have shown that this is, in fact, not the case. Prehospital care practitioners should consider providing analgesics to relieve pain as long as no contraindications exist. Splinting fractures and applying traction splints as appropriate based on the injury are extremely effective nonpharmacologic ways to control pain. The principle of pain management is discussed in Chapter 6, *Patient Assessment and Management,* and it is applied in nearly every chapter of this text. As discussed in Chapter 14, *Pediatric Trauma* and Chapter 15, *Geriatric Trauma,* although pain

management is different in some patient populations, it should not be withheld on the basis of the patient's age.

14. Provide Thorough and Accurate Communication Regarding the Patient and the Circumstances of the Injury to the Receiving Facility

Communication about a trauma patient with the receiving hospital involves three components:

- Prearrival warning
- Verbal report upon arrival
- Written documentation of the encounter in the patient care report (PCR)

Care of the trauma patient is a team effort. The response to a critical trauma patient begins with the prehospital care practitioner and continues in the hospital. Delivering information from the prehospital setting to the receiving hospital allows for notification and mobilization of appropriate hospital resources to ensure an optimal reception of the patient. Methods of ensuring effective communication with the receiving facility are discussed in Chapter 6, *Patient Assessment and Management* and apply to all patient care encounters.

Research

Historically, there has been a lack of meaningful research specific to prehospital care; however, in recent years that has started to change. Many of the established prehospital standards of care are being challenged by evidence-based research. For example, tourniquets are no longer considered a tool of last resort, advanced airways are increasingly contraindicated in the prehospital setting, and crystalloid resuscitation is now used sparingly and with defined goals. Although some of the literature is controversial, prehospital care is ever-changing secondary to evidence-based medicine for the best interest of the patient. Throughout this text, the evidence from these studies is described and discussed to enable you to make the best choices for your patients based on your knowledge, training, skills, and resources.

Reading the EMS Literature

A major goal of PHTLS has been to ensure that the practice recommendations presented in this text accurately represent the best medical evidence available at the time of publication. PHTLS began this process with the sixth edition and has continued it with subsequent editions. We continue to add, as references and suggested readings, those manuscripts, sources, and resources that are fundamental to the topics covered and the recommendations made in each chapter. (See Suggested Readings at the end of this chapter for further information on evaluating EMS literature.) Every healthcare practitioner, including EMS practitioners, should obtain, read, and critically evaluate the publications and sources that make up the basis for the components of daily practice.

To make optimal use of available reference material, an understanding of exactly what constitutes medical literature and how to interpret the various sources of information is essential. In many cases the first source that is accessed for information about a particular topic is a medical text. As our level of interest and sophistication grows, a search is undertaken to find the specific references that represent the source of the information communicated in those text chapters or to find what, if any, primary research studies have been performed and published. Then, after reviewing and analyzing the various sources, a decision can be made about the quality and strength of the evidence that will guide our decision making and patient care interventions.

Levels of Medical Evidence

Multiple systems are employed in medicine to evaluate and describe the quality of the medical evidence and to understand the strength of that evidence and how it should be used in medical decision making. For many years, the randomized controlled trial (RCT) was considered the gold standard for medical literature. In many ways it still is, but even that design has some limitations.[21]

In any study, when comparing one treatment group, or one patient population, or one intervention to another, there is a risk of introducing what is known as bias. For example, physicians could compare the use of needle thoracostomy for treatment of tension pneumothorax in the field to the use of positive-pressure ventilation and rapid transport. In a retrospective study design, one would look at patients who had tension pneumothorax and compare those who received no needle thoracostomy to those who did not. If those who received needle thoracostomy ultimately had a higher mortality rate than those treated with other methods, one could conclude that needle thoracostomy was dangerous. The problem with that approach is that the two treatment groups are dissimilar in this model. There is certainly a likelihood that those who were treated with needle thoracostomy started off worse in terms of their physiologic condition than those who were not. Stated differently, there was a reason those patients were treated with needle thoracostomy in the first place; namely, their underlying condition was worse, and they were more likely to die regardless of the type of intervention received.

An alternative design for such a study would be an RCT. In that study, practitioners would be presented with a patient with signs of tension pneumothorax, and they would intervene with needle thoracostomy or not based on where the patient fell in the process of randomization. That would eliminate the selection bias associated with the prior retrospective design.

While the RCT is often the best way to conduct studies because it limits the introduction of such bias, it is not always feasible. A good example of that principle is the epidemiologic population-based studies of sudden infant death syndrome (SIDS) in New Zealand. In those studies, investigators used an observational study design. They compared infants who died from SIDS to a group of control infants and identified the prone sleeping position as a risk factor.[22] Subsequent studies demonstrated that programs to teach parents not to put infants to sleep on their stomachs substantially reduced the incidence of SIDS. Conducting an RCT to compare prone to supine sleeping positions in children to assess the efficacy of that intervention in reducing the incidence of SIDS would clearly be unfeasible and unethical.

Furthermore, one of the problems with RCTs is that the results are often not very generalizable. Using the needle thoracostomy example, if one were to design such a study, one would want to clearly define patient characteristics that would lead to inclusion in the study or exclusion from the study. When the study includes only a narrow group of patients, the degree to which the results may or may not be generalizable to a broader group of patients becomes less clear. The pragmatic study designs often include very broad groups of patients in order to increase the generalizability of the results. Unfortunately, such studies are very hard to design and implement rigorously.

For all of these reasons, it is neither possible nor desirable to rely purely on RCTs when making medical decisions. Furthermore, there are not enough RCTs to address the plethora of medical decisions that EMS practitioners are asked to make on a day-to-day basis when caring for trauma patients.

It is therefore necessary for prehospital practitioners caring for trauma patients to be aware of and to understand the different types of studies and to be able to carefully evaluate the strengths and weaknesses of the evidence presented. **Table 2-2** describes several categories of study design that are commonly employed.

The most powerful information in the literature can be gleaned from systematic reviews and from synopses that synthesize evidence from combinations of RCTs, cohort studies, case-control studies, and case reports. Background information and expert opinion still play an important role. In summary, it is necessary to evaluate every piece of literature and understand the strength of the evidence within that literature, and it is not possible to make every decision in the care of trauma patients based purely on perfect science. That said, the goal is to use the highest quality of scientific evidence available and to understand the specific limitations of that evidence.

Table 2-2 Commonly Employed Research Study Designs	
Study Type	**Description**
Systematic review	Collects all available studies on a topic; reviews and analyzes their results
Meta-analysis	Combines results of multiple randomized controlled trials on the same topic
Randomized controlled trial	Study design that eliminates selection bias by randomly assigning eligible study subjects to different treatment or intervention arms
Cohort study	Prospective observational trial where two groups of patients are followed longitudinally and results assessed at time intervals
Case-control study	Observational study where two groups with known different outcomes are compared based on some postulated underlying causal factor(s)
Case report	Uncontrolled report describing an individual outcome or outcome of a group of similar patients after an intervention
Expert opinion	Scholarly summation of opinions of recognized clinical experts on a particular clinical topic or question

© National Association of Emergency Medical Technicians (NAEMT)

SUMMARY

- Principles (or the *science* of medicine) define the duties required of the prehospital care practitioner in optimizing patient survival and outcome.
- Preferences (or the *art* of medicine) are the methods of achieving the principle. Considerations for choosing the method include the following:
  - Situation that currently exists
  - Condition of the patient
  - Knowledge and experience
  - Equipment available
- Critical thinking in medicine is a process in which the healthcare practitioner assesses the situation, the patient, and the resources. This information is rapidly analyzed and combined to provide the best care possible to the patient.
- There are four principles of biomedical ethics (autonomy, nonmaleficence, beneficence, and justice). Prehospital professionals must develop ethical reasoning skills necessary to manage ethical conflict in the prehospital environment.
- The following are the Golden Principles of prehospital trauma care:

1. Ensure the safety of the prehospital care practitioners and the patient.
2. Assess the scene situation to determine the need for additional resources.
3. Control any significant external hemorrhage.
4. Use the primary survey approach to identify life-threatening conditions.
5. Recognize the physics of trauma/mechanism of injury.
6. Provide appropriate airway management while maintaining spinal motion restriction as indicated.
7. Support ventilation and deliver oxygen to maintain an SpO_2 greater than or equal to 94%.
8. Provide basic shock therapy, including appropriate splinting of musculoskeletal injuries and preserving normal body temperature.
9. Apply appropriate spinal motion restriction principles based on the patient's complaints and mental status and considering the mechanism of injury.

(continues)

SUMMARY (CONTINUED)

10. For critically injured trauma patients, initiate transport to the closest appropriate facility as soon as possible after EMS arrival on scene.
11. Initiate intravenous fluid replacement en route to the receiving facility only if indicated based on specific criteria.
12. Ascertain the patient's medical history and perform a secondary survey when life-threatening problems have been satisfactorily managed or have been ruled out.
13. Provide appropriate pain relief.
14. Provide thorough and accurate communication regarding the patient and the circumstances of the injury to the receiving facility.

- Research provides the foundation and basis for all medical practice, including prehospital care.
- The quality of research and the strength of the conclusions and recommendations will vary depending on the type of study.

SCENARIO RECAP

You and your partner arrive at the scene of a two-vehicle T-bone collision. You are currently the only available unit. In a pickup truck, there is a young unrestrained male driver who smells strongly of alcohol and has an obvious forearm deformity. The truck struck the passenger's side front door of a small passenger sedan, with significant intrusion into the passenger compartment. There is an elderly female in the front passenger seat who does not appear to be breathing; the windshield is starred directly in front of her. The female driver of the sedan is also injured but conscious and extremely anxious. In the rear seat, two children are restrained. The child on the passenger side appears to be approximately 3 years old and is unconscious and slumped over in a car seat. On the driver's side, a restrained 5-year-old boy is crying hysterically in a booster seat and appears to be uninjured.

The driver of the pickup truck is obviously injured with an open arm fracture, but he is belligerent and verbally abusive and is refusing treatment. Meanwhile, the driver of the sedan is frantically inquiring about her children and her mother.

- How would you manage this multiple-patient incident?
- Which of these patients is of highest priority?
- What would you tell the mother of the two children about their condition?
- How would you deal with the apparently intoxicated driver of the other vehicle?
- Would you allow the apparently intoxicated driver to refuse care?

SCENARIO SOLUTION

In this five-victim scenario, your ambulance crew, having no assistance available, faces a triage situation with the patients outnumbering the prehospital care practitioners. It is in this type of triage situation that the concept of justice becomes immediately applicable. Your available resources—two practitioners—are limited and must be distributed in a manner that will do the greatest good for the greatest number of people. This involves deciding who is treated first and by which practitioner.

In this scenario, a rapid decision must be made regarding whether to treat the older woman or the unconscious child first. Frequently a child has a higher likelihood of survival than an older adult when both patients have suffered similar traumatic injuries. However, additional assessment and medical history may change the clinical picture and the appropriateness of triaging decisions. For example, the mother may report that the unconscious minor child has a terminal condition, so making a triage decision based solely on age may not be the *just* action in this instance. While triage protocols generally provide direction in such situations and are

SCENARIO SOLUTION (CONTINUED)

based on concepts of justice, triage protocols cannot account for every unique situation encountered. Therefore, a basic understanding of the principle of justice can be helpful for situations in which "in the moment" triage decisions need to be made.

The appearance of the driver and his truck may lead to stereotyping behaviors and judgments on the part of the prehospital care practitioners. Stereotypes are often inaccurate, simplistic generalizations or beliefs about a group of people that allow others to categorize the people and treat them based on those beliefs. Preconceived notions about a patient's appearance and behaviors can interfere with fair and equitable treatment.

Although there is a duty to treat patients in a fair and consistent manner, prehospital care practitioners are a valuable resource and have no obligation to put themselves at undue risk. Practitioners have the right not only to protect themselves but also to protect their ability to care for others.

In addition to justice concerns, there are several challenges to autonomy raised by this scenario. You must assess the decision-making capacity of both the driver of the pickup truck and the female driver of the car. Both drivers are injured and emotionally distraught, and the male driver is potentially impaired by an intoxicant. Furthermore, the female driver may be asked to make medical decisions for herself and to act as a surrogate decision maker for her two children and her mother. If, upon assessing the decision-making capacity of the two drivers, you were to determine that either of the drivers is incapacitated, then you would proceed with providing emergency medical care based on established clinical protocols and the best interests of the patients.

The balancing of risks and benefits is an important part of medical decision making. In this case, the female driver is requesting information about her mother and children. Although you have an obligation to tell the truth, both to establish patient–practitioner trust and to help the driver to make informed consent decisions for the incapacitated occupants of her vehicle, you must bear in mind that this patient may be injured and is likely traumatized, with the possibility of impairment and lack of capacity to make decisions. A full and truthful disclosure about the conditions of her mother and unconscious child may further traumatize her or cause harm. Her potential reactions to such information may further impair her decision-making capacity and could be upsetting to her 5-year-old child, who is conscious and already hysterical. Depending on the potential level of harm or burden that an action may cause—in this case, telling the female driver about the conditions of her loved ones—the principles of nonmaleficence and beneficence might suggest that you consider postponement of full disclosure until the patient is in a more stable environment. That does not obviate the responsibility to respond truthfully.

As is clear in this scenario, ethics rarely gives black-and-white solutions to difficult situations. Rather, ethics can provide a framework, such as the four principles discussed in this chapter—autonomy, nonmaleficence, beneficence, and justice—in which to consider and reason through ethically difficult situations in an attempt to do the right thing.

References

1. Lyng J, Adelgais K, Alter R, et al. Recommended essential equipment for basic life support and advanced life support ground ambulances 2020: a joint position statement. *Prehosp Emerg Care.* 2021;25(3):451-459. doi: 10.1080/10903127.2021.1886382

2. Hendricson WD, Andrieu SC, Chadwick DG, et al. Educational strategies associated with development of problem-solving, critical thinking, and self-directed learning. *J Dent Educ.* 2006;70(9):925-936.

3. Cotter AJ. Developing critical-thinking skills. *EMS Mag.* 2007;36(7):86.

4. Carroll RT. *Becoming a Critical Thinker: A Guide for the New Millennium.* 2nd ed. Pearson Custom Publishing; 2005.

5. Beauchamp TL, Childress JF. *Principles of Biomedical Ethics.* 6th ed. Oxford University Press; 2009.

6. Banning M. Measures that can be used to instill critical-thinking skills in nurse prescribers. *Nurse Educ Pract.* 2006;6(2):98-105.

7. Bamonti A, Heilicser B, Stotts K. To treat or not to treat: identifying ethical dilemmas in EMS. *JEMS.* 2001;26(3):100-107.

8. Daniels N. *Just Health Care.* Cambridge University Press; 1985.

9. Derse AR. Autonomy and informed consent. In: Iserson KV, Sanders AB, Mathieu D, eds. *Ethics in Emergency Medicine.* 2nd ed. Galen Press; 1995:99-105.

10. Post LF, Bluestein J, Dubler NN. *Handbook for Health Care Ethics Committees.* The Johns Hopkins University Press; 2007.

11. University of Maryland Medical Center. History of the Shock Trauma Center: tribute to R Adams Cowley, MD. Updated December 16, 2013. Accessed October 17, 2021. http://umm.edu/programs/shock-trauma/about/history

12. Lerner EB, Moscati RM. The Golden Hour: scientific fact or medical "urban legend"? *Acad Emerg Med.* 2001;8:758.

13. Tsybuliak GN, Pavlenko EP. Cause of death in the early post-traumatic period. *Vestn Khir Im I I Grek.* 1975;114(5):75.

14. Gunst M, Ghaemmaghami V, Gruszecki A, Urban J, Frankel H, Shafi S. Changing epidemiology of trauma deaths leads to a bimodal distribution. *Proc (Bayl Univ Med Cent).* 2010;23(4):349-354.

15. Kalkwarf KJ, Drake SA, Yang Y, et al. Bleeding to death in a big city: an analysis of all trauma deaths from hemorrhage in a metropolitan area over one year. *J Trauma Acute Care Surg.* 2020;89(4):716-722.

16. Sobrino J, Shafi S. Timing and causes of death after injuries. *Proc (Bayl Univ Med Cent).* 2013;26(2):120-123.

17. Clarke JR, Trooskin SZ, Doshi PJ, Greenwald L, Mode CJ. Time to laparotomy for intra-abdominal bleeding from trauma does affect survival for delays up to 90 minutes. *J Trauma.* 2002 Mar;52(3):420-425. doi: 10.1097/00005373-200203000-00002

18. Meizoso JP, Ray JJ, Karcutskie CA 4th, et al. Effect of time to operation on mortality for hypotensive patients with gunshot wounds to the torso: the Golden 10 Minutes. *J Trauma Acute Care Surg.* 2016 Oct;81(4):685-691. doi: 10.1097/TA.0000000000001198

19. Niles SE, McLaughlin DF, Perkins JG, et al. Increased mortality associated with the early coagulopathy of trauma in combat casualties. *J Trauma.* 2008;64(6):1459-1463; discussion 1463-1465.

20. Brohi K, Singh J, Heron M, Coats T. Acute traumatic coagulopathy. *J Trauma.* 2003;54(6):1127-1130.

21. Frieden TR. Evidence for health decision making—beyond randomized, controlled trials. *N Engl J Med.* 2017;377:465-475. doi: 10.1056/NEJMra1614394

22. Mitchell EA, Scragg R, Stewart AW, et al. Results from the first year of the New Zealand Cot Death Study. *N Z Med J.* 1991;104:71-77.

Suggested Reading

Adams JG, Arnold R, Siminoff L, Wolfson AB. Ethical conflicts in the prehospital setting. *Ann Emerg Med.* 1992;21(10):1259.

Beauchamp TL, Childress JF. *Principles of Biomedical Ethics.* 7th ed. Oxford University Press; 2013.

Buchanan AE, Brock DW. *Deciding for Others: The Ethics of Surrogate Decision Making.* Cambridge University Press; 1990.

Fitzgerald DJ, Milzman DP, Sulmasy DP. Creating a dignified option: ethical consideration in the formulation of prehospital DNR protocol. *Am J Emerg Med.* 1995;13(2):223.

Iverson KV. Foregoing prehospital care: should ambulance staff always resuscitate? *J Med Ethics.* 1991;17:19.

Iverson KV. Withholding and withdrawing medical treatment: an emergency medicine perspective. *Ann Emerg Med.* 1996;28(1):51.

Marco CA, Schears RM. Prehospital resuscitation practices: a survey of prehospital providers. *Ethics Emerg Med.* 2003;24(1):101.

Mohr M, Kettler D. Ethical aspects of prehospital CPR. *Acta Anaesthesiol Scand Suppl.* 1997;111:298-301.

Sandman L, Nordmark A. Ethical conflict in prehospital emergency care. *Nurs Ethics.* 2006;13(6):592.

Travers DA, Mears G. Physicians' experiences with prehospital do-not-resuscitate orders in North Carolina. *Prehosp Disaster Med.* 1996;11(2):91.

Van Vleet LM. Between black and white: the gray area of ethics in EMS. *JEMS.* 2006;31(10):55-56, 58-63; quiz 64-65.

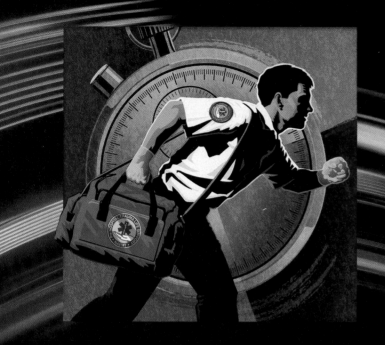

 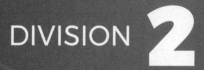

Assessment and Management

CHAPTER 3

© Ralf Hiemisch/Getty Images

Shock: Pathophysiology of Life and Death

Lead Editors
Samuel Galvagno, DO, PhD, FAMPA, FCCM
Jesse Shirki, DO, MS, FACEP

CHAPTER OBJECTIVES

At the completion of this chapter, you will be able to do the following:

- Define shock.
- Explain how preload, afterload, and contractility affect cardiac output.
- Classify shock on an etiologic basis.
- Explain the pathophysiology of shock and its progression through phases.
- Relate shock to acid–base status, energy production, etiology, prevention, and treatment.
- Describe the physical findings of shock.
- List practical assessment tools that define shock.
- Clinically differentiate the types of shock.

- Discuss the limitations of the field management of shock.
- Recognize the need for rapid transport and early definitive management in various forms of shock.
- Apply principles of management of shock in the trauma patient.
- List the components necessary for oxygen delivery (Fick principle).
- Discuss limitations of anaerobic metabolism in meeting cellular demands.

SCENARIO

You and your partner are dispatched to the scene of a motorcycle crash. The motorcycle veered off the road and rolled several times, ultimately impacting a telephone pole. Upon your arrival, you find a 29-year-old helmeted male driver lying supine approximately 50 feet (15 meters) from the motorcycle. The patient is in moderate distress with chief complaints of chest, sacral, and left hip pain.

Physical examination of the patient shows pale skin color, diaphoresis, decreased peripheral pulses, a contused chest, and an unstable pelvis. The patient is alert and oriented. His vital signs are as follows: pulse 110 beats/minute, blood pressure 82/56 millimeters of mercury (mm Hg), oxygen saturation (SpO_2) 92% on room air, and respiratory rate 28 breaths/minute, with diminished breath sounds on the right.

- What possible injuries do you expect to see after this type of mechanism?
- How would you manage these injuries in the field?
- What are the major pathologic processes occurring in this patient?
- How will you correct the pathophysiology causing this patient's presentation?
- You are working for a rural emergency medical services (EMS) system in a remote area distant from the nearest trauma center. How does this factor alter your management plans?

INTRODUCTION

Shock, derived from the French "choc," is defined as inadequate perfusion to the cells, resulting in widespread loss of oxygen delivery and dysfunction of the vital organs.[1] In 1872, shock was described by surgeon Samuel Gross as a "rude unhinging of the machinery of life."[2] In the 1970s, shock following trauma was subjected to further study, helping differentiate the pathophysiologic mechanisms responsible for inadequate perfusion of tissues and cells, leading to death.[3]

One of the fundamental goals of prehospital, emergency, and critical care is to promote tissue oxygenation. Shock is a pathologic state characterized by an imbalance between oxygen supply and demand. Therefore, prompt diagnosis, resuscitation, and definitive management of shock resulting from trauma are essential for preventing death and optimizing patient outcomes.

The assessment and management of trauma patients begins with the primary survey, which is focused on the identification and correction of problems affecting or interfering with the critical function of the delivery of oxygen to every cell in the body. Thus, an understanding of the physiology of life and pathophysiology that can lead to death is essential for the prehospital practitioner if abnormalities are to be identified and addressed.

In the prehospital setting, the therapeutic challenge posed by a patient in shock is compounded by the need to assess and manage these patients in a relatively austere, and sometimes dangerous, environment in which sophisticated diagnostic and management tools are either unavailable or impractical to apply. This chapter focuses on the causes of traumatic shock and describes the pathophysiologic changes present, to help direct management strategies.

Physiology of Shock

Metabolism

The human body consists of over 100 million cells. Each of these cells requires energy to function. Cells maintain their normal metabolic functions by producing and using energy in the form of adenosine triphosphate (ATP)—the energy currency for human metabolism. The most efficient method of generating this needed energy is via *aerobic metabolism*. The cells take in oxygen and glucose and metabolize them through a complex physiologic process that produces energy, along with the by-products of water and carbon dioxide. During this process, glucose is converted to pyruvate in the mitochondria and enters the citric acid cycle as acetyl coenzyme A.

When the aerobic metabolic pathway is disrupted by lack of oxygen, the steps leading to the entry of pyruvate into the citric acid cycle are disrupted and *anaerobic metabolism* occurs. Anaerobic metabolism, in contrast to aerobic metabolism, occurs without the use of oxygen. In anerobic metabolism, glucose is broken down into lactic acid (lactate) as a by-product. Even though some organs such as the brain, heart, liver, and skeletal muscle can use lactate as a temporary energy source, the energy yield is much lower than that of glucose. Lactate accumulation is a cause of metabolic acidosis, a condition defined by a decreased pH (increased hydrogen ions in the blood). When the pH falls below 7.20, myocardial contraction becomes severely depressed.[4]

If anaerobic metabolism is not reversed quickly, cells cannot continue to function and will die. If a sufficient number of cells in any one organ die, the entire organ ceases to function. Organ death can progress to patient death.

It is important to understand the difference between ischemia, hypoxemia, and hypoxia. *Ischemia* is defined as insufficient blood flow to provide oxygenation. Ischemia occurs when blood supply to tissue is interrupted. Following ischemia, a time-dependent relationship exists among low oxygen content in the blood (*hypoxemia*), low oxygen content in bodily tissues (*hypoxia*), and cellular death. The sensitivity of cells to the lack of oxygen varies from organ system to organ system. This sensitivity is called ischemic sensitivity, and it is greatest in the brain, heart, and lungs. It may take only 4 to 6 minutes of anaerobic metabolism before one or more of these vital organs is injured beyond repair. Skin and muscle tissue have a significantly longer ischemic sensitivity—as long as 4 to 6 hours. The abdominal organs generally fall between these two groups and are able to survive 45 to 90 minutes of anaerobic metabolism (**Table 3-1**).

Maintenance of normal function of the cells depends on the crucial relationship and interaction of several body systems. The patient's airway must be patent, and respirations must be of adequate volume and depth. The heart must be functioning and pumping normally. The circulatory system must have enough red blood cells (RBCs) available to deliver adequate amounts of oxygen

Table 3-1 Organ Tolerance to Ischemia	
Organ	**Warm Ischemia Time**
Heart, brain, lungs	4–6 minutes
Kidneys, liver, gastrointestinal tract	45–90 minutes
Muscle, bone, skin	4–6 hours

Modified from American College of Surgeons Committee on Trauma. *Advanced Trauma Life Support: Student Course Manual.* 7th ed. American College of Surgeons; 2004.

to tissue cells throughout the body, so these cells can produce energy.

Prehospital assessment and treatment of a trauma patient are directed at preventing or reversing anaerobic metabolism, thus avoiding cellular death and, ultimately, patient death. Ensuring that critical body systems are working together correctly—namely, that the patient's airway is patent and that breathing and circulation are adequate—is the major emphasis of the primary survey. These functions are managed in trauma patients by the following actions:

- Maintaining an adequate airway and ventilation, thus providing adequate oxygen to the RBCs
- Assisting ventilation with judicious use of supplemental oxygen
- Maintaining adequate circulation, thus perfusing tissue cells with oxygenated blood

Definition of Shock

The major complication of disruption of the normal physiology of life is known as *shock*. Shock is a state of change in cellular function from aerobic metabolism to anaerobic metabolism secondary to hypoperfusion of the tissue cells. As a result, the delivery of oxygen at the cellular level is inadequate to meet the body's metabolic needs. Shock is not defined as low blood pressure, rapid pulse rate, or cool, clammy skin; these are merely systemic manifestations of the entire pathologic process called shock. The correct definition of shock is insufficient tissue perfusion (oxygenation) at the cellular level, leading to anaerobic metabolism and loss of energy production needed to support life. Based on this definition, shock can be classified in terms of cellular perfusion and oxygenation. Understanding the cellular changes arising from this state of hypoperfusion, as well as the endocrine, microvascular, cardiovascular, tissue, and end-organ effects, will assist in directing treatment strategies.

Understanding this process is key to assisting the body in restoring aerobic metabolism and energy production. If prehospital care practitioners are going to understand this abnormal condition and be able to develop treatment plans to prevent or reverse shock, it is important that they know and understand what is happening to the body at a cellular level. The normal physiologic responses that the body uses to protect itself from the development of shock must be understood, recognized, and interpreted. Only then can a rational approach for managing the problems of the patient in shock be developed.

Shock can kill a patient in the field, the emergency department (ED), the operating room (OR), or the intensive care unit. Although actual physical death may be delayed for several hours or even several weeks, the most common cause of death is the failure of early and adequate resuscitation from shock. The lack of perfusion of cells by oxygenated blood results in anaerobic metabolism, decreased energy production, and eventually cellular death. Even when some cells in an organ are initially spared, death can occur later, because the remaining cells are unable to carry out the organ's functions indefinitely. The following section explains this phenomenon. Understanding this process is key to assisting the body in restoring aerobic metabolism and energy production.

Pathophysiology of Shock

Metabolism: The Human Motor

The cells take in oxygen and metabolize it through a complicated physiologic process, producing energy. At the same time, cellular metabolism requires energy, and cells must have fuel—glucose—to carry out this process. Each molecule of glucose yields 38 energy-storing ATP molecules when oxygen is available. As in any combustion event, a by-product is also produced. In the body, oxygen and glucose are metabolized to produce energy, with water and carbon dioxide as by-products.

The cellular metabolic process is similar to what occurs in a motor vehicle engine when gasoline and air are mixed and burned to produce energy and carbon monoxide is created as the by-product. The motor moves the car, the heater warms the driver, and the electricity generated is used for the headlights, all powered by the burning gasoline and air mixture in the vehicle's engine.

The same is true of the human motor. Aerobic metabolism is the main "driving" system, with anaerobic metabolism as the backup system. Unfortunately, it is not a strong backup. It produces much less energy than aerobic metabolism, and it cannot produce energy for a long period of time. In fact, anaerobic metabolism produces only two ATP molecules, a 19-fold decrease in energy. However, it can assist with survival for a short time while the body repairs itself with the assistance of the prehospital care practitioner.

The major by-product of anaerobic metabolism is lactic acid (lactate; **Figure 3-1**). If anaerobic metabolism is not reversed quickly, cells cannot continue to function in the increasingly acidic environment, and without adequate energy, they will die. If a sufficient number of cells in any one organ die, the entire organ ceases to function. If a large number of cells in an organ die, the organ's function will be significantly reduced, and the remaining cells in that organ will have to work even harder to keep the organ functioning. These overworked cells may or may not be able to continue to support the function of the entire organ, and the organ may still die.

A classic example is a patient who has suffered a heart attack. Blood flow and oxygen are cut off to one portion

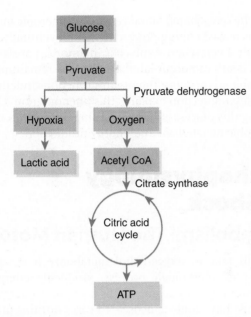

Figure 3-1 The formation of lactate during hypoxia. In the face of hypoxia, pyruvate is converted to lactic acid rather than processed by the citric acid cycle to make adenosine triphosphate (ATP).

© National Association of Emergency Medical Technicians (NAEMT)

of the myocardium (heart muscle), and some cells of the heart die. The loss of these cells impairs cardiac function, thus decreasing cardiac output and the oxygen supply to the rest of the heart. This in turn causes a further reduction in the oxygenation of the remaining heart cells. If too few cells remain viable or if the remaining cells are not strong enough to ensure the heart can continue to meet the body's blood flow needs, then heart failure can result. Unless major improvement in cardiac output occurs, the patient will not survive.

Another example of this deadly process occurs in the kidneys. When the kidneys are injured or are deprived of adequate oxygenated blood, some of the kidney cells begin to die and kidney function decreases. Other cells may be compromised yet continue to function for a while before they, too, die. If enough kidney cells die, the decreased level of kidney function results in the inadequate elimination of the toxic by-products of metabolism. The increased level of toxins further exacerbates cell death throughout the body. If this systemic deterioration continues, more cells and organs will die, and eventually the entire organism (the human) dies.

Depending on the organ initially involved, the progression from cell death to organism death can be rapid or delayed. It can take as little as 4 to 6 minutes or as long as 2 or 3 weeks before the damage caused by hypoxia or hypoperfusion in the first minutes after injury results in the patient's death. The effectiveness of a prehospital care practitioner's actions to reverse or prevent hypoxia and hypoperfusion in the critical prehospital

period may not be immediately apparent. However, these resuscitation measures are unquestionably necessary if the patient is to ultimately survive. These initial actions are a critical component of the Golden Hour of trauma care described by R Adams Cowley, MD,[5] and now often called the Golden Period because we know that the literal time frame within which critical abnormalities can be corrected is more variable than that conveyed by the figurative concept of the Golden Hour.

Oxygen Delivery (Fick Principle)

The Fick principle describes the components necessary for oxygenation of the cells in the body. These three components are as follows:

1. On-loading of oxygen to RBCs in the lung
2. Delivery of oxygenated RBCs to tissue cells
3. Off-loading of oxygen from RBCs to tissue cells

The Fick principle can be summarized by the following formula:

$$VO_2 = CO \times (CaO_2 - CvO_2)$$

VO_2 is the oxygen consumption (milliliters [mL] of O_2 consumed per minute) and is an index of the body's ability to do work. CO is the cardiac output, which is the product of the heart rate (beats per minute) multiplied by the stroke volume of blood (mL). CaO_2 is the concentration of oxygen in the arterial blood and CvO_2 is the concentration of oxygen in the venous blood. The concentration of oxygen in arterial or venous blood is dependent on the amount of hemoglobin, the amount of oxygen dissolved in blood, and the oxygen tension. The VO_2 is dependent on sex and level of activity; normal values for a resting man range between 35 and 40 mL/kilogram (kg)/minute (min), with average values for resting women ranging from approximately 27 to 30 mL/kg/min. Some men who are elite athletes have demonstrated VO_2 maxes of up to 85 mL/kg/min, and women who are elite runners have scored up to 77 mL/kg/min.

In addition to a patent airway and adequate respirations, a crucial part of this process is that the patient must have enough RBCs available to deliver adequate amounts of oxygen to tissue cells throughout the body so cells can produce energy.

This process is influenced by the patient's acid–base status. You may have a patient adequately ventilating and on supplemental oxygen with good saturation who is nonetheless deteriorating because of an inability to off-load oxygen at the cellular level caused by hypothermia. The prehospital treatment of shock is directed at ensuring that critical components of the Fick principle are maintained, with the goal of preventing or reversing anaerobic metabolism, and thus avoiding cellular death. These components are the major emphasis of the prehospital primary survey and are implemented in the management of the trauma patient by the following actions:

- Controlling exsanguinating extremity hemorrhage
- Maintaining an adequate airway and ventilation
- Administering supplemental oxygen
- Keeping the patient warm
- Maintaining adequate circulation

The first component of the Fick principle is oxygenation of the lungs and RBCs. This is covered in detail in Chapter 7, *Airway and Ventilation*. The second component involves perfusion, which is the delivery of blood to the tissue cells. A helpful analogy to use in describing perfusion is to think of the RBCs as transport cars on a train, the lungs as stations for receiving oxygen and offloading

carbon dioxide, the blood vessels as the railways, and the body tissue cells as the train stops. Normally, only 25% of oxygen is extracted in healthy humans. This is measured and monitored in the hospital as the mixed venous oxygen saturation (SvO$_2$; **Figure 3-2**).

An insufficient number of transport train cars, obstructions along the railways, and/or slow transport cars can all contribute to decreased oxygen delivery and the eventual starvation of the tissue cells.

Cellular Perfusion and Shock

The prime determinants of cellular perfusion are the heart (acting as the pump or the motor of the system), fluid volume (acting as the hydraulic fluid), the blood

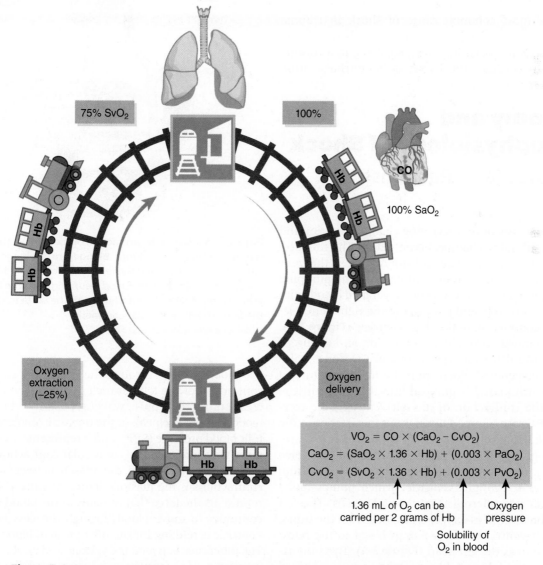

75% SvO$_2$

100%

CO

100% SaO$_2$

Oxygen extraction (−25%)

Oxygen delivery

$$VO_2 = CO \times (CaO_2 - CvO_2)$$
$$CaO_2 = (SaO_2 \times 1.36 \times Hb) + (0.003 \times PaO_2)$$
$$CvO_2 = (SvO_2 \times 1.36 \times Hb) + (0.003 \times PvO_2)$$

1.36 mL of O$_2$ can be carried per 2 grams of Hb

Oxygen pressure

Solubility of O$_2$ in blood

Figure 3-2 The concept of mixed venous oxygen saturation (SvO$_2$). Only 25% of the oxygen is used under normal circumstances, and approximately 70% to 75% is returned. A measure of the percentage returned is the SvO$_2$. A low SvO$_2$ indicates increased oxygen consumption and/or decreased oxygen supply.

vessels (serving as the conduits or plumbing), and, finally, the cells of the body. Based on these components of the perfusion system, shock may be classified into the following categories:

1. Hypovolemic—primarily hemorrhagic in the trauma patient, related to loss of circulating blood cells and fluid volume with oxygen-carrying capacity. This is the most common cause of shock in the trauma patient.
2. Distributive (or vasogenic)—related to abnormality in vascular tone arising from several different causes, including spinal cord injury, sepsis, and anaphylaxis.
3. Cardiogenic—related to interference with the pump action of the heart, often occurring after a heart attack.

By far the most common cause of shock in trauma patients is hypovolemia resulting from hemorrhage, and the safest approach in managing shock in a trauma patient is to consider the cause as hemorrhagic until proven otherwise.

Anatomy and Pathophysiology of Shock

Cardiovascular Response

Heart

The heart consists of two receiving chambers (atria) and two major pumping chambers (ventricles). The function of the atria is to accumulate and store blood so the ventricles can fill rapidly, minimizing delay in the pumping cycle. The right atrium receives deoxygenated blood from the veins of the body and pumps it to the right ventricle. With each contraction of the right ventricle (**Figure 3-3**), blood is pumped through the lungs for on-loading of oxygen to the RBCs and off-loading of CO_2 for exhalation. The oxygenated blood from the lungs is returned to the left atrium and is pumped into the left ventricle. Then, by the contraction of the left ventricle, the oxygenated RBCs are pumped throughout the arteries of the body to the tissue cells.

Although it is one organ, the heart actually has two subsystems. The right atrium, which receives blood from the body, and the right ventricle, which pumps blood to the lungs, are referred to as the right heart. The left atrium, which receives oxygenated blood from the lungs, and the left ventricle, which pumps blood to the body, are referred to as the left heart (**Figure 3-4**). Two important concepts to understand are **preload** (volume of blood entering into the right atrium) and **afterload** (pressure against which the blood has to push when it is squeezed out of the left ventricle).

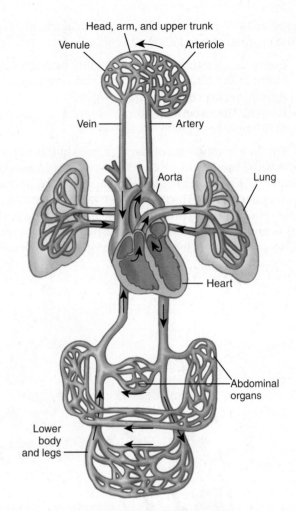

Figure 3-3 With each contraction of the right ventricle, blood is pumped through the lungs. Blood from the lungs enters the left side of the heart, and the left ventricle pumps it into the systemic vascular system. Blood returning from the lungs is pumped out of the heart and through the aorta to the rest of the body by left ventricular contraction.

© National Association of Emergency Medical Technicians (NAEMT)

Blood is forced through the circulatory system by the contraction of the left ventricle. This sudden pressure increase produces a pulse wave to push blood through the blood vessels. The peak of the pressure increase is the systolic blood pressure (SBP), and it represents the force of the pulse wave produced by ventricular contraction (**systole**). The resting pressure in the vessels between ventricular contractions is the diastolic blood pressure (DBP), and it represents the force that remains in the blood vessels that continues to move blood through the vessels while the ventricle is refilling for the next pulse of blood (**diastole**). The difference between the systolic and diastolic pressures is called **pulse pressure**. Pulse pressure is the pressure of the blood as it is being pushed out into the circulation. It is the pressure felt against the prehospital care practitioner's fingertip as the patient's pulse is checked.

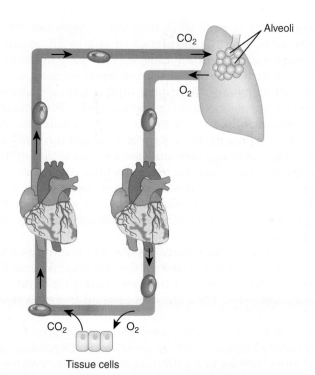

CO₂

Alveoli

O₂

CO₂   O₂

Tissue cells

Figure 3-4 Although the heart is considered to be one organ, it functions as if it were two organs. Deoxygenated blood is received into the right heart from the superior and inferior venae cavae and pumped through the pulmonary artery into the lungs. The blood is oxygenated in the lungs, flows back into the heart through the pulmonary vein, and is pumped out of the left ventricle.

© National Association of Emergency Medical Technicians (NAEMT)

Another term used in the discussion of blood pressure and shock but often not emphasized enough in the prehospital setting is **mean arterial pressure (MAP)**. This number gives a more realistic assessment of the overall pressure to produce blood flow than either the systolic or the diastolic pressures alone, and, in effect, it provides a numerical representation of end-organ perfusion. The MAP is the average pressure in the vascular system and is calculated as follows:

$$MAP = \text{Diastolic pressure} + 1/3 \text{ Pulse pressure}$$
or
$$MAP = \frac{(2 \times DBP) + SBP}{3}$$

For example, the MAP of a patient with a blood pressure of 120/80 mm Hg is calculated as follows:

$$MAP = 80 + ([120 - 80]/3)$$
$$= 80 + (40/3)$$
$$= 80 + 13.3$$
$$= 93.3, \text{ rounded to } 93$$

Many automatic noninvasive blood pressure (NIBP) devices automatically calculate and report the MAP in addition to the systolic and diastolic pressures. This is extremely helpful in guiding your treatment of trauma patients when using permissive hypotension strategies. Permissive hypotension strategies are covered in greater detail in the "Managing Volume Resuscitation" section of this chapter. A normal MAP is considered to be 70 to 100 mm Hg.

The **shock index (SI)** is another calculation that is often utilized to assess the level of shock. SI is calculated by dividing the heart rate by the systolic blood pressure. Both heart rate and blood pressure may appear normal during the early, compensatory stages of shock. Moreover, other confounding variables, such as medications, extremes of age, among other factors, may alter these vital signs. The SI has been studied in patients at risk for or suffering from shock from a wide variety of causes, including hemorrhage, myocardial infarction, pulmonary embolism, and sepsis.[6] The normal ratio of heart rate to systolic blood pressure is generally < 0.7.[7] Trauma patients with an SI ≥ 0.9 have been shown to have higher mortality and a higher risk for critical bleeding.[7,8]

The volume of fluid pumped into the circulatory system with each contraction of the ventricle is called the **stroke volume**, and the volume of blood pumped into the system over 1 minute is called the **cardiac output**. The formula for cardiac output is as follows:

$$\text{Cardiac output (CO)} = \text{Heart rate (HR)} \times \text{Stroke volume (SV)}$$
$$\text{Normal cardiac output} = 5-6 \text{ liters per minute}$$

Cardiac output is reported in liters per minute (lpm or L/min). Cardiac output is not measured in the prehospital environment; however, understanding cardiac output and its relationship to stroke volume is important in understanding shock. For the heart to work effectively, an adequate volume of blood must be present in the venae cavae and pulmonary veins to fill the ventricles.

Starling's law is an important concept that helps to explain how this relationship works. This pressure fills the heart (preload) and stretches the myocardial muscle fibers. The more the ventricles fill, the greater the stretch of the cardiac muscle fibers and the greater the strength of the contraction of the heart, until the point of overstretching. Significant hemorrhage or relative hypovolemia decreases cardiac preload, so a reduced volume of blood is present and the fibers are not stretched as much, resulting in a lower strength of contraction and a lower stroke volume; therefore, blood pressure will fall. If the filling pressure of the heart is too great, as can occur in fluid overloaded patients, the cardiac muscle fibers become overstretched and can fail to deliver a satisfactory stroke volume, and again blood pressure will decrease.

The resistance to blood flow that the left ventricle must overcome to pump blood out into the arterial system is called afterload, or **systemic vascular resistance**. As peripheral arterial vasoconstriction increases, the resistance to blood flow increases and the heart has to generate a greater force to pump blood into the arterial system. Conversely, widespread peripheral vasodilation decreases afterload.

The systemic circulation contains more capillaries and a greater length of blood vessels than the pulmonary circulation. Therefore, the left (or left-sided) heart system works at a higher pressure and bears a greater workload than the right (or right-sided) heart system. Anatomically, the muscle of the left ventricle is much thicker and stronger than that of the right ventricle.

Blood Vessels

The blood vessels contain the blood and route it to the various areas and cells of the body. They are the "highways" of the physiologic process of circulation. The aorta splits into multiple arteries of decreasing size, the smallest of which are the capillaries (**Figure 3-5**). A capillary

may be only one cell wide; therefore, oxygen and nutrients carried by RBCs and plasma are able to diffuse easily through the walls of the capillary into the surrounding tissue cells (**Figure 3-6**). Each cell has a covering called the cell membrane. Interstitial fluid is located between the cell membrane and the capillary wall. The amount of interstitial fluid varies tremendously. If little interstitial fluid is present, the cell membrane and the capillary wall are closer together, and oxygen can easily diffuse between them. When there is extra fluid (edema) forced into this space (such as occurs in over-resuscitation with crystalloid fluids), the cells move farther away from the capillaries, making transfer of oxygen and nutrients less efficient.

The size of the vascular "container" is controlled by smooth muscles in the walls of the arteries and arterioles and, to a lesser extent, by muscles in the walls of the venules and veins. These muscles respond to signals from the brain via the sympathetic nervous system, to the circulating hormones epinephrine and norepinephrine, and to other chemicals, such as nitric oxide. Depending on whether they are being stimulated to contract or allowed to relax, these muscle fibers in the walls of the vessels result in either the constriction or dilation of the blood vessels, thus changing the size of the container component of the cardiovascular system and thereby affecting the patient's blood pressure.

There are three fluid compartments: intravascular fluid (fluid inside the vessels), intracellular fluid (fluid inside the cells), and interstitial fluid (fluid between the cells and the vessels). When interstitial fluid is present

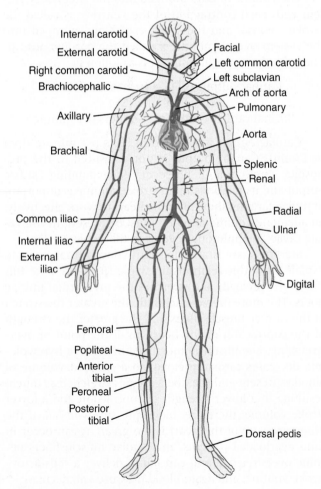

Figure 3-5 Principal arteries of the body.

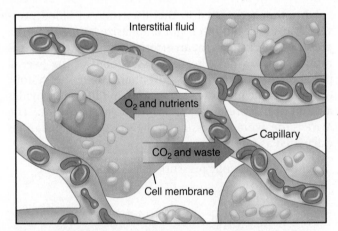

Figure 3-6 Oxygen from the RBCs and nutrients diffuse through the capillary wall, the interstitial fluid, and the cell membrane into the cell. Carbon dioxide and cellular waste products travel through the circulatory system to be eliminated by the lungs. By way of the buffer system of the body, this acid is converted into carbon dioxide and travels in the plasma along with the RBCs to be eliminated from the circulatory system by the lungs.

in excess amounts, it produces edema and causes the spongy, boggy feeling when the skin is compressed with a finger.

Hemodynamic Response

Blood

The fluid component of the circulatory system—the blood—contains (1) RBCs to carry oxygen, (2) infection-fighting factors (**white blood cells [WBCs]** and antibodies), and (3) platelets and clotting factors essential for blood clotting at times of vascular injury, protein for cellular rebuilding, nutrients such as glucose, and other substances necessary for metabolism and survival. The various proteins and minerals provide a high **oncotic pressure** to help keep water from leaking out through the walls of the vessels. The volume of fluid within the vascular system must equal the capacity of the blood vessels if it is to adequately fill the container and maintain perfusion. Any variance in the volume of the vascular system container compared to the volume of blood in that container will affect the flow of blood either positively or negatively.

The human body is 60% water, which is the base of all body fluids. A person who weighs 154 pounds (70 kg) contains approximately 40 liters of water. Body water is present in two components: intracellular and extracellular fluid. As noted previously, each type of fluid has specific important properties (**Figure 3-7**). **Intracellular fluid**, the fluid within the cells, accounts for approximately 45% of body weight. **Extracellular fluid**, the fluid outside the cells, can be further classified into two subtypes: interstitial fluid and intravascular fluid. **Interstitial**

fluid, which surrounds the tissue cells and also includes cerebrospinal fluid (found in the brain and spinal canal) and synovial fluid (found in the joints), accounts for approximately 10.5% of body weight. Intravascular fluid, which is found in the vessels and carries the formed components of blood as well as oxygen and other vital nutrients, accounts for approximately 4.5% of body weight.

A review of some key concepts is helpful in this discussion of how fluids move throughout the body. In addition to movement of fluid through the vascular system, there are two major types of fluid movements: (1) movement between the plasma and interstitial fluid (across capillaries) and (2) movement between the intracellular and interstitial fluid compartments (across cell membranes).

The movement of fluid through the capillary walls is determined by (1) the difference between the hydrostatic pressure within the capillary (which tends to push fluid out) and the hydrostatic pressure outside the capillary (which tends to push fluid in), (2) the difference in the oncotic pressure from protein concentration within the capillary (which keeps fluid in) and the oncotic pressure outside the capillary (which pulls fluid out), and (3) the "leakiness" or permeability of the capillary (**Figure 3-8**). Hydrostatic pressure, oncotic pressure, and capillary permeability are all affected by the shock state, as well as by the type and volume of fluid resuscitation, leading to alterations in circulating blood volume, hemodynamics, and tissue or pulmonary edema.

Movement of fluid between the intracellular and interstitial space occurs across cellular membranes, which is determined primarily by osmotic effects. **Osmosis** is the process by which solutes separated by a semipermeable membrane (permeable to water, relatively impermeable to solutes) govern the movement of water across that membrane based on the concentration of the solute. Water moves from the compartment of lower solute

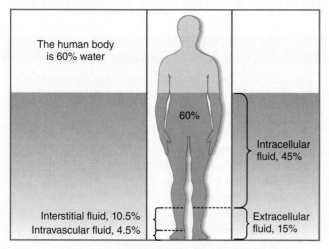

Figure 3-7 Body water represents 60% of body weight. This water is divided into intracellular and extracellular fluid. The extracellular fluid is further divided into interstitial and intravascular fluid.

© National Association of Emergency Medical Technicians (NAEMT)

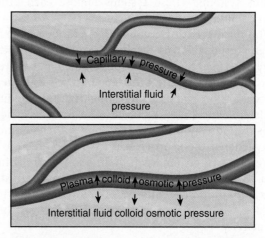

Figure 3-8 Forces governing fluid flux across capillaries.

© National Association of Emergency Medical Technicians (NAEMT)

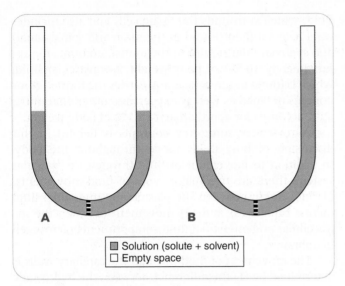

Figure 3-9 A. A U-tube, in which the two halves are separated by a semipermeable membrane, contains equal amounts of water and solid particles. **B.** If a solute that cannot diffuse through the semipermeable membrane is added to one side but not to the other, fluid will flow across the membrane to dilute the added particles. The pressure difference of the height of the fluid in the U-tube is known as osmotic pressure.

© National Association of Emergency Medical Technicians (NAEMT)

concentration to that of higher solute concentration to maintain osmotic equilibrium across the semipermeable membrane (**Figure 3-9**).

Endocrine Response

Nervous System

The **autonomic nervous system** directs and controls the involuntary functions of the body, such as respiration, digestion, and cardiovascular function. It is divided into two subsystems—the sympathetic and parasympathetic nervous systems. These systems oppose each other to keep vital body systems in balance.

The **sympathetic nervous system** produces the fight-or-flight response. This response simultaneously causes the heart to beat faster and stronger, increases the ventilatory rate, and constricts the blood vessels to nonessential organs (skin and gastrointestinal tract) while dilating vessels and improving blood flow to muscles. The goal of this response system is to maintain sufficient amounts of oxygenated blood to critical tissues so an individual can respond to an emergency situation while shunting blood away from nonessential areas. In contrast, the **parasympathetic nervous system** slows the heart rate, decreases the ventilatory rate, and increases gastrointestinal activity.

In patients who are hemorrhaging after sustaining trauma, the body attempts to compensate for the blood loss

and to maintain energy production. The cardiovascular system is regulated by the vasomotor center in the medulla. In response to a transient fall in blood pressure, stimuli travel to the brain via cranial nerves IX and X from stretch receptors in the carotid sinus and the aortic arch. These stimuli lead to increased sympathetic nervous system activity, with increased peripheral vascular resistance resulting from arteriolar constriction and increased cardiac output from an increased rate and force of cardiac contraction. Increased venous tone enhances circulatory blood volume. Blood is diverted from the extremities, bowel, and kidney to more vital areas—the heart and brain—in which vessels constrict very little under intense sympathetic stimulation. These responses result in cold, cyanotic extremities, decreased urine output, and decreased bowel perfusion.

A decrease in the left atrial filling pressure, a fall in blood pressure, and changes in plasma osmolality (the total concentration of all of the chemicals in blood) cause the release of antidiuretic hormone (ADH) from the pituitary gland and aldosterone from the adrenal glands, which enhances retention of sodium and water by the kidneys. This process helps to expand the intravascular volume; however, it requires many hours for this mechanism to make a clinical difference.

Classification of Traumatic Shock

The prime determinants of cellular perfusion are the heart (acting as the pump, or the motor of the system), fluid volume (acting as the hydraulic fluid), the blood vessels (serving as the conduits or plumbing), and, finally, the cells of the body. Based on these components of the perfusion system, shock may be categorized as shown in **Box 3-1**:

Box 3-1 Types of Traumatic Shock

The common types of shock seen after trauma in the prehospital setting include the following:

- Hypovolemic shock
  - Vascular volume smaller than normal vascular size
  - Result of blood and fluid loss
    - Hemorrhagic shock
- Distributive shock
  - Vascular space larger than normal
    - Neurogenic "shock" (hypotension as the result of severe vasodilation)
- Cardiogenic shock
  - Heart not pumping adequately
  - Result of cardiac injury

© National Association of Emergency Medical Technicians (NAEMT)

Types of Traumatic Shock

Hypovolemic Shock

Acute loss of blood volume from hemorrhage (loss of plasma and RBCs) causes an imbalance in the relationship of fluid volume to the size of the container. The container retains its normal size, but the fluid volume is decreased. Hypovolemic shock is the most common cause of shock encountered in the prehospital environment, and blood loss is by far the most common cause of hypovolemia and shock in trauma patients.

When blood is lost from the circulation, the heart is stimulated to increase cardiac output by increasing the strength and rate of contractions. This stimulus results from the release of **epinephrine** from the adrenal glands. At the same time, the sympathetic nervous system releases **norepinephrine** to constrict blood vessels to reduce the size of the container and bring it more into proportion with the volume of remaining fluid. Vasoconstriction results in closing of the peripheral capillaries, which reduces oxygen delivery to those affected cells and forces the switch from aerobic to anaerobic metabolism at the cellular level.

These compensatory defense mechanisms work well up to a point and will temporarily help maintain the patient's vital signs. A patient who has signs of compensation such as tachycardia and a rising SI is already in shock, not "going into shock." When the defense mechanisms can no longer compensate for the amount of blood lost, a patient's blood pressure will drop. This decrease in blood pressure marks the switch from compensated to decompensated shock—a sign of impending death. Unless aggressive resuscitation occurs, untreated shock leads to death.

Hemorrhagic Shock

The average 150-pound (70-kg) adult human has approximately 5 liters of circulating blood volume. Hemorrhage (hypovolemic shock resulting from blood loss) is categorized into four classes, depending on the severity and amount of hemorrhage, as follows (**Table 3-2**), with the proviso that the values and descriptions for the criteria listed for these classes should not be interpreted as absolute determinants of hemorrhage volume, as significant overlap exists (**Figure 3-10**):

1. *Class I hemorrhage* represents a loss of up to 15% of blood volume in the adult (up to 750 mL). This stage has few clinical manifestations. Tachycardia is often minimal, and no measurable changes in blood pressure, pulse pressure, or ventilatory rate occur. Most healthy

Table 3-2 Classification of Hemorrhage

	Class I	Class II	Class III	Class IV
Blood loss (mL)	< 750	750–1,500	1,500–2,000	> 2,000
Blood loss (% blood volume)	< 15%	15–30%	30–40%	> 40%
Pulse rate	↔	↔/↑	↑	↑/↑↑
Blood pressure	↔	↔	↔/↓	↓
Pulse pressure (mm Hg)	↔	↓	↓	↓
Central nervous system/mental status	Slightly anxious	Mildly anxious	Anxious, confused	Confused, lethargic
Base excess	0 to –2	–2 to –6	–6 to –10	More than –10
Need for blood	Monitor	Possible	Yes	Massive transfusion

↑ = increased, ↓ = decreased, ↔ = normal range

Note: The trends and descriptions for the criteria listed for these classes of shock should not be interpreted as absolute determinants of the class of shock, as significant overlap exists.

Data from American College of Surgeons Committee on Trauma. *Advanced Trauma Life Support for Doctors: Student Course Manual.* 8th ed. American College of Surgeons; 2008.

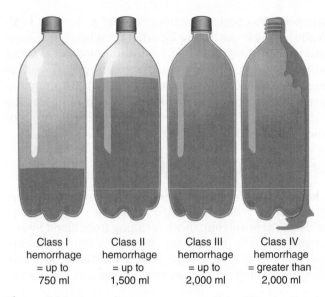

Class I
hemorrhage
= up to
750 ml

Class II
hemorrhage
= up to
1,500 ml

Class III
hemorrhage
= up to
2,000 ml

Class IV
hemorrhage
= greater than
2,000 ml

Figure 3-10 The approximate amount of blood loss for Class I, II, III, and IV hemorrhages.

© National Association of Emergency Medical Technicians (NAEMT)

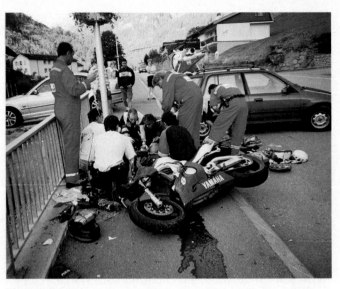

Figure 3-11 Massive blood loss, such as that sustained by the victim in this motorcycle crash, can rapidly lead to the onset of shock.

Photograph provided courtesy of Air Glaciers, Switzerland.

patients sustaining this amount of hemorrhage require only maintenance fluid as long as no further blood loss occurs. The body's compensatory mechanisms restore the intravascular container–fluid volume ratio and assist in the maintenance of blood pressure.

2. *Class II hemorrhage* may represent a loss of 15% to 30% of blood volume (approximately 750 to 1,500 mL). Most adults are capable of compensating for this amount of blood loss by activation of the sympathetic nervous system, which will maintain their blood pressure. Clinical findings include increased ventilatory rate, tachycardia, and a narrowed pulse pressure. The clinical clues to this phase are tachycardia, tachypnea, and normal systolic blood pressure. Because the blood pressure is normal, this response is called "compensated shock"; that is, the patient is in shock but is able to compensate for the time being. The SI may be elevated (> 0.9) in this stage. The patient often demonstrates anxiety or fright. Although not usually measured in the field, urine output drops slightly to between 20 and 30 mL/hour in an adult in the body's effort to preserve fluid. On occasion, these patients may require blood transfusion in the hospital.

3. *Class III hemorrhage* represents a loss of 30% to 40% of blood volume (approximately 1,500 to 2,000 mL). When blood loss reaches this point, most patients are no longer able to compensate for the volume loss, and hypotension occurs. The SI is > 1.0. The classic findings of shock are obvious and include tachycardia (heart rate greater

than 120 to 140 beats/minute), tachypnea (ventilatory rate of 30 to 40 breaths/minute), and severe anxiety or confusion. Urine output falls to 5 to 15 mL/hour. Many of these patients will require at least one blood transfusion and surgical intervention for adequate resuscitation and control of hemorrhage.

4. *Class IV hemorrhage* represents a loss of more than 40% of blood volume (greater than 2,000 mL). This amount of hemorrhage results in severe shock that is characterized by marked tachycardia (heart rate greater than 120 to 140 beats/minute), tachypnea (ventilatory rate greater than 35 breaths/minute), profound confusion or lethargy, and greatly decreased systolic blood pressure, typically in the range of 60 mm Hg. These patients truly have only minutes to live (**Figure 3-11**). Survival depends on immediate control of hemorrhage (surgery for internal hemorrhage) and aggressive resuscitation with blood and blood products, including a massive transfusion, defined by 3 or more units of packed red blood cells (PRBCs) in 1 hour, or more than 10 units of PRBCs in 24 hours.[9,10]

The rapidity with which a patient develops shock depends on how fast blood is lost from the circulation. A trauma patient who has lost blood needs to have the source of blood loss stopped, and, if significant blood loss has occurred, blood replacement needs to be accomplished. The fluid lost is whole blood, which includes all of its various components—RBCs with oxygen-carrying capacity, platelets, clotting factors, and proteins to maintain oncotic pressure.

Whole blood replacement, or even component therapy, is usually not available in the prehospital environment; therefore, in the field, when treating trauma patients with hemorrhagic shock, practitioners must take measures to control external blood loss, provide minimal intravenous (IV) electrolyte solution, blood products if appropriate and available, and transport rapidly to the hospital, where blood, plasma, and clotting factors are available and emergent interventions to control blood loss can be performed, as necessary. Tranexamic acid (TXA) is a clot-stabilizing medication that has been used for years to control bleeding and has started to make its way into the prehospital environment. TXA works by binding to plasminogen and preventing it from becoming plasmin, thereby preventing the breakdown of fibrin in a clot.

Prior shock research recommended a replacement ratio with electrolyte solution of 3 liters of replacement for each liter of blood lost.[11] This high ratio of replacement fluid was thought to be necessary because only about one-fourth to one-third of the volume of an isotonic crystalloid solution such as normal saline or lactated Ringer's solution remains in the intravascular space 30 to 60 minutes after infusing it.

More recent shock research has focused on the understanding that the administration of a limited volume of electrolyte solution before blood replacement is the correct approach while en route to the hospital. The result of administering too much crystalloid is increased interstitial fluid (edema), which potentially impairs oxygen transfer to the remaining RBCs and into the tissue cells. The goal is not to raise the blood pressure to normal levels but to provide only enough fluid to maintain perfusion and continue to provide oxygenated RBCs to the heart, brain, and lungs. Raising the blood pressure to normal levels may only serve to dilute clotting factors, disrupt any clot that has formed, and increase hemorrhage.

A common crystalloid solution for treating hemorrhagic shock is lactated Ringer's solution. Another isotonic crystalloid solution used for volume replacement is 0.9% "normal" saline; however, its use may produce hyperchloremia (marked increase in the blood chloride level), leading to acidosis in large volume resuscitation. Normosol and Plasma-Lyte are examples of balanced salt solutions that more closely match plasma concentrations of electrolytes, but they may also increase cost.

With significant blood loss, the optimal replacement fluid is ideally as near to whole blood as possible.[12-13] The first step is administration of PRBCs and plasma at a ratio of 1:1 or 1:2. Platelets, cryoprecipitate, and other clotting factors are added as needed. Plasma contains a large number of the clotting factors and other components needed to control blood loss from small vessels.

There are 13 identified factors in the coagulation cascade (**Figure 3-12**). In patients with massive blood loss requiring large volumes of blood replacement, most of the factors have been lost. Plasma transfusion is a reliable source of most of these factors. If major blood loss has occurred, the control of hemorrhage from large vessels requires operative management or, in some cases, endovascular placement of coils or clotting sponges for definitive management.

Distributive (Vasogenic) Shock

Distributive shock, or vasogenic shock, occurs when the vascular container enlarges without a proportional increase in fluid volume. After acute trauma, this is typically found in patients who have sustained a spinal cord injury.

Neurogenic "Shock"

Neurogenic "shock," or, more appropriately, neurogenic hypotension (hypotension in the absence of tachycardia), occurs when a spinal cord injury interrupts the sympathetic nervous system pathway. This usually involves injury to the cervical or upper thoracic levels. Because of the loss of sympathetic control of the vascular system, which controls the smooth muscles in the walls of the blood vessels, the peripheral vessels dilate below the level of injury. A marked decrease in systemic vascular resistance causes peripheral vasodilation. A patient with neurogenic shock is not hypovolemic—the normal blood volume is simply insufficient to fill an expanded (vasodilated) container.

Tissue oxygenation usually remains adequate (MAP > 65) in the neurogenic form of shock, and blood flow remains normal even though the blood pressure is low (neurogenic hypotension). In addition, energy production remains adequate in neurogenic hypotension.

Decompensated hypovolemic shock and neurogenic hypotension both result in decreased systolic blood pressure. However, the other vital and clinical signs, as well as the treatment for each condition, are different (**Table 3-3**). Hypovolemic shock is characterized by decreased systolic and diastolic pressures and a narrow pulse pressure. Neurogenic hypotension also displays decreased systolic and diastolic pressures, but the pulse pressure remains normal or is widened. Hypovolemia produces cold, clammy, pale, or cyanotic skin and delayed capillary refill time. In neurogenic hypotension the patient has warm, dry skin, especially below the area of injury. The pulse in patients with hypovolemic shock is weak, thready, and rapid. In neurogenic hypotension, because of unopposed parasympathetic activity on the heart, bradycardia is typically seen rather than tachycardia, but the pulse quality may be weak. Hypovolemia produces a decreased level of consciousness (LOC), or, at least, anxiety and often

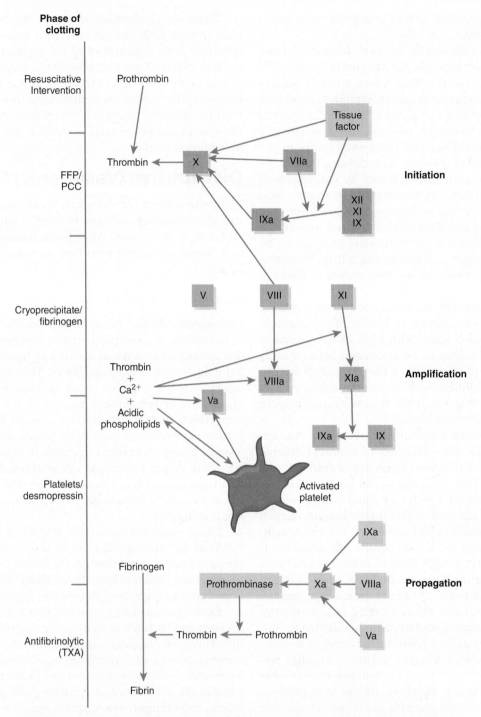

Figure 3-12 A contemporary visual description of the clotting cascade with clinical correlates (resuscitative interventions). A blood clot forms through three stages: initiation, amplification, and propagation. As formation of a blood clot is initiated, various clotting factors are activated and prothrombin is converted to thrombin. The clot is amplified by the activation of additional clotting factors and calcium. As the blood clot propagates, platelets play a central role, and additional clotting factors stimulate the generation of more thrombin and fibrin. The clot is eventually broken down; in trauma, clots are sometimes broken down too rapidly (fibrinolysis), requiring antifibrinolytics (e.g., tranexamic acid) to maintain clot strength. Recommended resuscitative interventions (i.e., replacement blood products) are listed, corresponding to the different stages of the clotting cascade.

Abbreviations: FFP, fresh frozen plasma; PCC, prothrombin complex concentrate.
© Jones & Bartlett Learning

Table 3-3 Signs Associated With Types of Shock

Vital Sign	Hypovolemic	Neurogenic Hypotension	Cardiogenic
Skin temperature/quality	Cool, clammy	Warm, dry	Cool, clammy
Skin color	Pale, cyanotic	Pink	Pale, cyanotic
Blood pressure	Drops	Drops	Drops
Level of consciousness	Altered	Lucid	Altered
Capillary refill time	Slowed	Normal	Slowed

© National Association of Emergency Medical Technicians (NAEMT)

Box 3-2 Neurogenic Hypotension Versus Spinal Shock

The term *neurogenic hypotension* refers to a disruption of the sympathetic nervous system, typically from injury to the spinal cord or a hemodynamic phenomenon, which results in significant dilation of the peripheral arteries. If untreated, this may result in shock and impaired perfusion to the body's tissues. Although typically lumped together, this condition should not be confused with *spinal shock*, a term that refers to an injury to the spinal cord that results in temporary loss of spinal cord reflex arc function.

© National Association of Emergency Medical Technicians (NAEMT)

combativeness. In the absence of a traumatic brain injury (TBI), the patient with neurogenic hypotension is usually alert, oriented, and lucid when in the supine position (**Box 3-2**).

Patients with neurogenic hypotension frequently have associated injuries that produce significant hemorrhage. Therefore, a patient who has neurogenic hypotension and potential physical signs of hypovolemia or any signs of shock other than hypotension, should first be treated as if blood loss is present. Stabilization of blood pressure with vasopressors may be helpful, but only after confirmation of adequate fluid resuscitation to address any hemorrhagic component should this be considered.

Cardiogenic Shock

Cardiogenic shock, or failure of the heart's ability to pump blood, results from causes categorized as either intrinsic (a result of direct damage to the heart) or extrinsic (related to a problem outside the heart).

Intrinsic Causes

Heart Muscle Damage

Any injury that damages the cardiac muscle may affect its output. The damage may result from a direct bruise to the heart muscle (as in a blunt cardiac injury causing cardiac contusion). In this type of injury, a recurring cycle will ensue: Decreased oxygenation causes decreased contractility, which results in decreased cardiac output and, therefore, decreased systemic perfusion. Decreased perfusion results in a continuing decrease in oxygenation and, thus, a continuation of the cycle. As with any muscle, the cardiac muscle does not work as efficiently when it becomes bruised or damaged.

Valvular Disruption

A sudden, forceful compressing blow to the chest or abdomen may damage the valves of the heart. Severe valvular injury results in acute valvular regurgitation, in which a significant amount of blood leaks back into the chamber from which it was just pumped. These patients often rapidly develop congestive heart failure, manifested by pulmonary edema and cardiogenic shock. The presence of a new heart murmur is an important clue in making this diagnosis.

Extrinsic Causes

Cardiac Tamponade

Fluid in the pericardial sac will prevent the heart from refilling completely during the diastolic (relaxation) phase of the cardiac cycle. In the case of trauma, blood leaks into the pericardial sac from a hole in the cardiac muscle. The blood accumulates, occupies space, and prevents the walls of the ventricle from expanding fully. This has two negative effects on cardiac output: (1) less volume is available for each contraction because the ventricle cannot expand fully, and (2) inadequate filling reduces the

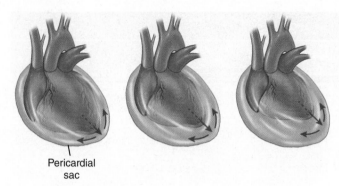

Pericardial
sac

Figure 3-13 Cardiac tamponade. As blood courses from a hole in the heart muscle into the pericardial space, it limits expansion of the ventricle. Therefore, the ventricle cannot fill completely. As more blood accumulates in the pericardial space, less ventricular space is available, and cardiac output is reduced.

© National Association of Emergency Medical Technicians (NAEMT)

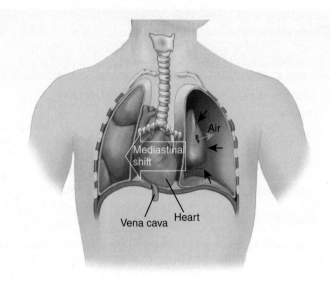

Figure 3-14 Tension pneumothorax. If the amount of air trapped in the pleural space continues to increase, not only does the lung on the affected side collapse, but the mediastinum shifts to the opposite side. The mediastinal shift impairs blood return to the heart through the venae cavae, thus affecting cardiac output, while at the same time compressing the opposite lung.

© National Association of Emergency Medical Technicians (NAEMT)

stretch of the cardiac muscle and results in diminished strength of the cardiac contraction. Additionally, more blood is forced out of the ventricle through the cardiac wound with each contraction and occupies more space in the pericardial sac, further compromising cardiac output (**Figure 3-13**). Severe shock and death may rapidly follow. (See Chapter 10, *Thoracic Trauma*, for additional information.)

Tension Pneumothorax

When either side of the thoracic cavity becomes filled with air that is under pressure, the lung becomes compressed and collapses. The involved lung is unable to re-fill with air from the outside through the nasopharynx. This produces at least four problems: (1) the tidal volume with each breath is reduced, (2) the collapsed alveoli are not available for oxygen transfer into the RBCs, (3) the pulmonary blood vessels are collapsed, reducing blood flow into the lung and heart, and (4) a greater force of cardiac contraction is required to force blood through the pulmonary vessels (pulmonary hypertension). If the volume of air and pressure inside the injured chest is great enough, the mediastinum is pushed away from the side of the injury. As the mediastinum shifts, the opposite lung becomes compressed, and compression and kinking of the superior and inferior venae cavae further impede venous return to the heart, producing a significant drop in preload (**Figure 3-14**). All of these factors reduce cardiac output, and shock rapidly ensues. (See Chapter 10, *Thoracic Trauma*, for additional information.)

Assessment

The assessment for the presence of shock begins by evaluating a patient for signs of poor blood perfusion to the vital organs. In the prehospital setting, this requires the assessment of organs and systems that are immediately accessible. Such systems are the brain and central nervous system (CNS), heart and cardiovascular system, respiratory system, skin and extremities, and kidneys. The signs of decreased perfusion and energy production and the body's response include the following:

- Decreased LOC, anxiety, disorientation, bizarre behavior (brain and CNS)
- Tachycardia, decreased systolic and pulse pressure (heart and cardiovascular system)
- Rapid, shallow breathing (respiratory system)
- Cold, pale, clammy, diaphoretic or even cyanotic skin with increased capillary refill time (skin and extremities)
- Decreased urine output (kidneys); identified rarely in the prehospital setting, but may be possible in situations of prolonged or delayed transport when a urinary catheter is present

Because hemorrhage is the most common cause of shock in trauma patients, hypotension in a trauma patient should be considered to be from hemorrhage until proven otherwise. The first priority is to examine for external sources of hemorrhage and control them as quickly and completely as possible. Controlling hemorrhage may involve such techniques as application of direct pressure, pressure dressings, pelvic binder, and tourniquets, or splinting of extremity fractures.

If there is no evidence of external hemorrhage, internal hemorrhage should be suspected. Because active control of internal hemorrhage is not practical in the prehospital setting, identification of an internal source of bleeding mandates rapid transport to the definitive care institution. Internal hemorrhage can occur in the chest, abdomen, or pelvis. Evidence of blunt or penetrating chest injury with decreased breath sounds would suggest a thoracic source. The abdomen and pelvis (either intraperitoneal or retroperitoneal portions) can be sources of bleeding with evidence of blunt trauma (e.g., ecchymosis) or penetrating trauma. Such evidence includes abdominal distension or tenderness, pelvic instability, leg-length inequality, pain in the pelvic area aggravated by movement, perineal ecchymosis, and blood at the urethral meatus. In some jurisdictions, prehospital ultrasound is used to perform an Extended Focused Assessment with Sonography for Trauma (eFAST) to evaluate for signs of internal hemorrhage.[14] The eFAST exam can identify intraperitoneal fluid (i.e., blood) or signs consistent with a pneumothorax after blunt trauma.

If the assessment does not suggest hemorrhage as the cause of the shock, nonhemorrhagic causes should be considered. These include cardiac tamponade and tension pneumothorax (both evident by distended neck veins versus collapsed neck veins in hemorrhagic shock) or neurogenic hypotension. Decreased breath sounds on the side of the chest injury, subcutaneous emphysema, respiratory distress (tachypnea), and tracheal deviation (a late finding rarely seen in the field) suggest tension pneumothorax. Presence of these signs suggests the need for immediate needle decompression of the involved side of the chest.

Different sources of cardiogenic shock may be suspected with blunt or penetrating chest trauma, muffled heart sounds suggesting cardiac tamponade (difficult to detect in the noisy prehospital environment), or dysrhythmias. Neurogenic hypotension may be suspected with signs of spinal trauma, bradycardia, and warm extremities. Most, if not all, of these features can be detected by an astute prehospital care practitioner who can determine the cause of the shock and the need for appropriate intervention when feasible in the field.

Areas of patient evaluation include status of the airway, ventilation, perfusion, skin color and temperature, capillary refill time, and blood pressure. Each one is presented separately here in the context of both the primary survey and the secondary survey. Simultaneous evaluation is an important part of patient assessment to gather and process information from different sources expeditiously.

Primary Survey

One of the first steps in patient assessment is to get an initial observation of the patient's condition as quickly as possible. The following signs identify the need for suspicion of life-threatening conditions:

- Mild anxiety, progressing to confusion or altered LOC
- Mild tachypnea, leading to rapid, labored ventilations
- Mild tachycardia, progressing to marked tachycardia
- Weakened radial pulse, progressing to an absent radial pulse
- Pale or cyanotic skin color
- Prolonged capillary refill time
- Loss of pulses in the extremities
- Hypothermia
- Sensation of thirst

Any compromise or failure of the airway, breathing, or circulatory system must be managed before proceeding. The following steps are described in an ordered series; however, all of these assessments are carried out more or less simultaneously (**Box 3-3** and **Box 3-4**).

Exsanguinating Hemorrhage

Bleeding patients die fast. It is possible to bleed to death in a few minutes from a significant arterial injury, and therefore this type of bleeding must be controlled immediately. The patient may be lying on the major source of the hemorrhage, or it may be hidden by the patient's clothes. The patient can lose a significant volume of blood from scalp lacerations because of the high concentration of blood vessels or from wounds that damage major blood vessels (subclavian, axillary, brachial, radial, ulnar, carotid, femoral, or popliteal). Rapidly scan the patient for any signs of severe bleeding from a major vessel and initiate appropriate interventions such as a tourniquet

---

Box 3-3 XABCDE

The primary survey of the trauma patient emphasizes control of life-threatening external bleeding as the first step in the sequence. Even though the steps of the primary survey are taught and displayed in a sequential manner, many of the steps can, and should when possible based on availability of help, be performed simultaneously. The steps can be remembered using the mnemonic XABCDE:

- **X**—Control of severe external (eXsanguinating) bleeding
- **A**—Airway management with cervical spine control when appropriate
- **B**—Breathing (ventilation and oxygenation)
- **C**—Circulation (perfusion and other hemorrhage)
- **D**—Disability
- **E**—Expose/environment

Box 3-4 MARCH

MARCH is an alternative patient assessment acronym similar to XABCDE and used by EMS practitioners working in trauma and tactical situations. MARCH stands for:

- **M**—Massive hemorrhage: Control the bleeding of a life-threatening hemorrhage with a tourniquet, pelvic binder, hemostatic dressing, or conventional pressure dressing.
- **A**—Airway: Assess for obstruction, and secure the casualty's airway with body positioning, nasopharyngeal airway, advanced airways, or surgical airway.
- **R**—Respirations: Assess and treat for penetrating chest wounds, sucking chest wounds, and tension pneumothoraces.
- **C**—Circulation: Assess and treat for shock. Establish intravenous or intraosseous access, and initiate fluid resuscitation if medically indicated.
- **H**—Head/hypothermia: Prevent secondary brain injury from hypotension, hypoxia, or elevated ICP. Protect the casualty from hypothermia. Heat, chemical, or toxic exposures may also be risk factors. Splint any major fracture, and provide spinal motion restriction for patients at risk (from the MARCH PAWS mnemonic).

The MARCH approach aligns closely with the XABCDE approach, which is the patient assessment acronym for trauma patients used by EMS practitioners. A side-by-side comparison shows the following parallel features:

Massive hemorrhage	e**X**sanguinating hemorrhage
Airway	**A**irway
Respirations	**B**reathing
Circulation	**C**irculation
Head/hypothermia	**D**isability
	Expose/environment

© National Association of Emergency Medical Technicians (NAEMT)

on a limb, pressure dressing on a scalp, or packing of a wound that is not amenable to any other therapy.

Airway

The airway should be evaluated quickly in all patients. A patent airway is a vital component of ensuring delivery of adequate amounts of oxygen to the cells of the body. Patients in need of immediate management of their airway include those with the following conditions, in order of importance:

1. Patients who are not breathing
2. Patients who have obvious airway compromise
3. Patients who have noisy sounds of ventilation
4. Patients who have markedly abnormal ventilatory rates

Breathing

The anaerobic metabolism associated with decreased cellular oxygenation produces an increase in lactic acid. The hydrogen ions produced from the acidosis are converted by the buffer system in the body into water and carbon dioxide. The brain's sensing system detects this abnormal increase in the amount of carbon dioxide and stimulates the respiratory center to increase the rate and depth of ventilation to remove the carbon dioxide. Thus, tachypnea is frequently one of the earliest signs of anaerobic metabolism and shock, even earlier than increased pulse rate. In the primary survey, time is not taken to measure a ventilatory rate. Instead, ventilations should be estimated to be slow, normal, fast, or very fast. A slow ventilatory rate, in conjunction with shock, generally indicates a patient who is in profound shock and may be moments away from cardiac arrest. A fast ventilatory rate is also a concern and should serve as an impetus to search for the cause of shock. It could also be a sign of a purely respiratory problem, such as a simple pneumothorax or early cardiac tamponade.

A patient who tries to remove an oxygen mask, particularly when such action is associated with anxiety and confusion, is displaying another sign of cerebral ischemia. This patient has "air hunger" and feels the need for more ventilation. The presence of a mask over the nose and mouth creates a psychological feeling of ventilatory restriction. This action should be a clue that the patient is not receiving enough oxygen and is hypoxemic.

Decreased oxygen saturation (SpO_2), as measured by the pulse oximeter, will confirm hypoxemia. Any pulse oximeter reading below 94% (at sea level) is worrisome and should serve as a stimulus to identify the cause of hypoxemia. Measurement and continuous monitoring of end-tidal carbon dioxide ($ETCO_2$) is a routine practice in EMS patients whose airway has been managed with procedures such as endotracheal intubation. While the correlation between the $ETCO_2$ and the partial pressure of carbon dioxide in arterial blood ($PaCO_2$) is good in patients who have adequate perfusion, the correlation is poor in patients in shock, thus limiting its utility to guide respirations. Monitoring $ETCO_2$ may still help to detect changes and trends in perfusion.

It is always important to remember to evaluate readings from machines in the context of the patient's appearance. If the appearance of the patient suggests hypoxemia, treat the patient for hypoxemia even if the machine would suggest otherwise. For example, note that peripheral pulse oximetry measurements are not reliable when patients are in decompensated shock. Because central pulse oximetry measurement is generally not available in the prehospital environment, the oximeter waveform should be used to determine the reliability of the reading. The waveform should be consistent with each pulse.

Circulation

The two components in the assessment of circulation are as follows:

- Hemorrhage and the amount of blood loss
- Perfusion with oxygenated blood
  - Total body
  - Regional

The data accumulated during the circulatory assessment help to make a quick initial determination of the patient's total blood volume and perfusion status and, secondarily, provide a similar assessment of specific regions of the body. For example, when checking the capillary refill time, the pulse, skin color (or nailbed color in dark pigmented patients), and temperature of a lower extremity may show compromised perfusion while the same signs may be normal in the upper extremity. This discrepancy does not mean the signs are inaccurate, only that one part is different from another. The immediate question to be answered is "Why?" It is important to check for the following circulatory and perfusion findings in more than one part of the body and to remember that the assessment of the total body condition should not be based on a single part.

Hemorrhage

Efforts at restoring perfusion will be less effective or completely ineffective in the face of ongoing hemorrhage. Severe external hemorrhage should be controlled as the first step in the primary survey. The prehospital care practitioner should reassess to ensure major bleeding remains under control and look for any additional sources of bleeding.

Loss of blood means loss of RBCs and a resulting loss of oxygen-carrying capacity. Thus, even though a patient who has been bleeding may have an SpO_2 that is "normal" due to a remaining blood volume that is fully saturated with oxygen, *total* oxygen delivery will be insufficient to supply all the cells of the body, leading to hypoxia.

Pulse

The next important assessment point for perfusion is the pulse. Initial evaluation of the pulse determines whether it is palpable at the artery being examined. In general, loss of a radial pulse indicates severe hypovolemia (or vascular damage to the arm), especially when a central pulse, such as the carotid or femoral artery, is weak, thready, and extremely fast, indicating the status of the total body circulatory system. If the pulse is palpable, its character and strength should be noted, as follows:

- Is the pulse rate strong, or is it weak and thready?
- Is the pulse rate normal, too fast, or too slow?
- Is the pulse rate regular or irregular?

Although many prehospital practitioners involved in the management of trauma patients focus on the patient's blood pressure, precious time should not be spent during the primary survey to obtain a precise blood pressure reading. The exact value of the blood pressure is much less important in the primary survey than other, earlier signs of shock. Significant information can be determined from the pulse rate and its character. In one series of trauma patients, a radial pulse characterized by practitioners as "weak" was associated with blood pressure that averaged 26 mm Hg lower than a pulse thought to be "normal." More importantly, trauma patients with a weak radial pulse were 15 times more likely to die than were patients with a normal pulse.[15] Although generally obtained at the beginning of the secondary survey, blood pressure can be palpated or auscultated earlier in the patient assessment if sufficient assistance is present, or once the primary survey has been completed and life-threatening issues are being addressed during transport.

Level of Consciousness

Mental status is part of the disability evaluation, but altered mental status may represent impaired cerebral oxygenation resulting from decreased perfusion. Assessment of mental status represents an assessment of end-organ perfusion and function. An anxious, confused patient should be assumed to have cerebral ischemia and anaerobic metabolism until another cause is identified. Drug and alcohol overdose and TBI are conditions that cannot be treated rapidly, but cerebral ischemia can be treated.

In addition to the concerns of the presence of hypoxemia and poor perfusion, altered mental status also suggests TBI. The presence of either hypoxemia and/or decreased blood pressure and TBI has a profound negative impact on patient survival. In a study of over 13,000 TBI cases, hypotension and/or hypoxemia were significantly associated with increased odds of death; the presence of both was linked with a mortality over 40%.[16] In a subsequent study by the same authors, statewide implementation of prehospital guidelines aimed at preventing hypoxemia and hypotension demonstrated a significant survival benefit for severely injured TBI patients.[17] Hence, prehospital practitioners should strive to prevent hypotension and hypoxemia in trauma patients with TBI.

Skin Color

Pale or mottled skin indicates unoxygenated hemoglobin and a lack of adequate oxygenation to the periphery. Pale, mottled, or cyanotic skin is the result of inadequate blood flow, resulting from one of the following three causes:

1. Peripheral vasoconstriction (most often associated with hypovolemia)
2. Decreased supply of RBCs (acute anemia)
3. Interruption of blood supply to that portion of the body, such as might be found with a fracture or injury of a blood vessel

Pale skin may be a localized or generalized finding with different implications. Other findings, such as tachycardia, should be used to resolve these differences and to determine whether the pale skin is a localized, regional, or systemic condition. Additionally, cyanosis may not develop in hypoxemic patients who have lost a significant number of RBCs from hemorrhage. In patients with dark-pigmented skin, cyanosis may be difficult to detect in the skin, but it can be noted in the lips, gums, nailbeds, and palms.

Skin Temperature

As the body shunts blood away from the skin to the vital organs, skin temperature decreases. Skin that is cool to the touch indicates vasoconstriction, decreased cutaneous perfusion, and decreased energy production and, therefore, shock. Because a significant amount of heat can be lost during the assessment phase, steps should be taken to preserve the patient's body temperature.

The environmental conditions in which the determination of body temperature is made can affect the results, as can an isolated injury that affects perfusion; therefore, the results of this assessment must be evaluated in the context of the entire situation.

Skin Quality

In addition to skin color and temperature, the skin is evaluated for dryness or moistness. Trauma patients in shock from hypovolemia typically have clammy (moist, diaphoretic) skin. In contrast, patients with hypotension from a spinal cord injury usually have dry skin.

Capillary Refill Time

The ability of the cardiovascular system to refill the capillaries after blood has been "removed" represents an important support system. Analyzing this support system's level of function by compressing capillaries to remove the blood and then measuring the refill time provides insight into perfusion of the capillary bed being assessed. Generally, the body shuts down circulation in the most distal parts first and restores this circulation last. Evaluation of the nail bed of the big toe or thumb provides an early indication that hypoperfusion is developing. Additionally, it provides a strong indication as to when resuscitation is complete. Nevertheless, several conditions—both environmental and physiologic—can alter the results. A measure of capillary refill time is the time required to reperfuse the skin and, therefore, an indirect measurement of the actual perfusion to that part of the body. It is not a diagnostic test of any specific disease process or injury.

Capillary refill time has been described as a poor test of shock. However, it is not a test of shock but rather a test of perfusion of the capillary bed being analyzed. Used along with other tests and components of the assessment, it is a good indicator of perfusion and suggestive of shock, but it is only a single piece of information and must be interpreted in the context of the overall situation and circumstances.

Shock may be the cause of poor perfusion and delayed capillary refill, but there are other causes, such as arterial interruption from a fracture, a vessel wounded by penetrating trauma (e.g., gunshot wound), hypothermia, and even arteriosclerosis. Another cause of poor capillary refill is decreased cardiac output resulting from hypovolemia (other than from hemorrhage).

Capillary refill time is a helpful diagnostic sign used as part of the process to help monitor the progress of resuscitation or progression of shock. If resuscitation of the patient is progressing in a positive manner and the patient's condition is improving, the capillary refill time will also show improvement.

Disability

One regional body system that can be readily evaluated in the field is brain function. At least six conditions can produce an altered LOC or change in behavior (combativeness or belligerence) in trauma patients:

1. Hypoxemia
2. Stroke
3. Shock with impaired cerebral perfusion
4. TBI
5. Intoxication with alcohol, drugs, or poisons
6. Metabolic processes such as diabetes, seizures, and eclampsia

Of these six conditions, the easiest to treat—and the one that will kill the patient most quickly if not treated—is hypoxemia. Any patient with an altered LOC should be treated as if decreased cerebral oxygenation is the cause. An altered LOC is usually one of the first visible signs of shock.

TBI may be considered primary (caused by direct trauma to brain tissue) or secondary (caused by the effects of hypoxemia, hypoperfusion, edema, loss of energy production, etc.). There is no effective treatment in the prehospital setting for the primary brain injury, but secondary brain injury can essentially be prevented or significantly reduced by maintaining oxygenation and perfusion.

The brain's ability to function decreases as perfusion and oxygenation drop and ischemia develops. This decreased function evolves through various stages as different areas of the brain become affected. Anxiety and belligerent behavior are usually the first signs, followed by a slowing of the thought processes and a decrease of the body's motor and sensory functions. The level of cerebral function is an important and measurable prehospital sign of shock. A belligerent, combative, anxious patient or one with a decreased LOC should be assumed to have a hypoxic, hypoperfused brain until another cause can be identified. Hypoperfusion and cerebral hypoxemia frequently accompany brain injury and make the long-term result even worse. Even brief episodes of hypoxemia and shock may worsen the original brain injury and result in poorer outcomes.

Expose/Environment

The patient's body is exposed to assess for less obvious sites of external blood loss and for clues indicating internal hemorrhage. The possibility of hypothermia is also considered. This exposure may be best performed in the heated patient compartment of the ambulance in order to protect the patient from a cold environment.

Secondary Survey

In any case when evidence of shock is present, do not take time to complete the secondary survey in the field. If time permits, the secondary survey can be done while en route to the hospital if no other issues need to be addressed.

Vital Signs

Measurement of an accurate set of vital signs is one of the first steps in the secondary survey or, after reassessing the primary survey, when a few minutes are available during transport.

Ventilatory Rate

The normal ventilatory rate for an adult is 12 to 20 breaths/minute. This rate will vary depending on age. (See Chapter 14, *Pediatric Trauma*.) A rate of 20 to 30 breaths/minute indicates a borderline abnormal rate; it suggests the onset of shock and the need for supplemental oxygen. A rate greater than 30 breaths/minute indicates a late stage of shock and the need for assisted ventilation. The physiologic drive for the increased ventilatory rate is the acidosis caused by shock, but it is usually associated with a decreased tidal volume. Both of these ventilatory rates indicate the need to search for potential sources of impaired perfusion. An accurate ventilatory rate can be obtained via $ETCO_2$ monitoring.

Pulse

In the secondary survey, the pulse rate is determined more precisely. The normal pulse range for an adult is 60 to 100 beats/minute. With lower rates, except in athletic individuals, an ischemic heart, medications, or a pathologic condition such as complete heart block should be considered. A pulse in the range of 100 to 120 beats/minute identifies a patient who has early shock, with an initial cardiac response of tachycardia. A pulse above 120 beats/minute is a definite sign of shock unless it is caused by pain or fear, and a pulse over 140 beats/minute is considered critical.

Blood Pressure

Blood pressure is one of the least sensitive signs of shock. Blood pressure does not begin to drop until a patient is profoundly hypovolemic (from either true fluid loss or container-enlarged relative hypovolemia). Decreased blood pressure indicates a patient can no longer effectively compensate for the hypovolemia and hypoperfusion. In otherwise healthy patients, blood loss may exceed 30% of blood volume before the patient's compensatory mechanisms fail and systolic blood pressure drops below 90 mm Hg. For this reason, ventilatory rate, pulse rate and character, capillary refill time, LOC, and the SI are more sensitive indicators of hypovolemia than is blood pressure.

When the patient's blood pressure has begun to drop, an extremely critical situation exists, and rapid intervention is required. In the prehospital environment, a patient who is found to be hypotensive has already lost a significant volume of blood, and ongoing blood loss is likely. The development of hypotension as a first sign of shock means that earlier signs may have been overlooked.

The severity of the situation and the appropriate type of intervention vary based on the cause of the condition. For example, low blood pressure associated with neurogenic hypotension is not nearly as critical as low blood pressure from hypovolemic shock. **Table 3-4** presents the

Table 3-4 Shock Assessment in Compensated and Decompensated Hypovolemic Shock		
Vital Sign	**Compensated**	**Decompensated**
Pulse	Increased; tachycardia	Greatly increased; marked tachycardia that can progress to bradycardia
Skin	Pale, cool, moist	Pale, cold, waxy
Blood pressure range	Normal	Decreased
Level of consciousness	Unaltered	Altered, ranging from disoriented to coma

signs used to assess compensated and decompensated hypovolemic shock.

An important pitfall to avoid involves equating systolic blood pressure with cardiac output and tissue perfusion. As previously emphasized, significant blood loss is typically required before the patient becomes hypotensive (Class III hemorrhage). Thus, patients will have decreased cardiac output and impaired tissue oxygenation when they have lost 15% to 30% of their blood volume, despite having a normal systolic blood pressure. Ideally, shock will be recognized and treated in the earlier stages before decompensation occurs.

Another possible source of error involves obtaining a single hypotensive blood pressure measurement and not believing it. The blood pressure is repeated and may return to normal (as a part of compensation). Additionally, a blood pressure may be obtained/attempted, and the noninvasive cuff is unable to produce a reading after multiple repeated attempts are cycled. Both of these issues should be concerning until proven otherwise.

Brain injuries do not cause hypotension until the brain begins to herniate. Therefore, a patient with a brain injury and hypotension should be assumed to have hypovolemia (usually blood loss) from other injuries and not from the brain injury. Young infants (younger than 6 months of age) are the exception to this rule, because they may bleed enough inside their head to produce hypovolemic shock as a result of open sutures and fontanelles that can spread apart and accommodate large amounts of blood.

Future Monitoring Capabilities

Current research has identified physiologic monitoring capabilities to assist in managing acutely injured patients. These advances are expected to enhance current capabilities, not replace physical examination skills. Using ultrasound to identify volume status and monitor tissue oxygenation, SI, and compensatory reserve index are methods that may evolve to assist prehospital practitioners in the future.

The compensatory reserve represents the body's capacity to compensate for blood loss. Compensatory reserve measurement (CRM) devices are able to noninvasively monitor a patient's arterial waveform each time the heart contracts and trend continuous changes in circulating blood volume that can predict impending decompensation.[18] Laboratory experiments in humans have shown CRM to have greater sensitivity and specificity than changes in heart rate, blood pressure, respiration rate, ETCO$_2$, SI, or SpO$_2$.[19] Data obtained from clinical studies suggest that CRM provides an accurate method to assess for shock in trauma patients with early warning signs of the patient's volume status.[20]

Musculoskeletal Injuries

Significant internal hemorrhage can occur with fractures, particularly multiple fractures. Fractures of the femur and pelvis are of greatest concern. Pelvic fractures, especially those resulting from significant falls or crushing mechanisms, can be associated with massive internal hemorrhage into the retroperitoneal space. Open fractures can be associated with a combination of internal and external hemorrhage that is substantial; however, supporting data for the amount of blood lost for any given fracture are lacking. A victim of blunt trauma can have multiple fractures and Class III or IV hemorrhage but no evidence of external blood loss, hemothoraces, intra-abdominal bleeding, or pelvic fracture. For example, an adult pedestrian struck by a vehicle and sustaining four rib fractures, a humerus fracture, a femur fracture, and bilateral tibia/fibula fractures may experience internal bleeding substantial enough for the patient to die from shock if it is unrecognized and inadequately treated.

Confounding Factors

Numerous factors can confound the assessment of trauma patients, obscuring or blunting the usual signs of shock. These factors may mislead unwary prehospital care practitioners into mistakenly thinking a trauma patient is stable.

Age

Patients at the extremes of life—the very young (neonates) and the elderly—have diminished capability to compensate for acute blood loss and other shock states. A relatively minor injury that would be tolerated without difficulty in a healthy adult may produce decompensated shock in these individuals. In contrast, children and young adults have a tremendous ability to compensate for blood loss and may appear relatively normal on a quick scan. They often appear to be doing well until they suddenly deteriorate into decompensated shock. A closer look may reveal subtle signs of shock, such as mild tachycardia and tachypnea, pale skin with delayed capillary refill time, and anxiety. Because of their powerful compensatory mechanisms, children found in decompensated shock represent dire emergencies. Elderly individuals may be more prone to certain complications of prolonged shock, such as acute renal failure.

Athletic Status

Well-conditioned athletes often have enhanced compensatory capabilities. Many have resting heart rates in the range of 40 to 50 beats/minute. A heart rate of 100 to

110 beats/minute or hypotension may a be warning sign indicating significant hemorrhage in a well-conditioned athlete. Similarly confusing, a heart rate of 50 in a well-conditioned athlete may be completely normal.

Pregnancy

During pregnancy, a woman's blood volume may increase by 45% to 50%. Heart rate and cardiac output during pregnancy are also increased. Thus, a pregnant woman may not demonstrate signs of shock until blood loss exceeds 30% to 35% of total blood volume. Also, well before a pregnant woman demonstrates signs of hypoperfusion, the fetus may be adversely affected because the placental circulation is more sensitive to the vasoconstrictive effects of catecholamines released in response to the shock state. During the third trimester, the gravid uterus may compress the inferior vena cava, greatly diminishing venous return to the heart and resulting in hypotension. Elevation of a pregnant patient's right side (i.e., left uterine displacement) may alleviate this compression. This positioning helps move the uterus away from the inferior vena cava, thereby allowing blood to return to the heart (i.e., preload). Hypotension in a pregnant woman persisting after performing this maneuver typically represents life-threatening blood loss.

Preexisting Medical Conditions

Patients with serious preexisting medical conditions, such as coronary artery disease, congestive heart failure, and chronic obstructive pulmonary disease, are typically less able to compensate for hemorrhage and shock. These patients may experience angina as their heart rate increases in an effort to maintain their blood pressure. Patients with implanted fixed-rate pacemakers are typically unable to develop the compensatory tachycardia necessary to maintain blood pressure. Patients with diabetes often have longer hospital and intensive care unit stays and more complications than patients without the underlying disease. Their blood vessels may be less compliant due to the long-term effects of hyperglycemia, and they also have decreased sensitivity and ability to respond to hemodynamic changes.

Medications

Numerous medications may interfere with the body's compensatory mechanisms. Beta-adrenergic blocking agents and calcium channel blockers used to treat hypertension may prevent an individual from developing a compensatory tachycardia to maintain blood pressure. Additionally, nonsteroidal anti-inflammatory drugs (NSAIDs), used in the treatment of arthritis and musculoskeletal pain, may impair platelet activity and blood clotting and may result in increased hemorrhage. Newer anticoagulant medications may prevent clotting for several days. Antiplatelet agents and anticoagulants ("blood thinners") may alter your choice of trauma center destination. If a history of medication use can be obtained from the patient or family members, this is important information to relay to the receiving trauma team.

Time Between Injury and Treatment

When the EMS response is rapid, prehospital practitioners may encounter patients who have life-threatening internal injury but have not yet lost enough blood to manifest severe shock (Class III or IV hemorrhage). Even patients with penetrating wounds to their aorta, venae cavae, or iliac vessels may arrive at the receiving facility with a normal systolic blood pressure if the EMS response, scene, and transport times are brief. The assumption that patients are not bleeding internally just because they "look good" is frequently wrong. The patient may "look good" because of compensated shock or because not enough time has elapsed for the signs of shock to manifest. It is important to remember that the majority of shock is compensated. Patients should be thoroughly assessed for even the subtlest signs of shock, and internal hemorrhage should be assumed to be present until it is definitively ruled out. The possibility of late-presenting internal hemorrhage is one reason why continued reassessment of trauma patients is essential.

Management

Steps in the management of shock are as follows:

1. Control any external severe hemorrhage.
2. Ensure oxygenation and ventilation (airway management).
3. Identify the source of hemorrhage. (Control external bleeding and recognize the likelihood of internal hemorrhage.)
4. Transport the patient to definitive care.
5. Administer blood component therapy when appropriate.

In addition to securing the airway and providing ventilation to maintain oxygenation, the prime goals of shock treatment include identifying the source or cause, treating the cause as specifically as possible, and supporting the circulation. By maintaining perfusion and oxygen delivery to the cells, energy production is supported, and cellular function assured.

In the prehospital setting, external sources of bleeding should be identified and directly controlled immediately. Internal causes of shock usually cannot be definitively treated in the prehospital setting; therefore, the approach is to transport the patient to the definitive care setting while supporting the circulation in the best way possible. Resuscitation in the prehospital setting includes the following:

- Control both external hemorrhage and internal hemorrhage to the extent possible in the prehospital setting. Every red blood cell counts.
- Improve oxygenation of the RBCs in the lungs through:
  - Appropriate airway management
  - Providing ventilatory support with a bag-mask device and delivering a high concentration of supplemental oxygen (fraction of inspired oxygen [FiO_2] greater than 0.85)
- Improve circulation to deliver the oxygenated RBCs more efficiently to the systemic tissues, and improve oxygenation and energy production at the cellular level.
  - Judicious use of crystalloids
  - Administration of blood products, if available and needed
- Prevent hypothermia.
- Reach definitive care as soon as possible for hemorrhage control and replacement of lost RBCs, plasma, coagulation factors, and platelets.

Without appropriate measures, a patient will continue to deteriorate rapidly until reaching the ultimate endpoint—death.

The following four questions need to be addressed when deciding what treatment to provide for a patient in shock:

1. What is the cause of the patient's shock?
2. What is the definitive care for the patient's shock?
3. Where can the patient best receive definitive care?
4. What interim steps can be taken to support the patient and manage the condition while the patient is being transported to definitive care?

Although the first question may be difficult to answer accurately in the field, identification of the possible source of the shock assists in defining which facility is best suited to meeting the patient's needs and what measures may be necessary during transport to improve the patient's chances of survival.

Exsanguinating Hemorrhage

Major hemorrhage must be controlled rapidly. A number of different tourniquets are available for use on extremity or junctional hemorrhage; several types of wound packing/clot-promoting materials are also available. Life-threatening hemorrhage must be treated promptly and aggressively.

Hemorrhage Control

The steps in the field management of external hemorrhage include the following:

- Hand-held direct pressure
- Compression dressings with wound packing and hemostatic agents, if possible
- Tourniquet
- Junctional tourniquets when indicated
- Pelvic binders for unstable pelvic fractures

Control of external hemorrhage should proceed in a stepwise fashion, escalating if initial measures fail to control bleeding (**Figure 3-15**). Some situations may require the need for tourniquet placement as the initial hemorrhage control maneuver.

Direct Pressure

Direct hand pressure or a pressure dressing, applied directly over a bleeding site, is the initial technique employed to control external hemorrhage. This application of pressure is based upon Bernoulli's principle and involves a number of considerations:

$$\text{Fluid leak} = \text{Transmural pressure} \times \text{Size of hole in vessel wall}$$

Transmural pressure is the difference between the pressure within the vessel and the pressure outside the vessel. The pressure exerted against the inside of the blood vessel walls by the intravascular fluids and blood pressure cycle is called the **intramural (intraluminal) pressure**. The force exerted against the wall of the blood vessel from

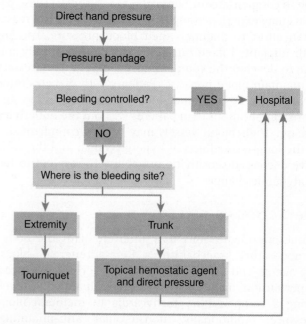

Figure 3-15 Hemorrhage control in the field.

the outside (such as by a hand or a dressing) is called the **extramural (extraluminal) pressure**. The following equation illustrates this relationship:

$$\text{Transmural pressure} = \text{Intramural pressure} - \text{Extramural pressure}$$

The higher the pressure inside the vessel, the faster that blood is forced out of the hole. The more pressure that the prehospital practitioner applies, the more slowly that blood will leak out. Direct pressure on the wound increases the extramural pressure, thus slowing the leak.

The ability of the body to respond to and control bleeding from a lacerated vessel is a function of the following:

- Size of the vessel
- Pressure within the vessel
- Presence of clotting factors
- Ability of the injured vessel to go into spasm and reduce the size of the hole and blood flow at the injury site
- Pressure of the surrounding tissue on the vessel at the injury site and any additional pressure provided by the prehospital care practitioner from the outside

Blood vessels, especially arteries, that are completely transected often retract and go into spasm. There is often less hemorrhage from the stump of an extremity with a complete amputation than from an extremity with severe trauma in which blood vessels are damaged but not completely transected.

Direct pressure over the site of hemorrhage increases the extraluminal pressure and, therefore, reduces the transmural pressure, helping to slow or stop bleeding. Direct pressure also serves a second and equally important function. Compressing the sides of the torn vessel reduces the size (area) of the opening and further reduces blood flow out of the vessel. Even if blood loss is not completely stemmed, it may be diminished to the point that the blood-clotting system can stop the hemorrhage. This is why direct pressure is almost always successful at controlling bleeding. Studies involving hemorrhage from femoral artery puncture sites after cardiac catheterization have documented that direct pressure is an effective technique.[21,22]

Following a leaky pipe analogy, if there is a small hole in the pipe, simply putting one's finger over the hole will stop the leak temporarily. Tape can then be wrapped around the pipe for a short-term fix of the leak. The same concept applies to the hemorrhaging patient. Direct pressure on the open wound is followed by a pressure dressing. However, for the pressure dressing to be most effective, the pressure must be placed directly on the injury in the vessel. A simple dressing placed on the skin over the wound does not impart any direct pressure on the bleeding site itself.

To achieve the most effective use of a pressure dressing, the dressing material must be packed tightly down into the wound and the elastic bandage placed on the outside. The effectiveness of wound packing may be augmented with the use of a hemostatic agent such as Combat Gauze, ChitoGauze, or Celox, or may be performed using a plain gauze roll.[23] The key is to place the packing material into the base of the wound, directly onto the bleeding site and then pack the entire roll into the wound. Direct pressure over the wound should be placed for a minimum of 3 minutes or per the manufacturer's instructions and for 10 minutes if using plain gauze.

THREE CRITICAL POINTS

Three additional points about direct pressure should be emphasized. First, when managing a wound with an impaled object, pressure should be applied on either side of the object rather than over the object. Impaled objects should not be removed in the field because the object may have damaged a vessel, and the object itself could be tamponading the bleeding. Removal of the object could result in uncontrolled internal hemorrhage.

Second, after controlling bleeding with direct pressure, a pressure dressing is still necessary since maintaining manual pressure during treatment of other conditions and transport is generally not possible.

Third, applying direct pressure to exsanguinating hemorrhage takes precedence over insertion of IV lines and fluid resuscitation. It would be a serious error to deliver a well-packaged trauma victim to the receiving facility with two IV lines inserted and neatly taped in place but who is dying from the hemorrhage of a wound that only has trauma dressings taped in place with no direct pressure applied.

Tourniquets

If external bleeding from an extremity cannot be immediately controlled by pressure, application of a tourniquet is the reasonable next step in hemorrhage control. Tourniquets had fallen out of favor because of concern about potential complications, including damage to nerves and blood vessels and potential loss of the limb if the tourniquet is left on too long. None of these concerns has been proven; in fact, data from the Iraq and Afghanistan wars have demonstrated just the opposite.[24-25] There were no limbs lost in these conflicts as a result of tourniquet placement by the U.S. military. Data from the military experience suggest that appropriately applied tourniquets could potentially have prevented 7 out of every 100 combat deaths.[26-27]

Tourniquet control of exsanguinating limb hemorrhage is 80% or better.[28-29] In addition, tourniquets occluding arterial inflow have been widely used in the OR by surgeons for many years with satisfactory results. Used properly, tourniquets are not only safe but also lifesaving.[30,31]

A study from the military in Iraq and Afghanistan showed a marked difference in survival when the tourniquet was applied before shock developed compared to instances when it was applied after blood pressure had dropped.[32] When the tourniquet was applied before the patient went into shock, survival was 96%; when it was placed after the patient developed shock, survival was 4%. There is no rationale for delaying tourniquet application in the face of exsanguinating hemorrhage.

DEVICE OPTIONS

Because of the U.S. military's interest in an effective (demonstrated arterial occlusion), easy-to-use tourniquet (especially one that a soldier could apply quickly with one hand should the other arm be injured), many commercial tourniquets have been developed and marketed. Through the Committee on Tactical Combat Casualty Care, the Department of Health Agency-Joint Trauma System identified eight tourniquets as recommended: Combat Application Tourniquet Generations 6 and 7 (C-A-T Gen 6, C-A-T Gen 7), Emergency and Military Tourniquet (EMT), Special Operations Force Tactical Tourniquet – Wide, Generation 3 (SOFTT-W), Tactical Mechanical Tourniquet (TMT), Ratcheting Medical Tourniquet-Tactical (RMT-T), SAM Extremity Tourniquet (SAM-XT), and Tactical Pneumatic Tourniquet, 2-inch (TPT2) (**Figure 3-16**).[33]

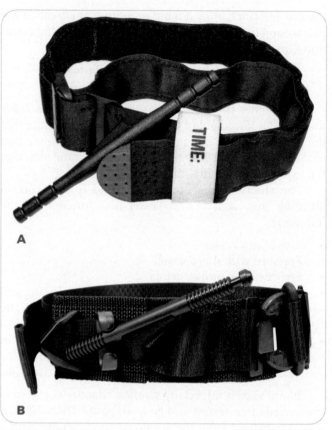

Figure 3-16 **A.** A C-A-T tourniquet. **B.** A SOF-T tourniquet.
A. © Looka/Shutterstock **B.** Courtesy of TacMed Solutions, LCC.

APPLICATION SITE

A tourniquet should be applied in the groin or axilla. If one tourniquet does not completely stop the hemorrhage, then another one should be applied just proximal to the first. By placing two tourniquets side by side, the area of compression is doubled and successful control of hemorrhage is more likely. Once applied, the tourniquet site should remain uncovered, so it can be easily seen and monitored.

Previously, some sources recommended application nearer to the site of hemorrhage, at a specified distance proximal to the site of bleeding, as opposed to primary application at the groin or axilla. In a civilian setting, when transport times to definitive care are relatively short, there are several reasons why this does not make sense:

1. Operative experience in elective settings strongly suggests that proximal applications are highly safe and effective.
2. The site of bleeding externally may not be representative of the extent of bleeding internally. This is true with both blunt and penetrating trauma. The zone of injury may actually extend more proximal than the site of tourniquet application, leading to ongoing bleeding from the injury despite tourniquet inflation to adequate pressure

levels at a more distal site. Thus, the most proximal application site possible is preferred.
3. There is at least theoretically, a greater risk of injury in areas where important nervous structures are close to the skin and to underlying bony prominences (e.g., the common peroneal nerve at the fibular neck or the ulnar nerve at the cubital tunnel). Severe nerve injury could result from application in these locations.
4. Bleeding control is harder to achieve in certain locations along the length of the extremity where bony prominences are close to the skin, impeding soft tissue and therefore arterial compression.

APPLICATION TIGHTNESS

A tourniquet should be applied tight enough to block arterial flow and occlude the distal pulse. A device that occludes only venous outflow from a limb will actually increase hemorrhage from a wound. A direct relationship exists between the amount of pressure required to control hemorrhage and the size of the limb. Thus, on average, a tourniquet will need to be placed more tightly on a leg to achieve hemorrhage control than on an arm.

TIME LIMIT

Arterial tourniquets are regularly used safely for up to 150 minutes in the operating room without significant nerve or muscle damage to achieve bleeding control during elective extremity surgery. Even in suburban or rural settings, most EMS transport times are significantly less than this. In general, a tourniquet placed in the prehospital setting should remain in place until the patient reaches definitive care at the closest appropriate hospital. U.S. military use has not shown significant deterioration with prolonged application times.[33] If application of a tourniquet is required, the patient will most likely need emergency surgery to control the hemorrhage. Thus, the ideal receiving facility for such a patient is a trauma center or, at a minimum, a nontrauma hospital with immediately available surgical capabilities.

In the past, it was often recommended that a tourniquet be loosened every 10 to 15 minutes to allow for some blood flow back into the injured extremity; it was thought that this blood flow would help preserve the limb and prevent subsequent amputation. This practice, however, serves only to increase the blood loss sustained by the patient and often does nothing for the limb itself. Current recommendations are that once applied, a tourniquet should be left in place until the limb can be evaluated at a center capable of definitive treatment. A tourniquet may need to be removed in a few, limited situations, but these are rare circumstances and whenever possible should only be performed in the context of online medical direction.

A tourniquet can be painful for a conscious patient to tolerate, and pain management should be considered. **Box 3-5** provides a sample protocol for tourniquet application.

Hemostatic Agents

The U.S. Food and Drug Administration (FDA) has approved a number of topical hemostatic agents for use. Hemostatic agents are designed to be placed or packed into a wound to enhance clotting and promote control of life-threatening hemorrhage that cannot be stopped with direct pressure alone in areas of the body that are not amenable to tourniquet placement. These agents generally come in the form of a gauze impregnated with the hemostatic material that is applied to or packed into the wound (**Figure 3-17**).

For hemorrhage from locations not amenable to placement of a tourniquet, such as on the abdomen or groin, it is reasonable to use hemostatic agents. Combat Gauze, Celox, and ChitoGauze are hemostatic dressings designed to be tightly packed into a wound. XStat (best for deep, narrow-tract junctional wounds) uses an applicator with multiple small hemostatic sponges that are injected deep into a wound. The iTClamp is a polycarbonate

---

Box 3-5 Protocol for Tourniquet Application

Tourniquets should be used if controlling the hemorrhage with direct pressure or a pressure dressing is not effective. The steps in applying a tourniquet are as follows:

1. Apply a commercially manufactured tourniquet to the extremity at the level of the groin for the lower extremity or the axilla for the upper extremity.
2. Tighten the tourniquet until hemorrhage ceases and until distal pulses disappear, and then secure it in place.
3. Write the time of tourniquet application on a piece of tape and secure it to the tourniquet. For example, "TK 2145" indicates that the tourniquet was applied at 2145 hours.
4. Leave the tourniquet uncovered so the site can be seen and monitored. If bleeding continues after application and tightening of the initial tourniquet, a second tourniquet can be applied just above the first.
5. Anticipate the need for pain management.
6. Transport the patient, ideally to a trauma center that has surgical capability.

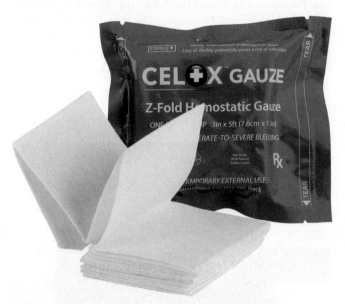

Figure 3-17 Hemostatic gauze is designed to be placed or packed into wounds in areas of the body that are not amenable to tourniquet placement.

clamp with metallic teeth used for temporarily closing a bleeding wound to obtain a tamponade effect.[34] Hemostatic dressings and sponges are best applied with a minimum of 3 minutes of direct pressure. The hemostatic dressing should be applied directly into the wound; it should not be applied as merely a dressing to cover the open injury. These dressings have different mechanisms of action, so if one type of dressing fails to control hemorrhage, a different dressing may be applied. The XStat device is unique insofar as it is not designed to be removed in the field, so once applied, this dressing should be left in place. Additional XStat dressings or other dressings can be applied if necessary.[34]

The newest generation hemostatic dressings have demonstrated a survival and blood loss difference when utilizing a lethal injury model in multiple large animal studies.[35-37]

Junctional Hemorrhage Control

Wounds located in the so-called junctional areas of the body, locations where the extremities and head join the trunk (groin, axilla and shoulder, and neck), may injure major blood vessels that can bleed profusely. In particular, wounds of the lower extremities from improvised explosive devices (IEDs) often result in high amputations and wounds that cannot accommodate tourniquet placement. A number of devices have been used by the U.S. military in combat theaters to control severe bleeding (**Figure 3-18**). These devices include the Combat Ready Clamp (CRoC; Combat Medical Systems), the Junctional Emergency Treatment Tool (JETT; North American Rescue Products, LLC), and the SAM Junctional Tourniquet (SJT; SAM Medical Products). There is little experience with these devices in civilian settings and minimal evidence that they might be effective in most civilian situations where junctional hemorrhage occurs.

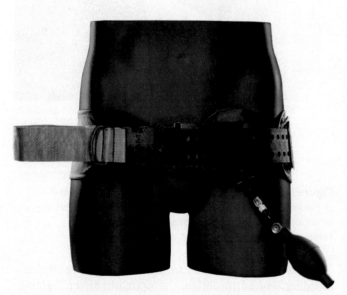

Figure 3-18 The SAM Junctional Tourniquet.
Used with permission from SAM Medical.

Elevation and Pressure Points

In the past, emphasis was placed on elevation of an extremity and compression on a pressure point (proximal to the bleeding site) as intermediate steps in hemorrhage control. No research has been published on whether elevation of a bleeding extremity slows hemorrhage. If a bone in the extremity is fractured, this maneuver could potentially result in increased internal hemorrhage. The use of pressure points for hemorrhage control has not been studied, and the likelihood that even if effective, such pressure could be maintained effectively throughout transport is low. Thus, in the absence of compelling data, these interventions are no longer recommended.

Airway

Advanced techniques for securing the airway and maintaining ventilation may be required in the prehospital setting. (See Chapter 7, *Airway and Ventilation*.) The importance of essential airway skills, especially when transport times are brief, should not be underestimated.

Breathing

Once a patent airway is ensured, patients in shock or those at risk for developing shock (almost all trauma patients) should initially receive supplemental oxygen in a concentration as close to 100% (FiO_2 of 1.0) as possible. This level of oxygenation can be achieved only with a device with a reservoir attached to the oxygen source. A nasal cannula, or a simple face mask do not meet this requirement. SpO_2 should be monitored by pulse oximetry in virtually all trauma patients and maintained at or above 94% and correlated with the patient's condition.

A nonbreathing patient, or one who is breathing without an adequate depth and rate, needs ventilatory assistance by opening the airway and using adjunct airway devices such as oropharyngeal and nasopharyngeal airways. If there is no response to these maneuvers, use a bag-mask device immediately.

It is critical to pay close attention to the quality of your assisted ventilations. Hyperventilation during assisted ventilation produces a negative physiologic response, especially in the patient with hypovolemic shock or with TBI. Ventilating too deeply or too quickly can make the patient alkalotic. This chemical response increases the affinity of hemoglobin for oxygen, resulting in decreased oxygen delivery to the tissue. In addition, hyperventilation may increase the intrathoracic pressure, leading to impaired venous return to the heart and hypotension. The increase in intrathoracic pressure could result either from large tidal volumes (10 to 12 mL/kg body weight) or from the creation of "auto-PEEP" (positive end-expiratory pressure) when ventilated too quickly (inadequate exhalation leads to air trapping in the lungs). In the patient with TBI, inadvertent hyperventilation can lead to cerebral vasoconstriction and decreased cerebral blood flow. This will exacerbate the secondary injury occurring in the brain. Several studies have demonstrated worse outcomes for TBI patients who are hyperventilated.[16,17,38] For an adult patient, administering a reasonable tidal volume (350 to 500 mL) at a rate of 10 ventilations/minute is likely sufficient.

ETCO$_2$ monitoring is often used in conjunction with pulse oximetry to maintain the patient in a **eucapnic state** (normal blood carbon dioxide level) with satisfactory oxygenation; however, in a patient with compromised perfusion, the correlation of ETCO$_2$ with PaCO$_2$ may be altered and cannot be relied upon to accurately judge ventilation.

Circulation

Although severe external hemorrhage was addressed first, addressing impending circulatory failure requires understanding how to recognize and intervene to control internal hemorrhage. Restoring functional circulation also may involve volumetric resuscitation in appropriate patients.

Internal Hemorrhage

Internal hemorrhage from fracture sites should also be considered. Rough handling of an injured extremity could potentially convert a closed fracture to an open one, although this is rare. What is more common is that such maneuvers can significantly increase internal bleeding from bone ends and increase injury to adjacent muscle and other soft tissues or vessels. All suspected extremity fractures should be stabilized to minimize this type of secondary injury. Time may be taken to splint several fractures individually if the patient has no evidence of life-threatening conditions such as shock. If the primary survey identifies threats to the patient's life, however, the patient should be immobilized rapidly on an appropriate device, thereby stabilizing all of the extremities in an anatomic manner, and transported to a medical facility. Pelvic binders have been shown to splint and approximate fractures and other disruptions of the pelvic ring. Although no studies have been done to show any change in outcome if used in the prehospital setting, there is good reason to believe that judicious early use of pelvic binders can limit hemorrhage from pelvic fractures and potentially limit mortality. In addition, there is no evidence that use of such devices in the prehospital setting or elsewhere is at all dangerous.

Hypotensive Resuscitation

From a vascular and patient perspective, the MAP (intraluminal pressure) and the pressure in the tissue surrounding the vessel (extraluminal pressure) have a direct relationship in controlling the rate of blood loss from the vessel as well as the size of the hole in the vessel. Of note, when a patient's blood pressure has been reduced by blood loss, it is appropriate not to increase it back to normal levels; rather, blood loss should be stopped and blood pressure maintained at a level sufficient to perfuse vital organs. This level generally occurs when the patient's systolic blood pressure is between 80 and 90 mm Hg. This means avoiding overinfusion of IV fluids into the patient and maintaining a modest degree of hypotension. Raising the blood pressure back to normal levels by administering large volumes of IV crystalloid fluids produces the exact opposite of the desired effect, increasing hemorrhage as a result of "popping" any clot that has formed over an opening in a blood vessel.

Multiple studies have demonstrated that withholding fluid resuscitation until hemorrhage control does not increase mortality.[39-44] Hypotensive resuscitation has been shown to be feasible and safe, with trends indicating improved survival in some patient populations, such as penetrating trauma patients.[39,40] An exception is a patient with a traumatic brain injury or spinal cord injury. Patients with these injuries and concomitant hypotension from hemorrhage should be supported more aggressively with fluid, blood products, or vasopressors to maintain a systolic blood pressure of at least 110 mm Hg.[43,45]

The steps in managing hemorrhage are to (1) increase external pressure (direct hand pressure), which decreases the size of the hole in the lumen of the blood vessel and decreases the differential between internal and external pressure, both of which contribute to retarding blood flow out of the injured vessel, and (2) use the technique of hypotensive resuscitation to ensure that the intraluminal pressure is not raised extensively.

Disability

There are no unique, specific interventions for altered mental status in the shock patient. If the patient's abnormal neurologic status is the result of cerebral hypoxia and poor perfusion, efforts to correct hypoxia and restore perfusion throughout the body should result in improved mental status. In assessing a patient's condition after TBI, an "initial" Glasgow Coma Scale (GCS) score is typically considered to be the score established following adequate resuscitation and restoration of cerebral perfusion. Assessing a patient's GCS score while still in shock may result in an overly grim prognosis.

Expose/Environment

Maintaining the patient's body temperature within a normal range is critically important. Hypothermia results from exposure to colder environments by convection, conduction, and other physical means (see Chapter 19, *Environmental Trauma I: Heat and Cold*). and from loss of energy production with anaerobic metabolism. The greatest concern regarding hypothermia is its effect on blood clotting. As the body cools, clotting is impaired. In addition, hypothermia worsens coagulopathy, myocardial dysfunction, hyperkalemia, vasoconstriction, and a host of other problems that negatively affect a patient's chance of survival.[46] Although cold temperatures preserve tissue for a short time, the temperature drop must be very rapid and very low for preservation to occur. Such a rapid change has not been proven effective for patients in shock after trauma.

In the prehospital setting, increasing the core temperature once hypothermia has developed can be difficult; therefore, all steps that can be taken in the field to preserve normal body temperature should be initiated. Once exposed and examined, the patient must be protected from the environment in an attempt to maintain core body temperature. Any wet clothing, including that saturated with blood, should be removed because wet clothing increases heat loss. Cover the patient with warm blankets. The need for warming should be anticipated, and blankets should be placed near heater vents in the ambulance en route to the call. An alternative to blankets involves covering the patient with plastic sheets, such as heavy, thick garbage bags. They are inexpensive, easily stored, disposable, and effective devices for heat retention. Heated, humidified oxygen, if available, may help preserve body heat, especially in intubated patients.

Once assessed and packaged, the patient in shock is moved into the warmed patient compartment of the ambulance. Ideally, the patient compartment of an ambulance is kept at 85°F (29°C) or more when transporting a severely injured trauma patient. The patient's rate of heat loss into a cold compartment is very high. The conditions must be ideal for the patient, not for the prehospital care practitioners, because the patient is the most important person in any emergency. A good general rule is that if the practitioner is comfortable in the patient compartment, it is too cold for the patient.

Patient Transport

Because effective treatment of severe hemorrhagic shock requires resources not normally available in the prehospital setting (an OR and blood products), rapid evaluation and emergent transport to a facility capable of managing the patient's injuries is important. Rapid transport does not mean doing the old-fashioned "scoop and run" and disregarding or neglecting the treatment modalities that are important in patient care. The prehospital practitioner must quickly institute critical, potentially lifesaving measures, such as hemorrhage control, airway management, and ventilatory support. Time must not be wasted on an

inappropriate assessment or with unnecessary immobilization maneuvers. When caring for a critically injured patient, many steps, such as warming the patient, starting intravascular therapy, and even performing the secondary survey, are accomplished in the ambulance while en route to the appropriate trauma facility.

Patient Positioning

In general, trauma patients who are in shock should typically be transported in the supine position. Special positioning, such as the Trendelenburg position (placed on an incline with the feet elevated above the head) or the "shock" position (head and torso supine with legs elevated), although used for 150 years, has not been proven to be effective. The Trendelenburg position may aggravate already impaired ventilatory function, may present an aspiration/airway obstruction risk, and may increase intracranial pressure in patients with TBI. More important, patients who are in severe hypovolemic shock are, generally, maximally vasoconstricted.[47] Patients with isolated TBI should typically be transported on an incline with the head of the bed elevated to 30 degrees.[48] This position facilitates improvement in cerebral perfusion pressure and decreases intracranial pressure. Additionally, if a patient is intubated, there is a benefit to inclining the stretcher or board to elevate the head relative to the feet by 30 degrees to decrease risk of aspiration and later stage ventilator-associated pneumonia. Importantly, this positioning must be achieved by elevating the head without causing the patient to flex at the waist, thus potentially aggravating a thoracolumbar spinal column injury (**Figure 3-19**).

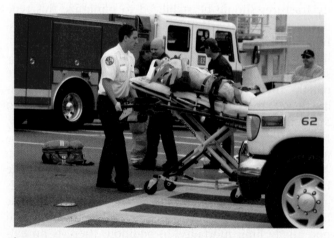

Figure 3-19 The head of the bed is elevated relative to the foot and the rest of the body by tilting the stretcher on an incline (reverse Trendelenburg position) or by elevating the backboard or vacuum mattress. It should NOT be accomplished by flexing the patient at the waist and thus moving the patient to a sitting position until thoracolumbar spinal injury has been excluded as a possibility.
© Michael Ledray/Shutterstock

Vascular Access

Intravenous Route

Intravascular access is obtained in a trauma patient who has known or suspected serious injuries so the prehospital care practitioner can initiate resuscitation if appropriate. Except in unusual circumstances, such as a patient undergoing extrication from a vehicle or when practitioners are awaiting the arrival of a helicopter, IV access should be obtained after the patient has been placed in the ambulance and transport has been initiated to the closest appropriate facility. Gaining IV access should not delay transport to the hospital for a severely injured patient.

Although volume resuscitation of a trauma patient in shock makes empiric sense, no research has demonstrated improved survival rates of critically injured trauma patients when IV fluid therapy was initiated in the prehospital setting. Transport of trauma patients should never be delayed to initiate IV lines. In fact, several studies failed to demonstrate any benefit from administration of intravenous crystalloids before hemorrhage was controlled.[39,40]

For patients in shock or with potentially serious injuries, one, or preferably two, large-bore (18-gauge or larger), short (1-inch [25-mm]) IV catheters should be inserted by percutaneous puncture as time permits. The rate of fluid administration is directly proportional to the fourth power of the radius of the catheter and inversely proportional to its length (meaning more fluid will rapidly flow through a shorter, larger diameter catheter than through a longer, smaller diameter catheter). The preferred site for percutaneous access is a vein of the forearm. Alternative sites for IV access are the veins of the antecubital fossa, the hand, and the upper arm (cephalic vein).

Intraosseous Route

An alternative for vascular access in adults is the intraosseous (IO) route.[49,50] The intraosseous route of giving IV fluids is not new and was described by Dr. Walter E. Lee in 1941.[49] This method of vascular access can be accomplished in a number of ways. It is most commonly established in sites such as the distal femur, humeral head, or proximal or distal tibia. Studies show best flow rates are through the humeral head and distal femur sites. It can also be established via the sternal technique, using appropriately designed devices (**Figure 3-20**, **Figure 3-21**, and **Figure 3-22**).[50-52] These techniques are commonly used in the prehospital setting, but the focus should be on rapid transport rather than IV fluid administration. For delayed or prolonged transport to definitive care, intraosseous vascular access may have a role in adult trauma patients. Fluid administration via the interosseous route in an awake patient may be painful. Appropriate analgesia should be considered in accordance with local policy.

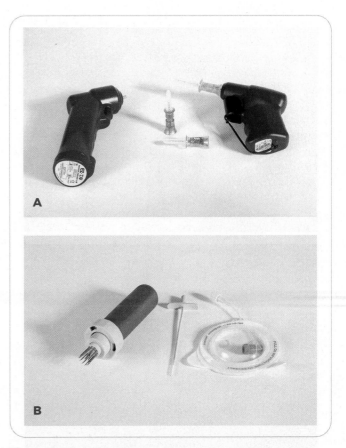

Figure 3-20 A. IO needles and IO gun for manual insertion (various sizes shown). **B.** IO sternal driver.

© Jones & Bartlett Learning. Photographed by Darren Stahlman.

Volume Resuscitation

There are two general categories of fluid resuscitation products that have been used in the past 50 years for the management of trauma patients—blood and IV solutions.[53] These products can be further subdivided as follows:

- Blood
  - Whole blood
  - Reconstituted whole blood as blood products
  - PRBCs
  - Plasma (e.g., thawed, lyophilized [freeze dried])
  - Additional blood component therapy (i.e., cryoprecipitate)
- IV solutions
  - Crystalloid solutions (e.g., lactated Ringer's, 0.9% saline)
  - Hypertonic fluid
    - 3% saline
  - Colloid solutions (e.g., dextran, Hextend, albumin)
  - Hypotensive or restricted fluid strategies (e.g., 5% dextrose in water)
  - Blood substitutes

Each of these products has advantages and disadvantages.

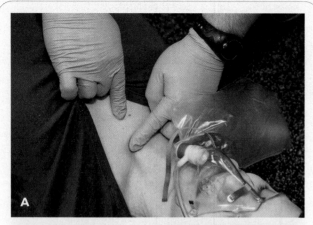

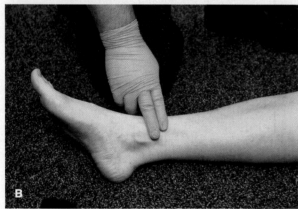

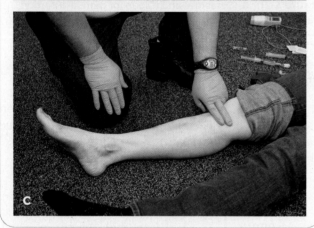

Figure 3-21 **A.** Sternal insertion site in the manubrium below the suprasternal notch. Note that the EZ-IO device cannot be used at the sternal site. **B.** Distal tibia insertion site above the ankle. **C.** Proximal tibia insertion site below the knee.

© National Association of Emergency Medical Technicians (NAEMT)

Blood

Because of its ability to transport oxygen, blood or various blood products remain the fluid of choice for the resuscitation of a patient in severe hemorrhagic shock. Experience gained by the U.S. military as a result of the

Iraq and Afghanistan wars has demonstrated the importance of administration of whole blood, PRBCs, and plasma to the survival of injured soldiers. This "reconstituted" blood replaces the lost oxygen-carrying capacity, clotting factors, and proteins needed to maintain oncotic pressure to prevent fluid loss from the vascular system. Unfortunately, blood, for the most part, is challenging for use in many current civilian prehospital settings primarily because blood and its subcomponents are perishable if not kept refrigerated or frozen until the moment of use. Nevertheless, several EMS systems have established protocols for prehospital blood transfusions.[54,55]

Lyophilized plasma is being used in the field in several countries. Lyophilized plasma is human plasma that has been freeze dried. It has a stable shelf life of approximately 2 years, does not require refrigeration, and must be reconstituted prior to use. Liquid plasma is being carried by a few EMS and HEMS (helicopter EMS) systems in the United States, and in one study that included over 500 patients, the prehospital administration of thawed plasma was associated with a significant improvement in 30-day mortality for trauma patients at risk for hemorrhagic shock.[56]

Intravenous Solutions

Alternative solutions for volume resuscitation fall into one of four categories: (1) isotonic crystalloids, (2) hypertonic crystalloids, (3) synthetic (artificial) colloids, and (4) blood substitutes.

Isotonic Crystalloid Solutions

Isotonic crystalloids are balanced salt solutions composed of electrolytes (substances that separate into charged ions when dissolved in solutions). They act as effective volume expanders for a short time, but they possess no oxygen-carrying capacity. Immediately after infusion, crystalloids fill the vascular space depleted by blood loss, improving preload and cardiac output. **Lactated Ringer's solution** remains the isotonic crystalloid solution of choice for the management of shock because its composition is most similar to the electrolyte composition of blood plasma. It contains specific amounts of sodium, potassium, calcium, chloride, and lactate ions. **Normal saline** (0.9% sodium chloride [NaCl] solution with a pH of 5.5) remains an alternative, although hyperchloremia (a marked increase in the blood chloride level) and metabolic acidosis may occur with large volume resuscitation with normal saline administration. Normosol and Plasma-Lyte are alternative options intended to provide more "balanced" acid–base solutions (pH 7.4) than normal saline. These solutions have been shown to be associated with less renal dysfunction when used in critically ill adults.[57] Solutions of dextrose in water (i.e., D_5W) are not effective volume expanders and have no place in the resuscitation of trauma patients.

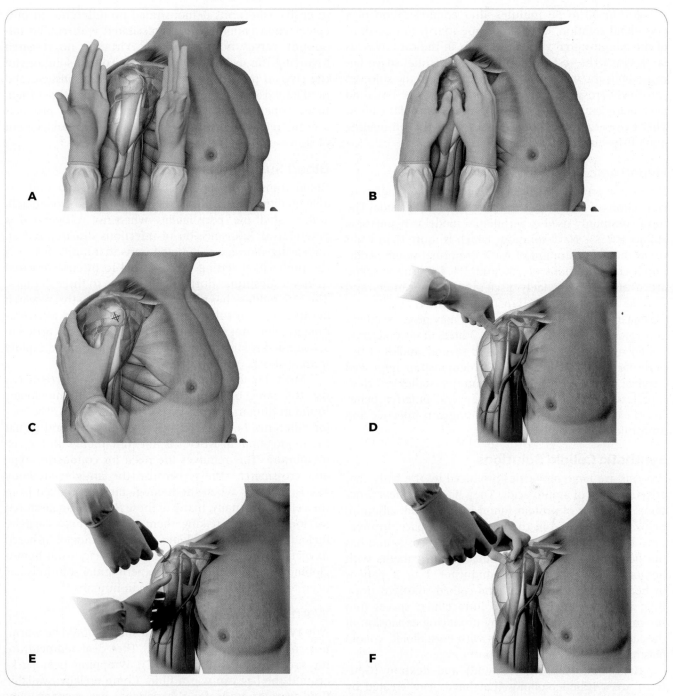

Figure 3-22 Proximal humerus insertion of the EZ-IO® device. **A.** Locate the insertion site by placing the ulnar aspect of your hands vertically over the axilla. The ulnar aspect of the other hand is placed along the midline of the upper arm laterally. **B.** Place your thumbs together over the arm. This identifies the vertical line of insertion on the proximal humerus. **C.** Palpate the surgical neck of the humerus. This should feel like a golf ball on a tee, the spot where the "ball" meets the "tee" is the surgical neck. The insertion site is 1 to 2 centimeters (cm) above the surgical neck. **D.** Keep a thumb on the insertion site. **E.** With the other hand, press the needle through the skin until the tip touches the bone. Squeeze the trigger while applying gentle, steady pressure. **F.** Stabilize the hub of the needle once inserted, and apply a stabilization device. Placement is confirmed with a flush of normal saline (5–10 mL for adults; 2–5 mL for infants/children).

Within 30 to 60 minutes after administration of a crystalloid solution, only about one-fourth to one-third of the administered volume remains in the cardiovascular system. The rest shifts into the interstitial space because both the water and the electrolytes in the solution can freely cross the capillary membranes. The lost fluid becomes edema in the soft tissues and organs of the body. This extra fluid causes difficulties with the on-loading and off-loading of oxygen to the RBCs.

Hypertonic Crystalloid Solutions

Hypertonic crystalloid solutions have extremely high concentrations of electrolytes compared to blood plasma. The most commonly used experimental model is **hypertonic saline**, a 7.5% NaCl solution, which is more than eight times the concentration of NaCl in normal saline. Additional concentrations of 2% and 3% hypertonic saline are available and widely used in trauma centers and neurocritical care units. Hypertonic saline is an effective plasma expander; a 250-mL infusion may produce effects equivalent to the infusion of 2 to 3 liters of isotonic crystalloid solution.[58,59] An analysis of several studies of hypertonic saline failed, however, to demonstrate improved survival rates over the use of isotonic crystalloids.[60] Nevertheless, hypertonic saline has several putative benefits in experimental models, including anti-infective and anti-inflammatory effects.[61]

Synthetic Colloid Solutions

Proteins are large molecules produced by the body that are composed of amino acids. They have countless functions. One type of protein found in the blood, albumin, helps maintain fluid in the intravascular space. Intravenous administration of human albumin is costly and has not been shown to improve outcomes in patients with hemorrhagic shock. When administered to a patient in hemorrhagic shock, synthetic colloid solutions draw fluid from the interstitial and intracellular spaces into the intravascular space, thereby producing expansion of the blood volume; however, as with crystalloids, colloid plasma expanders do not transport oxygen.

Hetastarch (Hespan, Hextend) and dextran (Gentran) are synthetic colloids that have been created by linking numerous starch (amylopectin) or dextrose molecules together until they are similar in size to an albumin molecule. These solutions are moderately expensive compared to crystalloids and have been associated with allergic reactions and impairment of blood typing. Two meta-analyses of the literature related to the use of hetastarch have raised concerns about an increased incidence of acute kidney injury and increased mortality related to administration of these compounds.[62,63]

The use of crystalloids versus colloids has caused a long-standing debate in the management of trauma patients.[64] A study of nearly 7,000 patients admitted to intensive care units demonstrated no difference in outcome when patients were resuscitated with colloid (albumin) versus normal saline.[65] Virtually no research involving the use of these synthetic colloid solutions in the civilian prehospital setting has been published, and no data exist from their use in hospitals that show them to be superior to crystalloid solutions. These products are not recommended for the prehospital management of shock.

Blood Substitutes

Blood transfusion has several limitations and undesirable qualities, including the need to type and crossmatch, a short shelf life, perishability when not refrigerated, a potential for transmission of infectious disease, and an increasing shortage of donated units that limits its use in the prehospital setting. This has led to intense research in blood substitutes during the past two to three decades. The U.S. military has played a central role in this research because a blood substitute that does not need refrigeration and does not require blood typing could be carried to a wounded soldier on the battlefield and infused rapidly to treat shock.

Most hemoglobin-based oxygen carriers (HBOCs) use the same oxygen-carrying molecule (hemoglobin) found in human, bovine, or porcine blood cells. The major difference between HBOCs and human blood is that the hemoglobin in HBOCs is not contained within a cell membrane. This removes the need for conducting type and crossmatch studies because the antigen–antibody risk is removed when the hemoglobin is extracted from the cell. Additionally, many of these HBOCs can be stored for long periods, making them ideal for mass-casualty incidents. Early problems with hemoglobin-based oxygen-carrying solutions included toxicity from hemoglobin. To date, none of these experimental solutions has been found to be safe or effective in humans.[61]

Warming Intravenous Fluids

Any IV fluid given to a patient in shock should be warm, not room temperature or cold. The ideal temperature for such fluids is 102°F (39°C). Wrapping heat packs around the bag can warm fluid. Commercially available fluid-warmer units for the patient care compartment provide an easy and reliable means to keep fluids at the correct temperature. These units are costly but justifiable for prolonged transports or when transfusing cold stored products. For acute routine transport of trauma patients, the emphasis on limited volume resuscitation and rapid transport makes these warmers less relevant.

Managing Volume Resuscitation

As noted earlier, significant controversy surrounds prehospital fluid administration for a trauma patient who is in shock.[66] When Prehospital Trauma Life Support (PHTLS) was first introduced in the United States, prehospital care practitioners adopted the approach used by emergency physicians and surgeons in most trauma centers: Administer an IV crystalloid solution until the vital signs return to normal (typically, pulse less than 100 beats/minute and systolic blood pressure greater than 100 mm Hg). When sufficient crystalloid solution is infused to restore vital signs to normal, the patient's perfusion should be improved. At the time, experts believed such rapid intervention would clear lactic acid and restore energy production in the cells of the body and decrease the risk of developing irreversible shock and kidney failure. However, no study of trauma patients in the prehospital setting has shown that the administration of IV fluid decreases complications and death.

A major contribution of PHTLS over the past two decades has been to establish the conceptual change that, in the critically injured trauma patient, transport should never be delayed while IV lines are placed and fluid is infused. In a study from the National Trauma Data Bank that included over 776,000 patients, prehospital IV fluid administration was associated with increased odds of death. IV lines can be placed in the back of the ambulance en route to the closest appropriate facility. A critically injured trauma patient who is in shock generally requires blood transfusion and intervention to control internal hemorrhage, neither of which can be accomplished in the field in most systems. Almost nothing should delay the expeditious transport of a bleeding patient to an OR or ED where the hemorrhage can be controlled.

Prehospital volume resuscitation should be tailored to the clinical situation, as described in the following discussion (**Figure 3-23**).

Uncontrolled Hemorrhage

For patients with suspected internal hemorrhage in the chest, abdomen, or pelvis, sufficient IV crystalloid solution (if blood products are not available) should be titrated to maintain a systolic blood pressure above 80 mm Hg, which will provide a MAP of 60 to 65 mm Hg. This blood pressure level should maintain adequate perfusion to the kidneys with less risk of worsening internal hemorrhage. A large fluid bolus should not be administered because this may "overshoot" the target blood pressure range, resulting in recurrent intrathoracic, intra-abdominal, or intrapelvic bleeding.

The current philosophy of restricted crystalloid administration in the prehospital setting and during initial hospital care has been called by several names, including permissive hypotension, hypotensive resuscitation, and "balanced" resuscitation, meaning that a balance must be struck between the amount of fluid administered and the degree of blood pressure elevation. Once the patient arrives at the hospital, fluid administration continues by giving plasma and blood (1:1 ratio) or whole blood until the hemorrhage is controlled. Blood pressure is then returned to normal values with ongoing transfusion with restricted crystalloid administration.

Central Nervous System Injuries

Hypotension has been associated with increased mortality in the setting of TBI.[16] Patients with certain conditions (e.g., TBI or spinal cord injury) require a higher blood pressure in order to maintain perfusion and decrease secondary neurologic injury. Guidelines published by the Brain Trauma Foundation recommend maintaining the systolic blood pressure above 110 mm Hg in patients with suspected TBI.[43,45] Consensus guidelines focusing on the management of acute spinal cord injury recommend not only avoiding hypotension (systolic blood pressure less than 90 mm Hg) but also maintaining a MAP of at least 85 to 90 mm Hg in the hopes of improving spinal cord perfusion. To accomplish this goal, more aggressive volume resuscitation may be indicated, at the expense of increasing the risk of recurrent bleeding from associated internal injuries.

Controlled Hemorrhage

Patients with significant external hemorrhage that has been controlled can be managed with a more aggressive volume resuscitation strategy, provided the prehospital practitioner has no reason to suspect associated intrathoracic, intra-abdominal, or intrapelvic injuries and hemorrhage. Examples include a large scalp laceration or a wound in an extremity involving major blood vessels but with the bleeding controlled with a pressure dressing or tourniquet. Adult patients who fall into this category and present with Class II, III, or IV hemorrhage may receive an initial bolus of 250 mL of crystalloid fluid repeated up to a total of 1 liter, or to achieve a systolic blood pressure of 90 mm Hg. Pediatric patients should receive a bolus of 20 mL/kg of warmed crystalloid solution. As noted previously, fluid administration should always occur during transport to the closest appropriate facility. Vital signs—including pulse and ventilatory rates, as well as blood pressure—should be monitored to assess the patient's response to the initial fluid therapy. In most urban settings, the patient will be delivered to the receiving facility before the initial fluid bolus is completed.

The initial fluid bolus elicits three possible responses, as follows:

1. *Rapid response.* The vital signs return to and remain normal. This typically indicates the patient has lost less than 20% of blood volume and that the hemorrhage has stopped.
2. *Transient response.* The vital signs initially improve (pulse slows and blood pressure increases); however, during reassessment, these patients show deterioration with recurrent signs of shock. These patients have typically lost

Managing Volume Resuscitation

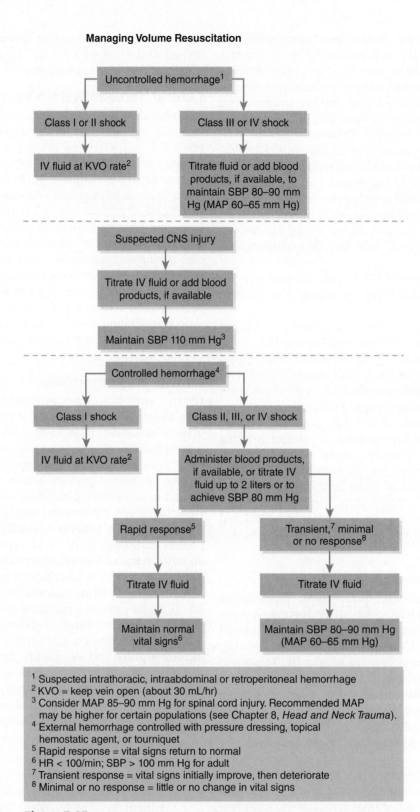

¹ Suspected intrathoracic, intraabdominal or retroperitoneal hemorrhage
² KVO = keep vein open (about 30 mL/hr)
³ Consider MAP 85–90 mm Hg for spinal cord injury. Recommended MAP
   may be higher for certain populations (see Chapter 8, *Head and Neck Trauma*).
⁴ External hemorrhage controlled with pressure dressing, topical
   hemostatic agent, or tourniquet
⁵ Rapid response = vital signs return to normal
⁶ HR < 100/min; SBP > 100 mm Hg for adult
⁷ Transient response = vital signs initially improve, then deteriorate
⁸ Minimal or no response = little or no change in vital signs

Figure 3-23 A. Algorithm for managing volume resuscitation in trauma patients.

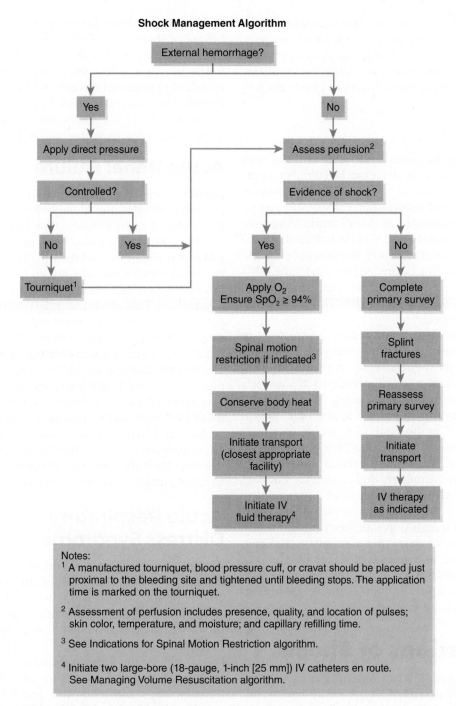

Figure 3-23 (*continued*) **B.** Algorithm for managing shock.

© National Association of Emergency Medical Technicians (NAEMT)

between 20% and 40% of their blood volume and may be experiencing ongoing hemorrhage

3. *Minimal or no response.* These patients show virtually no change in the profound signs of shock after a 1-liter bolus. They likely have sustained massive hemorrhage, are experiencing ongoing hemorrhage, or both.

Patients who have a rapid response are candidates for continued volume resuscitation, until vital signs have returned to normal and all clinical indicators of shock have resolved. Patients who fall into either the transient response or minimal/no response groups have ongoing hemorrhage that is probably internal. These patients are best managed in a state of relative hypotension, and IV fluid should be titrated to systolic blood pressure in the range of 80 to 90 mm Hg (MAP of 60 to 65 mm Hg), barring any evidence of a TBI or spinal cord injury. The concept of transient response is receiving less emphasis, but the underlying physiology remains an important process to understand.

Tranexamic Acid

TXA is an analog of the amino acid lysine and has been used for many decades to decrease bleeding in gynecologic patients with severe uterine bleeding, patients undergoing cardiac and orthopaedic surgery, and hemophiliacs for such procedures as dental work. When the coagulation cascade (see Figure 3-12) is activated to form a blood clot as a result of an injury, the process of breaking down the blood clot begins at the same time. TXA interferes with the breakdown process to maintain and stabilize the newly formed blood clot. TXA also has an anti-inflammatory effect.[67]

Multiple studies have shown that TXA may improve survival for severely injured trauma patients.[68-70] TXA appears to be most effective when given early (i.e., < 3 hours after injury) and when patients are severely injured (i.e., hypotensive, tachycardic). Additional research is underway to determine appropriate indications for the use of prehospital TXA, including use in TBI patients, because not all studies have demonstrated a definitive benefit.[71,72] Current tactical casualty care guidelines for use in the military and civilian tactical EMS communities endorse a one-time dose of 2 grams (g) of TXA given slowly via IV or IO push for patients who will likely need a blood transfusion (i.e., hemorrhagic shock, elevated lactate, one or more major amputations, penetrating torso trauma, or evidence of severe bleeding) or have signs of a significant TBI (i.e., altered mental status associated with blast injury or blunt trauma), and present no later than 3 hours after injury.[73]

Complications of Shock

The symptoms of hypothermia, coagulopathy, and acidosis are frequently described as the lethal triad. While not actually causes of death, they are findings that are worrisome for impending death. They are markers of anaerobic metabolism and loss of energy production, and they describe the interventions needed to reverse anaerobic metabolism that must be provided quickly. Several complications may result in patients with persistent or inadequately resuscitated shock, which is why early recognition and aggressive management of shock are essential. The quality of care delivered in the prehospital setting can affect a patient's hospital course and outcome. Recognizing shock and initiating proper treatment in the prehospital setting may shorten hospital length of stay and improve chances for survival. The following complications of shock are not often seen in the prehospital setting, but they are a result of shock both in the field and in the ED. In addition, they may be encountered when transferring patients between facilities. Knowing the outcome of the process of shock helps in the understanding of the severity of the condition, the importance of rapid hemorrhage control, and appropriate fluid replacement.

Acute Renal Failure

Impaired circulation to the kidneys changes the aerobic metabolism in the kidney to anaerobic metabolism. The reduced energy production leads to renal cellular swelling, which decreases renal perfusion, thus causing additional anaerobic metabolism. The cells that make up the renal tubules are sensitive to ischemia and may die if their oxygen delivery is impaired for more than 45 to 60 minutes. This condition, referred to as **acute tubular necrosis (ATN)** or acute renal failure, reduces the filtration efficiency of the renal tubules. The result is decreased renal output and reduced clearing of toxic products and electrolytes. Because the kidneys are no longer functioning, excess fluid is not excreted, and volume overload may result. Also, the kidneys lose their ability to excrete metabolic acids and electrolytes, leading to a metabolic acidosis and hyperkalemia (increased blood potassium). These patients often require dialysis for several weeks or months. Most patients who develop ATN resulting from shock eventually recover normal renal function.

Acute Respiratory Distress Syndrome

Acute respiratory distress syndrome (ARDS) results from damage to the alveolar cells of the lung and decreased energy production to maintain the metabolism of these cells. This injury, combined with fluid overload produced by too much crystalloid administration during resuscitation, leads to leakage of fluid into the interstitial spaces and alveoli of the lungs, making it much more difficult for oxygen to diffuse across the alveolar walls and into the capillaries and bind with the RBCs. This problem was first described during World War II but was formally recognized during the Vietnam War where it was called Da Nang lung (after the location of the hospital that saw many of these cases). Although these patients do have pulmonary edema, it is not the result of impaired cardiac function, as in congestive heart failure (cardiogenic pulmonary edema). ARDS represents a noncardiogenic form of pulmonary edema. The change of the resuscitative process to restricted crystalloid, permissive hypotension, and damage control resuscitation (RBCs-to-plasma ratio of 1:1) has significantly reduced ARDS in the immediate trauma period (24 to 72 hours).

Hematologic Failure

The term **coagulopathy** refers to impairment in the normal clotting capabilities of blood. This abnormality may result from hypothermia (decreased body temperature), dilution of clotting factors from administration of fluids, or depletion of the clotting substances as they are used up in an effort to control bleeding (consumptive coagulopathy). The normal blood-clotting cascade involves several enzymes and factors that eventually result in the creation of fibrin molecules that serve as a matrix to trap platelets and form a plug in a vessel wall to stop bleeding (**Figure 3-24**). This process is most effective within a narrow temperature range (i.e., near-normal body temperature). As the core temperature of the body falls (even just a few degrees) and energy production lessens, blood clotting is compromised, leading to continued hemorrhage. The blood-clotting factors may also be used up as they form blood clots in an effort to slow and control hemorrhage. The decreased body temperature worsens the clotting problems, which exacerbates hemorrhage, which further reduces the ability of the body to maintain its temperature. With inadequate resuscitation, this becomes an ever-worsening cycle.

Hepatic Failure

Severe damage to the liver may occur, although it is a less common result of prolonged shock. Evidence of damage to the liver from shock typically does not become manifest for several days, until laboratory results document elevated liver function tests. Liver failure is manifested by persistent hypoglycemia (low blood sugar), persistent lactic acidosis, and jaundice. Because the liver produces many of the clotting factors necessary for hemostasis, a coagulopathy may accompany liver failure.

Overwhelming Infection

There is increased risk of infection associated with severe shock. This increased risk is attributed to the following causes:

- Marked decrease in the number of WBCs, predisposing the shock patient to infection, is another manifestation of hematologic failure.
- Ischemia and reduction in energy production in the cells of the shock patient's bowel wall may allow bacteria to leak out into the bloodstream.
- Decreased function of the immune system in the face of ischemia and loss of energy production.
- Increased permeability of the capillary membranes in the lung secondary to ischemic injury and to circulating inflammatory factors leads to fluid buildup in the alveoli. This leads to respiratory insufficiency and need for intubation. The combination of these factors

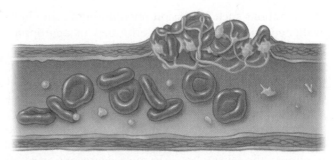

Figure 3-24 Blood clotting involves several enzymes and factors that eventually result in the creation of fibrin molecules, which serve as a matrix to trap platelets and form a plug in a vessel wall to stop bleeding.
© Jones & Bartlett Learning

predisposes shock patients to pneumonia episodes, which can cause systemic sepsis.
- Most important, multiple procedures, vascular intrusion, and indwelling catheters increase the risk of infections in critically injured patients.

Multiple Organ Failure

Shock, if not successfully treated, can lead to dysfunction first in one organ, then in several organs simultaneously, with sepsis as a common accompaniment, leading to *multiple organ dysfunction syndrome* (MODS).

Failure of one major body system (e.g., lungs, kidneys, blood-clotting cascade, liver) is associated with a mortality rate of about 40%. Cardiovascular failure, in the form of cardiogenic and septic shock, can only occasionally be reversed. By the time four organ systems fail, the mortality rate is essentially 100%.[74]

Prolonged Transport

During prolonged transport of a trauma patient in shock, it is important to maintain perfusion to the vital organs. Airway management should be optimized before a long transport, and an airway stabilization procedure such as endotracheal intubation or supraglottic airway placement should be performed if there is any question regarding airway patency. Ventilatory support is provided, with care taken to ensure ventilations are of a reasonable tidal volume and rate (maintaining minute volume) so as not to compromise preload and therefore cardiac output in a patient with already tenuous perfusion. Pulse oximetry should be monitored continuously. Capnography provides information regarding the position of the endotracheal tube, as well as information on the patient's perfusion status. A marked drop in $ETCO_2$ indicates that the airway has become dislodged or the patient has experienced a significant drop in perfusion. Additional considerations such as tension pneumothorax should be evaluated and interventions performed in appropriate patients.

Direct pressure by hand is impractical during a long transport, so significant external hemorrhage should be controlled with pressure dressings. If these efforts fail, a tourniquet should be applied. In situations in which a tourniquet has been applied and transport time is expected to exceed 4 hours, attempts should be considered to remove the tourniquet after more aggressive attempts at local hemorrhage control. The tourniquet should be slowly loosened while observing the dressing for signs of hemorrhage. If bleeding does not reoccur, the tourniquet is completely loosened but left in place in case hemorrhage reoccurs. Conversion of a tourniquet back to a dressing should not be attempted in the following situations: (1) presence of Class III or IV hemorrhage, (2) complete amputation, (3) inability to observe the patient for reoccurrence of bleeding, and (4) tourniquet in place longer than 6 hours.[26] External hemorrhage control should be optimized by splinting all fractures.

Techniques for maintaining normal body temperature, as previously described, are even more important in the case of prolonged transport time. In addition to a warmed patient compartment, the patient should be covered with blankets or materials that preserve body heat; even large, plastic garbage bags help prevent loss of heat. Intravenous fluids should be warmed before administration. Use of room temperature intravenous fluids in trauma patients, particularly in large volumes, can lead to hypothermia, which, in turn, can affect the patient's ability to form clots.

In prolonged transport circumstances, vascular access for fluid administration may be needed, and two large-bore IV lines should be established. For both children and adults, inability to obtain peripheral vascular access may necessitate use of the intraosseous route, as described previously.

For patients with suspected ongoing hemorrhage, maintaining systolic blood pressure in the range of 80 to 90 mm Hg or MAP of 60 to 65 mm Hg can usually accomplish the goal of maintaining perfusion to vital organs with less risk of renewing internal hemorrhage. Patients with suspected TBIs or spinal cord injuries should have systolic blood pressure maintained above 110 mm Hg.

Vital signs should be reassessed frequently to monitor response to resuscitation. The following should be documented at serial intervals: ventilation rate, pulse rate, blood pressure, skin color and temperature, capillary refill, GCS score, SpO_2, and $ETCO_2$, if available.

Although insertion of a urinary catheter is not usually required in rapid transport circumstances, monitoring urine output is an important tool to help guide decisions regarding the need for additional fluid therapy during prolonged transport. Insertion of a urinary catheter, if local protocols permit, should be considered so urine output can be monitored. Adequate urine outputs include 0.5 mL/kg/hour for adults, 1 mL/kg/hour for pediatric patients, and 2 mL/kg/hour for infants younger than 1 year. Urine output of less than these amounts may be a key indicator that the patient requires further volume infusion.

If time and local protocols permit during prolonged transport, placement of an orogastric or nasogastric tube should be considered for intubated patients. If midfacial fractures are present, placement of an orogastric catheter instead should be considered. Gastric distension may cause unexplained hypotension and dysrhythmias, especially in children. Placement of a nasogastric or orogastric tube may also decrease the risk of vomiting and aspiration.

SUMMARY

- In trauma patients, hemorrhage is the most common cause of shock.
- Humans produce the energy needed to sustain life via a complex system, called aerobic metabolism, using glucose and oxygen. This entire process depends on the respiratory system to provide adequate amounts of oxygen to the circulatory system, which must be able to deliver the oxygen to the cells of the body.
- The backup system to aerobic metabolism is called anaerobic metabolism. It does not require oxygen, but it is inefficient and only creates a small amount of energy.
- Shock is a state of generalized change in cellular function from aerobic metabolism to anaerobic metabolism secondary to hypoperfusion of the tissue cells, in which the delivery of oxygen at the cellular level is inadequate to meet metabolic needs. As a result, cellular energy production falls, and, over a relatively short period of time, cellular functions become impaired, eventually leading to cell death.
- Shock may be classified into the following categories:
  - Hypovolemic—primarily hemorrhagic in the trauma patient, related to loss of circulating

SUMMARY (CONTINUED)

blood cells and fluid volume with oxygen-carrying capacity (the most common cause of shock in the trauma patient)

- Distributive (or vasogenic)—related to abnormality in vascular tone
- Cardiogenic—related to interference with the pump action of the heart, often occurring after a heart attack

■ Care of the patient in shock, or one who may go into shock, begins with an assessment of the patient, beginning with a history of the event and a quick visual examination of the patient looking for obvious signs of shock and blood loss.

■ Steps in the management of shock are as follows:
1. Control any external severe hemorrhage.
2. Ensure oxygenation and ventilation (airway management).
3. Identify source of hemorrhage.
4. Transport to definitive care.
5. Administer blood component therapy when appropriate.

■ External hemorrhage should be controlled with direct pressure, followed by application of a pressure dressing. If this is not rapidly effective, a tourniquet should be applied to the extremity at the level of the groin or axilla. A topical hemostatic agent may also provide additional hemorrhage control. Consider the use of a pelvic binder for suspected pelvic fracture.

■ In some cases, nonhemorrhagic sources of shock in trauma patients (e.g., tension pneumothorax) can be rapidly corrected.

■ All trauma patients in shock, in addition to maintenance of adequate oxygenation, require rapid extrication and expeditious transport to a definitive care institution where the cause of the shock can be specifically identified and treated.

■ Transport should not be delayed for measures such as IV access and volume infusion. These interventions should be done in the ambulance during transport.

■ Overaggressive fluid infusion should be avoided to minimize further bleeding and edema formation in patients with hemorrhagic shock after trauma.

SCENARIO RECAP

You and your partner are dispatched to the scene of a motorcycle crash. The motorcycle veered off the road and rolled several times, ultimately impacting a telephone pole. Upon your arrival, you find a 29-year-old helmeted male driver lying supine approximately 50 feet (15 meters) from the motorcycle. The patient is in moderate distress with chief complaints of chest, sacral, and left hip pain.

Physical examination of the patient shows pale skin color, diaphoresis, decreased peripheral pulses, a contused chest, and an unstable pelvis. The patient is alert and oriented. His vital signs are as follows: pulse 110 beats/minute, blood pressure 82/56 mm Hg, oxygen saturation (SpO_2) 92% on room air, and respiratory rate 28 breaths/minute, with diminished breath sounds on the right.

- What possible injuries do you expect to see after this type of mechanism?
- How would you manage these injuries in the field?
- What are the major pathologic processes occurring in this patient?
- How will you correct the pathophysiology causing this patient's presentation?
- You are working for a rural EMS system in a remote area distant from the nearest trauma center. How does this factor alter your management plans?

SCENARIO SOLUTION

You recognize that this patient is demonstrating signs of hemorrhagic shock (increased heart rate, decreased blood pressure, and increased ventilatory rate). You asses the airway, breathing, and circulation. You are concerned about internal hemorrhage secondary to a pelvic fracture. You establish spinal motion restriction, immediately apply a commercial pelvic binder, transfer the patient to the ambulance, and begin transport to the closest trauma center.

While en route, you apply oxygen at 2 L/min via non-rebreather mask with $ETCO_2$ monitoring. You also place two 18-gauge IV lines, giving only enough fluid to maintain an SBP of > 90 mm Hg. Due to the patient's hemodynamics and the potential for internal hemorrhage, you note the patient is a candidate for TXA administration, especially given that you are in a remote area some distance from the nearest trauma center. Additionally, you warm the fluids that are administered and prevent heat loss of the patient by applying appropriate environmental controls such as turning up the heat in the patient compartment and layering blankets. En route to the trauma center, you provide your report via radio. You inform the trauma center that the patient takes anticoagulants. Upon arrival at the receiving facility, the patient is transferred to trauma staff with the patient still in stable condition.

References

1. Janssens U, Graf J. Shock—what are the basics? *Internist (Berl)*. 2004;45(3):258-266.
2. Gross SD. *A System of Surgery: Pathological, Diagnostic, Therapeutic, and Operative*. Blanchard and Lea; 1859.
3. Knisely MH, Cowley RA, Hawthorne I, Garris D. Separation of shock types: experimental and clinical separation of hypovolemic and septic shock. *Angiology*. 1970;21(11):728-744.
4. Galvagno SM. *Emergency pathophysiology*. Teton NewMedia, 2004.
5. Cowley RA. A total emergency medical system for the state of Maryland. *Md State Med J*. 1975;45:37-45.
6. Koch E, Lovett S, Nghiem T, et al. Shock index in the emergency department: utility and limitations. *Emerg Med*. 2019;11:179-199.
7. Cannon CM, Braxton CC, Kling-Smith M, et al. Utility of the shock index in predicting mortality in traumatically injured patients. *J Trauma Acute Care Surg*. 2009;67(6):1426-1430.
8. Olaussen A, Blackburn T, Mitra B, et al. Shock index for prediction of critical bleeding post-trauma: A systematic review. *Emerg Med Austral*. 2014;26:223-228.
9. Savage SA, Sumislawski JJ, Zarzaur BL, Dutton WP, Croce MA, Fabian TC. The new metric to define large-volume hemorrhage: results of a prospective study of the critical administration threshold. *J Trauma Acute Care Surg*. 2015;78(2):224-229.
10. Meyer DE, Cotton BA, Fox EE, et al. A comparison of resuscitation intensity and critical administration threshold in predicting early mortality among bleeding patients: a multicenter validation in 680 major transfusion patients. *J Trauma Acute Care Surg*. 2018;85(4):691-696.
11. McClelland RN, Shires GT, Baxter CR, et al. Balanced salt solutions in the treatment of hemorrhagic shock. *JAMA*. 1967;199:830-834.
12. Duchesne JC, Hunt JP, Wahl G, et al. Review of current blood transfusion strategies in a mature level I trauma center: were we wrong for the last 60 years? *J Trauma*. 2008;65(2):272-276; discussion 276-278.
13. Holcomb JB, Jenkins D, Rhee P, et al. Damage control resuscitation: directly addressing the early coagulopathy of trauma. *J Trauma*. 2007;62(2):307-310.
14. Amaral CB, Ralston DC, Becker TK. Prehospital point-of-care ultrasound: a transformative technology. *SAGE Open Medicine*. 2020;8:1-6.
15. McManus J, Yershov AL, Ludwig D, Holcomb JB, Salinas J, Dubick MA, Convertino VA, Hinds D, David W, Flanagan T, Duke JH. Radial pulse character relationships to systolic blood pressure and trauma outcomes. *Prehosp Emerg Care*. 2005 Oct-Dec;9(4):423-8. doi: 10.1080/10903120500255891. PMID: 16263676.
16. Spaite DW, Hu C, Bobrow BJ, et al. The effect of combined out-of-hospital hypotension and hypoxia on mortality in major traumatic brain injury. *Ann Emerg Med*. 2017;69(1):62-72. doi: 10.1016/j.annemergmed.2016.08.00
17. Spaite DW, Bobrow BJ, Keim SM, et al. Association of statewide implementation of the prehospital traumatic brain injury treatment guidelines with patient survival following traumatic brain injury: the Excellence in Prehospital Injury Care (EPIC) study. *JAMA Surg*. 2019;154(7):e191152.
18. Convertino VA, Koons NJ, Suresh M. Physiology of human hemorrhage and compensation. *Compr Physiol*. 2021;11:1531-1574.
19. Convertino VA, Schauer SG, Weitzel EK, et al. Wearable sensors integrated with compensatory reserve monitoring in critically injured trauma patients. *Sensors*. 2020;20(22):6463.

20. Convertino VA, Johnson MC, Alarhayem A, et al. Compensatory reserve detects subclinical phases of shock with more expeditious prediction for need of life-saving interventions compared to vital signs and arterial lactate. *Transfusion.* 2021;61:S167-S173.

21. Koreny M, Riedmuller E, Nikfardjam M, et al. Arterial puncture closing devices compared with standard manual compression after cardiac catheterization: systematic review and meta-analysis. *JAMA.* 2004;291:350-357.

22. Walker SB, Cleary S, Higgins M. Comparison of the FemoStop device and manual pressure in reducing groin puncture site complications following coronary angioplasty and coronary stent placement. *Int J Nurs Pract.* 2001;7:366-375.

23. Peng HT. Hemostatic agents for prehospital hemorrhage control: a narrative review. *Military Med Res.* 2020;7:13. doi: 10.1186/s40779-020-00241-z

24. Butler FK. The US Military Experience with Tourniquets and Hemostatic Dressings in the Afghanistan and Iraq Conflicts. *Bull Am College Surg.* 2015:100: September Supplement: 60-65.

25. Kragh JF, Walters TJ, Baer DG, et al. Survival with emergency tourniquet use to stop bleeding in major limb trauma. *Ann Surg.* 2009;249(1):1-7.doi:10.1097/SLA.0b013e31818 842ba.

26. Beekley AC, Sebesta JA, Blackbourne LH, et al. Prehospital tourniquet use in Operation Iraqi Freedom: effect on hemorrhage control and outcomes. *J Trauma.* 2008;64(2):S28-S37.

27. Kragh JF Jr, Walters TJ, Baer DG, et al. Practical use of emergency tourniquets to stop bleeding in major limb trauma. *J Trauma.* 2008;64(2):S38-S50.

28. Bellamy RF. The causes of death in conventional land warfare: implications for combat casualty care research. *Mil Med.* 1984;149:55-62.

29. Mabry RL, Holcomb JB, Baker AM, et al. United States Army Rangers in Somalia: an analysis of combat casualties on an urban battlefield. *J Trauma.* 2000;49:515-528.

30. Lakstein D, Blumenfeld A, Sokolov T, et al. Tourniquets for hemorrhage control on the battlefield: a 4-year accumulated experience. *J Trauma.* 2003;54:S221-S225.

31. Eilertsen KA, Winberg M, Jeppesen E, Hval G, Wisborg T. Prehospital tourniquets in civilians: a systematic review. *Prehosp Disaster Med.* 2021;36(1):86–94.

32. Kragh JF, Walters TJ, Baer DG, et al. Survival with emergency tourniquet use to stop bleeding in major limb trauma. *Ann Surg.* 2009;249(1):1-7.

33. Montgomery HR, Hammesfahr R, Fisher AD, et al. 2019 recommended limb tourniquets in tactical combat casualty care. *J Spec Ops Med.* 19(4):27-50.

34. Joint Trauma System. Tactical Combat Casualty Care Guidelines 2020. Accessed September 30, 2021. https:// deployedmedicine.com/content/40

35. Kheirabadi BS, Scherer MR, Estep JS, Dubick MA, Holcomb JB. Determination of efficacy of new hemostatic dressings in a model of extremity arterial hemorrhage in swine. *J Trauma.* 2009 Sep;67(3):450-459; discussion 459-460. doi: 10.1097/TA.0b013e3181ac0c99

36. Kheirabadi BS, Edens JW, Terrazas IB, et al. Comparison of new hemostatic granules/powders with currently deployed hemostatic products in a lethal model of extremity arterial hemorrhage in swine. *J Trauma.* 2009 Feb;66(2):316-326; discussion 327-328. doi: 10.1097 /TA.0b013e31819634a1

37. Kunio NR, Riha GM, Watson KM, Differding JA, Schreiber MA, Watters JM. Chitosan based advanced hemostatic dressing is associated with decreased blood loss in a swine uncontrolled hemorrhage model. *Am J Surg.* 2013 May;205(5):505-510. doi: 10.1016/j .amjsurg.2013.01.014

38. Dumont TM, Visioni AJ, Rughani AI, et al. Inappropriate prehospital ventilation in severe traumatic brain injury increases in-hospital mortality. *J Neurotrauma.* 2010;27(7):1233-1241.

39. Bickell WH, Wall MJ Jr, Pepe PE, et al. Immediate versus delayed fluid resuscitation for hypotensive patients with penetrating torso injuries. *N Engl J Med.* 1994 Oct 27;331(17):1105-1109.

40. Dutton RP, Mackenzie CF, Scalea TM. Hypotensive resuscitation during active hemorrhage: impact on in-hospital mortality. *J Trauma.* 2002 Jun;52(6):1141-1146.

41. Schreiber MA, Meier EN, Tisherman SA, et al.; ROC Investigators. A controlled resuscitation strategy is feasible and safe in hypotensive trauma patients: results of a prospective randomized pilot trial. *J Trauma Acute Care Surg.* 2015 Apr;78(4):687-695; discussion 695-697.

42. Carrick MM, Morrison CA, Tapia NM, et al. Intraoperative hypotensive resuscitation for patients undergoing laparotomy or thoracotomy for trauma: early termination of a randomized prospective clinical trial. *J Trauma Acute Care Surg.* 2016 Jun;80(6):886-896.

43. Woolley T, Thompson P, Kirkman E, et al. Trauma Hemostasis and Oxygenation Research Network position paper on the role of hypotensive resuscitation as part of remote damage control resuscitation. *J Trauma Acute Care Surg.* 2018 Jun;84(6 Suppl 1):S3-S13.

44. Woodward L, Alsabri M. Permissive hypotension vs. conventional resuscitation in patients with trauma or hemorrhagic shock: a review. *Cureus.* 2021 Jul 19;13(7):e16487.

45. Carney N, Totten AM, O'Reilly C, et al. Guidelines for the management of severe traumatic brain injury, fourth edition. *Neurosurgery.* 2017 Jan 1;80(1):6-15.

46. Gentilello LM. Advances in the management of hypothermia. *Surg Clin North Am.* 1995;75(2):243-256.

47. Marino PL. *The ICU Book.* 4th ed. Lippincott Williams & Wilkins, 2014.

48. Johnson S, Henderson SO. Myth: The Trendelenburg position improves circulation in cases of shock. *Can J Emerg Med.* 2004;6:48.

49. Deboer S, Seaver M, Morissette C. Intraosseous infusion: not just for kids anymore. *J Emerg Med Serv.* 2005;34:56-63.

50. Sawyer RW, Bodai BI, Blaisdell FW, et al. The current status of intraosseous infusion. *J Am Coll Surg.* 1994; 179:353-360.

51. Macnab A, Christenson J, Findlay J, et al. A new system for sternal intraosseous infusion in adults. *Prehosp Emerg Care.* 2000;4:173.

52. Glaeser PW, Hellmich TR, Szewczuga D, et al. Five-year experience in prehospital intraosseous infusions in children and adults. *Ann Emerg Med.* 1993;22:1119.

53. Marino PL, Galvagno SM. *The Little ICU Book*. Wolters Kluwer; 2017.

54. Shand S, Curtis K, Dinh M, et al. Prehospital blood transfusion in New South Wales, Australia: a retrospective cohort study. *Prehosp Emerg Care*. 2021;25(3):404-411.

55. Roehl A, Grottke O. Prehospital administration of blood and plasma products. *Curr Opin Anaesthesiol*. 2021;34(4):507-513.

56. Sperry JL, Guyette FX, Brown JB, et al. Prehospital plasma during air medical transport in trauma patients at risk for hemorrhagic shock. *N Engl J Med*. 2018;379(4):315-326.

57. Semler MW, Self WH, Wanderer JP, et al. Balanced crystalloids versus saline in critically ill adults. *N Engl J Med*. 2018;378:829-839.

58. Vassar MJ, Fischer RP, Obrien PE, et al. A multicenter trial of resuscitation of injured patients with 7.5% sodium chloride: the effect of added dextran 70. *Arch Surg*. 1993;128:1003-1013.

59. Vassar MJ, Perry CA, Holcroft JW. Prehospital resuscitation of hypotensive trauma patients with 7.5% NaCl versus 7.5% NaCl with added dextran: a controlled trial. *J Trauma*. 1993;34:622-633.

60. Wade CE, Kramer GC, Grady JJ. Efficacy of hypertonic 7.5% saline and 6% dextran in treating trauma: a meta-analysis of controlled clinical trials. *Surgery*. 1997;122:609-616.

61. Galvagno SM, Mackenzie CF. New and future resuscitation fluids for trauma patients using hemoglobin and hypertonic saline. *Anesthesiol Clin*. 2013;31:1-19.

62. Zarychanski R, Abou-Setta AM, Turgeon AF, et al. Association of hydroxyethyl starch with mortality and acute kidney injury in critically ill patients requiring volume resuscitation. *JAMA*. 2013;309:678-688.

63. Lewis SR, Pritchard MW, Evans DJW, et al. Colloids versus crystalloids for fluid resuscitation in critically ill people. Cochrane Database Syst Rev. 2018;8:CD000567. doi: 10.1002/14651858.CD000567.pub7

64. Rizoli SB. Crystalloids and colloids in trauma resuscitation: a brief overview of the current debate. *J Trauma*. 2003;54:S82-S88.

65. SAFE Study Investigators. A comparison of albumin and saline for fluid resuscitation in the intensive care unit. *N Engl J Med*. 2004;350:2247-2256.

66. Haut ER, Kalish BT, Cotton BA, et al. Prehospital intravenous fluid administration is associated with higher mortality in trauma patients: a National Trauma Data Bank analysis. *Ann Surg*. 2011;253(2):371-377.

67. Jimenez JJ, Iribarren JL, Lorente L, et al.: Tranexamic acid attenuates inflammatory response in cardiopulmonary bypass surgery through blockade of fibrinolysis: a case control study followed by a randomized double-blind controlled trial. *Crit Care*. 2007;11:R117.

68. Guyette FX, Brown JB, Zenati MS, et al. Tranexamic acid during prehospital transport in patients at risk for hemorrhage after injury: a double-blind, placebo-controlled, randomized clinical trial. *JAMA Surg*. 2020;156(10):11-20.

69. The CRASH-2 Collaborators. Effects of tranexamic acid on death, vascular occlusive events, and blood transfusion in trauma patients with significant haemorrhage (CRASH-2): a randomised, placebo-controlled trial. *Lancet*. 2010;376:23-32.

70. Morrison JJ, Dubose JJ, Rasmussen TE, Midwinter MJ. Military Application of Tranexamic Acid in Trauma Emergency Resuscitation (MATTERs) study. *Arch Surg*. 2012;147:113-119.

71. Bossers SM, Loer SA, Bloemers FW, et al. Association between prehospital tranexamic acid administration and outcomes of severe traumatic brain injury. *JAMA Neurol*. 2021;78(3):338-345.

72. CRASH-3 Trial Collaborators. Effects of tranexamic acid on death, disability, vascular occlusive events and other morbidities in patients with acute traumatic brain injury (CRASH-3): a randomised, placebo-controlled trial. *Lancet*. 2019;394(10210):1713-1723.

73. Drew B, Auten J, Donham B, et al. The use of tranexamic acid in tactical combat casualty care. *J Spec Oper Med*. 2020;20(3):36-43.

74. Marshall JC, Cook DJ, Christou NV, et al. The multiple organ dysfunction score: a reliable descriptor of a complex clinical syndrome. *Crit Care Med*. 1995;23:1638-1652.

Suggested Reading

American College of Surgeons (ACS) Committee on Trauma. Shock. In: *Advanced Trauma Life Support Student Course Manual*. 10th ed. ACS; 2018.

Hemorrhage and hypovolemia. In: Marino PL, Galvagno SM. The Little ICU Book. Wolters-Kluwer, 2017.

Hypoperfusion. In: Bledsoe B, Porter RS, Cherry RA, eds. *Essentials of Paramedic Care*. 2nd ed. Brady-Pearson Education; 2011:257-265.

Revell M, Greaves I, Porter K. Endpoints for fluid resuscitation in hemorrhagic shock. *J Trauma*. 2003;54:S637.

Shock. In: Bledsoe B, Porter RS, Cherry RA, eds. *Essentials of Paramedic Care*. 2nd ed. Brady-Pearson Education; 2011:837-849.

Somand DM, Ward KR. Approach to traumatic shock. In: Tintinalli J, ed. *Emergency Medicine: A Comprehensive Study Guide*. 9th ed. McGraw-Hill; 2019:63-68.

SPECIFIC SKILLS

Intraosseous Vascular Access

Principle: To establish a vascular access site for fluids and medications when traditional IV access is unobtainable.

This technique may be performed in both adult and pediatric patients, using a variety of commercially available devices.

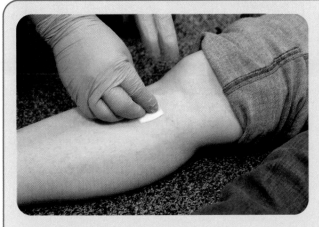

1 Assemble the equipment, which includes an intraosseous infusion needle, syringe filled with at least 5 mL of sterile saline, antiseptic, IV fluid and tubing, and tape. Ensure standard precautions and proper body substance isolation (BSI). Place the patient in a supine position.

The choice of insertion site may be the humeral head, distal femur, tibia, or sternum. For pediatric patients, a common insertion site is the anterior-medial proximal tibia just below the tibial tuberosity. The prehospital care practitioner identifies the tibia is the insertion site; the lower extremity is stabilized by another practitioner. Clean the insertion site area with an antiseptic.

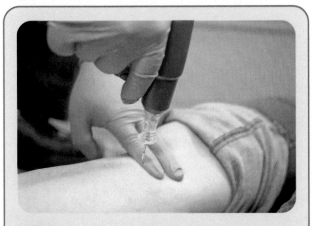

2 Holding the drill and needle at a 90-degree angle to the selected bone, activate the drill and insert the rotating needle through the skin and into the bone cortex. A "pop" will be felt upon entering the bone cortex.

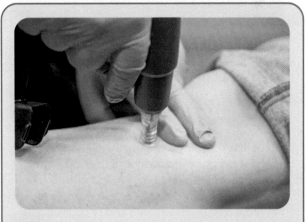

3 When you feel a lack of resistance against the needle, release the trigger of the drill. While holding the needle, remove the drill from the needle.

(continues)

Intraosseous Vascular Access (continued)

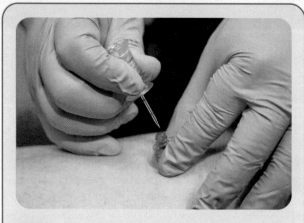

4 Release and remove the trocar from the center of the needle.

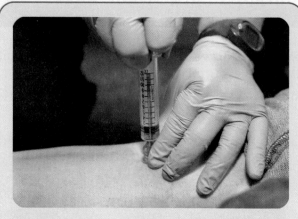

5 Attach the syringe with saline to the needle hub. Draw back with the syringe plunger slightly, looking for fluid from the marrow cavity to mix with the saline. "Dry" taps are not uncommon.

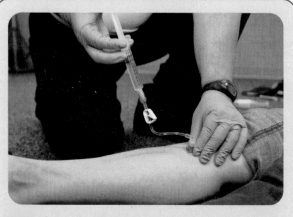

6 Next, inject 5 mL of the saline, observing for signs of infiltration. If there are no signs of infiltration, remove the syringe from the needle hub, attach the IV tubing, and set the flow rate. Secure the needle and IV tubing.

Tourniquet Application

C-A-T Application to an Upper Extremity

The Combat Application Tourniquet (C-A-T) is demonstrated in these photos. Any approved tourniquet may be used.

Note: A patient with bleeding severe enough to warrant tourniquet application is at risk for lightheadedness and loss of consciousness, and, therefore, should be rapidly placed in a supine position. In this example, the model is sitting upright to facilitate demonstration of the tourniquet application procedure.

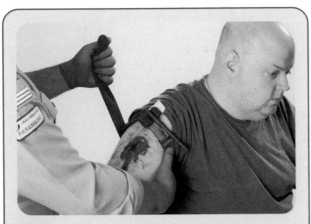

1 Insert the wounded extremity through the loop of the self-adhering band.

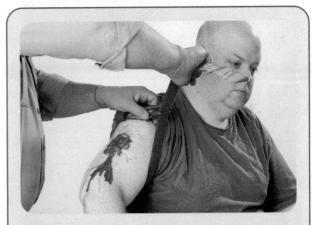

2 Pull the self-adhering band tight, and securely fasten it back on itself.

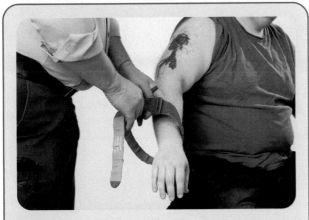

3 Adhere the band around the arm. Do not adhere the band past the clip.

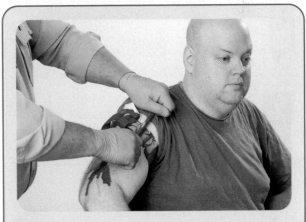

4 Twist the windlass rod until the bleeding stops (usually no more than three 180-degree turns).

(continues)

Tourniquet Application (continued)

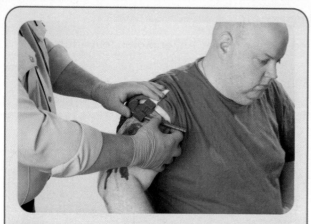

5   Lock the rod in place with the windlass clip.

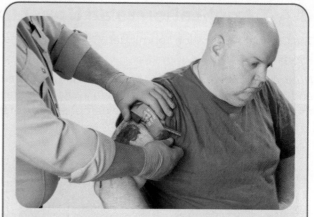

6   Adhere the band over the windlass rod. For small extremities, continue to adhere the band around the extremity.

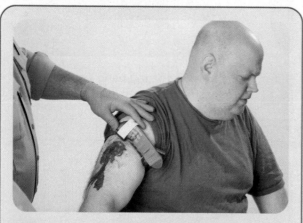

7   Secure the rod and band with the windlass strap. Grasp the strap, pull it tight, and adhere it to the opposite hook on the windlass clip.

Tourniquet Application (*continued*)

C-A-T Application to a Lower Extremity

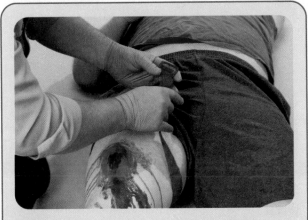

1 Place the tourniquet at the most proximal possible location on the thigh.

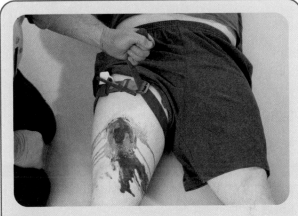

2 Pass the band through the outside slit of the friction adapter buckle, which will lock the band in place.

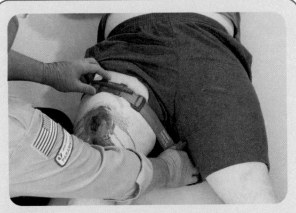

3 Pull the self-adhering band tight, and securely fasten it back on itself.

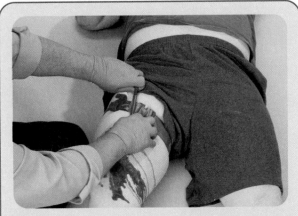

4 Twist the windlass rod until the bleeding stops (usually no more than three 180-degree turns).

(*continues*)

Tourniquet Application (continued)

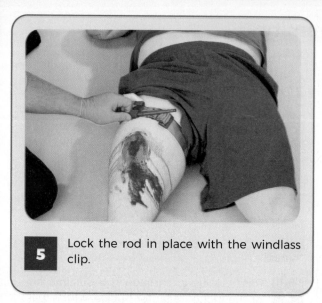

5 Lock the rod in place with the windlass clip.

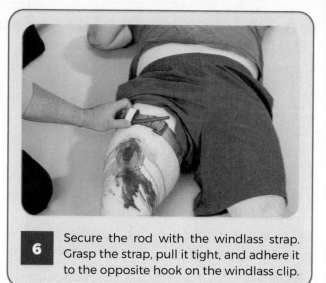

6 Secure the rod with the windlass strap. Grasp the strap, pull it tight, and adhere it to the opposite hook on the windlass clip.

On occasion, multiple tourniquets may be required to manage hemorrhage. Place the additional tourniquet immediately adjacent (just proximal, if possible) the previous application.

Wound Packing With Topical Hemostatic Dressing or Plain Gauze

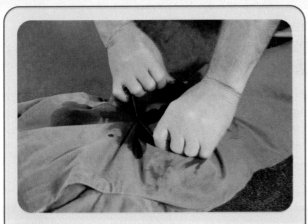

1 Expose the wound.

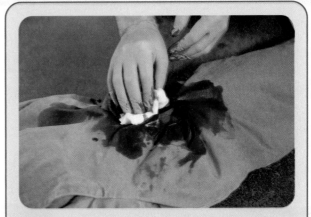

2 Gently remove excess blood from the wound site while trying to preserve any clots that have formed. Locate the source of active bleeding in the wound (often at the base of the wound).

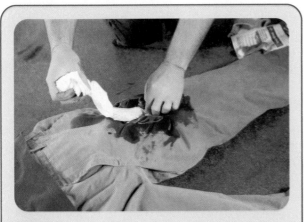

3 Remove the selected dressing from its packaging, and pack the entire dressing tightly into the wound, directly over the most active point of bleeding.

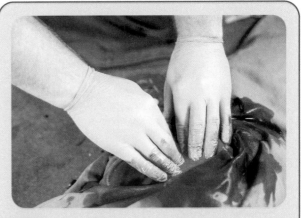

4 Apply direct pressure onto the wound and packing for a minimum of 3 minutes (if using a hemostatic agent and per the manufacturer's instructions) or 10 minutes if using plain gauze.

(continues)

Wound Packing With Topical Hemostatic Dressing or Plain Gauze *(continued)*

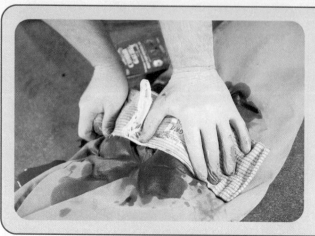

5 Reassess to ensure that bleeding has stopped. Wound may be repacked or a second dressing inserted into the wound if needed to control continued bleeding. If bleeding is controlled, leave packing in place and apply a compression wrap around the wound to secure the dressing.

Pressure Dressing Using Israeli Trauma Bandage

Principle: To provide mechanical circumferential pressure and dressing to an open wound of an extremity with uncontrolled hemorrhage.

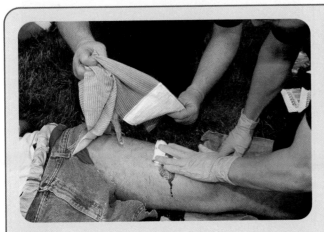

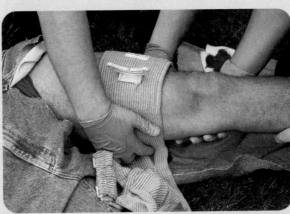

1 Ensure proper BSI, and place the dressing pad over the wound.

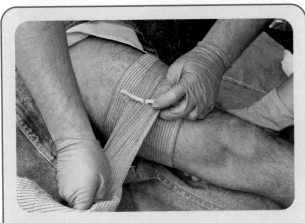

2 Wrap the elastic bandage around the extremity at least once.

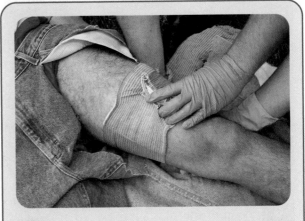

3 Loop the elastic bandage through the bar.

(continues)

Pressure Dressing Using Israeli Trauma Bandage (continued)

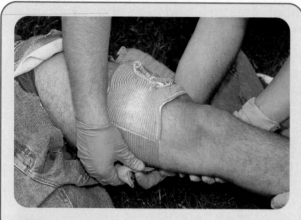

4 Wrap the bandage tightly around the wounded extremity in the opposite direction, applying enough pressure to control the bleeding.

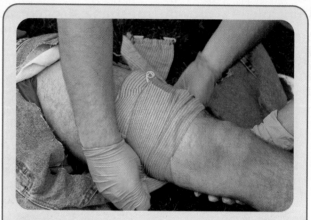

5 Continue wrapping the bandage around the extremity.

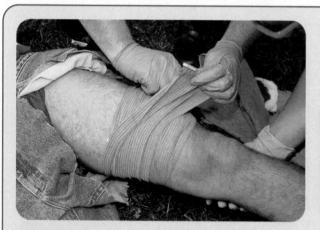

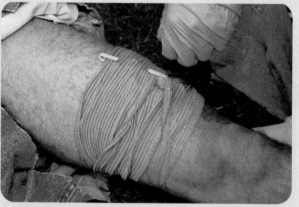

6 Secure the distal end of the bandage to maintain continued pressure to control the hemorrhage.

CHAPTER **4**

The Physics of Trauma

Lead Editors
Andrew Schmidt, MD
Kelsey Wise, MD
Brandon Kelly, MD

CHAPTER OBJECTIVES

At the completion of this chapter, you will be able to do the following:

- Define energy in the context of producing injury.
- Explain the association between the laws of motion, energy, and the physics of trauma.
- Describe the relationship of injury and energy exchange to speed.
- Discuss energy exchange and cavitation.
- Given the description of a motor vehicle crash, use the physics of trauma to predict the likely injury pattern for an unrestrained occupant.
- Describe the specific injuries and their causes as related to interior and exterior vehicle damage.
- Discuss the function of restraint systems for vehicle occupants.

- Relate the laws of motion and energy to mechanisms other than motor vehicle crashes (e.g., blasts, falls).
- Define the five phases of blast injury and the injuries produced in each phase.
- Explain the differences in the production of injury with low-, medium-, and high-energy weapons.
- Discuss the relationship of the frontal surface of an impacting object to energy exchange and injury production.
- Integrate principles of the physics of trauma into trauma patient assessment.

SCENARIO

Before first light on a cold winter morning, you and your partner are dispatched to a single-vehicle crash. On arrival, you find a single vehicle that has crashed into a tree on a rural road. The front end of the vehicle appears to have impacted the tree, and the car has spun around the tree and backed into a drainage ditch on the side of the road. The driver appears to be the only occupant. The airbag has deployed and the driver is moaning, still restrained by his seat belt. You note damage to the front end of the car where it impacted the tree as well as rear-end damage from spinning around and going into the ditch backward.

- What is the potential for injury for this patient based on the physics of trauma of this event?
- How would you describe the patient's condition based on the physics of trauma?
- What injuries do you expect to find?

INTRODUCTION

In the United States, 36,096 people were killed in vehicle crashes in 2019. This represents a 2% decrease (739 fewer casualties) compared to 2018, but 1,000 more deaths than in 2015.[1] The estimated number of injuries occurring on our roads increased just over 1% to 2.74 million in 2019.[1] The most recent World Health Organization (WHO) report estimates that 1.35 million people are killed each year in car crashes around the world, and further, states that road traffic injuries are the leading cause of death worldwide among people ages 5 to 29 years.[2] On a per capita basis, the worldwide rate of deaths from road traffic accidents has remained fairly constant since 2000, despite a rise in the number of vehicles on the world's roads during that same period. More than 90% of these deaths occur in low-income and middle-income countries, and primarily affect pedestrians, cyclists, and motorcyclists.[2]

In the United States, firearms are a major cause of death, accounting for 39,707 deaths in 2019. The two primary causes of firearm-related death were suicide, accounting for 60% of the firearm deaths, and homicide (75% of which are caused by firearm injuries).[3] Blast injuries are a major cause of injuries in many countries, whereas penetrating injuries from knives are prominent in others.

Successful management of trauma patients depends on the identification of both obvious and hidden injuries, and it demands the use of good assessment skills that are informed by an understanding of the mechanism of injury. Although it is difficult in the prehospital setting to determine the exact set of injuries produced in a given scenario, understanding the potential for injury and the potential for significant blood loss will allow the prehospital care practitioner to use their critical-thinking skills to recognize this likelihood and make appropriate triage, management, and transport decisions.

The management of any patient begins (after initial resuscitation) with taking the history of the patient's injury. In trauma, the history is the story of the impact and the energy exchange that resulted from this impact.[4] An understanding of the energy exchange process allows prehospital care practitioners to anticipate a high percentage of potential injuries encountered.

The physics of trauma deals with the motion of objects without reference to the forces that cause the motion.[4] Any injury that results from a force applied to the body is related directly to the interaction between the host and a moving object that impacts the host. When the prehospital care practitioner, at any level of care, does not understand the principles of the physics of trauma or the mechanisms involved, injuries may be missed. An understanding of these principles will increase the level of suspicion for certain injuries that are likely to be encountered given a specific mechanism. This information and the suspected injuries can be used to properly assess the patient on the scene and can be transmitted to the physicians and nurses in the emergency department (ED). At the scene and en route, these suspected injuries can be managed to provide the most appropriate patient care and "do no further harm."

Injuries that are not obvious but still severe can be fatal if they are not recognized at the scene and communicated to the medical team on arrival at the trauma center or appropriate hospital. Knowing where to look and how to assess for injuries is just as important as knowing what to do after finding injuries. A complete, accurate history of a traumatic incident and proper interpretation of these data will provide this information. Many of a patient's injuries can be predicted by a proper survey of the scene, even before examining the patient.

This chapter discusses the general principles of understanding the physics of trauma. The general principles begin with the laws of mechanics that govern energy exchange and the general effects of the energy exchange. Mechanical principles address the interaction of the human body with the components of a crash. A crash is the interaction that occurs when an object with energy, usually something solid, impacts another. Though we often associate the word *crash* with a motor vehicle impact, it can also refer to the crash of a falling body onto the pavement, the impact of a bullet on the external and internal tissues of the body, and the overpressure and debris of a blast. All of these events involve energy exchange, result in injury, can result in potentially life-threatening conditions, and require correct treatment by a knowledgeable and insightful prehospital care practitioner.

General Principles

A traumatic event can be divided into three phases: pre-event, event, and post-event. Simply stated, the *pre-event* phase is the prevention phase (**Box 4-1**). The *event* phase is that portion of the traumatic event that involves the exchange of energy or the physics of trauma (mechanics of energy). Last, the *post-event* phase is the patient care phase.

Whether the injury results from a car crash, a weapon, a fall, or a building collapse, energy is transformed into injury when it is absorbed into the body.

Pre-event

The *pre-event phase* includes all of the events that preceded the incident. Conditions that were present before the incident occurred and that are important in the management of the patient's injuries are assessed as part of the pre-event history. These considerations include the patient's acute or preexisting medical conditions (and medications to treat those conditions), ingestion of recreational substances (illegal and prescription drugs, alcohol, etc.), and the patient's state of mind.

Typically, young trauma patients do not have chronic illnesses. With older patients, however, medical conditions that are present before the trauma event can cause serious complications in the prehospital assessment and management of the patient and can significantly influence the outcome. For example, a 75-year-old driver of a vehicle that has struck a utility pole may have chest pain indicative of a myocardial infarction (heart attack). Did the driver hit the utility pole and have a heart attack, or did they have a heart attack and then strike the utility pole? Does the driver take medication (e.g., beta blocker) that will prevent elevation of the pulse in response to shock? Most of these conditions not only directly influence the assessment and management strategies (discussed in Chapter 5, *Scene Management* and Chapter 6, *Patient Assessment and Management*), but they are also important in overall patient care, even if they do not necessarily influence the physics of trauma of the crash.

Event

The *event phase* begins at the time of impact between one moving object and a second object. The second object can be moving or stationary and can be either an object or a person. Using a vehicle crash as an example, three impacts occur in most vehicular crashes:

1. The impact of the two objects
2. The impact of the occupants into the vehicle
3. The impact of the vital organs inside the occupants

For example, when a vehicle strikes a tree, the first impact is the collision of the vehicle with the tree. The second impact is the occupant of the vehicle striking the steering wheel or windshield. If the occupant is restrained, an impact occurs between the occupant and the seat belt. The third impact is between the occupant's internal organs and their chest wall, abdominal wall, or skull.

As stated, while the term *crash* typically brings to mind a motor vehicle incident, it does not necessarily refer to a vehicular crash. The impact of a vehicle into a pedestrian, a projectile into the abdomen, and a construction worker onto asphalt after a fall are all examples of a crash. Note that in a fall, only the first and third types of impacts are involved.

In all collisions, energy is exchanged between a moving object and the tissue of the human body or between the moving human body and a stationary object. The direction in which the energy exchange occurs, the amount of energy that is exchanged, and the effect that these forces have on the patient are all important considerations as assessment begins.

Post-event

During the *post-event phase*, the information gathered about the crash and pre-event phase is used to assess and manage a patient. This phase begins as soon as the energy from the crash is absorbed. The onset of the complications from life-threatening trauma can be slow or fast (or these complications can be prevented or significantly reduced), depending in part on the care provided at the scene and en route to the hospital. In the post-event phase, the understanding of the physics of trauma, the index of suspicion regarding injuries, and strong assessment skills all become crucial to the practitioner's ability to influence patient outcome.

To understand the effects of the forces that produce bodily injury, the prehospital care practitioner first needs to understand two components—energy exchange and human anatomy. For example, in a motor vehicle collision (MVC), what does the scene look like? Who hit what and at what speed? How long was the stopping time? Were the occupants using appropriate restraint devices such as seat belts? Did the airbag deploy? Were the children restrained properly in child seats, or were they unrestrained and thrown about the vehicle? Were any occupants ejected from the vehicle? Did they strike objects? If so, how many objects and what was the nature of those objects? These and many other questions must be answered if the prehospital care practitioner is to understand the exchange of forces that took place and translate this information into a prediction of injuries and appropriate patient care.

The astute prehospital care practitioner will use knowledge of the physics of trauma in the process of surveying the scene to determine what forces and motion were involved and what injuries might have resulted from those forces. Because the physics of trauma is based on fundamental principles of physics, an understanding of the pertinent laws of physics is necessary.

Energy

The initial steps in obtaining a history include evaluating the events that occurred at the time of the crash (**Figure 4-1**), estimating the energy that was exchanged with the human body, and making a gross approximation of the specific conditions that resulted.

Laws of Energy and Motion

Newton's first law of motion states that a body at rest will remain at rest and a body in motion will remain in motion unless acted on by an outside force. In **Figure 4-2**, the skier was stationary until unopposed gravitational forces moved him down the slope. Once in motion, although he leaves the ground, he will remain in motion until he hits something or returns to the ground and comes to a stop.

As previously mentioned, in any collision, when the body of the potential patient is in motion, there are three collisions:

1. The vehicle of the crash hitting an object, moving or stationary
2. The potential patient hitting the inside of the vehicle, crashing into an object, or being struck by energy in an explosion
3. The internal organs interacting with the walls of a compartment of the body or being torn loose from their supporting structures

An example is an occupant sitting in the front seat of a vehicle who is not wearing any restraint devices. When the vehicle hits a tree and stops, the unrestrained occupant continues in motion—at the same rate of speed—until they hit the steering column, dashboard, and windshield. The impact with these objects stops the forward motion of the torso or head, but the internal organs of the occupant remain in motion until the organs hit the inside of the chest wall, abdominal wall, or skull, halting the forward motion.

Newton's second law of motion, also known as the law of conservation of energy, states that energy can neither be created nor destroyed but can be changed in form. The motion of the vehicle is a form of energy. To start the vehicle, energy from the engine is transferred by a set of gears to the wheels, which grasp the road as they turn and impart motion to the vehicle. To stop the vehicle, the energy of its motion must be changed to another form, such as by heating up the brakes or crashing into an object and bending the frame. When a driver applies the brakes, the energy of motion is converted into the heat of friction (thermal energy) by the brake pads on the brake drums/discs and by the tires on the roadway. The vehicle thus decelerates.

Newton's third law of motion is perhaps the most well-known of Newton's three laws. It states that for every action or force there is an equal and opposite reaction. As we walk across the ground, the earth is exerting

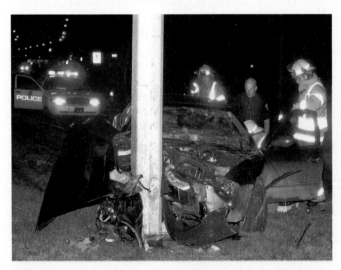

Figure 4-1 Evaluating the scene of an incident is critical. Information such as direction of impact, passenger-compartment intrusion, and amount of energy exchange provides insight into the possible injuries of the occupants.
© Jack Dagley Photography/Shutterstock

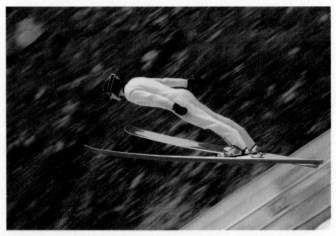

Figure 4-2 The skier was stationary until the energy from gravity moved him down the slope. Once in motion, although he leaves the ground, the momentum will keep him in motion until he hits something or returns to the ground, and the transfer of energy (friction or a collision) causes him to come to a stop.
© technotr/iStock/Getty Images

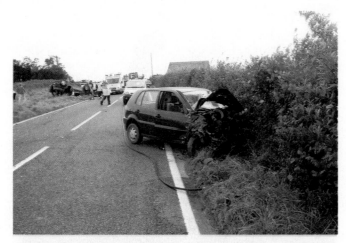

Figure 4-3 Energy is dissipated by deformation of the vehicle frame.
© Peter Seyfferth/imageBROKER/age fotostock

a force against us equal to the force we are applying upon the earth. Those who have fired a shotgun have felt the third law as the impact of the butt of the gun against their shoulder.

Just as the mechanical energy of a vehicle that crashes into a wall is dissipated by the bending of the frame or other parts of the vehicle (**Figure 4-3**), the energy of motion of the organs and the structures inside the body must be dissipated as these organs stop their forward motion. The same concepts apply to the human body when it is stationary and comes into contact and interacts with an object in motion such as a knife, a bullet, or a baseball bat.

Kinetic energy is a function of an object's mass and velocity. Although they are not technically the same, a victim's weight may be used to represent their mass. Likewise, speed is used to represent velocity (which is really speed plus direction). The relationship between weight and speed as it affects kinetic energy is as follows:

Kinetic energy = One-half the mass times the velocity squared
$$KE = 1/2 \ (mv^2)$$

Thus, the kinetic energy involved when a 150-pound (lb) (68-kilogram [kg]) person travels at 30 miles per hour (mph) (48 kilometers per hour [km/hr]) is calculated as follows:

$$KE = 150/2 \times 30^2 = 67{,}500 \ \textbf{units}$$

For the purpose of this discussion, no specific physical unit of measure (e.g., foot-pounds, joules) is used. The units are used merely to illustrate how this formula affects the change in the amount of energy. As just shown, a 150-lb (68-kg) person traveling at 30 mph (48 km/hr) would have 67,500 units of energy that must

be converted to another form when the person stops. This change takes the form of damage to the vehicle and injury to the occupant unless the energy dissipation can take some less harmful form, such as on a seat belt or into an airbag.

It is helpful to know which factor in the formula—mass or velocity—has the greatest effect on the amount of kinetic energy produced. To determine this, consider adding 10 lb (4.5 kg) to the 150-lb (68-kg) person traveling at 30 mph (48 km/hr) in the prior example, making the mass equal to 160 lb (73 kg):

$$KE = 160/2 \times 30^2 = 72{,}000 \ \textbf{units}$$

This 10-lb increase has resulted in a 4,500-unit increase in kinetic energy. Next, using the same example of a 150-lb (68-kg) person, let us see how increasing the velocity by 10 mph (16 km/hr) affects the kinetic energy:

$$KE = 150/2 \times 40^2 = 120{,}000 \ \textbf{units}$$

This velocity increase has resulted in a 52,500-unit increase in kinetic energy.

These calculations demonstrate that increasing the velocity (speed) increases the kinetic energy much more than does increasing the mass. Much more energy exchange will occur (and, therefore, produce greater injury to either the occupant, the vehicle, or both) in a high-speed crash than in a crash at a slower speed. The velocity is exponential and the mass is linear, making velocity the more critical factor even when there is a great mass disparity between two objects.

In anticipating the injuries sustained during a high-speed crash, it can be helpful to bear in mind that the force involved in initiating an event is equal to the force transferred or dissipated at the end of that event.

Mass × Acceleration = Force = Mass × Deceleration

Force (energy) is required to put a structure into motion. This force (energy) is required to create a specific speed. The speed imparted is dependent on the weight (mass) of the structure. Once this energy is passed on to the structure and it is placed in motion, the structure will remain in motion until the energy is given up (Newton's first law of motion). This loss of energy will place other components in motion (tissue particles) or be lost as heat (dissipated into the brake discs on the wheels). An example of this process is gun-related trauma. The chamber of a gun holds a cartridge that contains gunpowder. When this gunpowder is ignited, it burns rapidly, creating energy that pushes the bullet out of the barrel at a great speed. This speed is equivalent to the weight of the bullet and the amount of energy produced by the burning of the gunpowder or force. To slow down (Newton's first law of motion), the bullet must give up its energy into the structure that it hits. This transfer of energy will produce an explosion in the tissue that is equal to the explosion that occurred in the chamber of the gun when the initial speed was given to the bullet. The same phenomenon occurs in the moving automobile, the patient falling from a building, or the explosion of an improvised explosive device (IED).

Another important factor in a crash is the **stopping distance**. The shorter the stopping distance and the quicker the rate of that stop, the more energy is transferred to the occupant and the more damage or injury is done to the patient. Consider a vehicle that stops against a brick wall versus one that stops when the brakes are applied. Both dissipate the same amount of energy, just in a different manner. The rate of energy exchange (into the vehicle body or into the brake discs) is different and occurs over a different distance and time. In the first instance, the energy is absorbed in a very short distance and amount of time by the bending of the vehicle's frame. In the latter case, the energy is absorbed over a longer distance and period of time by the heat of the brakes. The forward motion of the occupant of the vehicle (energy) is absorbed in the first instance by damage to the soft tissue and bones of the occupant. In the second instance, the energy is dissipated, along with the energy of the vehicle, into the brakes.

This inverse relationship between stopping distance and injury also applies to falls. People have a better chance of surviving falls if they land on a compressible surface, such as snow or a deep pool of water. A fall from the same height terminating on a hard surface, such as concrete, can produce more severe injuries. The compressible material (i.e., the snow or water) increases the stopping distance and absorbs at least some of the energy rather than allowing all of the energy to be absorbed by the body. The result is decreased injury and damage to the body. This principle also applies to other types of crashes. An unrestrained driver will be more severely injured than a restrained driver because the restraint system, rather than the body, absorbs a significant portion of the energy transfer.

Therefore, once an object is in motion and has energy in the form of motion, in order for it to come to a complete rest, the object must lose all of its energy by converting the energy to another form or transferring it to another object. For example, if a vehicle strikes a pedestrian, the pedestrian is knocked away from the vehicle (**Figure 4-4**). Although the vehicle is somewhat slowed by the impact, the greater force of the vehicle imparts much more acceleration to the lighter-weight pedestrian than it loses in speed because of the mass difference between the two. The softer body parts of the pedestrian versus the harder body parts of the vehicle also means more damage to the pedestrian than to the vehicle.

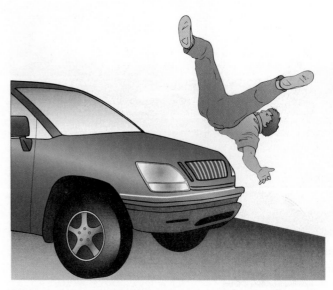

Figure 4-4 The energy exchange from a moving vehicle to a pedestrian crushes tissue and imparts speed and energy to the pedestrian, knocking the victim away from the point of impact. Injury to the victim can occur as the pedestrian is hit by the vehicle and as the pedestrian is thrown to the ground or into another vehicle.

© National Association of Emergency Medical Technicians (NAEMT)

Energy Exchange Between a Solid Object and the Human Body

When the human body collides with a solid object, or vice versa, the number of body tissue particles that are impacted by the solid object determines the amount of energy exchange that takes place. This transfer of energy produces the amount of damage (injury) that occurs to the patient. The number of tissue particles affected is determined by (1) the density (particles per volume) of the tissue and (2) the size of the contact area of the impact.

Density

The denser the tissue (measured in particles per volume), the greater the number of particles that will be impacted by a moving object and, therefore, the greater the rate and the total amount of energy exchanged. Driving a fist into a pillow and driving a fist at the same speed into a brick wall will produce different effects on the hand. The fist absorbs more energy colliding with the dense brick wall than with the less dense pillow, thus leading to more significant injury to the hand (**Figure 4-5**).

Simplistically, the body has three different types of tissue densities: **air density** (much of the lung and some portions of the intestine), **water density** (muscle and most solid organs; e.g., liver, spleen), and **solid density** (bone). Therefore, the amount of energy exchange (with resultant injury) will depend on which type of tissue is impacted.

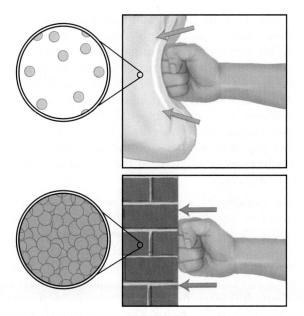

Figure 4-5 The human fist absorbs more energy colliding with the dense brick wall than with the less dense pillow, which dissipates the force.

© National Association of Emergency Medical Technicians (NAEMT)

Contact Area

Wind exerts pressure on a hand when it is extended out of the window of a moving vehicle. When the palm of the hand is horizontal and parallel to the direction of the flow through the wind, some backward pressure is exerted on the front of the hand (fingers) as the particles of air strike the hand. Rotating the hand 90 degrees to a vertical position places a larger surface area into the wind; thus, more air particles make contact with the hand, increasing the amount of force on it.

For trauma events, the energy imparted and the resulting damage can be modified by any change in the size of the impact surface area. Examples of this effect on the human body include the front of an automobile, a baseball bat, or a rifle bullet. The automobile's front surface contacts a large portion of the victim, a baseball bat contacts a smaller area, and a bullet contacts a very small area. The amount of energy exchange that would produce damage to the patient depends on the energy of the object and the density of the tissue in the path of the energy exchange.

If all of the impact energy is in a small area and this force exceeds the resistance of the skin, the object is forced through the skin. Consider the difference between striking a wooden table with a hammer and striking a nail held to the surface of the table with that same hammer. When you strike the table with the hammer, the force of the hammer striking the table is spread out across the surface of the table and the entire head of the hammer,

limiting penetration and creating only a dent. In contrast, striking the head of a nail with the hammer using the same amount of force drives the nail into the wood as all of that force is applied over a very small area. When the force is spread out over a larger area and the skin is not penetrated (like the hammer striking the table), the injury is defined as **blunt trauma**. If the force is applied over a small area and the object penetrates the skin and underlying tissues (like the hammer driving the nail through the table), the injury is defined as **penetrating trauma**. In either instance, a cavity in the patient is created by the force of the impacting object.

Even with an object such as a bullet, the impact surface area can be different based on such factors as bullet size, its motion (tumble) within the body, deformation ("mushroom"), and fragmentation. These factors are discussed later in this chapter.

Cavitation

The basic mechanics of energy exchange are relatively simple. The impact on the tissue particles accelerates those tissue particles away from the point of impact. These tissues then become moving objects themselves and crash into other tissue particles, producing a "falling domino" effect. Similarly, when a solid object strikes the human body or when the human body is in motion and strikes a stationary object, the tissue particles of the human body are knocked out of their normal position, creating a hole or cavity. Thus, this process is called **cavitation**. A common example that provides a visual illustration of cavitation is the game of pool (i.e., billiards).

The cue ball is driven down the length of a pool table by the force of the muscles in the arm. The cue ball crashes into the racked balls at the other end of the table. The energy from the arm into the cue ball is thus transferred onto each of the racked balls (**Figure 4-6**). The cue ball gives up its energy to the other balls. The other balls begin to move while the cue ball, which has lost its energy, slows or even stops. The other balls take on this energy as motion and move away from the impact point. A cavity has been created where the rack of balls once was. The same kind of energy exchange occurs when a bowling ball rolls down the alley, hitting the set of pins at the other end. The result of this energy exchange is a cavity. This same type of energy exchange occurs in both blunt and penetrating trauma.

Two types of cavities are created as follows:

- A *temporary cavity* is caused by the stretching of the tissues that occurs at the time of impact. Because of the elastic properties of the body's tissues, some or all of the contents of the temporary cavity return to their previous position. The size, shape, and portions of the cavity that become part of the permanent damage depend on the tissue type, the

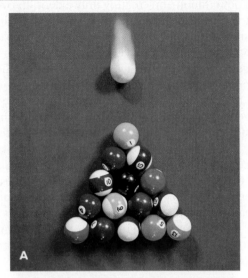

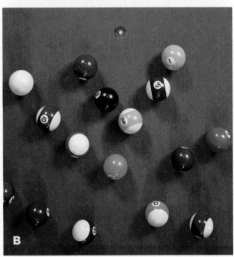

Figure 4-6 A. The energy of a cue ball is transferred to each of the other balls. **B.** The energy exchange pushes the balls apart to create a cavity.

© National Association of Emergency Medical Technicians (NAEMT)

elasticity of the tissue, and how much rebound of tissue occurs. The extent of this cavity usually is not visible when the prehospital care or hospital practitioner examines the patient, even seconds after the impact.

- A *permanent cavity* is left after the temporary cavity collapses and is the visible part of the tissue destruction. In addition, a crush cavity is produced by the direct impact of the object on the tissue. Both of these cavities can be seen when the patient is examined (**Figure 4-7**).[5]

The amount of the temporary cavity that remains as a permanent cavity is related to the elasticity (stretchability) of the tissue involved. For example, forcefully swinging a baseball bat into a steel drum leaves a dent, or cavity, in its side. Swinging the same baseball bat with the same force into a mass of foam rubber of similar size and shape will leave no dent once the bat is removed. The difference is **elasticity**. The foam rubber is more elastic than the steel drum. The human body is more like the foam rubber than the steel drum. If a person punches another person's abdomen, they would feel the fist go in. However, when the person pulls the fist away, no dent is left. Similarly, a baseball bat swung into the chest will leave no obvious cavity in the thoracic wall, but it would cause damage, both from direct contact and the cavity created by the energy exchange (**Figure 4-8**). The history of the incident and the interpretation of energy transfer will provide the information needed to determine the potential size of the temporary cavity at the time of impact. The organs or the structures involved predict injuries.

When the trigger of a loaded gun is pulled, the firing pin strikes the cap and produces an explosion in the cartridge. The energy created by this explosion is applied to the bullet, which speeds from the muzzle of the weapon. The bullet now has energy, or force (acceleration × mass = force). Once such force is imparted, the bullet cannot

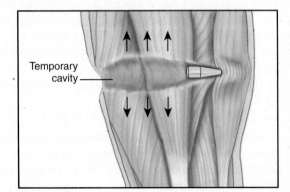

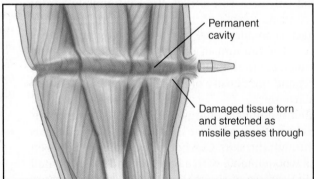

Figure 4-7 Damage to tissue is greater than the permanent cavity that remains from a missile injury. The faster or heavier the missile, the larger the temporary cavity and the greater the zone of tissue damage.

© National Association of Emergency Medical Technicians (NAEMT)

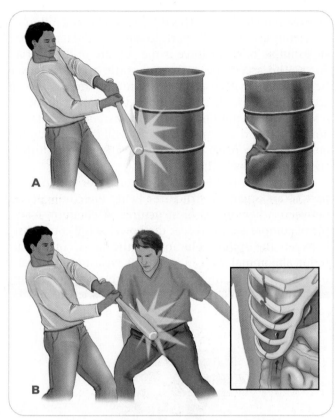

Figure 4-8 A. Swinging a baseball bat into a steel drum leaves a dent, or cavity, in its side. **B.** Swinging a baseball bat into a person usually leaves no visible cavity; the elasticity of the trunk usually returns the body to its normal shape even though damage has occurred.

© National Association of Emergency Medical Technicians (NAEMT)

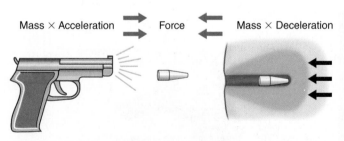

Mass × Acceleration → Force ← Mass × Deceleration

Figure 4-9 As a bullet travels through tissue, its kinetic energy is transferred to the tissue with which it comes in contact, accelerating the tissue away from the bullet.

© National Association of Emergency Medical Technicians (NAEMT)

slow down until acted on by an outside force (Newton's first law of motion). For the bullet to stop inside the human body, the energy of the bullet must be absorbed by body tissues in the amount that is equivalent to the explosion in the weapon (acceleration × mass = force = mass × deceleration; **Figure 4-9**). This absorbed energy causes movement of the tissue particles out of their normal position, creating a cavity.

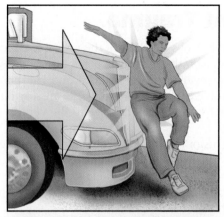

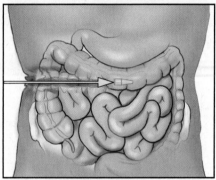

Figure 4-10 The force from the collision of a vehicle with a person is generally distributed over a large area, whereas the force of a collision between a bullet and a person is localized to a small area and results in penetration of the body and underlying structures.

© National Association of Emergency Medical Technicians (NAEMT)

Blunt and Penetrating Trauma

Trauma is generally classified as either blunt or penetrating. However, the energy exchanged and the injuries produced are similar in both types of trauma. Cavitation occurs in both; only the type and direction are different, along with the resulting penetration (or not) of the skin. If an object's entire energy is concentrated on one small area of skin, the skin likely will tear, and the object will enter the body and create a more concentrated energy exchange along its path. This can result in greater destructive power to one localized area. A larger object whose energy is dispersed over a larger area of skin may not penetrate the skin. The damage will be distributed over a larger area of the body, and the injury pattern will be less localized. An example is the difference in the impact of a large truck into a pedestrian versus a gunshot impact (**Figure 4-10**).

The cavitation in blunt trauma is frequently only a temporary cavity and is directed away from the point of impact. Penetrating trauma creates both a permanent and a temporary cavity. The temporary cavity that is created will spread away from the path of this missile in both frontal and lateral directions.

Blunt Trauma

The on-scene observations of the probable circumstances that led to a crash resulting in blunt trauma provide clues as to the severity of the injuries and the potential organs involved. The factors to assess are (1) direction of the impact, (2) external damage to the vehicle (type and severity), (3) internal damage (e.g., occupant compartment intrusion, steering wheel/column bending, fracture in the windshield, mirror damage, dashboard–knee impacts), (4) location of occupants within the vehicle, and (5) restraint devises employed or deployed at the time of the crash.

In blunt trauma, two forces are involved in the impact—**shear** and **compression**—both of which may result in cavitation. *Shear* is the result of one organ or structure (or part of an organ or structure) changing speed faster than another organ or structure (or part of

an organ or structure). This difference in acceleration (or deceleration) causes the parts to separate and tear. A classic example of shear force is the rupture of the thoracic aorta. The ascending aorta and aortic arch are loosely held in place within the mediastinum, whereas the descending aorta is tightly bound to the spinal column. In a sudden deceleration incident, the ascending aorta and aortic arch can continue moving while the descending aorta is held in place, leading to shearing and rupture of the aorta (**Figure 4-11**).

Compression is the result of an organ or structure (or part of an organ or structure) being directly squeezed between other organs or structures. A common example of compression involves the bowel being compressed between the spinal column and the inside of the anterior abdominal wall in a patient wearing only a seat belt (**Figure 4-12**). Injury can result from any type of impact, such as MVCs (vehicle or motorcycle), pedestrian

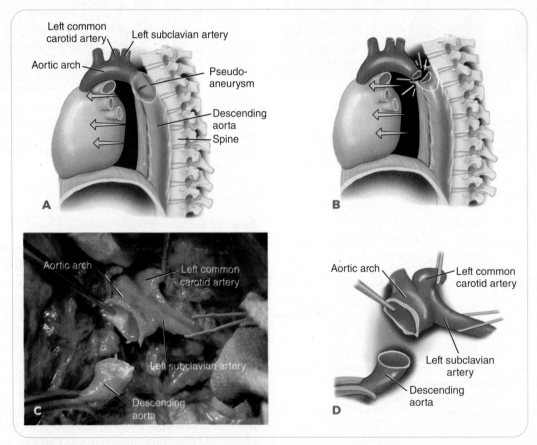

Figure 4-11 **A.** The descending aorta is a fixed structure that moves with the thoracic spine. The arch, aorta, and heart are freely mobile. Acceleration of the torso in a lateral-impact collision or rapid deceleration of the torso in a frontal-impact collision produces a different rate of motion between the arch–heart complex and the descending aorta. This motion may result in a tear of the inner lining of the aorta that is contained within the outermost layer, producing a pseudo-aneurysm. **B.** Tears at the junction of the arch and descending aorta may also result in a complete rupture, leading to immediate exsanguination in the chest. **C.** Operative photograph of a traumatic aortic tear. **D.** Illustration of a traumatic aortic tear.

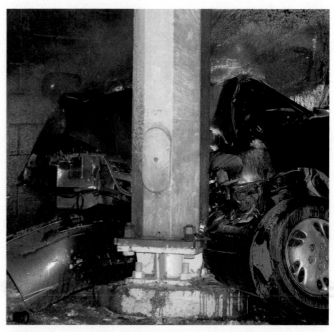

Figure 4-13 As a vehicle impacts a utility pole, the front of the car stops, but the rear portion of the vehicle continues traveling forward, causing deformation of the vehicle.

© Jack Dagley Photography/Shutterstock

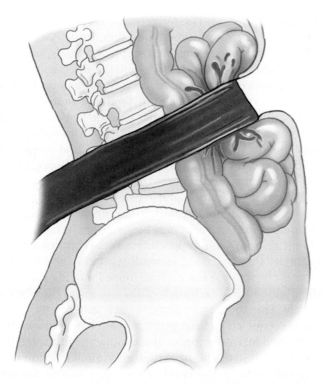

Figure 4-12 A seat belt that is incorrectly positioned above the brim of the pelvis allows the abdominal organs to be trapped between the moving posterior spinal column and the belt. Injuries to the pancreas and other retroperitoneal organs result, as well as blowout ruptures of the small intestine and colon.

© National Association of Emergency Medical Technicians (NAEMT)

collisions with vehicles, falls, sports injuries, or blast injuries. All of these mechanisms are discussed separately, followed by the results of this energy exchange on the specific anatomy in each of the body regions.

As discussed previously in this chapter, three collisions occur in blunt trauma. The vehicle striking an object, the occupant striking the vehicle, and the occupant's organs striking the body cavity. The first of these collisions will be discussed as it relates to MVCs, falls, and explosions. The latter two will be discussed in the context of the specific body regions involved.

Motor Vehicle Crashes

Many forms of blunt trauma occur, but MVCs (including motorcycle crashes) are the most common.[6] In 2019 in the United States, 36,096 people died, and an estimated 2.74 million people were injured in MVCs.[1] This number is likely associated with an increase in distracted driving episodes, despite the increased availability of hands-free technology to operate phones and electronic devices. This also represents a clear opportunity to increase education and preventive efforts in this area. Whereas the majority of the injuries were to occupants of the vehicles, over 230,000 of the injuries were to motorcyclists,

over 460,000 were to bicyclists, and over 180,000 were to pedestrians.[6]

MVCs can be divided into the following five types:

1. Frontal impact
2. Rear impact
3. Lateral impact
4. Rotational impact
5. Rollover[6]

Although each pattern has variations, accurate identification of the five patterns can provide insight into other, similar types of crashes.

One method to estimate the potential for injury to the occupant is to look at the vehicle and determine which of the five types of collisions occurred, the energy exchange involved, and the direction of the impact. The occupant is vulnerable to the same type of force as the vehicle from the same direction as the vehicle, and the potential injuries can be predicted.[6] The amount of force exchanged with the occupant, however, will be reduced by the absorption of energy by the vehicle.

Frontal Impact

In **Figure 4-13**, the vehicle has hit a utility pole in the center of the car. The impact point stopped its forward motion, but the rest of the car continued forward until the energy was absorbed by the bending of the car. The same type of motion occurs to the driver, resulting in injury. The stable steering column is impacted by the chest, perhaps in the center of the sternum. Just as the car continued in forward motion, significantly deforming the front of the vehicle, so too did the driver's chest. As the sternum stops forward motion against the dash, the posterior thoracic wall continues until the energy is absorbed by the bending and possible fracture of the ribs. This process may also crush the heart and the lungs, which are trapped between the sternum and the vertebral column and the posterior thoracic wall.

The amount of damage to the vehicle is related to the approximate speed of the vehicle at the time of impact. The greater the intrusion into the body of the vehicle, the greater the likely speed at the time of impact. The greater the vehicle speed, the greater the energy exchange and the more likely the occupants are to be injured.

Although the vehicle suddenly ceases to move forward in a frontal impact, the occupant continues to move and will follow one of two possible paths: up and over or down and under.

The use of a seat belt and the deployment of an airbag or restraint system will absorb some or most of the energy, thus reducing the injury to the victim. For clarity and simplicity of discussion, the occupant in these examples is assumed to be unrestrained.

Up-and-Over Path

In this sequence, the body's forward motion carries it up and over the steering wheel (**Figure 4-14**). The head is usually the lead body portion striking the windshield, windshield frame, or roof. The head then stops its forward motion. The torso continues in motion until its energy/force is absorbed along the spine. The cervical spine is the least protected segment of the spine. The chest or abdomen then collides with the steering column, depending on the position of the torso. The impact of the chest into the steering column produces thoracic cage, cardiac, lung, and aortic injuries (see the Regional Effects of Blunt Trauma section). The impact of the abdomen into the steering column can compress and crush the solid organs, produce overpressure injuries (especially to the diaphragm), and rupture the hollow organs.

The kidneys, spleen, and liver are also subject to shear injury as the abdomen strikes the steering wheel and abruptly stops. An organ may be torn from its normal anatomic restraints and supporting tissues (**Figure 4-15**). For example, the continued forward motion of the kidneys after the vertebral column has stopped moving produces shear along the attachment of the organs at their blood supply. The aorta and vena cava are tethered tightly to the posterior abdominal wall and vertebral column. The continued forward motion of the kidneys can stretch the renal vessels to the point of rupture. A similar action may tear the aorta in the chest at the point where the unattached arch becomes the tightly adhered descending aorta (see Figure 4-11).

Down-and-Under Path

In a down-and-under path, the occupant moves forward, downward, and out of the seat into the dashboard

Displaced liver, spleen, and bowel

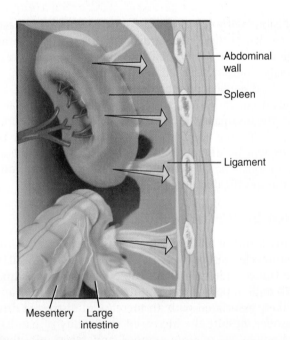

Abdominal wall

Spleen

Ligament

Mesentery   Large intestine

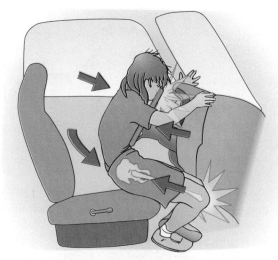

Figure 4-16 The occupant and the vehicle travel forward together. The vehicle stops, and the unrestrained occupant continues forward until something stops that motion.

© National Association of Emergency Medical Technicians (NAEMT)

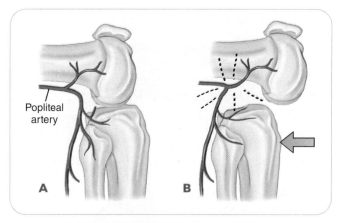

Figure 4-17 A. The knee has two possible impact points in a motor vehicle crash: the tibia and the femur. **B.** The popliteal artery lies close to the joint, tightly tied to the femur above and tibia below. Separation of these two bones stretches, kinks, and tears the artery.

© National Association of Emergency Medical Technicians (NAEMT)

(**Figure 4-16**). The importance of understanding the physics of trauma is illustrated by the injuries produced to the lower extremity in this path. Because many of the injuries are difficult to identify, an understanding of the mechanism of injury is important.

The foot, if planted on the floor panel or on the brake pedal with a straight knee, can twist as the continued torso motion angulates and fractures the ankle joint. More often, however, the knees are already bent, and the force is not directed to the ankle. Therefore, the knees strike the dashboard.

The knee has two possible impact points against the dashboard, the tibia and the femur (**Figure 4-17A**). If the tibia hits the dashboard and stops first, the femur remains in motion and overrides it. A dislocated knee, with torn ligaments, tendons, and other supporting structures, can result. Because the popliteal artery lies close to the knee joint, dislocation of the joint is frequently associated with injury to this vessel.[7] The artery can be completely disrupted, or the lining alone (*intima*) may be damaged (**Figure 4-17B**). In either case, a blood clot may form in the injured vessel, resulting in significantly decreased blood flow to the leg tissues below the knee. Early recognition of the knee injury and the potential for vascular injury should prompt the prehospital practitioner to alert ED physicians to the need for assessment of the vessel in this area.

Early identification and treatment of such a popliteal artery injury significantly decrease the complications of distal limb ischemia. Perfusion to this tissue needs to be reestablished within about 6 hours. Delays could occur because the prehospital care practitioner failed to consider the physics of trauma of the injury or overlooked important clues during assessment of the patient.

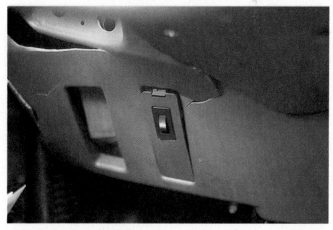

Figure 4-18 An imprint on the dashboard where the knee impacted is a key indicator that significant energy was focused on this joint and adjacent structures.

Courtesy of Norman McSwain, MD, FACS, NREMT-P.

Although most of these patients have evidence of injury to the knee, an imprint on the dashboard where the knee impacted is a key indicator that significant energy was focused on this joint and adjacent structures (**Figure 4-18**). Further investigation is needed in the hospital to better define the possible injuries.

When the femur is the point of impact, the energy is absorbed by the shaft of the bone, which can then break (**Figure 4-19**). If the femur remains intact, the continued forward motion of the pelvis onto the femur can dislocate the femoral head from the acetabulum (**Figure 4-20**).

After the knees and legs stop their forward motion, the upper body will bend forward into the steering column or dashboard. The unrestrained occupant may then sustain many of the same injuries described previously for the up-and-over path.

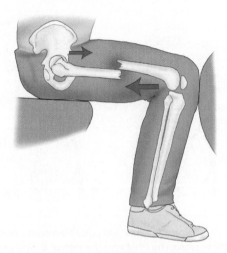

Figure 4-19 When the femur is the point of impact, the energy is absorbed by the femoral shaft, which can then break.

© National Association of Emergency Medical Technicians (NAEMT)

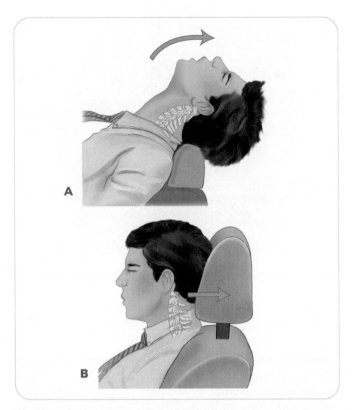

Figure 4-21 **A.** A rear-impact collision forces the torso forward. If the headrest is improperly positioned, the head is hyperextended over the top of the headrest. **B.** If the headrest is up, the head moves with the torso, and neck injury is prevented or reduced.

© National Association of Emergency Medical Technicians (NAEMT)

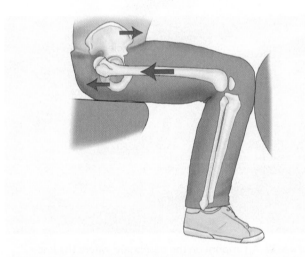

Figure 4-20 The continued forward motion of the pelvis relative to the femur can result in a posterior dislocation of the hip joint.

© National Association of Emergency Medical Technicians (NAEMT)

Recognizing these potential injuries and relaying the information to the ED physicians can result in long-term benefits to the patient.

Rear Impact

Rear-impact collisions occur when a slower-moving or stationary vehicle is struck from behind by a vehicle moving at a faster speed. For ease of understanding, the more rapidly moving vehicle is called the "bullet vehicle," and the slower-moving or stopped object is called the "target vehicle." In such collisions, the energy of the bullet vehicle at the moment of impact is converted to acceleration of the target vehicle, and damage results to both vehicles. The greater the difference in the momentum of the

two vehicles, the greater the force of the initial impact and the more energy is available to create damage and acceleration.

During a rear-impact collision, the target vehicle (in front) is accelerated forward. Everything that is attached to the frame will move forward at the same speed. This includes the seats in which the occupants are riding. The unattached objects in the vehicle, including the occupants, will begin forward motion only after something in contact with the frame begins to transmit the energy of the forward motion to them. As an example, the torso is accelerated by the back of the seat after some of the energy has been absorbed by the springs in the seats. If the headrest is improperly positioned behind and below the occiput of the head, the head will begin its forward motion after the torso, resulting in hyperextension of the neck. Shear and stretching of the ligaments and other support structures, especially in the anterior part of the neck, can result in injury (**Figure 4-21A**).

If the headrest is properly positioned, the head moves at approximately the same time as the torso without hyperextension (**Figure 4-21B** and **Box 4-2**). If the target vehicle is allowed to move forward without interference until it slows to a stop, the occupant will probably not suffer significant injury because most of the body's motion is supported by the seat, similar to an astronaut launching into orbit.

However, if the vehicle strikes another vehicle or object or if the driver slams on the brakes and stops suddenly, the occupants will continue forward, following the characteristic pattern of a frontal-impact collision. The collision then involves two impacts—rear and frontal. The double impact increases the likelihood of injury.

Lateral Impact

Lateral-impact mechanisms come into play when the vehicle is involved in an intersection (T-bone) collision or when the vehicle veers off the road and impacts sideways into a utility pole, tree, or other obstacle on the roadside. If the collision is at an intersection, the target vehicle is accelerated from the impact in the direction away from the force created by the bullet vehicle. The side of the vehicle or the door that is struck is thrust against the side of the occupant. The occupants may be injured as they are accelerated laterally (**Figure 4-22**) or as the passenger compartment is bent inward by the door's projection (**Figure 4-23**). Injury caused by the vehicle's movement is less severe if the occupant is restrained and moves with the initial motion of the vehicle.[9]

The following five body regions can sustain injury in a lateral impact:

- *Clavicle.* The clavicle can be compressed and fractured if the force is against the shoulder (**Figure 4-24A**).
- *Chest.* Compression of the thoracic wall inward can result in fractured ribs, pulmonary contusion, or compression injury of the solid organs beneath the rib cage, as well as overpressure injuries (e.g., pneumothorax) (**Figure 4-24B**). Shear injuries of the aorta can result from the lateral acceleration (25% of aortic shear injuries occur in lateral-impact collisions).[10,11]
- *Abdomen and pelvis.* The intrusion compresses and fractures the pelvis and pushes the head of the femur through the acetabulum (**Figure 4-24C**). Occupants on the driver's side are vulnerable to spleen injuries because the spleen is on the left side of the body, whereas occupants on the passenger side are more likely to receive an injury to the liver.

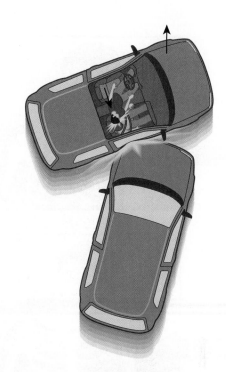

Figure 4-22 Lateral impact of the vehicle pushes the entire vehicle into the unrestrained passenger. A restrained passenger moves laterally with the vehicle.
© National Association of Emergency Medical Technicians (NAEMT)

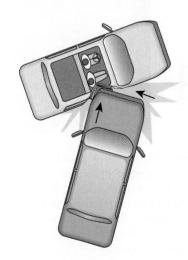

Figure 4-23 Intrusion of the side panels into the passenger compartment provides another source of injury.
© National Association of Emergency Medical Technicians (NAEMT)

- *Neck.* The torso can move out from under the head in lateral collisions as well as in rear impacts. The attachment point of the head is posterior and inferior to the center of gravity of the head. Therefore, the motion of the head in relationship to the neck is lateral flexion and rotation. The contralateral side of the spine will be opened (distraction) and the ipsilateral side compressed. This motion can fracture

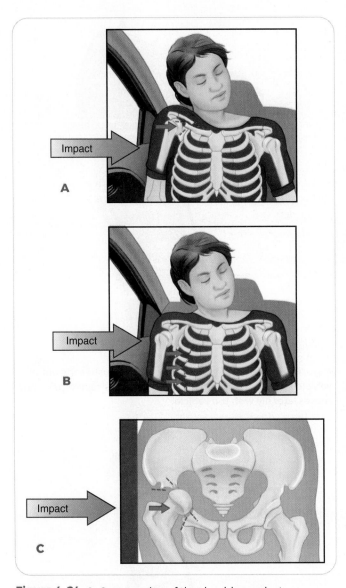

Figure 4-24 A. Compression of the shoulder against the clavicle produces midshaft fractures of this bone. **B.** Compression against the lateral chest and abdominal wall can fracture ribs and injure the underlying spleen, liver, and kidney. **C.** Lateral impact on the femur pushes the head through the acetabulum or fractures the pelvis.

© National Association of Emergency Medical Technicians (NAEMT)

the vertebrae, or more likely, produce jumped (dislocated) facets and possible dislocation as well as spinal cord injury (**Figure 4-25**).

- *Head.* The head can impact the frame of the door and the side window. Near-side impacts produce more injuries than far-side impacts.

Rotational Impact

Rotational-impact collisions occur when one corner of a vehicle strikes an immovable object, the corner of another vehicle, or a vehicle moving slower or in the opposite direction of the first vehicle. Following Newton's first law of motion, this corner of the vehicle will stop while the rest of the vehicle continues its forward motion until all its energy is completely transformed.

Rotational-impact collisions result in injuries that are a combination of those seen in frontal impacts and lateral collisions. The occupant continues to move forward and then is hit by the side of the vehicle (as in a lateral collision) as the vehicle rotates around the point of impact (**Figure 4-26**).

With multiple occupants, the patient closest to the point of impact will likely have the worst injuries because all of the energy of the impact is transferred into their body. Additional occupants may benefit from the deformation and rotation of the vehicle, which use up some of the energy before it can be absorbed by their bodies.

Rollover

During a rollover, a vehicle may undergo several impacts at many different angles, as may the unrestrained occupant's body and internal organs (**Figure 4-27**). Injury and damage can occur with each of these impacts. In rollover collisions, a restrained occupant is at risk for shearing-type injuries because of the significant forces created by a rolling vehicle. Although the occupants are held securely by restraints, the internal organs still move and can tear at the connecting tissue areas. More serious injuries result from being unrestrained. In many cases, the occupants are ejected from the vehicle as it rolls and are either crushed as the vehicle rolls over them or sustain injuries from the impact with the ground. If the occupants are ejected onto the roadway, they can be struck by oncoming traffic. The National Highway Traffic Safety Administration (NHTSA) reports that in crashes involving fatalities in the year 2017, 83% of occupants who were totally ejected from a vehicle were killed.[12]

Vehicle Incompatibility

The types of vehicles involved in the crash play a significant role in the potential for injury and death to the occupants. For example, in a lateral impact between two cars that lack airbags, the occupants of the car struck on its lateral aspect are more likely to die than are the occupants in the vehicle that strikes the car. This disproportionate risk to the occupants of the struck vehicle can be explained largely by the relative lack of protection on the side of a car. In comparison, a large amount of deformation can occur to the front end of a vehicle before there is intrusion into the passenger compartment. When the vehicle that is struck in a lateral collision (by a car) is a sport utility vehicle (SUV), van, or pickup truck rather than a car, the risk of death to occupants in both vehicles is

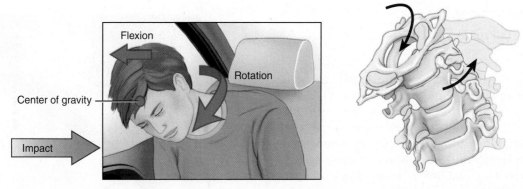

Figure 4-25 The center of gravity of the skull is anterior and superior to its pivot point between the skull and cervical spine. During a lateral impact, when the torso is rapidly accelerated out from under the head, the head turns toward the point of impact, in both lateral and anterior–posterior angles. Such motion separates the vertebral bodies from the side opposite the impact and rotates them apart. Jumped facets, ligament tears, and lateral compression fractures result.
© National Association of Emergency Medical Technicians (NAEMT)

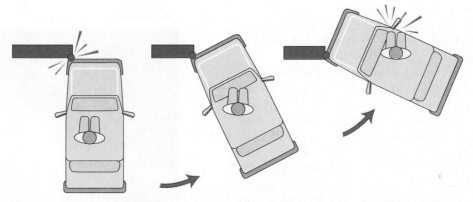

Figure 4-26 The occupant in a rotational-impact crash first moves forward and then laterally as the vehicle pivots around the impact point.
© National Association of Emergency Medical Technicians (NAEMT)

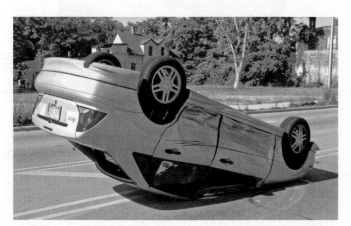

Figure 4-27 During a rollover, the unrestrained occupant can be wholly or partially ejected from the vehicle or can bounce around inside the vehicle. This action produces multiple and somewhat unpredictable injuries that are often severe.
© Rechitan Sorin/Shutterstock

almost the same. This is because the passenger compartments of SUVs, vans, and pickup trucks sits higher off the ground than does that of a car, meaning the occupants sustain less of a direct blow in a lateral impact.

More serious injuries and a greatly increased risk of death to vehicle occupants have been documented when a car is struck on its lateral aspect by a van, SUV, or pickup. In a lateral-impact collision between a van and a car, the occupants of the car struck broadside are more likely to die than are those in the van. If the striking vehicle is a pickup truck or SUV, the occupants of the car struck broadside are more likely to die than are those in the pickup truck or SUV. This tremendous disparity results from the higher center of gravity and increased mass of the van, SUV, or pickup truck. Knowledge of vehicle types in which occupants were located in a crash may lead the prehospital care practitioner to have a higher index of suspicion for serious injury.

Occupant Protective and Restraining Systems

Seat Belts

In the injury patterns described previously, the occupants were assumed to be unrestrained. The NHTSA has reported a steady increase in seat belt use since 2000, and only 9.7% of front-seat passengers were unrestrained in 2020.[13] Seat belt use is lower among males (88.4%) than females (92.8%); lower in those aged 16- to 24-years (86.9%), and lower among Black occupants (85.2%) than White occupants (90.5%) or members of other races (92.8%).[13] Ejection from vehicles accounts for approximately one-fourth of vehicular deaths. About 83% of passenger vehicle occupants who were totally ejected were killed; 1 in 13 ejection victims sustained a spine fracture.[12] After ejection from a vehicle, the body is subjected to a second impact as it strikes the ground (or another object) outside the vehicle. This second impact can result in injuries that are even more severe than the initial impact. The risk of death for ejected victims is six times greater than for those who are not ejected. Clearly, seat belts save lives.[14,15]

The NHTSA reports that 49 states and the District of Columbia have seat belt legislation for both adults and minors. The only exception is New Hampshire, which has regulations for minors but not adults. Research has found that seat belts, when used, reduce the risk of fatal injury to front-seat car occupants by 45% and the risk of serious injury by 50%.[16] In 2017, seat belts saved an estimated 14,955 lives.[15] Of the 22,215 passenger vehicle occupants who died in car crashes in 2019, 47% were not wearing seat belts.[17]

What occurs when the occupants are restrained? If a seat belt is positioned properly, the pressure of the impact is absorbed by the pelvis and the chest, resulting a decreased risk of serious injuries (**Figure 4-28**). The proper use of restraints transfers the force of the impact from the occupant's body to the restraint belts and restraint system. With restraints, the chance of sustaining life-threatening injuries is greatly reduced.[14,18,19]

Seat belts must be worn properly to be effective. An improperly worn belt may not protect against injury in the event of a crash, and it may even cause injury. When lap belts are worn loosely or are strapped above the pelvis, compression injuries of the soft abdominal organs can occur. Injuries of the soft intra-abdominal organs (spleen, liver, and pancreas) result from compression between the seat belt and the posterior abdominal wall or spinal column (see Figure 4-12). Increased intra-abdominal pressure can cause diaphragmatic rupture and herniation of abdominal organs. Lap belts should be worn in combination with a shoulder restraint. Anterior compression fractures of the lumbar spine can occur as the upper and lower parts of the torso pivot over the lap belt and the

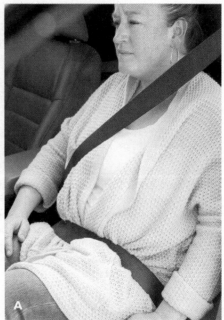

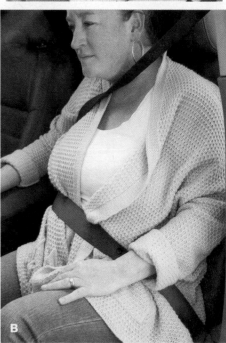

Figure 4-28 A. A properly positioned seat belt is located below the anterior-superior iliac spine on each side, above the femur, and is tight enough to remain in this position. The bowl-shaped pelvis protects the soft intra-abdominal organs. **B.** Improperly placed restraints can result in significant injury in the event of a crash.

© Jones & Bartlett Learning. Photographed by Darren Stahlman.

restrained twelfth thoracic (T12), first lumbar (L1), and second lumbar (L2) vertebrae. Occasionally vehicle occupants place the diagonal strap under the arm and not over the shoulder, decreasing its effectiveness.

With the passage and enforcement of mandatory laws on seat belt use in the United States, the overall severity of injuries has decreased, and the number of fatal crashes has been significantly reduced.

Airbags

Airbags (in addition to seat belts) provide supplemental protection to the vehicle occupant. Originally, front-seat driver and passenger airbag systems were designed to cushion the forward motion of only the front-seat occupants. The airbags absorb energy slowly by increasing the body's stopping distance. They are extremely effective in the first collision of frontal and near-frontal impacts (the 65% to 70% of crashes that occur within 30 degrees of the headlights). However, airbags deflate immediately after the impact and, therefore, are not effective in multiple-impact or rear-impact collisions. An airbag deploys and deflates within 0.5 second. As the vehicle veers into the path of an oncoming vehicle or off the road into a fixed object after the initial impact, no airbag protection is left. Side airbags do add to the protection of occupants.

When airbags deploy, they can produce minor but noticeable injuries that the prehospital care practitioner needs to identify (**Box 4-3**). These injuries include abrasions of the arms, chest, and face (**Figure 4-29**); foreign bodies to the face and eyes; and injuries caused by the occupant's eyeglasses (**Figure 4-30**).

Airbags that do not deploy can still be dangerous to both the patient and the prehospital care practitioner. Airbags can be deactivated by an extrication specialist trained to do so properly and safely. Such deactivation should not delay patient care or extrication of the critical patient.

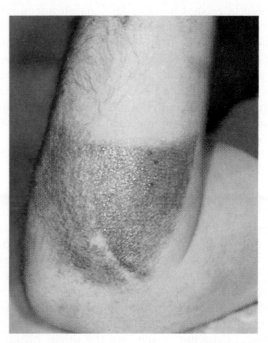

Figure 4-29 Abrasions of the forearm are secondary to rapid expansion of the airbag when the hands are tight against the steering wheel.
Courtesy of Norman McSwain, MD, FACS, NREMT-P.

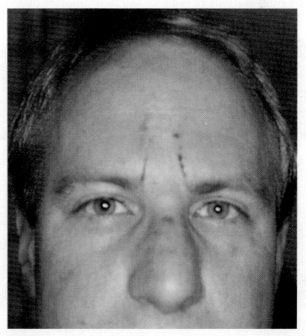

Figure 4-30 Expansion of the airbag into eyeglasses produces abrasions.
Courtesy of Norman McSwain, MD, FACS, NREMT-P.

Box 4-3 Airbag Hazards

Front-seat passenger airbags have been shown to be dangerous to children and small adults, especially when children are placed in incorrect positions in the front seat or in incorrectly installed child seats. Children age 12 years and younger should always be in the proper restraint device for their size and should be in the back seat. It is estimated that 46% of all car seats and booster seats are used incorrectly in one or more ways. By seat type, misuse of forward-facing car seats is 61%, rear-facing infant car seats is 49%, rear-facing convertible car seats is 44%, backless belt-positioning boosters is 24%, and high-back belt-positioning boosters is 16%.[20]

Drivers should always be at least 10 inches (25 centimeters [cm]) from the airbag cover, and front-seat passengers should be at least 18 inches (45 cm) away. In most cases, when the proper seating arrangements and distances are used, airbag injuries are limited to simple abrasions.

Many vehicles now have airbags in the sides and tops of the doors.

Airbags pose a significant hazard to infants and children if the child is either unrestrained or placed in a rear-facing child seat in the front-passenger compartment.

Motorcycle Crashes

Motorcycle crashes account for a significant number of the motor vehicle deaths each year. Although the laws of physics for motorcycle crashes are the same, the mechanism of injury varies from automobile and truck crashes. This variance occurs in each of the following types of impacts: head on, angular, and ejection. An additional factor that leads to increased death, disability, and injury is the lack of structural framework around the rider that is present in other motor vehicles.

Head-On Impact

A head-on collision into a solid object stops the forward motion of a motorcycle (**Figure 4-31**). Because the motorcycle's center of gravity is above and behind the front axle, which often becomes a pivot point in such a collision, the motorcycle will tip forward, and the rider may crash into the handlebars. The rider may receive injuries to the head, chest, abdomen, or pelvis, depending on which part of the anatomy impacts with the handlebars or another object first. If the rider's feet remain on the pegs of the motorcycle and the thighs hit the handlebars, the forward motion may be absorbed by the midshaft of the femur, sometimes resulting in bilateral femoral fractures (**Figure 4-32**). The interaction between the rider's pelvis and the handlebars can result in various combinations of bone or ligament injuries that may

disrupt the anterior pubic symphysis while the posterior pelvic ring opens like the hinge of a book (thus the term *open-book* pelvis injuries). Such injuries may result in life-threatening intra-pelvic hemorrhage, and the immediate application of a pelvic binder of some sort could be a lifesaving measure. This is a great example of the application of kinematic assessment leading to a potentially lifesaving intervention in the field.

Angular Impact

In an angular-impact collision, the motorcycle hits an object at an angle. The motorcycle will then collapse on the rider or cause the rider to be crushed between the motorcycle and the object that was struck. Injuries to the upper or lower extremities can occur, resulting in fractures and extensive soft-tissue injury (**Figure 4-33**). Injuries can also occur to organs of the abdominal cavity as a result of energy exchange.

Ejection Impact

Because of the lack of restraints, the rider is susceptible to ejection. The rider will continue in flight until the head, arms, chest, abdomen, or legs strike another object, such as a motor vehicle, a utility pole, or the road. Injury will occur at the point of impact and will radiate to the rest of the body as the energy is absorbed.[21]

Injury Prevention

Many motorcycle riders do not use proper protection. Protection for motorcyclists includes boots, leather clothing, and helmets. Of the three, the helmet affords the best protection. It is built similarly to the skull: strong and supportive externally and energy-absorbent internally.

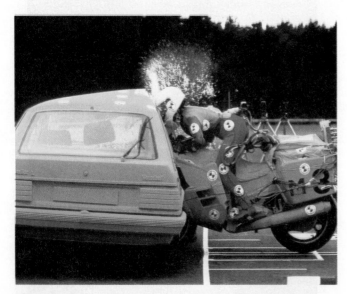

Figure 4-31 The position of a motorcycle rider is above the pivot point of the front wheel as the motorcycle impacts an object head on.
© TRL Ltd./Science Source

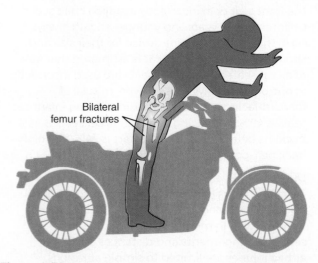

Bilateral femur fractures

Figure 4-32 The body travels forward and over the motorcycle, and the thighs and femurs impact the handlebars. The rider can also be ejected.
© National Association of Emergency Medical Technicians (NAEMT)

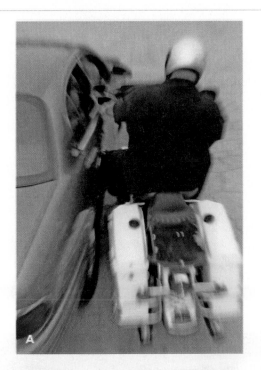

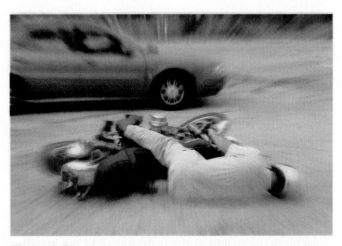

Figure 4-34 To prevent being trapped between two pieces of steel (motorcycle and vehicle), the rider "lays the bike down" to dissipate the injury. This tactic often causes abrasions ("road rash") as the rider's speed is slowed on the asphalt.
© National Association of Emergency Medical Technicians (NAEMT)

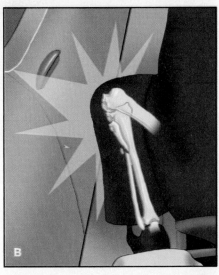

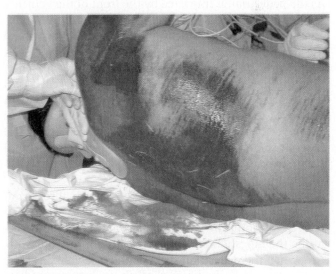

Figure 4-35 Road "burns" (abrasions) after a motorcycle crash without protective clothing.
Courtesy of Dr. Jeffrey Guy.

Figure 4-33 A. If the motorcycle does not hit an object head-on, it collapses like a pair of scissors. **B.** This collapse traps the rider's lower extremity between the object that was impacted and the motorcycle.
© National Association of Emergency Medical Technicians (NAEMT)

The helmet's structure absorbs much of the impact, thereby decreasing injury to the face, skull, and brain. The helmet provides only minimal protection for the neck but does not cause neck injuries. Mandatory helmet laws are effective in increasing the use of helmets by riders. Use of motorcycle helmets is highly effective in reducing the risk of head injury and death in those riders involved in motorcycle crashes. [22]

"Laying the bike down" is a protective maneuver used by riders to separate themselves from the motorcycle in an impending crash (**Figure 4-34**). The rider turns the motorcycle sideways and drags the inside leg on the ground. This action slows the rider more than the motorcycle so that the motorcycle moves out from under the rider. The rider will slide along on the pavement but will not be trapped between the motorcycle and any object it hits. Using this maneuver, riders usually receive abrasions ("road rash") and minor fractures but generally avoid the severe injuries associated with the other types of impacts, unless they directly strike another object (**Figure 4-35**).

Pedestrian Injuries

One common scenario in collisions in which motor vehicles impact pedestrians involves three separate phases, each with its own injury pattern, as follows:

1. The initial impact is to the legs and sometimes the hips (**Figure 4-36A**).
2. The torso rolls onto the hood of the vehicle (and may strike the windshield) (**Figure 4-36B**).
3. The pedestrian then falls off the vehicle and onto the ground, usually headfirst, with possible cervical spine trauma (**Figure 4-36C**).

The injuries produced in pedestrian crashes vary according to the height of the pedestrian and the height of the vehicle (**Figure 4-37**). A child and an adult standing in front of a vehicle present different anatomic impact points to the vehicle.

Adults are usually struck first by the vehicle's bumper in the lower legs, fracturing the tibia and fibula. As the pedestrian is impacted by the front of the vehicle's hood, depending on the height of the hood, the abdomen and thorax are struck by the top of the hood and the windshield. This substantial second strike can result in fractures of the upper femur, pelvis, ribs, and spine, producing intra-abdominal or intrathoracic crush and shear. If the victim's head strikes the hood or if the victim continues to move up the hood so that the head strikes the windshield, injury to the face, head, and cervical and thoracic spine can occur. If the vehicle has a large frontal area (such as with trucks and SUVs), the entire pedestrian is hit simultaneously.

The third impact occurs as the victim is thrown off the vehicle and strikes the pavement. The victim can receive a significant blow on one side of the body, injuring the hip, shoulder, and head. Head injury often occurs when the pedestrian strikes either the vehicle or the pavement. Similarly, because all three impacts produce sudden, violent movement of the torso, neck, and head, an unstable spine fracture may result. After falling, the victim may be struck by a second vehicle traveling next to or behind the first.

Because they are shorter, children are initially struck higher on the body than adults (**Figure 4-38A**). The first impact generally occurs when the bumper strikes the child's legs (above the knees) or pelvis, damaging the femur or pelvic girdle. The second impact occurs almost instantly afterward as the front of the vehicle's hood continues forward and strikes the child's thorax. Then, the head and face strike the front or top of the vehicle's hood (**Figure 4-38B**). Because of the child's smaller size and weight, the child may not be thrown clear of the vehicle, as usually occurs with an adult. Instead, the child may be dragged by the vehicle while partially under the vehicle's front end. If the child falls to the side, the lower limbs

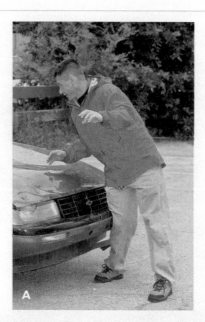

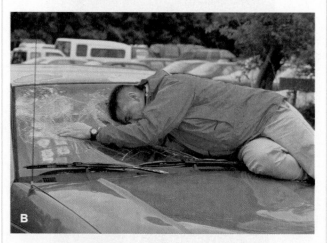

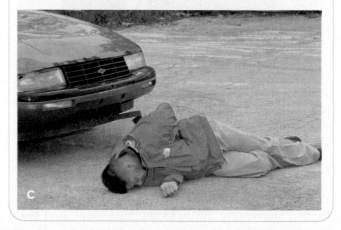

Figure 4-36 Phases of vehicle–pedestrian crashes. **A.** Phase 1: Initial impact is to the legs and sometimes to the hips.
B. Phase 2: The torso of the pedestrian rolls onto the hood of the vehicle. **C.** Phase 3: The pedestrian falls off the vehicle and hits the ground.

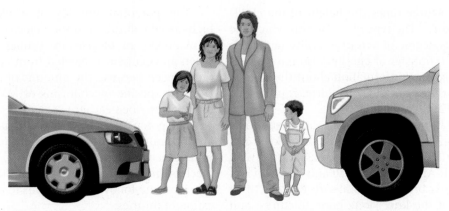

Figure 4-37 The injuries resulting from vehicle–pedestrian crashes vary according to the height of the pedestrian and the height of the vehicle.

© National Association of Emergency Medical Technicians (NAEMT)

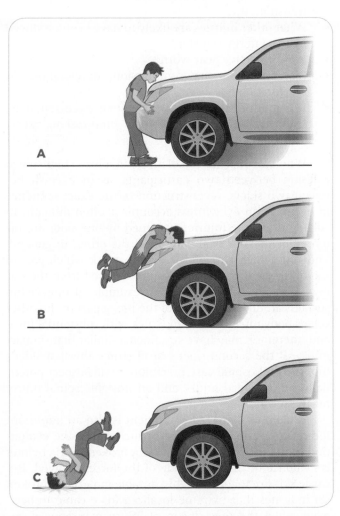

Figure 4-38 A. The initial impact with a child occurs when the vehicle strikes the child's upper leg or pelvis. **B.** The second impact occurs when the child's head and face strike the front or top of the vehicle's hood. **C.** A child may be thrown clear of a vehicle, as shown here, but also may be trapped and dragged by the vehicle.

© National Association of Emergency Medical Technicians (NAEMT)

may also be run over by a front wheel (**Figure 4-38C**). If the child falls backward, ending up completely under the vehicle, almost any injury can occur (e.g., being dragged, struck by projections, or run over by a wheel).

If the foot is planted on the ground at the time of impact, the child will receive energy exchange at the upper leg, hip, and abdomen. This will force the hips and abdomen away from the impact. The upper part of the torso will come along later, as will the planted foot. The energy exchange moving the torso but not the feet will fracture the pelvis and shear the femur, producing severe angulation at the point of impact and possible spine injury as well.

To complicate these injuries further, a child will likely turn toward the car out of curiosity, exposing the anterior body and face to injuries, whereas an adult will attempt to escape and will be hit in the back or the side.

As with an adult, any child struck by a vehicle can receive some type of head injury. Because of the sudden, violent forces acting on the head, neck, and torso, cervical spine injuries are high on the suspicion list.

Knowing the specific sequence of multiple impacts in a vehicle–pedestrian collision and understanding the multiple underlying injuries that they can produce are keys to making an initial assessment and determining the appropriate management of a patient.

Falls

Victims of falls can sustain injury from multiple impacts. The estimated height from which the victim fell, the surface on which the victim landed, and the part of the body impacted first are important factors to determine because they indicate the level of energy involved and, thus, the energy exchange that occurred. Victims who fall from greater heights have a higher incidence of injury because their velocity increases as they fall. Falls from greater than 20 feet (ft; [6.1 m]) in adults and 10 ft (3 m) in children (two to three times the height of the child) are frequently severe.[23] The type of surface on which the victim lands and its degree of **compressibility** (ability to be deformed by the transfer of energy) also have an effect on stopping distance. Information about the unique physics of trauma of fall injuries in children is presented in Chapter 14, *Pediatric Trauma*.

In real life, bilateral fractures of the calcaneus (heel bone), compression or shear fractures of the ankles, and distal tibial or fibular fractures are often associated with landing on the feet. After the feet land and stop moving, the legs are the next body part to absorb energy. Tibial plateau fractures of the knee, long-bone fractures, and hip fractures can result. The body is compressed by the weight of the head and torso, which are still moving, and can cause compression fractures of the spinal column in the thoracic and lumbar areas. Hyperflexion occurs at each concave bend of the S-shaped spine, producing compression injuries on the concave side and distraction injuries on the convex side.

If a victim falls forward onto the outstretched hands, the result can be fractures of one or both the wrists. If the victim did not land on the feet, the prehospital care practitioner will assess the part of the body that struck first, evaluate the path of energy displacement, and determine the injury pattern.

If the falling victim lands on the head with the body almost in-line, as often occurs in shallow-water diving injuries, the entire weight and force of the moving torso, pelvis, and legs compress the head and cervical spine. A fracture of the cervical spine may be a result, as with the up-and-over path of the frontal-impact vehicle collision.

Sports Injuries

Severe injury can occur during many sports or recreational activities, such as skiing, diving, baseball, and contact sports such as football. These injuries can be caused by sudden deceleration forces or by excessive compression, twisting, hyperextension, or hyperflexion. In recent years, various sports activities have become available to a wide spectrum of occasional, recreational participants who often lack the necessary training and conditioning or the proper protective equipment. Recreational sports and activities include participants of all ages. Sports such as downhill skiing, waterskiing, bicycling, and skateboarding are all potentially high-velocity activities. Other sports, such as trail biking, all-terrain vehicle riding, and snowmobiling, can produce velocity deceleration, collisions, and impacts similar to motorcycle crashes or MVCs. Protective equipment worn in sports can provide some protection but may have the potential to create injury, such as when a helmeted football player drives his head into another player.

The potential injuries of a victim who is in a high-speed collision and then ejected from a skateboard, snowmobile, or bicycle are similar to those sustained when an occupant is ejected from an automobile at the same speed because the amount of energy is the same. (See the specific mechanisms of MVCs and motorcycle crashes described earlier.)

The potential mechanisms associated with each sport are too numerous to list in detail. However, the general principles are the same as for MVCs. While assessing the mechanism of injury, the prehospital care practitioner considers the following questions to assist in the identification of injuries:

- What forces acted on the victim and how?
- What are the apparent injuries?
- To what object or part of the body was the energy transmitted?
- What other injuries are likely to have been produced by this energy transfer?
- Was protective gear worn?
- Was there sudden compression, deceleration, or acceleration?
- What injury-producing movements occurred (e.g., hyperflexion, hyperextension, compression, excessive lateral bending)?

When the mechanism of injury involves a high-speed collision between two participants, as in a crash between two skiers, reconstruction of the exact sequence of events from eyewitness accounts is often difficult. In such crashes, the injuries sustained by one skier are often guidelines for examination of the other. In general, knowing which part of one victim struck which part of the other victim, and what injury resulted from the energy transfer, is important. For example, if one victim sustains an impact fracture of the hip, a part of the other skier's body must have been struck with substantial force and, therefore, may have sustained a similar high-impact injury. If the second skier's head struck the first skier's hip, the prehospital care practitioner will suspect potentially serious head injury and an unstable spinal injury for the second skier.

Broken or damaged equipment is also an important indicator of injury and must be included in the evaluation of the mechanism of injury. A broken sports helmet is evidence of the magnitude of the force involved. Because skis are made of highly durable material, a broken ski indicates that extreme localized force came to bear, even when the mechanism of injury may appear unimpressive. A snowmobile with a severely dented front end indicates the force with which it struck a tree. The presence of a broken stick after an ice hockey skirmish raises the questions of whether it was broken as a result of a fight or whether it broke as a result of normal hockey playing.

Victims of significant crashes who do not complain of injury must be thoroughly assessed, as severe yet occult injuries may exist. The steps are as follows:

1. Evaluate the patient for life-threatening injury.
2. Evaluate the patient for mechanism of injury. (What happened and exactly how did it happen?)
3. Determine how the forces that produced injury in one victim may have affected any other person.
4. Determine whether any protective gear was worn. (It may have already been removed.)
5. Assess damage to the protective equipment. (What are the implications of this damage relative to the patient's body?)
6. Assess whether the damage was caused by this incident or whether it was preexisting and worsened.
7. Thoroughly assess the patient for possible associated injuries.

High-speed falls, collisions, and falls from heights without serious injury are common in many contact sports. The ability of athletes to experience incredible collisions and falls and sustain only minor injury—largely as a result of impact-absorbing equipment—may be confusing. The potential for injury in sports participants may be overlooked. The principles of the physics of trauma and careful consideration of the exact sequence and mechanism of injury provide insight into sports collisions in which greater forces than usual came to bear. The physics of trauma is an essential tool in identifying possible underlying injuries and determining which patients require further evaluation and treatment at a medical facility.

Regional Effects of Blunt Trauma

The body can be divided into several regions: head, neck, thorax, abdomen, pelvis, and extremities. Each body region is subdivided into (1) the external part of the body, usually composed of skin, bone, soft tissue, vessels, and nerves, and (2) the internal part of the body, usually vital internal organs. The injuries produced as a result of compression and shear forces are used to provide an overview in each component and region for potential injuries.

Head

The only external indication that compression and shear injuries have occurred to the patient's head may be a soft-tissue injury to the scalp, a contusion of the scalp, or a bull's-eye fracture of the windshield (**Figure 4-39**).

Compression

When the body is traveling forward with the head leading the way, as in a frontal vehicular crash or a headfirst

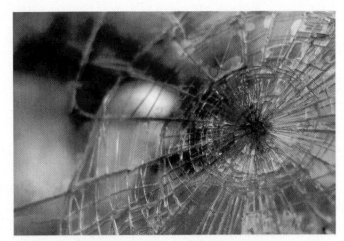

Figure 4-39 A bull's-eye fracture of the windshield is a major indication of skull impact and energy exchange to both the skull and the cervical spine.

© Kristin Smith/Shutterstock

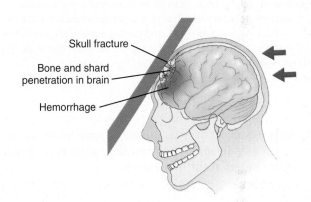

Figure 4-40 As the skull impacts an object, pieces of bone may be fractured and pushed into the brain.

© National Association of Emergency Medical Technicians (NAEMT)

fall, the head is the first structure to receive the impact and the energy exchange. The continued momentum of the torso then compresses the head. The initial energy exchange occurs on the scalp and the skull. The skull can be compressed and fractured, pushing the broken, bony segments of the skull into the brain (**Figure 4-40**).

Shear

After the skull stops its forward motion, the brain continues to move forward, compressing against the intact or fractured skull with resultant concussion, contusions, or lacerations. The brain is soft and compressible; therefore, its length is shortened. The posterior part of the brain can continue forward, pulling away from the skull, which has already stopped moving. As the brain separates from the skull, stretching or breaking (shearing) of brain tissue itself or any blood vessels in the area occurs (**Figure 4-41**). Hemorrhage into the epidural, subdural, or subarachnoid

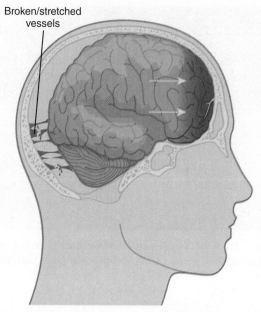

Figure 4-41 As the skull stops its forward motion, the brain continues to move forward. The part of the brain nearest the impact is compressed, bruised, and perhaps even lacerated. The portion farthest from the impact is separated from the skull, with tearing and lacerations of the vessels involved.

© National Association of Emergency Medical Technicians (NAEMT)

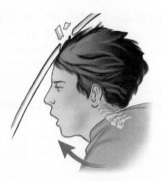

Figure 4-42 The skull frequently stops its forward motion, but the torso does not. The torso continues its forward motion until its energy is absorbed. The weakest point of this forward motion is the cervical spine.

© National Association of Emergency Medical Technicians (NAEMT)

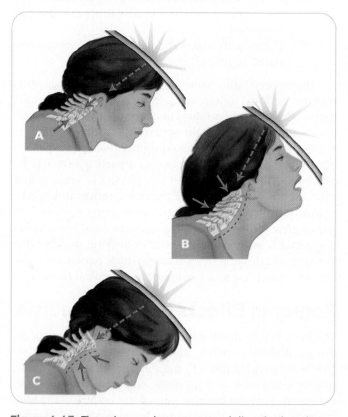

Figure 4-43 The spine can be compressed directly along its own axis **(A)**, angled in hyperextension **(B)**, or hyperflexion **(C).**

© National Association of Emergency Medical Technicians (NAEMT)

space can result, as well as diffuse axonal injury of the brain. If the brain separates from the spinal cord, it will most likely occur at the brain stem.

Neck

Compression

The dome of the skull is fairly strong and can absorb the impact of a collision; however, the cervical spine is much more flexible. The continued pressure from the momentum of the torso toward the stationary skull produces angulation or compression (**Figure 4-42**). Hyperextension or hyperflexion of the neck may result in fracture or dislocation of one or more vertebrae and injury to the spinal cord. The result can be jumped facets, fractures, spinal cord compression, or soft-tissue (ligament) injuries (**Figure 4-43**). Direct in-line compression crushes the bony vertebral bodies. Both angulation and in-line compression can result in an unstable spine.

Shear

The skull's center of gravity is anterior and cephalad to the point at which the skull attaches to the bony spine. Therefore, a lateral impact on the torso when the neck is unrestrained will produce lateral flexion and rotation of the neck (see Figure 4-24). Extreme flexion or hyperextension may also cause stretching injuries to the soft tissues of the neck.

Thorax

Compression

If the impact of a collision is centered on the anterior part of the chest, the sternum will receive the initial energy exchange. When the sternum stops moving, the posterior thoracic wall (muscles and thoracic spine) and the organs in the thoracic cavity continue to move forward until the organs strike and are compressed against the sternum.

The continued forward motion of the posterior thorax bends the ribs. If the tensile strength of the ribs is exceeded, fractured ribs and a flail chest can develop (see Chapter 10, *Thoracic Trauma*; **Figure 4-44**). Flexion injury with resultant compression or burst fracture to the thoracolumbar spine can occur. This injury is similar to what happens when a vehicle stops suddenly against a dirt embankment (see Figure 4-3). The frame of the vehicle bends, which absorbs some of the energy. The rear of the vehicle continues to move forward until the bending of the frame absorbs all the energy. In the same way, the posterior thoracic wall continues to move until the ribs absorb all the energy.

Compression of the chest wall is common with frontal and lateral impacts and produces an interesting phenomenon called the "paper bag effect," which may result in a pneumothorax. A victim instinctively takes a deep breath and holds it just before impact. This closes the glottis, effectively sealing off the lungs. With a significant energy exchange on impact and compression of the chest wall, the lungs may then burst, like a paper bag full of air that is popped (**Figure 4-45**). The lungs can also become compressed and contused, compromising ventilation.

Compression injuries of the internal structures of the thorax may include cardiac contusion, which occurs as the heart is compressed between the sternum and the spine and can result in significant dysrhythmias. Perhaps a more frequent injury is compression of the lungs

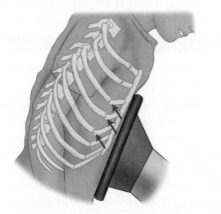
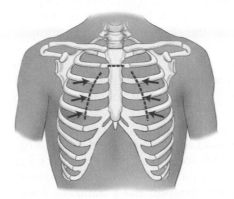

Figure 4-44 Ribs forced into the thoracic cavity by external compression usually fracture in multiple places, sometimes producing the clinical condition known as flail chest.

© National Association of Emergency Medical Technicians (NAEMT)

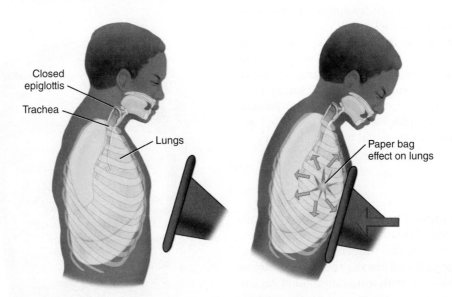

Closed epiglottis

Trachea

Lungs

Paper bag effect on lungs

Figure 4-45 Compression of the lung against a closed glottis, by impact on either the anterior or the lateral chest wall, produces an effect similar to compressing a paper bag when the opening is closed tightly by the hands. The paper bag ruptures, as does the lung.

© National Association of Emergency Medical Technicians (NAEMT)

leading to pulmonary contusion. Although the clinical consequences may develop over time, the patient may immediately lose the ability to properly ventilate. Pulmonary contusion can have consequences in the field for the prehospital care practitioner and for the physicians during resuscitation after arrival in the hospital. In situations in which long transport times are required, this condition can play a role en route.

Shear

The heart, ascending aorta, and aortic arch are relatively unrestrained within the thorax. The descending aorta, however, is tightly adherent to the posterior thoracic wall and the vertebral column. The resultant motion of the aorta is similar to holding the flexible tubes of a stethoscope just below where the rigid tubes from the earpiece end and swinging the acoustic head of the stethoscope from side to side. As the skeletal frame stops abruptly in a collision, the heart and the initial segment of the aorta continue their forward motion. The shear forces produced can tear the aorta at the junction of the portion that moves freely with the tightly bound portion (see Figure 4-14).

An aortic tear may result in an immediate, complete transection of the aorta followed by rapid exsanguination. Some aortic tears are partial, where one or more layers of tissue remain intact. However, the remaining layers are under great pressure, and a traumatic aneurysm can develop, similar to a bubble that forms on a weak part of a tire. The aneurysm can eventually rupture within minutes, hours, or days after the original injury. It is important that the prehospital care practitioner recognize the potential for such injuries and relay this information to the hospital personnel.

Shear injury can occur to the thoracolumbar spine resulting in fractures and fracture-dislocations that can be associated with neurologic compromise and may place the patient at risk for secondary neurologic injury with further motion. Similarly, excess extension anywhere along the thoracolumbar spine can produce unstable fracture(s) or dislocation with potential neurologic injury.

Abdomen

Compression

Internal organs compressed by the vertebral column into the steering wheel or dashboard during a frontal collision may rupture. The effect of this sudden increase in pressure is similar to the effect of placing the internal organ on an anvil and striking it with a hammer. Solid organs frequently injured in this manner include the spleen, liver, and kidneys.

Injury may also result from overpressure within the abdomen. The diaphragm is a ¼-inch-thick (5-mm-thick) muscle located across the top of the abdomen

that separates the abdominal cavity from the thoracic cavity. Its contraction causes the pleural cavity to expand for ventilation. The anterior abdominal wall comprises two layers of fascia and one very strong muscle. Laterally, there are three muscle layers with associated fascia, and the lumbar spine and its associated muscles provide strength to the posterior abdominal wall. The diaphragm is the weakest of all the walls and structures surrounding the abdominal cavity. It may be torn or ruptured as the intra-abdominal pressure increases (**Figure 4-46**). This injury has the following four common consequences:

- The "bellows" effect that is usually created by the diaphragm is lost, and ventilation is impaired.
- The abdominal organs can enter the thoracic cavity and reduce the space available for lung expansion.
- The displaced organs can become ischemic from compression of their blood supply.
- If intra-abdominal hemorrhage is present, the blood can also cause a hemothorax.

Another injury caused by increased abdominal pressure is from sudden retrograde blood flow up the aorta and against the aortic valve. This force against the valve can rupture it. This injury is rare but can occur when a collision with the steering wheel or involvement in another type of incident (e.g., ditch or tunnel cave-in) has produced a rapid increase in intra-abdominal pressure. This rapid pressure increase results in a sudden increase of aortic blood pressure. Blood is pushed back (retrograde) against the aortic valve with enough pressure to cause rupture of the valve cusps.

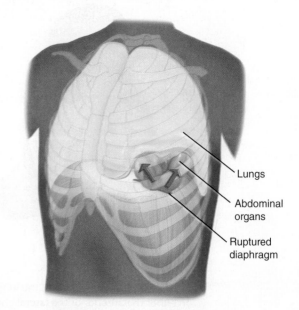

Lungs

Abdominal organs

Ruptured diaphragm

Figure 4-46 With increased pressure inside the abdomen, the diaphragm can rupture.

© National Association of Emergency Medical Technicians (NAEMT)

Shear

Injury to the abdominal organs occurs at their points of attachment to the mesentery. During a collision, the forward motion of the body stops, but the organs continue to move forward, causing tears at the points where the organs attach to the abdominal wall. If the organ is attached by a pedicle (a stalk of tissue), the tear can occur where the pedicle attaches to the organ, where it attaches to the abdominal wall, or anywhere along the length of the pedicle (see Figure 4-13). Organs that can shear in this manner are the kidneys, small intestine, large intestine, and spleen.

Another type of injury that often occurs during deceleration is laceration of the liver caused by its impact with the *ligamentum teres*. The liver is suspended from the diaphragm but is only minimally attached to the posterior abdomen near the lumbar vertebrae. The ligamentum teres attaches to the anterior abdominal wall at the umbilicus and to the left lobe of the liver in the midline of the body (the bulk of the liver is to the right of the midline). A down-and-under path in a frontal impact or a feet-first fall causes the liver to bring the diaphragm with it as it descends into the ligamentum teres (**Figure 4-47**). The ligamentum teres will fracture or transect the liver, analogous to pushing a cheese-cutting wire into a block of cheese.

Pelvic fractures are the result of damage to the external abdomen and may cause injury to the bladder or lacerations of the blood vessels in the pelvic cavity. Between 4% and 15% of patients with pelvic fractures also have a genitourinary injury.[24]

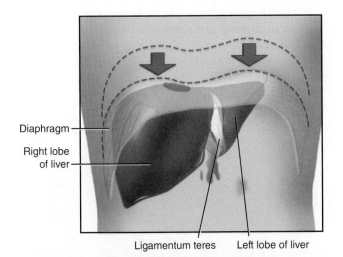

Figure 4-47 The liver is not supported by any fixed structure. Its major support is from the diaphragm, which moves freely. As the body travels in the down-and-under path, so does the liver. When the torso stops but the liver does not, the liver continues downward onto the ligamentum teres, tearing the liver. This is much like pushing a cheese-cutting wire into a block of cheese.

Diaphragm

Right lobe of liver

Ligamentum teres   Left lobe of liver

Pelvic fractures resulting from compression from the side, usually due to a lateral-impact collision, have two components. One is the compression of the proximal femur into the pelvis, which pushes the head of the femur into the acetabulum. This frequently produces fractures that involve the hip joint. Further compression of the femur and/or of the lateral walls of the pelvis produce compression fractures of the pelvic bones or the ring of the pelvis. Because a circular structure generally cannot be broken in only one place, there is typically a second fracture of the pelvis that occurs somewhere else along the pelvic ring.

The other type of compression fracture occurs anteriorly when the compression force is directly over the symphysis pubis. This force will either break the symphysis by pushing in on both sides or break one side and push it back toward the sacroiliac joint. This latter mechanism opens the joint, producing the so-called open-book fracture.

Shear fractures usually involve the ilium and the sacral area. This shearing force tears the joint open. Because joints in a ring, such as the pelvis, generally must be fractured in two places, frequently there will be a fracture somewhere else along the pelvic ring.

For more detailed information about pelvic fractures, Andrew Burgess and his coauthors have discussed these mechanisms of injury.[25]

Penetrating Trauma
Physics of Penetrating Trauma

The principles of physics discussed earlier are equally important when dealing with penetrating injuries. Again, the kinetic energy that a striking object transfers to body tissue is represented by the following formula:

$$KE = 1/2 \ (mv^2)$$

Energy can neither be created nor destroyed, but it can be transformed. This principle is important in understanding penetrating trauma. For example, although a lead bullet is in the brass cartridge casing that is filled with explosive powder, the bullet has no force. However, when the primer explodes, the powder burns, producing rapidly expanding gases that are transformed into force. The bullet then moves out of the gun and toward its target.

According to Newton's first law of motion, after this force has acted on the missile, the bullet will remain at that speed and force until it is acted on by an outside force. When the bullet hits something, such as a human body, it strikes the individual tissue cells. The energy (speed and mass) of the bullet's motion is exchanged for the energy that crushes these cells and moves them away (cavitation) from the path of the bullet:

$$\textbf{Mass} \times \textbf{Acceleration} = \textbf{Force} = \textbf{Mass} \times \textbf{Deceleration}$$

Factors That Affect the Size of the Frontal Area

The larger the frontal surface area of the moving missile, the greater the number of particles that will be hit—therefore, the greater the energy exchange that occurs and the larger the cavity that is created. The size of the frontal surface area of a projectile is influenced by three factors: profile, tumble, and fragmentation. Energy exchange or potential energy exchange can be analyzed based on these factors.

Profile

Profile describes an object's initial size and whether that size changes at the time of impact. The profile, or frontal area, of an ice pick is much smaller than that of a baseball bat, which, in turn, is much smaller than that of a truck. Of these three items, much less energy is required to pass the ice pick through a layer of tissue. A hollow-point bullet flattens and spreads on impact (**Box 4-4**). The larger the frontal area of a projectile traveling at a specific velocity with a specific mass, the more tissue cells are struck and a greater energy exchange occurs. As a result, a larger cavity forms and more injury occurs.

In general, a bullet should remain aerodynamic as it travels through the air en route to the target. Low resistance while passing through the air (hitting as few air particles as possible) is a good thing. It allows the bullet to maintain most of its speed. To avoid resistance, the frontal area is kept small, using a conical shape. A lot of drag (resistance to travel) is a bad thing. A good bullet design would have little drag while passing through the air but much more drag when passing through the body's tissues. If that missile strikes the skin and becomes deformed, covering a larger area and creating much more drag, then a much greater energy exchange from the bullet to the tissue will occur. Therefore, the ideal bullet is designed to keep its shape while in the air and deform only on impact.

Tumble

Tumble describes a situation in which the object turns over and over and assumes a different angle inside the body than the angle it assumed as it entered the body, thus creating more drag inside the body than in the air. A wedge-shaped bullet's center of gravity is located nearer to the base than to the nose of the bullet. When the nose of the bullet strikes something, it slows rapidly. Momentum continues to carry the base of the bullet forward, with the center of gravity seeking to become the leading point of the bullet. A slightly asymmetric shape causes an end-over-end motion, or tumble. As the bullet tumbles, the normally horizontal sides of the bullet become its leading edges, and strike many more particles than when the bullet was in the air (**Figure 4-48**). More energy exchange is produced, and therefore, greater tissue damage occurs.

Fragmentation

Fragmentation describes whether the object breaks up to produce multiple parts or rubble and, therefore, more drag and more energy exchange. There are two types of fragmentation rounds: (1) fragmentation on leaving the weapon (e.g., shotgun pellets) (**Figure 4-49**) and (2) fragmentation after entering the body. Fragmentation inside the body can be active or passive. Active fragmentation involves a bullet that has an explosive inside it that detonates inside the body. In contrast, bullets with soft noses or vertical cuts in the nose and safety slugs that contain many small fragments to increase body damage by breaking apart on impact are examples of passive fragmentation. The resulting mass of fragments creates a larger frontal area than a single solid bullet, and energy is dispersed rapidly into the tissue. If the missile shatters, it will

---

Box 4-4 Expanding Bullets

A munitions factory in Dum Dum, India, manufactured a bullet that expanded when it hit the skin. Ballistic experts recognized this design as one that would cause more damage than is necessary in war; therefore, these bullets were prohibited in military conflicts. The Petersburg Declaration of 1868 and the Hague Convention of 1899 affirmed this principle, denouncing these "Dum-Dum" projectiles and other expanding missiles, such as silver-tipped bullets, hollow-point bullets, scored-lead cartridges or jackets, and partially jacketed bullets, and outlawing their use in war.

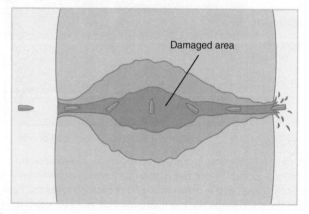

Figure 4-48 The tumble motion of a missile maximizes its damage at 90 degrees.

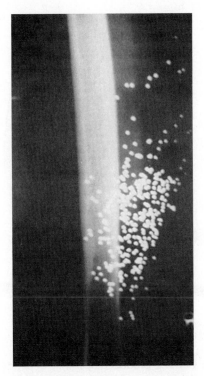

Figure 4-49 Shotgun pellets disperse upon exiting the weapon resulting in fragmentation. Maximum damage is inflicted at close range when fragmentation is least.

© National Association of Emergency Medical Technicians (NAEMT)

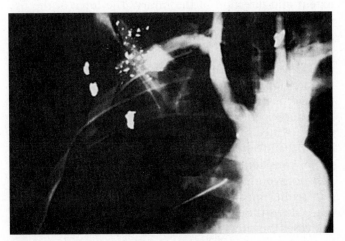

Figure 4-50 Bullet fragmentation that occurs on impact increases the frontal projection of the missile and distributes injury over a larger portion of the body.

Courtesy of Norman McSwain, MD, FACS, NREMT-P.

spread out over a wider area, with two results: (1) more tissue particles will be struck by the larger frontal projection, and (2) the injuries will be distributed over a larger portion of the body because more organs will be struck (**Figure 4-50**). The multiple pieces of shot from a shotgun blast produce similar results. Shotgun wounds are an excellent example of the fragmentation injury pattern.

Damage and Energy Levels

Knowing the energy capacity of a penetrating object helps to predict the damage caused in a penetrating injury. Weapons that cause penetrating injuries can be categorized by their energy capacity as low-, medium-, and high-energy weapons.

Low-Energy Weapons

Low-energy weapons include hand-driven weapons such as a knife or an ice pick. These weapons produce damage only with their sharp points or cutting edges. Because these are low-velocity injuries, they are usually associated with less secondary trauma (i.e., less cavitation will occur). Injury in these patients can be predicted by tracing the path of the weapon into the body. If the weapon has been removed, the prehospital care practitioner should try to identify the type of weapon used, if time permits.

The trajectory of the knife may be a reflection of the position of the attacker's hand on the knife handle. If the attacker grasps the weapon with the thumb on the top, the trajectory will be upward. If the grasp is with the small finger on top, the resultant trajectory is downward (**Figure 4-51**).

An attacker may stab a victim and then move the knife around inside the body. A simple-appearing entrance wound may produce a false sense of security. The entrance wound may be small, but the damage inside may be extensive. The potential scope of the movement of the inserted blade is an area of possible damage (**Figure 4-52**).

Evaluation of the patient for associated injury is important. For example, the diaphragm can reach as high as the nipple line on deep expiration. A stab wound to the lower chest can injure intra-abdominal as well as intra-thoracic structures, and a wound of the upper abdomen may involve the lower chest.

Penetrating trauma can result from impaled objects such as fence posts and street signs in vehicle crashes and falls, ski poles in snow sports, and handlebar injuries in bicycling.

Medium-Energy and High-Energy Weapons

Firearms fall into two groups: medium energy and high energy. Medium-energy weapons include handguns and some rifles whose muzzle velocity is 1,000 feet per second (ft/sec) (305 m/sec). The temporary cavity created by this weapon is three to five times the caliber of the bullet. High-energy weapons have muzzle velocity in excess of 2,000 ft/sec (610 m/sec) and significantly greater muzzle energy. They create a temporary cavity that is 25 or more times the caliber of the bullet. As the amount of

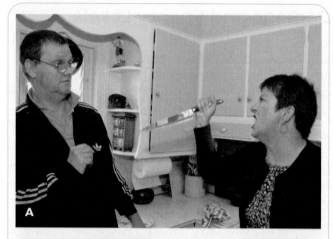

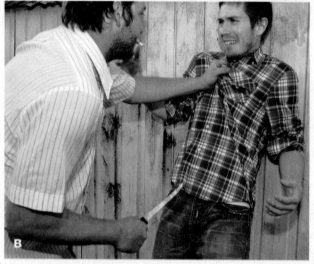

Figure 4-51 The trajectory of the knife is determined by the position of the hand on the handle. **A.** If the fingers are on the top of the handle, a downward trajectory results. **B.** If the thumb is on the top, the trajectory is upward.

© National Association of Emergency Medical Technicians (NAEMT)

gunpowder in the cartridge increases and the size of the bullet increases, the speed and mass of the bullet and, therefore, its kinetic energy increase (**Figure 4-53**). The mass of the bullet is an important, but smaller, contributor to the kinetic energy imparted than is the velocity ($KE = \frac{1}{2}[mv^2]$).

However, the bullet mass should not be discounted. In the American Civil War, the Kentucky long rifle 0.55-caliber Minié ball had almost the same muzzle energy as the modern M16 rifle. The mass of the missile becomes more important when considering the damage produced by a 12-gauge shotgun at close range or an IED.

In general, medium-energy and high-energy weapons damage not only the tissue directly in the path of the missile but also the tissue involved in the temporary cavity on each side of the missile's path. The variables of missile profile, tumble, and fragmentation influence

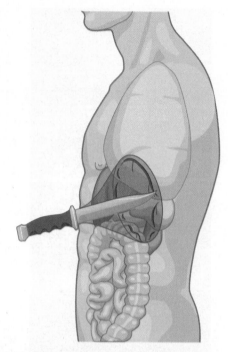

Figure 4-52 Damage produced by a knife depends on the movement of the blade inside the victim.

© National Association of Emergency Medical Technicians (NAEMT)

the rapidity of the energy exchange and, therefore, the extent and direction of the injury. The force of the tissue particles moved out of the direct path of the missile compresses and stretches the surrounding tissue (**Figure 4-54**).

High-energy weapons discharge high-velocity missiles (**Figure 4-55**). Tissue damage is much more extensive with a high-energy penetrating object than it is from a medium-energy penetrating object. The vacuum created in the cavity created by a high-speed missile can pull clothing, bacteria, and other debris from the surface into the wound.

A consideration in predicting the damage from a gunshot wound is the range or distance from which the gun (either medium or high energy) is fired. Air resistance slows the bullet; therefore, increasing the distance decreases the energy at the time of impact and will result in less injury. Most shootings with handguns are done at close range, so the probability of serious injury is related to both the anatomy involved and the energy of the weapon rather than loss of kinetic energy.

High-Energy Weapons

Cavitation

The unusual injury pattern of an AK-47 is described by Fackler and Malinowski. Because of its eccentricity, the bullet tumbles and travels at almost a right angle to the area of entrance. During this tumbling action, the rotation carries it over and over so that there are two or sometimes

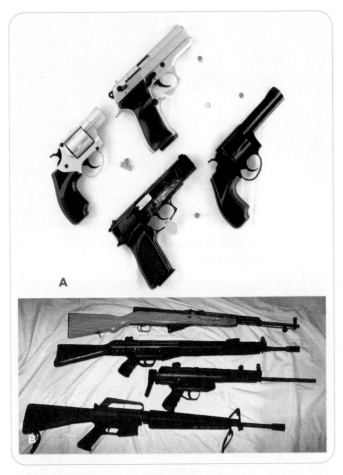

Figure 4-53 A. Medium-energy weapons are usually guns that have short barrels and contain cartridges with less power. **B.** High-energy weapons.

A. © National Association of Emergency Medical Technicians (NAEMT). B. Courtesy of Norman McSwain, MD, FACS, NREMT-P.

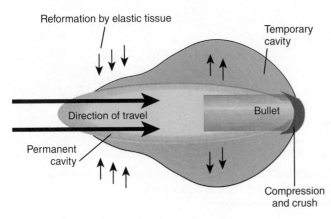

Figure 4-54 A bullet crushes tissues directly in its path. A cavity is created in the wake of the bullet. The crushed part is permanent. The temporary expansion also produces injury.

© National Association of Emergency Medical Technicians (NAEMT)

even three (depending on how long the bullet stays in the body) cavitations.[26] The very high energy exchange produces the cavitation and a significant amount of damage.

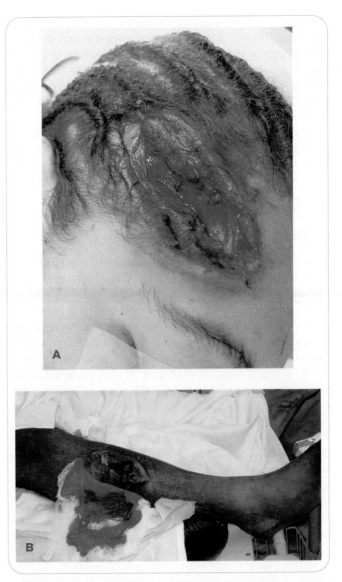

Figure 4-55 A. Graze wound to the scalp created by a projectile from a high-velocity weapon. The skull was not fractured. **B.** High-velocity gunshot wound to the leg demonstrating the large, permanent cavity.

Courtesy of Norman McSwain, MD, FACS, NREMT-P.

The size of the permanent cavity is associated with the elasticity in the tissue struck by the missile. For example, if the same bullet going the same speed penetrates muscle or the liver, the result is very different. Muscle has much more elasticity and will expand and return to a relatively small permanent cavity. The liver, however, has little elasticity; it develops fracture lines and a much larger permanent cavity than is produced by the same energy exchange in muscle.[27,28]

Fragmentation

The combination of a high-energy weapon with fragmentation can produce significant damage. If the high-energy missile fragments on impact (many do not), the initial entrance site may be large and may involve significant soft-tissue injury. If the bullet fragments when it hits a hard structure in the body (such as bone), a large cavitation occurs at this impact point, and the bony fragments themselves become part of the damage-producing component. Significant destruction to the bone and nearby organs and vessels may result.[26]

Emil Theodor Kocher, a surgeon living in the latter part of the 19th century, was extremely active in the understanding of ballistics and the damage produced by the weapons. He was a strong advocate of not using the "Dum-Dum" bullet.[29]

Entrance and Exit Wounds

Tissue damage occurs at the site of missile entry into the body, along the path of the penetrating object, and upon exit from the body. Knowledge of the victim's position, the attacker's position, and the weapon used is helpful in determining the path of injury. If the entrance wound and the exit wound can be related, the anatomic structures that would likely be in this path can be approximated.

Evaluating wound sites provides valuable information to direct the management of the patient and to relay to the receiving facility. Do two holes in the victim's abdomen indicate that a single missile entered and exited or that two missiles entered and are both still inside the patient? Did the missile cross the midline (usually causing more severe injury) or remain on the same side? In what direction did the missile travel? What internal organs are likely to have been in its path?

Entrance and exit wounds usually, but not always, produce identifiable injury patterns to soft tissue. Evaluation of the apparent trajectory of a penetrating object is helpful to the clinician. This information should be given to the physicians in the hospital. That said, prehospital care practitioners (and most physicians) do not have the experience or the expertise of a forensic pathologist; therefore, the assessment of which wound is an entrance wound and which is an exit wound is fraught with uncertainty. Such information is intended solely to assist in patient care to try to gauge the trajectory of the missile and not for legal purposes to determine specifics about the incident. These two issues should not be confused. Prehospital care practitioners must have as much information as possible to determine the potential injuries sustained by the patient and to best decide how the patient should be managed. The legal issues related to the specifics of entrance and exit wounds are best left to others.

An entrance wound from a gunshot lies against the underlying tissue, but an exit wound has no support. The former is typically a round or oval wound, depending on the entry path, and the latter is usually a **stellate (starburst) wound** (**Figure 4-56**). Because the missile

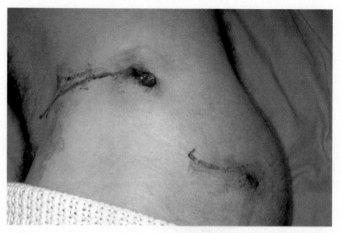

Figure 4-56 An entrance wound is round or oval in shape, and an exit wound is often stellate or linear.
© Mediscan/Alamy Stock Photo

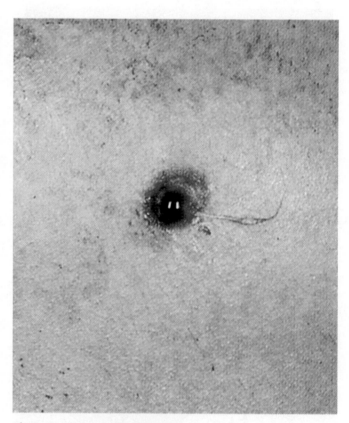

Figure 4-57 The abraded edge indicates that the bullet traveled from top right to bottom left.
Courtesy of Norman McSwain, MD, FACS, NREMT-P.

is spinning as it enters the skin, it leaves a small, pink area of abrasion (1 to 2 mm in size) (**Figure 4-57** and **Figure 4-58**). Abrasion is not present on the exit side. If the muzzle was placed directly against the skin at the time of discharge, the expanding gases will enter the tissue and produce crepitus on examination (**Figure 4-59**). If the muzzle is within 2 to 3 inches (5 to 7 cm), the

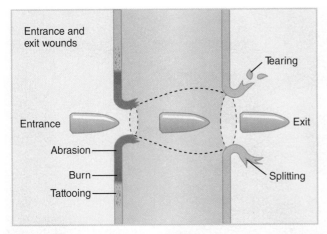

Figure 4-58 Spin and compression of the bullet on entrance produce round or oval holes. On exit, the wound is pressed open.

© National Association of Emergency Medical Technicians (NAEMT)

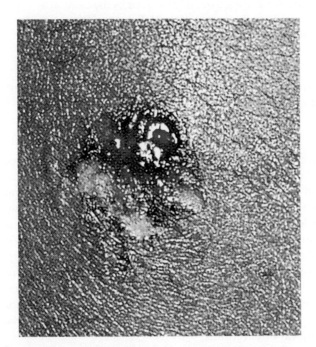

Figure 4-59 Hot gases coming from the end of a muzzle held in proximity to the skin produce partial-thickness and full-thickness burns on the skin.

Courtesy of Norman McSwain, MD, FACS, NREMT-P.

hot gases that exit will burn the skin; at 2 to 6 inches (5 to 15 cm) the smoke will adhere to the skin; and inside 10 inches (25 cm) the burning cordite particles will tattoo the skin with small (1- to 2-mm) burned areas.

Regional Effects of Penetrating Trauma

This section discusses the injuries sustained by various parts of the body during penetrating trauma.

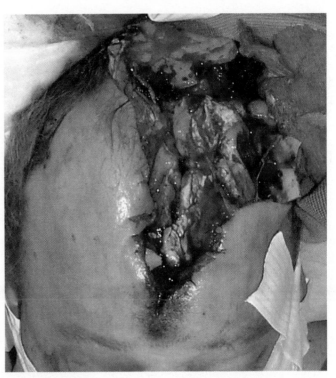

Figure 4-60 After a missile penetrates the skull, its energy is distributed within a closed space. It is like putting a firecracker in a closed container. If the forces are strong enough, the container (the skull) may explode from the inside out.

Courtesy of Norman McSwain, MD, FACS, NREMT-P.

Head

After a missile penetrates the skull, its energy is distributed within a closed space. Particles accelerating away from the missile are forced against the unyielding skull, which cannot expand as can skin, muscle, or even the abdomen. Thus, the brain tissue is compressed against the inside of the skull, producing more injury than would otherwise occur if it could expand freely. It is similar to putting a firecracker in an apple and then placing the apple in a metal can. When the firecracker explodes, the apple will be destroyed against the wall of the can. In the case of a missile penetrating the skull, if the forces are strong enough, the skull may explode from the inside out (**Figure 4-60**).

A bullet may follow the curvature of the interior of the skull if it enters at an angle and has insufficient force to exit the skull. This path can produce significant damage (**Figure 4-61**). Because of this characteristic, small-caliber, medium-velocity weapons, such as the 0.22-caliber or 0.25-caliber pistol, have been called the "assassin's weapon." They go in and exchange all of their energy into the brain.

Thorax

Three major groups of structures are inside the thoracic cavity: the pulmonary system, vascular system, and

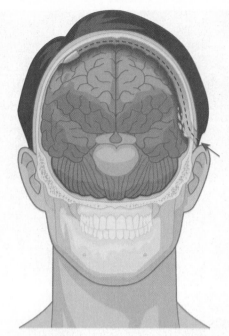

Figure 4-61 The bullet may follow the curvature of the skull.
© National Association of Emergency Medical Technicians (NAEMT)

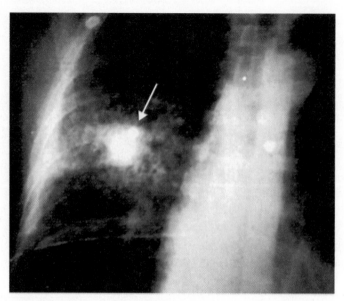

Figure 4-62 Lung damage produced by the cavity at a distance from the point of impact. The arrow shows a bullet fragment.
Courtesy of Norman McSwain, MD, FACS, NREMT-P.

gastrointestinal tract. The bones and muscles of the chest wall and spine make up the outer structure of the thorax. One or more of the anatomic structures of these systems may be injured by a penetrating object.

Pulmonary System

Lung tissue is less dense than blood, solid organs, or bone; therefore, a penetrating object will hit fewer particles, exchange less energy, and do less damage to lung tissue. Damage to the lungs can be clinically significant (**Figure 4-62**), but fewer than 15% of patients will require surgical exploration.[30]

Vascular System

Smaller vessels that are not attached to the chest wall may be pushed aside without significant damage. However, larger vessels, such as the aorta and venae cavae, are less mobile because they are tethered to the spine or the heart. They cannot move aside easily and are more susceptible to damage.

The myocardium (almost totally muscle) stretches as the bullet passes through and then contracts, leaving a smaller defect. The thickness of the muscle may control the bleeding from a low-energy penetration, such as by a knife, or even a small, medium-energy 0.22-caliber bullet. This closure can prevent immediate exsanguination and allow time to transport the victim to an appropriate facility.

Gastrointestinal Tract

The **esophagus**, the part of the gastrointestinal tract that traverses the thoracic cavity, can be penetrated and can leak its contents into the thoracic cavity. The signs and symptoms of such an injury may be delayed for several hours or several days.

Abdomen

The abdomen contains structures of three types: air filled, solid, and bony. Penetration by a low-energy missile may not cause significant damage; only 30% of knife wounds penetrating the abdominal cavity require surgical exploration to repair damage. A medium-energy injury (e.g., handgun wound) is more damaging; most require surgical repair. However, in injuries caused by medium-energy missiles, the damage to solid and vascular structures frequently does not produce immediate exsanguination. This enables prehospital care practitioners to transport the patient to an appropriate facility in time for effective surgical intervention.

Extremities

Penetrating injuries to the extremities can include damage to bones, muscles, nerves, or vessels. When bones are hit, bony fragments become secondary missiles, lacerating surrounding tissue (**Figure 4-63**). Muscles often expand away from the path of the missile, causing hemorrhage. The missile may penetrate blood vessels, or a near miss may damage the lining of a blood vessel, causing clotting and obstruction of the vessel within minutes or hours.

Shotgun Wounds

Although shotguns are not high-velocity weapons, they are high-energy weapons, and, at close range, they can

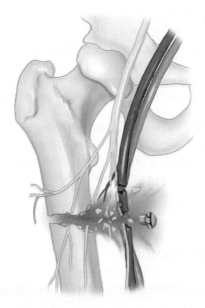

Figure 4-63 Bone fragments become secondary missiles themselves, producing damage by the same mechanism as the original penetrating object.
© National Association of Emergency Medical Technicians (NAEMT)

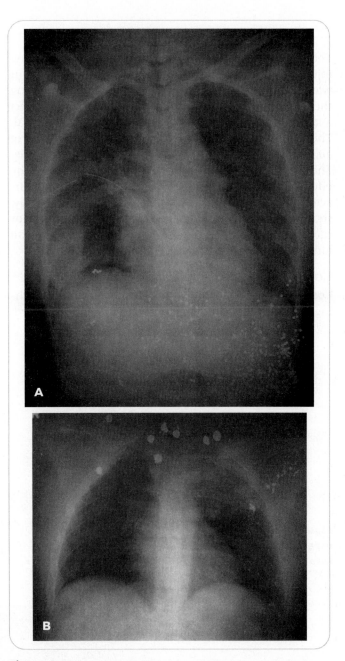

Figure 4-64 A. An average birdshot shell may contain 200 to 2,000 pellets. **B.** A buckshot shell may contain 6 to 20 pellets.
Courtesy of Norman McSwain, MD, FACS, NREMT-P.

be more lethal than some of the highest energy rifles. Handguns and rifles predominantly use **rifling** (grooves) on the inside of the barrel to spin a single missile in a flight pattern toward the target. In contrast, most shotguns possess a smooth, cylindrical-tube barrel that directs a load of missiles in the direction of the target. Devices known as **chokes** and **diverters** can be attached to the end of a shotgun barrel to shape and form the column of missiles into specific patterns (e.g., cylindrical or rectangular). Regardless, when a shotgun is fired, a large number of missiles are ejected in a **spread**, or **spray**, pattern. The barrels may be shortened ("sawed off") to prematurely widen the trajectory of the missiles.

Although shotguns may use various types of ammunition, the structure of most shotgun shells is similar. A typical shotgun shell contains gunpowder, wadding, and projectiles. When discharged, all of these components are propelled from the muzzle and can inflict injury on the victim. Certain types of gunpowder can **stipple** ("tattoo") the skin in close-range injuries. Wadding, which is usually lubricated paper, fibers, or plastic used to separate the shot (missiles) from the charge of gunpowder, can provide another source of infection in the wound if not removed. The missiles can vary in size, weight, and composition. A wide variety of missiles are available, from compressed metal powders to *birdshot* (small metal pellets), *buckshot* (larger metal pellets), *slugs* (a single metal missile), and, more recently, plastic and rubber alternatives. The average shell is loaded with 1 to 1.5 ounces (28 to 43 g) of shot. Fillers that are placed within the shot (polyethylene or polypropylene

granules) can become embedded in the superficial layers of the skin.

An average birdshot shell may contain 200 to 2,000 pellets, whereas a buckshot shell may contain 6 to 20 pellets (**Figure 4-64**). It is important to note that as the size of the pellets increases, they approach the wounding characteristics of 0.22-caliber missiles in regard to effective range and energy transfer characteristics. Larger, or *magnum* shells are also available. These shells may contain more shot and a larger charge of gunpowder or only the larger powder charge to boost the muzzle velocity.

Categories of Shotgun Wounds

The type of ammunition used is important in gauging injuries, but the range (distance) at which the patient was shot is the most important variable when evaluating the shotgun-injury victim (**Figure 4-65**). Shotguns eject a large number of missiles, most of which are spherical. These projectiles are especially susceptible to the effects of air resistance, quickly slowing once they exit the muzzle. The effect of air resistance on the projectiles decreases the effective range of the weapon and changes the basic characteristics of the wounds that it generates. Consequently, shotgun wounds have been classified into four major categories: contact, close-range, intermediate-range, and long-range wounds (**Figure 4-66**).

Contact Wounds

Contact wounds occur when the muzzle is touching the victim at the time the weapon is discharged.

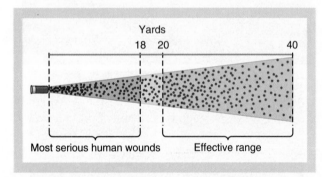

Figure 4-65 The diameter of the spread of a shot column expands as range increases.

Data from DeMuth WE Jr. The mechanism of shotgun wounds. *J Trauma.* 1971;11:219–229; Sherman RT, Parrish RA. Management of shotgun injuries: a review of 152 cases. *J Trauma.* 1963;3:76–86.

Discharge at this range typically results in circular entrance wounds, which may or may not have soot or an imprint of the muzzle. Searing or burning of the wound edges is common, secondary to the high temperatures and the expansion of hot gases as the missiles exit the muzzle (see Figure 4-59). Some contact wounds may be more stellate in appearance, caused by the superheated gases from the barrel escaping from the tissue. Contact wounds usually result in widespread tissue damage and are associated with high mortality. The length of a standard shotgun barrel makes it difficult to commit suicide with this weapon because it is difficult to reach and pull the trigger. Such attempts usually result in a split face without the shot reaching the brain.

Close-Range Wounds

Close-range wounds (less than 6 ft [1.8 m]), although still typically characterized by circular entrance wounds, will likely have more evidence of soot, gunpowder, or filler stippling around the wound margins than contact wounds. Additionally, abrasions and markings from the impact of the wadding that coincide with the wounds from the missiles may be found. Close-range wounds create significant damage in the patient; missiles fired from this range retain sufficient energy to penetrate deep structures and exhibit a slightly wider spread pattern. This pattern increases the extent of injury as missiles travel through soft tissue.

Intermediate-Range Wounds

Intermediate-range wounds are characterized by the appearance of satellite pellet holes emerging from the border around a central entrance wound. This pattern is a result of individual pellets spreading from the main column of shot and generally occurs at a range of 6 to 18 ft

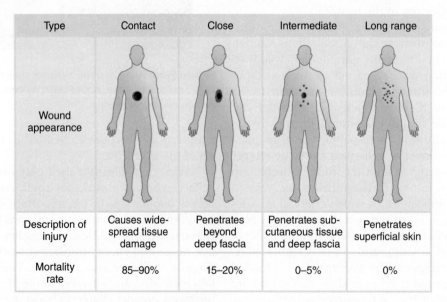

Type	Contact	Close	Intermediate	Long range
Wound appearance				
Description of injury	Causes widespread tissue damage	Penetrates beyond deep fascia	Penetrates subcutaneous tissue and deep fascia	Penetrates superficial skin
Mortality rate	85–90%	15–20%	0–5%	0%

Figure 4-66 Patterns of shotgun injury.

© Jones & Bartlett Learning

(1.8 to 5.5 m). These injuries are a mixture of deep, penetrating wounds and superficial wounds and abrasions. Because of the deep, penetrating components of this injury, however, mortality rate for victims with mixed wound patterns may be similar to that of close-range injuries.

Long-Range Wounds

Long-range wounds are rarely lethal. These wounds are typically characterized by the classic spread of scattered pellet wounds and result from a range of greater than 18 ft (5.5 m). However, even at these slower velocities, the pellets can cause significant damage to certain sensitive tissues (e.g., eyes). In addition, larger buckshot pellets can retain sufficient velocity to inflict damage to deep structures, even at long range. The prehospital care practitioner needs to consider the cumulative effects of many small missile wounds and their locations, focusing on sensitive tissues. *Adequate exposure* is essential when examining patients involved in trauma, and shotgun injuries are no exception.

Assessment of Shotgun Wounds

These varying characteristics need to be taken into account when evaluating injury patterns in patients with shotgun injuries. For example, a single circular shotgun wound could represent a contact or close-range injury with birdshot or buckshot in which the missiles have retained a tight column or grouping. Conversely, this may represent an intermediate-range to long-range injury with a slug or solitary missile. Only detailed examination of the wound will allow differentiation of these injuries, which can involve significant damage to internal structures despite strikingly different missile characteristics.

Contact and close-range wounds to the chest may result in a large, visually impressive wound resulting in an open pneumothorax, and bowel may eviscerate from such wounds to the abdomen. On occasion, a single pellet from an intermediate-range wound may penetrate deep enough to perforate the bowel, leading eventually to peritonitis, or may damage a major artery, resulting in vascular compromise to an extremity or organ. Alternatively, a patient who exhibits multiple small wounds in a spread pattern may have dozens of entrance wounds. However, none of the missiles may have retained enough energy to penetrate through fascia, let alone produce significant damage to internal structures.

Although immediate patient care must always remain the priority, any information (e.g., shell type, suspected range of the patient from the weapon, number of shots fired) that prehospital care practitioners can gather from the scene and relay to the receiving facility can assist with appropriate diagnostic evaluation and treatment of the shotgun-injured patient. Furthermore, recognition of various wound types can aid practitioners in maintaining a high index of suspicion for internal injury regardless of the initial impression of the injury.

Blast Injuries

Injury From Explosions

Explosive devices are the most frequently used weapons in combat and by terrorists. Explosive devices cause human injury by multiple mechanisms, some of which are exceedingly complex. The greatest challenges for clinicians at all levels of care in the aftermath of an explosion are the large numbers of casualties and the presence of multiple penetrating injuries (**Figure 4-67**).[31]

Physics of Blast

Explosions are physical, chemical, or nuclear reactions that result in the almost instantaneous release of large amounts of energy in the form of heat and rapidly expanding, highly compressed gas, capable of projecting fragments at extremely high velocities. The energy associated with an explosion can take multiple forms: kinetic and heat energy in the **blast wave**, kinetic energy of fragments formed by the breakup of the weapon casing and surrounding debris, and electromagnetic energy.

Blast waves can travel at greater than 16,400 ft/sec (5,000 m/sec) and are composed of static and dynamic components. The static component (**blast overpressure**) surrounds objects in the flow field of the explosion, loading them on all sides with a discontinuous rise in pressure called the **shock front** or **shock wave**, up to a **peak overpressure value**. Following the shock front, the overpressure drops down to ambient pressure, and then a partial vacuum is often formed as a result of air being sucked back (**Figure 4-68**). The dynamic component (**dynamic pressure**) is directional and is experienced as

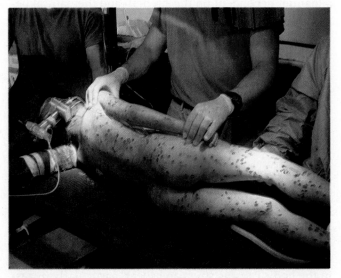

Figure 4-67 Patient with multiple fragment wounds from a bomb blast.

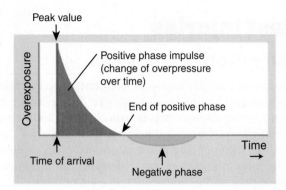

Figure 4-68 Pressure–time history of a blast wave. This graph shows the sudden massive increase in pressure (blast overpressure) following the decrease in pressure and negative pressure phase.

From Federal Emergency Management Agency. Primer to Design Safe School Projects in Case of Terrorist Attacks: Providing Protection to People and Buildings. Author; 2003:Chapter 4. https://www.fema.gov/pdf/plan/prevent/rms/428/fema428_ch4.pdf

a **blast wind**. The primary significance of the blast wind is that it propels fragments at speeds in excess of several thousand meters per second (faster than standard ballistic weapons such as bullets and shells).[32] Whereas the effective range of both the static and dynamic pressure is measured in tens of feet, the fragments accelerated by the dynamic pressure will quickly outpace the blast wave to become the dominant cause of injury out to ranges of thousands of feet.

Interaction of Blast Waves With the Body

Blast waves interact with the body and other structures by transmitting energy from the blast wave into the structure. This energy causes the structure to deform in a manner dependent on the strength and the natural period of oscillation of the structure being affected. Changing density interfaces within a structure cause complex re-formations, convergences, and couplings of the transmitted blast waves. Such interactions can be seen particularly in large-density interfaces such as solid tissue to air or liquid (e.g., lung, heart, liver, and bowel).

Explosion-Related Injuries

Injuries from explosions are generally classified as primary, secondary, tertiary, quaternary, and quinary after the injury taxonomy described in Department of Defense Directive 6025.21E24 (**Table 4-1**). Detonation of an explosive device sets off a chain of interactions in the objects and people in its path.[30] If an individual is close enough, the initial blast wave increases pressure in the body, causing stress and shear, particularly in gas-filled organs such as the ears, lungs, and (rarely) bowels.

Morbidity and mortality associated with primary blast injury decrease as the distance from the blast location increases and is proportionate to the magnitude of the explosive force (**Figure 4-69**). These primary blast injuries are more prevalent when the explosion occurs in an enclosed space because the blast wave bounces off surfaces, thus enhancing the destructive potential of the pressure waves.[33]

Immediate death from pulmonary barotrauma (blast lung) occurs more often in enclosed-space than in open-air bombings.[29-36] Most (95%) blast injuries in Iraq and Afghanistan have resulted from open-space explosions.[37]

The most common form of primary blast injury is tympanic membrane rupture.[38,39] Tympanic membrane rupture, which may occur at pressures as low as 5 pounds per square inch (psi; 35 kilopascals [kPa]),[38-40] is often the only significant overpressure injury experienced. The next major injury occurs at less than 40 psi (276 kPa), a threshold known to be associated with pulmonary injuries, including pneumothorax, air embolism, interstitial and subcutaneous emphysema, and pneumomediastinum.[41] Data from burned soldiers from Operation Iraqi Freedom confirm that tympanic membrane rupture is not predictive of lung injury.

The shock front of the blast wave quickly dissipates and is followed by the blast wind, which propels fragments to create multiple penetrating injuries. Although these injuries are termed *secondary*, they are usually the predominant wounding agent.[42] The blast wind also propels large objects into people or people onto hard surfaces (whole or partial body translocation), creating blunt (tertiary blast) injuries. This category of injury includes crush injuries caused by structural collapse.[41] Heat, flames, gas, and smoke generated during explosions cause quaternary injuries that include burns and toxicity from fuel, inhalation injury, and asphyxiation.[42] Quinary injuries are produced when bacteria, chemicals, radioactive materials, or projectiles are added to the explosive device and released upon detonation.

Injury From Fragments

Conventional explosive weapons are designed to maximize damage caused by fragments. With initial velocities of many thousands of feet per second, the distance that fragments may be thrown for a 50-lb (23-kg) bomb will be well over 1,000 ft (0.3 km), whereas the lethal radius of the blast overpressure is approximately 50 ft (15 m). The developers of both military and terrorist weapons, therefore, design weapons to maximize fragmentation injury to significantly increase the damage radius of a free-field explosive.

Few explosive devices cause injury solely by blast overpressure, and serious primary blast injury is relatively rare compared to the predominant numbers of

Table 4-1 Blast Injury Categories

Category	Description	Typical Injuries
Primary	▪ Produced by contact of blast shock wave with body ▪ Stress and shear waves occur in tissues ▪ Waves reinforced/reflected at tissue density interfaces ▪ Gas-filled organs (lungs, bowel, ears, etc.) at particular risk	▪ Tympanic membrane rupture ▪ Blast lung/pulmonary barotrauma ▪ Eye injuries ▪ Concussion ▪ Abdominal hemorrhage

Secondary	▪ Ballistic wounds produced by:
	  · Primary fragments (pieces of exploding weapon)
	  · Secondary fragments (environmental fragments [e.g., glass])
	▪ Threat of fragment injury extends farther than that from blast wave
		▪ Penetrating injuries
		▪ Traumatic amputations
		▪ Lacerations
		▪ Closed or open head injuries

Tertiary	▪ Blast wave propels individuals onto surfaces/objects or objects onto individuals, causing whole body translocation ▪ Crush injuries caused by structural damage or building collapse	▪ Blunt injuries ▪ Crush syndrome ▪ Compartment syndrome ▪ Fractures
Quaternary	▪ Other explosion-related injuries, illnesses, or diseases	▪ Burns ▪ Toxic gas and other inhalation injury ▪ Injury or infection from environmental contamination
Quinary	▪ Injuries resulting from specific additives such as bacteria, chemicals, and radiation ("dirty bombs")	▪ Chemical burns ▪ Bacterial infections ▪ Radiation exposure

Data from Pennardt A. Blast injuries. *Medscape*. Updated August 6, 2021. Accessed October 26, 2021. https://emedicine.medscape.com/article/822587-overview; U.S. Department of Defense, Blast Injury Research Coordinating Office. Blast Injury 101. June 18, 2019. Accessed October 26, 2021. https://blastinjuryresearch.amedd.army.mil/index.cfm/blast_injury_101; Department of Defense. Taxonomy of Injuries from Explosive Devices. Department of Defense Directive (DoDD) 6025.21E. Accessed October 26, 2021. https://www.esd.whs.mil/Portals/54/Documents/DD/issuances/dodd/602521p.pdf?ver=2018-10-24-112151-983; National Association of Emergency Medical Technicians. *PHTLS: Prehospital Trauma Life Support*. Military 9th ed. Jones & Bartlett Learning; 2021.

secondary and tertiary injuries. Thus, few patients have injuries dominated by primary blast effects. The entire array of explosion-related injuries is often referred to en masse as "blast injuries," leading to major confusion regarding what constitutes a blast injury. Because energy from the blast wave dissipates rapidly, most explosive devices are constructed to cause damage primarily from fragments. These may be primary fragments generated through the breakup of the casing surrounding the explosive device or secondary fragments created from debris in the surrounding environment. Regardless of whether the fragments are created from shattered munitions casing,

flying debris, or embedded objects that terrorists often pack into homemade bombs, they exponentially increase the range and lethality of explosives and are the primary cause of explosion-related injury.

Multi-etiology Injury

In addition to the direct effects of an explosion, prehospital care practitioners must be mindful of the other causes of injury from attacks with explosions. For instance, an IED that targets a vehicle may result in minimal initial damage to the vehicle occupants. However, the vehicle

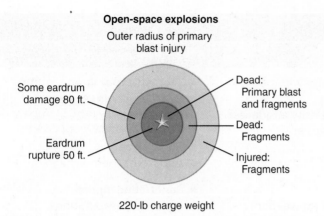

Open-space explosions
Outer radius of primary blast injury

Some eardrum damage 80 ft.

Eardrum rupture 50 ft.

Dead: Primary blast and fragments

Dead: Fragments

Injured: Fragments

220-lb charge weight

Figure 4-69 Morbidity and mortality as a function of distance from open-space detonation of a 220-lb (100-kg) explosive.
© National Association of Emergency Medical Technicians (NAEMT)

Using the Physics of Trauma in Assessment

The assessment of a trauma patient must involve knowledge of the physics of trauma. For example, a driver who hits the steering wheel (blunt trauma) will have a large cavity in the anterior chest at the time of impact; however, the chest rapidly returns to, or near to, its original shape as the driver rebounds from the steering wheel. If two prehospital care practitioners examine the patient separately—one who understands the physics of trauma and another who does not—the one without knowledge of the physics of trauma will be concerned only with the bruise visible on the patient's chest. The practitioner who understands the physics of trauma will recognize that a large cavity was present at the time of impact, that the ribs had to bend in for the cavity to form, and that the heart, lungs, and great vessels were compressed by the formation of the cavity. Therefore, the knowledgeable practitioner will suspect injury to the heart, lungs, great vessels, and chest wall. The other practitioner will not be aware of these possibilities.

The knowledgeable prehospital care practitioner, suspecting serious intrathoracic injuries, will assess for these potential injuries, manage the patient, and initiate transport more aggressively, rather than react to what would otherwise appear to be a minor closed soft-tissue injury. Early identification, adequate understanding, and appropriate treatment of underlying injury will significantly influence whether a patient lives or dies.

itself may be displaced vertically or vectored off course resulting in occupant blunt trauma from collision, from flipping upside down as part of the vertical displacement process, or from rollover, for instance, down an embankment or culvert. In these circumstances, occupants sustain injury based on the mechanisms previously described for blunt trauma.

In the military setting, a vehicle's occupants may be afforded some protection from blunt injury by virtue of their body armor. Furthermore, the occupants of a vehicle that is disabled following an IED attack are subject to ambush and may be attacked with gunfire as they exit the vehicle, thus potentially becoming victims of penetrating injury.

SUMMARY

- Integrating the principles of the physics of trauma into the assessment of the trauma patient is key to discovering the potential for severe or life-threatening injuries.
- Most injuries can be anticipated by understanding the energy exchange that occurs with the human body at the time of a collision. Knowledge of the physics of trauma allows for injuries that are not immediately apparent to be identified and treated appropriately. Left unsuspected, undetected, and therefore untreated, these injuries can contribute significantly to morbidity and mortality resulting from trauma.
- Energy can be neither created nor destroyed, only changed in form. The kinetic energy of an object, expressed as a function of both velocity (speed) and mass (weight), is transferred to another object on contact.

- Damage to the object or body tissue impacted is not only a function of the amount of kinetic energy applied to it but also a function of the tissue's ability to tolerate the forces applied to it.

Blunt Trauma

- The direction of the impact determines the pattern of and potential for injury: frontal, lateral, rear, rotational, rollover, or angular.
- Ejection from a car reduces the protection on impact afforded by the vehicle.
- Energy-absorbing protective devices are important. These devices include seat belts, airbags, drop-down engines, and energy-absorbing auto parts, such as bumpers, collapsible steering wheels, dashboards, and helmets. The damage to the vehicles and the direction of the impact will indicate which occupants are most likely to have been more severely injured.

SUMMARY (CONTINUED)

- Pedestrian injuries vary according to the height of the victim and which part of the patient had direct contact with the vehicle.

Falls

- The distance traveled before impact affects the severity of the injury sustained.
- The energy-absorbing capability of the surface at the end of the fall (e.g., concrete versus soft snow) affects the severity of the injury.
- The part of the patient's body that impacts the surface and progression of the energy exchange through the patient's body are important.

Penetrating Trauma

- The energy varies depending on the primary injuring agent:
  - Low energy—hand-driven cutting devices
  - Medium energy—most handguns
  - High energy—high-powered rifles, assault weapons, etc.

- The distance of the victim to the perpetrator and the objects that the bullet might have struck affect the amount of energy at the time of impact with the body and, therefore, the available energy to be dissipated into the patient to produce damage to the body parts.
- Organs in proximity to the path of the penetrating object determine the potential life-threatening conditions.
- The path of the penetrating trauma is determined by the wound of entrance and the wound of exit.

Blasts

- There are five types of injuries in a blast:
  - Primary—blast shock wave
  - Secondary—projectiles (the most common source of injury from blasts)
  - Tertiary—propulsion of the body into another object
  - Quaternary—heat and flames
  - Quinary—radiation, chemicals, bacteria

SCENARIO RECAP

Before first light on a cold winter morning, you and your partner are dispatched to a single-vehicle crash. On arrival, you find a single vehicle that has crashed into a tree on a rural road. The front end of the vehicle appears to have impacted the tree, and the car has spun around the tree and backed into a drainage ditch on the side of the road. The driver appears to be the only occupant. The airbag has deployed and the driver is moaning, still restrained by his seat belt. You note damage to the front end of the car where it impacted the tree as well as rear-end damage from spinning around and going into the ditch backward.

- What is the potential for injury for this patient based on the physics of trauma of this event?
- How would you describe the patient's condition based on the physics of trauma?
- What injuries do you expect to find?

SCENARIO SOLUTION

As you approach the patient, your understanding of the physics of trauma of this event leads you to be concerned about the potential for head, neck, chest, and abdominal injuries. The patient is responsive, but his speech is slurred and he smells of alcohol. While providing manual stabilization of his head and neck, you note a small laceration on the bridge of his nose as you continue to assess him for injury. He admits that he has been drinking and is unsure of the time of day or where he was going.

Releasing the seat belt and shoulder harness, you note tenderness and an abrasion over his left clavicle. He also complains of some tenderness of his face, neck, anterior chest, and mid-abdomen. Due to his admitted alcohol use, slurred speech, and confusion, you cannot rule out more serious injuries, so you establish spinal motion restriction as you remove him from the vehicle.

Continuing your exam en route to the trauma center, you note that the patient has significant tenderness to both lower abdominal quadrants, and you are concerned that there may be hollow organ injury.

References

1. U.S. Department of Transportation, National Highway Traffic Safety Administration. 2015 motor vehicle crashes overview. Published December 2020. Accessed October 1, 2021. https://crashstats.nhtsa.dot.gov/Api/Public/View Publication/813060

2. World Health Organization. Global Status Report on Road Safety 2018. Published June 7, 2018. Accessed October 1, 2021. https://www.who.int/publications/i/item /9789241565684

3. Centers for Disease Control and Prevention/National Center for Health Statistics. All firearm deaths. Accessed October 1, 2021. https://www.cdc.gov/nchs/fastats/injury .htm

4. Hunt JP, Marr AB, Stuke LE. Kinematics. In: Mattox KL, Moore EE, Feliciano DV, eds. *Trauma*. 7th ed. McGraw-Hill; 2013.

5. Hollerman JJ, Fackler ML, Coldwell DM, et al. Gunshot wounds: 1. bullets, ballistics, and mechanisms of injury. *Am J Roentgenol*. 1990;155(4):685-690.

6. Centers for Disease Control and Prevention. Leading causes of death. Updated April 20, 2017. Accessed May 30, 2017. https://www.cdc.gov/injury/wisqars/index.html

7. Boyce RH, Singh K, Obremskey WT. Acute management of traumatic knee dislocations for the generalist. *J Am Acad Orthop Surg*. 2015 Dec;23(12):761-768.

8. Hernandez IA, Fyfe KR, Heo G, et al. Kinematics of head movement in simulated low velocity rear-end impacts. *Clin Biomech*. 2005;20(10):1011-1018.

9. Kumaresan S, Sances A, Carlin F, et al. Biomechanics of side-impact injuries: evaluation of seat belt restraint system, occupant kinematics, and injury potential. *Conf Proc IEEE Eng Med Biol Soc*. 2006;1:87-90.

10. Siegel JH, Yang KH, Smith JA, et al. Computer simulation and validation of the Archimedes lever hypothesis as a mechanism for aortic isthmus disruption in a case of lateral impact motor vehicle crash: a Crash Injury Research Engineering Network (CIREN) study. *J Trauma*. 2006;60(5):1072-1082.

11. Horton TG, Cohn SM, Heid MP, et al. Identification of trauma patients at risk of thoracic aortic tear by mechanism of injury. *J Trauma*. 2000;48(6):1008-1013; discussion 1013-1014.

12. Insurance Information Institute. Facts + Statistics: Highway Safety. Accessed October 1, 2021. https://www.iii .org/fact-statistic/facts-statistics-highway-safety

13. Enriquez J. Occupant restraint use in 2020: Results from the NOPUS controlled intersection study (Report No. DOT HS 813 186). National Highway Traffic Safety Administration. Published September 2021. Accessed October 1, 2021. https://crashstats.nhtsa.dot.gov/Api/Public /ViewPublication/813186

14. U.S. Department of Transportation, National Highway Traffic Safety Administration. 2011 motor vehicle crashes: overview. Published December 2012. Accessed September 29, 2017. http://www-nrd.nhtsa.dot.gov/Pubs/811701.pdf

15. Insurance Institute for Highway Safety. Seat belts. Accessed October 2, 2021. https://www.iihs.org/topics/seat -belts#laws

16. Kahane CJ. Lives saved by vehicle safety technologies and associated Federal Motor Vehicle Safety Standards, 1960 to 2012 – Passenger cars and LTVs – With reviews of 26 FMVSS and the effectiveness of their associated safety technologies in reducing fatalities, injuries, and crashes. (Report No. DOT HS 812 069). National Highway Traffic Safety Administration. Published January 2015. Accessed October 2, 2021. https://crashstats.nhtsa.dot.gov/Api /Public/ViewPublication/812069

17. National Highway Traffic Safety Administration. Seat belts. Accessed October 2, 2021. https://www.nhtsa.gov /risky-driving/seat-belts

18. U.S. Department of Transportation, National Highway Traffic Safety Administration. Lives saved in 2008 by restraint use and minimum drinking age laws. *Traffic Safety Facts*. Published May 2010. Accessed September 29, 2017. https://crashstats.nhtsa.dot.gov/Api/Public/View Publication/811153

19. National Center for Statistics and Analysis U.S. Department of Transportation, National Highway Traffic Safety Administration. Seat belt use in 2020: use rates in the states and territories. *Traffic Safety Facts*. Report No. DOT HS 813 109. Published April 2021. Accessed January 4, 2022. https://crashstats.nhtsa.dot.gov/Api/Public/View Publication/813109

20. Greenwell NK. *Results of the National Child Restraint Use Special Study* (Report No. DOT HS 812 142). National Highway Traffic Safety Administration; May 2015.

21. Rogers CD, Pagliarello G, McLellan BA, et al. Mechanism of injury influences the pattern of injuries sustained by patients involved in vehicular trauma. *Can J Surg*. 1991;34(3):283-286.

22. Mayrose J. The effects of a mandatory motorcycle helmet law on helmet use and injury patterns among motorcyclist fatalities. J Safety Res. 2008;39(4):429-32. Published August 6, 2008. Accessed February 25, 2022. https:// pubmed.ncbi.nlm.nih.gov/18786430/

23. Centers for Disease Control and Prevention. Guidelines for field triage of injured patients: recommendations of the National Expert Panel on Field Triage. *MMWR*. 2012;61:1-20.

24. Pedersen A, Stinner DJ, McLaughlin HC, Bailey JR, Walter JR, Hsu JR. Characteristics of genitourinary injuries associated with pelvic fractures during Operation Iraqi Freedom and Operation Enduring Freedom. *Mil Med*. 2015 Mar;180(3 Suppl):64-67.

25. Burgess AR, Eastridge BJ, Young JW, et al. Pelvic ring disruptions: effective classification system and treatment protocols. *J Trauma*. 1990;30(7):848-856.

26. Fackler ML, Malinowski JA. Internal deformation of the AK-74: a possible cause for its erratic path in tissue. *J Trauma*. 1998;28(Suppl 1):S72-S75.

27. Fackler ML, Surinchak JS, Malinowski JA, et al. Wounding potential of the Russian AK-74 assault rifle. *J Trauma*. 1984;24(3):263-266.
28. Fackler ML, Surinchak JS, Malinowski JA, et al. Bullet fragmentation: a major cause of tissue disruption. *J Trauma*. 1984;24(1):35-39.
29. Fackler ML, Dougherty PJ. Theodor Kocher and the Scientific Foundation of Wound Ballistics. *Surg Gynecol Obstet*. 1991;172(2):153-160.
30. American College of Surgeons (ACS) Committee on Trauma. *Advanced Trauma Life Support Course*. ACS; 2002.
31. Wade CE, Ritenour AE, Eastridge BJ, et al. Explosion injuries treated at combat support hospitals in the Global War on Terrorism. In: Elsayed N, Atkins J, eds. *Explosion and Blast-Related Injuries*. Elsevier; 2008.
32. Department of Defense. Directive Number 6025:21E: Medical Research for Prevention, Mitigation, and Treatment of Blast Injuries. Published July 5, 2006. Accessed October 2, 2021. https://www.esd.whs.mil/Portals/54/Documents/DD/issuances/dodd/602521p.pdf?ver=2018-10-24-112151-983
33. Leibovici D, Gofrit ON, Stein M, et al. Blast injuries: bus versus open-air bombings—a comparative study of injuries in survivors of open-air versus confined-space explosions. *J Trauma*. 1996;41:1030-1035.
34. Gutierrez de Ceballos JP, Turégano-Fuentes F, Perez-Diaz D, et al. The terrorist bomb explosions in Madrid, Spain—an analysis of the logistics, injuries sustained, and clinical management of casualties treated at the closest hospital. *Crit Care Med*. 2005;9:104-111.
35. Gutierrez de Ceballos JP, Turégano Fuentes F, Perez Diaz D, et al. Casualties treated at the closest hospital in the Madrid, March 11, terrorist bombings. *Crit Care Med*. 2005;34(Suppl 1):S107-S112.
36. Avidan V, Hersch M, Armon Y, et al. Blast lung injury: clinical manifestations, treatment, and outcome. *Am J Surg*. 2005;190:927-931.
37. Ritenour AE, Blackbourne LH, Kelly JF, et al. Incidence of primary blast injury in U.S. military overseas contingency operations: a retrospective study. *Ann Surg*. 2010;251(6):1140-1144.
38. Ritenour AE, Wickley A, Ritenour JS, et al. Tympanic membrane perforation and hearing loss from blast overpressure in Operation Enduring Freedom and Operation Iraqi Freedom wounded. *J Trauma*. 2008;64:S174-S178.
39. Zalewski T. Experimentelle Untersuchungen uber die Resistenzfahigkeit des Trommelfells. *Z Ohrenheilkd*. 1906;52:109.
40. Helling ER. Otologic blast injuries due to the Kenya embassy bombing. *Mil Med*. 2004;169:872-876.
41. Nixon RG, Stewart C. When things go boom: blast injuries. *Fire Engineering*. May 1, 2004.
42. National Association of Emergency Medical Technicians. Explosions and weapons of mass destruction. In: Pollak AN, ed. *PHTLS: Prehospital Trauma Life Support*. 9th ed. Jones & Bartlett Learning; 2018.

Suggested Reading

Alderman B, Anderson A. Possible effect of air bag inflation on a standing child. In: *Proceedings of 18th American Association of Automotive Medicine*. American Association of Automotive Medicine; 1974.

American College of Surgeons (ACS) Committee on Trauma. *Advanced Trauma Life Support Course*. ACS; 2018.

Anderson PA, Henley MB, Rivara P, et al. Flexion distraction and chance injuries to the thoracolumbar spine. *J Orthop Trauma*. 1991;5(2):153.

Anderson PA, Rivara FP, Maier RV, et al. The epidemiology of seatbelt-associated injuries. *J Trauma*. 1991;31(1):60.

Bartlett CS. Gunshot wound ballistics. *Clin Orthop*. 2003;408:28.

DePalma RG, Burris DG, Champion HR, et al. Current concepts: blast injuries. *N Engl J Med*. 2005;352:1335.

Di Maio VJM. *Gunshot Wounds: Practical Aspects of Firearms, Ballistics and Forensic Techniques*. CRC Press; 1999.

Garrett JW, Braunstein PW. The seat belt syndrome. *J Trauma*. 1962;2:220.

Huelke DF, Mackay GM, Morris A. Vertebral column injuries and lap-shoulder belts. *J Trauma*. 1995;38:547.

Huelke DF, Moore JL, Ostrom M. Air bag injuries and occupant protection. *J Trauma*. 1992;33(6):894.

Hunt JP, Marr AB, Stuke LE. Kinematics. In: Mattox KL, Moore EE, Feliciano DV, eds. *Trauma*. 7th ed. McGraw-Hill; 2013.

Joksch H, Massie D, Pichler R. *Vehicle Aggressivity: Fleet Characterization Using Traffic Collision Data*. Department of Transportation; 1998.

McSwain NE Jr, Brent CR. Trauma rounds: lipstick sign. *Emerg Med*. 1998;21:46.

McSwain NE Jr, Paturas JL. *The Basic EMT: Comprehensive Prehospital Patient Care*. 2nd ed. Mosby; 2001.

Ordog GJ, Wasserberger JN, Balasubramaniam S. Shotgun wound ballistics. *J Trauma*. 1922;28:624.

Oreskovich MR, Howard JD, Compass MK, et al. Geriatric trauma: injury patterns and outcome. *J Trauma*. 1984;24:565.

Rutledge R, Thomason M, Oller D, et al. The spectrum of abdominal injuries associated with the use of seat belts. *J Trauma*. 1991;31(6):820.

States JD, Annechiarico RP, Good RG, et al. A time comparison study of the New York State Safety Belt Use Law utilizing hospital admission and police accident report information. *Accid Anal Prev*. 1990;22(6):509.

Swierzewski MJ, Feliciano DV, Lillis RP, et al. Deaths from motor vehicle crashes: patterns of injury in restrained and unrestrained victims. *J Trauma*. 1994;37(3):404.

Sykes LN, Champion HR, Fouty WJ. Dum-dums, hollowpoints, and devastators: techniques designed to increase wounding potential of bullets. *J Trauma*. 1988;28:618.

CHAPTER **5**

Scene Management

Lead Editor
Matthew Levy, DO

CHAPTER OBJECTIVES

At the completion of this chapter, you will be able to do the following:

- Identify potential threats to human life and safety that are common to all emergency scenes.
- Be familiar with threats that are unique to a given scenario.
- Integrate analysis of scene safety, scene situation, and the physics of trauma into assessment of the trauma patient to make patient care decisions.

- Describe appropriate steps that need to be taken to mitigate threats to safety.
- Given a mass-casualty incident (MCI) scenario (hazardous materials, weapons of mass destruction), discuss the use of a triage system in managing the scene, and make triage decisions based on assessment findings.

SCENARIO

You are dispatched to the scene of a domestic altercation. It is 0245 hours on a hot summer night. As you arrive on the scene of a single-family dwelling, you can hear two people arguing loudly and the sounds of children crying in the background. Police have been dispatched to this call but have not yet arrived to the location.

- What are your concerns about the scene?
- What considerations are important before you contact the patient?

INTRODUCTION

There are a number of concerns that prehospital practitioners should consider while responding to a call and when arriving at a scene:

1. Preliminary assessment of scene safety is initiated while en route based on prearrival information from the dispatcher. This assessment should take into consideration prior responses to the same location, the need for other public safety emergency responders, such as law enforcement, additional emergency medical services (EMS) units, and other resources, including fire suppression or specialty rescue team.

2. The first priority upon arriving at the scene of an incident is performing an overall assessment.

This assessment involves (1) identifying any threats that require immediate mitigation to establish that the scene is safe enough for EMS practitioners to enter, (2) ensuring practitioner and patient safety, and (3) determining the need (if any) for alterations in patient care based on the current conditions. Issues identified in this evaluation must be addressed before beginning the assessment of individual patients. In some situations, such as situations involving assailants or hazardous materials exposures, this evaluation process becomes even more critical and can alter the methods and types of patient care to be performed.

Scene assessment and reassessment is an ongoing process, not a one-time event. Continuous attention must be paid to environment and situation occurring around the emergency responders. A scene initially deemed safe can change rapidly, and responders must be ready to take appropriate steps to ensure their continued safety, should the conditions change.

3. The overall scene assessment will help determine if multiple patients are present. If the scene involves more than one patient, the situation is classified as either a multiple-patient incident or a mass-casualty incident (MCI). MCIs are discussed further in Chapter 17, *Disaster Management*. In an MCI, the number of patients exceeds available resources and the immediate priority shifts from focusing all resources on the most injured patient to saving the maximum number of patients. An initial abbreviated form of triage (discussed in the final section of this chapter) helps to identify and prioritize the patients to be treated first when there are multiple victims. The prioritization of patient management is (a) conditions that may result in the immediate loss of life, (b) conditions that may result in the loss of limb, and (c) all other conditions that do not threaten life or limb.

Scene Assessment

Scene assessment begins when dispatch either gathers and processes information by questioning the caller or obtains information provided by other public safety units already on the scene. The dispatcher then relays the initial information about the incident and the patient to the responding EMS unit.

While traveling to the scene, taking the time to prepare and practicing good communication skills may be the difference between a well-managed scene and a chaotic scene. Maintaining situational awareness is key and involves good observation, perception, and communication skills.

The on-scene information-gathering process begins as the EMS practitioner arrives at the incident. Before making contact with the patient, the practitioner should evaluate the scene by doing the following:

1. Obtaining a general impression of the situation for scene safety, by observing for any immediate threats of harm to the crew or patient
2. Looking at the cause (mechanism) and results of the incident (such as a weakened structure, number of victims)
3. Observing family members and bystanders

The scene's appearance helps to create an impression that influences the global assessment and serves as a basis for situational awareness purposes. A wealth of information is gathered by simply looking, listening, and cataloguing as much information as possible.

It is essential to realize that scene conditions can change quickly, just as the patient's condition can improve or deteriorate, so ongoing monitoring of the scene is key. Failing to reassess how the scene may change can result in serious consequences for both the prehospital care personnel and the patient.

Scene assessment comprises the following two major components: safety and situation.

Safety

The primary consideration when approaching any scene is the safety of *all* emergency responders. *When EMS personnel become victims, they can no longer assist other injured people, and they add to the number of patients.* Patient care may need to wait until the scene is safe enough that EMS can enter without undue risk. Safety concerns vary from commonplace events, such as exposure to body fluids and infectious materials, to rare events, such as exposure to chemical weapons used in warfare. Clues to potential risks and hazards on scene include not only the obvious, such as vehicles operating on a busy highway, or the sound of gunshots, or the presence of blood and other body fluids, but also more subtle findings, such as odors or smoke.

Scene safety encompasses both emergency responder safety and patient safety. In general, patients in a hazardous situation should be moved to a safe area before assessment and treatment begin and may require some type of intervention, such as decontamination, prior to comprehensive assessment. Conditions that pose a threat to patient or emergency responder safety include slippery surfaces, fire, downed electrical lines, explosives, hazardous materials (including body fluids, traffic, floodwater, and weapons), and environmental conditions. Also, an assailant may still be on the scene and may pose a threat to the patient, emergency responders, or bystanders. It is important to note, however, that in situations involving an active shooter, having EMS work in a coordinated fashion with law enforcement to enter a scene as soon as it is reasonably possible improves patient survival.

Situation

Assessment of the situation follows the safety assessment. The situational survey includes both issues that may affect how the prehospital care practitioner manages the patient and incident-specific concerns related to the patient directly. Questions to consider when assessing the issues posed by a given situation include the following:

- What really happened at the scene? What were the circumstances that led to the injury? Was it intentional or unintentional?
- Why was help summoned, and who summoned it?
- What was the mechanism of injury? (See Chapter 4, *The Physics of Trauma*.) The majority of patient injuries can be predicted based on evaluating and understanding the physics of trauma involved in the incident.
- How many people are involved, and what are their ages?
- Are additional EMS units needed for scene management, patient treatment, or transport?
- Are any other personnel or resources needed (e.g., law enforcement, fire department, power company)?
- Is special extrication or rescue equipment needed?
- Is helicopter transport necessary?
- Is a physician needed to assist with triage or on-scene medical care issues?
- Could a medical problem be the instigating factor that led to the trauma (e.g., a vehicle collision that resulted from the driver's heart attack or stroke)?

Issues related to safety and situation have significant overlap; many safety topics are also specific to certain situations, and certain situations pose serious safety hazards. These issues are discussed in further detail in the following sections.

Safety Issues

Traffic Safety

The majority of EMS personnel who are killed or injured each year were involved in motor vehicle–related incidents (**Figure 5-1**).[1] Although most of these fatalities and injuries are related to direct ambulance collisions during the response phase, a subset occurs while working on the scene of a motor vehicle crash (MVC). Many factors can result in prehospital care practitioners being injured or

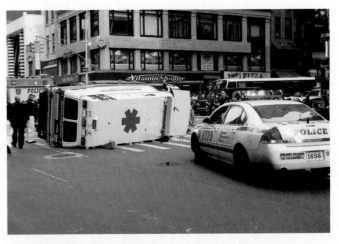

Figure 5-1 The majority of EMS personnel who are killed or injured each year were involved in motor vehicle–related incidents.
© Robert Brenner/PhotoEdit

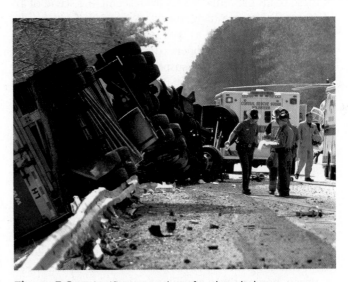

Figure 5-2 A significant number of prehospital care practitioners who are injured or killed were working at the scene of an MVC.
© Jeff Thrower (Web Thrower)/Shutterstock

killed on the scene of an MVC (**Figure 5-2**). Some factors, such as weather conditions or road design, cannot be changed; however, the practitioner should be aware that these conditions exist and act appropriately to mitigate the dangers present at these situations.

Weather/Light Conditions

Many prehospital care responses to MVCs take place in adverse weather conditions and at night. Added complexities may include ice and snow during the winter months, or other weather conditions such as fog, rainstorms, or sandstorms in which oncoming traffic may not see or be able to stop in time to avoid emergency vehicles or EMS personnel parked on the scene.

Highway Design

High-speed, limited-access highways have made moving large amounts of traffic efficient, but when a crash occurs, the resulting traffic backups create dangerous situations for all emergency responders. Elevated roadways and overpasses may limit an oncoming driver's vision of what lies ahead, and the driver may suddenly encounter stopped vehicles and emergency responders on the road upon reaching the apex of the overpass. Law enforcement may be reluctant to completely shut down a limited-access highway and effort is made to keep the flow of traffic moving. Although this approach may appear to produce further danger to emergency responders, it may prevent additional rear-end collisions caused by the backup of vehicles.

Rural roads present a unique set of problems. Although the volume of traffic is much less than on urban roadways, the winding, narrow, and hilly nature of some of these roads prevents drivers from seeing the scene of an MVC until they are dangerously close to it. Additionally, rural roads may not be as well maintained as those in urban areas, resulting in slippery conditions long after a storm has passed and catching unsuspecting drivers off guard. Isolated areas of snow, ice, or fog that caused the original MVC may still be present, may hinder EMS arrival, and may result in suboptimal conditions for oncoming drivers.

Risk Mitigation Strategies

Prehospital care practitioners must respond at all times of day and in any weather condition. As such, steps must be taken to reduce the risks of becoming a victim while working at the scene of an MVC. The best way is to limit the number of responders, particularly on limited-access highways. The number of people on the scene should be only what is needed to accomplish the tasks at hand. For example, having three ambulances and a supervisor's vehicle at a scene that has one patient dramatically increases the risk of a practitioner being hit by a passing vehicle.

Reflective Clothing

In most cases when EMS responders are struck by oncoming vehicles, drivers state that they did not see the practitioner in the road. To enhance visibility, high-visibility safety apparel should be worn at all MVC scenes, day or night. Some agencies have a "boots on the ground, wear high visibility vests" policy requiring EMS personnel to wear their high visibility vests when exiting their vehicle on all responses. The National Fire Protection Association (NFPA), the Occupational Safety and Health Administration (OSHA), and the International Safety Equipment Association all have standards for reflective warning garments to be worn when working on highways. OSHA has three levels of protection for workers on highways, with the highest level (level 3) to be used at night on high-speed roadways. The Federal Highway

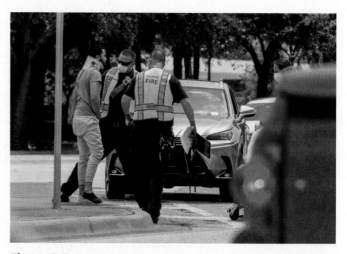

Figure 5-3 American National Standards Institute class 2 and class 3 reflective vests provide a measure of safety for those responding to a roadway incident.
© YES Market Media/Shutterstock

Administration has mandated that all workers, including all emergency responders, wear American National Standards Institute (ANSI) Class 2 or Class 3 reflective vests (**Figure 5-3**) when responding to an incident on a highway funded by federal aid. The ANSI standards can be met either by affixing reflective material to the outer jacket or by wearing an approved reflective vest.

Vehicle Positioning and Warning Devices

The location of equipment in the ambulance also plays a role in safety. Equipment should be placed so that it can be gathered without stepping into traffic. EMS agencies will often have specific policies and procedures regarding how and where to park vehicles on scene. In some coordinated EMS systems, a "buffer" vehicle, such as fire engine might be used to block a lane.

The incident commander or the safety officer should ensure that responding vehicles are placed in the best positions to protect prehospital care practitioners. It is important for the first-arriving emergency vehicles to "take the lane" of the accident (**Figure 5-4**). Although placement of the ambulance behind the scene will not facilitate the loading of the patient, it will protect practitioners and patient(s) from oncoming traffic. As additional emergency vehicles arrive, they should generally be placed on the same side of the road as the incident. These vehicles should be placed farther from the incident to give increased warning time to oncoming drivers.

Headlights, especially emergency warning systems that incorporate flashing the vehicle's high beams, should be turned off to avoid blinding approaching drivers unless needed to illuminate the scene. The number of warning lights at the scene should be evaluated; too many lights may only serve to confuse oncoming drivers. Many

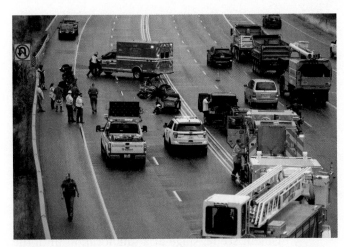

Figure 5-4 The correct positioning of an emergency vehicle.
© VDB Photos/Shutterstock

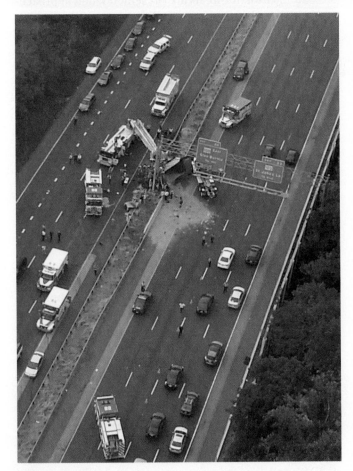

Figure 5-5 The placement of traffic delineation devices.
Courtesy of Andrew Pollak, MD.

departments use warning signs stating "accident ahead" to give ample warning for drivers. Light sticks or flares may be arranged to warn and direct traffic flow; however, care should be used in dry conditions to prevent grass fires. Reflective cones can serve to direct traffic flow away from the lane taken up by the emergency (**Figure 5-5**).

Practitioners should remain vigilant about safety during all phases of roadway operations. This includes clearing all directions before exiting a vehicle. Never exit an ambulance from the rear compartment using the side door along active traffic lanes. If you must, use the back door and look out the window before opening the door. Always maintain three points of contact when exiting an emergency vehicle, much like exiting a ladder. Three points of contact are the handrail, door, and step = 2 hands + 1 foot = 3 points of contact with vehicle.

If traffic needs to be directed, law enforcement or personnel with special training in traffic control should handle this task so that EMS can focus on patient management. Confusing or contradicting instructions given to drivers create additional safety risks. The best situations are created when traffic is not impeded, and vehicle flow can be maintained around the emergency.

Traffic Safety Education

Several educational programs are available that are designed to educate emergency responders about safe operations at the scene of an MVC. Each EMS agency should check with its state EMS agency, the National Highway Traffic Safety Administration (NHTSA), or OSHA about the local availability of these programs and incorporate them into their annual required training programs. The National Association of Emergency Medical Technicians (NAEMT) EMS Safety Course prepares emergency responders to develop a safety mindset and to promote a culture of safety within their agencies, whether practitioners are responding to and operating at the scene of MVCs or during routine community calls.

Violence

Each call has the potential to take the prehospital care practitioner into an emotionally charged environment. Some EMS agencies have a policy that requires the presence of law enforcement before practitioners enter a scene of known violence. Even a scene that appears nonthreatening has the potential to deteriorate into violence; therefore, practitioners must always be alert to subtle clues that suggest a changing situation. The patient, family, or others on the scene may not be able to perceive the situation rationally. These individuals may think the response time was too long, may be overly sensitive to words or actions, and may misunderstand the standardized and systematic approach to patient assessment. Maintaining a confident and professional manner while demonstrating respect and concern is important to gaining the patient's trust and achieving control of the scene.

It is important that EMS personnel train themselves to *observe* the scene. This includes learning to notice the numbers and locations of individuals when arriving on the scene, the movement of bystanders into or out of the scene, any indicators of stress or tension, unexpected or unusual reactions to EMS presence, or other intuitive feelings that may develop. Always watch the patient's and bystanders' hands, as it is someone's hands that pose one of the greatest risks to safety. Look for signs that someone is carrying a weapon, clothing that is worn out of season, or oversized clothing that could easily hide a weapon. Follow people when necessary to find a patient as opposed to letting them get behind you where you cannot easily observe their actions. If a developing threat is perceived, immediately prepare to leave the scene. An assessment or a procedure may need to be completed in the ambulance. The safety of prehospital care practitioners is the highest priority. It is essential to always have an exit or egress strategy that, when possible, includes an alternate way to evacuate the scene.

Consider the following situation: You and your partner are in the living room of a patient's home. While your partner is checking the patient's blood pressure, an apparently intoxicated individual enters the room from the back of the house. He looks angry, and you notice what appears to be the handle of a gun sticking out of the waistband of his pants. Your partner does not see or hear this person enter the room because he is focused on the patient. The suspicious person begins to question your presence and is extremely agitated about your uniform and your badge. His hands repeatedly move toward, then away from, his waist. He begins to pace and mumble. How can you and your partner prepare for this sort of situation?

Managing the Violent Scene

Partners need to discuss and agree on methods to handle a violent patient or bystander. Attempting to develop a process during the event is prone to failure. Partners can use a hands-on/hands-off approach, as well as predetermined code words and hand signals, for emergencies.

- The role of the *hands-on* prehospital care practitioner is to take charge of the patient assessment, giving necessary attention to the patient. The *hands-off* practitioner stands back to observe the scene, interact with family or bystanders, collect necessary information, and create better access and egress. In essence, the hands-off practitioner is monitoring the scene for both practitioners, so that the hands-on person can focus solely on the patient. If both prehospital care practitioners have all their attention focused on the patient, the scene can quickly become threatening, and early clues may be missed. When one practitioner begins interacting with and assessing the patient, the other practitioner can maintain situational awareness, observe the scene, and intervene early should a safety concern develop. Maintaining a heightened situational awareness can gain time for prehospital practitioners when deciding how to respond in a violent situation.
- A predetermined *code word* and *hand signals* allow partners to communicate a threat without alerting

others of their concerns. For example, one EMS practitioner notices that the patient's partner is suspiciously reaching into a cabinet to retrieve something and uses a code word to communicate potential danger to the other EMS practitioner. Such advance notice could give both practitioners time to react and to subtly signal for help or escape without raising the suspicion of the potential perpetrator. This is only effective if both EMS providers recall the code word and have practiced implementation.

There are various methods for dealing with a scene that has become dangerous, including the following:

1. *Don't be there.* When responding to a known violent scene, stage at a safe location until the scene has been rendered safe by law enforcement and clearance to respond has been given.
2. *Retreat.* If threats are presented when approaching the scene, tactfully retreat to the vehicle and leave the scene. Stage at a safe location and notify appropriate personnel.
3. *Defuse.* If a scene becomes threatening during patient care, use verbal skills to reduce tension and aggression (while preparing to leave the scene).
4. *Defend.* As a last resort, prehospital care practitioners may find it necessary to defend themselves. It is important that such efforts are to "disengage and get away." Do not attempt to chase or subdue an aggressive party. Ensure that law enforcement personnel have been notified and are responding.

The Active Assailant

Situations involving an active shooter or *assailant* have become all too frequent. To improve patient outcomes from injuries sustained during this type of incident, there is a growing trend for EMS agencies to partner with law enforcement colleagues to enter these scenes much earlier than would normally occur. In these cases, a contact team of officers enters the scene to engage and neutralize the threat. A joint EMS and law enforcement team follows the contact team to identify and begin treating victims quickly. (See Chapter 22, *Civilian Tactical Emergency Medical Support (TEMS)* for more information.) It is important to note that such programs require extensive planning, training, and coordination. The formation of impromptu hybrid teams of EMS and law enforcement personnel who have not been specially trained and exercised is discouraged.

Situation Issues

There are a number of situation issues that can profoundly affect the medical care that prehospital practitioners are able to offer a patient.

Crime Scenes

Trauma patients encountered by prehospital care practitioners may have suffered intentional injuries. In addition to shootings and stabbings, patients may be victims of assaults with fists, blunt objects, or attempted strangulation. In other cases, victims may have been intentionally struck by a vehicle or pushed off of a structure or out of a moving vehicle, resulting in significant injury. Even an MVC can be considered a crime scene if one of the drivers is thought to have been driving under the influence of alcohol or drugs, driving recklessly, speeding, or texting while driving.

When managing these types of patients, prehospital care personnel often interact with law enforcement personnel (**Figure 5-6**). Although both EMS and law enforcement share the goal of preserving life, these parties occasionally find that their duties at a crime scene come into conflict. EMS personnel focus on the need to assess a victim for signs of life and viability, whereas law enforcement personnel are concerned with preserving evidence at a crime scene or bringing a perpetrator to justice. Law enforcement and criminal investigation should never preclude proper patient care. Should the scene need to be disrupted in any way for patient assessment or care, documentation and follow-up communication with the investigating law enforcement agency are imperative. Effort should be made to minimize any unnecessary disruption of a crime scene but never in a way that compromises or delays patient care.

By developing awareness of the general approach taken by law enforcement personnel at a crime scene, prehospital care practitioners may not only aid their patient, they may also cooperate more effectively with law enforcement personnel, leading to the arrest of their patient's assailant. At the scene of a major crime (e.g., homicide, suspicious death, rape, traffic death), most law enforcement agencies collect and process evidence. Law enforcement personnel typically perform the following duties:

- Canvass the scene to identify all evidence, including weapons and shell casings.
- Photograph the scene.
- Sketch the scene.
- Create a log of everyone who has entered the scene.
- Conduct a more thorough search of the entire scene, looking for all potential evidence.
- Look for and collect trace evidence, ranging from fingerprints to items that may contain DNA evidence (e.g., cigarette butts, strands of hair, fibers).

Police investigators believe that everyone who enters a crime scene brings some type of evidence into a scene and, unknowingly, removes some evidence from the scene. To solve the crime, a detective's goal is to identify the evidence deposited and removed by the perpetrator. To accomplish this, the investigators must account for any evidence left or removed by other law enforcement officers, EMS personnel, citizens, and anyone else who may have entered the scene. Prehospital practitioners at a crime scene who are not careful may disrupt, destroy, or contaminate vital evidence, hampering a criminal investigation.

On occasion, prehospital care practitioners arrive at a potential crime scene before law enforcement officers. If the victim is obviously dead, practitioners should carefully back out of the location without touching any items and await the arrival of law enforcement. Although they would prefer that a crime scene not be disturbed, investigators realize that in some circumstances, practitioners need to turn a body or move objects at a crime scene to access a patient and determine viability. If practitioners need to transport a patient or move a body or other objects in the area before the arrival of law enforcement, investigators will typically ascertain the following:

- When were the alterations made to the scene?
- What was the purpose of the movement?
- Who made the alterations?
- At what time was the patient's death identified by EMS personnel?

If prehospital care practitioners entered a crime scene before law enforcement personnel, investigators may want to interview and take a formal statement from the practitioners regarding their actions or observations. Practitioners should never be alarmed or concerned about such a request. The purpose of the interview is not to critique the actions of the practitioners; the purpose is to gain information that may prove helpful to the investigator in solving the case. Investigators may request to

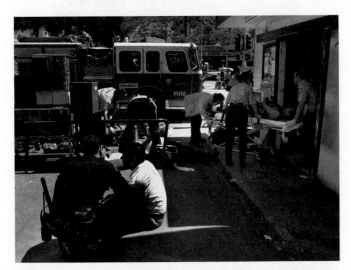

Figure 5-6 Prehospital care practitioners often are called to manage patients at the scene of a crime and need to collaborate with law enforcement to preserve evidence. Avoid disruption of a crime scene but never at the expense of delivery of patient care.

© Steve Osman/Contributor/Los Angeles Times/Getty Images

take fingerprints of the practitioners if items in the crime scene were touched or handled by the practitioners without gloves.

Proper handling of a patient's clothing may preserve valuable evidence. If a patient's clothing needs to be removed, law enforcement officers and medical examiners prefer that prehospital care practitioners refrain from cutting through bullet or knife holes in the clothing. If the clothing is cut, investigators may ask what alterations were made to the clothing, who made the alterations, and the reason for alterations. Any clothing that is removed should be placed in a paper (not plastic) bag and turned over to investigators.

One final important issue involving victims of violent crimes is the value of any statements made by the patient while under the care of prehospital care practitioners. Some patients, realizing the critical nature of their injuries, may tell practitioners who inflicted their injuries. This information should be documented and passed on to investigators. If possible, practitioners should inform officers of the critical nature of a patient's injuries so that a sworn officer can be present if the patient is capable of providing any information regarding the perpetrator. This is called a "dying declaration."

Hazardous Materials

The risk of exposure to hazardous materials is not as simple as recognizing environments with potential for hazardous material exposure. Hazardous materials are widespread in the modern world. Increasingly, vehicles, buildings, and homes contain hazardous materials. In addition to hazardous materials, this discussion applies equally to weapons of mass destruction. Because these dangers exist in such varied forms, all practitioners must obtain a minimum of awareness-level hazardous materials training. Hazardous materials is often abbreviated to *HazMat*.

There are four common levels of hazardous materials training:

- **Awareness.** This is the first of four levels of training available to emergency responders, and it is designed to provide a basic level of knowledge on hazardous materials incidents.
- **Operations.** Operations-level training is helpful for all emergency responders, as it provides the training and knowledge to help control the hazardous materials event. These emergency responders are trained to set up perimeters and safety zones, limiting the spread of the event.
- **Technician.** Technicians are trained to work within the hazardous area and stop the release of hazardous materials.
- **Specialist.** This advanced level indicates that the emergency responder has achieved expertise in the management of and response to a hazardous materials event.

Scene Evaluation

Because the first priority at any scene is the safety of prehospital care practitioners, an important first step is to evaluate the site for the potential of hazardous materials exposure. The information given by dispatch may establish a high index of suspicion of hazardous materials. A call that involves a large number of patients who are presenting with similar symptoms (such as respiratory distress or seizures) should raise the possibility of a hazardous material exposure.

Once a scene has been determined to involve a hazardous material, focus must shift to securing the scene and summoning appropriate help to safely isolate the involved area and remove and decontaminate exposed patients and individuals. The general rule is, "If the scene is not safe, make it safe." If the prehospital care practitioner cannot make the scene safe, help should be summoned. The *Emergency Response Guidebook* (*ERG*), produced by the U.S. Department of Transportation, or contact with a chemical emergency response service, is useful to identify potential hazards (**Figure 5-7**). The guidebook (and related app) uses a simple system that allows identification of a material by its name or identification placard number. The text

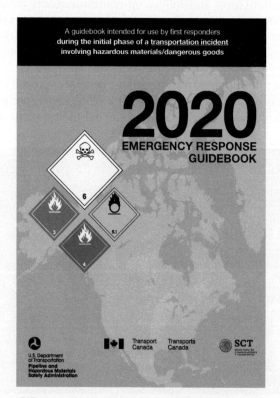

Figure 5-7 The *Emergency Response Guidebook* produced by the U.S. Department of Transportation provides critical information at the scene of a potential hazardous materials incident. The *ERG* is also available as an app for smartphones.

Reproduced from U.S. Department of Transportation, Transport Canada, and Secretariat of Communications and Transport of Mexico. 2020 Emergency Response Guidebook. Pipeline and Hazardous Materials Safety Administration, U.S. Department of Transportation, 2020. https://www.phmsa.dot.gov/sites/phmsa.dot.gov/files/2021-01/ERG2020-WEB.pdf

then refers the reader to a page that provides basic information about safe distances for emergency responders, life and fire hazards, and the patient's likely complaints.

Use binoculars to read labels from a distance; if labels can be read without the use of viewing devices, the prehospital care practitioner is too close and likely to be exposed. A good rule is that if your extended thumb held at arm's length does not cover the entire incident scene, then you are too close.

At a hazardous materials scene, security of the site must be ensured: "Nobody in, nobody out." The staging area should be established upwind and upgrade at a safe distance from the hazard. Entry into and exit from the scene should be denied until the arrival of hazardous materials specialists. In most cases, patient care begins when a decontaminated patient is delivered to the prehospital care practitioner.

It is important for the prehospital care practitioner to understand the command system and structure of the work zones in a hazardous materials operation (**Figure 5-8**). The scene of an incident involving a weapon of mass destruction or hazardous material is generally divided into

hot (direct threat), warm (indirect threat), and cold zones. For a description of the functions of each zone, see Chapter 18, *Explosions and Weapons of Mass Destruction.*

On the scene of large, more complex HazMat incidents, EMS personnel will also often be requested to provide emergency medical standby and support services for members of the HazMat team who will be making entry into the hot zone.

Weapons of Mass Destruction

The response to a scene involving a weapon of mass destruction (WMD) has safety and other concerns similar to the response to a scene involving hazardous materials, as discussed earlier.

Every scene that involves multiple victims, especially if they complain of similar symptoms or findings, or that was reported to have resulted from an explosion should trigger two questions: (1) Was a WMD involved? (2) Could there be a secondary device intended to harm emergency responders? (For greater detail, see Chapter 18, *Explosions and Weapons of Mass Destruction.*)

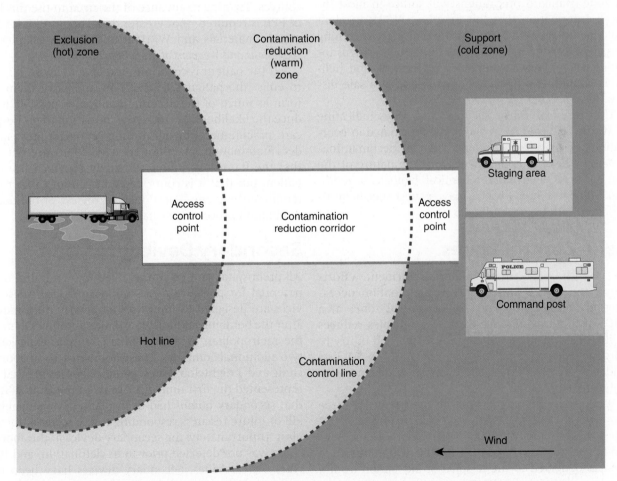

Figure 5-8 The scene of an incident involving a weapon of mass destruction or hazardous material is generally divided into hot, warm, and cold zones.

© National Association of Emergency Medical Technicians (NAEMT)

To avoid becoming a victim, the prehospital care practitioner needs to approach such scenes with extreme caution and resist the urge to rush in to care for the victims. Instead, the practitioner should approach the scene from an upwind position and take a moment to stop, look, and listen for clues indicating the possible presence of a WMD. Obvious spills of wet or dry material, visible vapors, and smoke should be avoided until the nature of the material has been ascertained. Enclosed or confined spaces should never be entered without the appropriate training and personal protective equipment (PPE). (For greater detail about PPE for hazardous materials and WMD incidents, see Chapter 18, *Explosions and Weapons of Mass Destruction*.)

Once a WMD has been included as a possible cause, the prehospital care practitioner needs to take all appropriate steps for self-protection and protection of other responders arriving at the scene. These steps include the use of PPE appropriate to the function and level of training of the individual practitioner. For example, emergency responders responsible for entering the hot zone must wear the highest level of skin and respiratory protection; in the cold zone, standard precautions will suffice in most instances. Information that this may be a WMD incident should be relayed back to dispatch to alert incoming emergency responders from all services. Staging areas for additional equipment, emergency responders, and helicopters should be established upwind and at a safe distance from the site.

The scene should be secured, and zones indicating hot, warm, and cold areas should be designated in coordination with law enforcement. Sites for decontamination should also be established. Once the nature of the agent has been determined (chemical, biologic, or radiologic), subject matter experts may request specific antidotes, medications, or antibiotics.

Scene Control Zones

Just as with a hazardous materials incident, efforts to limit the spread and further contamination necessitates the designation and use of control zones at a WMD incident. Adherence to these principles reduces the likelihood of spread of contamination and injury to emergency responders and bystanders. **Table 5-1** lists mandatory and preferred safe evacuation distances for bomb threats.

While these zones are typically illustrated as three concentric circles (see Figure 5-7), in reality, at most scenes, these zones will likely be irregularly shaped depending on the geography and wind conditions. If a patient is delivered to the hospital or aid station from a hazardous materials or WMD scene, it is most prudent to reevaluate whether that patient has been decontaminated and to mimic the concepts of these zones.

Decontamination

Whether the incident involves a hazardous material or a WMD, decontamination of an exposed individual is often required. **Decontamination** is the reduction or removal of hazardous chemical, biologic, or radiologic agents. The first priority is ensuring personal safety if there is any question of a continued exposure. Decontamination of the patient by appropriately trained hazardous materials technician-level personnel is the next priority. This will minimize the exposure risk to the prehospital care practitioner during assessment and treatment of the patient and will prevent contamination of equipment and vehicles.

OSHA provides regulatory guidelines for PPE used by prehospital care practitioners during the emergency care of victims in a potentially hazardous environment. Individuals providing medical care within environments of an unknown hazard must have a minimum level of appropriate training and be supplied and trained with level B protection. Level B protection consists of splash-protective, chemical-resistant clothing and self-contained breathing sources. Training in advance of the need to use this level of PPE is required. (For greater detail about PPE for hazardous materials and WMD incidents, see Chapter 18, *Explosions and Weapons of Mass Destruction*.)

If the patient is conscious and able to assist, it is best to enlist the patient's cooperation and have them perform as much of the decontamination as possible to reduce the likelihood of cross-contamination to prehospital care practitioners. In performing or overseeing patient decontamination, practitioners need to ensure not only that the hazardous product is safely removed from the patient but that it is controlled and cannot further contaminate the scene. For a detailed review of the decontamination process, see Chapter 13, *Burn Injuries*.

Secondary Devices

All prehospital care personnel need to be mindful of the potential for presence of a secondary device; these devices are designed to injure responders. Within months after the bombing at the 1996 Atlanta Summer Olympics, the metropolitan area of Atlanta, Georgia, experienced two additional bombings. These bombings, at an abortion clinic and a nightclub, had secondary bombs planted and represented the first time in 17 years in the United States that secondary bombs had been planted, presumably to kill or injure rescuers responding to the scene of the first blast. Unfortunately, the secondary device at the abortion clinic was not detected prior to its detonation, and there were six casualties. Secondary devices have been used with regularity by terrorists worldwide.

After these incidents, the Georgia Emergency Management Agency developed the following guidelines for

Table 5-1 Bomb Threats: Safe Evacuation Distances

Threat Description	Explosives Capacity (TNT Capacity)	Mandatory Evacuation Distance	Preferred Evacuation Distance
 © Jones & Bartlett Learning Pipe bomb/pressure cooker	5 lb (2.3 kg)	70 ft (21.3 m)	1,200 ft (365.8 m)
 © Jones & Bartlett Learning IED suicide vest	20 lb (9.1 kg)	110 ft (33.5 m)	1,700 ft (518 m)
 © Jones & Bartlett Learning Briefcase/suitcase bomb	50 lb (22.7 kg)	150 ft (45.7 m)	1,850 ft (564 m)
 © Jones & Bartlett Learning Car	500 lb (227 kg)	320 ft (97.5 m)	1,900 ft (579 m)
 © Jones & Bartlett Learning SUV/van	1,000 lb (454 kg)	400 ft (122 m)	2,400 ft (731.5 m)
 © Jones & Bartlett Learning Small moving van, delivery truck	4,000 lb (1,814 kg)	640 ft (195 m)	3,800 ft (1,158 m)

(continues)

Table 5-1 Bomb Threats: Safe Evacuation Distances (*continued*)

Threat Description	Explosives Capacity (TNT Capacity)	Mandatory Evacuation Distance	Preferred Evacuation Distance
© Jones & Bartlett Learning Moving van, small tank truck	10,000 lb (4,536 kg)	860 ft (262 m)	5,100 ft (1,554.5 m)
© Jones & Bartlett Learning Semitrailer	60,000 lb (27,216 kg)	1,570 ft (479 m)	9,300 ft (2,835 m)

Note: lb = pounds; kg = kilograms; ft = feet; m = meters; IED, improvised explosive device.

Data from the U.S. Department of Homeland Security.

rescuers and prehospital care personnel responding to the scene of a bombing at which a secondary bomb might be planted:

1. *Refrain from use of electronic devices.* Sound waves from cell phones and radios may cause a secondary device to detonate, especially if used close to the bomb. Equipment used by the news media may also trigger a detonation.
2. *Ensure sufficient standoff distance for the scene.* The hot zone should extend 1,000 feet (ft; 305 meters [m]) in all directions (including vertically) from the original blast site. As more powerful bombs are created, fragments may travel farther. The initial bomb blast may damage infrastructure, including gas lines and power lines, which may further jeopardize the safety of emergency responders. Access to and exit from the hot zone should be carefully controlled.
3. *Provide rapid evacuation of victims from the scene and hot zone.* An EMS command post should be established 2,000 to 4,000 ft (610 to 1,219 m) from the scene of the initial bombing. Emergency responders can rapidly evacuate victims from the bombing site with minimal interventions until victims and emergency responders are out of the hot zone.
4. *Coordinate with law enforcement personnel on preserving and recovering evidence.* Bombing events constitute crime scenes, and emergency responders should disrupt the scene only as necessary to evacuate victims. Any potential evidence that is inadvertently removed from the scene with a victim should be documented and turned over to law enforcement personnel

to ensure proper chain of custody. Prehospital care personnel can document exactly where they were in the scene and which items they touched.

Command Structure

An ambulance responding to a call will typically have one prehospital care practitioner in charge and another assisting in a support role. As an incident grows larger and more emergency responders from other agencies respond to the scene, the need for a formal system and structure to oversee and control the response becomes increasingly important.

Incident Command

The **incident command system (ICS)** has developed over the years as an outgrowth of planning systems used by firefighting services for multiple-service responses to major fire situations. In 1987, the NFPA published NFPA Standard 1561, *Standard on Fire Department Incident Command Management System.* NFPA 1561 was later revised as the *Standard on Emergency Services Incident Management System and Command Safety.* This version can be implemented and adjusted to any type or size of event by any agency managing an incident. In the 1990s, the National Fire Incident Management System (IMS) was created, which further refined the single-incident management approach.

Dealing with any incident, large or small, is enhanced by the precise command structure afforded by the ICS. At the core of the ICS is the establishment of centralized command at the scene and the subsequent buildup of divisional responsibilities. The first-arriving unit establishes the command center, and communications are established through command for the buildup of the response. The five key elements of the ICS are:

1. *Command* provides overall control of the event and the communications that will coordinate the movement of resources in and patients out of the incident scene.
2. *Operations* includes divisions to handle the tactical needs of the event. Fire suppression, EMS, and rescue are examples of operational branches.
3. *Planning* is a continuous process of evaluating immediate and potential needs of the incident and planning the response. Throughout the event, this element will be used to evaluate the effectiveness of operations and to make suggested alterations in the response and tactical approach.
4. *Logistics* handles the task of acquiring resources identified by the planning section and moving them to where they are needed. These resources include personnel, shelter, vehicles, and equipment.
5. *Finance* tracks the money. Response personnel from all involved agencies as well as contractors, personnel, and vendors brought into service in the incident are tracked so that the cost of the event can be determined and these groups can be paid for goods, supplies, equipment, and services.

Unified Command

An expansion of the ICS is the unified command system. This expansion takes into account the need to coordinate numerous agencies and disciplines (such as EMS, firefighting, and law enforcement). The technical aspects of bringing resources to bear from multiple communities, counties, and states are covered by this additional coordinating structure.

National Incident Management System

On February 28, 2003, President George W. Bush directed the secretary of Homeland Security through Presidential Directive HSPD-5 to produce a National Incident Management System (NIMS). The goal of this directive is to establish a consistent, nationwide approach for federal, state, and local governments to work effectively together to prepare for, respond to, and recover from domestic incidents regardless of cause, size, or complexity. The Department of Homeland Security established NIMS on March 1, 2004, after collaborating with detailed working groups consisting of state and local government

officials and representatives of the National Association of Emergency Medical Technicians (NAEMT), Fraternal Order of Police (FOP), International Association of Fire Chiefs (IAFC), and International Association of Emergency Managers (IAEM), as well as a wide range of other public safety organizations.[2]

NIMS focuses on the following incident management characteristics:

- Common terminology (as well as speaking in "plain English")
- Modular organization
- Management by objectives
- Reliance on an incident action plan
- Manageable span of control
- Predesignated "incident mobilization center" locations and facilities
- Comprehensive resource management
- Integrated communications
- Establishment of transfer of command
- Chain of command and unity of command
- Unified command
- Accountability of resources and personnel
- Deployment
- Information and intelligence management

The key components of NIMS are as follows:

1. Preparedness
2. Communications and information management
3. Resource management
4. Command and management
5. Ongoing management and maintenance

Command

Command comprises the **incident commander (IC)** and command staff. Every incident should have an identified commander who oversees the response. Command staff positions to assist the IC are assigned as appropriate to the size and nature of the event and may include public information officer, safety officer, and liaison officer. Other positions can be created as deemed necessary by the IC.

As described earlier, unified command is an enhancement to incident command in situations involving multiple jurisdictions. In a single-command situation, the IC is solely responsible for the incident management. In a unified command structure, individuals representing various agencies jointly determine objectives, plans, and priorities. The unified command system seeks to solve problems involving differences in communications and operational standards (**Figure 5-9**).

One element not included in the ICS that is added with unified command and NIMS is *intelligence*. Based on the size of the event, intelligence and information gathering

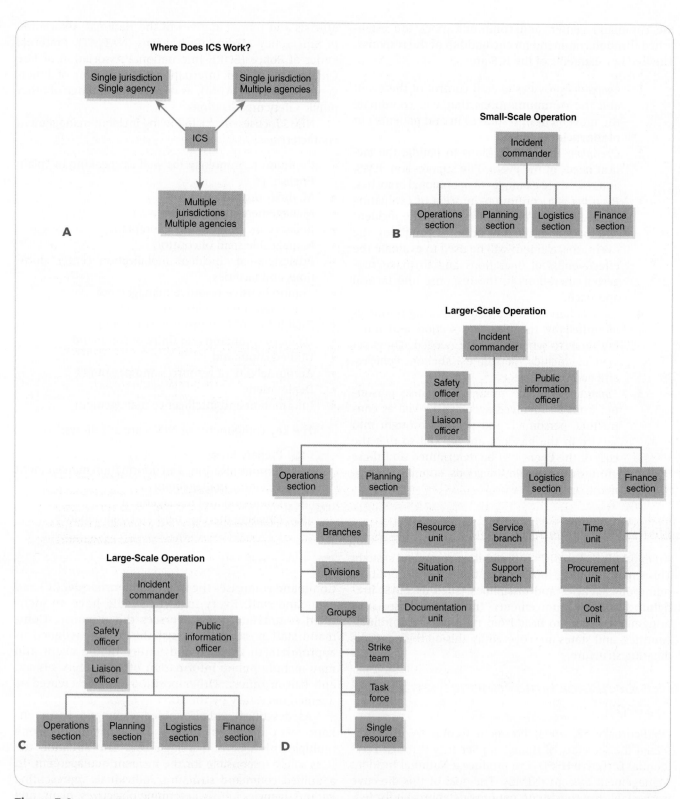

Figure 5-9 The incident command structure is flexible and scalable, meaning that it can be expanded or decreased based on the complexity of the event. The five key elements of ICS (Command, Operations, Planning, Logistics, and Finance) are operationalized as sections. The operational functions of each of the sections under incident command are organized into branches. The Medical Branch is the operational component responsible for coordinating and providing medical services needed to meet the tactical objectives of the incident. Depending upon the incident size, these services may be operationalized into elements called **units** that include equipment and personnel management, triage, communications with medical facilities, and transport.

related to national security may include risk-management assessment, medical intelligence, weather information, structural design of buildings, and information on toxic containment. Although these functions are typically handled in the planning section, the IC may separate information gathering from planning in certain situations.

In NIMS, the IC can assign intelligence and information gathering as follows:

- Within the command staff
- As a unit of the planning section
- As a branch of operations
- As a separate general staff function

Incident Action Plans

Incident action plans (IAPs) include overall incident objectives and strategies established by the IC or unified command personnel. The planning section develops and documents the IAP. The IAP addresses the tactical objectives and support activities for a designated operational period, which is generally 12 to 24 hours. The planning section provides an ongoing critique, or "lessons learned" process, to ensure the response meets the needs of the event.

In very large incidents, multiple ICS organizations may be established. Area command may be established to manage multiple ICS organizations. Area command does not have operational responsibilities; however, it performs the following duties:

- Sets overall incident-related priorities for the agency
- Allocates critical resources according to established priorities
- Ensures that incidents are managed properly
- Ensures effective communications
- Ensures that incident management objectives are met and do not conflict with each other or with agency policies
- Identifies critical resource needs and reports to the Emergency Operations Center(s)
- Ensures that short-term emergency recovery is coordinated to assist in the transition to full-recovery operations
- Provides for personnel accountability and safe operating environments

Hazardous Materials Training & Research Institute. *Emergency and Disaster Response to Chemical Releases*. January 2006. https://tools.niehs.nih.gov/wetp/public/Course_download2.cfm?tranid=6020

Detailed information and training programs regarding the ICS and NIMS can be found on the Federal Emergency Management Agency (FEMA) website (**Box 5-1**).

Bloodborne Pathogens

Before the recognition of acquired immunodeficiency syndrome (AIDS) in the early 1980s, healthcare workers, including healthcare practitioners, sterile processing

technicians, and prehospital care practitioners, showed little concern regarding exposure to body fluids. Despite knowledge that blood could transmit certain hepatitis viruses, practitioners and others involved in emergency medical care often viewed contact with a patient's blood as an inconvenience rather than an occupational hazard. Because of the high mortality rate associated with contracting AIDS and the recognition that the human immunodeficiency virus (HIV)—the causative agent of AIDS—could be transmitted in blood, healthcare workers became much more concerned about the patient as a vector of disease. Federal agencies, such as the Centers for Disease Control and Prevention (CDC) and OSHA, developed guidelines and mandates for healthcare workers to minimize exposure to bloodborne pathogens, including HIV and hepatitis. The primary infectious agents transmitted through blood include the hepatitis B virus (HBV), hepatitis C virus (HCV), and HIV. Although this issue became a concern because of HIV, it is important to note that hepatitis infection occurs much more easily and requires much less inoculum than does HIV infection.

Epidemiologic data demonstrate that healthcare workers are much more likely to contract bloodborne illness from their patients than their patients are to contract disease from healthcare workers. Exposures to blood are typically characterized as either **percutaneous** or **mucocutaneous**. Percutaneous exposures occur when an individual sustains a puncture wound from a contaminated sharp object, such as a needle or scalpel, with the risk of transmission directly related to both the contaminating agent and the volume of infected blood introduced by the injury. Mucocutaneous exposures typically are less likely to result in transmission and include exposure of blood to nonintact skin, such as a soft-tissue wound (e.g., abrasion, superficial laceration) or a skin condition (e.g., acne) or to mucous membranes (e.g., conjunctiva of eye).

Viral Hepatitis

Hepatitis can be transmitted to healthcare workers through needlesticks and mucocutaneous exposures on nonintact skin. As stated earlier, the rate of infection after exposure to blood from patients with hepatitis is much greater than the rate of infection with HIV. Specifically, the infection rates following exposure to HBV-infected needles is 37% to 62%. Infection with HCV is approximately 1.8% (1 in 50).[3] The probable explanation for the varying rates of infection is the relative concentration of virus particles found in infected blood. In general, HBV-positive blood contains 100 million to 1 billion virus particles/mL, whereas HCV-positive blood contains 1 million particles/mL, and HIV-positive blood contains 100 to 10,000 particles/mL.

Although a number of hepatitis viruses have been identified, HBV and HCV are of most concern to healthcare workers experiencing a blood exposure. Viral hepatitis causes acute inflammation of the liver (**Box 5-2**). The incubation period (time from exposure to manifestation of symptoms) is generally 60 to 90 days. Up to 30% of those infected with HBV may have an asymptomatic course.[3]

A vaccine derived from the hepatitis B surface antigen (HBsAg) can immunize individuals against HBV infection.[6] Before the development of this vaccine, more than 10,000 healthcare workers became infected with HBV annually, and several hundred died each year from either severe hepatitis or complications of chronic HBV infection.[7] OSHA now requires employers to offer HBV vaccine to healthcare workers in high-risk environments. All prehospital care practitioners should be immunized against HBV infection. Almost everyone who completes the series of three vaccines will develop antibody (Ab) to HBsAg, and immunity can be determined by testing the healthcare worker's blood for the presence of HBsAb. If a healthcare worker is exposed to blood from a patient who is potentially infected with HBV before the healthcare worker has developed immunity (i.e., before completing the vaccine series), passive protection from HBV can be conferred to the healthcare worker by the administration of hepatitis B immune globulin (HBIG).

At present, no immune globulin or vaccine is available to protect healthcare workers from exposure to HCV, emphasizing the need for using standard precautions. Direct-acting oral agents are capable of curing HCV infection. These drugs were approved in the United States in 2011. The treatment regimen depends on the genotype, viral load, and level of cirrhosis. The cost of these new agents limits universal accessibility.

Human Immunodeficiency Virus

After infection, HIV targets the immune system of its new host. Over time, the number of certain types of white blood cells falls dramatically, leaving the individual prone to developing unusual infections or cancers (**Box 5-3**).

Only about 0.3% (about 1 in 300) of needlestick exposures to HIV-positive blood leads to infection.[4] The risk of infection appears higher with exposure to a larger quantity of blood, exposure to blood from a patient with

---

Box 5-2 Hepatitis

The clinical manifestations of viral hepatitis are right upper-quadrant pain, fatigue, loss of appetite, nausea, vomiting, and alteration in liver function. Jaundice, a yellowish coloration of the skin, results from an increased level of bilirubin in the bloodstream. Although most individuals with hepatitis recover without serious problems, a small percentage of patients develop acute fulminant hepatic failure and may die. A significant number of those who recover develop a carrier state in which their blood can transmit the virus.

As with HBV infection, infection with HCV can range from a mild, asymptomatic course to liver failure and death. The incubation period for hepatitis C is somewhat shorter than for hepatitis B, typically 6 to 9 weeks. Chronic infections with HCV are much more common than with HBV, and about 75% to 85% of those who contract HCV will develop persistently abnormal liver function, predisposing them to hepatocellular carcinoma.[4] Hepatitis C is primarily transmitted through blood, whereas hepatitis B can be transmitted through blood or sexual contact. The risk of intravenous drug users becoming infected with HCV increases with the duration of intravenous drug use.[5] Before routine testing of donated blood for the presence of HBV and HCV, blood transfusion was the primary reason patients contracted hepatitis.

Box 5-3 Human Immunodeficiency Virus

Two serotypes of HIV have been identified. HIV-1 accounts for virtually all AIDS in the United States and equatorial Africa, and HIV-2 is found almost exclusively in Western Africa. Although early victims of HIV were male homosexuals, intravenous drug users, or hemophiliacs, HIV disease is now found in many teenage and adult heterosexual populations, with the fastest growing numbers in minority communities. The screening test for HIV is very sensitive, but false-positive tests occasionally occur. All positive screening tests should be confirmed with a more specific technique (e.g., Western blot electrophoresis).

After infection with HIV, when patients develop one of the characteristic opportunistic infections or cancers, they transition from being considered HIV positive to having AIDS. In the past decade, significant advances have been made in the treatment of HIV disease, primarily in developing new drugs to combat its effects. This progress has enabled many individuals with HIV infection to lead fairly normal lives because the progression of the disease is slowed dramatically.

Although healthcare workers typically are more concerned about contracting HIV for a variety of reasons, they are actually at greater risk of contracting HBV or HCV.

a more advanced stage of disease, a deep percutaneous injury, or an injury from a hollow-bore, blood-filled needle. HIV is primarily transmitted through infected blood or semen, but vaginal secretions and pericardial, peritoneal, pleural, amniotic, and cerebrospinal fluids are all considered potentially infected. Unless obvious blood is present, tears, urine, sweat, feces, and saliva are generally considered noninfectious. Timely prophylactic treatment in the context of high-risk exposure has been shown to reduce the risk of seroconversion and chronic infection. Immediate referral to a local needlestick and exposure hotline or your service's infection control officer is therefore warranted in the context of occupational exposure.

Standard Precautions

Because clinical examination cannot reliably identify all patients who pose a potential infection threat to healthcare workers, standard precautions were developed to prevent healthcare workers from coming into direct contact with any patient's body fluid. At the same time, these precautions help protect the patient from infections the prehospital care practitioner may have. OSHA has developed regulations that mandate that employers and their employees follow standard precautions in the workplace. Standard precautions consist of both physical barriers to blood and body fluid and exposure as well as safe-handling practices for needles and other "sharps." Because trauma patients often have external hemorrhage and because blood is an extremely high-risk body fluid, appropriate protective equipment should be worn by practitioners while caring for patients.

Physical Barriers

Gloves

Gloves should be worn when touching nonintact skin, mucous membranes, or areas contaminated by gross blood or other body fluids. Because perforations may readily occur in gloves while caring for a patient, gloves should be examined regularly for defects and changed immediately if a problem is noted (**Figure 5-10**). Gloves should also be changed between contact with each patient at a multiple-casualty incident.

Masks and Face Shields

Masks serve to protect the healthcare worker's oral and nasal mucous membranes from exposure to infectious agents, especially in situations in which droplet or airborne pathogens are known or suspected. Masks and face shields should be changed immediately if they become wet or soiled.

Surgical-style face masks are useful for protecting against droplet-borne illnesses. Examples of conditions requiring droplet precautions include seasonal influenza and *Bordetella pertussis*.

For certain other types of illnesses, including tuberculous, chickenpox, and the virus that causes COVID-19, airborne precautions are needed. The use of an N95 respirator or a powered air purifier are needed for protection against airborne illness. N95 respirators require fit-testing to ensure that a proper mask seal is obtained.

Eye Protection

Eye protection should universally be worn by EMS practitioners. Eye protection must be worn in circumstances in which droplets of potentially infected fluid or blood may be splattered, such as while providing airway management to a patient with blood in the oropharynx or when managing a patient with any open wounds or any time a face mask is being worn.

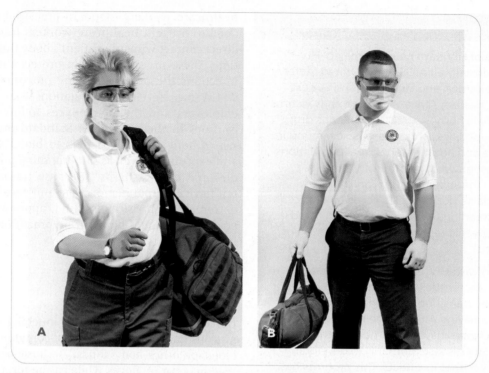

Figure 5-10 At a minimum, PPE for prehospital care practitioners should consist of gloves, mask, and eye protection. **A.** Goggles, face mask, and gloves. **B.** Face shield, face mask, and gloves.

© Jones & Bartlett Learning. Photographed by Darren Stahlman.

Gowns

Disposable gowns with impervious plastic liners offer the best protection, but they may be extremely uncomfortable and impractical in the prehospital environment. Gowns or clothing should be changed immediately if significant soilage occurs.

Resuscitation Equipment

Healthcare workers should have access to bag-mask devices or mouthpieces to protect them from direct contact with a patient's saliva, blood, and vomit. Resuscitation equipment used for positive-pressure ventilation of patients should also have in-line viral filters to provide additional protections to personnel.

Hand Washing

Hand washing is a fundamental principle of infection control. Hands should be washed with soap and running water if gross contamination with blood or body fluid occurs. Alcohol-based hand antiseptics are useful toward preventing transmission of many infectious agents but are not appropriate for situations in which obvious soiling has occurred. They can, however, provide some cleansing and protective effect in situations in which running water and soap are not available. Hands should be cleansed with either soap and water or an alcohol-based antiseptic prior to putting on and after removing gloves.

Preventing Sharps Injuries

As previously described, percutaneous exposure to a patient's blood or body fluid constitutes a significant manner in which infections could be transmitted to healthcare workers. Many percutaneous exposures are caused by injuries from needlesticks with contaminated needles or other sharps. Eliminate unnecessary needles and sharps, never recap a used needle, and implement safety devices such as needleless intravenous systems when possible (**Box 5-4**).

Management of Occupational Exposure

In the United States, OSHA mandates that every organization providing health care have a control plan for managing occupational exposures of its employees to blood and body fluids. Each exposure should be thoroughly documented, including the type of injury and estimation of the volume of inoculate. If a healthcare worker has a mucocutaneous or percutaneous exposure to blood or sustains an injury from a contaminated sharp, efforts are taken to prevent infection, including

Box 5-4 Preventing Sharps Injuries

Prehospital care practitioners are at significant risk for injury from needles and other sharps. Strategies for reducing sharps injuries include the following:

- Use safety devices, such as shielded or retracting needles and scalpels and automatically retracting lancets.
- Use "needleless" systems that allow injection of medication at ports without needles.
- Refrain from recapping needles and other sharps.
- Immediately dispose of contaminated needles into rigid sharps containers rather than setting them down or handing them to someone else for disposal.
- Use prefilled medication syringes rather than drawing medication from an ampule.
- Be familiar with your agency's written exposure control plan, and ensure that all employees are aware of the plan.
- Maintain a sharps injury log.

tetanus, HBV, and HIV infection. No prophylactic therapy to prevent HCV infection is currently approved or available. **Box 5-5** describes a typical blood and body-fluid exposure protocol.

Patient Assessment and Triage

Once all the preceding issues have been addressed, the actual process of assessing and treating patients can begin. The greatest challenge occurs when the prehospital care practitioner is faced with multiple victims.

Triage is a French word meaning "to sort." Triage is a process that is used to assign priority for treatment and transport. In the prehospital environment, triage is used in two different contexts:

1. *Sufficient resources are available to manage all patients.* In this triage situation, the most severely injured patients are treated and transported first, and those with lesser injuries are treated and transported later.

2. *The number of patients exceeds the immediate capacity of on-scene resources.* The objective in such triage situations is to ensure survival of the largest possible number of injured patients. Patients are sorted into categories, and care must be rationed

Box 5-5 Sample Exposure Protocol

After a percutaneous or mucocutaneous exposure to blood or other potentially infected body fluids, taking the appropriate actions and instituting appropriate postexposure prophylaxis (PEP) can help minimize the potential for acquiring viral hepatitis or HIV infection. Appropriate steps include the following:

1. Prevent bacterial infection.
   - Cleanse exposed skin thoroughly with germicidal soap and water; exposed mucous membranes should be irrigated with *copious* amounts of water.
   - Administer a tetanus toxoid booster, if not received in the previous 5 years.
2. Perform baseline laboratory studies on both the exposed healthcare worker and the source patient, if known.
   - Healthcare worker: Hepatitis B surface antibody (HBsAb), HCV, and HIV tests.
   - Source patient: Hepatitis B and C serology and HIV test (rapid, if possible).

3. Prevent HBV infection.
   - If the healthcare worker has not been immunized against hepatitis B, the first dose of HBV vaccine is administered along with HBIG.
   - If the healthcare worker has begun but not yet completed the HBV vaccine series or if the healthcare worker has completed all HBV immunizations, HBIG is given if the HBsAb test fails to show the presence of protective antibodies and the source patient's tests demonstrate active infection with HBV. HBIG may be administered up to 7 days after an exposure and still be effective.
4. Prevent HIV infection.
   - PEP depends upon the route of exposure and the likelihood and severity of HIV infection in the source patient. If the source patient is known to be negative, PEP is not indicated regardless of exposure route. It is recommended that an expert evaluate an exposed prehospital care practitioner to determine the most appropriate PEP regimen, based on the circumstances of the exposure.

because the number of patients exceeds the available resources. Relatively few prehospital care practitioners ever experience an MCI with 50 to 100 or more simultaneously injured patients, but many will be involved in MCIs with 10 to 20 patients, and most practitioners have managed an incident with 2 to 10 patients.

Incidents that involve sufficient emergency responders and medical resources allow for the treatment and transport of the most severely injured patients first. In a large-scale MCI, limited resources require that patient treatment and transport be prioritized to salvage the victims with the greatest chance of survival. These victims are prioritized for treatment and transport (**Figure 5-11**).

The goal of patient management at the MCI scene is to do the greatest good for the most patients with the resources available. It is the responsibility of the prehospital care practitioner to make decisions about who should be managed first. The usual rules about saving lives are different in MCIs. The decision is always to save the most lives; however, when the available resources are not sufficient for the needs of all of the injured patients present, these resources should be used for the patients who have the best chance of surviving. In a choice between a patient with a catastrophic injury, such as severe brain

trauma, and a patient with acute intra-abdominal hemorrhage, the proper course of action in an MCI is to first manage the patient with a survivable injury—the patient with the abdominal hemorrhage. Treating the patient with severe head trauma first will potentially result in the loss of both patients.

In a triage MCI situation, the catastrophically injured patient may need to be considered "lower priority," with treatment deferred until more help and equipment become available. These are difficult decisions and circumstances, but a prehospital care practitioner must respond quickly and properly. EMS personnel should not make efforts to resuscitate a traumatic cardiac arrest patient with little or no chance of survival while three other patients die because of airway compromise or external hemorrhage.

One unique scenario, however, where the rules of triage do not necessarily apply is when there are multiple victims following a lightning strike. In this situation, care should be focused on those in cardiopulmonary arrest (typically the opposite in an MCI). This is because under most circumstances, those who are conscious and with vital signs after a lightning strike have reasonably good outcomes absent immediate interventions. Conversely, the cause of cardiac arrest in most lightning strikes is cardiopulmonary arrest due to temporary autonomic nervous shutdown. This can be effectively treated with

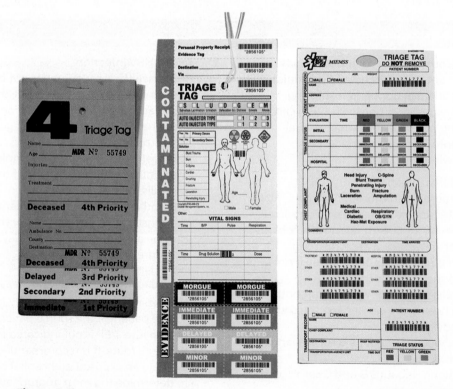

Figure 5-11 Examples of triage tags.
© File of Life Foundation, Inc.

Box 5-6 START Triage

In 1983, medical personnel from Hoag Memorial Hospital and firefighter–paramedics from the Newport Beach Fire Department created a triage process for emergency medical responders called Simple Triage and Rapid Treatment (START) (see Figure 5-12). This triage process was designed to identify critically injured patients easily and quickly. START does not establish a medical diagnosis but instead provides a rapid and simple sorting process. START uses three simple assessments to identify those victims most at risk to die from their injuries. Typically, the process takes 30 to 60 seconds per victim. START requires no tools, specialized medical equipment, or special knowledge.

How Does START Work?

The first step is to direct anyone who can walk to a designated safe area. If the victims can walk and follow commands, their condition is categorized as minor, and they will be further triaged and tagged when more rescuers arrive. This initial sorting leads to a smaller group of presumably more seriously injured victims remaining to triage. The mnemonic "30-2-can do" is used as the START triage prompt (see Figure 5-13). The "30" refers to the victim's respiratory rate, the "2" refers to capillary refilling time, and the "can do" refers to the ability of the victim to follow commands. Any victim with respirations fewer than 30 per minute,

capillary refilling time of less than 2 seconds, and the ability to follow verbal commands and to walk is categorized as minor. When victims meet these criteria but cannot walk, they are categorized as delayed. Victims who are unconscious *or* have rapid breathing, *or* who have delayed capillary refilling time *or* absent radial pulse are categorized as immediate.

While at the victim's side, two basic lifesaving measures can be performed: opening the airway and controlling external hemorrhage. For those victims who are not breathing, the prehospital care practitioner should open the airway, and if breathing resumes, the victim is categorized as immediate. No cardiopulmonary resuscitation (CPR) should be attempted. If the victim does not resume breathing, the victim is categorized as dead. Bystanders or the "walking wounded" can be directed by the practitioner to help maintain the airway and hemorrhage control.

Retriage is also needed if lack of transportation prolongs the time the victims remain at the scene. Using START criteria, significantly injured victims may be categorized as delayed. The longer they remain without treatment, the greater the chance their condition will deteriorate. Therefore, repeat evaluation and triage are appropriate over time.

Courtesy of Hoag Hospital Newport Beach and the Newport Beach Fire Department.

ventilation and chest compressions in many cases. (See Chapter 21, *Wilderness Trauma Care*.)

The "sorting scheme" most often used divides patients into five categories based on need of care and chance of survival:

1. *Immediate (Red Tag)*—Patients whose injuries are critical but who require only minimal time or equipment to manage and who have a good prognosis for survival. An example is the patient with a compromised airway or massive external hemorrhage.
2. *Delayed (Yellow Tag)*—Patients whose injuries are debilitating but who do not require immediate management to salvage life or limb. An example is the patient with a long-bone fracture.
3. *Minor (Green Tag)*—Patients, often called the "walking wounded," who have minor injuries that can wait for treatment or who may even

assist in the interim by comforting other patients or helping as litter bearers.
4. *Expectant (Gray Tag)*—Patients whose injuries are so severe that they have a minimal chance of survival. An example is the patient with a 90% full-thickness burn and thermal pulmonary injury.
5. *Dead (Black Tag)*—Patients who are unresponsive, pulseless, and breathless. In a disaster, resources rarely allow for attempted resuscitation of cardiac arrest patients.

Box 5-6, **Figure 5-12**, and **Figure 5-13** describe a commonly used triage scheme known as START, which uses only four categories: immediate, delayed, minor, and dead. (For more information on the START triage system, see Chapter 17, *Disaster Management*.)

A triage system developed specifically with MCIs in mind is the SALT triage system (**Box 5-7** and **Figure 5-14**).[8]

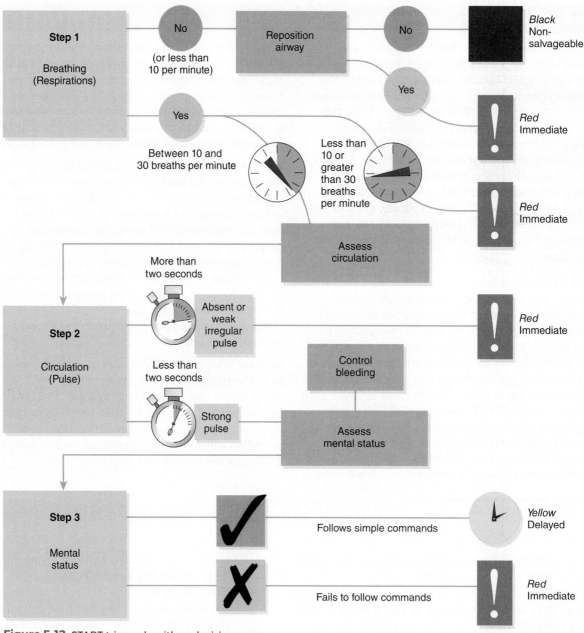

Figure 5-12 START triage algorithm: decision map.

Courtesy of Hoag Hospital Newport Beach and the Newport Beach Fire Department.

Respirations **30**

Perfusion **2**

Mental status **CAN DO**

Figure 5-13 START triage algorithm: "30-2-can do."

Courtesy of Hoag Hospital Newport Beach and the Newport Beach Fire Department.

Box 5-7 SALT Triage

The CDC, in conjunction with an expert panel representing a large constituency of medical organizations, developed the SALT triage scheme. The intent of the project was to develop a triage methodology that would serve as a basis for a nationally agreed-upon triage system. This system begins by using a global sorting process: asking victims to walk or wave (follow commands). Those victims who do not respond are then assessed for life threats and subsequently categorized into immediate, delayed, minimal, expectant, or dead (see Figure 5-14).

SALT Mass Casualty Triage

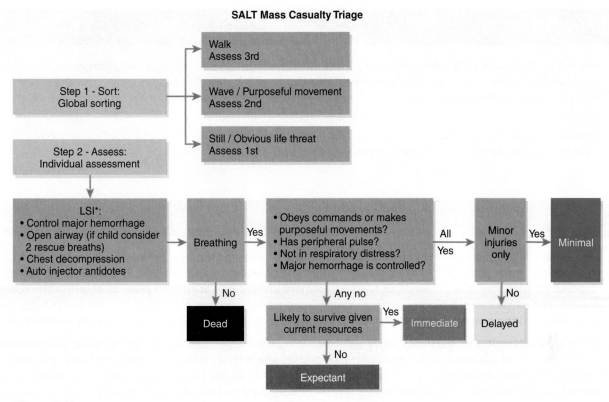

Figure 5-14 SALT triage algorithm.

*Note: LSI stands for lifesaving interventions.

Modified from Chemical Hazards Emergency Medical Management, U.S. Department of Health and Human Services. SALT mass casualty triage algorithm (sort, assess, lifesaving interventions, treatment/transport). Accessed December 14, 2021. https://chemm.hhs.gov/salttriage.htm

SUMMARY

- As a part of assessing the scene for safety, it is important to assess for hazards of all types such as traffic issues, environmental concerns, violence, bloodborne pathogens, and hazardous materials.
- An ongoing assessment of the scene will assure that EMS personnel and equipment are not compromised and unavailable for others and ensure that other emergency responders are protected from hazards that are not isolated or removed.
- Sometimes hazards can be excluded quickly, but if they are not assessed for, they will not be seen.
- Prehospital care practitioners should have a plan in place to mitigate risk at potentially dangerous scenes. For example, they should wear reflective clothing and park strategically at motor vehicle crashes; at a scene that involves a hostile person, partners should have a plan in place to prevent violence.

- Certain situations, such as crime scenes or intentional acts, including the use of weapons of mass destruction, will affect how the prehospital care practitioner responds to the scene.
- Incidents are managed using an incident command system (ICS) structure. Prehospital care practitioners must know and understand the ICS and their role within that system.
- Prehospital care practitioners must take precautionary steps to avoid contamination by infectious materials including bloodborne pathogens, such as hepatitis viruses and HIV. Key considerations include using standard precautions, employing physical barriers, washing hands, and preventing sharps injury.
- Prehospital care practitioners faced with multiple victims must be prepared to triage patients based on the severity of their condition and resources available.

SCENARIO RECAP

You are dispatched to the scene of a domestic altercation. It is 0245 hours on a hot summer night. As you arrive on the scene of a single-family dwelling, you can hear two people arguing loudly and the sounds of children crying in the background. Police have been dispatched to this call but have not yet arrived at the location.

- What are your concerns about the scene?
- What considerations are important before you contact the patient?

SCENARIO SOLUTION

Assessment of the scene reveals several potential hazards. Domestic violence incidents are among the most hazardous to emergency responders. These incidents often escalate and can lead to assault of emergency responders. Therefore, the presence of law enforcement should be considered prior to entering the scene. As with all trauma cases, a bloody patient exposes prehospital care practitioners to the risks of bloodborne infections, and the practitioners should wear physical barriers, including gloves, masks, and eye protection.

In this case, you wait until the police arrive before entering the home. Upon entering the house, you note that one of the individuals has obvious multiple facial bruises and a small laceration over one cheek. The officers take the other individual into custody and make arrangements for the care of the children. You perform your primary survey, which reveals no life threats. The secondary survey does not reveal any additional injuries. You transport the patient to the closest hospital without incident.

References

1. Miller A. Emergency medical service personnel injury and fatality in the United States. *J Epidemiol Res.* 2018;4(2): 9-18.
2. Federal Emergency Management Agency, U.S. Department of Homeland Security. *National Incident Management System.* 3rd ed. October 2017. Accessed October 17, 2021. https://www.fema.gov/sites/default/files/2020-07/fema_nims_doctrine-2017.pdf
3. Kuhar DT, Henderson DK, Struble KA, et al. Updated US Public Health Service guidelines for the management of occupational exposures to human immunodeficiency virus and recommendations for postexposure prophylaxis [published correction appears in *Infect Control Hosp Epidemiol.* 2013 Nov;34(11):1238. Dosage error in article text]. *Infect Control Hosp Epidemiol.* 2013;34(9):875-892. doi:10.1086/672271
4. Chen SL, Morgan TR. The natural history of hepatitis C virus (HCV) infection. *Int J Med Sci.* 2006;3(2):47-52.
5. Bell J, Batey RG, Farrell GC, Crewe EB, Cunningham AL, Byth K. Hepatitis C virus in intravenous drug users. *Med J Aust.* 1990 Sep 3;153(5):274-276.
6. Poland GA, Jacobson RM. Prevention of hepatitis B with the hepatitis B vaccine. *N Engl J Med.* 2004;351:2832.
7. U.S. Department of Health and Human Services, Centers for Disease Control and Prevention. Exposure to blood: what healthcare personnel need to know. July 2003. Accessed October 17, 2021. https://www.cdc.gov/hai/pdfs/bbp/exp_to_blood.pdf
8. Lerner EB, Schwartz RB, Coule PL, et al. Mass casualty triage: an evaluation of the data and development of a proposed national guideline. *Disaster Med Pub Health Prep.* 2008;2:S25-S34.

Suggested Reading

Centers for Disease Control and Prevention: See website for information on standard precautions and postexposure prophylaxis, www.cdc.gov.
National Institute for Occupational Safety and Health. Workplace solutions: preventing exposure to bloodborne pathogens among paramedics. DHHS (NIOSH) Publication No. 2010-139.
Rinnert KJ. A review of infection control practices, risk reduction, and legislative regulations for blood-borne disease: applications for emergency medical services. *Prehosp Emerg Care.* 1998;2(1):70.
Rinnert KJ, O'Connor RE, Delbridge T. Risk reduction for exposure to blood-borne pathogens in EMS: National Association of EMS Physicians. *Prehosp Emerg Care.* 1998;2(1):62.

CHAPTER 6

Patient Assessment and Management

Lead Editors
Vince Mosesso, MD, FACEP
Michael Holtz, MD

© Ralf Hiemisch/Getty Images

CHAPTER OBJECTIVES

At the completion of this chapter, you will be able to do the following:

- Relate the significance of patient assessment in the context of overall management of the trauma patient.
- Explain how to perform a rapid primary survey, as well as how assessment and management are integrated during the primary survey.
- Describe the components of the secondary survey and when it is used in the assessment of the trauma patient.
- Utilize the Field Triage Decision Scheme to determine the destination for a trauma patient.

SCENARIO

It is a Saturday morning in early November. The weather is clear, with an outside temperature of 42°F (5.5°C). Your squad is dispatched to a residential area for a person who has fallen from the roof of a two-story building. Upon arrival at the scene, you are met by an adult family member who leads you around the house to the backyard. The family member states the patient was cleaning leaves from the rain gutters with a leaf blower when he lost his balance and fell approximately 12 feet (ft; 3.6 meters [m]) from the roof, landing on his back. The patient initially lost consciousness for a "brief period" but was conscious by the time the family member called 911.

Approaching the patient, you observe an approximately 40-year-old male lying supine on the ground with two bystanders kneeling by his side. The patient is conscious and talking with the bystanders. You do not see any signs of severe bleeding. As your partner provides manual stabilization to the patient's head and neck, you ask the patient where he hurts. The patient states both his upper and lower back hurt the most.

Your initial questioning serves the multiple purposes of obtaining the patient's chief complaint, determining his initial level of consciousness, and assessing his ventilatory effort. Detecting no obvious respiratory distress, you proceed with the patient assessment. The patient answers your questions appropriately to establish that he is oriented to person, place, and time.

- Based on the physics of trauma as they relate to this incident, what potential injuries do you anticipate finding during your assessment?
- What are your next priorities?
- How will you proceed with this patient?

INTRODUCTION

Assessment is the cornerstone of all patient care. For the trauma patient, as for other critically ill patients, assessment is the foundation on which all management and transport decisions are based. An overall impression of a patient's status is developed, and baseline values for the status of the patient's respiratory, circulatory, and neurologic systems are established. When life-threatening conditions are identified, immediate intervention and resuscitation are initiated. If time and the patient's condition allow, a secondary survey is conducted for injuries that are not life or limb threatening. Often this secondary survey occurs during patient transport.

All of these steps are performed quickly and efficiently with a goal of minimizing time spent on the scene. Critical patients should not remain in the field for care other than to manage immediate life threats, unless they are trapped or other complications exist that prevent early transport. By applying the principles learned in this course, on-scene delay can be minimized, and patients can be moved rapidly to an appropriate medical facility. Successful assessment and intervention require a strong knowledge base of trauma physiology and a well-developed plan of management that is carried out quickly and effectively.

The trauma management literature frequently mentions the need to transport the trauma patient to definitive surgical care within a minimum amount of time after the onset of the injury. This urgency is because a critical trauma patient may have injuries that simply cannot be managed in the prehospital setting, such as internal bleeding. Definitive hemorrhage control for most serious bleeding is accomplished in the hospital setting, primarily in the operating room (OR).

The primary concerns for assessment and management of the trauma patient are (1) major hemorrhage control, (2) airway, (3) oxygenation, (4) ventilation, (5) perfusion, and (6) neurologic function. This sequence protects both the ability of the body to oxygenate and the ability of the red blood cells (RBCs) to deliver oxygen to the tissues.

R Adams Cowley, MD developed the concept of the "Golden Hour" of trauma. He believed that the time between injury occurrence and definitive care was critical. During this period, when bleeding is uncontrolled and inadequate tissue oxygenation is occurring because of decreased perfusion, damage occurs throughout the body.

The Golden Hour is better thought of as the "Golden Period," because this critical period is not exactly 1 hour. Some patients have less than an hour in which to receive care, whereas others have more time. The prehospital care practitioner is responsible for recognizing the urgency of a given situation and transporting a patient as quickly as possible to a facility in which definitive

care can be accomplished. To deliver the trauma patient to definitive care, the seriousness of the patient's life-threatening injuries must be quickly identified; only essential, lifesaving care provided at the scene; and rapid transport initiated to an appropriate medical facility. In many urban prehospital systems, the average time between activation of emergency services and arrival to the scene is 8 to 9 minutes, not including the time between the injury and the call to the public safety answering point. Usually, another 8 to 9 minutes are spent transporting the patient. If the practitioners spend only 10 minutes on the scene, over 30 minutes of time will have already passed by the time a patient arrives at the receiving facility. Every additional minute spent on the scene is additional time that the patient is bleeding, and valuable time is ticking away from the Golden Hour, or Period.

To address this critical trauma management issue, rapid, efficient evaluation and management of the patient are the ultimate objectives. Scene time should be minimized, and while the "platinum 10 minutes" is not directly supported by research, there is evidence to support expeditious care.[1] There is good evidence that delays in reaching the OR from the emergency department (ED) result in increased mortality[2-4] for patients with hemorrhagic shock due to trauma. It is therefore logical that delays in arriving in the ED in the first place would also be detrimental. It is further inherently logical and indisputable that bleeding control is an essential element in the treatment of hemorrhagic shock. There is also a lack of evidence that prolonged scene times are beneficial or that they improve patient care in any way.

The longer the trauma patient is kept on scene, the greater the potential for blood loss and death. Extended scene times should occur only for extenuating circumstances, such as prolonged extrication, scene hazards, and other unexpected situations. Almost nothing should impede the progress of the bleeding trauma patient in moving toward the OR.

This chapter covers the essentials of patient assessment and initial management in the field and is based on the approach taught to physicians in the Advanced Trauma Life Support (ATLS) program.[5] In addition, the approach taught in Prehospital Trauma Life Support (PHTLS) reflects the differences in prehospital care versus the in-hospital care taught in ATLS. The principles described are identical to those learned in initial basic- or advanced-level training programs, although different terminology may occasionally be used. For example, the phrase *primary survey* is used in the ATLS program to describe the patient assessment activity known as *primary assessment* in the National EMS Education Standards. For the most part, the activities performed in this phase are the same; various courses simply use different terminology.

Establishing Priorities

There are three immediate priorities on arrival to a scene:

1. The first priority for everyone involved at a trauma incident is assessment of the scene and scene safety. Personal protective equipment (PPE) appropriate to the situation should be donned, and standard precautions (for protection from blood and body fluids) should be followed. Droplet and/or airborne precautions for contagious diseases should be used if appropriate depending on the current situation with regard to aerosolized disease spread in your community. Chapter 5, *Scene Management*, discusses this topic in detail.

2. Identify the need for additional resources. Responders must recognize the potential for multiple-patient incidents and mass-casualty incidents (MCIs). In an MCI, the priority shifts from focusing all resources on the most injured patient to saving the maximum number of patients (providing the greatest good to the greatest number). Factors that may impact the triage decisions when there are multiple patients include severity of the injuries and the resources (manpower and equipment) available to care for the patients. Chapter 5, *Scene Management*, and Chapter 17, *Disaster Management*, also discuss triage.

3. Once a brief scene assessment has been performed and pertinent needs addressed, attention can be turned to evaluating individual patients. The assessment and management process begins by focusing on the patient or patients who have been identified as most critical, as resources allow. Emphasis is placed on the following, in this order: (1) conditions that may result in the loss of life, (2) conditions that may result in the loss of limb, and (3) all other conditions that do not threaten life or limb. Depending on the severity of the injury, the number of injured patients, and the proximity to the receiving facility, conditions that do not threaten life or limb may never be addressed at the scene.

Most of this chapter focuses on the critical-thinking skills required to conduct a proper assessment, interpret the findings, and set priorities for proper patient care. This process will allow for the appropriate provision of needed interventions.

Primary Survey

In the critical multisystem trauma patient, the priority for care is the rapid identification and management of life-threatening conditions (Box 6-1). The majority of

---

> **Box 6-1** Multisystem Versus Single-System Trauma Patient
>
> - A **multisystem trauma patient** has injuries involving more than one body system, such as the pulmonary, circulatory, neurologic, gastrointestinal, musculoskeletal, and integumentary systems. An example would be a patient involved in a motor vehicle crash who has a traumatic brain injury (TBI), pulmonary contusions, a splenic injury with shock, and a femur fracture.
> - A **single-system trauma patient** has injury to only one body system. An example would be a patient with an isolated ankle fracture and no evidence of blood loss or shock. Patients often have more than one injury within that single system.
>
> © National Association of Emergency Medical Technicians (NAEMT)

---

trauma patients have injuries that involve only one system (e.g., an isolated limb fracture). For these single-system trauma patients, there is more often time to be thorough in both the primary and the secondary surveys. For the physiologically unstable patient with multisystem injuries, the prehospital care practitioner may not be able to conduct more than just a primary survey. In these critical patients, the emphasis is on rapid evaluation, initiation of resuscitation, and transport to an appropriate medical facility. The emphasis on rapid transport does not eliminate the need for prehospital treatment. Rather, treatment should be initiated immediately for life threats and continued while simultaneously moving to the closest appropriate trauma center.

Quick establishment of priorities and the initial evaluation and recognition of life-threatening injuries must become ingrained in the prehospital care practitioner. Therefore, the components of the primary and secondary surveys need to be memorized and the logical progression of priority-based assessment and treatment understood and performed the same way every time, regardless of the severity of the injury. The practitioner must think about the pathophysiology of a patient's injuries and conditions.

One of the most common life-threatening conditions in trauma is lack of adequate tissue oxygenation (shock), which leads to anaerobic (without oxygen) metabolism. Metabolism is the mechanism by which cells produce energy. Four conditions are necessary for normal metabolism: (1) an adequate number of RBCs, (2) oxygenation of RBCs in the lungs, (3) delivery of RBCs to the cells throughout the body, and (4) off-loading of oxygen to these cells. The activities involved in the primary survey are aimed at identifying and correcting problems with these conditions. Anaerobic metabolism leads to less efficient energy production and lactic acidosis.

General Impression

The primary survey begins with a rapid global overview of the status of a patient's respiratory, circulatory, and neurologic systems to identify obvious threats to life or limb, such as evidence of severe hemorrhage; airway, breathing, or circulation compromise; or gross deformities. When initially approaching a patient, the prehospital care practitioner looks for severe external hemorrhage and observes whether the patient appears to be moving air effectively, is awake or unresponsive, and is moving spontaneously. Once at the patient's side, practitioners should introduce themselves to the patient and ask the patient's name. A reasonable next step is to ask the patient, "What happened to you?" If the patient appears comfortable and answers with a coherent explanation in complete sentences, the practitioner can conclude that the patient has a patent airway, sufficient respiratory function to support speech, adequate cerebral perfusion, and reasonable neurologic functioning; that is, there are probably no immediate threats to this patient's life.

If a patient is unable to provide such an answer or appears in distress, a detailed primary survey to identify life-threatening problems is begun. Within a few seconds, a general impression of the patient's overall condition has been obtained. By rapidly assessing vital functions, the primary survey serves to establish whether the patient is presently or imminently in a critical condition.

Sequence of Primary Survey

The primary survey must proceed rapidly and in a logical order. If the prehospital care practitioner is alone, some key interventions may be performed as life-threatening conditions are identified. If the problem is easily correctable, such as by suctioning an airway or placing a tourniquet, the practitioner may opt to address the issue before moving on to the next step. Conversely, if the problem cannot be quickly addressed at the scene, such as shock resulting from suspected internal hemorrhage, the remainder of the primary survey is expeditiously completed. If more than one practitioner is present, one practitioner may complete the primary survey while others initiate care for the problems identified. When several critical conditions are identified, the primary survey allows the practitioner to establish treatment priorities. In general, compressible external hemorrhage is managed first, an airway issue is managed before a breathing problem, and so forth.

The same primary survey approach is utilized regardless of the patient type. All patients, including elderly, pediatric, or pregnant patients, are assessed in a similar fashion to ensure that all components of the assessment are covered and that no significant pathology is missed.

The primary survey of the trauma patient emphasizes control of life-threatening external bleeding as the first step in the sequence. Even though the steps of the primary survey are taught and displayed in a sequential manner, many of the steps can, and should, be performed simultaneously. The steps can be remembered using the mnemonic XABCDE:

- X—eXsanguinating hemorrhage (control of severe external bleeding)
- A—Airway management and spinal motion restriction
- B—Breathing (ventilation and oxygenation)
- C—Circulation (perfusion and other hemorrhage)
- D—Disability
- E—Expose/environment

X—Exsanguinating Hemorrhage (Control of Severe External Bleeding)

In the primary survey of a trauma patient, life-threatening external hemorrhage must be immediately identified and managed. If exsanguinating external hemorrhage is present, it must be controlled even before assessing the airway (or simultaneously, if adequate assistance is present at the scene) or performing other interventions, such as spinal immobilization. This type of hemorrhage typically involves arterial bleeding from an extremity but may also occur from the scalp or at the junction of an extremity with the trunk (junctional bleeding) and other sites.

Exsanguinating arterial hemorrhage from an extremity is best managed by immediately placing a tourniquet as proximal as possible (i.e., near the groin or axilla) on the affected extremity. Other bleeding control measures, such as direct pressure and hemostatic agents, may also be used but should not delay or take the place of tourniquet placement in such cases. Direct pressure and hemostatic packing and dressings should be applied in cases of nonarterial severe bleeding in extremities and severe bleeding from truncal sites. Occasionally, bleeding from distal or smaller arteries can be controlled with focal direct compression of the artery. However, this is generally a temporizing maneuver until a tourniquet can be applied proximally. Severe bleeding from junctional areas may be managed by placing an appropriate junctional tourniquet or clamp, if available, or packing with hemostatic gauze and placing a pressure dressing (**Box 6-2**).

A—Airway Management and Spinal Motion Restriction

Airway

The patient's airway is quickly checked to ensure that it is **patent** (open and clear) and that no danger of obstruction exists. If the airway is compromised, it will have to

Box 6-2 Severe Bleeding at Junctional Locations

Junctional hemorrhage is defined as bleeding that occurs at the junction of the torso with an extremity, including the base of the neck. Examples of junctional areas include the groin, buttocks, and axilla (**Figure 6-1**). The use of a tourniquet or pressure dressing in these areas is often both impractical and ineffective.

The key treatment for junctional hemorrhage is direct compression of the large vessels that span the area proximal to the injury. In the prehospital setting, a significant amount of direct pressure to the femoral, iliac, or axillary arteries may be necessary to slow the bleeding. A variety of commercial devices are available for this purpose. This is often combined with the use of externally applied hemostatic agents and pressure dressings. Additionally, evidence supports the empiric application of a pelvic binder in the patient with traumatic amputation of the lower extremity above the level of the knee to aid in bleeding control.[6] The significant forces encountered in these traumatic injuries often damage the adjoining structures, such as the pelvic and shoulder girdle; thus, stabilization of these areas should also be considered.

The Committee on Tactical Combat Casualty Care (CoTCCC) recommends three tourniquets purpose-built for use at junctional hemorrhage sites. These include the Combat Ready Clamp (CRoC), Junctional Emergency Treatment Tool (JETT), and SAM Junctional Tourniquet (SJT). Various advantages and disadvantages have been identified in studies comparing these devices in the laboratory setting, all of which should be taken into consideration when choosing a device with which to equip field personnel.[6-10]

The most important concepts to consider when attempting to control bleeding at junctional sites are (1) that a large amount of direct pressure and compression to the blood vessels spanning the area will be necessary, and (2) a direct pressure dressing, ideally with a hemostatic agent, should be placed on the open surface of the wound. When these two techniques are combined, they offer increased chances for survival in what is otherwise often a fatal traumatic injury.[11] The bottom line is: You need to get a pressure dressing on the injury and pressure on bleeding arterial points as soon as possible.

© National Association of Emergency Medical Technicians (NAEMT)

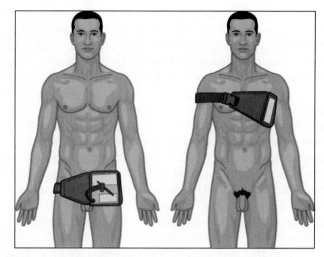

Figure 6-1 The junctional areas at the axillae and inguinal regions.
© Jones & Bartlett Learning

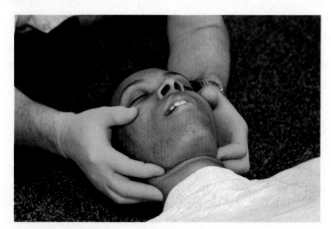

Figure 6-2 If the airway appears compromised, it must be opened while continuing to protect the spine.
© National Association of Emergency Medical Technicians (NAEMT)

be opened, initially using manual methods (trauma chin lift or trauma jaw thrust) (**Figure 6-2**), and cleared of blood, body substances, and foreign bodies, if necessary. Eventually, as equipment and more personnel become available, airway management can advance to include suction and mechanical means (oral airway, nasal airway, supraglottic airways, and endotracheal intubation or transtracheal methods). Numerous factors play a role in determining the method of airway management, including available equipment, the skill level of the prehospital care practitioner, and the distance from the trauma center. Some airway injuries, such as a laryngeal fracture or incomplete airway transection, can be aggravated by attempts at endotracheal intubation. Airway management is discussed in detail in Chapter 7, *Airway and Ventilation*.

Spinal Motion Restriction

Spinal injury should be suspected in every trauma patient with a significant blunt mechanism of injury until spinal injury is conclusively ruled out. It is particularly important to maintain a high index of suspicion for spinal injury in elderly or chronically debilitated patients, even with more minor mechanisms of injury. (See Chapter 9, *Spinal Trauma,* for a complete list of indications for spinal motion restriction.) While establishing an open airway takes precedence, the possibility of cervical spine injury must always be considered. Excessive movement in any direction could either produce or aggravate neurologic damage because bony compression of the spinal cord may occur in the presence of a fractured spine. Therefore, the patient's head and neck should be manually maintained (stabilized) in the neutral position during the entire assessment process, especially when opening the airway and administering necessary ventilation. This need for stabilization does not mean that necessary airway maintenance procedures cannot be applied. Instead, it means that the procedures will be performed while protecting the patient's spine from unnecessary movement. If spinal motion restriction devices that were placed need to be removed to reassess the patient or perform some necessary intervention, manual stabilization of the head and neck is employed until the device can be re-applied. There is no role for spinal motion restriction in patients with only penetrating trauma.[12]

B—Breathing (Ventilation and Oxygenation)

Breathing functions to effectively deliver oxygen to a patient's lungs to help maintain the aerobic metabolic process. Hypoxia can result from inadequate ventilation of the lungs and leads to lack of oxygenation of the patient's tissues. Once the patient's airway is open, the quality and quantity of the patient's breathing (ventilation) can be evaluated as follows:

1. Check to see if the patient is breathing by looking for chest motion and feeling for air movement from the mouth or nose.
2. If the patient is not breathing (i.e., is **apneic**), immediately begin ventilating the patient with a bag-mask device before continuing the assessment. Provide supplemental oxygen when available and maintain spinal motion restriction when indicated.
3. Ensure that the patient's airway is patent, continue providing or assisting ventilation, and insert an oral or nasal (if no severe facial trauma) airway if tolerated. If the patient remains unresponsive, consider whether a more definitive airway should be placed based on patient condition and proximity to a trauma center. This may involve placement of a supraglottic airway (if no signs of severe oropharyngeal trauma) or endotracheal intubation (for experienced

practitioners). Be prepared to suction blood, vomitus, or other fluids from the airway.
4. Although commonly referred to as the "respiratory rate," a more correct term for how fast a patient is breathing is "ventilatory rate." Ventilation refers to the process of inhalation and exhalation, whereas respiration best describes the physiologic process of gas exchange between the capillaries and the alveoli. If the patient is breathing, estimate the adequacy of the ventilatory rate and depth to determine whether the patient is moving enough air (recall that minute ventilation is rate × depth). (See Chapter 7, *Airway and Ventilation.*)
5. Ensure that the patient is not hypoxic and that the oxygen saturation is greater than or equal to 94%. Supplemental oxygen (and assisted ventilation) should be provided as needed to maintain an adequate oxygen saturation.
6. If the patient is conscious, see if the patient can speak a full sentence without difficulty.

The ventilatory rate can be divided into the following five categories:

1. *Apneic.* The patient is not breathing. This includes occasional agonal gasps, which do not effectively result in air exchange.
2. *Slow.* A very slow ventilatory rate, below 10 breaths/minute (**bradypnea**), may indicate severe injury to or ischemia (decreased supply of oxygen) of the brain. In these cases, the practitioner must assure adequate volume of air exchange is occurring. Often it will be necessary to either assist or completely take over the patient's breathing with a bag-mask device. Assisted or total ventilatory support with the bag-mask device should include supplemental oxygen to ensure an oxygen saturation greater than or equal to 94% (**Figure 6-3**).
3. *Normal.* If the ventilatory rate is between 10 and 20 breaths/minute, the prehospital practitioner should ensure that there is adequate ventilatory volume and oxygen saturation. Supplemental oxygen should be applied if indicated.
4. *Fast.* If the ventilatory rate is between 20 and 30 breaths/minute (**tachypnea**), the patient must be watched closely for improvement or deterioration. The drive for increasing the ventilatory rate is increased accumulation of carbon dioxide in the blood or a decreased level of blood oxygen (due to hypoxia or anemia). Pain or anxiety may also cause elevated ventilatory rate. When a patient displays an abnormal ventilatory rate, the cause must be investigated. A rapid rate may indicate that not enough oxygen is reaching the body tissue. This lack of oxygen

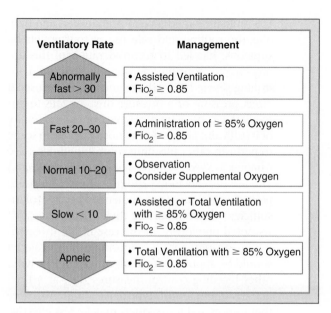

Ventilatory Rate	Management
Abnormally fast > 30	• Assisted Ventilation • $Fio_2 \geq 0.85$
Fast 20–30	• Administration of ≥ 85% Oxygen • $Fio_2 \geq 0.85$
Normal 10–20	• Observation • Consider Supplemental Oxygen
Slow < 10	• Assisted or Total Ventilation with ≥ 85% Oxygen • $Fio_2 \geq 0.85$
Apneic	• Total Ventilation with ≥ 85% Oxygen • $Fio_2 \geq 0.85$

Figure 6-3 Airway management based on spontaneous ventilation rate.

© Jones & Bartlett Learning

initiates anaerobic metabolism (see Chapter 3, *Shock: Pathophysiology of Life and Death*) and, ultimately, an increase in the carbon dioxide level in the blood leading to metabolic acidosis. The body's detection system recognizes this increased level of carbon dioxide and tells the ventilatory system to increase depth and volume to eliminate this excess. Therefore, an increased ventilatory rate may indicate that the patient needs better perfusion or oxygenation, or both. Supplemental oxygen should be administered to achieve an oxygen saturation of 94% or greater. The prehospital practitioner should monitor the patient closely for any deterioration in overall condition.

5. *Extremely fast.* A ventilatory rate greater than 30 breaths/minute (severe tachypnea) indicates hypoxia, anaerobic metabolism, or both, with a resultant **acidosis**. A search for the cause of the rapid ventilatory rate should begin at once to ascertain if the etiology is a primary ventilatory problem or an oxygen delivery problem such as inadequate perfusion or severe blood loss. Injuries that can produce major impairment in oxygenation and ventilation include tension pneumothorax, flail chest with pulmonary contusion, massive hemothorax, and open pneumothorax. Once the cause is identified, the intervention must occur immediately to correct the problem. (See Chapter 10, *Thoracic Trauma.*) Patients with ventilatory rates greater than 30 breaths/minute should be placed on oxygen. Carefully monitor these patients for fatigue or signs of inadequate ventilation such

as decreasing mental status, elevation of end-tidal carbon dioxide levels, or low oxygen saturation, and assist ventilations with a bag-mask device as needed to obtain adequate minute ventilation and oxygen saturation.

In the patient with abnormal ventilation, the chest must be exposed, observed, and palpated rapidly. Then, auscultation of the lungs will identify abnormal, diminished, or absent breath sounds. Injuries that may impede ventilation include tension pneumothorax, flail chest, spinal cord injuries, and TBIs. These injuries should be identified or suspected during the primary survey and require that ventilatory support be initiated at once. Needle decompression should be performed immediately if tension pneumothorax is suspected.

When assessing the trauma patient's ventilatory status, the ventilatory *depth* as well as the rate is assessed. A patient can be breathing at a normal ventilatory rate of 16 breaths/minute but have a greatly decreased ventilatory depth. Conversely, a patient can have a normal ventilatory depth but an increased or decreased ventilatory rate. The tidal volume is multiplied by the ventilatory rate to calculate the patient's minute ventilation volume. (See Chapter 7, *Airway and Ventilation*.)

C—Circulation (Perfusion and Other Hemorrhage)

Assessing for circulatory system compromise or failure is the next step in caring for the trauma patient. Oxygenation of the RBCs without delivery to the tissue cells is of no benefit to the patient. In the first step of the sequence, life-threatening bleeding was identified and controlled. After subsequently assessing the patient's airway and breathing status, the prehospital practitioner should obtain an overall estimate of the patient's cardiac output and perfusion status. Hemorrhage—either external or internal—is the most common cause of preventable death from trauma. Control of less severe bleeding occurs during this phase of the primary survey after airway and breathing have been addressed.

Hemorrhage Control

External exsanguinating hemorrhage is identified and controlled as the first step in the primary survey because if severe bleeding is not controlled as soon as possible, the potential for the patient's death increases dramatically. The three types of external hemorrhage are capillary, venous, and arterial, which are described as follows:

1. *Capillary bleeding* is caused by abrasions that have scraped open the tiny capillaries just below the skin's surface. Capillary bleeding is generally not life threatening and may have slowed or even stopped before the arrival of prehospital care practitioners.

2. *Venous bleeding* is caused by laceration or other injury to a vein, which leads to steady flow of dark red blood from the wound. This type of bleeding is usually controllable with direct pressure. Venous bleeding is usually not life threatening unless bleeding is prolonged or a large vein is involved.

3. *Arterial bleeding* is caused by an injury that has lacerated an artery. This is the most important and most difficult type of blood loss to control. It is generally characterized by spurting blood that is bright red in color. However, arterial bleeding may also present as blood that rapidly "pours out" of a wound if a deep artery is injured. Even a small, deep arterial puncture wound can produce life-threatening blood loss.

Rapid control of arterial exsanguinating bleeding is one of the most important goals in the care of a trauma patient. The primary survey cannot advance unless exsanguinating hemorrhage is controlled during the very first phase. Capillary and venous bleeding are generally addressed later in the primary survey when Circulation is addressed.

Hemorrhage can be controlled in the following ways:

1. *Direct pressure.* Direct pressure is exactly what the name implies—applying pressure to the site of bleeding. This is accomplished by placing a dressing (hemostatic gauze is preferred) directly over the site of bleeding (if it can be identified) and applying pressure. Pressure should be applied as precisely and focally as possible. A finger on a visible compressible artery is effective. Pressure should be applied continuously for at a minimum of 3 minutes or per the manufacturer's instructions for hemostatic gauze and for 10 minutes if using plain gauze; prehospital care practitioners should avoid the temptation to remove pressure to check if the wound is still bleeding before that time period. The application and maintenance of direct pressure will require all of one prehospital care practitioner's attention, preventing that practitioner from participating in other aspects of patient care. Alternatively, or if assistance is limited, a pressure dressing can be applied. There are multiple commercial options (e.g., Israeli bandage), or a pressure dressing can be fashioned out of gauze pads and an elastic bandage. If bleeding is not controlled, it will not matter how much oxygen or fluid the patient receives; perfusion will not improve in the face of large volume hemorrhage.

2. *Tourniquets.* Tourniquets were often described in the past as the technique of last resort. U.S. military experience in Afghanistan and Iraq, plus the routine and safe use of tourniquets by surgeons, has led to reconsideration of this approach.[13-15] Tourniquets are effective for controlling severe hemorrhage and should be used if direct pressure or a pressure dressing fails to immediately control hemorrhage from an extremity or if sufficient personnel are not available on scene to perform other bleeding control methods. (See Chapter 3, *Shock: Pathophysiology of Life and Death.*) The use of "elevation" and pressure on "pressure points" is no longer recommended because of insufficient data supporting their effectiveness.[16,17] As noted previously, in the case of life-threatening or exsanguinating hemorrhage, a tourniquet should be applied instead of, or concurrent with, other bleeding control measures (i.e., as a first-line treatment for this type of bleeding). Also note that improvised tourniquets may be less effective than commercially available verisons.[18]

Perfusion

The patient's circulatory status can be determined by checking peripheral pulses and evaluating skin color, temperature, and moisture, and, in the absence of severe TBI, the patient's mental status (**Box 6-3**). Assessment of perfusion may be challenging in elderly or pediatric patients or in those who are well conditioned or on certain medications. Shock in trauma patients is almost always

---

Box 6-3 Capillary Refill Time

The capillary refill time is checked by pressing over the nail beds and then releasing the pressure. This downward pressure removes the blood from the visible capillary bed. The rate of return of blood to the nail beds after releasing pressure (refill time) is a tool for estimating blood flow through this most distal part of the circulation. A capillary refill time of greater than 2 seconds may indicate that the capillary beds are not receiving adequate perfusion. However, capillary refill time by itself is a poor indicator of shock because it is influenced by many other factors. For example, peripheral vascular disease (arteriosclerosis), cold temperatures, the use of pharmacologic vasodilators or constrictors, or the presence of neurogenic shock can skew the results. Measuring the capillary refill time becomes a less useful check of cardiovascular function in these cases. Capillary refill time has a place in the evaluation of circulatory adequacy, but it should always be used in conjunction with other physical examination findings (e.g., blood pressure).

due to hemorrhage. (Refer to Chapter 3, *Shock: Pathophysiology of Life and Death*.)

The potential sites of massive internal hemorrhage include the chest (both pleural cavities), the abdomen (peritoneal cavity), the pelvis, the retroperitoneal space, and the extremities (primarily the thighs). If internal hemorrhage is suspected, the thorax, abdomen, pelvis, and thighs are exposed to quickly inspect and palpate for signs of injury. Hemorrhage in these areas is not easy to control outside the hospital. If indicated and available, a pelvic binder should be applied rapidly to address potential "open book" pelvic injuries. The overall goal is rapid delivery of the patient to a facility equipped and appropriately staffed for rapid control of hemorrhage in the OR.

Pulse

The pulse is evaluated for presence, quality, and regularity. A quick check of the pulse reveals whether the patient has tachycardia, bradycardia, or an irregular rhythm. In the past, the presence of a radial pulse has been thought to indicate a systolic blood pressure of at least 80 mm Hg, with the presence of a femoral pulse indicating blood pressure of at least 70 mm Hg, and the presence of only a carotid pulse indicating blood pressure of 60 mm Hg. Evidence has shown this theory to be inaccurate and to overestimate blood pressures.[19] While the absence of peripheral pulses in the presence of central pulses likely represents profound hypotension, the presence of peripheral pulses should not be overly reassuring regarding the patient's blood pressure.

In the primary survey, determination of an exact pulse rate is not necessary. Instead, a rough estimate is rapidly obtained, and the actual pulse rate is obtained later in the process. In trauma patients, it is important to consider treatable causes of abnormal vital signs and physical findings. For example, the combination of compromised perfusion and impaired breathing should prompt the prehospital care practitioner to consider the presence of a tension pneumothorax. If clinical signs are present, needle decompression can be lifesaving. (See Chapter 10, *Thoracic Trauma*.)

Skin

The skin examination can reveal a great deal about a patient's circulatory status.

- *Color*. Skin becomes pale when blood is shunted away from an area. Pale coloration is associated with poor perfusion. Bluish coloration indicates poor oxygenation. The bluish color is caused by perfusion with deoxygenated blood to that region of the body. Skin pigmentation can often make this determination difficult. In patients with deeply pigmented skin, examination of the color of nail beds, palms/soles, and mucous membranes—particularly the palpebral conjunctiva—helps overcome this challenge because changes in color usually first appear in the eyelids, lips, gums, or fingertips due to relative lack of pigmentation in these areas.

- *Temperature*. As with overall skin evaluation, skin temperature is influenced by environmental conditions. Cool skin indicates decreased perfusion, regardless of the cause. Skin temperature can be assessed with a simple touch of the patient's skin with the back of the hand. Normal skin temperature is warm to the touch, neither cool nor hot.

- *Condition*. Under normal circumstances, skin is usually dry. Moist, cool skin can occur in patients with poor perfusion due to sympathetic stimulation (diaphoresis). However, it is important to consider ambient conditions when evaluating skin findings. A patient in a hot or humid environment may have moist skin at baseline, regardless of severity of injury.

D—Disability

After evaluating and correcting, to the extent possible, the factors involved in delivering oxygen to the lungs and circulating it throughout the body, the next step in the primary survey is assessment of cerebral function, which is an indirect measurement of cerebral oxygenation. This begins with determining the patient's level of consciousness (LOC).

The prehospital care practitioner should assume that a confused, belligerent, combative, or uncooperative trauma patient is hypoxic or has suffered a TBI until proved otherwise. Most patients want help when their lives are medically threatened. If a patient refuses help, the reason must be questioned. Does the patient feel threatened by the presence of a practitioner on the scene? If so, further attempts to establish rapport will often help to gain the patient's trust. If nothing in the situation seems to be threatening, the source of the behavior should be considered physiologic and reversible conditions should be identified and treated. During the assessment, the history can help determine whether the patient lost consciousness at any time since the injury occurred, whether toxic substances might be involved (and what they might be), and whether the patient has any preexisting conditions that may produce a decreased LOC or aberrant behavior. Careful observation of the scene can provide invaluable information in this regard.

A decreased LOC alerts a prehospital care practitioner to the following possibilities:

1. Decreased cerebral oxygenation (caused by hypoxia/hypoperfusion) or severe hypoventilation (carbon dioxide narcosis)
2. Central nervous system (CNS) injury (e.g., TBI)
3. Drug or alcohol overdose or toxin exposure
4. Metabolic derangement, in particular hypoglycemia (e.g., caused by diabetes, seizure, or cardiac arrest)

A more in-depth discussion about altered mental status can be found in Chapter 8, *Head and Neck Trauma*, including a thorough explanation of the Glasgow Coma Scale (GCS).

The GCS score is a tool used for determining LOC and is preferred over the AVPU classification (**Box 6-4**).[20] It is a quick, simple method for determining cerebral function and is predictive of patient outcome, especially the best motor response. It also provides a baseline of cerebral function for serial neurologic evaluations. The GCS score is divided into three sections: (1) *eye* opening, (2) *verbal* response, and (3) *motor* response. The patient is assigned a score according to the *best* response to each component of the GCS (**Figure 6-4**). For example, if a patient's right eye is so severely swollen that the patient cannot open it,

Eye Opening	Points
Spontaneous eye opening	4
Eye opening on command	3
Eye opening to pressure	2
No eye opening	1
Best Verbal Response	
Answers appropriately (oriented)	5
Gives confused answers	4
Inappropriate words	3
Makes unintelligible noises	2
Makes no verbal response	1
Best Motor Response	
Follows command	6
Localizes	5
Normal flexion response	4
Abnormal flexion response	3
Extension response	2
Gives no motor response	1
Total	

Figure 6-4 Glasgow Coma Scale (GCS).
© Jones & Bartlett Learning

but the left eye opens spontaneously, the patient receives a 4 for the best eye movement. If a patient lacks spontaneous eye opening, the prehospital care practitioner should use a verbal command (e.g., "Open your eyes"). If the patient does not respond to a verbal stimulus, a painful stimulus, such as pressing the nail bed with a pen or squeezing the axillary tissue, can be applied.

The patient's verbal response is determined by using a question such as, "What happened to you?" If fully oriented, the patient will supply a coherent answer. Otherwise, the patient's verbal response is scored as confused, inappropriate, unintelligible, or absent. If a patient is intubated, the GCS score includes a 1 to reflect the lack of a verbal response, the eye and motor scales are calculated and added, and the letter T is added to note the inability to assess the verbal response (e.g., 8T).

The third component of the GCS is the motor score. A simple, unambiguous command, such as, "Hold up two fingers" or "Show me a thumbs-up," is given to the patient. If the patient complies with the command, the highest score of 6 is given. A patient who squeezes or grasps the finger of a prehospital care practitioner may simply be demonstrating a grasping reflex and not purposefully following a command. If the patient fails to follow a command, a painful stimulus, as noted previously, should be used, and the patient's best motor response should be scored. A patient who attempts to push away a painful stimulus is considered to be *localizing*. Other possible responses to pain include withdrawal from the stimulus, abnormal flexion (*decorticate posturing*) or extension (*decerebrate posturing*) of the upper extremities, or absence of motor function.

The maximum GCS score is 15, indicating a patient with no disability. The lowest score of 3 is generally an ominous sign. A score of less than 8 indicates a major injury, 9 to 12 a moderate injury, and 13 to 15 a minor injury. A GCS score of 8 or less is an indication to carefully evaluate the need for active airway management of the patient. The prehospital care practitioner can easily calculate and relate the individual components of the score and should include them in the verbal report to the receiving facility as well as in the patient care report. Often, it is preferable to communicate individual components of the GCS rather than just the total score, as specific changes can then be documented. A patient care report that states that "the patient is E4, V4, M6" indicates that the patient is confused but follows commands.

Although the GCS score is almost ubiquitous in the evaluation of trauma patients, there are several issues that may limit its usefulness in the prehospital setting. For example, it has poor interrater reliability, meaning practitioners may score the same patient differently and thus provide different management.[21-23] Also, as noted previously, scores are skewed in intubated patients. Therefore, there has been a search for a simpler scoring system, which still has predictive value for patient severity and outcomes. Evidence suggests that the motor component of the GCS alone is essentially as useful in evaluating a patient as the entire score.[24] It has been shown to accurately predict outcomes such as a patient's need for intubation and survival to hospital discharge.[25] One study even suggests that whether a patient can follow commands (i.e., has a motor score of 6) or not predicts severity of injury as well as total GCS score.[26]

If a patient is not awake, oriented, or able to follow commands, the prehospital care practitioner can quickly assess spontaneous extremity movement as well as the patient's pupils. Are the pupils equal and round, reactive to light (PERRL)? Are the pupils equal to each other? Is each pupil round and of normal appearance, and does it appropriately react to light by constricting, or is it unresponsive and dilated? Is the gaze conjugate? A GCS score of less than 14 in combination with an abnormal pupil examination can indicate the presence of a life-threatening TBI.

E—Expose/Environment

An early step in the assessment process is to remove a patient's clothes because exposure of the trauma patient is critical to finding all injuries (**Figure 6-5**). The saying, "The one part of the body that is not exposed will be the most severely injured part," may not always be true, but it is true often enough to warrant a total body examination. Also, blood can collect in and be absorbed by clothing and go unnoticed. After seeing the patient's entire body, the prehospital care practitioner can then cover the patient again to conserve body heat.

Although it is important to expose a trauma patient's body to complete an effective assessment, **hypothermia** is a serious problem in the management of a trauma patient. Only what is necessary should be exposed to the outside environment. Once the patient has been moved

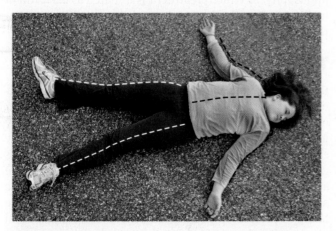

Figure 6-5 Clothing can be quickly removed by cutting, as indicated by the dotted lines.
© National Association of Emergency Medical Technicians (NAEMT)

inside the warm emergency medical services (EMS) unit, the complete examination can be accomplished, and the patient covered again as quickly as possible.

The amount of the patient's clothing that should be removed during an assessment varies depending on the conditions or injuries found. A general rule is to remove as much clothing as necessary to determine the presence or absence of a suspected condition or injury. If a patient has normal mental status and an isolated injury, only the area around the injury generally needs to be exposed. Patients with a serious mechanism of injury or altered mental status should be fully exposed to evaluate for injuries. The prehospital care practitioner need not be afraid to remove clothing if it is the only way to complete the assessment and treatment properly. On occasion, patients can sustain multiple mechanisms of injury, such as experiencing a motor vehicle crash after being shot. Life-threatening injuries may be missed if the patient is inadequately examined. Injuries cannot be treated if they are not identified.

Special care should be taken when cutting and removing clothing from a victim of a crime so as not to inadvertently destroy evidence (**Box 6-5**).

To maintain body temperature and prevent hypothermia, the patient should be covered as soon as practical

---

Box 6-5 Forensic Evidence

Unfortunately, some trauma patients are victims of violent crimes. In these situations, it is important to do everything possible to preserve evidence for law enforcement personnel. When cutting clothing from a crime victim, care should be taken not to cut through holes in the clothing made by bullets (projectiles), knives, or other objects because this can compromise valuable forensic evidence. If clothing is removed from a victim of a potential crime, it should be placed in a paper (not plastic) bag and turned over to law enforcement personnel on scene before patient transport. Any weapons, drugs, or personal belongings found during patient assessment should also be turned over to law enforcement personnel. If the patient's condition warrants transport before the arrival of law enforcement, these items should be brought with the patient to the hospital. The local law enforcement agency should be notified of the destination facility. Document the turnover of the patient's belongings to law enforcement or the hospital per local protocols. Note, however, that patient care always comes first. No procedure or intervention should be delayed or altered in the name of a pending criminal investigation.

© National Association of Emergency Medical Technicians (NAEMT)

after assessment and treatment. In cold environments, prehospital care practitioners should consider using thermal blankets. Once in the ambulance, practitioners should adjust the vehicle heater to adequately warm the patient compartment, even though this may feel uncomfortably hot to practitioners.

Simultaneous Evaluation and Management

As mentioned earlier in this chapter, even though the primary survey is presented and taught in a stepwise fashion, many steps can be assessed simultaneously. By asking questions such as "Where do you hurt?", airway patency is assessed and respiratory function observed. This questioning can occur while the prehospital care practitioner is palpating the radial pulse and feeling the temperature and moistness of the skin. The patient's LOC and mentation can be determined by the appropriateness of the patient's verbal responses. Then the practitioner can rapidly scan the patient from head to foot looking for signs of hemorrhage or other injury. The second practitioner could be directed to apply direct pressure or a tourniquet to an external hemorrhage while the first practitioner continues to assess the patient's airway and breathing. By using this approach, a rapid evaluation for life-threatening injuries is achieved. The primary survey should be repeated frequently, especially in patients with serious injury.

Adjuncts to Primary Survey

Several adjuncts may be useful in monitoring the patient's condition, including the following:

- *Pulse oximetry.* A pulse oximeter should be applied during the primary survey or as soon as available. Oxygen can then be titrated to maintain oxygen saturation (SpO_2) of greater than or equal to 94%. A pulse oximeter also alerts the prehospital care practitioner to the patient's heart rate. Any drop in SpO_2 should prompt a repeat of the primary survey to identify the underlying cause. It is important to remember that pulse oximetry is subject to a "lag time" between the true blood oxygen saturation and what is displayed on the monitor because the signal is averaged, generally over 5 to 30 seconds. In patients with poor peripheral perfusion or peripheral vasoconstriction, the latency period becomes significantly longer, up to 120 seconds or more.[27] Therefore, a patient can (temporarily, at least) have a normal oximetry reading without adequate oxygenation, and vice versa. Other factors, such as carbon monoxide, can also affect the reliability of pulse oximetry readings.
- *End-tidal carbon dioxide ($ETCO_2$) monitoring.* Monitoring the $ETCO_2$ can be useful in confirming proper placement of an endotracheal tube and supraglottic airway as well as indirectly measuring the patient's arterial carbon dioxide level ($PaCO_2$).[28] Although $ETCO_2$ may not always correlate well with the patient's $PaCO_2$, especially in multisystem trauma patients, trending of $ETCO_2$ may be useful in guiding ventilatory rate.
- *Electrocardiographic (ECG) monitoring.* ECG monitoring is less useful than monitoring pulse oximetry, as the presence of an organized cardiac electrical pattern on the monitor does not always correlate with adequate perfusion. Monitoring of the pulse and/or blood pressure is still required to assess for perfusion. An audible signal can alert the prehospital care practitioner of a change in the patient's heart rate or rhythm.
- *Blood pressure monitoring.* In general, obtaining blood pressure is not part of the primary survey; however, in a critically injured patient whose condition does not permit a more thorough secondary survey, obtaining an initial manual blood pressure followed by application of an automated blood pressure monitor for trending purposes during transport can provide additional information regarding the patient's degree of shock. Whenever time permits, the practitioner should attempt to obtain a blood pressure reading by auscultation rather than by automated means as automated blood pressure measurements are less accurate than manual readings in trauma.[29] Nonetheless, trending using automated measurements provides useful information while preserving manpower.

Resuscitation

Resuscitation describes treatment steps taken to correct life-threatening problems as identified in the primary survey. PHTLS assessment is based on a "treat as you go" philosophy, in which treatment is initiated as each threat to life is identified or at the earliest possible moment (**Figure 6-6**).

Transport

If life-threatening conditions are identified during the primary survey, the patient should be rapidly packaged after initiating limited field intervention. Transport of critically injured trauma patients to the closest appropriate facility should be initiated as soon as possible (**Box 6-6**). Unless complicating circumstances exist, scene time should be as short as possible for these patients. Limited scene time and initiation of rapid transport to the closest appropriate facility—preferably a trauma center—are fundamental aspects of prehospital trauma resuscitation.

Research has found that worse outcomes occurred in severely injured trauma patients when the on-scene time

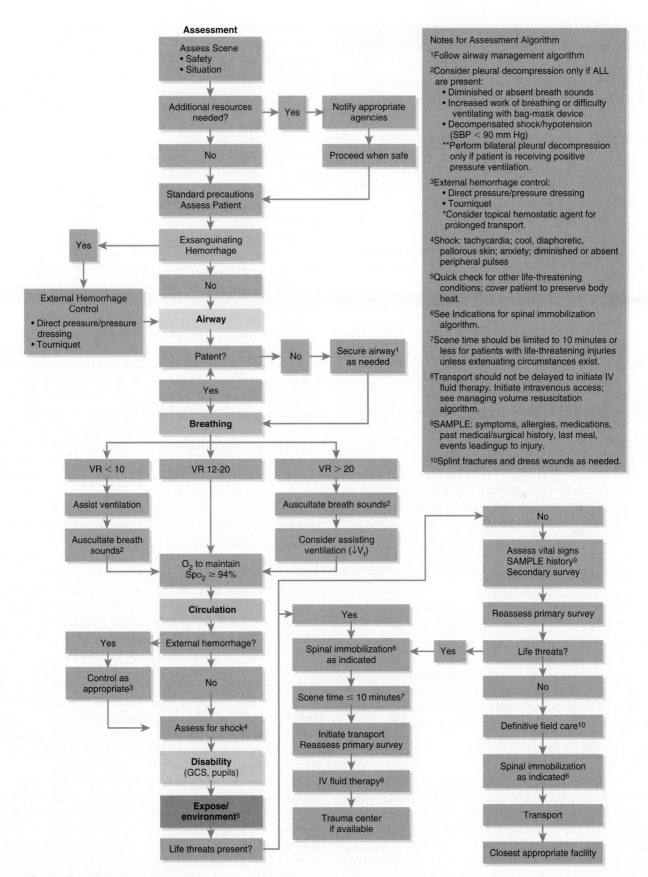

Figure 6-6 Assessment algorithm.

© National Association of Emergency Medical Technicians (NAEMT)

Box 6-6 Critical Trauma Patient

Keep scene time as brief as possible (ideally 10 minutes or less) when any of the following life-threatening conditions is present:

1. Inadequate or threatened airway
2. Impaired ventilation, as demonstrated by the following:
   - Abnormally fast or slow ventilatory rate
   - Hypoxia (SpO$_2$ < 94% even with supplemental oxygen)
   - Dyspnea
   - Open pneumothorax or flail chest
   - Suspected closed or tension pneumothorax
3. Significant external hemorrhage or suspected internal hemorrhage
4. Abnormal neurologic status
   - GCS score ≤ 13 or motor component < 6
   - Seizure activity
   - Sensory or motor deficit
5. Penetrating trauma to the head, neck, or torso or proximal to the elbow or knee in the extremities
6. Amputation or near-amputation proximal to the fingers or toes
7. Any significant trauma in the presence of the following:
   - History of serious medical conditions (e.g., coronary artery disease, chronic obstructive pulmonary disease, bleeding disorder)
   - Age > 55 years
   - Hypothermia
   - Burns
   - Pregnancy

© National Association of Emergency Medical Technicians (NAEMT)

was extended compared to the response and transport intervals. This finding was particularly true for patients with hypotension, flail chest, or penetrating injury. The finding further supports the concept that time on scene should be as short as possible, with only interventions for reversible life-threatening conditions performed on scene.[30]

Fluid Therapy

Another important step in resuscitation is the restoration of the perfusing volume within the cardiovascular system as quickly as possible. This step does not involve restoring blood pressure to normal but rather providing enough fluid to ensure that vital organs are perfused. Although a few ground EMS agencies now have blood available for prehospital administration,[31] blood products are usually only found on critical care and helicopter EMS units.

Crystalloid fluids such as lactated Ringer's or normal saline solution are most commonly used for trauma resuscitation in the prehospital setting. In addition to sodium and chloride, lactated Ringer's solution contains small amounts of potassium, calcium, and lactate, making it less acidotic than saline. However, crystalloid fluids do not replace the oxygen-carrying capacity of the lost RBCs nor do they replace the platelets that are necessary for clotting. Therefore, rapid transport of a severely injured patient to an appropriate facility is an absolute necessity. Furthermore, given the risks of excessive crystalloid resuscitation, these fluids must be used judiciously and titrated to specific clinical targets.

En route to the receiving facility, one or two 18-gauge intravenous (IV) catheters may be placed in the patient's forearm or antecubital veins, if possible, as time permits. Prehospital care practitioners should be cognizant of the increased risk of needlestick injury while starting an IV in a moving ambulance and should take steps to minimize this risk. If attempts at IV access are not quickly successful, intraosseous (IO) access should be initiated. The proximal humerus site allows for faster fluid flow rates than the proximal tibia.[32] In general, central IV lines (subclavian, internal jugular, or femoral) are not appropriate for the field management of trauma patients. The appropriate amount of fluid administration depends on the clinical scenario, primarily whether the patient's hemorrhage has been controlled when the IV fluid is initiated, if the patient is hypotensive, or whether the patient has evidence of TBI. One study suggests that prehospital IV fluid is beneficial for patients with hypotension but may be harmful in those without hypotension.[33] Chapter 3, *Shock: Pathophysiology of Life and Death*, and Chapter 8, *Head and Neck Trauma*, provide more detailed guidelines for fluid resuscitation.

Starting an IV line at the scene only prolongs on-scene time and delays transport. As addressed previously, the definitive treatment for the trauma patient with internal hemorrhage or significant blood loss can be accomplished only in the hospital. For example, a patient with an injury to the spleen who is losing 50 milliliters of blood per minute will continue to bleed at that rate until intervention in the OR or angiography suite. Initiating IV lines on the scene instead of early transport will not only increase blood loss but also may decrease the patient's chance of survival. Exceptions exist, such as entrapment, when a patient cannot be moved immediately.

External hemorrhage should be controlled prior to initiation of IV fluid. Aggressive administration of IV fluids should be avoided as this approach may "pop the clot" and lead to further hemorrhage by increasing blood pressure and diluting platelets and clotting factors. More important, continual volume replacement is not a substitute for manual control of external hemorrhage and initiation of transport for internal hemorrhage.

Basic Versus Advanced Prehospital Care Practitioner Levels

The key steps in resuscitating a critically injured trauma patient are the same at both the basic and the advanced levels of prehospital care practitioner. They include (1) immediately controlling major external hemorrhage, (2) opening and maintaining the airway, (3) ensuring adequate ventilation, (4) rapidly packaging the patient for transport, and (5) quickly initiating rapid, but safe, transport of the patient to the closest appropriate facility. If transport time is prolonged, it may be appropriate for the basic-level practitioner to call for assistance from a nearby advanced life support (ALS) service that can rendezvous with the basic unit en route. Helicopter evacuation to a trauma center is another option. Both the ALS service and the flight service can provide advanced airway management and IV fluid replacement. Air medical services may also carry blood, fresh frozen plasma, and other therapies beyond typical ground ALS unit.

Secondary Survey

The secondary survey is a more detailed head-to-toe evaluation of a patient. It is performed only after the primary survey is completed, all identified life-threatening injuries have been treated, and resuscitation has been initiated. The objective of the secondary survey is to identify injuries or problems that were not identified during the primary survey. Because a well-performed primary survey will identify all immediately life-threatening conditions, the secondary survey, by definition, deals with less serious problems. Therefore, a critical trauma patient is transported as soon as possible after conclusion of the primary survey and not held in the field for either IV initiation or a secondary survey.

The secondary survey uses a "look, listen, and feel" approach to evaluate the patient. The practitioner identifies injuries and correlates physical findings region by region, beginning at the head and proceeding through the neck, chest, and abdomen to the extremities, concluding with a detailed neurologic examination (**Figure 6-7**).

While examining the patient, all available information is used to formulate a patient care plan.

See

- Examine all the skin of each region.
- Be attentive for external hemorrhage or signs of internal hemorrhage, such as distension of the abdomen, swollen and tense extremity, or an expanding hematoma.
- Note soft-tissue injuries, including abrasions, burns, contusions, hematomas, lacerations, and puncture wounds.

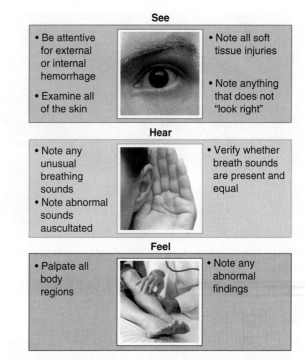

Figure 6-7 The physical assessment of a trauma patient involves careful observation, auscultation, and palpation (look, listen, and feel).

Eye photo: © REKINC1980/iStock/Getty Images; ear photo: © vvs1976/iStock/Getty Images; hands photo: © Image Point Fr/Shutterstock. © National Association of Emergency Medical Technicians (NAEMT)

- Note any masses or swelling or deformation of bones (deformities).
- Note abnormal indentations on the skin and the skin's color.
- Note anything that does not "look right."

Hear

- Note any unusual sounds when the patient inhales or exhales. Normal breathing is quiet.
- Note any abnormal sounds when auscultating the chest.
- Auscultate whether the breath sounds are equal in both lung fields (**Figure 6-8**).
- Auscultate over the carotid arteries and note any unusual sounds (bruits) over the vessels that would indicate vascular damage (often not realistic on a trauma scene).

Feel

- Firmly palpate the entire body. Note whether anything moves that should not, whether there is any crepitus or subcutaneous emphysema, whether the patient complains of tenderness, whether all pulses are present, and whether pulsations are felt that should not be present.
- Carefully move each joint in the region. Note any resulting crepitus, pain, or limitation of range of motion, or unusual movement, such as laxity.

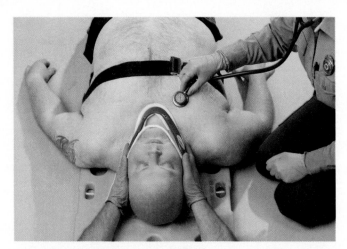

Figure 6-8 Check whether the breath sounds are equal in all lung fields.

© Jones & Bartlett Learning. Photographed by Darren Stahlman.

Vital Signs

The first step of the secondary survey is measuring the vital signs. The rate and quality of the pulse, rate and depth of ventilation, and the other components of the primary survey are continually reevaluated and compared to previous findings because significant changes can occur rapidly. Depending on the situation, a second prehospital care practitioner may obtain vital signs while the first practitioner completes the primary survey, to avoid further delay. However, exact "numbers" for pulse rate, ventilatory rate, and blood pressure are not critical in the initial management of the patient with severe multisystem trauma. Therefore, the measurement of the exact numbers can be delayed until completion of the essential steps of resuscitation and stabilization.

A set of complete vital signs includes blood pressure, pulse rate and quality, ventilatory rate and depth, oxygen saturation (pulse oximetry), and temperature (skin temperature and body temperature). For the critical trauma patient, a complete set of vital signs is evaluated and recorded every 3 to 5 minutes, if possible; the time of any change in condition or medical problem should also be noted. Even if an automated, noninvasive blood pressure device is available, the initial blood pressure reading should be taken manually. Automated blood pressure devices may be inaccurate when the patient is significantly hypotensive; therefore, in these patients, all blood pressure measurements should be obtained manually, or at least correlation of an automated reading with a manual reading should be confirmed.

SAMPLER History

A quick history is obtained on the patient. This information should be documented on the patient care report and passed on to the medical personnel at the receiving facility.

The mnemonic SAMPLER serves as a reminder of the key components:

- *Symptoms.* What is the patient's main complaint? Pain? Trouble breathing? Numbness? Tingling?
- *Allergies.* Does the patient have any known allergies, particularly to medications?
- *Medications.* What prescription or nonprescription drugs (including vitamins, supplements, and other over-the-counter medications) does the patient regularly take? What recreational substance does the patient use regularly and, in particular, today?
- *Past medical and surgical history.* Does the patient have any significant medical problems requiring ongoing medical care? Has the patient undergone any prior surgeries?
- *Last meal/last menstrual period.* How long has it been since the patient last ate? Many trauma patients will require surgery, and recent food intake increases the risk of aspiration during induction of anesthesia. For female patients of childbearing age, when was their last menstrual period? Is there a possibility of pregnancy?
- *Events.* What events preceded the injury? Immersion in water (drowning or hypothermia) and exposure to hazardous materials should be included.
- *Risk factors.* Is the patient living alone and at higher risk for falls? Did the weather or other environmental hazard add to patient's risk for traumatic injury? Are there special population risk factors to consider (e.g., pediatric, geriatric, bariatric, or obstetric patients)?

Assessing Anatomic Regions

Head

Visual examination of the head and face will reveal contusions, abrasions, lacerations, bone asymmetry, hemorrhage, bony defects of the face and supportive skull, and abnormalities of the eye, eyelid, external ear, mouth, and mandible. The following steps are included during a head examination:

- Search thoroughly through the patient's hair for any soft-tissue injuries of the scalp.
- Check pupil size for reactivity to light, equality, accommodation, roundness, and irregular shape.
- Carefully palpate the bones of the face and skull to identify focal tenderness, crepitus, deviation, depression, or abnormal mobility. (This is extremely important in the nonradiographic evaluation for head injury.) **Figure 6-9** reviews the bony anatomy of the skull.
- Care should be exercised when attempting to open and examine the eyes of an unconscious trauma patient who has evidence of facial injury. Even small amounts of pressure may further damage an eye that has a blunt or penetrating injury.

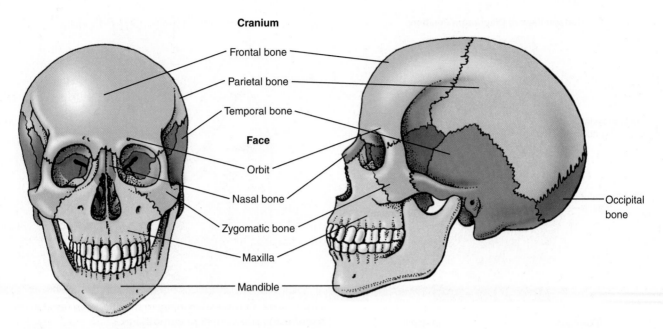

Figure 6-9 Normal anatomic structure of the face and skull.
© National Association of Emergency Medical Technicians (NAEMT)

Fractures of the bones of the midface are often associated with a fracture of the portion of the skull base called the cribriform plate. If the patient has midface trauma (e.g., injury between the upper lip and orbits), a gastric tube, if used, should be inserted through the mouth rather than through the nose.

Neck

Visual examination of the neck for contusions, abrasions, lacerations, hematomas, and deformities will alert the prehospital care practitioner to the possibility of underlying injuries. Palpation may reveal subcutaneous emphysema from a laryngeal, tracheal, or pulmonary origin. Crepitus of the larynx, hoarseness, and subcutaneous emphysema constitute a triad classically indicative of laryngeal fracture. Lack of tenderness of the cervical spine may help rule out cervical spine fractures (when combined with strict criteria), whereas tenderness may frequently indicate the presence of a fracture, dislocation, or ligamentous injury. Such palpation is performed carefully, ensuring that the cervical spine remains in a neutral, in-line position. Absence of a neurologic deficit does not exclude the possibility of an unstable cervical spine injury. Reevaluation may reveal expansion of a previously identified hematoma or shifting of the trachea. **Figure 6-10** reviews the normal anatomic structure of the neck.

Chest

Because the thorax is strong, resilient, and elastic, it can absorb a significant amount of trauma. Close visual examination of the chest for deformities, puncture and penetrating wounds, contusions, and abrasions is necessary

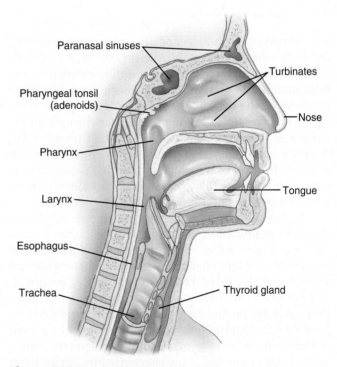

Figure 6-10 Normal anatomy of the neck.
© National Association of Emergency Medical Technicians (NAEMT)

to identify underlying injuries. Other signs for which the prehospital care practitioner should watch closely include splinting and guarding, unequal bilateral chest excursion, areas of paradoxical movement, and intercostal, suprasternal, or supraclavicular bulging or retraction.

A contusion over the sternum may be the only indication of an underlying cardiac injury. Penetrating wounds may affect body areas remote from the entry site.

Lateral View of Diaphragm Position

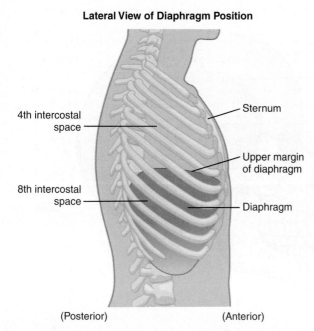

(Posterior)   (Anterior)

Figure 6-11 Lateral view of diaphragm position at full expiration.

© National Association of Emergency Medical Technicians (NAEMT)

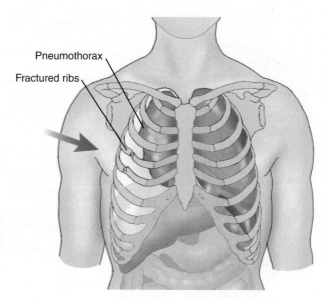

Figure 6-12 Compression injury to the chest can result in rib fracture and subsequent pneumothorax.

© National Association of Emergency Medical Technicians (NAEMT)

It is important to understand the relationship between the body surface and underlying organs, such as the diaphragm and its variable position during exhalation and inhalation. A line traced from the fourth intercostal space anteriorly to the sixth intercostal space laterally and to the eighth intercostal space posteriorly defines the upward excursion of the diaphragm at full expiration (**Figure 6-11**). A penetrating injury that occurs below this line (which is about the level of the nipples) or with a path that may have taken it below this line should be considered to have traversed both the thoracic and abdominal cavities.

Auscultation with a stethoscope is an essential part of the chest examination. A patient will most often be in a supine position so that only the anterior and lateral chest is available for auscultation. It is important to recognize normal and decreased breath sounds with a patient in this position. Diminished or absent breath sounds indicate a possible pneumothorax, tension pneumothorax, or hemothorax. Crackles heard posteriorly (when the patient is logrolled) or laterally may indicate pulmonary contusion. Cardiac tamponade is characterized by distant heart sounds; however, these may be difficult to ascertain given the commotion at the scene or road noise during transport.

A small area of rib fractures may indicate a severe underlying pulmonary contusion. Any type of compression injury to the chest can result in a pneumothorax (**Figure 6-12**). The thorax is palpated for the presence of subcutaneous emphysema (air in the soft tissue).

Abdomen

The abdominal examination begins, as with the other parts of the body, by visual evaluation. Abrasions and ecchymosis indicate the possibility of underlying injury; in particular, periumbilical and flank ecchymosis is associated with retroperitoneal bleeding. In the case of a motor vehicle collision, the abdomen should be examined carefully for a telltale transverse red stripe across the lower abdomen, which suggests that a seat belt may have caused underlying injury. A significant portion of patients with this sign will have underlying injury, most frequently small bowel injury.[34-36] Lumbar spine fractures may also be associated with this "seat belt sign."

Examination of the abdomen also includes palpation of each quadrant to evaluate for tenderness, abdominal muscle guarding, and masses. When palpating, the prehospital care practitioner notes whether the abdomen is soft or whether rigidity or guarding is present. There is no need to continue palpating after discovering abdominal tenderness or pain. Additional information will not alter prehospital management, and the only outcomes of a continued abdominal examination are further discomfort to the patient and delayed transport to the receiving facility. Similarly, auscultation of the abdomen adds virtually nothing to the assessment of a trauma patient. The peritoneal cavity can hide a large volume of blood, often with minimal or no abdominal distension.

Altered mental status resulting from a TBI or intoxication with alcohol or other drugs often obscures evaluation of the abdomen.

Pelvis

The pelvis is evaluated by observation and palpation. The pelvis is first visually examined for abrasions, contusions, hematomas, lacerations, open fractures, and signs of distension. Pelvic fractures can produce massive internal hemorrhage, resulting in rapid deterioration of a patient's hemodynamic status.

Palpation of the pelvis in the prehospital setting provides minimal information that will affect the management of the patient. When examined, the pelvis is palpated only once for tenderness and instability as part of the secondary survey. Because palpation of the unstable pelvis can move fractured segments and disrupt any clot that has formed, thus aggravating hemorrhage, this examination step should be performed only once and not repeated. Palpation is accomplished by gently applying anterior-to-posterior pressure with the heels of the hands on the symphysis pubis and then medial pressure to the iliac crests bilaterally, evaluating for pain and abnormal movement. Any evidence of instability should preclude further palpation of the pelvis and prompt placement of a pelvic binder, if available.

Genitals

In general, genitalia are not examined in detail in the prehospital setting. However, note should be made of bleeding from the external genitalia, obvious blood at the urethral meatus, or presence of priapism in males. Additionally, clear fluid from a pregnant patient may represent amniotic fluid from rupture of the amniotic membranes.

Back

The back should be examined for evidence of injury. This is best accomplished when logrolling the patient for placement onto or removal from the long backboard or other transfer device. Breath sounds should be auscultated over the posterior thorax; the back should be observed for contusions, abrasions, and deformities; and the spine should be palpated for tenderness.

Extremities

The examination of the extremities begins at the clavicle in the upper extremity and the pelvis in the lower extremity and then proceeds toward the most distal portion of each extremity. Each individual bone and joint is evaluated by visual inspection for deformity, hematoma, or ecchymosis and by palpation to determine the presence of crepitus, pain, tenderness, or unusual movements. Any suspected fracture should be immobilized. Circulation and motor and sensory nerve function at the distal end of each extremity are also checked. If an extremity is immobilized, pulses, movement, and sensation should be checked both before and after splinting.

Neurologic Examination

As with the other regional examinations described, the neurologic examination in the secondary survey is conducted in much greater detail than in the primary survey. Calculation of the GCS score, evaluation of motor and sensory function, and observation of pupillary response are all included. A gross examination of sensory capability and motor response

will determine the presence or absence of weakness or loss of sensation in the extremities, suggesting brain or spinal cord injury, and will identify areas that require further examination. When examining a patient's pupils, equality of response in addition to equality of size are evaluated. A small but significant portion of the population has pupils of differing sizes (*anisocoria*) as a normal condition. Even in these patients, however, the pupils should react to light in a similar manner. Pupils that react at differing speeds to the introduction of light are considered to be unequal. Unequal pupils in an unconscious trauma patient may indicate increased intracranial pressure or pressure on the third cranial nerve, caused by either cerebral edema or a rapidly expanding intracranial hematoma (**Figure 6-13**). Direct eye injury can also cause unequal pupils.

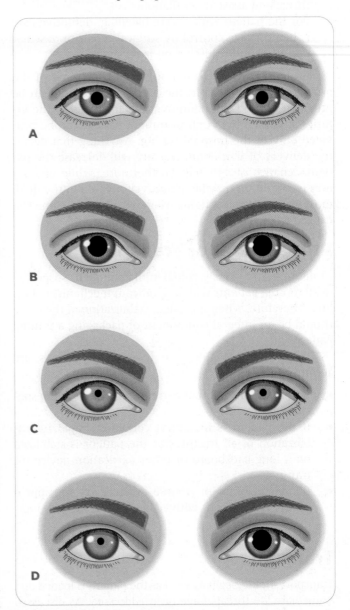

Figure 6-13 A. Normal pupils. **B.** Pupil dilation. **C.** Pupil constriction. **D.** Unequal pupils.
© Jones & Bartlett Learning.

Definitive Care in the Field

Definitive care is an intervention that completely corrects a particular condition. The following are examples of definitive care:

- For a patient with cardiac arrest in ventricular fibrillation, definitive care is defibrillation resulting in return of spontaneous circulation (ROSC).
- For a patient in a diabetic hypoglycemic coma, definitive care is glucose administration and a return to normal blood glucose levels.
- For a patient with an obstructed airway, definitive care is relief of the obstruction, which may be accomplished by a maneuver as simple as the trauma jaw thrust and assisted ventilation.
- For the patient with severe bleeding, definitive care is hemorrhage control by surgical repair or vascular occlusion and resuscitation from shock.

In general, whereas definitive care for some of the problems encountered in the prehospital setting can be provided in the field, definitive care for many of the injuries sustained by a critical trauma patient can be provided only in the hospital setting. Anything that delays the delivery of that definitive care will decrease the patient's chance of survival. Furthermore, while one injury or condition may be definitively treated in the field, most major trauma patients will have others that must be treated in the hospital.

Preparation for Transport

As discussed previously, spinal injury should be suspected in all trauma patients with a significant mechanism of injury. Therefore, when indicated, stabilization of the spine should be an integral component of packaging a trauma patient.

If time is available, the following measures are accomplished:

- Careful stabilization of extremity fractures using specific splints
- If the patient is in critical condition, rapid immobilization of all fractures as the patient is stabilized on a long backboard or other extrication device for transport
- Bandaging of major wounds as necessary and appropriate (i.e., wounds with active hemorrhage, abdominal evisceration)

Transport

Transport should begin as soon as the patient is loaded and immediate life threats have been addressed. As discussed previously, delay at the scene to start an IV line or to complete the secondary survey only extends the period before the receiving facility can administer blood and control hemorrhage. Continued evaluation and further resuscitation occur en route to the receiving facility. *For some critically injured trauma patients, initiation of transport is the single most important aspect of definitive care in the field.*

A patient whose condition is not critical can receive attention for individual injuries before transport, but even for this patient, transportation should be initiated before a hidden condition becomes critical.

Field Triage of Injured Patients

Selection of the proper destination facility for a critically injured patient can be every bit as important as other lifesaving interventions provided in the prehospital setting, and it is based on the assessment of the patient's injuries or suspected injuries (**Box 6-7**). For more than 40 years, numerous articles published in the medical literature have documented that facilities that have made the commitment to be prepared to care for injured patients—i.e., trauma centers—have better outcomes.[37-41] A study funded by the Centers for Disease Control and Prevention (CDC), published in 2006, demonstrated that patients were 25% more likely to survive their injuries if they received care at a level I trauma center than if they were cared for in a nontrauma center.[42] Although 82.1% of the U.S. population lives within 60 minutes of a trauma center, slightly more than half of all persons injured did not receive their care from a designated trauma center, including 36% of major trauma victims.[43-45] The data are clear: The mortality rate from serious injury is significantly reduced by transporting injured patients to designated trauma centers.

One of the more challenging decisions faced by a prehospital care practitioner involves determining which injured patients are best cared for in trauma centers. Proper

---

Box 6-7 National Guideline for the Field Triage of Injured Patients

The American College of Surgeons Committee on Trauma National Guideline for the Field Triage of Injured Patients (previously published by the Centers for Disease Control and Prevention) segregate trauma patients into groups that are at high versus moderate risk of serious injury. High-risk patients (red criteria) should be transported to the highest-level trauma center available. Moderate-risk patients (yellow criteria) can be safely transported to any trauma center. In both cases, the geographic constraints of the regional trauma system must be considered.[46]

Data from American College of Surgeons. COT releases updated national guideline for field triage of injured patients. Reviewed May 3, 2022. Accessed June 1, 2022. https://www.facs.org/for-medical-professionals/news-publications/news-and-articles/acs-brief/may-10-2022-issue/cot-releases-updated-national-guideline-for-field-triage-of-injured-patients

selection of which patients to transport to a trauma center involves a balance between "overtriage" and "undertriage." Transporting all trauma patients to trauma centers may result in overtriage, meaning that a significant number of these injured patients will not need the specialized services offered by these facilities. Overtriage could result in worse care to patients who have more serious injuries, because the trauma center's resources become overwhelmed by patients who have less serious injuries. At the opposite end of the spectrum is undertriage, in which a seriously injured patient is taken to a nontrauma center. Undertriage can also result in worse patient outcomes, as the facility may lack the capabilities to properly care for the patient. Some degree of undertriage seems inevitable, as some life-threatening conditions may not be identifiable in the prehospital setting. To minimize undertriage, experts estimate that an overtriage rate of 30% to 50% is necessary, meaning that 30% to 50% of injured patients transported to a trauma center will not need the specialized care available there.[47]

The commonly recognized definition for a "major trauma patient" is a patient with an Injury Severity Score (ISS) of 16 or higher (**Box 6-8**). Unfortunately, an ISS can be calculated only when all of the patient's injuries are diagnosed, including those found through advanced imaging (e.g., computed tomography) or surgery. Thus, the patient's ISS cannot be calculated in the prehospital setting. Alternative definitions have been proposed that include trauma patients who (1) die in the ED or within 24 hours of admission, (2) need massive transfusion of blood products, (3) need admission to an intensive care unit, (4) require urgent surgery for their injuries, or (5) require control of internal hemorrhage using interventional angiography. Although all these definitions are useful for research purposes, none can be identified by prehospital care practitioners.

In an effort to identify patients who would most benefit from transport to and care at a trauma center, the American College of Surgeons Committee on Trauma (ACS-COT) updated the National Guidelines for the Field Triage of Injured Patients in May 2022 (**Figure 6-14**). This document provides guidelines to assist EMS practitioners in making appropriate decisions about the transport destination of individual trauma patients.[49,50]

The National Field Triage Guidelines contain four sections for consideration:

- *Injury Patterns*. This section describes those injury patterns most likely to be associated with life-threatening conditions such as flail chest, pelvic fracture, or active bleeding. Patients with these injury patterns warrant transfer to the highest-level trauma center available.
- *Mental Status and Vital Signs*. These patients have an altered mental status and/or other evidence of physiologic instability that indicates transport to the highest-level trauma center available is warranted.

Box 6-8 ISS Assessment

Various scoring systems are used to analyze and categorize patients who suffer traumatic injury in the hospital setting. Scoring systems may also be used to predict patient outcomes based on the severity of their traumatic injury. These scoring systems generally are not calculated until the patient has been fully evaluated at the trauma center. They offer limited use in the initial triage of injured patients in the field, but they do have significant value in the overall quality assessment and quality improvement (QA/QI) process of trauma care delivery.

One of the most commonly discussed scoring systems is the **Injury Severity Score (ISS)**. The ISS categorizes injuries into six anatomically distinct body regions:

1. Head and neck
2. Face
3. Chest
4. Abdomen
5. Extremities
6. External

Only the most severe injury in any one region is taken into account. After the most severe injuries in all six regions have been identified, they are assigned a value from 1 to 6 using the **Abbreviated Injury Scale (AIS)**:

1. Minor
2. Moderate
3. Serious
4. Severe
5. Critical
6. Unsurvivable

The highest three values are then squared to give additional weight to the highest scores and minimize the lowest scores. These values are then added together to calculate the final ISS.[48]

Higher ISS scores correlate linearly with mortality, morbidity, length of stay in the hospital, and other measures of severity. The major limitations of the ISS are that AIS scoring errors are amplified when calculated into the ISS, and there is no consideration given to the fact that injuries to certain areas of the body may inherently be more severe than injuries to other areas. Although of limited use in the field triage of trauma patients, an understanding of how injury severity scores are calculated is highly valuable for the EMS practitioner when reading research articles and practice updates.

National Guideline for the Field Triage of Injured Patients

RED CRITERIA
High Risk for Serious Injury

Injury Patterns	Mental Status & Vital Signs
• Penetrating injuries to head, neck, torso, and proximal extremities • Skull deformity, suspected skull fracture • Suspected spinal injury with new motor or sensory loss • Chest wall instability, deformity, or suspected flail chest • Suspected pelvic fracture • Suspected fracture of two or more proximal long bones • Crushed, degloved, mangled, or pulseless extremity • Amputation proximal to wrist or ankle • Active bleeding requiring a tourniquet or wound packing with continuous pressure	**All Patients** • Unable to follow commands (motor GCS < 6) • RR < 10 or > 29 breaths/min • Respiratory distress or need for respiratory support • Room-air pulse oximetry < 90% **Age 0–9 years** • SBP < 70mm Hg + (2 x age in years) **Age 10–64 years** • SBP < 90 mmHg or • HR > SBP **Age ≥ 65 years** • SBP < 110 mmHg or • HR > SBP

Patients meeting any one of the above RED criteria should be transported to the highest-level trauma center available within the geographic constraints of the regional trauma system

YELLOW CRITERIA
Moderate Risk for Serious Injury

Mechanism of Injury	EMS Judgment

• High-Risk Auto Crash
  - Partial or complete ejection
  - Significant intrusion (including roof)
    • >12 inches occupant site OR
    • >18 inches any site OR
    • Need for extrication for entrapped patient
  - Death in passenger compartment
  - Child (age 0–9 years) unrestrained or in unsecured child safety seat
  - Vehicle telemetry data consistent with severe injury
• Rider separated from transport vehicle with significant impact (eg, motorcycle, ATV, horse, etc.)
• Pedestrian/bicycle rider thrown, run over, or with significant impact
• Fall from height > 10 feet (all ages)
	Consider risk factors, including:
	
	• Low-level falls in young children (age ≤ 5 years) or older adults (age ≥ 65 years) with significant head impact
	
	• Anticoagulant use
	
	• Suspicion of child abuse
	
	• Special, high-resource healthcare needs
	
	• Pregnancy > 20 weeks
	
	• Burns in conjunction with trauma
	
	• Children should be triaged preferentially to pediatric capable centers
	
	If concerned, take to a trauma center

Patients meeting any one of the YELLOW CRITERIA WHO DO NOT MEET RED CRITERIA should be preferentially transported to a trauma center, as available within the geographic constraints of the regional trauma system (need not be the highest-level trauma center)

Figure 6-14 Deciding where to transport a patient is critical, requiring consideration of the type and location of available facilities and the geographic restraints of the regional trauma system.

- *Mechanism of Injury.* These criteria identify additional patients who may have occult injury not manifested with physiologic derangement or obvious external injury.
- *EMS Judgement.* These criteria identify how factors such as use of anticoagulants, or the presence of burns or pregnancy may affect the decision to transport to a trauma center.

Patients who meet injury criteria based on injury patterns or mental status and vital signs should be transported to the highest level of trauma care available in the region. Patients who meet mechanism of injury criteria or EMS judgement criteria should be transported to the closest appropriate, but not necessarily highest level, trauma center in the region. As with any decision tool, however, it should be used as guidance and not as a replacement for good judgment. When in doubt, transportation to a trauma center is recommended.

Duration of Transport

As discussed previously, the prehospital care practitioner should choose a receiving facility according to the severity of the patient's injury. In simple terms, the patient should be transported to the closest appropriate facility (i.e., the closest facility capable of managing the patient's problems). If the patient's injuries are severe or indicate the possibility of continuing hemorrhage, the practitioner should take the patient to a facility that will provide definitive care as quickly as possible (i.e., a trauma center, if available).

For example, an EMS unit responds to a call in 8 minutes, and the prehospital team spends 6 minutes on the scene to package and load the patient into the transporting unit. So far 14 minutes have passed. The closest hospital is 5 minutes away, and the trauma center is 14 minutes away. In scenario 1, the patient is taken to the trauma center. On arrival, the surgeon is in the emergency department (ED) with the emergency physician and the entire trauma team. The OR is staffed and ready. After 10 minutes in the ED for resuscitation, necessary radiographs, and blood work, the patient is taken to the OR. The total time since the incident is now 38 minutes. In scenario 2, the patient is taken to the closest hospital, which is 9 minutes closer than the trauma center. It has an available emergency physician, but the surgeon and OR team are out of the hospital. The patient's 10 minutes in the ED for resuscitation could stretch to 45 minutes by the time the surgeon arrives and examines the patient. Another 30 minutes could elapse while waiting for the OR team to arrive once the surgeon has examined the patient and decided to operate. The total time for scenario 2 is 94 minutes, or 2½ times longer than the trauma center scenario. The 9 minutes saved by the shorter transport to the closest hospital actually cost 56 minutes to the patient, during which time operative management could have been started and hemorrhage control achieved at the trauma center.

In a rural community, the transport time to an awaiting trauma team may be 45 to 60 minutes or even longer. In this situation, the closest hospital with an on-call trauma team is the appropriate receiving facility.

Another consideration is that many nontrauma centers do not provide definitive care for severely injured patients and so will transfer these patients to a trauma center. If such were the case in scenario 2, the delay to definitive care would be even longer in many instances.

Method of Transport

Another aspect of the patient assessment and transport decision is the transportation method. Some systems have air transport available. Air medical services may offer a higher level of care than ground units for critically injured trauma victims. Air transport may also be quicker and smoother than ground transport in some circumstances. As previously mentioned, if air transport is available in a community and is appropriate for the specific situation, the earlier in the assessment process that the decision is made to call for air transport, the greater the likely benefit to the patient. Helicopter EMS should be considered for those patients meeting guideline criteria for transport to the hospital with the highest level of care in the region.

Monitoring and Reassessment (Ongoing Assessment)

After the primary survey and initial care are complete, the patient must be continuously monitored, the vital signs reassessed, and the primary survey repeated several times while en route to the receiving facility or at the scene if transport is delayed. Continuous reassessment of the components of the primary survey will help ensure that vital functions do not deteriorate or are immediately corrected if they do. The practitioner should pay particular attention to any significant change in a patient's condition and reconsider management options if such a change is noted. Furthermore, the continued monitoring of a patient helps reveal conditions or problems that were overlooked during the primary survey or that are only now presenting. Often the patient's condition will not be obvious, and looking at and listening to the patient provides much information. How the information is gathered is not as important as ensuring that all the information is gathered. Reassessment should be conducted as quickly and thoroughly as possible. Monitoring during a prolonged transport situation is described later.

Communication

Communication between prehospital practitioners and hospital personnel is a critical part of quality patient care and consists of multiple components: prearrival notification, verbal report on arrival at bedside, and the formal written patient care report. Notification to the receiving facility should be made as soon as possible. Early communication allows the facility to assemble the appropriate personnel and equipment necessary to best care for the patient, often by way of a trauma alerting system. During transport, a member of the prehospital care team should provide a brief patient care report to the receiving facility that includes the following information:

- Patient sex and exact or estimated age
- Mechanism of injury
- Life-threatening injuries, conditions identified, and anatomic location of injuries
- Current vital signs
- Interventions that have been performed, and the patient's response to treatment
- Estimated time of arrival (ETA)

If time permits, additional information can be included, such as pertinent medical conditions and medications, other non–life-threatening injuries, characteristics of the scene including protective gear used by the patient (seat belt, helmet, etc.), and information about additional patients. Otherwise, this can be given at the bedside.

The prehospital care practitioner also verbally transfers responsibility for a patient (often called "sign off," "report," or "transfer") to the physician or nurse who takes over the patient's care at the receiving facility. This verbal report is typically more detailed than the radio report but less detailed than the written PCR, providing an overview of the significant history of the incident, the action taken by the practitioners, and the patient's response to this action. Both the verbal and written reports must highlight any significant changes in the patient's condition that have taken place since transmitting the radio report. Transfer of important prehospital information further emphasizes the team concept of patient care.

Some trauma centers have formalized this process to avoid miscommunication and misunderstandings between prehospital and hospital personnel. Upon arrival of the patient in the trauma bay, the trauma team leader will do a rapid primary survey to assure the patient is breathing and has a pulse and then pause to listen to a "20-second shout-out" from the EMS team leader. This verbal report should include the following elements:

1. Age, sex, mechanism of injury, and time of event
2. Prehospital vital signs, including any instance of systolic blood pressure (SBP) < 90 mm Hg

3. Injuries identified
4. Prehospital interventions
5. Changes in patient status, particularly neurologic or hemodynamic
6. Patient medical history, allergies, and medications, particularly blood thinners

For severely injured patients, the trauma team will not be able to hold their assessment for longer than this 20- to 30-second period, and additional information can be given to a nurse or other member of the trauma team not involved in direct assessment or procedures with the patient.

Also important is the written **patient care report (PCR)**. A good PCR is valuable for the following two reasons:

1. It gives the receiving facility staff a thorough understanding of the events that occurred and of the patient's condition should any questions arise after the prehospital care practitioners have left.
2. It helps ensure quality control throughout the prehospital system by making case review possible.

For these reasons, it is important that the prehospital care practitioner fill out the PCR accurately and completely and provide it to the receiving facility. The PCR should stay with the patient; it is of little use if it does not arrive until hours or days after the patient arrives. If an agency uses an electronic record program, a written summary of key information can be left at bedside, and the full record should be transmitted to the hospital when complete.

The PCR is a part of the patient's medical record. It is a legal record of what was found and what was done and can be used as part of a legal action. The report is the official record of the injuries found and the actions taken in the prehospital setting. As such, it should be thorough and accurate. Another important reason for providing a copy of the PCR to the receiving facility is that most trauma centers maintain a "trauma registry," a database of all trauma patients admitted to their facility. The prehospital information is an important aspect of this database and may aid in valuable research.

Special Considerations
Traumatic Cardiopulmonary Arrest

Cardiopulmonary arrest resulting from trauma differs from that caused by medical problems in several significant ways. First, medical cardiac arrest is generally the result of either a respiratory problem (e.g., foreign body airway obstruction) or a cardiac dysrhythmia. These are best managed with attempts at resuscitation at the scene. Traumatic cardiac arrest is most often due to exsanguination or severe brain injury. These patients generally cannot be appropriately resuscitated in the field. Survival rates from traumatic cardiac arrest are low, with less than 4% overall survival and less than 2% surviving with good neurologic status.[51]

The decisions regarding the management of traumatic cardiac arrest in the prehospital setting are often complex and must take a variety of factors into consideration. Guidelines and position statements developed by the National Association of EMS Physicians (NAEMSP) and American College of Surgeons Committee on Trauma, as well as the European Resuscitation Council represent the best understanding of the available evidence. However, emerging research and local factors must be considered, and thus some local protocols may deviate from these guidelines.

General Principles

Unless obvious signs of death (e.g., exposed brain matter) are immediately apparent or the patient clearly meets the criteria for withholding resuscitation described in the next section, resuscitation should be initiated while performing further assessment and preparing for transport. External hemorrhage should be immediately controlled. Even though many protocols include the use of closed chest compressions in algorithms for the management of traumatic cardiopulmonary arrest, the effectiveness of cardiopulmonary resuscitation (CPR) in the setting of severe trauma/exsanguination is questionable. Despite this reservation, it is reasonable to attempt CPR in patients who may be salvageable while prioritizing management of reversible causes of traumatic arrest. As with all CPR attempts, prehospital care practitioners should limit interruptions to compressions.[52]

If an ALS practitioner is available, ALS is provided while maintaining basic life support (BLS) techniques. The airway is secured with an appropriate airway device (while maintaining in-line stabilization of the cervical spine), such as an endotracheal tube or supraglottic device. Breath sounds should be auscultated, and tension pneumothorax should be considered if a decrease in breath sounds or inadequate chest excursion during ventilation is noted. If any doubt exists that the patient may have a tension pneumothorax, chest decompression should be performed. Appropriate venous access is obtained and isotonic crystalloid solution is delivered through a wide-open line. ECG monitoring is performed and cardiac rhythm assessed. Defibrillation should be provided for ventricular fibrillation.

In general, patients with severe trauma are best served by short scene times and rapid transport to a trauma center. However, for patients in traumatic cardiac arrest, the decision on when to transport (or whether to transport at all) is much more complex. Aeromedical services may be able to provide more advanced capabilities on scene, such as blood transfusion, and their speed may allow them to reach a hospital faster than ground transportation. However, many aeromedical services do not transport patients who are in cardiac arrest.

If cardiac arrest is witnessed by EMS personnel, or if prehospital care practitioners have reason to believe that cardiac arrest has occurred within several minutes prior to their arrival on scene, and the patient can be transported to an appropriate receiving facility within 10 to 15 minutes, consider immediate transport with further treatment and resuscitation efforts performed en route. If the patient cannot arrive at an appropriate hospital, preferably a trauma center, within this time frame, practitioners may consider providing resuscitation efforts on scene followed by termination of resuscitation, if appropriate.

Withholding Resuscitation

Resuscitation attempts in patients who are extremely unlikely to survive put prehospital care practitioners at unjustifiable risk from exposure to blood and body fluids as well as injuries sustained in motor vehicle crashes during transport. Such unsuccessful attempts at resuscitation may also divert resources away from patients who are viable and have a greater likelihood of survival. For these reasons, good judgment needs to be exercised regarding the decision to initiate resuscitation attempts for victims of traumatic cardiopulmonary arrest.

The NAEMSP collaborated with the ACS-COT to develop guidelines for withholding or terminating resuscitation in the prehospital setting.[53] Victims of drowning, lightning strike, or hypothermia, as well as pediatric or pregnant patients deserve special consideration before a decision is made to withhold or terminate resuscitation. A patient found in cardiopulmonary arrest at the scene of a traumatic event may have experienced the arrest because of a medical problem (e.g., myocardial infarction), especially if the patient is elderly or evidence of injury is minimal. In such patients, for whom a medical cause of cardiac arrest is deemed more likely than a traumatic cause, standard guidelines for out-of-hospital cardiac arrest should be followed.

For patients with traumatic injuries that are believed to be the most likely cause of cardiac arrest and who meet the following criteria, resuscitation may be withheld, and the patient declared dead[53]:

- Presence of an obviously fatal injury (e.g., decapitation, exposed brain matter) or when evidence of irreversibility exists (dependent lividity, rigor mortis, or decomposition).

Table 6-1 Considerations for Choosing to Withhold Resuscitation in Traumatic Cardiac Arrest

Consideration	Presentation	Recommendation
Death is the most likely outcome even when resuscitation is initiated.	▪ The patient is pulseless, apneic, lacks organized ECG activity, and has no spontaneous movement or pupillary reflexes	Withhold resuscitation STOP
The injuries present are not compatible with life.	▪ Decapitation ▪ Traumatic separation of the torso (hemicorporectomy)	Withhold resuscitation STOP
There is evidence of prolonged cardiac arrest.	▪ Rigor mortis ▪ Dependent lividity ▪ Evidence of decay	Withhold resuscitation STOP
There is evidence of a nontraumatic cause of arrest.*	▪ Minor vehicle damage with a patient who appears uninjured ▪ A fall from an otherwise nonfatal height without evidence of significant injury	Initiate resuscitation GO

*These are patients in whom there is suspicion that the traumatic event was a result of preceding cardiac arrest and not the cause of the cardiac arrest (e.g., falling from a ladder after suffering a major heart attack, crashing a vehicle after suffering a stroke, etc.).

© National Association of Emergency Medical Technicians (NAEMT)

- For victims of blunt trauma, resuscitation efforts may be withheld if the patient is pulseless and apneic and without organized electrocardiographic activity on arrival of prehospital care practitioners.
- For victims of penetrating trauma, resuscitation efforts may be withheld if the patient is pulseless, apneic, and there are no other signs of life (no pupillary reflexes, no spontaneous movement, no organized electrocardiographic activity) on the arrival of prehospital practitioners.

Extreme caution must be exercised when assessing a potentially dead victim, as the decision to withhold resuscitation is medically justifiable only when proper assessment has been performed. There are reports every year of a trauma patient who was incorrectly presumed to be deceased only to be found later to have vital signs. Nearly all these patients go on to succumb to their injuries, but such incidents can be embarrassing to both the prehospital care practitioners and their agencies. In the excitement of a scene with multiple patients, a practitioner may not adequately assess for presence of a pulse. Dying trauma patients may be profoundly bradycardic and hypotensive, thus contributing to the difficulty in identifying a preterminal condition. Prior to making the decision to withhold resuscitation in a patient without obvious signs of death, the EMS practitioner must perform adequate assessment, including palpating for a pulse (preferably at multiple sites), evaluation of the patient's neurologic status (e.g., pupillary reflexes, assessing for spontaneous movement or response to painful stimuli, etc.), and application of an ECG monitor.

Considerations for choosing to withhold resuscitation in traumatic cardiac arrest are presented in **Table 6-1**.

Terminating Resuscitation

The NAEMSP and the ACS-COT have published revised guidelines for termination of resuscitation in the prehospital setting.[54] Termination of resuscitation for trauma patients should be considered when there are no signs of life and no ROSC despite appropriate field EMS treatment that includes minimally interrupted CPR and treatment of reversible causes of arrest (**Table 6-2**). The appropriate duration of resuscitation of a patient in traumatic cardiac

Table 6-2 Considerations for Terminating Resuscitation in Traumatic Cardiac Arrest

Consideration	Presentation	Recommendation
Signs of life are present	■ Spontaneous respirations, movement, a pulse, or measurable blood pressure is present	Do not terminate resuscitation GO
PEA with organized ECG activity is present	■ Narrow-complex PEA with normal or tachycardic rhythm (more likely to survive) ■ Wide-complex PEA with bradycardic rhythm (less likely to survive)	Do not terminate resuscitation GO
The patient may benefit from ED thoracotomy	■ Penetrating chest trauma with witnessed signs of life ■ Narrow-complex PEA with normal or tachycardic rate on ECG	Do not terminate resuscitation GO
The patient is progressing into less-favorable ECG activity despite effective CPR	■ Narrow-complex PEA with a normal rate decompensates into wide-complex PEA with a bradycardic rate	Consider terminating resuscitation STOP
The duration of resuscitation is consistent with poor prognosis	■ Generally accepted to be no longer than 15 minutes ■ Certain patient considerations may extend this 15-minute duration	Consider terminating resuscitation STOP

Abbreviations: CPR, cardiopulmonary resuscitation; ECG, electrocardiogram; ED, emergency department; PEA, pulseless electrical activity.

© National Association of Emergency Medical Technicians (NAEMT)

arrest before termination of resuscitation should be considered is still unclear. A reasonable guideline is 15 minutes of resuscitative efforts; however, local protocols may dictate different periods of time. Termination of resuscitation is generally not feasible after transport has been initiated.

Pain Management

In the distant past, pharmacologic pain management (*analgesia*) had a limited role in the management of trauma patients, primarily because of the concern that side effects (decreased ventilatory drive and vasodilation) of opioids may cause or exacerbate hypotension or hypoxia. This concern resulted in pain relief being denied to some patients for whom pain management was otherwise indicated. That practice was followed

by a period of time where pharmacologic pain management employing opiate-derived medications was administered fairly liberally with a goal of pain elimination. This practice throughout medicine was associated with a national epidemic of narcotic addiction and fatal overdosages. A more balanced approach using appropriate pain management, avoiding narcotics whenever possible, and employing nonpharmacologic options frequently should be employed instead.[55] The pain management option selected should be chosen based on efficacy and safety and should not interfere with lifesaving treatments or rapid transport to an appropriate receiving facility.[56]

Nonpharmacologic analgesia options include immobilization/splinting, cold packs, and verbal calming techniques. There are many available options for pharmacologic analgesia, including nonopioid medications such as acetaminophen, ketamine, and nonsteroidal anti-inflammatory drugs (NSAIDs). Opioid medications such as fentanyl, morphine, and hydromorphone are also available but should be used sparingly. Fentanyl is often a first-line agent due to speed of onset, short duration of action, and minimal effect on hemodynamics. Another attractive option is a subdissociative dose (analgesic dose) of ketamine, because of its favorable safety profile that maintains hemodynamic stability and respiratory drive when appropriately administered.[57]

If any analgesic medications are administered, the patient should be closely monitored both for analgesic effect as well as for any potential side effects or complications. Monitoring should include pulse oximetry, heart rate, mental status, and frequent blood pressure checks. $ETCO_2$ monitoring should also be used, if available.

Injury Due to Interpersonal Abuse

A prehospital care practitioner is often the first person on the scene, allowing for assessment for a potentially abusive situation. The practitioner inside a house can observe and then relay the details of the scene to the receiving facility so that the appropriate social services in the area can be alerted of the concern for abuse. The practitioner is often the only medically trained person able to observe, suspect, and relay information about this silent danger. Note that some states have legislation that mandates EMS practitioners to report potential abuse to the appropriate law enforcement agency, even if they have already notified hospital personnel of their concern.

Anyone at any age can be a potential victim of abuse or an abuser. A pregnant woman, infant, toddler, child, adolescent, young adult, middle-aged adult, and older adult are all at risk for abuse. Several different types of abuse exist, including physical, psychological (emotional), sexual, and financial. Abuse may occur by **commission**, in which a purposeful act results in an injury (i.e., physical violence or sexual abuse), or by **omission** (e.g., neglectful care of a dependent). This section does not discuss types of abuse and merely introduces the general characteristics and heightens a prehospital care practitioner's awareness and suspicion of abuse.

Some common characteristics of a potential abuser include a description of events (the "story") that does not correlate with the injuries, minimizing the patient's injuries, a negative attitude, appearing overly confident, abrasiveness with prehospital care practitioners, or (in the case of a young patient) lack of parental interest and/or not wanting to answer any questions. Some common characteristics of a patient who is experiencing abuse include quietness, reluctance to elaborate on details of the

incident, constant eye contact or lack of eye contact with someone at the scene, minimization of personal injuries, and refusal to remove clothing that might reveal injuries. Abuse, abusers, and the abused can take many different forms, and practitioners need to keep their level of suspicion high if the scene and the story do not correlate.

Prolonged Transport and Interfacility Transfers

Although most urban or suburban EMS transports take 30 minutes or less, transport times may be prolonged because of weather conditions, traffic congestion, trains that block a crossing, or bridges that may be up to allow a ship to pass. These sorts of delays should be documented on the patient care report to explain prolonged transport times to the trauma center. Many prehospital care practitioners in rural and frontier settings routinely manage patients for much longer periods of time during transport. Additionally, practitioners are called on to manage patients during transfer from one medical facility to another, either by ground or air. These transfers may take up to several hours.

Special preparations need to be taken when prehospital care practitioners are involved in the prolonged transport of a trauma patient, particularly interfacility transfers. The issues that must be considered before undertaking such a transport can be divided into those that concern the patient, the prehospital crew, and the equipment.

Patient Issues

Of preeminent importance is providing a safe, warm, and secure environment for patient transport. The gurney should be appropriately secured to the ambulance and the patient properly secured to the gurney. As emphasized throughout this text, hypothermia is a potentially deadly complication in a trauma patient, and the patient compartment must be sufficiently warm. If you, as a fully clothed prehospital care practitioner, are comfortable with the temperature in the patient compartment, it is likely too cold for the patient who has been exposed.

The patient should be secured in a position that allows maximum access to the patient, especially the injured areas. Before transport, the security of any airway devices placed must be confirmed, and equipment (e.g., monitors, oxygen tanks) should be placed and secured so that they do not become projectiles if the ambulance has to swerve in an evasive action or is involved in a motor vehicle crash. Equipment should not rest on the patient because it may be dropped or covered if the patient moves, may be uncomfortable for the patient, and even may cause pressure wounds during a prolonged transport. During transport, all IV lines and catheters must be securely fastened to prevent loss of the venous access. If prolonged transport time is anticipated and a backboard was used to transfer the patient to the gurney, consider removing the patient from the backboard prior to transport by carefully logrolling the patient off the board while maintaining appropriate spinal motion restriction. This will increase patient comfort and decrease the risk of decubitus ulcer formation associated with immobilization on a hard surface.

The patient should undergo serial assessments of the primary survey and vital signs at frequent intervals. Pulse oximetry and ECG are monitored continuously for virtually all seriously injured patients, as well as $ETCO_2$, if available. Note that for nonintubated patients, capnography can be obtained using the naso-oral cannula. The prehospital care practitioners accompanying the patient should be trained at a level appropriate to the anticipated needs of the patient. Critically injured patients should generally be managed by practitioners with advanced training. If the patient is anticipated to require blood transfusion during transport, an individual should be in attendance whose scope of practice allows this procedure; in the United States, this generally requires a critical care trained practitioner, registered nurse, advanced care practitioner, or physician.

Two management plans should be devised. The first, a medical plan, is developed to manage either anticipated or unexpected problems with the patient during transport. Necessary equipment, medications, and supplies should be readily available. The second, a transport plan, involves identifying the most expeditious route to the receiving hospital. Weather conditions, road conditions (e.g., construction), and traffic concerns should be identified and anticipated. Additionally, the prehospital care practitioners should be knowledgeable about the medical facilities along the transport route in case a problem arises that cannot be managed in the field while en route to the primary destination.

Adjuncts to the care of the patient during prolonged transport, or performed at the referring facility prior to transfer, may include the following:

- *Gastric tube.* If trained in proper insertion, a nasogastric or orogastric tube can be inserted into the patient's stomach. Suctioning out gastric contents can decrease abdominal distension and potentially decrease the risk of vomiting and aspiration.
- *Urinary catheter.* If trained on proper insertion, a urinary catheter may be inserted into the patient's bladder. Urine output can be a sensitive measure of

the patient's renal perfusion and a marker of the patient's volume status.

- *Arterial or venous blood gas monitoring via point-of-care testing.* While the pulse oximeter gives valuable information regarding the oxyhemoglobin saturation, a blood gas reading may give useful information regarding the patient's partial pressure of carbon dioxide (PCO_2), pH, and the base deficit, an indicator of the severity of shock.

Crew Issues

The safety of the prehospital care crew is as important as that of the patient. The prehospital care crew should be adequately rested and fed, particularly for long-duration transfers. A recent evidence-based review recommends a number of fatigue management strategies, including use of caffeinated drinks, napping, and avoidance of shifts that are 24 hours or longer in duration.[58] The crew should have and use appropriate safety devices, including seat belts in both the driver and patient compartments. The prehospital care crew members must use standard precautions and ensure that sufficient gloves and other PPE to avoid body fluids, blood, and other possible exposures are available for the trip.

Equipment Issues

Equipment issues during prolonged transport involve the vehicle, supplies, medications, monitors, and communications. The ambulance or medical transport helicopter must be in good working order, including an adequate amount of fuel. The prehospital care crew must make sure sufficient supplies and medications are available and accessible for the transport, including gauze and pads for reinforcing dressings, IV fluids, oxygen, and pain medications. Medication supplies are based on anticipated patient needs and include sedatives, paralytic agents, analgesics, and antibiotics. A good general rule is to stock the ambulance with about 50% more supplies and medications than the anticipated need in case a significant delay is encountered. Patient care equipment must be in good working order, including monitors (with functioning alarms), oxygen regulators, ventilators, and suction devices. Adequate power supply for all equipment, including charged and spare batteries, should be assured. Also, success of a prolonged transport may depend on functional communications, including the ability to communicate with other crew members, medical control, and the destination facility.

The management of specific injuries during prolonged transport is discussed in the subsequent corresponding chapters of this text.

SUMMARY

- The likelihood of survival for a patient with traumatic injuries depends on the immediate identification and mitigation of conditions that interfere with tissue perfusion.
- The identification of these conditions requires a systematic, prioritized, logical process of collecting information and acting on it. This process is referred to as patient assessment.
- Patient assessment begins with assessment of the scene including a safety evaluation and includes the formation of a general impression of the patient, a primary survey, and, when the patient's condition and availability of additional EMS personnel permit, a secondary survey.
- The information obtained through this assessment process is analyzed and used as the basis for patient care and transport decisions.
- In the care of the trauma patient, a missed problem is a missed opportunity to potentially aid in an individual's survival.
- After the simultaneous determination of scene safety and general impression of the situation, practitioners initiate the primary survey, following the XABCDE format:
  - X—eXsanguinating hemorrhage (control of severe external bleeding)
  - A—Airway management and spinal motion restriction
  - B—Breathing (ventilation and oxygenation)
  - C—Circulation (perfusion and other hemorrhage)
  - D—Disability
  - E—Expose/environment
- Despite the sequential presentation of this mnemonic, the actions of the primary survey occur in rapid order, essentially at the same time.
- Immediate threats to the patient's life are quickly corrected in a "find and fix" manner. Once the prehospital care practitioner controls exsanguinating hemorrhage and manages the patient's airway and breathing, the practitioner packages the patient and begins transport without additional treatment at the scene. The limitations of field management of trauma require the safe, expedient delivery of the patient to definitive care.
- The primary and secondary surveys should be repeated frequently to identify any changes in the patient's condition and new problems that demand prompt intervention.
- The patient's outcome can be greatly improved when the prehospital care practitioner selects the most appropriate destination for the patient, communicates with the receiving facility, and thoroughly documents the patient's condition and the actions performed in the prehospital setting.

SCENARIO RECAP

It is a Saturday morning in early November. The weather is clear, with an outside temperature of 42°F (5.5°C). Your squad is dispatched to a residential area for a person who has fallen from the roof of a two-story building. Upon arrival at the scene, you are met by an adult family member who leads you around the house to the backyard. The family member states the patient was cleaning leaves from the rain gutters with a leaf blower when he lost his balance and fell approximately 12 ft (3.6 m) from the roof, landing on his back. The patient initially lost consciousness for a "brief period" but was conscious by the time the family member called 911.

Approaching the patient, you observe an approximately 40-year-old male lying supine on the ground with two bystanders kneeling by his side. The patient is conscious and talking with the bystanders. You do not see any signs of severe bleeding. As your partner provides manual stabilization to the patient's head and neck, you ask the patient where he hurts. The patient states both his upper and lower back hurt the most.

Your initial questioning serves the multiple purposes of obtaining the patient's chief complaint, determining his initial level of consciousness, and assessing his ventilatory effort. Detecting no shortness of breath, you proceed with the patient assessment. The patient answers your questions appropriately to establish that he is oriented to person, place, and time.

- Based on physics of trauma as they relate to this incident, what potential injuries do you anticipate finding during your assessment?
- What are your next priorities?
- How will you proceed with this patient?

SCENARIO SOLUTION

You have been on the scene for 1 minute, yet you have obtained much important information to guide further assessment and treatment of the patient. In the first 15 seconds of patient contact, you have developed a general impression of the patient, determining that resuscitation is not necessary. With a few simple actions, you have evaluated the X, A, B, C, and D of the primary survey. There was no severe external bleeding. The patient spoke to you without difficulty, indicating that his airway is open and he is breathing with no signs of distress. At the same time, with an awareness of the mechanism of injury, you have stabilized the cervical spine. Your partner has assessed the radial pulse, and you have observed the patient's skin color, temperature, and moisture. These findings indicate no immediate threats to the patient's circulatory status. Additionally, you have simultaneously found no initial evidence of disability because the patient is awake and alert, answers questions appropriately, and can move all extremities. This information, along with information about the fall, will help you determine the need for additional resources, the type of transport indicated, and the type of facility to which you should deliver the patient.

Now that you have completed these steps and no immediate lifesaving intervention is necessary, you will proceed with step E of the primary survey early in the evaluation process and then obtain vital signs. You will expose the patient to look for additional injuries and bleeding that may have been concealed by clothing and then cover the patient to protect him from the environment. During this process, you will perform a more detailed examination, noting less serious injuries.

The next steps you will take are packaging the patient, including motion restriction of the entire spine, splinting extremity injuries, initiating transport; and communicating with medical direction and the receiving facility. During the trip to the hospital, you will continue to reevaluate and monitor the patient, obtain IV access, administer safe and appropriate analgesia as indicated, and dress open wounds as time allows. Your knowledge of the physics of trauma and the patient's witnessed loss of consciousness will generate a high index of suspicion for TBI, lower extremity injuries, and injuries to the spine.

References

1. Brown JB, Rosengart MR, Forsythe RM, et al. Not all prehospital time is equal: influence of scene time on mortality. *J Trauma Acute Care Surg.* 2016;81:93-100.

2. Meizoso JP, Ray JJ, Karcutskie CA 4th, et al. Effect of time to operation on mortality for hypotensive patients with gunshot wounds to the torso: the golden 10 minutes. *J Trauma Acute Care Surg.* 201;81(4):685-691. doi: 10.1097/TA.0000000000001198

3. Clarke JR, Trooskin SZ, Doshi PJ, Greenwald L, Mode CJ. Time to laparotomy for intra-abdominal bleeding from trauma does affect survival for delays up to 90 minutes. *J Trauma.* 2002;52(3):420-425. doi: 10.1097/00005373-200203000-00002

4. Brown E, Tohira H, Bailey P, et al. Longer prehospital time was not associated with mortality in major trauma: a retrospective cohort study, *Prehosp Emerg Care.* 2019;23(4):527-537. doi: 10.1080/10903127.2018.1551451

5. Advanced Trauma Life Support (ATLS) Subcommittee, Committee on Trauma. Initial assessment and management. In: *Advanced Trauma Life Support Course for Doctors, Student Course Manual.* 10th ed. American College of Surgeons; 2018.

6. Kotwal RS, Butler FK, Gross KR, et al. Management of junctional hemorrhage in Tactical Combat Casualty Care: TCCC guidelines–proposed change 13-03. *J Spec Oper Med.* 2013;13:85-93.

7. Kragh JF Jr, Mann-Salinas EA, Kotwal RS, et al. Laboratory assessment of out-of-hospital interventions to control junctional bleeding from the groin in a manikin model. *Am J Emerg Med.* 2013;31:1276-1278.

8. Kragh JF Jr, Parsons DL, Kotwal RS, et al. Testing of junctional tourniquets by military medics to control simulated groin hemorrhage. *J Spec Oper Med.* 2014;14:58-63.

9. Kragh JF, Kotwal RS, Cap AP, et al. Performance of junctional tourniquets in normal human volunteers. *Prehosp Emerg Care.* 2015;19:391-398.

10. Chen J, Benov A, Nadler R, et al. Testing of junctional tourniquets by medics of the Israeli Defense Force in control of simulated groin hemorrhage. *J Spec Oper Med.* 2016;16:36-42.

11. Bulger EM, Snyder D, Schoelles K, et al. An evidence-based prehospital guideline for external hemorrhage control: American College of Surgeons Committee on Trauma. *Prehosp Emerg Care.* 2014;18(2):163-173.

12. Fischer PE, Perina DG, Delbridge TR, et al. Spinal motion restriction in the trauma patient: a joint position statement. *Prehosp Emerg Care.* 2018;22(6):659-661. doi: 10.1080/10903127.2018.1481476

13. Kragh JF, Littrel ML, Jones JA, et al. Battle casualty survival with emergency tourniquet use to stop limb bleeding. *J Emerg Med.* 2011;41:590-597.

14. Beekley AC, Sebesta JA, Blackbourne LH, et al. Prehospital tourniquet use in Operation Iraqi Freedom: effect on hemorrhage control and outcomes. *J Trauma.* 2008;64:S28-S37.

15. Doyle GS, Taillac PP. Tourniquets: a review of current use with proposals for expanded prehospital use. *Prehosp Emerg Care.* 2008;12:241-256.

16. First Aid Science Advisory Board. First aid. *Circulation.* 2005;112(III):115.

17. Swan KG Jr, Wright DS, Barbagiovanni SS, et al. Tourniquets revisited. *J Trauma.* 2009;66:672-675.

18. King DR, Larentzakis A, Ramly EP; Boston Trauma Collaborative. Tourniquet use at the Boston Marathon bombing: lost in translation. *J Trauma Acute Care Surg.* 2015;78(3):594-599.

19. Deakin CD, Low JL. Accuracy of the advanced trauma life support guidelines for predicting systolic blood pressure using carotid, femoral, and radial pulses: observational study. *Br Med J.* 2000;321(7262):673-674.

20. Teasdale G, Jennett B. Assessment of coma and impaired consciousness: a practical scale. *Lancet.* 1974;2:81-84. doi: 10.1016/s0140-6736(74)91639-0

21. Bledsoe B, Casey M, Feldman J, et al. Glasgow Coma Scale scoring is often inaccurate. *Prehosp Disaster Med.* 2015;30(1):46-53.

22. Gill MR, Reiley DG, Green SM. Interrater reliability of Glasgow Coma Scale scores in the emergency department. *Ann Emerg Med.* 2004;43(2):215-223.

23. Kerby JD, Maclennan PA, Burton JN, Mcgwin G, Rue LW. Agreement between prehospital and emergency department Glasgow Coma scores. *J Trauma.* 2007;63(5):1026-1031.

24. Healey C, Osler TM, Rogers FB, et al. Improving the Glasgow Coma Scale score: motor score alone is a better predictor. *J Trauma.* 2003;54:671-678.

25. Beskind DL, Stolz U, Gross A, et al. A comparison of the prehospital motor component of the Glasgow Coma Scale (mGCS) to the prehospital total GCS (tGCS) as a prehospital risk adjustment measure for trauma patients. *Prehosp Emerg Care.* 2014;18(1):68-75.

26. Kupas DF, Melnychuk EM, Young AJ. Glasgow Coma Scale motor component ("patient does not follow commands") performs similarly to total Glasgow Coma Scale in predicting severe injury in trauma patients. *Ann Emerg Med.* 2016;68(6):744-750.

27. Aguilar SA, Davis DP. Latency of pulse oximetry signal with use of digital probes associated with inappropriate extubation during prehospital rapid sequence intubation in head injury patients: case examples. *J Emerg Med.* 2012;42(4):424-428.

28. Vithalani VD, Vlk S, Davis SQ, Richmond NJ. Unrecognized failed airway management using a supraglottic airway device. *Resuscitation.* 2017;119:1-4.

29. Davis JW, Davis IC, Bennink LD, Bilello JF, Kaups KL, Parks SN. Are automated blood pressure measurements accurate in trauma patients? *J Trauma.* 2003;55(5):860-863.

30. Brown JB, Rosengart MR, Forsythe RM, et al. Not all prehospital time is equal: influence of scene time on mortality. *J Trauma Acute Care Surg.* 2016;81:93-100.

31. Pokorney DM, Braverman MA, Edmundson PM, et al. The use of prehospital blood products in the resuscitation of trauma patients: a review of prehospital transfusion practices and a description of our regional whole blood program in San Antonio, TX. *IBST Sci Ser.* 2019;14(3):332-342.

32. Pasley J, Miller CH, Dubose JJ, et al. Intraosseous infusion rates under high pressure: a cadaveric comparison of anatomic sites. *J Trauma Acute Care Surg.* 2015;78(2):295-299.

33. Brown JB, Cohen MJ, Minei JP, et al. Goal directed resuscitation in the prehospital setting: a propensity adjusted analysis. *J Trauma Acute Care Surg.* 2013;74(5):1207-1214.

34. Biswas S, Adileh M, Almogy G, Bala M. Abdominal injury patterns in patients with seatbelt signs requiring laparotomy. *J Emerg Trauma Shock.* 2014;7(4):295-300.

35. Bansal V, Conroy C, Tominaga GT, Coimbra R. The utility of seat belt signs to predict intra-abdominal injury following motor vehicle crashes. *Traffic Inj Prev.* 2009;10(6):567-572.

36. Chandler CF, Lane JS, Waxman KS. Seatbelt sign following blunt trauma is associated with increased incidence of abdominal injury. *Am Surg.* 1997;63(10):885-888.

37. Moylan JA, Detmer DE, Rose J, Schulz R. Evaluation of the quality of hospital care for major trauma. *J Trauma.* 1976;16(7):517-523.

38. West JG, Trunkey DD, Lim RC. Systems of trauma care: a study of two counties. *Arch Surg.* 1979;114(4):455-460.

39. West JG, Cales RH, Gazzaniga AB. Impact of regionalization: the Orange County experience. *Arch Surg.* 1983;118(6):740-744.

40. Shackford SR, Hollingworth-Fridlund P, Cooper GF, Eastman AB. The effect of regionalization upon the quality of trauma care as assessed by concurrent audit before and after institution of a trauma system: a preliminary report. *J Trauma.* 1986;26(9):812-820.

41. Waddell TK, Kalman PG, Goodman SJ, Girotti MJ. Is outcome worse in a small volume Canadian trauma centre? *J Trauma.* 1991;31(7):958-961.

42. MacKenzie EJ, Rivara FP, Jurkovich GJ, et al. A national evaluation of the effect of trauma-center care on mortality. *N Engl J Med.* 2006;354(4):366-378.

43. Branas CC, MacKenzie EJ, Williams JC, et al. Access to trauma centers in the United States. *JAMA.* 2005;293(21):2626-2633.

44. Nathens AB, Jurkovich GJ, Rivara FP, Maier RV. Effectiveness of state trauma systems in reducing injury-related mortality: a national evaluation. *J Trauma.* 2000;48(1):25-30; discussion 30-31.

45. Report Card Task Force Members, American College of Emergency Physicians (ACEP) Staff. America's emergency care environment, a state-by-state report card: 2014 edition. *Ann Emerg Med.* 2014;63(2):97-242.

46. American College of Surgeons. *COT Releases Updated National Guideline for Field Triage of Injured Patients.* Reviewed May 3, 2022. Accessed June 1, 2022. https://www.facs.org/for-medical-professionals/news-publications/news-and-articles/acs-brief/may-10-2022-issue/cot-releases-updated-national-guideline-for-field-triage-of-injured-patients/

47. American College of Surgeons. *Resources for the Optimal Care of the Injured Patient.* 6th ed. American College of Surgeons; 2014.

48. Baker SP, O'Neill B, Haddon W Jr, Long WB. The injury severity score: a method for describing patients with multiple injuries and evaluating emergency care. *J Trauma.* 1974;14(3):187-196.

49. McCoy CE, Chakravarthy B, Lotfipour S. Guidelines for field triage of injured patients: in conjunction with the *Morbidity and Mortality Weekly Report* published by the Centers for Disease Control and Prevention. *West J Emerg Med.* 2013;14(1):69-76.

50. Centers for Disease Control and Prevention. Guidelines for field triage of injured patients: recommendations of the national expert panel on field triage 2011. *Morb Mortal Wkly Rep.* 2012;61:1-21.

51. Truhlar A, Deakin CD, Soar J, et al. European Resuscitation Council Guidelines for Resuscitation 2015. Section 4: cardiac arrest in special circumstances. *Resuscitation.* 2015;95:148-201.

52. American Heart Association. 2015 guidelines for cardiopulmonary resuscitation and emergency cardiovascular care. *Circulation.* 2015;132:S313-S314.

53. National Association of EMS Physicians and American College of Surgeons Committee on Trauma. NAEMSP position statement: withholding of resuscitation for adult traumatic cardiopulmonary arrest. *Prehosp Emerg Care.* 2013;17:291.

54. The National Association of EMS Physicians (NAEMSP) and the American College of Surgeons Committee on Trauma (ACS-COT). Termination of resuscitation for adult traumatic cardiopulmonary arrest. *Prehosp Emerg Care.* 2012;16(4):571.

55. U.S. Department of Health and Human Services. *What is the U.S. opioid epidemic?* Reviewed October 27, 2021. Accessed February 11, 2022. https://www.hhs.gov/opioids/about-the-epidemic/index.html

56. Alonso-Serra HM, Wesley K. Prehospital pain management. *Prehosp Emerg Care.* 2003;7(4):482-488. doi: 10.1080/312703002260

57. Morgan MM, Perina DG, Acquisto NM, et al. Ketamine use in prehospital and hospital treatment of the acute trauma patient: a joint position statement. *Prehosp Emerg Care.* 2021;25(4):588-592, doi: 10.1080/10903127.2020.1801920

58. Patterson DP, Higgins JS, Van Dongen HPA, et al. Evidence-based guidelines for fatigue risk management in emergency medical services. *Prehosp Emerg Care.* 2018;22(1):89-101.

Suggested Reading

Merchant RM, Topjian AA, Panchal AR, et al. Part 1: executive summary: 2020 American Heart Association guidelines for cardiopulmonary resuscitation and emergency cardiovascular care. *Circulation.* 2020;142:S337-S357.

CHAPTER **7**

Airway and Ventilation

Lead Editors
Jean-Cyrille Pitteloud, MD
Jay Johannigman, MD, FACS, FCCM

CHAPTER OBJECTIVES

At the completion of this chapter, you will be able to do the following:

- Integrate the principles of ventilation and gas exchange.
- Recognize the way traumatic injuries impair the normal processes of ventilation and oxygenation.
- Articulate the impact of impaired oxygenation and ventilation on perfusion and the progression of traumatic shock.
- Understand how trauma affects minute volume and oxygenation.
- Distinguish the difference between ventilation and oxygenation.
- Explain the mechanisms by which supplemental oxygen and ventilatory support may be beneficial to an injured patient.

- Present a scenario that involves a trauma patient, select the most effective means of providing a patent airway.
- Given varying scenarios, develop appropriate responses and interventions of airway management, oxygenation, and ventilation.
- Recognize current research initiatives and understand the risks and benefits of various invasive procedures.
- Discuss the indications and limitations of end-tidal carbon dioxide ($ETCO_2$) monitoring in trauma patients.

SCENARIO

You are called to the scene of a motorcycle crash on a busy freeway. As you arrive on scene, you see the patient lying supine about 50 feet (ft; 15 meters [m]) from a heavily damaged motorcycle. The patient is a young male who still has his helmet on. He is not moving, and you see from a distance that he is breathing rapidly. As you approach the patient, you see a pool of blood around his head, and you notice that his breathing is noisy, with snoring and gurgling sounds.

You are 15 minutes from a trauma center, and the dispatch center informs you that the helicopter emergency medical services (HEMS) cannot fly due to bad weather.

- What indicators of airway compromise are evident in this patient?
- What other information, if any, would you seek from witnesses or the emergency medical responders?
- What are the important signs and symptoms of compromise of oxygenation and ventilation that should be sought and observed during the initial rapid assessment in the field?
- Describe the sequence of actions you would take to manage this patient before and during transport.

INTRODUCTION

Two of the most important prehospital skills are those that provide and maintain airway patency and gas exchange. Failure to adequately maintain a patent airway and provide adequate oxygenation and ventilation rapidly compromises key organ systems and may result in irreversible injury. The ability to recognize airway compromise and inadequate oxygenation and ventilation are critical steps in minimizing the overall burden of injury.

For purposes of definition, the following may be considered:

- Oxygenation refers to the process by which inspired molecular oxygen crosses the alveolar membrane and is bound to hemoglobin for subsequent delivery to the tissues of the body.
- Ventilation refers to the process of gaseous exchange resulting from inspiration and expiration.

Aerobic metabolism is the most efficient form of energy conversion in the human body. In this process oxygen is a critical element in the transition of fuel sources into cellular energy to sustain the machinery of life.

The two primary functions of the respiratory system are as follows:

1. *To deliver oxygen for uptake by hemoglobin for transport to the cell.* The body has virtually no oxygen reserves; therefore, lack of oxygen can lead to cell death within minutes.
2. *To eliminate carbon dioxide* produced by the process of metabolism in the body. If ventilation is inadequate, CO_2 accumulates, leading to acidosis and coma.

An appropriately functioning respiratory system must deliver both oxygenation and ventilation to sustain life.

Anatomy

The respiratory system is comprised of the upper airway and the lower airway, including the lungs (**Figure 7-1**). Each component of the respiratory system plays an important role in ensuring gas exchange.

Upper Airway

The upper airway consists of the nasal cavity and the oral cavity (**Figure 7-2**). It has the dual function of food and water intake as well as ventilation. For that reason, it has a robust but elaborate anatomy and a sophisticated nerve supply. Air entering the nasal cavity is warmed, humidified, and filtered. Beyond the mouth and the nasal cavity is the area known as the **pharynx**, which extends from the soft palate to the upper end of the esophagus. The pharynx is a muscular structure lined with mucous membranes and is divided into three distinct sections: the **nasopharynx** (upper portion), the **oropharynx** (middle portion), and the **hypopharynx** (lower or distal end of the pharynx). Below the pharynx is the **esophagus**, leading to the stomach, and the trachea, the beginning of the lower airway. At the junction of the hypopharynx and the trachea is the **larynx** (**Figure 7-3**), which contains the vocal cords and the muscles that coordinate their function. The larynx is housed in a strong and protective cartilaginous box. The vocal cords are folds of tissue projecting into the airway that produce sound. The vocal cords have a range of motion that creates and modifies sound as well as the ability to meet in the midline to protect the airway from aspiration. The false cords, or **vestibular folds**, direct the airflow through the vocal cords. Supporting the cords posteriorly are the arytenoid cartilages. Directly above the larynx is a leaf-shaped structure called the **epiglottis**. The epiglottis functions as a gate or flapper valve directing air into the trachea and solids and liquids into the esophagus.

Lower Airway

The lower airway consists of the trachea, its branches, and the lungs. The function of the lower airway is to provide filtration (trachea, bronchi, and bronchioles) as well as a pathway for gas exchange in the alveoli. The lining of the trachea is delicate and highly sensitive to anything other than air. On inspiration, air travels through the upper airway and into the lower airway before reaching the alveoli, where the actual gas exchange occurs.

The trachea divides into the right and left main bronchi. The right main bronchus is shorter, wider, and more vertically oriented than the left. The right main bronchus comes off the trachea at approximately a 25-degree angle, whereas the left has a 45-degree angulation. This anatomic difference explains why right main bronchus placement of an endotracheal tube is a common complication of intubation. Each of the main bronchi repeatedly divides into multiple primary and then secondary branches before ending in the terminal bronchioles. The **bronchioles** (very small bronchial tubes) usher gas into, and out of, the **alveoli**. Alveoli are the functional units of the lung and are comprised of tiny air sacs surrounded by blood-containing capillaries. The alveoli are the site of gas exchange where the respiratory and circulatory systems meet.

Pulmonary tissue may be compared to a sponge containing millions of little balloons (the alveoli), each of which consists of a thin wall full of blood vessels, providing a huge surface for air exchange to occur. In the adult, the total surface area of the alveoli is approximately 100 square meters (m^2) (more than 1,000 square feet [ft^2]), which is 50 times the surface area of the skin. The lung has no musculature of its own; rather, it is the elastic recoil of

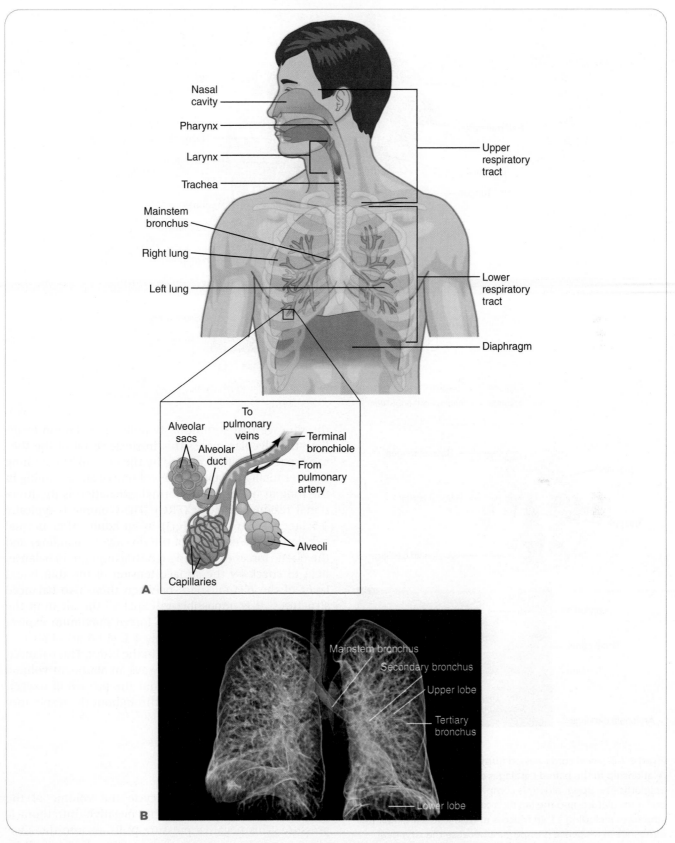

Figure 7-1 **A.** Organs of the respiratory system: upper respiratory tract and lower respiratory tract. **B.** Cross-section of the lower respiratory tract.

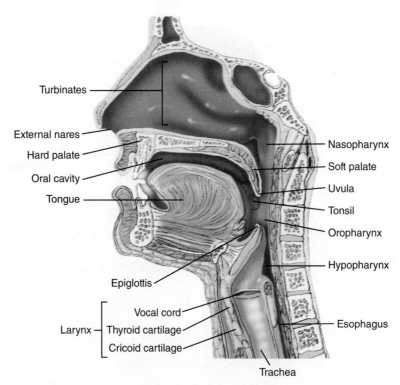

Figure 7-2 Sagittal section through the nasal cavity and pharynx.
© National Association of Emergency Medical Technicians (NAEMT)

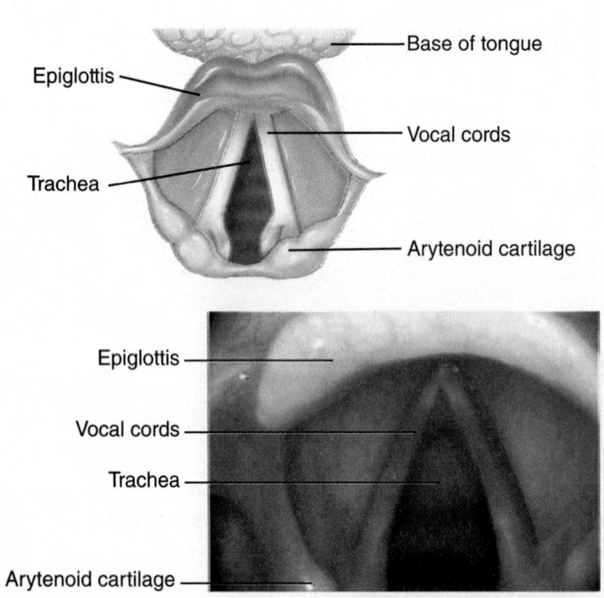

Figure 7-3 Vocal cords viewed from above, showing their relationship to the paired cartilages of the larynx and the epiglottis. The upper airway is comprised of the rigid teeth and oral musculature, and the larynx is composed of more delicate structures including a thin mucosa and delicate cartilage. This difference in resilience is important because the laryngeal structures are more susceptible to injury during therapeutic interventions.

A: © National Association of Emergency Medical Technicians (NAEMT); B: Courtesy of James P. Thomas, M.D., www.voicedoctor.net

the rib cage that continuously pulls in expansion to inflate the alveolar space. This intrinsic recoil of the thoracic space helps to explain why the normal human lung is never totally collapsed. The volume of air remaining in the lung at the end of a normal exhalation is the functional residual capacity (FRC). This volume is typically 2.5 liters (L; 2.6 quarts [qt]) in an adult. After normal exhalation, the elasticity of the rib cage (expanding) and the elastic forces of the lung (contracting) are in balance, held in check by the surface tension of the thin liquid layer of the pleural space between these two balanced structures. It is impossible to expel all the air from the lungs. Even after an absolute forced maximum expiration, there is still approximately 1 L (1.06 qt) of air that remains (the residual volume) in the lungs. This balanced system assures that there is always an abundant volume of functional alveoli to carry out the process of oxygen and carbon dioxide exchange throughout the respiratory cycle.

Physiology

During a normal breathing cycle the volume of the chest cavity expands, creating negative intrathoracic pressure. This negative pressure pulls air into the alveoli. Conversely, during expiration, the elasticity of the rib cage and the resultant elastic recoil of the lungs promotes the movement of air to the outside environment.

The following three components work in synchrony to expand the volume of the chest cavity:

- The **diaphragm** contracts and displaces in a downward direction, acting like the plunger of a syringe, to increase the volume of the chest and create a negative pressure gradient moving air to the alveoli (**Figure 7-4A**). The diaphragm is activated by the phrenic nerve (C3-C5). During normal, quiet breathing, diaphragmatic excursion creates the necessary pressure gradients to carry out the task of ventilation.
- When additional respiratory volume is needed to increase oxygen intake, release carbon dioxide, or overcome increasing airway resistance, the ribs move actively outward at the articulations with the sternum and vertebrae, forming the shape of a bucket handle, expanding the volume of the chest (**Figure 7-4B**). At this stage of breathing, chest wall movements become more visible.
- When additional tidal volume is required, the neck muscles (i.e., sternocleidomastoid muscle) become engaged, expanding the rib cage upwards, further expanding the volume of the thoracic cavity (**Figure 7-4C**). These accessory muscles of respiration are innervated by the cervical C2-C7 roots.
- Normal exhalation occurs as a result of the passive elasticity of the rib cage. If a more rapid expiration process is required, the intercostal and abdominal muscles may be recruited to actively augment the process of exhalation (**Table 7-1**).

The generation of pressure changes to promote inhalation and exhalation requires an intact chest wall. Damage or compromise of the chest wall may compromise the patient's ability to generate the required pressure gradients to promote adequate ventilation. A wound that breaches the normally intact thoracic cavity introduces an alternative pathway for the entry of air between the atmosphere and the thoracic cavity. This breach may result in air being introduced into the thoracic cavity but outside of the alveolar domain. This alternative pathway to the thoracic cavity is one mechanism by which a pneumothorax may be created. (See Chapter 10, *Thoracic Trauma*.)

The presence of air within the alveoli promotes the movement of oxygen across the capillary-alveolar interface and into the vascular space where it comes into contact with the hemoglobin of the red blood cell (RBC). Oxygen fills the O_2 bonding sites on the hemoglobin molecules (three out of four oxygen binding sites [75%] occupied prior to oxygenation versus four out of four after oxygenation [98–100%]; **Figure 7-5A**). At the same time, carbon dioxide that was produced as a by-product of cellular metabolism is delivered to the alveolar capillary interface and moves in the opposite direction (bloodstream to alveoli). Carbon dioxide, which is carried

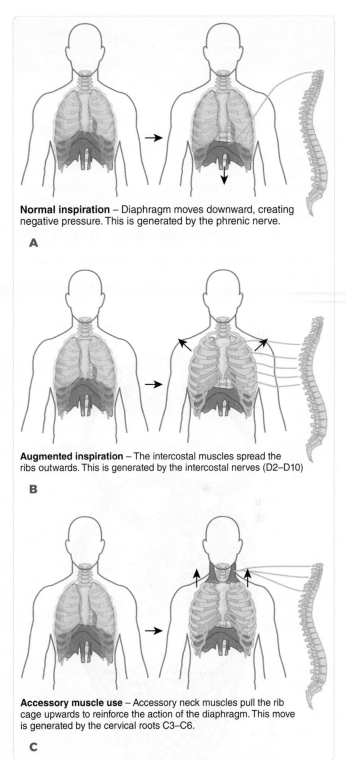

Normal inspiration – Diaphragm moves downward, creating negative pressure. This is generated by the phrenic nerve.

A

Augmented inspiration – The intercostal muscles spread the ribs outwards. This is generated by the intercostal nerves (D2–D10)

B

Accessory muscle use – Accessory neck muscles pull the rib cage upwards to reinforce the action of the diaphragm. This move is generated by the cervical roots C3–C6.

C

Figure 7-4 A. Normal inspiration. **B.** Augmented inspiration. **C.** Accessory muscle use.
© National Association of Emergency Medical Technicians (NAEMT)

dissolved in the plasma (approximately 10%), bound to proteins (mostly hemoglobin in the RBCs [approximately 20%]), and as bicarbonate (approximately 70%), moves from the bloodstream, across the alveolar–capillary

Table 7-1 Respiratory Mechanics

	Inspiration	Expiration
Normal respiration	Diaphragm	Passive
Increased respiratory effort	Diaphragm and intercostal muscles	Intercostal muscles
Extreme respiratory effort	Diaphragm, intercostal muscles, and accessory muscles	Intercostal muscles and abdominal muscles

© National Association of Emergency Medical Technicians (NAEMT)

membrane, and into the alveoli, where it is eliminated during exhalation (**Figure 7-5B**). On completion of this exchange, the oxygenated RBCs and plasma with a low carbon dioxide level return to the left side of the heart to be pumped to all the cells in the body.

How Is Ventilation Regulated?

Ventilation is regulated by the brainstem and as a function of the pH of arterial blood. Oxygen and glucose produce energy and CO_2. CO_2 is dissolved in blood as bicarbonate (HCO_3^-), which is a weak acid (pH = 6.3). This makes the arterial blood more acidic. When the blood PCO_2 rises, CO_2 diffuses into the cerebrospinal fluid. This liberates H+ ions in the cerebrospinal fluid, which stimulates the central chemoreceptors in the midbrain, triggering an increase in respiratory rate and tidal volume,

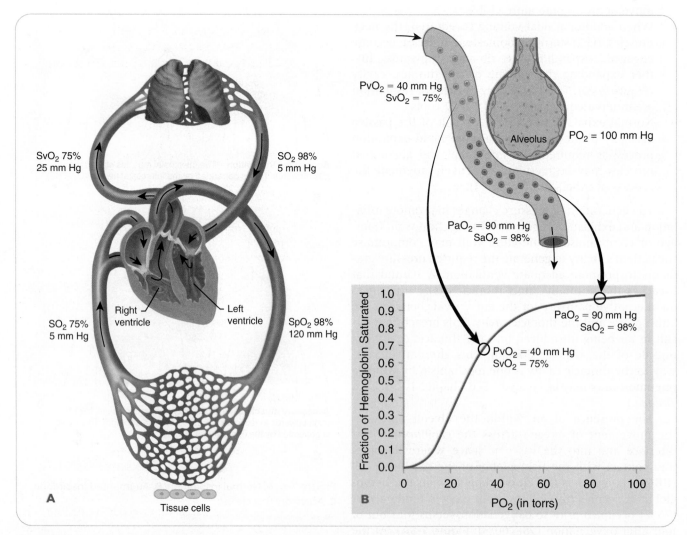

Figure 7-5 A. Venous blood is drawn toward the heart via the low-pressure venous system (5 mm Hg in the vena cava just prior to entering the heart) and pumped by the right heart into the lungs (25 mm Hg after exiting the right ventricle). Oxygen is absorbed from the alveoli into the red blood cells, while CO_2 dissolved in the plasma is excreted into the lungs. Fully oxygenated blood is then pumped in the high-pressure arterial system toward the body's tissues. **B.** As RBCs pass through the lung, they are exposed to oxygen molecules, which bind to hemoglobin molecules, resulting in the oxygen binding sites on the hemoglobin molecules becoming increasingly filled (oxygen saturation [SO_2] increases) and the partial pressure of oxygen within the blood (PO_2) progressively increasing.

© National Association of Emergency Medical Technicians (NAEMT)

which results in the exhalation of more CO_2. There are also peripheral chemoreceptors located in the carotid bodies that respond to arterial PCO_2, but this accounts for less than 20% of ventilatory response. Blood pH is a far more potent stimulus of respiration than oxygen level, which starts to stimulate respiration only in the face of marked hypoxemia. While this might seem illogical at first, it allows the brain to respond proactively to oxygen consumption rather than reactively to oxygen shortage.

Dead Space

The alveoli are filled with very thin capillary vessels that are separated from alveolar air only by a thin membrane through which gas exchange occurs. Prior to reaching the lung, air first travels across the mouth, pharynx, and bronchi, which do not participate in gas exchange. This results in a volume of approximately 150 mL (5 ounces [oz]) in the adult where no air exchange takes place, referred to as dead space. This means that with each breath, the last 150 mL of air never actually reaches the alveoli. While this is not a concern during normal breathing, it can become more significant when ventilation is impaired. Dead space volume also increases with large inspirations.

Alveoli must be constantly replenished with a fresh supply of air that contains an adequate amount of oxygen. This replenishment of air, known as *ventilation*, is also essential for the elimination of carbon dioxide. Ventilation is measurable. The size of each breath, called the tidal volume, multiplied by the ventilatory rate for 1 minute equals the **minute volume**:

$$\textbf{Minute volume} = \textbf{Tidal volume} \times \textbf{Ventilatory rate}$$
$$\textbf{per minute}$$

During normal resting ventilation, about 500 mL (16.5 oz) of air is taken into the lungs. As mentioned previously, part of this volume, 150 mL (5 oz), remains in the airway system (the trachea and bronchi) as dead space and does not participate in gas exchange. Only 350 mL (12 oz) is available for gas exchange in the alveoli. If the tidal volume is 500 mL and the ventilatory rate is 14 breaths/minute, the minute volume can be calculated as follows:

$$\textbf{Minute volume} = \textbf{500 mL} \times \textbf{14 breaths/minute}$$
$$= \textbf{7,000 mL/minute, or 7 L/minute}$$

However, by factoring in dead space, it becomes clear that only 4.9 L/minute encounters the alveoli and therefore takes part in gas exchange. That is:

$$\textbf{500 mL} - \textbf{150 mL} = \textbf{350 mL}$$
$$\textbf{350 mL} \times \textbf{14 breaths/minute} = \textbf{4,900 mL/minute,}$$
$$\textbf{or 4.9 L/minute}$$

This second calculation identifies the **effective ventilation**, which is total minute ventilation minus dead space ventilation.

If the minute volume fails to meet increased demand, the patient has inadequate ventilation, a condition called *hypoventilation*. Hypoventilation leads to a fall in oxygen supply within the alveoli as well as a buildup of carbon dioxide in the alveoli and then in the body. Hypoventilation is common when head or chest trauma causes an altered breathing pattern or an inability to move the chest wall adequately.

For example, a patient with rib fractures who is breathing quickly and shallowly because of the pain of the injury may have a tidal volume of 200 mL and a ventilatory rate of 30 breaths/minute. This patient's minute volume can be calculated as follows:

$$\textbf{Minute volume} = \textbf{200 mL} \times \textbf{30 breaths/minute}$$
$$= \textbf{6,000 mL/minute, or 6 L/minute}$$

If 7 L/minute is necessary for adequate gas exchange in an uninjured person at rest, 6 L/minute is less than the body requires to absorb enough oxygen and to eliminate carbon dioxide effectively, therefore O_2 concentration in the lung will decrease and CO_2 will begin to accumulate. Furthermore, calculating the effective minute ventilation reveals the true severity of the patient's condition:

$$\textbf{200 mL} - \textbf{150 mL} = \textbf{50 mL}$$
$$\textbf{50 mL} \times \textbf{30 breaths/minute} = \textbf{1,500 mL/minute, or}$$
$$\textbf{1.5 L/minute}$$

At this stage almost no oxygenated air will reach the alveoli; most of the air will get only as far as the trachea and bronchi. If left untreated, this hypoventilation will quickly lead to severe hypoxemia, acidosis, multiple organ failure, and, ultimately, death (**Figure 7-6**).

You can see from the previous example that the patient with rib fractures is hypoventilating even though the ventilatory rate is 30 breaths/minute. Thus, respiratory rate by itself does not accurately describe the adequacy of the ventilation. Prehospital care practitioners must take tidal volume into account and never simply assume that a patient with a normal or fast ventilatory rate is ventilating adequately.

Assessment of ventilatory function always includes an evaluation of how well a patient is taking in, diffusing, and delivering oxygen to the tissue cells. Without proper intake, delivery of oxygen to the tissue cells, and processing of oxygen within these cells to maintain aerobic metabolism and energy production is impaired. If left uncorrected, cellular metabolism converts to the anaerobic pathway. The anaerobic pathway is markedly less efficient in converting fuel to energy (about 18 times less efficient). In addition, lactic acid is a byproduct of the pathway. Excessive accumulation of lactic acid has its own (negative) consequences and impact on the physiology of cellular metabolism.

The Oxygen Pathway

While CO_2 is highly soluble in plasma, oxygen solubility in plasma is very limited. That is why oxygen must

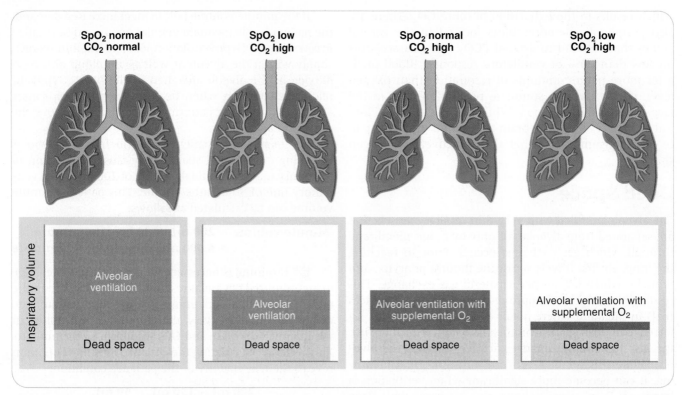

Figure 7-6 As inspiratory volume progressively decreases, the ability to maintain sufficient saturation of hemoglobin molecules with oxygen decreases, and the ability to adequately clear CO_2 from the lungs is impaired.
© National Association of Emergency Medical Technicians (NAEMT)

be transported by hemoglobin (Hb) within the RBCs. Each hemoglobin molecule has four binding sites for oxygen. The affinity of hemoglobin for oxygen varies with the gaseous partial pressure of O_2. In the oxygen-rich environment of the lung, each O_2 binding site is bound to an individual oxygen molecule. In the tissues, where the O_2 pressure is much lower, the conformation of the hemoglobin molecule changes, resulting in the release of O_2 from the hemoglobin molecule into the tissues.

The ability of oxygen to dissolve within the plasma of the bloodstream is very limited. That is why most of the oxygen delivery to cellular tissue is determined by the saturation of the hemoglobin molecules within the RBCs.

The three phases of oxygenation are external respiration, oxygen delivery, and internal (cellular) respiration. Adequate oxygenation depends on all three of these phases:

1. *External respiration* is the transfer or diffusion of oxygen molecules from air to the blood. Air contains oxygen (20.95%), nitrogen (78.1%), argon (0.93%), and carbon dioxide (0.031%), but for practical purposes, the content of air is

oxygen 21% and nitrogen 79%. All alveolar oxygen exists as free gas; therefore, each oxygen molecule exerts pressure. Increasing the percentage of oxygen in the inspired air will increase alveolar oxygen pressure or tension. When supplemental oxygen is provided, the ratio of oxygen in each inspiration increases, causing an increase in the amount of oxygen in each alveolus. This, in turn, will increase the amount of gas that gets transferred to blood because the amount of gas that will enter a liquid is directly related to the pressure it exerts. The greater the partial pressure of the gas, the greater the amount of that gas that will be absorbed into the fluid (plasma) component of the circulatory system.

2. *Oxygen delivery* is the process of the provision of oxygen to the end point of utilization (the cell). Oxygen delivery is dependent on three key components: cardiac output, hemoglobin, and oxygen saturation. It can be calculated with the following formula: $CO \times CaO_2$ ($CaO_2 = 1.31 \times Hgb \times O_2$ Sat).

3. *Internal (cellular) respiration* is the movement of oxygen from the RBCs into the cell's

mitochondria where oxygen is utilized as the main oxidizing agent. There are multiple catabolic reactions that release energy to fuel cellular activity, primarily glycolysis and the tricarboxylic acid (TCA) cycle (also known as the Krebs cycle or citric acid cycle). Understanding the specific details of these processes is not necessary; however, it is important to have a general understanding of the role of oxygen in energy production.

Pathophysiology

Trauma can affect the respiratory system's ability to adequately provide oxygen and eliminate carbon dioxide in many ways. Clinical conditions may have multiple causes of hypoxia. While there is some overlap, the terms hypoxemia and hypoxia are not synonymous. Hypoxemia refers to a decrease in the partial pressure of oxygen in the blood, while hypoxia is defined as reduced tissue oxygenation.

Causes of hypoxemia and examples of traumatic etiology include:

- Decreased ambient or inspired partial pressure of oxygen
  - Trauma at altitude or transport of the patient to altitude
- Hypoventilation
  - Obstructed airway
  - Decreased respiratory drive such as intoxication or head injury
  - Paralysis such as high cervical spinal cord injury
  - Pain such as caused from rib fractures
- Ventilation perfusion mismatch: V/Q mismatch refers to an imbalance between ventilation (V) and perfusion (Q); typically, hypoxemia is seen with low V/Q states due to decreasing alveolar oxygen levels. Hypoxemia can also be seen in circumstances of high V/Q ratio or "physiologic dead space" when the lung is ventilated but not perfused. Shunt is the other extreme of low V/Q mismatch, when the lung is perfused but not ventilated.
  - Low V/Q and shunt:
    - Damage of lung tissue, such as pulmonary contusion
    - Poor lung aeration such as aspiration, atelectasis, or lung collapse
  - High V/Q or physiologic dead space:
    - Pulmonary embolism
    - Shock
- Diffusion abnormalities (gas transport across the capillary–alveoli membrane is impaired)
  - Pulmonary edema

- Profound anemia (due to decreased capacity to uptake oxygen)

Tissue hypoxia can be caused by any hypoxemia unless there is enough of a compensatory increase in cardiac output to mitigate. In addition, hypoxia can be caused in the absence of hypoxemia if the cells or tissues are unable to normally utilize oxygen:

- Decreased oxygen utilization due to toxins or poisons, which impair this process, such as cyanide poisoning.

Causes and Sites of Airway Obstruction in the Trauma Patient

The most common cause of mechanical obstruction of the upper airway is the tongue falling backward and obstructing the hypopharynx (**Figure 7-7A**). The tongue may become an obstruction from any process that alters the upper airway protective reflexes (intoxication is a common example) or creates a mechanical situation that allows the tongue to move rearward and obstruct the hypopharynx (mandibular fractures are a common example). Obstruction of the airway by the tongue at the level of the hypopharynx is characterized by snoring and sonorous sounds as well as abnormal thoracic excursions. In a trauma patient, this obstruction is often further complicated by blood and secretions accumulating in the upper airway. This condition can be corrected by positioning and simple airway maneuvers, such as the trauma jaw thrust or chin lift.

Another common cause of upper airway obstruction is accumulation of secretions, blood, and debris in the hypopharynx whenever patients are unable to clear their airways due to decreased level of consciousness (LOC) or due to extensive trauma (**Figure 7-7B**). A gurgling respiration is a sure sign of inability to clear the airway and of aspiration risk and/or airway obstruction with the very next breath. This condition can be corrected, at least temporarily, by logrolling the patient to the side or/and by suctioning the upper airway.

The third most common location of upper airway obstruction is the larynx, where obstruction can be caused either by direct trauma to the laryngeal cartilage or by inhalation burns with swelling of the mucosa (**Figure 7-7C**). This condition may manifest with hoarseness and stridor and is much more complicated to correct. It usually will require an advanced airway (**endotracheal (ET) tube** or surgical airway). Even if you are not an advanced practitioner, it is critical to recognize this condition and expedite transport to the hospital or obtain support from an advanced life support (ALS) unit.

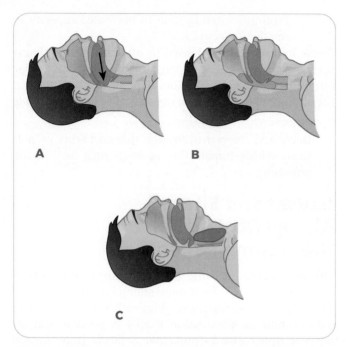

Figure 7-7 Common causes of upper airway obstruction.
A. Tongue blocking the airway. **B.** Vomitus, blood, or other
secretions. **C.** Direct trauma to the larynx or inhalation injury.

© National Association of Emergency Medical Technicians (NAEMT)

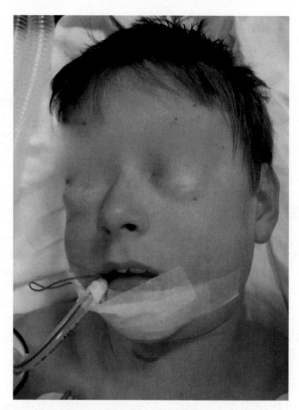

Figure 7-8 A patient who sustained trauma to the anterior
neck, causing rupture of the trachea and subcutaneous
emphysema of the neck and face. If you just look in the patient's
mouth and not at the neck, you are likely to miss a vital piece
of information.

Courtesy of J.C. Pitteloud MD, Switzerland.

In the face of partial obstruction of the upper airway, increased effort of inspiratory muscles is required
to overcome resistance and maintain adequate tidal
volume. This often results in noisy inspiration. If the
patient is unable to provide that additional effort, tidal
volume drops and breathing sometimes stops alto-
gether. This is especially common in children. The best
treatment is to manually open the patient's airway and
to consider positioning adjuncts such as the lateral decubitus (rescue) position or by allowing the patient to
sit up and lean forward. In patients whose inspiratory
effort is limited as a result of chest wall or spinal cord
injury, opening the airway to improve patency may be
helpful in allowing the patient to breathe more effectively. Supplemental oxygen never makes up for an obstructed airway.

Assessment of the Airway

The ability to assess the airway is a prerequisite for effectively managing it. Prehospital care practitioners perform many aspects of assessing the airway automatically.
Trauma patients who are alert and talking with a normal
voice likely have an open and patent airway. In these
situations, a thorough systematic evaluation can still help
identify any impending airway problems (**Figure 7-8**).
When the patient's LOC is decreased, it is even more essential to thoroughly assess the airway prior to moving

to other, lower priority injuries. The following should be
performed as part of the primary assessment:

- Assess airway patency.
- Look in the mouth for fluids or solids.
- Look for any deformity or swelling of the mandible
  and the anterior part of the neck.
- Listen for any abnormal sounds.
- Look for abnormal chest movements/retractions.

Position of the Airway and Patient

As you make visual contact with the patient, it is important to observe the patient's position. Patients in a
supine position with a decreased LOC are at risk for airway obstruction from the tongue falling back into the airway. Most trauma patients with a decreased LOC will be
placed in the supine position on a backboard or vacuum
mattress for spinal motion restriction, so any patient exhibiting signs of decreased LOC will need constant reex-
amination for airway obstruction, and placement of an
adjunctive device (oral or nasopharyngeal airway) may

be necessary to ensure an open airway. Patients who present with an open airway while lying on their side may obstruct their airways when placed supine.

Position is an important consideration in patients with massive facial trauma and active bleeding. These patients may need to be maintained in the position in which they are found if they are maintaining their own airway. In some cases, this may mean allowing the patient to sit in an upright position if the airway is being maintained. Placing these patients supine as opposed to inclined may cause obstruction of the airway and possible aspiration of blood. In such cases, if the patients are maintaining their own airways, the best course of action may be to let them maintain the position that has allowed them to survive. Suction should be available if needed to remove blood and secretions. If necessary, stabilization of the cervical spine may be accomplished by manually holding the head in the position needed to allow for maintenance of an open airway. Stabilization of the thoracolumbar spine is harder to accomplish in an upright position, but if the choice is between increased protection of the thoracolumbar spine versus inability to maintain an open airway in a patient who was found in an upright position, maintaining airway patency must take priority. Remember that this concept applies to patients who are found in a partially upright position. This does not necessarily mean that it is safe to move a patient who is found in a supine position into an upright position. Doing so risks displacing an unstable fracture at the thoracolumbar spine.

Upper Airway Sounds

Noises other than normal speech coming from the upper airway may be a sign of airway obstruction or distress. These noises may often be heard as you approach the patient. They are usually a result of a partial airway obstruction caused by the tongue, blood, or foreign bodies in the upper airway.

The type of sound you hear can give you clues as to the cause and location of upper airway obstruction. Snoring is caused by the base of the tongue and the soft palate falling backward and obstructing the upper airway. Gurgling occurs when blood, vomit, or secretions are present in the pharynx and signals an inability to clear and protect the airway. Stridor comes from narrowing at the level of the vocal cords. This may be heard on either inspiration or expiration. Stridor is typically caused by direct trauma, foreign body, or swelling of the mucosa, as in inhalation burns. Swelling is a challenging situation because it occurs at the narrowest point of the upper airway and demands quick action to prevent total airway obstruction. Steps must be taken immediately to alleviate the obstruction and maintain an open airway.

Examine the Airway for Obstructions

Because the upper airway extends from the tip of the nose to the sternal notch, simply looking in the mouth is not enough. Look in the mouth for any obvious foreign matter, such as vomit, blood, or debris, or any gross anatomic malformations, such as hematoma or swelling, and then look along the anterior neck down to the sternal notch (see Figure 7-7 and Figure 7-8). A thorough evaluation of the airway is important because some especially dangerous airway obstructions occur in the anterior neck. If found, remove any foreign bodies.

Look for Chest Rise and Retractions

Limited chest rise may be a sign of an obstructed airway. Additional signs, such as retractions, use of accessory muscles, or/and the appearance of increased work of breathing, should lead to a high index of suspicion for airway compromise.

When a patient is working hard to move air across a partially obstructed airway, a greater degree of negative intrathoracic pressure will develop within the chest. As a result, the soft tissue of the chest wall and intercostal spaces will be drawn inward, creating retractions between the ribs and at the jugular notch as muscle and soft tissues are pulled into the chest with inspiratory efforts. These retractions are especially visible in children. The presence of retractions indicate that the patient is struggling to breathe and should prompt you to actively search for, and relieve, airway obstruction.

In severe partial airway obstructions, "seesaw breathing" or "rocking boat breathing" is likely to occur. As the patient attempts to breathe through the obstructed airway, the diaphragm descends, causing the abdomen to lift (as in normal inspiration) and the chest to sink (not normal). The reverse happens as the diaphragm relaxes. Prehospital care practitioners observing this pattern of breathing should suspect and aggressively rule out an airway obstruction.

Management
Airway Control

After controlling any severe hemorrhage, ensuring a patent airway is the next priority of trauma management and resuscitation. Ideally, the airway of a trauma patient should be both open for air entry and protected against aspiration and occlusion from swelling. However, ensuring an *open* airway is the priority, and most of the time this can be accomplished quickly with no equipment other than the prehospital care practitioner's gloved hands. Regardless of how the airway is managed, a cervical spine injury must be considered if the mechanism of injury suggests the potential for one and the patient's LOC or other factors preclude definitively excluding the presence of such an injury. The use of any of these described methods of airway control requires simultaneous manual stabilization of the cervical spine in a neutral position until the patient has been completely immobilized. The exception to this rule is penetrating neck trauma, because data have shown that spinal immobilization is not necessary in these patients and can be detrimental from a time perspective.[1-3] (See Chapter 10, *Spinal Trauma*.)

Essential Skills

Management of the airway in a trauma patient can range from relatively simple to challenging, but in most patients, manual or simple procedures are sufficient during the initial phases of care. All prehospital care practitioners, regardless of level of training, need to maintain their ability to perform these simple and essential manual skills. Depending on the clinical situation, most airway issues are addressed in a simple manner that then progresses to more complex if the obstruction is not relieved. Manual and simple procedures often lead to a better patient outcome than more complex techniques, which require increased time, personnel, and equipment; have a higher risk of failure; and can be damaging if used improperly. Practitioners always need to weigh the risks versus the benefits of performing highly invasive, complex procedures. Advanced procedures require a high degree of skill proficiency and close oversight by the medical director. They should not be used unnecessarily.

Airway maintenance skills can be broken into four different levels: manual, simple, advanced, and definitive. The application of these skills, if they are within the prehospital care practitioner's scope of practice, should be patient driven, dependent on the situation and the severity of the patient.

Manual Clearing of the Airway

The first step in airway management is a quick visual inspection of the oropharyngeal cavity. Foreign material (e.g., pieces of food), broken teeth or dentures, and blood may be found in the mouth of a trauma patient. These objects should be swept out of the mouth using a gloved finger or suctioned away. A bite block or oral airway may then be a valuable adjunct to securing the upper airway.

In addition, positioning of the patient on the side (or in a sitting position when not contraindicated by possible spinal trauma) will allow for gravity-assisted clearing of secretions, blood, and vomitus, especially if there are large amounts. If spinal trauma is suspected, the patient can be logrolled onto the side to allow clearing of blood and vomit.

Simple Manual Maneuvers

In unresponsive patients, the tongue becomes flaccid, falling back and blocking the hypopharynx. This is the most common cause of airway obstruction. Manual methods to clear this type of obstruction can easily be accomplished because the tongue is attached to the mandible (jaw) and moves forward with it. Any maneuver that moves the mandible forward will pull the tongue away from the back of the hypopharynx:

- **Trauma jaw thrust**. In patients with suspected head, neck, or facial trauma, the cervical spine is maintained in a neutral in-line position. The trauma jaw thrust maneuver allows the prehospital care practitioner to open the airway with little or no movement of the head and cervical spine (**Figure 7-9A**). The mandible is thrust forward by placing the thumbs on each zygoma (cheekbone), placing the index and long fingers on the mandible, and at the same angle, pushing the mandible forward. This maneuver can be applied from the head or from the front position by a single practitioner. Because it allows a single practitioner to both clear the airway and maintain cervical spine alignment, it is an "all in one" technique and should become second nature for every trauma care practitioner.
- **Trauma chin lift**. While a first practitioner holds the head to maintain cervical spine alignment, the second practitioner grasps the chin and opens the mouth and then pulls the chin forward (**Figure 7-9B**). As opposed to the trauma jaw thrust, two practitioners are needed to safely use this method. Please note that the older version with the practitioner putting a thumb into the patient's mouth is dangerous, as a reactive patient can bite the practitioner's thumb.

Both techniques result in movement of the lower mandible anteriorly (upward) and slightly caudal (toward the feet), pulling the tongue forward, away from the posterior airway, and opening the mouth. The trauma jaw thrust *pushes* the mandible forward, whereas the trauma chin lift *pulls* the mandible. The trauma jaw thrust and the trauma chin lift are modifications of the conventional jaw thrust and chin lift. The modifications provide protection to the patient's cervical spine while opening the airway by displacing the tongue from the posterior pharynx.

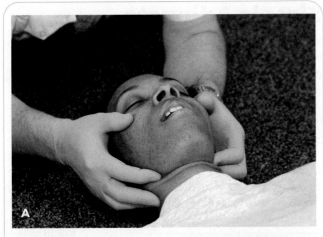

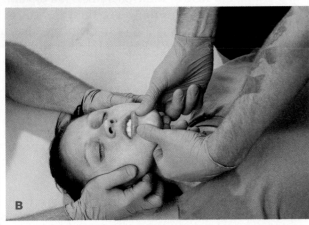

Figure 7-9 **A.** Trauma jaw thrust. A thumb is placed on each zygoma, with the index and long fingers at the angle of the mandible. The mandible is lifted superiorly. **B.** Trauma chin lift. The chin lift performs a function similar to that of the trauma jaw thrust. It moves the mandible forward displacing the tongue.

A: © National Association of Emergency Medical Technicians (NAEMT); B: © Jones & Bartlett Learning. Photographed by Darren Stahlman.

Suctioning

A trauma patient may not be capable of effectively clearing the buildup of secretions, vomitus, blood, or foreign objects from the trachea. Providing suction is an important part of maintaining a patent airway.

A trauma patient whose airway has not yet been managed may require aggressive suctioning of the upper airway. Large amounts of blood and vomit may have already accumulated in the airway before the arrival of emergency medical services (EMS) practitioners, and this may have already compromised ventilation and oxygen transport into the alveoli. In case of massive vomiting or bleeding, the amount of fluid may be more than a simple suction unit can quickly clear. If so, the patient may be logrolled onto the side while maintaining cervical spine alignment; gravity will assist in clearing the airway.

A rigid large-bore suction device is preferred to clear the oropharynx, and should be introduced laterally into the mouth since this will be much better tolerated by a reactive patient.

Although it is true that hypoxia can result from prolonged suctioning, a totally obstructed airway will provide no air exchange, so aggressive suctioning and patient positioning are continued until the airway is at least partially clear. At that point, hyperoxygenation is performed, followed by repeated suctioning if needed. Hyperoxygenation, like preoxygenation, may be accomplished with either a nonrebreathing mask or a bag-mask device running attached to a high flow of oxygen. The goal when hyperoxygenating is to maintain an oxygen saturation as close to 100% as achievable for a short period of time.

Selection of Adjunctive Device

Airway issues noted during the primary survey require immediate action to establish and maintain a patent airway. These initial steps are the manual maneuvers, such as a trauma jaw thrust or chin lift. Once opened, the airway must be maintained, typically with the aid of some type of adjunctive device. The particular device should be selected based on the prehospital care practitioner's level of training and proficiency with that device and a risk–benefit analysis for the use of various adjuncts and techniques that relate to the patient. (See Chapter 2, *Golden Principles, Preferences, and Critical Thinking*.) The choice of airway adjunct should be patient driven: "What is the best airway for this particular patient in this particular situation?" (**Box 7-1**).

During initial training as well as during continuing education, prehospital care practitioners at various levels are exposed to a range of adjunctive devices to help maintain an open airway. The amount of training directly relates to the difficulty in placement of the device. At the emergency medical responder level, practitioners are trained to place oropharyngeal airways. At the other end of the spectrum, advanced practitioners have been trained to use complex airway devices, with some protocols allowing surgical airway procedures.

Box 7-1 Factors in Selecting Airway Adjuncts

- Does the method maintain an open airway?
- Training
- Available equipment and assistance
- Transport time
- Perceived difficulty

© National Association of Emergency Medical Technicians (NAEMT)

With complex skills such as intubation or surgical cricothyrotomy, the more times a skill is performed, the better the chance for a successful outcome. A new paramedic who has performed these procedures only in the classroom setting has less of a chance of intubating a difficult patient successfully compared to a 10-year veteran who has performed this intervention numerous times. The more steps there are in a procedure, the more difficult the procedure is to learn and master. Complex skills also lend themselves to a greater probability of failure, because greater knowledge is required and more steps are involved in completing the intervention. As a skill increases in difficulty, so do the educational requirements, both in initial training and ongoing skill maintenance. Generally, the more difficult a procedure is to perform, the greater the penalty to the patient for failure or error. This is particularly true with airway procedures.

The following are several types of airway devices that may be selected, depending on the needs or potential needs of the patient:

- **Simple adjuncts** (devices that lift the tongue from the back of the pharynx only)
  - Oropharyngeal airway
  - Nasopharyngeal airway
  - Ventilation requires a mask (usually with bag-mask device)
- **Advanced airways** (devices that are placed at the level of the oral pharynx and meant to secure the airway above the vocal cords; also called supraglottic airways)
  - Laryngeal mask airway
  - Laryngeal tube (LT; e.g., King LT)
- **Definitive airways** (devices that isolate the trachea with some form of seal and allow for the management of the airway at a level below the vocal cords)
  - Endotracheal (ET) tube
  - Surgical airway

Simple Adjuncts

When manual airway maneuvers are unsuccessful or when continued maintenance of an open airway is necessary, the use of an artificial airway is the next step (**Figure 7-10**). After placement of a simple adjunctive device, a decision to escalate to an advanced airway may be appropriate, depending on the patient and situation. Simple airway adjuncts are discussed next.

There are two kinds of basic life support (BLS) airways, the oropharyngeal airway and the nasopharyngeal airway. They are called BLS devices because BLS practitioners are typically credentialed to insert them. They are basic devices that simply keep the back of the tongue from blocking the airway. If the pharynx is full of vomit, or if the larynx swells shut however, these devices will not help the patient to establish or to maintain a patent airway. Still, they are quick and useful tools to relieve most airway obstructions.

Oropharyngeal Airway

The most frequently used artificial airway is the **oropharyngeal airway (OPA)** (see **Figure 7-11A**). The OPA is inserted in either a direct or an inverted manner.

Indications
- Patient who is unable to independently maintain a patent airway because of posterior displacement of the base of the tongue
- To prevent an intubated patient from biting an ET tube

Contraindications
- Patient who is conscious or semiconscious
- Patient with a gag reflex

Complications
- Because the OPA presses against the posterior aspect of the tongue, its use may lead to gagging, vomiting, and laryngospasm in patients who are conscious.

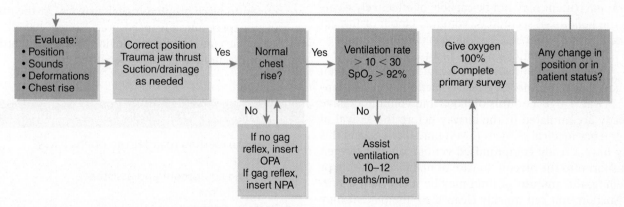

Figure 7-10 Basic airway management algorithm.

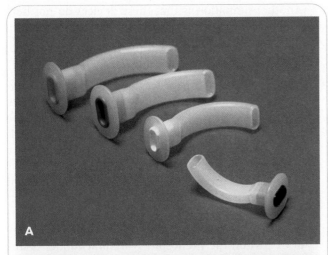

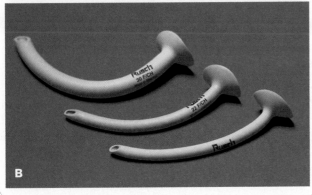

Figure 7-11 **A.** Oropharyngeal airways. **B.** Nasopharyngeal airways.

© Jones & Bartlett Learning. Courtesy of MIEMSS.

- For patients who are truly unconscious, the most common complication is failure to completely establish and maintain a patent airway, in which case additional chin lift may be necessary.

Nasopharyngeal Airway

The **nasopharyngeal airway (NPA)** is a soft, rubberlike device that is inserted through one of the nares and then along the curvature of the posterior wall of the nasopharynx and oropharynx to keep the back of the tongue from blocking the upper airway (**Figure 7-11B**).

Indications
- Patient who is unable to independently maintain an open airway

Contraindications
- Although there have been some case reports[1] of intracranial insertion of an NPA, evidence has not supported the claim that facial/basilar skull fractures are a contraindication to placement of an

NPA if one is needed. However, if signs of a fracture to the base of the skull are present, caution is advised. Correct insertion technique should minimize the risks.[4]

Complications
- Bleeding caused by insertion

Supraglottic Airways

The principle of advanced airways is that they keep the upper airway open and separated from the digestive tract while providing a tight seal, which facilitates positive-pressure ventilation. **Supraglottic airways (SGAs)** are the simplest advanced airways. They can be useful in a patient whose airway is difficult to maintain or in patients who need positive-pressure ventilation and in whom tight mask seal is difficult to achieve (**Figure 7-12**).

Types of supraglottic airways include the **laryngeal mask airway (LMA)**, which builds a seal around the larynx while its tip occludes the esophagus, and the **laryngeal tube airway (LTA)**, which seals the oropharynx while the end of the tube seals the esophagus (**Table 7-2**).

Because both devices press on the back of the throat, they can only be used in unconscious patients, and because a false placement can potentially occlude the airway, placement should be confirmed by chest inspection, auscultation, and continuous waveform $ETCO_2$ monitoring. The LMA comes in varying sizes and must be matched to the patient's anatomy for correct use.

Their advantages are easy and quick placement (less than 20 seconds in most studies)[5]; excellent skill retention[6]; and the ability to be inserted independent of the patient's position, which may be especially important in trauma patients when there are access and extrication difficulties or when there is a high suspicion of cervical spinal injury. They can be useful if positive-pressure ventilation is needed and obtaining a tight mask seal is difficult (**Figure 7-13**).

When in place, these devices provide an airway seal of 16–26 centimeters of water (cm H_2O) even in pediatric patients,[7] which is enough to allow for very effective positive-pressure ventilation. They also provide an esophageal seal (about 16 cm H_2O) that can help to prevent passive regurgitation. Most of these devices have a lumen through which a suction catheter can be inserted down through the esophagus, which makes it possible to partially decompress the stomach, further reducing the risk of regurgitation and improving the effectiveness of ventilations. However, be aware that active vomiting can produce pressures up to 300 cm H_2O in an adult and may therefore dislodge the device. So, while SGAs offer a relatively high degree of airway protection, they do not offer complete airway protection.

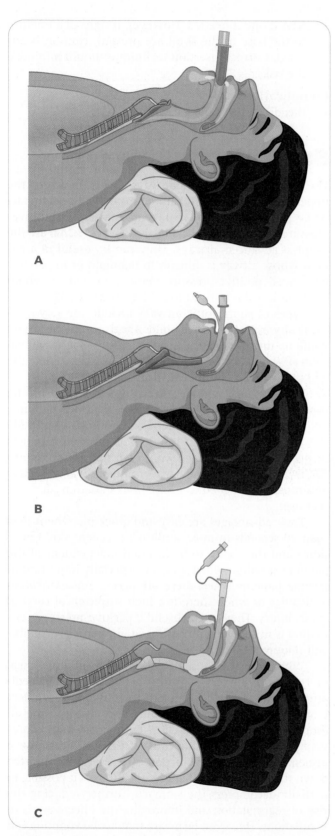

Figure 7-12 **A.** The i-gel is a polymer ring adapted to provide a seal around the larynx. **B.** The laryngeal mask has an inflatable ring that provides a seal around the larynx. **C.** The laryngeal tube has an opening that faces the larynx, while the proximal cuff seals the oropharynx.

Another limitation is that these devices do not help to address laryngeal edema because that occurs distal to the terminal end of the SGA device.

Indications

- If the prehospital care practitioner is trained and authorized, a supraglottic airway is an efficient device to maintain the airway in an unconscious trauma patient who lacks a gag reflex. Its insertion is typically faster than ET intubation and more reliable as a primary airway management tool. Because it allows positive-pressure ventilation, it is useful in a patient who is apneic or ventilating at a rate of less than 10 breaths/minute.
- A supraglottic airway is often the alternative airway device when the prehospital care practitioner is unable to perform endotracheal intubation and cannot easily ventilate the patient with a bag-mask device and an OPA or NPA.

Contraindications

- Intact gag reflex
- Known esophageal disease (This contraindication is especially relevant for the King LT airway; the risk is reduced with the LMA because it does not enter the esophagus.)
- Recent ingestion of caustic substances

Complications

- Gagging and vomiting (if gag reflex is intact)
- Aspiration
- Damage to the esophagus
- Hypoxia and hypoventilation if placement is incorrect

Laryngeal Mask Airway

The LMA is the most widely used of the supraglottic devices. The device comprises an inflatable silicone ring attached diagonally at the distal end of a silicone tube (**Figure 7-14**). When inserted, the ring creates a low-pressure seal between the LMA and the glottic opening, without direct insertion of the device into the larynx itself.

Different brands and designs of LMAs are available, including some models with a rigid, anatomically curved conduit. One special model is the i-gel LMA, which is made from a medical-grade thermoplastic elastomer. It has been designed to create a noninflatable, anatomic seal of the pharyngeal, laryngeal, and perilaryngeal structures while avoiding compression trauma. This eliminates the need for a syringe, which makes it particularly valuable in military or other tactical environments.

Advantages of the LMA include the following:

- The LMA is designed for blind insertion. Direct visualization of the trachea and vocal cords is unnecessary.

Table 7-2 Supraglottic Airways

	Airway Seal	Inflatable Cuff	Gastric Decompression	Possibility to Pass an Endotracheal Tube
Classic laryngeal mask	Around larynx	Yes	No	Yes
Supreme laryngeal mask (intubating laryngeal mask)	Around larynx	Yes	Yes	No
i-gel laryngeal mask	Around larynx	No	Yes	Yes
Laryngeal tube	Oropharynx	Yes	In some models	No

© National Association of Emergency Medical Technicians (NAEMT)

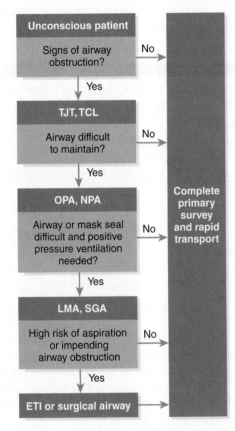

Figure 7-13 Basic techniques to establish and maintain a patent airway are adequate for many unconscious patients. Advanced techniques are valuable when maintaining mask seal is difficult, when aspiration risk is high, or to establish a secure route for the provision of positive pressure ventilation. Establishing priorities requires an organized approach.

Abbreviations: TCL, trauma chin lift; TJT, trauma jaw thrust.
© National Association of Emergency Medical Technicians (NAEMT)

- The LMA is available in a range of sizes to accommodate both pediatric and adult patient groups.

Currently, there is vast experience using the LMA in the prehospital environment in Europe, in North America, and in the military. A more sophisticated version of the device is the "intubating LMA." This device is inserted similarly to the original LMA, but a flexible ET tube can then be inserted though the LMA into the trachea.

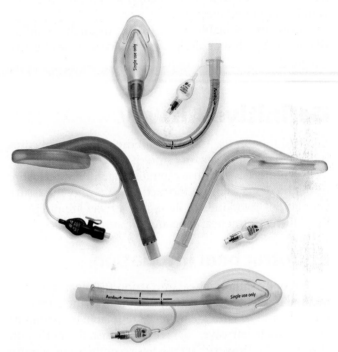

Figure 7-14 Laryngeal mask airway.
Courtesy of Ambu, Inc.

Intubating Laryngeal Mask Airway

The intubating laryngeal mask airway (ILMA) device is similar in design to the LMA and is inserted the same way. It allows for secondary insertion of an ET tube and directs the tube into the trachea. Once endotracheal tube position within the trachea has been confirmed, the ILMA is typically left in place throughout transport to help stabilize the ET tube and to and serve as a backup.

The device is available only in adult sizes. It may be valuable as a tool to achieve temporizing airway control prior to patient extrication with addition of the ET tube attempted once better access to the patient is possible.

I-gel Device

The i-gel device creates a seal using a noninflatable mechanism and a blind insertion technique. Although the seal forms around the glottic opening, it is not as inclusive as that of an ET tube. Aspiration remains a concern.

Sizes are available from neonatal through adult. Advantages include less risk of trauma to the airway and relative ease of insertion.

Laryngeal Tube Airway

The laryngeal tube airway (LTA) is a double lumen tube with cuffs distally and proximally. The primary lumen is intended for ventilation. The second is meant to facilitate insertion of an aspiration catheter for gastric decompression. The device provides less protection from aspiration than does an ET tube, but it allows for positive-pressure ventilation nonetheless.

Sizes are available from infant through to adult. Given the dual lumen design, the device may be effective in aiding tracheal intubation.

Definitive Airway

A cuffed tube in the trachea underneath the vocal cords is called a definitive airway since it provides the most effective protection against aspiration and airway closure through edema and the most effective positive-pressure ventilation. Two kinds of definitive airway are discussed here: the endotracheal tube and the surgical airway.

Endotracheal Intubation

Traditionally, endotracheal intubation (ETI) was the ideal method for achieving maximum control of the airway in trauma patients who are apneic, are unable to maintain/protect their airways, or require assisted ventilation (**Figure 7-15**). However, its use has recently become more controversial, because in terms of patient survival, the results of using this technique have been variable.[8]

Unlike intubation in the operating room (OR), which is a safe procedure with few complications, emergency intubation of a critical patient in the prehospital environment is a very risky procedure and it has been associated with serious complications. Even in a well-equipped and staffed emergency department (ED) or ICU, emergency intubation of a critical patient was linked with 40% cardiovascular instability, 9% severe hypoxia, and up to 3% risk of cardiac arrest.[9] This can explain why, although some prehospital studies show an intubation success rate of more than 97%, impact on patient survival remains less clear. Studies have shown that in an urban environment, critically injured trauma patients with ETI had no better outcome than those transported with a bag-mask device and OPA.[10] As a result, the role of ETI has increasingly come into question and, to date, few studies have demonstrated any actual benefit to the use of the technique.[11]

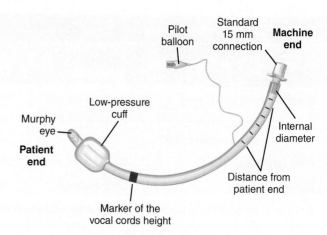

Figure 7-15 Characteristic features of an endotracheal tube.
© National Association of Emergency Medical Technicians (NAEMT)

However, a better understanding of the indications and optimization of the technique might lead to a more positive impact on patient survival.

Advantages
- Definitive and tight seal of the airway
- Allows positive-pressure ventilation
- Optimal protection against bronchoaspiration

Disadvantages
- Time consuming
- Intravenous (IV) line, drugs, and monitoring needed (**Table 7-3**)
- Skilled and experienced practitioner necessary
- High incidence of complications

The decision to perform ETI or to employ an alternative device should be made after a global evaluation of risk and benefit, including the probable difficulty and the practitioner's level of experience. Consideration should also be given to the effect of the increase in scene time necessary to perform the procedure. Average additional on-scene time for patients undergoing ETI was 8 minutes in one large European study.[12]

What is certain is that intubation in the field will always be more difficult than in the hospital and will add to on-scene time, no matter how skilled or efficient the crew is. As such, while there might be good reasons to intubate a patient with airway burns for a 30-minute flight to the hospital, those reasons are less compelling if the patient is unconscious and hypotensive with no facial trauma and is 5 minutes from a well-equipped and well-staffed trauma center.[13]

Prediction of Potentially Difficult Endotracheal Intubation

Prior to performing ETI, it is imperative that an assessment of the difficulty of the intubation be done. Many

- Facilitates deep tracheal suctioning
- Prevents gastric insufflation

Indications
- Patients who are unable to protect their airways, classically patients with a Glasgow Coma Scale score < 8, although this indication has been challenged recently[15]
- Patient with significant oxygenation problems, requiring administration of high concentrations of oxygen
- Patient with significant ventilatory impairment requiring assisted or positive-pressure ventilation
- Relatively prolonged transport time to a hospital capable of achieving definitive airway control
- Inability to adequately achieve and maintain airway control using less invasive maneuvers

Contraindications
- Lack of training or maintenance of training in technique
- Lack of proper indications
- Proximity to receiving facility (relative contraindication)
- High probability of failed airway
- Intravascular hypovolemia and/or hemorrhagic shock

Complications
- Hypoxemia from prolonged intubation attempts
- Hypercarbia from prolonged intubation attempts
- Vagal stimulation causing bradycardia
- Increased intracranial pressure
- Trauma to the airway with resultant hemorrhage and edema
- Right main bronchus intubation
- Esophageal intubation
- Vomiting leading to aspiration
- Loose or broken teeth
- Injury to the vocal cords
- Conversion of a cervical spine injury without neurologic deficit to one with neurologic deficit
- Conversion of a simple pneumothorax to a tension pneumothorax due to positive-pressure ventilation
- Circulatory collapse because of sedative medications combined with positive-pressure ventilation

As with all procedures, the prehospital care practitioner, along with the medical director, makes a risk–benefit judgment when employing ETI. Performing procedures simply because "the protocols allow it" is inappropriate. Think of the possible benefits and the possible risks, and form a plan based on the clinical scenario and the physical findings of the patient. Situations differ dramatically based on transport time, location (urban vs. rural), and the practitioner's level of experience in performing a given procedure (**Box 7-3**). Keep in mind that the intubation success rate is not the sole measure of success. Time to achieving airway control and number of attempts have been shown to correlate significantly with morbidity and mortality.[16]

Table 7-3 Equipment and Setup for Endotracheal Intubation

Ventilation and Oxygenation	Intubation	Rescue Plan
Bag-mask device	Endotracheal tube with cuff	Laryngeal mask
Oxygen tank	Syringe	Surgical airway set
Mask	Stylet	
OPA and NPA	Laryngoscope	
	Rigid, large-bore suction catheter	
Monitoring with ECG, NIBP, SpO$_2$, and ETCO$_2$		
IV access with sedative drugs, muscle relaxants, and vasopressors		

Abbreviations: ECG, electrocardiogram; ETCO$_2$, end-tidal carbon dioxide; IV, intravenous; NIBP, noninvasive blood pressure; NPA, nasopharyngeal airway; OPA, oropharyngeal airway; SpO$_2$, peripheral oxygen saturation.

© National Association of Emergency Medical Technicians (NAEMT)

factors can result in a difficult intubation of the trauma patient. Some of these are directly related to the trauma that has been sustained, others are due to anatomic anomalies of the face and upper airway, and still others to positioning of the patient.

HEAVEN is a set of criteria to predict difficult intubation[14] that seems to be better adapted to trauma patients in the prehospital environment than traditional, hospital, or office-based evaluation methods (**Box 7-2**).

Transport time may also be a factor when deciding on the appropriate modality; an example may be a patient who is being maintained effectively with an OPA and bag-mask device with a short transport time to the trauma center. The prehospital care practitioner may elect not to intubate but rather transport while maintaining the airway using simple airway techniques. Practitioners need to assess the risks versus the benefits when making the decision to use complex airway procedures.

Despite the potential challenges of this procedure, ETI often remains a preferred method of airway control because it does the following:

- Isolates the airway
- Allows for ventilation with 100% oxygen (FiO$_2$ of 1.0)
- Eliminates the need to maintain an adequate mask-to-face seal
- Significantly decreases the risk of aspiration (vomitus, foreign material, blood)

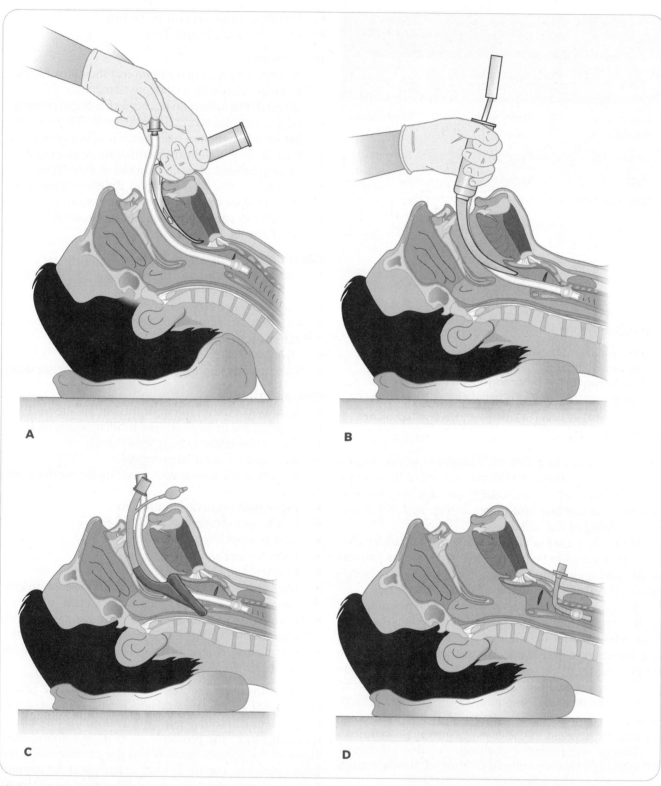

Figure 7-16 A definitive airway is a tube with a cuff in the trachea underneath the vocal cords. It is the definitive protection against bronchoaspiration and airway closure through swelling. Establishing a definitive airway in a conscious or semiconscious patient requires an IV line, sedative drugs, and monitoring. **A.** Orotracheal intubation under direct visualization with a laryngoscope. **B.** Orotracheal intubation under indirect visualization using a video laryngoscope. This puts less pressure on the patient's cervical spine. **C.** Intubation with a laryngeal mask. **D.** A surgical airway provides rapid access with basic equipment and local anesthesia, but requires extensive training.

Box 7-2 HEAVEN Criteria

- Hypoxemia: oxygen saturation value $\leq$ 93% at the time of initial laryngoscopy
- Extremes of size: pediatric patient $\leq$ 8 years of age or clinical obesity
- Anatomic challenge: includes trauma, mass, swelling, foreign body, or other structural abnormality limiting laryngoscopic view
- Vomit/blood/fluid: clinically significant fluid present in the pharynx/hypopharynx at the time of laryngoscopy
- Exsanguination: suspected anemia that could potentially accelerate desaturation during rapid-sequence intubation–associated apnea
- Neck: limited cervical range of motion

Reproduced from Davis D, Olvera DJ. HEAVEN criteria: derivation of a new difficult airway prediction tool. *Air Med J.* 2017;36(4):195-197. https://doi.org/10.1016/j.amj.2017.04.001

Box 7-3 Practice Improves Intubation Success Rate

Research studies have shown that practice increases the likelihood of success when intubating. Although no correlation was found between success rate and length of time as a paramedic, there was a correlation between the number of patients intubated by the paramedic and the success rate. Experience with the procedure increases the likelihood of successful performance.[17] One hospital study has shown that it takes operators in the OR 70 intubations to achieve a 90% success rate. In the prehospital trauma setting, in a patient with immobilized cervical spine, this number is likely to be even higher.[18]

In assessing success rate, speed and number of attempts are important considerations; both factors have been shown to correlate significantly with morbidity and mortality.[19] Prehospital care practitioners must keep in mind that the patient's oxygenation and perfusion, not the kind of airway used, will determine the outcome.

Box 7-4 Problems and Solutions With Endotracheal Intubation

Problems
- Hypoxia during intubation attempts is frequent and often unrecognized, as SpO_2 signal changes may lag in patients with poor circulation.
- Number of complications is proportional to the number of attempts.
- Overzealous ventilation is frequent despite $ETCO_2$ monitoring and is especially detrimental in patients with traumatic brain injury.
- Positive-pressure ventilation and anesthetic drugs can both cause a drop in blood pressure

Possible Solutions
- Optimize preoxygenation and wait until SpO_2 is at least 93%.
- Optimize preconditions and aim for first-pass success.
- Use apneic oxygenation and observe vital signs during intubation

should aim at optimizing preconditions, using the best technique first, watching vital parameters, and abandoning the technique early in the face of failure (**Box 7-4**).

Methods of ETI

Several alternative methods are available for performing endotracheal intubation. The method of choice depends on such factors as the patient's needs, the level of urgency, patient positioning, or training and scope of practice. Regardless of the method selected, the patient's head and neck should be stabilized in a neutral position during the procedure and spinal motion restriction should be maintained throughout. In general, if intubation is not successful after two attempts, consider trying another method of airway control. Going back to a more basic method often is the best option. It is better to bring a well-oxygenated patient into the ED without an ET tube than an intubated patient with additional brain damage after multiple prolonged episodes of hypoxia.

Orotracheal Intubation

Orotracheal intubation involves placing an ET tube into the trachea through the mouth. The nontrauma patient is often placed in a "sniffing" position to facilitate intubation. Because this position hyperextends the cervical spine at C1-C2 (the second most common site for cervical spine fractures) and hyperflexes it at C5-C6 (the most common site for cervical spine fractures), it should not be used for patients with blunt trauma (**Figure 7-17**). However, numerous studies have shown that orotracheal intubation with cervical spine protection is easier when performed using a video laryngoscope.

Studies in the early 2000s raised concerns about the incidence and impact of hypoxemia during prehospital intubation.[20] More recent publications have highlighted the physiologic aspects of intubation, and suggested that both the number of complications and mortality may increase with the number of attempts.[21] Older approaches advocated for multiple attempts, using a new tool every step of the way. Unfortunately, even when the approach eventually led to a high intubation success rate, it was often disastrous in terms of mortality.[22] That is why practitioners

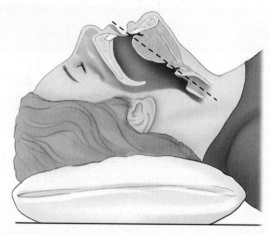

Figure 7-17 Placing the patient's head in the "sniffing" position provides ideal visualization of the larynx through the mouth. However, such positioning hyperextends the patient's neck at C1 and C2 and hyperflexes it at C5 and C6. These are the two most common points of fracture of the cervical spine.

© National Association of Emergency Medical Technicians (NAEMT)

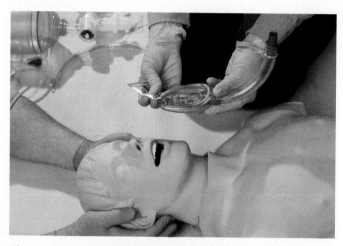

Figure 7-18 Intubating laryngeal mask.

© Jones & Bartlett Learning. Photographed by Darren Stahlman.

Nasotracheal Intubation

In conscious trauma patients or in those with an intact gag reflex, ETI may be difficult to accomplish. If spontaneous ventilations are present, **blind nasotracheal intubation (BNTI)** may be attempted if the benefit outweighs the risk. Although nasotracheal intubation is often more difficult to perform than direct visualization and oral intubation, a high success rate has been reported in trauma patients by practitioners skilled in this technique.[23,24] During BNTI, the patient must be breathing to ensure that the ET tube is passed through the vocal cords. Many texts suggest that BNTI is contraindicated in the presence of midface trauma or fractures, but an exhaustive literature search reveals only rare evidence of risk of an ET tube entering the cranial vault.[25] Apnea is a contraindication specific to BNTI, because the procedure takes some time, during which the patient cannot be effectively ventilated. Furthermore, the procedure itself is enabled by the patient's breathing. This facilitating factor is absent in an apneic patient.

Face-to-Face Intubation

Face-to-face intubation is indicated when standard trauma intubation techniques cannot be used because of the inability of the prehospital care practitioner to assume the standard position at the head of the trauma patient. These situations include but are not limited to the following:

- Vehicle entrapment
- Pinning of the patient in rubble

This technique has traditionally been attempted with a Macintosh laryngoscope held in the right hand;

however, intubation with ILMA seems to be both easier and more reliable, allowing ventilation between intubation attempts.

Intubation With Intubating Laryngeal Mask

The ILMA is a modified version of the LMA and is designed to allow the passage of an ET tube. It is a rigid, anatomically curved tube that is wide enough to accept an ET tube and short enough that the end of the ET tube enters the trachea (**Figure 7-18**). Several studies have shown a high success rate in difficult intubation cases (i.e., patients in whom intubation by direct laryngoscopy had failed).[26] Added benefits of the ILMA include that it is possible to ventilate the patient intermittently during intubation attempts and that a backup plan is already in place if the intubation fails.

Intubation With Video Laryngoscope

Video laryngoscopes are devices that allow for videoscopic visualization of the larynx. Intubation using video laryngoscopy appears to be especially useful in situations where patient anatomy (short neck, anterior cords, or other anatomic challenges) is a challenge and direct laryngoscopy is difficult. Some studies have demonstrated that video laryngoscopy use may improve intubation success rates.[27] This appears especially true in trauma patients where cervical spine alignment must be maintained, or blood and secretions are obscuring the practitioner's vision. Video laryngoscopy may be difficult in outdoor or bright settings as the video screen becomes difficult to see in these conditions.[28]

Video laryngoscopes are either unchanneled or channeled (**Figure 7-19**). With unchanneled video laryngoscopes, the ET tube must be brought into the field of view freehand, whereas with the channeled type, the ET tube is inserted into the laryngoscope blade and advanced

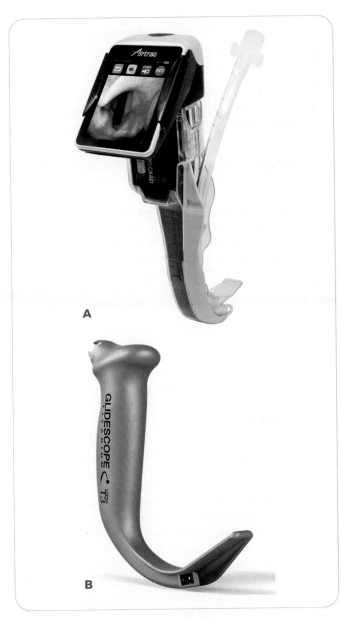

Figure 7-19 **A.** Channeled video laryngoscope. **B.** Unchanneled laryngoscope blade.

A: Courtesy of Airtraq LLC a subsidiary of Prodol Meditec S.A.; B: Courtesy of Verathon Inc.

through the channel once good visualization of the larynx is obtained. Unlike conventional laryngoscopes, which must displace the tissues to provide a clear line of sight, channeled video laryngoscopes can slide under the soft tissues until the lens and the intubating channel are aligned with the vocal cords.

Drug-Assisted Intubation

Several studies have shown that drug-assisted intubation (DAI) or pharmacologically assisted intubation increases the success rate of intubation; however, this comes at a cost.[29] Pharmacologic sedation and relaxation bring the risk of respiratory depression, apnea, and circulatory

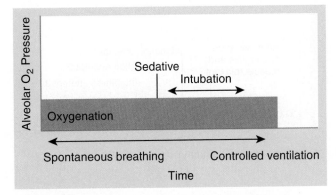

Figure 7-20 Drug-assisted intubation. The patient is given a sedative/anesthetic to facilitate intubation. The patient continues to breathe throughout the procedure, reducing desaturation risk.

© National Association of Emergency Medical Technicians (NAEMT)

collapse. When muscular paralytic agents are used, they will block every muscle except the heart; thus, from the moment the paralytic is injected into the patient, all the patient's breathing and airway control becomes the responsibility of the practitioner. Nonetheless, in skilled hands, this technique can facilitate effective airway control when other methods fail or are otherwise not acceptable. To maximize the effectiveness of this procedure and ensure patient safety, prehospital care practitioners need to be familiar with applicable local protocols, medications, and indications for use of the technique. Different sequences of DAI are currently in use, the most widely known being **rapid-sequence intubation (RSI)** and **delayed-sequence intubation (DSI)**. RSI is an anesthesia technique focused on preventing aspiration, whereas DSI focuses on preventing desaturation and hypoxia. However, the use of medications to assist with intubation, particularly RSI, does have risks above and beyond those of intubation alone. Intubation using medications falls into the following three categories:

1. *Intubation using only sedatives or narcotics.* Anesthetic medications such as ketamine, etomidate, or propofol; barbiturates such as diazepam or midazolam; or narcotics such as fentanyl or morphine, may be used alone or in combination, with the goal being to relax the patient enough to permit intubation but not to abolish protective reflexes or breathing (**Figure 7-20**). Ketamine is an excellent first-line induction agent. It causes less circulatory depression than the other induction agents and has a strong analgesic effect. Still, the success rate seems to be less than when using paralytic agents, and the complications more frequent.[29]

2. *RSI using paralytic agents.* The aim of RSI is to minimize the period at risk for aspiration. To that purpose, sedative medications and a

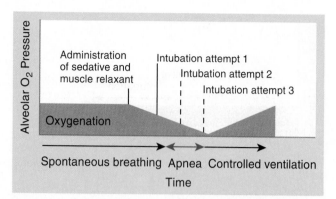

Figure 7-21 Rapid-sequence intubation. RSI is a technique aimed at preventing bronchoaspiration. The patient is given a sedative and a rapid-acting muscle relaxant simultaneously, and then intubated. This method has a high rate of success, but there is an increased risk of hypoxia during the apnea period if the patient is not well oxygenated at the start of the procedure or if intubation attempts are prolonged.

© National Association of Emergency Medical Technicians (NAEMT)

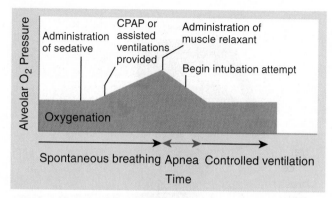

Figure 7-22 Delayed-sequence intubation. DSI is a technique developed to reduce the risk of desaturation and hypoxia in high-risk patients. The patient is given a sedative to make preoxygenation with continuous positive airway pressure (CPAP) and/or assisted ventilations possible before the muscle relaxant is given. This method has a high rate of success and added safety, but additional time is needed to optimize preoxygenation.

© National Association of Emergency Medical Technicians (NAEMT)

fast-acting paralytic are given simultaneously, as opposed to the traditional sequence in which sedation is given first (**Figure 7-21**). The aim of RSI is to smoothly and quickly render the patient unconscious and to induce skeletal muscle paralysis, thereby facilitating the passage of the endotracheal tube across the upper airway and into the trachea. This results in facilitating intubation while maintaining stable cerebral perfusion pressure and cardiovascular hemodynamics. This method provides complete muscle paralysis, removes all protective reflexes, and produces apnea, making intubation much easier. However, this procedure is not without risk, because from the moment the patient's ventilation stops, there is definite risk of hypoxia if the patient cannot be effectively ventilated.

Studies of this method of airway management have demonstrated successful performance of the technique in the field, with intubation success rates reported in the mid-90% range. However, few studies have critically evaluated whether patient outcome is affected.[30] One center reported its experience with RSI in the field and documented those patients with TBI who underwent RSI had a worse outcome than those who did not require RSI.[31] Subsequent analysis has shown that unrecognized hyperventilation leading to hypocarbia and unrecognized hypoxia were major contributors to the poor outcome. Another study showed a better outcome at 6 months for patients with TBI who were intubated in the field when compared to

those intubated in the hospital.[32] There is increasing evidence that some, if not most, of the adverse mortality associated with ETI in trauma patients is the result of the rather profound fall in perfusion pressure (MAP and CPP) which accompanies ETI; particularly in hypovolemic patients (i.e., patients in hemorrhagic or traumatic shock).[33] So, the final answer to the important question of whether long-term patient outcome is positively or negatively impacted by prehospital RSI has not yet been answered by the available research. What is certain is that this technique is for highly trained prehospital care practitioners only and that efficient ventilation and perfusion are the aim no matter what technique is used.

3. *DSI.* DSI, a newer technique of medication-assisted intubation emphasizing preoxygenation with continuous positive airway pressure (CPAP) and apneic oxygenation during intubation, has shown some promising results (**Figure 7-22**). The patient is preoxygenated under ketamine sedation, then paralytic agents are administered and the patient is intubated, with a nasal cannula providing apneic oxygenation during the procedure. This technique takes longer to accomplish and may delay time to definitive care; this risk should be assessed and considered (**Box 7-5**).[34]

What to Look For During Intubation

Even short episodes of hypoxemia have been shown to have devastating impacts on the survival of TBI patients.[39,40] Single episodes of SpO_2 < 90% have been correlated with a significant increase in hospital and intensive care length of stay. What is more, desaturation below 70% puts the patient at serious risk for cardiac decompensation. That is why attention should be paid to preoxygenation before any intubation attempts, especially if paralytics are used. As a rule, SpO_2 should be greater than 93% before intubation can be safely attempted.[41] During the intubation attempts, one team member should keep a close eye on the monitor and, if the SpO_2 is approaching 93%, intubation attempts should be stopped and the patient ventilated again. Another helpful tip is to set the monitor so that the oxygen saturation tone is clearly audible to the team members during the attempted airway procedures.

Bradycardia is another sign team members should look for. Remember that cerebral hypoxia does not happen at the fingertips. In fact, peripheral SpO_2 has been demonstrated to drop much later than cerebral SpO_2; this has been described as the "pulse ox lag."[42] That is why the team should be on the lookout for bradycardia episodes during intubation, as these can be a sign of cerebral hypoxemia. Human factor seems to play a role, as studies have demonstrated that such episodes were often not recognized by the practitioners.[43] Don't let this happen to your team (**Box 7-6**). Make certain that a team member is assigned to monitor vital signs—including oxygenation levels—while you intubate (**Box 7-7**).

Last, but not least, remember that sedative drugs as well as positive-pressure ventilation will impact venous return and can lead to a drop in blood pressure, which dramatically increases mortality in TBI patients. That is why checking the vital signs, including blood pressure, after intubation is a vital part of postintubation control. The practitioner should be prepared to address postintubation hypotension with the use of appropriate volume-loading strategies in the hypovolemic patient.

Getting the tube into the trachea is not enough. Optimizing the patient's physiologic status must be the goal.[45]

Indications

- A patient who requires a secure airway and is difficult to intubate because of uncooperative behavior (as induced by hypoxia, TBI, hypotension, or intoxication)

Relative Contraindications
- Availability of an alternative airway (e.g., supraglottic)
- Severe facial trauma that would impair or preclude successful intubation
- Neck deformity or swelling that complicates or precludes placement of a surgical airway
- Medical problems that would preclude use of indicated medications

Absolute Contraindications
- Inability to intubate
- Inability to maintain airway with bag-mask device and OPA
- Known allergies to indicated medications

Complications
- Inability to insert the ET tube in a sedated or paralyzed patient no longer able to protect the airway or breathe spontaneously; patients who are medicated and then cannot be intubated require prolonged bag-mask ventilation until the medication wears off
- Development of hypoxia or hypercarbia during prolonged intubation attempts

- Aspiration
- Hypotension—virtually all the medications have the side effect of decreasing blood pressure

Patients who are mildly or moderately hypovolemic but compensating may experience a profound drop in blood pressure associated with the intravenous administration of many of the medications used in ETI. Exercise caution whenever the use of medications for intubation is considered (**Table 7-4**). Furthermore, patients who are volume depleted will often become hypotensive when transitioning from spontaneous breathing (negative intrathoracic pressure during active inspiration) to positive-pressure ventilation.

Verification of Endotracheal Tube Placement

Following intubation, prehospital care practitioners must take specific measures to ensure that the ET tube has been properly placed in the trachea. Once a patient is intubated and relaxed, ventilation and oxygenation depend completely on the practitioner, so monitoring of ventilation, oxygenation, and vital signs must be meticulous.

Table 7-4 Common Drugs Used for Pharmacologically Assisted Intubation

	Dosage (adult)	Duration	Effect	Side Effects	Tricks of the Trade
Sedation					
Midazolam	0.1–0.3 mg/kg IV	1–2 hours	Long-acting sedation, amnesia	Respiratory depression, apnea, hypotension	Classic induction agent, onset somewhat slow (up to 3 minutes)
Etomidate	0.2–0.3 mg/kg IV	3–10 minutes	Induced anesthesia	Apnea, hypotension, vomiting	Fast onset, causes only moderate hypotension. Suppression of the adrenal cortex
Ketamine	1–2 mg/kg IV	10 minutes	Sedation, induced anesthesia, analgesia	Tachycardia, hypertension, increased intracranial pressure (?)	Provides both anesthesia and analgesia. Best choice in shock patient Caution advised if SBP is above normal
Propofol	1–2 mg/kg IV	5–10 minutes	Sedation, induced anesthesia	Apnea, hypotension	Very popular anesthetic but causes profound hypotension Use in trauma patients tricky even in experienced hands

	Dosage (adult)	Duration	Effect	Side Effects	Tricks of the Trade
Analgesia					
Fentanyl	2–3 mcg/kg IV	20–30 minutes	Analgesia	Respiratory depression, apnea, hypotension	Classic analgesic for RSI, powerful and fast acting
Morphine	0.01 mg/kg IV	2–3 hours	Analgesia	Respiratory depression, apnea, hypotension	Not well adapted for rapid RSI because of very slow onset (up to 5 minutes)
Ketamine*	0.1–0.3 mg/kg	10 minutes		Hallucinations, especially at doses above 0.5 mg/kg	An "all in one" analgesic and anesthetic In low doses, provides excellent analgesia with normal muscle tone and without respiratory depression
Relaxation					
Succinylcholine	1–2 mg/kg IV	3–5 minutes	Fast (30–60 seconds) and short-acting muscle relaxation	Hyperkalemia, muscle fasciculation	Quick, cheap, and efficient Contraindicated in patients with neuromuscular diseases
Rocuronium	0.6–1.2 mg/kg IV	30 minutes	Fast and long-acting muscle relaxation		Quick and efficient Antidote (sugammadex) available
Vecuronium	0.1 mg/kg IV	30–40 minutes	Muscle relaxation	Slow onset	Slow onset (up to 5 minutes) makes it second choice for RSI

*Caveat for tactical practitioners: *Never* give ketamine before the patient has been disarmed!

Abbreviations: IV, intravenous; kg, kilogram; mcg, microgram; mg, milligram; RSI, rapid-sequence intubation; SBP, systolic blood pressure.

© National Association of Emergency Medical Technicians (NAEMT)

Inadvertent esophageal placement of an ET tube, if unrecognized for only a brief period, may result in profound hypoxia, with resultant brain injury (hypoxic encephalopathy) and even death. Therefore, it is important that proper placement be confirmed. Techniques to verify intubation include the use of both clinical assessments and adjunct devices.[41] Clinical assessments include the following:

- Direct visualization of the ET tube passing through the vocal cords

- Presence of bilateral breath sounds (auscultate laterally below the axilla) and absence of air sounds over the epigastrium
- Visualization of the chest rising and falling during ventilation
- Fogging (water vapor condensation) in the ET tube on expiration

Unfortunately, none of these techniques is 100% reliable *by itself* for verifying proper ET tube placement. Therefore, prudent practice involves assessing and documenting all these clinical signs, if possible. On rare occasions, because of difficult anatomy, visualization of the ET tube passing through the vocal cords may not be possible. In a moving vehicle (ground or aeromedical), engine noise may make auscultation of breath sounds almost impossible. Obesity and chronic obstructive pulmonary disease may interfere with the ability to see chest movement during ventilation.

Monitoring devices include the following:

- $ETCO_2$ monitoring (capnography)
- Colorimetric carbon dioxide detector
- Pulse oximetry

In a patient with a perfusing rhythm, $ETCO_2$ monitoring (capnography) serves as the "gold standard" for confirming ET tube placement. This technique should be used in the prehospital setting whenever available. Patients in cardiopulmonary arrest may not produce sufficient carbon dioxide, even with CPR in progress. It is for this reason that colorimetric detectors or capnography are of limited use in patients who lack a perfusing cardiac rhythm.

Because *none* of these techniques is universally reliable, *all* the clinical assessments noted previously should be performed as possible. Clinical assessment should be followed by use of at least *one* of the monitoring devices. If any of the techniques used to verify proper placement suggests that the ET tube may not be properly positioned, the ET tube should be immediately removed and reinserted, with placement verified again. All the techniques used to verify ET tube placement should be appropriately documented in the patient care report.

Securing an Endotracheal Tube

Once ETI has been performed, the ET tube must be secured in place and proper tube placement verified; the depth of tube insertion at the central incisors (front teeth) should be noted. Several commercially available products may serve to secure the ET tube adequately. A study identified that umbilical tape (twill tape) held the ET tube as effectively as commercial devices; however, it needs to be tied around the ET tube using appropriate knots and technique.[46] Ideally, if sufficient EMS personnel are present, someone should be assigned the task of manually holding the ET tube in proper position to ensure that it does not move.

Continuous pulse oximetry should be considered mandatory for all patients who require ETI. Any decline in the pulse oximetry reading (i.e., oxygen saturation [SpO_2]) or development of cyanosis requires reverification of ET tube placement. Additionally, an ET tube may become dislodged during any movement of the patient. Reverify ET tube position after every move of a patient, such as logrolling to a backboard, loading or unloading

into or from the ambulance, or carrying the patient down a staircase. It is particularly important to assign a team member to maintenance and monitoring of the ET position during all patient movement evolutions.

Suctioning the Intubated Patient

When suctioning intubated patients through the ET tube, a standard, commercially available tracheal suction tube should be used to limit trauma to the tracheal mucosa and to minimize frictional resistance. It needs to be long enough to pass the tip of the artificial airway (20 to 22 inches, or 50 to 55 centimeters [cm]). The soft catheter will probably not be effective in suctioning copious amounts of foreign material or fluid from the pharynx of a trauma patient, in which case the device of choice will be one with a tonsil-tip or Yankauer design. Under no circumstances should a tonsil-tip or Yankauer rigid suction device be placed in the end of the ET tube.

When suctioning an intubated patient, aseptic procedures are vital. This technique includes the following steps:

1. Preoxygenate the trauma patient with 100% oxygen (fraction of inspired oxygen [FiO_2] of 1.0).
2. Prepare the equipment while maintaining sterility.
3. Insert the catheter without suction. Suctioning is then initiated and continued for up to 10 seconds while withdrawing the catheter.
4. Reoxygenate the patient, and ventilate for at least five assisted ventilations.
5. Repeat as necessary, allowing time for reoxygenation to take place between procedures.

Alternate Techniques

If ETI has been unsuccessful after three attempts, it is appropriate to consider airway management using the manual and simple skills described previously and ventilating with a bag-mask device. If the receiving facility is reasonably close, these techniques may be the most prudent option for airway management when faced with a brief transport time. If the nearest appropriate facility is more distant, a surgical cricothyrotomy may be considered. Again, it is better to bring a well-oxygenated patient to the ED without an ET tube than an intubated patient with additional brain damage following a long episode of hypoxia. Remember, it is hypoxia that will further damage the injured brain, not the lack of an ET tube.

Surgical Airway

Surgical cricothyrotomy involves the creation of a surgical opening in the *cricothyroid membrane*, which lies between the larynx (thyroid cartilage) and the cricoid cartilage, through which a tube is directed into the tracheal lumen. In most patients, the skin is very thin in this location, making it amenable to immediate access to the airway.[15] Furthermore, it requires relatively little additional equipment.

However, achieving correct anatomic placement of the tube has proven to be difficult in many cases, with inaccurate placement being as high as 40% in some studies,[47] and complications are frequent.[48]

The use of this surgical airway in the prehospital arena is controversial. Complications are common with this procedure.[34] Conversely, the traditional view of surgical airway as a last resort has been questioned by a study, which reported a cricothyrotomy success rate of 97%. The mortality rate in this study, however, was a staggering 89%.[22] Thus the literature is at best unclear regarding the benefits and efficacy of this technique in the prehospital arena. To date, insufficient data exist to support a recommendation that surgical cricothyrotomy be established as a national standard for routine use in prehospital airway management.

For this technique to be successful in actual field practice, training must be done on real tissue. Current manikins and other simulation devices do not replicate actual human tissue and the feel of the anatomy in a patient. The prehospital care practitioner's first exposure to real tissue should not be a dying patient. In addition, this skill, perhaps more than other airway interventions, requires frequent practice in order to maintain the anatomic familiarity and skills needed to perform

it correctly in only seconds during a true emergency. Usually there is not a second chance to get it right. The value of spending additional time in training for this technique must be weighed against the potential benefit of using that time to train in ETI, as proficient ETI skills should dramatically minimize the need to even consider surgical cricothyrotomy for most patients (**Figure 7-23**).

Indications
- Massive midface and/or oral trauma precluding the use of a bag-mask device
- Inability to control the airway using less invasive maneuvers

Contraindications
- Any patient who can be safely intubated, either orally or nasally
- Patients with laryngotracheal injuries
- Children under 10 years of age
- Patients with acute laryngeal disease of traumatic or infectious origin
- Insufficient training

Complications
- Prolonged procedure time
- Hemorrhage
- Aspiration
- Misplacement or false passage of the ET tube
- Injury to neck structures or vessels
- Perforation of the esophagus

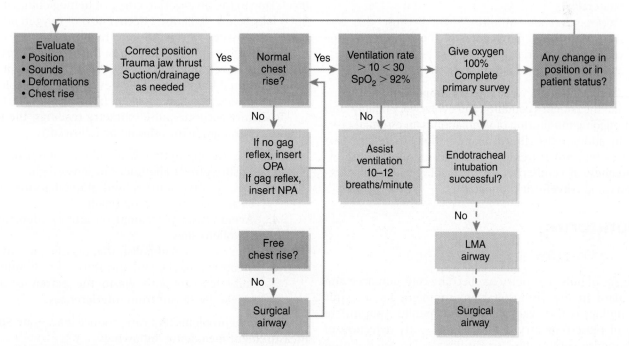

Figure 7-23 The surgical airway in the airway management system.
© National Association of Emergency Medical Technicians (NAEMT)

Ventilation

After securing the airway, the next step is to ensure adequate ventilation. As a reminder, the four things you need to breathe are an open airway, an intact rib cage, functional respiratory muscles, and a healthy lung to absorb oxygen.

The most immediate effect of most traumatic conditions, such as an unstable chest wall, a significant pneumothorax, or respiratory muscle weakness, is an acute reduction in tidal volume. More complex problems like reduced oxygen diffusion mostly occur later in the ICU, and while they are challenging to manage, they are rarely problematic in the prehospital phase. Acute reduction in tidal volume is the primary ventilatory challenge encountered in the field.

To assess ventilation during primary survey, it is important to check the following:

- *Tidal volume.* Look at the thorax. How effectively is the patient moving air? How is the chest expanding? If the patient is conscious, what is the quality of speech (i.e., are full sentences possible or only a few words at a time)?
- *Inspection of the rib cage.* Is there a deformity, any instability, or any open wounds? Is there symmetric expansion of both the right and left hemithorax? Is there paradoxical chest wall motion?
- *Respiratory rate.* Get a rough estimate of the respiratory rate. Is it normal, fast, very fast, or slow?
- *Auscultation on both sides.* Are breath sounds audible bilaterally?
- *Oxygen saturation.* Monitor SpO_2, because this is a measure of the effectiveness of the respiratory process. If the arterial blood is not becoming oxygenated, successful resuscitation is not possible.

After the initial evaluation, it is important to remember that the patient's condition can evolve very rapidly, and that ongoing monitoring of ventilation is an essential task.

In addition to clinical examination, there are two devices that are extremely useful in monitoring the effectiveness of ventilation on an ongoing basis: pulse oximetry and waveform capnography.

Monitoring

Pulse Oximetry

The use of pulse oximetry has become commonplace and standard in the prehospital environment. In fact, this technology is also available to the lay public. Appropriate use of pulse oximetry devices allows early detection of pulmonary compromise or cardiovascular deterioration before other physical signs are evident. **Pulse oximeters** are particularly useful in prehospital applications because

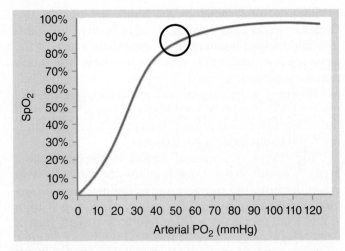

Figure 7-24 Pulse oximetry. Most pulse oximeters will display the SpO_2 value as well as the pulse rate. It is important to realize that 90% SpO_2 is not merely 100% minus 10%. Rather, it represents the flipping point beyond which desaturation progresses very quickly.
© National Association of Emergency Medical Technicians (NAEMT)

of their high reliability, portability, ease of application, and applicability across all age ranges and races.

Pulse oximeters provide measurements of oxygen saturation (SpO_2) and pulse rate. SpO_2 is determined by measuring the absorption ratio of red and infrared light passed through tissue. A small microprocessor correlates changes in light absorption caused by the passage of blood through vascular beds to determine arterial saturation and pulse rate. Normal SpO_2 is greater than 94% at sea level. Due to the dissociation curve of hemoglobin, when SpO_2 falls below 90%, the effectiveness of oxygen delivery to the tissues can deteriorate rapidly (**Figure 7-24**). When operating at higher altitudes, the acceptable levels of SpO_2 are lower than at sea level. Prehospital care practitioners should know what SpO_2 levels are acceptable at higher altitudes, if practicing in such settings.

To ensure accurate pulse oximetry readings, the following general guidelines should be followed:

1. Use the appropriate size and type of sensor.
2. Ensure proper alignment of sensor light.
3. Ensure that sources and photodetectors are clean, dry, and in good repair.
4. Avoid sensor placement on grossly edematous (swollen) sites.
5. Remove any nail polish that may be present.
6. Wrap the finger and the sensor in aluminum foil, this can both warm the extremity and shield the sensor from interferences.

Common problems that can produce inaccurate SpO_2 measurement include the following:

- Excessive motion
- Moisture in SpO_2 sensors

- Improper sensor application and placement
- Poor patient perfusion or vasoconstriction from hypothermia/hypovolemia
- Anemia
- Carbon monoxide poisoning

In a critical trauma patient, pulse oximetry may be less than accurate because of poor capillary perfusion status and because of anemia related to acute blood loss. Therefore, pulse oximetry is a valuable addition to the prehospital care practitioner's "toolbox" only when combined with a thorough knowledge of trauma pathophysiology and strong assessment and intervention skills. A prehospital practitioner caring for a trauma patient should immediately question a pulse oximeter that does not appear to be functioning on an extremity and consider if the issue is the oximeter or poor tissue perfusion (shock).

Capnography

Capnography, or end-tidal carbon dioxide ($ETCO_2$) monitoring, has been used in critical care units for many years and is commonly employed in most EMS programs.

Detecting CO_2 in expired air confirms that the patient has an active metabolism that is able to generate CO_2 as a byproduct of that metabolism. In addition, the presence of CO_2 in expired air confirms that there is sufficient ongoing circulation to bring CO_2 to the lungs and that effective alveolar ventilation and air exchange are taking place (**Figure 7-25**).

$ETCO_2$ can be measured in the context of a tight airway seal when the patient is intubated or when a supraglottic airway adjunct is employed. In that case, the waveform capnography display will show a precise curve (**Figure 7-26A**).

On the other hand, if it is measured in a spontaneously breathing patient without a tight contact to the airway (i.e., nasal capnography), the curve will be less precise (**Figure 7-26B**). Nonetheless, nasal capnography can provide an approximation of perfusion and ventilatory effectiveness. In addition, it provides a tool to assist with monitoring respiratory rate.

Recent advances in technology have allowed smaller, more durable units to be produced for prehospital use. Capnography measures the *fraction* of carbon dioxide (PCO_2) in a sample of gas, with the machine converting this fraction (%) to partial pressure of CO_2 (in millimeters of mercury [mm Hg]). If this sample is taken at the end of exhalation ($ETCO_2$) in a patient with good peripheral

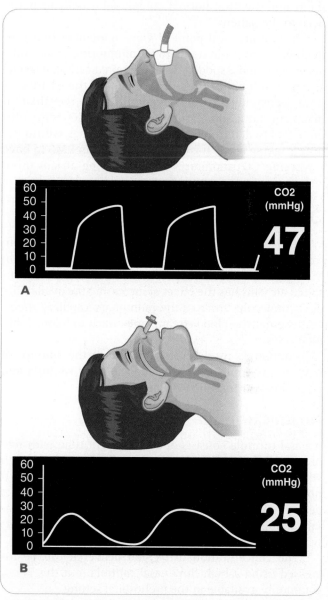

Figure 7-26 **A.** When capnography is used with a tight seal to the airway (as in intubated patients), you obtain a precise curve with four phases. **B.** When used with a nasal cannula during spontaneous ventilation, the CO_2 is diluted, so the curve is rounded. However, the shape of the curve can confirm that air exchange is taking place and provide an estimation of the ventilatory rate. In addition, if the baseline is not down to zero, this can indicate that oxygen flow is insufficient and rebreathing is occurring.

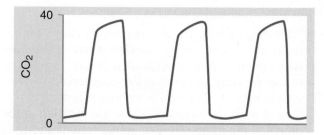

Figure 7-25 Normal end-tidal capnography waveform.

© National Association of Emergency Medical Technicians (NAEMT)

perfusion, it correlates closely to arterial PCO_2 ($PaCO_2$). However, in the multiple trauma patient with compromised perfusion, the correlation of $ETCO_2$ to arterial $PaCO_2$ is much less reliable.[36,37]

In the critical patient, the $PaCO_2$ is generally 2 to 5 mm Hg higher than the $ETCO_2$. (A normal $ETCO_2$ reading is 30 to 40 mm Hg.) Although these readings may not totally reflect the patient's $PaCO_2$, working to maintain the readings within normal ranges will usually be beneficial to the patient.

From a practical point of view, remember that capnography is the gold standard for monitoring proper tube placement, and a sudden drop in expired carbon dioxide, as may result either from dislodgment of the ET tube or from decreased perfusion, should prompt a reevaluation of patient status and ET tube position.[48] $ETCO_2$ is the ultimate tool to determine whether air exchange within the lung is taking place. It is standard practice in EMS to have a working CO_2 monitor when employing an advanced airway management technique.

Optimizing Oxygenation

Whenever the lung is not getting enough oxygen from room air, one method to increase oxygen pressure in the lung is to increase the fraction of oxygen in the inspired air. This has the effect of increasing the availability of O_2 molecules to cross the pulmonary capillary membrane, enter the blood stream, and attach to hemoglobin molecules.

Commonly used devices to increase the amount of oxygen a patient inhales include the nasal cannula and nonrebreather mask (NRB).

Nasal Cannula

A nasal cannula consists of a lightweight tube with two prongs that are placed into the nostrils and through which a mixture of air and supplemental oxygen flows. It normally delivers O_2 flow rates ranging from 2 to 6 liters per minute, which provides a maximum FiO_2 of 0.4. Nasal capnography is potentially of less benefit in patients who breathe through their mouths.

The concentration of oxygen delivered can be increased using a high-flow nasal cannula, but this is not commonly available in the prehospital setting.

Nonrebreather Mask

The NRB consists of a face mask completely covering the nose and mouth connected to an oxygen source. It can be fitted with a variety of adaptors (e.g., Venturi adaptor) that allow it to deliver a more precise fraction of oxygen.

The NRB can also be used with a reservoir. In this case, the mask is connected to a plastic reservoir bag filled with a high concentration of oxygen, with a one-way valve that prevents exhaled air from reentering the oxygen reservoir. The nonrebreather mask itself is fitted with valves preventing expired air from reentering the mask. It is important to ensure that the reservoir bag is always filled with oxygen or the patient will not be able to inhale a full volume of air; this can result in increased respiratory difficulty, and often the patient will attempt to remove the mask to breathe more easily. Studies suggest that while the NRB is better tolerated than assisted ventilation in conscious patients, it is less effective in improving oxygenation.[49]

Optimizing Ventilation

The goal of supplemental oxygen is to increase the fraction of O_2 inside the lung to improve alveolar oxygenation and to increase SpO_2. However, in the context of insufficient ventilation, CO_2 will continue to accumulate. As a result, $PaCO_2$ will increase, and so will the respiratory rate. This increase in respiratory rate is a sign that overall ventilatory function is inadequate, even in the context of an improved PaO_2.

In cases of severe hypoventilation, insufficient air exchange occurs to maintain alveolar ventilation, and oxygenation starts to decrease even in the context of 100% inspired oxygen. It is not possible to compensate adequately if the inspired oxygen does not sufficiently traverse the dead space to the alveoli. Decreasing SpO_2 in a patient receiving an FiO_2 of 100% with an increasing ventilatory rate is a warning of impending ventilatory collapse. Similarly, if the respiratory rate is too low (less than 10 breaths/minute) to provide sufficient minute ventilation, it is necessary to increase the tidal volume to get oxygen to the alveoli. This requires either actively assisting ventilations or completely converting to positive-pressure ventilation.

Checking tidal volume is an important part of evaluating ventilations. Normal breathing has an unremarkable appearance. Patients breathing normally are generally able to speak in full sentences; in patients unable to speak in complete sentences or for whom breathing appears labored, evaluating chest expansion is important.

You can partially correct ventilation with the following:

- *Optimizing position.* The sitting position allows for optimal use of respiratory muscles—there is a reason why athletes sit up to catch their breath. Sitting can reduce pressure on the diaphragm, especially in overweight patients. Use of this technique is of relatively limited utility in trauma, because hypotension or the potential for thoracolumbar spinal trauma limits its applicability. However, placement of the patient in

reverse Trendelenburg position may often offload the diaphragm and improve respiratory excursion
- *Recognizing and sealing an open pneumothorax.* (See Chapter 10, *Thoracic Trauma*.)
- *Treating a tension pneumothorax.* This is a key intervention to relieve the pressure that blocks pulmonary expansion. (See Chapter 10, *Thoracic Trauma*.)

If the tidal volume is still insufficient, ventilatory assistance becomes necessary.

Assisted Ventilation

As opposed to ventilating a cardiac arrest patient who is completely apneic, trauma patients often continue to attempt to breathe even when the breathing efforts are ineffective because of chest or brain injury. Complete control of ventilation typically can only be achieved in sedated patients or patients with profound brain injury. In most cases, assisting ventilations for a patient whose breathing is inadequate is necessary, and this task can be challenging (**Figure 7-27**). During normal inspiration, chest expansion lowers the pressure inside the chest below atmospheric pressure, creating a pressure gradient that draws air into the airway. With assisted ventilation, in the context of good timing, the pressure created by squeezing the bag is added to the negative pressure gradient created by the patient's inspiratory attempt to result in sufficient cumulative pressure to inflate the lung.

However, if your timing is not accurate and the pressure delivered by squeezing the bag is applied against the gradient associated with the patient's attempts to exhale, the lungs will fail to inflate, air exchange will not occur in the alveoli, and air will be forced into the esophagus and the stomach, leading to regurgitation and vomiting and potentially aspiration.

Therefore, timing and coordination are important factors in successfully assisting ventilations.

Bag-Mask Ventilation

The first-line intervention to optimize ventilation in the prehospital setting after (or in conjunction with the three techniques described earlier) is the bag-mask device.

The bag-mask device consists of a self-inflating bag and a nonrebreathing valve; it can be used with a simple face mask with an OPA or NPA, or the bag and valve can be detached from the mask and used with more advanced (LMA, endotracheal, nasotracheal) airway devices. Most bag-mask devices have a volume of 1,600 mL and can deliver an oxygen concentration of 90% to 100%. Some models also have a built-in colorimetric carbon dioxide detector, or these detectors may be added between the mask and the valve or the tube and the valve. However, a single prehospital care practitioner attempting to

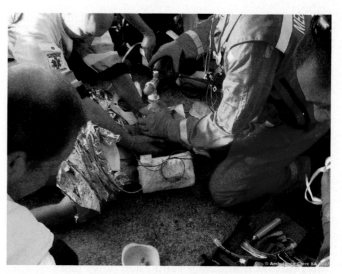

Figure 7-27 The task of assisting ventilations in a trauma patient who is breathing inadequately can be challenging. The rescuer must focus on simultaneously maintaining an adequate seal and squeezing the bag to coincide with the patient's respiratory cycle to avoid forcing air into the esophagus and increasing risk of aspiration. Ongoing practice of the skill is necessary to ensure that patients receive effective ventilatory support.
Courtesy of J.C. Pitteloud MD, Switzerland.

ventilate a patient while maintaining a sufficient mask seal on a noninvasive mask is rarely, if ever, able to provide effective ventilation.[50] Ongoing practice of this skill is necessary to ensure that the technique is effective and that the patient receives appropriate ventilatory support.

Controlled ventilation is typically necessary in a sedated or anesthetized patient who lacks spontaneous respiratory efforts. Studies have shown that the most frequent error made by prehospital practitioners is hyperventilating these patients, both by using excessive tidal volumes and by employing high ventilatory rates, leading to hypocapnia, decreased venous return, elevated mean airway pressures, and potentially gastric inflation if the patient is not intubated.

Those responsible for providing bag-mask ventilation should be carefully trained. Inflation volume should be just enough to obtain a visible chest rise, and the ventilatory rate and $ETCO_2$ should be carefully monitored.

The rate should be 10–12 breaths per minute in the adult, 25 breaths per minute in children, and 30 breaths per minute for infants.

Positive-Pressure Ventilators

Positive-pressure volume ventilators during prolonged transport have long been used in the prehospital and aeromedical environments. In most civilian settings involving short transport times, simple, relatively inexpensive volume ventilators are used. These ventilators do not need to be as sophisticated as those used in the hospital and only have a few simple modes of ventilation, as described in the following sections.

Assist Control Ventilation

Assist control (A/C) ventilation is probably the most widely used mode of ventilation in prehospital transport from the scene to the ED. The A/C setting delivers ventilations at a preset rate and tidal volume. If patients initiate a breath on their own, an additional ventilation of the full tidal volume is delivered, which may lead to breath-stacking and overinflation of the lungs.

Intermittent Mandatory Ventilation

Intermittent mandatory ventilation (IMV) delivers a set rate and tidal volume to patients. If patients initiate their own breath, only the amount that they pull on their own will be delivered.

Positive End-Expiratory Pressure

Positive end-expiratory pressure (PEEP) provides an elevated level of pressure at the end of expiration, thereby decreasing alveolar collapse at the end of the expiratory cycle. This intervention promotes improved oxygenation. However, by increasing the end-expiratory pressure and, therefore, the overall intrathoracic pressure, very high levels of PEEP may decrease blood return to the heart. In patients who are hypovolemic due to blood loss, high levels of PEEP may further decrease blood pressure. High PEEP levels should also be avoided in patients with TBIs. The increase in thoracic pressure can cause an elevation in intracranial pressure. Conversely, patients with TBI are also particularly sensitive to hypoxia, and judicious use of PEEP in these patients can be beneficial.

Initial Settings for Mechanical Ventilations

RATE

The rate is set initially at between 10 and 12 breaths/minute in nonbreathing adult patients. Patients should be closely monitored to ensure that $ETCO_2$ levels are within normal limits.

TIDAL VOLUME

The tidal volume should be set using 5 to 7 mL/kg of the patient's ideal body weight. Idealized body weight is calculated by patient sex and height, not body mass. This should be used as a guide and may need to be adjusted in the trauma patient.

PEEP

When employed, PEEP should be set initially at 5 cm H_2O. This setting will maintain what is known as physiologic PEEP, which is the amount of PEEP that is normally present in the airway prior to intubation. Once intubated, this amount of positive pressure is theoretically taken away. Although increased levels of PEEP may be needed as the traumatic insult worsens, this rarely ever takes place in the first few hours following injury. Prehospital care practitioners may encounter patients requiring high levels of PEEP during interhospital transfer calls. The hospital staff prior to the transfer will have established these levels of PEEP. Normal physiologic PEEP values range from 5 to 10 cm H_2O. The more PEEP that is used, the greater the risk of untoward effects. Careful monitoring is necessary if PEEP is increased, as there can be adverse complications, such as the following:

- Decreased blood pressure caused by decreased venous return
- Increased intracranial pressure
- Increased intrathoracic pressure leading to pneumothorax or tension pneumothorax

OXYGEN CONCENTRATION

The oxygen concentration should be set to maintain a saturation of 94% or greater at sea level in trauma patients. It is prudent to start with 100% FiO_2 and decrease to the minimal concentration needed to achieve an SpO_2 between 93% and 98% saturation. It has been increasingly recognized that prolonged hyperoxemia (O_2 saturation 100% and PaO_2 greater than 150 mm Hg) may result in oxidation injuries and should also be avoided.

HIGH-PRESSURE ALARM/POP-OFF

The high-pressure alarm and pressure relief pop-off should be set at no more than 10 cm H_2O above the pressure needed to normally ventilate the patient (peak inspiratory pressure). Care should be taken when setting the alarm above 40 cm H_2O. Levels above this have been shown to produce barotrauma and a higher possibility of a pneumothorax. Should more than 40 cm H_2O be needed to deliver the desired tidal volume, reassessment of the airway and preset tidal volume is warranted. Decreasing the tidal volume and increasing the rate to maintain the same alveolar minute ventilation may be the prudent action in this case.

As with any alarm, if the high-pressure alarm continues to activate for more than a few breaths, the patient should be removed from the ventilator and manually ventilated with a bag-mask device while the ventilator circuit and ET tube are evaluated. The patient should also be reevaluated for a decrease in compliance (moving less air for the same given pressure). This decrease in compliance may be caused by many factors. A common, early cause of decreased compliance in a

Box 7-8 Basic Ventilator Settings

- Tidal volume: 5 to 7 mL/kg of idealized body weight
- Ventilatory rate: 10 to 12 breaths/minute
- FiO_2: 100% initially, then reduce gradually to maintain SpO_2 > 94%
- Peak pressure alarm: 28 cm H_2O
- Low-pressure alarm: 5 cm H_2O below normal peak pressure to have an early warning of circuit disconnection

© National Association of Emergency Medical Technicians (NAEMT)

Box 7-9 Ventilator Troubleshooting: DOPE

- *Check the patient first*. Disconnect the patient from the ventilator and ventilate manually. Then check using the DOPE mnemonic:
  - *Displacement*. Look at the depth of the tube. The distance from teeth arcade should be three times the tube's length.
  - *Obstruction*. Get a suction catheter down the tube all the way in to make sure the tube is neither kinked nor obstructed.
  - *Pneumothorax*. Rule out pneumothorax by auscultating both lung fields.
  - *Equipment*. Ventilate the patient manually while checking the respirator.
- *Remember the old saying*. Most problems involving a $30,000 ventilator can be solved with a $30 bag. Always check the patient first!

© National Association of Emergency Medical Technicians (NAEMT)

trauma patient may be an evolving tension pneumothorax. The tension pneumothorax should be treated with chest decompression as indicated. A patient coughing or "fighting" the ventilator is demonstrating asynchrony with the ventilator and may require additional sedation or modification of the ventilator settings. Other potential problems include displacement or obstruction of the ET tube. In no case should the prehospital care practitioner simply continue to increase the upper pressure limit and alarm. A listing of basic ventilator settings can be found in **Box 7-8**.

LOW-PRESSURE ALARM

The low-pressure alarm alerts prehospital care practitioners if the connection between the patient and the ventilator is disconnected or is losing significant volume through a leak in the ventilator circuit, or if the airway device has become dislodged. In most transport ventilators, this alarm is preset and cannot be adjusted. See **Box 7-9** for ventilator troubleshooting.

The Negative Impact of Positive-Pressure Ventilation

Under physiologic conditions, pressure inside the chest oscillates between negative during inspiration and neutral or slightly positive during expiration. When the patient is intubated and placed on positive-pressure ventilation (with either a bag-valve device or mechanical ventilation), the measured intrathoracic pressure will become markedly positive. It is extremely important for the practitioner to recognize this change, understand its consequences, and to be prepared to respond to the patient's change in physiology. The primary component of venous blood returning to the heart is the negative pressure generated within the chest during the normal inspiratory cycle. Intubation and positive pressure swing this pressure gradient in the opposite direction and can immediately and significantly impact venous return and cardiac

performance. The usual manifestation of this wide swing in thoracic pressure is hypotension accompanying intubation. While having a constant positive pressure in the lungs and in the chest is well tolerated in the healthy, volume-loaded patient, the same may not be true in the setting of trauma. If a trauma patient is hypovolemic from hemorrhagic losses or intravascular volume shifts, the process of intubation can result in profound hypotension. In severe cases the sequence of intubation of the hypovolemic patient may result in hypovolemic cardiac arrest as the negative effects of anesthetic agents utilized for intubation (negative cardiac inotropic effects) are combined with marked decrease in venous return to the heart (preload) (**Figure 7-28**):

- Continuous positive pressure in the chest reduces venous return to the heart. This is particularly problematic in a patient who is also experiencing hypovolemia due to acute blood loss.
- If a pneumothorax is present, adding positive pressure inside the lung markedly increases the risk of increasing the size and severity of the pneumothorax and the potential for developing a tension pneumothorax.
- If a patient who is not intubated attempts to exhale during the delivery of a positive-pressure breath, the pressure inside the airway will rise and the delivered breath will take the path of least resistance and be directed into the stomach.
- There is at least a theoretical risk of air embolism if lung laceration is present, as often occurs with penetrating thoracic trauma.

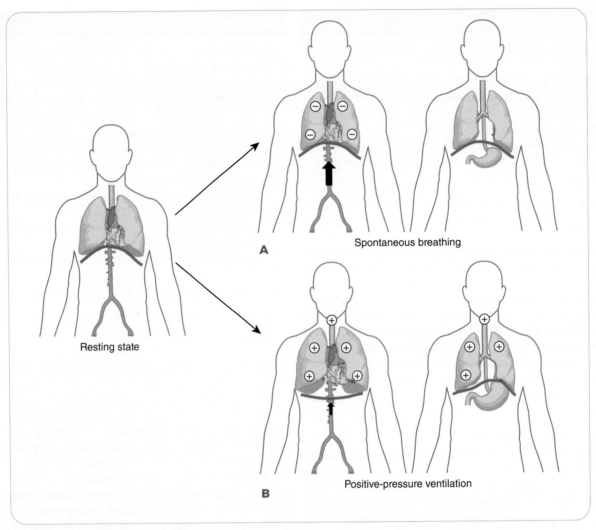

A Spontaneous breathing

Resting state

B Positive-pressure ventilation

Figure 7-28 Physiologic and anatomic responses to negative-pressure versus positive-pressure ventilation. **A.** During normal inspiration, the lowering of the diaphragm and expansion of the rib cage create negative pressure inside the chest, which draws blood from the vena cava to the heart. **B.** When positive-pressure ventilation is applied, positive pressure is created in the chest, decreasing venous return. In addition, air can be forced into the stomach, resulting in overinflation and displacing the diaphragm upward.

© National Association of Emergency Medical Technicians (NAEMT)

Continuous Quality Improvement in Intubation

Because the efficacy of prehospital intubation of trauma patients remains in question, it is important that the administrative oversight of any prehospital system continuously review all out-of-hospital intubations or episodes involving use of an invasive airway technique. This is especially true if medications have been used to facilitate the intubation attempt. Specific points include the following:

- Adherence to protocol and procedures
- Number of intubation attempts
- Confirmation of tube placement and the procedures used for verification
- Outcome and complications
- Proper indications for the use of induction agents if used
- Proper documentation of medication dosage routes and monitoring of the patient during and after intubation
- Vital signs before, during, and after intubation

An effective continuous quality improvement (CQI) program is the means to ensure that the system of care is functioning to provide a safe, effective, and high-value opportunity for the patient. A properly functioning CQI program should not be perceived as a "punishment," but rather as an opportunity for the prehospital care practitioners, administrative managers, and medical director to ensure that the system is functioning to provide an optimal environment for success for the provider and quality care and outcomes for the patient. The foundation of an appropriately functioning CQI program is a standard chart review process combined with an aggressive surveillance program that identifies unanticipated events. Issues identified by the CQI process become the target for future educational initiatives as well as system changes to address identified areas of improvement. Once education and system changes have been completed, the final step of the CQI process is to re-evaluate the problem to see if correction has occurred. The CQI process is a never-ending cycle of identify, analyze, implement, and reanalyze. Appropriately functioning CQI programs have been demonstrated to improve both quality and outcome of patients undergoing intubation.[45] The primary target of the CQI program is the system. Individual action of a provider occurs when educational gaps are identified. Individual disciplinary action arising from the CQI process should be reserved for extremely rare situations where the practitioner *knowingly and intentionally* ignored protocols and procedures, recklessly placing the patient's safety in jeopardy.

Prolonged Transport

Airway management of a patient prior to and during a prolonged transport often requires complex decision making on the part of the prehospital care practitioner. Interventions to control and secure the airway, especially the employment of advanced techniques, requires consideration of numerous factors. These factors include but are not limited to the patient's injuries, the clinical skills of the practitioner, the equipment available, and the distance and transport time to definitive care. Risks and benefits of all the airway options available should be considered prior to making a final airway decision. Transport distance and an anticipated longer transport time lower the threshold for securing the airway prior to transport. For transports of 15 to 20 minutes, essential skills, including an oral airway and bag-mask ventilation, may be sufficient. Use of air medical transport also lowers the threshold to perform ETI, as a cramped, noisy environment makes ongoing airway assessment and management difficult.

Patients requiring airway management or ventilatory support during transport require an elevated level of continuous monitoring during transport. Continuous pulse oximetry monitoring should be used for all trauma patients during transport, and capnography should be considered mandatory for all intubated patients. Loss of $ETCO_2$ indicates that the ventilator circuit has become disconnected, the ET tube has been dislodged, or the patient's perfusion has decreased significantly. All of these possible causes require immediate action.

Vital signs should be monitored on a continuous basis and presented in a graphical fashion to allow the practitioner the opportunity to identify potential issues at an earlier juncture. Confirmation of ETI, as described previously, should be performed each time the patient is moved or repositioned. It is also a good idea to frequently confirm the security of any airway device.

Patients requiring an increasing FiO_2 or PEEP to maintain oxygenation must be carefully reevaluated. Possible etiologies include the development of a pneumothorax or worsening pulmonary function. Any recognized or suspected pneumothorax must be monitored closely for evolution into a tension pneumothorax. Pleural decompression should be performed if hemodynamic compromise occurs that cannot be explained by other causes such as ongoing hemorrhage, hypovolemia, or neurogenic shock. If the patient is receiving positive-pressure ventilation, this process may convert a simple pneumothorax to a tension pneumothorax. If the patient has had an open pneumothorax covered with an occlusive seal, the dressing should be opened intermittently to assure that any potential accumulation of excessive intrathoracic pressure (pneumothorax) is vented to the atmosphere.

Burn patients should receive supplemental oxygen to maintain SpO_2 greater than 94%, whereas those with known or suspected carbon monoxide poisoning should receive 100% oxygen, or be monitored with a pulse oximeter capable of measuring carboxyhemoglobin saturation. (See Chapter 13, *Burn Injuries*, for more information.)

Prior to embarking on a prolonged transport of a patient, potential oxygen needs should be calculated, and sufficient amounts of oxygen should be made available for the transport. The patient should be maintained on the lowest inspired oxygen concentration that assures a saturation > 94%. This strategy is medically optimal and assures oxygen conservation. A good general rule is to bring 50% more oxygen than the anticipated need (**Table 7-5**).

Intubated patients should be sedated for the transport according to local protocols. Ventilator modalities that minimize ventilator–patient dyssynchrony should be sought. Ventilator dyssynchrony occurs when the patient attempts to breathe in a pattern that is not recognized appropriately, or in a timely fashion, by the ventilator. Patients who are said to be "fighting the ventilator" are usually struggling because the ventilator is not providing adequate access to flow and volume from the ventilator

Table 7-5 Oxygen Tank Size and Duration

Flow Rate (L/min)	Tank Size and Duration (hours)				
	D	**E**	**M**	**G**	**H/K**
2	2.5	4.4	24.7	38.2	49.7
5	1	1.8	9.9	15.3	19.9
10	0.5	0.9	4.9	7.6	9.9
15	0.3	0.6	3.3	5.1	6.6

Note: This table shows the approximate duration in hours of various sizes of oxygen tanks and flow rates. The numbers assume that the oxygen tank is completely full at 2,100 pounds per square inch (psi).

© National Association of Emergency Medical Technicians (NAEMT)

as a result of unrecognized triggering cues or tachypnea. Sedation may improve the situation but does not necessarily address the underlying issue. Sedation agents of choice are short acting and readily reversible and include propofol, etomidate, Precedex, and ketamine. The use of neuromuscular blocking agents may be considered if the patient is significantly combative, the airway is secured with an ET tube, and prehospital care personnel are properly trained and credentialed. However, patients should *not* receive neuromuscular blocking agents without proper sedation.

SUMMARY

- The provision of adequate cerebral oxygenation and oxygen delivery at the cellular level of the body as accomplished by adequate airway management and ventilation is among the most important components of prehospital patient care.
- The prehospital practitioner must be able to integrate the principles of ventilation and gas exchange with the pathophysiology of trauma to provide appropriate care of a trauma patient.
- Effective ventilation is defined as total minute ventilation minus dead space ventilation. As effective minute ventilation begins to fall below normal levels, the patient may demonstrate inadequate ventilation, which is termed *hypoventilation.*
- Decreased effective ventilation may be the result of many factors. The most common prehospital factors associated with this condition include mechanical obstruction (usually the tongue), a decreased level of consciousness, or other trauma conditions that compromise the mechanics of effective ventilation (flail chest, open chest wounds, etc.).
- Audible respiratory sounds emanating from the upper airway may indicate partial airway obstruction. Causes of partial airway obstruction include physical obstruction of the airway by the tongue, blood, or foreign bodies in the upper airway. Practitioners must listen and look for signs of obstruction.

- Hypoxemia (decreased oxygen saturation) should be avoided in trauma patients. This is particularly true for patients with traumatic brain injuries. It is important that prehospital care practitioners be alert to any condition that may compromise the oxygenation of a trauma patient. If identified, the practitioner must then decide which method or equipment is appropriate to reverse this condition.
- Categories for airway adjuncts and procedures include the following:
  - *Manual methods* are the simplest and require no additional equipment; they include the trauma chin lift and the trauma jaw thrust.
  - *Simple airway management* involves the use of adjunctive devices that require only one piece of equipment, and the technique for inserting the device necessitates minimal training; they include oropharyngeal and nasopharyngeal airways.
  - *Advanced airways* include supraglottic airway adjuncts; these require additional training but provide the added benefit of more complete control of the oral pharynx.
  - *Definitive airways* include endotracheal tubes and surgical airways. These methods require extensive training and practice, can be time and resource intensive, and have a higher rate of complications. These techniques also provide the most secure airway.
- The decision to perform endotracheal intubation or to use an alternative device should be made

SUMMARY (CONTINUED)

after assessment of the airway has defined the problem. It constitutes a risk–benefit judgment that accounts for factors such as the skill and experience of the provider and transport time to the nearest trauma center.

- End-tidal carbon dioxide ($ETCO_2$) monitoring (capnography) serves as the "gold standard" for confirming ET tube placement. This technique should be used in the prehospital setting whenever available.

- Managing the airway is not without risks. When applying certain skills and modalities, the risk must be weighed against the potential benefit for that patient. What may be the best choice for one patient in a certain situation may not be for another with a similar presentation.
- Sound critical-thinking skills need to be in place to make the best judgments for the trauma patient.

SCENARIO RECAP

You are called to the scene of a motorcycle crash on a busy freeway. As you arrive on scene, you see the patient lying supine about 50 feet (ft; 15 meters [m]) from a heavily damaged motorcycle. The patient is a young male who still has his helmet on. He is not moving, and you see from a distance that he is breathing rapidly. As you approach the patient, you see a pool of blood around his head, and you notice that his breathing is noisy, with snoring and gurgling sounds.

You are 15 minutes from a trauma center, and the dispatch center informs you that the helicopter emergency medical services (HEMS) cannot fly due to bad weather.

What indicators of airway compromise are evident in this patient?

- What other information, if any, would you seek from witnesses or the emergency medical responders?
- What are the important signs and symptoms of compromise of oxygenation and ventilation that should be sought and observed during the initial rapid assessment in the field?
- Describe the sequence of actions you would take to manage this patient before and during transport.

SCENARIO SOLUTION

Bystanders confirm that the patient was alone, and while checking that traffic has been stopped, you observe that the patient is lying 50 ft (15 m) from his destroyed motorcycle, which indicates a significant mechanism of injury. His breathing pattern, as well as the pool of blood around his head, are highly suggestive of an airway problem. Snoring and gurgling sounds confirm your suspicion as you approach the patient.

You and your partner remove the helmet while maintaining cervical spine protection. The snoring sounds disappear once you apply a trauma jaw thrust and suction the airway; still, the breathing remains fast and superficial. Auscultation on both sides is normal, but SpO_2 is 80% so you decide to place supplemental oxygen via a nonrebreather face mask. This maneuver is only partially successful, and saturation improves to the 87% range. Because of concern for a traumatic brain injury, you attempt to achieve an oxygen saturation level of > 94%. The next maneuver is assisted bag-valve mask ventilation timed with the patient's spontaneous breathing. You ensure a secured upper airway through the placement of an oral airway and you and your partner are able to rapidly improve saturations to 96%. Your partner informs you that the pulse is fast and thready. His Glasgow Coma Scale score is 7 without lateralizing signs.

(continues)

SCENARIO SOLUTION (CONTINUED)

Because the HEMS is not available, you immediately prepare for transport to the hospital. Once inside the ambulance you rapidly reassess your options for maintaining the patient's oxygenation and ventilation. With intermittent suctioning and with the oral airway in place the patient appears to have a strong and symmetrical respiratory drive and saturations are maintained above 94%. You ask for additional assistance from your EMS service so that there will be two advanced life support practitioners during transport and your partner stays with you once an ambulance operator is available. You continue to provide assisted ventilation enroute via a bag-valve mask while your partner establishes an IV line and connects the patient to a monitor. The vital signs read SpO$_2$ 95%, heart rate 100 beats/minute, and blood pressure 110/60 mm Hg as you hand over the patient to the trauma team 15 minutes later.

References

1. Vanderlan WB, Tew BE, McSwain NE. Increased risk of death with cervical spine immobilisation in penetrating cervical trauma. *Injury.* 2009;40:880-883.

2. Barkana Y, Stein M, Scope A, et al. Prehospital stabilization of the cervical spine for penetrating injuries of the neck—is it necessary? *Injury.* 2000;31:305-309.

3. Brown JB, Bankey PE, Sangosanya AT, Cheng JD, Stassen NA, Gestring ML. Prehospital spinal immobilization does not appear to be beneficial and may complicate care following gunshot injury to the torso. *J Trauma.* 2009;67:774-778.

4. Roberts K, Whalley H, Bleetman A. The nasopharyngeal airway: dispelling myths and establishing the facts. *Emerg Med J.* 2005;22:394-396.

5. Liti A, Giusti GD, Gili A, et al. Insertion of four different types of supraglottic airway devices by emergency nurses: a mannequin-based simulation study. *Acta Biomed.* 2020 Nov 30;91(12-S):e2020016. doi: 10.23750/abm.v91i12-S.10832

6. Ruetzler K, Roessler B, Potura L, et al. Performance and skill retention of intubation by paramedics using seven different airway devices: a manikin study. *Resuscitation.* 2011 May;82(5):593-597. doi: 10.1016/j.resuscitation.2011.01.00

7. Kleine-Brueggeney M, Gottfried A, Nabecker S, Greif R, Book M, Theiler L. Pediatric supraglottic airway devices in clinical practice: a prospective observational study. *BMC Anesthesiol.* 2017 Sep 2;17(1):119. doi: 10.1186/s12871-017-0403-6

8. Carney N, Cheney T, Totten AM, et al. *Prehospital Airway Management: A Systematic Review* [Internet]. Report No.: 21-EHC023. Agency for Healthcare Research and Quality; 2021. Accessed April 22, 2022. https://www.ncbi.nlm.nih.gov/books/NBK571440/

9. Mort TC. The incidence and risk factors for cardiac arrest during emergency tracheal intubation: a justification for incorporating the ASA Guidelines in the remote location. *J Clin Anesth.* 2004 Nov;16(7):508-516. doi: 10.1016/j.jclinane.2004.01.007

10. Stockinger ZT, McSwain NE Jr. Prehospital endotracheal intubation for trauma does not improve survival over bag-mask ventilation. *J Trauma.* 2004;56(3):531-536.

11. Davis DP, Koprowicz KM, Newgard CD, et al. The relationship between out-of-hospital airway management and outcome among trauma patients with Glasgow Coma Scale scores of 8 or less. *Prehosp Emerg Care.* 2011;15(2):184-192.

12. Gravesteijn BY, Sewalt CA, Stocchetti N, et al; CENTER-TBI collaborators. Prehospital management of traumatic brain injury across Europe: a CENTER-TBI study. *Prehosp Emerg Care.* 2021;25(5):629-643. Epub 2020 Oct 1. doi: 10.1080/10903127.2020.1817210

13. Brown CVR, Inaba K, Shatz DV, et al. Western Trauma Association critical decisions in trauma: airway management in adult trauma patient. *Trauma Surg Acute Care Open.* 2020;5:e000539.

14. Davis DP, Olvera DJ. HEAVEN criteria: derivation of a new difficult airway prediction tool. *Air Med J.* 2017;36(4):195-197.

15. American College of Surgeons (ACS) Committee on Trauma. *Advanced Trauma Life Support Course.* ACS; 2018.

16. Sakles JC, Chiu S, Mosier J, Walker C, Stolz U. The importance of first pass success when performing orotracheal intubation in the emergency department. *Acad Emerg Med.* 2013 Jan;20(1):71-78. doi: 10.1111/acem.12055

17. Garza AG, Gratton MC, Coontz D, et al. Effect of paramedic experience on orotracheal intubation success rates. *J Emerg Med.* 2003;25(3):251.

18. Buis ML, Maissan IM, Hoeks SE, Klimek M, Stolker RJ. Defining the learning curve for endotracheal intubation using direct laryngoscopy: a systematic review. *Resuscitation.* February 2016;99:63-71.

19. Warner KJ, Sharar SR, Copass MK, Bulger EM. Prehospital management of a difficult airway: a prospective cohort study. *J Emerg Med.* 2008;36(3):257-265.

20. Dunford JV, Davis DP, Ochs M, Doney M, Hoyt DB. Incidence of transient hypoxia and pulse rate reactivity during paramedic rapid sequence intubation. *Ann Emerg Med.* 2003 Dec;42(6):721-728. doi: 10.1016/s0196-0644(03)00660-7

21. Walls RM, Brown CA, Bair AE, Pallin DJ. Emergency airway management: a multi-center report of 8937 emergency department intubations. *J Emerg Med.* 2011;41(4):347-354.

22. Aziz S, Foster E, Lockey DJ, Christian MD. Emergency scalpel cricothyroidotomy use in a prehospital trauma service: a 20-year review. *Emerg Med J.* 2021 May;38(5):349-354. doi: 10.1136/emermed-2020-210305

23. Weitzel N, Kendall J, Pons P. Blind nasotracheal intubation for patients with penetrating neck trauma. *J Trauma.* 2004 May;56(5):1097-1101. doi: 10.1097/01.ta.0000071294.21893.a4

24. O'Brien DJ, Danzl DF, Hooker EA, Daniel LM, Dolan MC. Prehospital blind nasotracheal intubation by paramedics. *Ann Emerg Med.* 1989 Jun;18(6):612-617. doi: 10.1016/s0196-0644(89)80512-8

25. Marlow TJ, Goltra DD Jr, Schabel SI. Intracranial placement of a nasotracheal tube after facial fracture: a rare complication. *J Emerg Med.* 1997;15(2):187-191. doi: 10.1016/s0736-4679(96)00356-3

26. Tentillier E, Heydenreich C, Cros AM, Schmitt V, Dindart JM, Thicoïpé M. Use of the intubating laryngeal mask airway in emergency pre-hospital difficult intubation. *Resuscitation.* 2008 Apr;77(1):30-34.

27. Theiler L, Hermann K, Schoettker P, et al. SWIVIT—Swiss video-intubation trial evaluating video-laryngoscopes in a simulated difficult airway scenario: study protocol for a multicenter prospective randomized controlled trial in Switzerland. *Trials.* 2013 Apr 4;14:94. doi:10.1186/1745-6215-14-94

28. Nabecker S, Greif R, Kotarlic M, Kleine-Brueggeney M, Riggenbach C, Theiler L. Outdoor performance of different videolaryngoscopes on a glacier: a manikin study. *Emergencias* [Spanish]. 2016;28(4):216-222.

29. Driver BE, Prekker ME, Reardon RF, et al. Success and complications of the ketamine-only intubation method in the emergency department. *J Emerg Med.* 2021 Mar;60(3):265-272. doi: 10.1016/j.jemermed.2020.10.042

30. Wang HE, Davis DP, O'Connor RE, et al. Drug-assisted intubation in the prehospital setting. *Prehosp Emerg Care.* 2006;10(2):261-271.

31. Davis DP, Hoyt DB, Ochs M, et al. The effect of paramedic rapid sequence intubation on an outcome in patients with severe trauma brain injury. *J Trauma.* 2003;54:444-453.

32. Bernard SA, Nguyen V, Cameron P, et al. Prehospital rapid sequence intubation improves functional outcome for patients with severe traumatic brain injury: a randomized controlled trial. *Ann Surg.* 2010;252(6):959-965.

33. Galbiati G, Paola C. Effects of open and closed endotracheal suctioning on intracranial pressure and cerebral perfusion pressure in adult patients with severe brain injury: a literature review. *J Neurosci Nurs.* 2015 Aug;47(4):239-46. doi: 10.1097/JNN.0000000000000146.

34. Weingart SD, Trueger NS, Wong N, Scofi J, Singh N, Rudolph SS. Delayed sequence intubation: a prospective observational study. *Ann Emerg Med.* 2015 Apr;65(4):349-355. doi: 10.1016/j.annemergmed.2014.09.025

35. Smith KJ, Dobranowski J, Yip G, Dauphin A, Choi PT. Cricoid pressure displaces the esophagus: an observational study using magnetic resonance imaging. *Anesthesiology.* 2003;99(1):60-64.

36. Werner SL, Smith CE, Goldstein JR, Jones RA, Cydulka RK. Pilot study to evaluate the accuracy of ultrasonography in confirming endotracheal tube placement. *Ann Emerg Med.* 2007;49(1):75-80.

37. Butler J, Sen A. Best evidence topic report: cricoid pressure in emergency rapid sequence induction. *Emerg Med J.* 2005;22(11):815-816.

38. O'Connor RE, Swor RA. Verification of endotracheal tube placement following intubation. *Prehosp Emerg Care.* 1999;3:248-250.

39. Weingart SD, Levitan RM. Preoxygenation and prevention of desaturation during emergency airway management. *Ann Emerg Med.* 2012;59(3):165-175.

40. Jeremitsky E, Omert L, Dunham CM, Protetch J, Rodriguez A. Harbingers of poor outcome the day after severe brain injury: hypothermia, hypoxia, and hypoperfusion. *J Trauma.* 2003;54:312–319.

41. Davis DP, Hwang JQ, Dunford JV. Rate of decline in oxygen saturation at various pulse oximetry values with prehospital rapid sequence intubation. *Prehosp Emerg Care.* 2008 Jan–Mar;12(1):46-51. doi: 10.1080/10903120701710470

42. Davis DP, Aguilar S, Sonnleitner C, Cohen M, Jennings M. Latency and loss of pulse oximetry signal with the use of digital probes during prehospital rapid-sequence intubation. *Prehosp Emerg Care.* 2011;15(1):18-22.

43. Cemalovic N, Scoccimarro A, Arslan A, Fraser R, Kanter M, Caputo N. Human factors in the emergency department: is physician perception of time to intubation and desaturation rate accurate? *Emerg Med Australas.* 2016 Jun;28(3):295-299. doi: 10.1111/1742-6723.12575

44. Jensen M, Barmaan B, Orndahl CM, Louka A. Impact of suction-assisted laryngoscopy and airway decontamination technique on intubation quality metrics in a helicopter emergency medical service: an educational intervention. *Air Med J.* 2020 Mar-Apr;39(2):107-110. doi: 10.1016/j.amj.2019.10.005

45. Jarvis JL, Gonzales J, Johns D, Sager L. Implementation of a clinical bundle to reduce out-of-hospital peri-intubation hypoxia. *Ann Emerg Med.* 2018 Sep;72(3):272-279.e1. doi: 10.1016/j.annemergmed.2018.01.044

46. Kupas DF, Kauffman KF, Wang HE. Effect of airway-securing method on prehospital endotracheal tube dislodgment. *Prehosp Emerg Care.* 2020;14(1):26-30. doi: 10.3109/10903120903144932

47. Moroco AE, Armen SB, Goldenberg D. Emergency cricothyrotomy: a 10-year single institution experience. *Am Surg.* 2021 Feb 10:3134821995075. doi: 10.1177/0003134821995075

48. Mabry RL, Frankfurt A. An analysis of battlefield cricothyrotomy in Iraq and Afghanistan. *J Spec Oper Med.* 2012;12(1):17-23.

49. Warner KJ, Cuschieri J, Garland B, et al. The utility of early end-tidal capnography in monitoring ventilation status after severe injury. *J Trauma.* 2009;66:26-31.

50. Groombridge CJ, Ley E, Miller M, Konig T. A prospective, randomised trial of pre-oxygenation strategies available in the pre-hospital environment. *Anaesthesia.* 2017 May;72(5):580-584. doi: 10.1111/anae.13852. Epub 2017 Mar 14.

51. Johannigman JA, Branson RD, Davis K Jr, Hurst JM. Techniques of emergency ventilation: a model to evaluate tidal volume, airway pressure, and gastric insufflation. *J Trauma.* 1991 Jan;31(1):93-8.

Specific Airway Management Techniques

Trauma Jaw Thrust

Principle: To open the airway without moving the cervical spine.

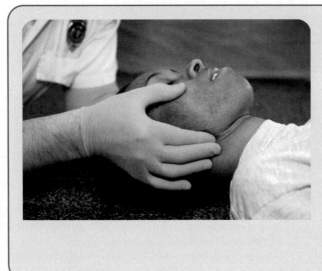

1 In both the trauma jaw thrust and the trauma chin lift, manual neutral in-line stabilization of the head and neck is maintained while the mandible is moved anteriorly (forward). This maneuver moves the tongue forward, away from the hypopharynx while holding the mouth slightly open.

From a position above the patient's head, the prehospital care practitioner positions the hands on either side of the patient's head, fingers pointing **caudad** (toward the patient's feet) and the thumb on the cheekbone. Gentle pressure is applied with the ring finger to lift the mandible upward while the thumbs rest on the cheekbones. The palms of the hands stabilize the head in the process.

© National Association of Emergency Medical Technicians (NAEMT)

Alternate Trauma Jaw Thrust

Principle: To open the airway from the front without moving the cervical spine.

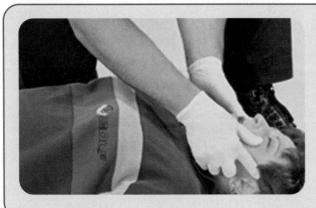

1 The trauma jaw thrust can also be performed while the practitioner is positioned beside the patient, facing the patient's head. The thumbs rest on the cheekbones, while the index finger is "hooked" behind the angle of the mandible to move it forward. Having the forearms resting on the patient's clavicles provides additional stability. Gentle equal pressure is applied with the ring finger to lift the mandible, while the thumb presses on the cheekbone and the other fingers help to stabilize the mandible. The practitioner then checks for air entry and chest movement.

© National Association of Emergency Medical Technicians (NAEMT)

Trauma Chin Lift

Principle: To open the airway without moving the cervical spine.

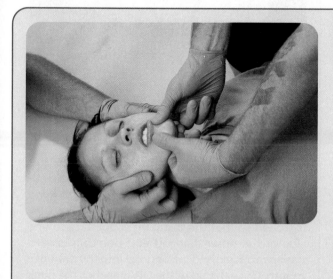

1 From a position above the patient's head, the patient's head and neck are moved into a neutral in-line position, and manual stabilization is maintained. The first practitioner is at the head, while the second practitioner is kneeling in front of the patient. While a first practitioner stabilizes the patient's head, the second practitioner grabs the patient's chin with both hands, with the index fingers hooked under the patient's chin and the thumbs on the patient's chin. The practitioner then opens the patient's mouth and pulls the mandible forward. For this move to be successful, it is necessary to open the patient's mouth first.

This technique avoids insertion of the thumb into the patient's mouth, which can be dangerous should the patient bite down or have a seizure.

© Jones & Bartlett Learning. Photographed by Darren Stahlman.

Oropharyngeal Airway

Principle: An adjunct used to maintain an open airway mechanically in a patient without a gag reflex.

The oropharyngeal airway (OPA) is designed to hold the back of patient's tongue anteriorly out of the pharynx. The OPA is available in various sizes. Proper sizing to the patient is required to ensure a patent airway. Placement of an OPA in the hypopharynx is *contraindicated* in patients who have an intact gag reflex. Two methods for insertion of the OPA are effective: the tongue jaw lift insertion method and the tongue blade insertion method. Regardless of which method is used, the first prehospital care practitioner stabilizes the patient's head and neck in a neutral in-line position, while the second practitioner measures and inserts the OPA.

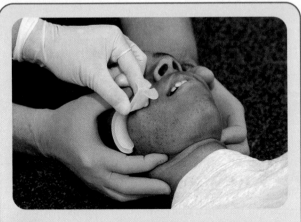

1 The first practitioner brings the patient's head and neck into a neutral in-line position and maintains stabilization while opening the patient's airway with a trauma jaw thrust maneuver. The second practitioner selects and measures for a properly sized OPA. The distance from the corner of the patient's mouth to the earlobe is a good estimate for proper size.

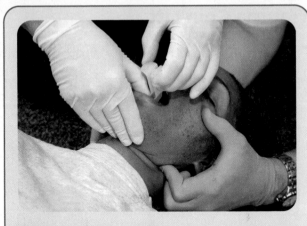

2 While the second practitioner stabilizes the head from the front, the first practitioner opens the patient's mouth with the left hand and introduces the OPA. The OPA is turned so that the distal tip is pointing to one side or the other (flanged end pointing toward patient's cheek) and introduced into the patient's mouth. Once the tip of the OPA reaches the back of the throat, it is rotated to fit the contours of the patient's anatomy.

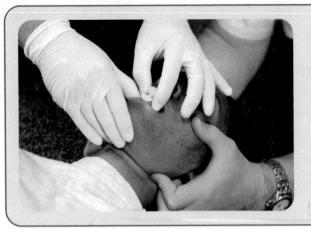

3 The OPA is rotated until the inside curve is resting against the tongue, holding it out of the posterior pharynx. The flanges of the OPA should be resting against the outside surface of the patient's teeth. Air entry and chest movements are checked.

Oropharyngeal Airway: Tongue Blade Insertion Method

The tongue blade insertion method is probably a safer method than the tongue jaw lift because it allows the practitioner to check with the tongue blade if some degree of gag reflex is still present. It also carries less risk of dislodging loose teeth in the case of facial trauma. It is the recommended technique in pediatric patients because the tip of a rotating cannula can injure the soft palate.

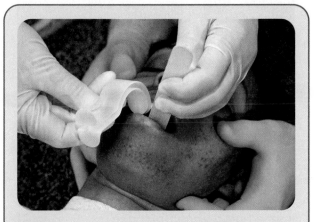

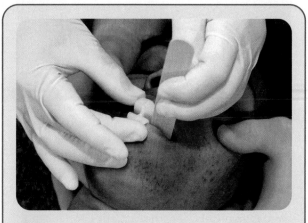

1 The first practitioner brings the patient's head and neck into a neutral in-line position and maintains stabilization while opening the patient's airway with the trauma jaw thrust maneuver. The second practitioner selects and measures for a properly sized OPA. The second practitioner pulls the patient's mouth open by the chin and places a tongue blade into the patient's mouth to move the tongue forward in place. At the same time, the second practitioner checks for any protective reflex or loose structure.

2 The device is inserted with the flanged end pointing toward the patient's feet and the distal tip pointing into the patient's mouth, following the curvature of the airway. The OPA is advanced until the flanged end of the OPA rests against the outside surface of the patient's teeth. Check air entry and chest movements to assess the effectiveness of your intervention.

© National Association of Emergency Medical Technicians (NAEMT)

Nasopharyngeal Airway

Principle: An adjunct used to maintain an open airway mechanically in a patient with or without a gag reflex or in a patient with clenched teeth.

The nasopharyngeal airway (NPA) is a simple airway adjunct that provides an effective way to maintain a patent airway in patients who may still have an intact gag reflex. Most patients will tolerate the NPA if properly sized. NPAs are available in a range of diameters (internal diameters of 5 to 9 mm), and the length varies appropriately with the size of the diameter. NPAs are usually made of a flexible, rubberlike material.

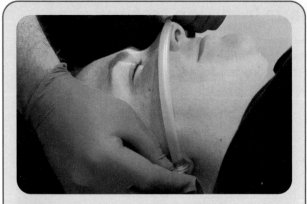

1 The practitioner who will be inserting the NPA selects the appropriately sized device for the patient's nostril, a size slightly smaller in diameter than the size of the nostril opening (frequently the diameter of the patient's little finger). The length of the NPA is important. The NPA needs to be long enough to supply an air passage between the patient's tongue and the posterior pharynx. The distance from the patient's nose to the earlobe is a good estimate for proper size. (*Note:* The NPA must not be stretched out when measuring this distance.)

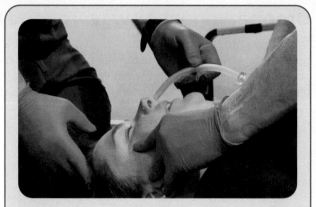

2 The first practitioner brings the patient's head and neck into a neutral in-line position and maintains stabilization while opening the patient's airway with the trauma jaw thrust maneuver. A second lubricates the distal tip (nonflanged end) and the outside of the NPA with a water-soluble jelly. The NPA is then slowly inserted into the nostril of choice. Insertion should be in an anterior-to-posterior direction along the floor of the nasal cavity, not in a superior-to-inferior direction. The NPA is advanced along the soft palate. If resistance is met at the posterior end of the nostril, a gentle back-and-forth rotation of the NPA between the fingers will usually aid in passing it beyond the turbinate bones of the nasal cavity without damage. Should the NPA continue to meet with resistance, the NPA should not be forced past the obstruction, but rather withdrawn, and the distal tip should be relubricated and inserted into the other nostril.

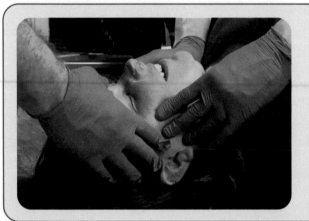

3 The second practitioner continues insertion until the flange end of the NPA is next to the anterior nares or until the patient gags. If the patient gags or coughs, it can be a sign that the end of the NPA tube is in contact with the upper part of the larynx and must be withdrawn slightly. Again, check air entry and chest movements to assess the effectiveness of your intervention.

Bag-Mask Ventilation

Ventilation using a bag-mask device has an advantage over other ventilatory support systems because it gives a prehospital care practitioner feedback from the feel of the bag (compliance). Positive feedback ensures the operator of successful ventilations; changes in the feedback indicate a loss of mask seal, the presence of an obstructed airway, or a thoracic problem interfering with the delivery of successful ventilations. This "feel" and the control it provides also make the bag-mask device suitable for assisting ventilations. The bag-mask device's portability and readiness for immediate use make it useful for immediate delivery of ventilations when needed.

Without supplemental oxygen, however, a bag-mask device provides an oxygen concentration of only 21%, or a fraction of inspired oxygen (FiO_2) of 0.21; as soon as time allows, an oxygen reservoir and high-concentration supplemental oxygen should be connected to the bag-mask. When oxygen is connected without a reservoir, the FiO_2 is limited to 0.50 or less; with a reservoir, the FiO_2 is 0.85 or greater.

If the patient being ventilated is unconscious without a gag reflex, a properly sized OPA should be inserted before attempting to ventilate with the bag-mask device. If the patient has an intact gag reflex, a properly sized NPA should be inserted before attempting to assist ventilations. Various bag-mask devices are available, including disposable single-patient-use models that are relatively inexpensive. Different brands have varying bag, valve, and reservoir designs. All of the parts used should be of the same model and brand because these parts are usually not safely interchangeable.

Bag-mask devices are available in adult, pediatric, and neonatal sizes. Although an adult bag can be used with the properly sized pediatric mask in an emergency, use of the correct bag size is recommended as a safe practice. Adequate ventilations of an adult patient are being delivered when normal chest rise is achieved.

When ventilating with any positive-pressure device, inflation should stop once a normal tidal volume has been achieved, that is, when visible chest rise is achieved. When using the bag-mask device, the chest should be visualized and the bag felt to recognize any marked increased resistance in the bag. Adequate time for exhalation is needed (1:3 ratio between time for inhalation and time for exhalation). If enough time is not allowed, "stepped or stacked breaths" occur, providing a greater volume of inspiration than expiration. Stepped breaths produce poor air exchange and result in hyperinflation, increased pressure, opening of the esophagus, and gastric distension. It is very important to pay attention to proper ventilation rate and to allow normal expiration.

Assisting ventilation with a bag-mask device is easier with two or more prehospital care practitioners than with only one practitioner. The first practitioner can focus attention on maintaining an adequate mask seal, while the second provides good delivery volume by using both hands to squeeze (deflate) the bag.

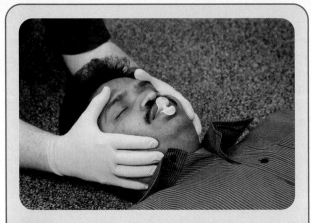

1 The first practitioner kneels above the patient's head and maintains manual stabilization of the patient's head and neck in a neutral in-line position.

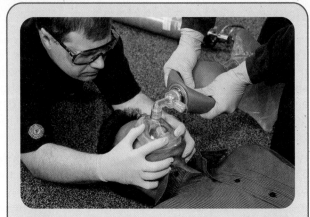

2 The face mask is placed over the patient's nose and mouth, and the mask is held in place with the thumbs on the lateral portion of the mask while pulling the mandible up into the mask. The other fingers provide the manual stabilization and maintain a patent airway. The second practitioner kneels at the side of the patient and squeezes the bag with both hands to inflate the lungs, paying attention to proper ventilatory rate and adequate tidal volume.

© National Association of Emergency Medical Technicians (NAEMT)

Supraglottic Airways

Supraglottic airways should not be used as a first technique to open the airway. The patient should be preoxygenated to a SpO$_2$ of at least 93% (preferably 100%) before insertion of an SGA is attempted. As a rule, an unconscious patient who tolerates an OPA is likely to tolerate an SGA.

Laryngeal Tube Airway

Principle: A blindly inserted double-lumen airway used to provide ventilation of a trauma patient.

The laryngeal tube airway (LTA) is a double-lumen tube with both a distal and oral (proximal) cuff. The second lumen is meant to facilitate the insertion of an aspiration catheter for gastric decompression. It should be noted that the LTA does not provide complete protection from aspiration. In fact, the manufacturer lists lack of fasting as a contraindication to its use, as well as "situations where gastric contents may be present [that] include, but are not limited to . . . multiple or massive injury, acute abdominal or thoracic injury." While these contraindications apply to the OR setting, they should be a reminder that the LTA provides only limited protection from aspiration in an emergency. Therefore, significant care must be taken to avoid aspiration when the LTA is used in these situations.

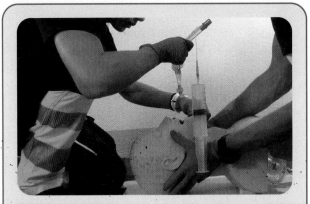

1 The prehospital practitioner chooses the correct LTA size, based on patient height. The cuff-inflation system is tested by injecting the maximum recommended volume of air into the cuff using a large syringe. The second practitioner preoxygenates the patient.

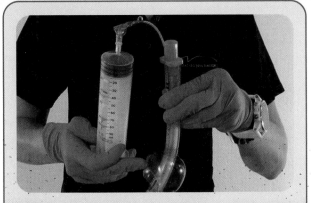

2 The first practitioner applies a water-based lubricant to the beveled distal tip and posterior aspect of the tube and holds the LTA in the dominant hand. With the nondominant hand, the first practitioner opens the patient's mouth using the scissor technique. The second practitioner maintains cervical spine stabilization as necessary.

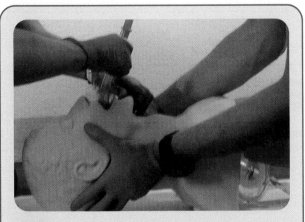

3 The first practitioner introduces the tip into the patient's mouth and advances it behind the base of the tongue.

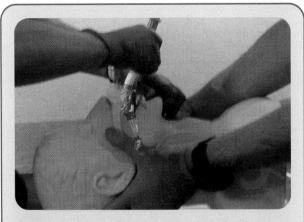

4 The first practitioner advances the LTA until the base of the connector is aligned with the patient's teeth. Reference marks are provided at the proximal end of the LTA, which, when aligned with the upper teeth, give an indication of the depth of insertion.

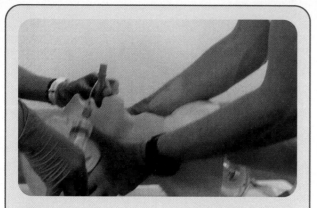

5 The first practitioner inflates the cuff with a large syringe. The required inflation volume is indicated on a color coded syringe, and should allow a tight seal of the airway. The airway opening should face the larynx (white circle), while the distal cuff should rest at the entrance of the esophagus.

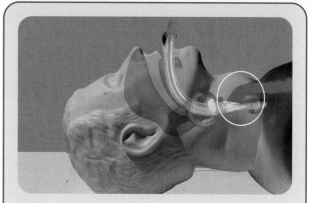

6 The first practitioner attaches a bag-mask device to the LTA. While gently ventilating the patient to assess ventilation, the first practitioner simultaneously withdraws the airway until ventilation is easy and free-flowing (large tidal volume with minimal airway pressure). This image demonstrates ideal final placement of the LTA device with the large balloon inflated in the oropharynx, the small balloon inflated in the esophagus, and the proximal lumen positioned immediately proximal to the esophagus.

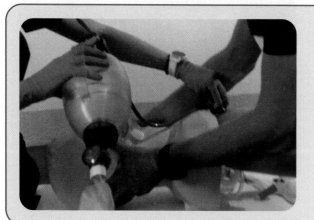

7 The first practitioner confirms proper position by auscultation, chest movement, and verification of carbon dioxide by capnography. The first practitioner readjusts the cuff inflation to 60 cm H_2O (or to seal volume). The first practitioner secures the LTA to the patient using tape or other accepted means. A bite block can also be used, if desired.

Courtesy of J.C. Pitteloud MD, Switzerland.

I-Gel Laryngeal Mask Airway

Principle: A mechanical device used to maintain an open airway without direct visualization of the airway.

The i-gel is an airway device that can be inserted by a prehospital care practitioner without the need for direct visualization of the vocal cords. This blind insertion technique has advantages over endotracheal intubation, as initial training requirements are less and skill retention is easier to accomplish.

The objective of the i-gel is creation of a noninflatable seal of the pharyngeal, laryngeal, and perilaryngeal structures while avoiding compression trauma. A limitation of the i-gel is that although it forms a seal around the glottic opening, this seal is not as occlusive as that of an endotracheal tube cuff. Aspiration remains a potential problem. As with any airway in a trauma patient, cervical stabilization must be maintained for the duration of the procedure.

The i-gel LMA is available in a range of sizes to accommodate both pediatric and adult patient groups.

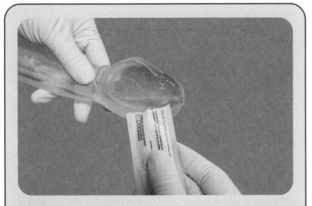

1 The prehospital care practitioner takes out the protective cradle and applies a water-soluble lubricant to the posterior surface. The i-gel is held along the bite block in the dominant hand. A second practitioner stabilizes the head from the front.

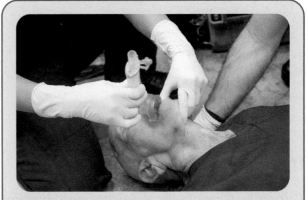

2 The first practitioner at the head gently presses the chin down, then introduces the leading soft tip into the mouth toward the hard palate. Pressing the tip against the hard palate will facilitate rotation downward.

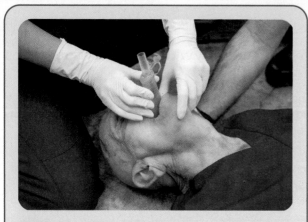

3 The first practitioner continues to advance the i-gel into the hypopharynx until a definite resistance is felt. At this point, the tip is in the upper esophagus and the cuff around the larynx. The incisors should be resting on the bite block.

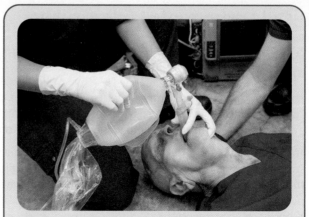

4 The first practitioner attaches a bag-mask device to the i-gel and ventilates the patient while the second practitioner confirms breath sounds. Once confirmed, the second practitioner applies a commercial strap or a tape to fix the device at the desired depth (not shown). A suction catheter can then be measured and introduced in the suction port to decompress the stomach.

© Jones & Bartlett Learning. Photographed by Glen Ellman.

Intubating Laryngeal Mask

Principle: A mechanical device used to maintain an open airway without direct visualization of the airway.

The laryngeal mask is inserted in the usual way. Once normal chest rise shows that the opening is in front of the larynx, and the patient is preoxygenated, the ET tube is introduced into the intubating laryngeal mask (ILMA) and then down into the trachea. Note that the laryngeal mask should be left in place during transport, first, because it provides excellent fixation for the ET tube, and second, because it can be used as a backup should anything go wrong with the ET tube. As with any airway in a trauma patient, cervical stabilization must be maintained for the duration of the procedure (this is not shown on the pictures for the sake of clarity).

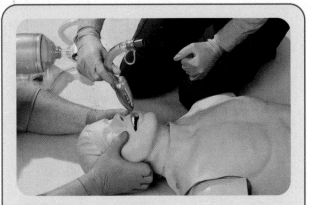

1 The first practitioner deflates the cuff and places water-soluble lubricant on the posterior surface of the ILMA.

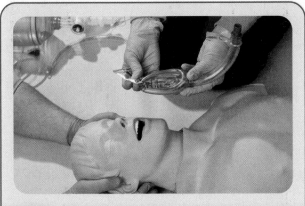

2 The second practitioner stabilizes the patient's head, while the first practitioner holds the ILMA between thumb and index finger, with the connector pointing downward toward the patient's chest and the tip of the distal end toward the hard palate.

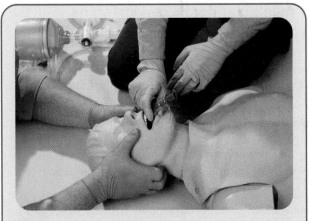

3 The first practitioner introduces the tip into the patient's mouth, and while maintaining pressure, continues to rotate the mask downward in a circular motion, following the contour of the hard palate until a definite resistance is felt.

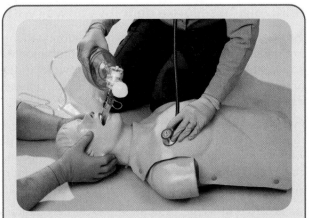

4 The first practitioner attaches a bag-mask device to the LMA and confirms breath sounds while ventilating the patient to ensure the mask is in front of the tracheal opening. Do not proceed to the next step until this is achieved and the patient has been adequately ventilated.

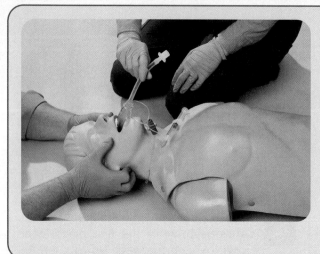

5 The first practitioner introduces the ET tube into the proximal opening of the ILMA. Keep in mind that the opening of the ILMA is at 4 to 5 cm at the teeth. It is necessary to add this distance to the standard insertion depth of the ET tube. The cuff is then inflated by the first practitioner. While the patient is ventilated via the ET tube, breath sounds are auscultated to confirm proper placement.

If the ET tube cannot be inserted or otherwise becomes dislodged, ventilating the patient with the ILMA is still possible. In that situation, tape the ET tube to the ILMA and do not remove the ILMA until at the hospital.

© Jones & Bartlett Learning. Photographed by Darren Stahlman.

Visualized Orotracheal Intubation of the Trauma Patient

Principle: To secure a definitive airway without manipulating the cervical spine.

Visualized orotracheal intubation of a trauma patient is done with the patient's head and neck stabilized in a neutral in-line position. Orotracheal intubation while maintaining manual in-line stabilization requires additional training and practice beyond that for intubation of nontrauma patients. As with all skills, training requires observation, critique, and certification initially and at least twice a year by the medical director or designee.

In hypoxic trauma patients who are not in cardiac arrest, intubation should *never* be the initial airway maneuver. The prehospital care practitioner should perform intubation only after preoxygenating the patient with a high concentration of oxygen using a simple airway adjunct or manual maneuver. The prehospital care practitioner should not interrupt ventilation for more than 20 seconds when intubating the patient. Ventilation should never be interrupted for more than 30 seconds for any reason.

Visualized orotracheal intubation is extremely difficult in conscious patients or patients with an intact gag reflex and, as a rule, should not be attempted. The prehospital care practitioner should consider use of drug-assisted intubation agents after additional training, protocol development, and approval by the EMS medical director.

Because the success rate of intubation is often related to the practitioner's comfort with a given design, the style of blade selection for the laryngoscope remains a matter of individual preference.

Note: The cervical collar will limit forward motion of the mandible and complete opening of the mouth. Therefore, after adequate spinal immobilization is ensured, the cervical collar is removed, manual stabilization of the cervical spine is held, and intubation is attempted. Once intubation is accomplished, the collar is reapplied. Before attempting intubation, the prehospital care practitioners should assemble and test all required equipment and follow standard precautions. The first practitioner kneels at the patient's head and ventilates the patient with a bag-mask device and high-concentration oxygen. As a rule, an SpO_2 of at least 93% should be achieved if possible before any attempt at intubation.

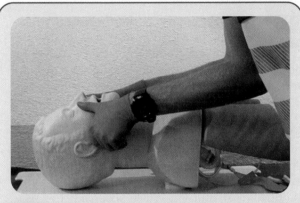

1 The second practitioner, kneeling at the patient's side, provides manual stabilization of the patient's head and neck. The second practitioner holds the head with the thumb resting on the patient's cheekbones and the fingers behind the head. Improper hand positioning can block the mouth opening and make laryngoscopy impossible. After preoxygenation, the first practitioner stops ventilations and grasps the laryngoscope in the left hand and the ET tube (with syringe attached to pilot valve) in the right hand. If a stylet is used, this should have been inserted when the equipment was inspected and tested. The distal end of the stylet should be inserted just short of the ET tube's distal opening.

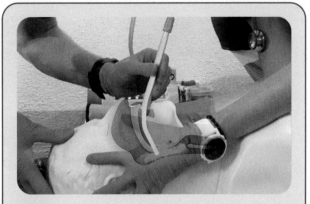

2 An essential difference between prehospital intubation and intubation on a manikin is that suctioning the airway first drastically improves your chances of first-pass success, even more so if you use a video laryngoscope. Use a rigid large-bore catheter and a reverse grip technique to clear the back of the throat, and then leave your catheter in place with the tip on the back of the oropharynx, moving it to the left to make room for your blade. If attached to a suction device, it will continue clearing any ongoing secretions, giving you a great view of the larynx (Du Canto technique).

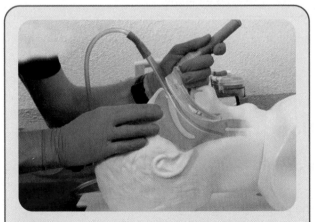

3 The laryngoscope blade is inserted with the left hand into the right side of the patient's airway to the correct depth, sweeping toward the center of the airway while observing the desired landmarks.

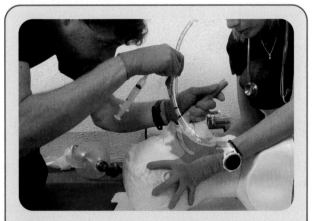

4 After identification of desired landmarks, the ET tube is inserted between the patient's vocal cords to the desired depth.

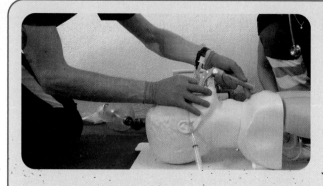

5 The laryngoscope is then removed while holding the ET tube in place; the depth marking on the side of the ET tube is noted. If a malleable stylet has been used, it should be removed at this time. The pilot valve is inflated with enough air to complete the seal between the patient's trachea and the cuff of the ET tube (usually 5 mL of air), and the syringe is removed from the pilot valve. The first practitioner attaches the bag-mask device with a reservoir attached to the proximal end of the ET tube, and ventilation is resumed while observing the rise of the patient's chest with each delivered breath. Manual stabilization of the patient's head and neck is maintained throughout the process (this is not shown on the pictures for the sake of clarity). Bilateral breath sounds and absence of air sounds over the epigastrium, along with other indications of proper ET tube placement, including waveform capnography, are checked (see earlier discussion in this chapter, in the "Verification of Endotracheal Tube Placement" section). Once placement has been confirmed, the ET tube is secured in place. Although the use of tape or other commercially available device is adequate in controlled situations in which the patient is not moved, the *best* way to guard against displacement of the ET tube in the prehospital situation is to physically hold onto the tube at all times.

Courtesy of J.C. Pitteloud MD, Switzerland.

Face-to-Face Orotracheal Intubation

Principle: An alternative method of securing a definitive airway when patient positioning limits use of traditional methods.

Situations may arise in the prehospital setting in which the prehospital care practitioner cannot take a position above the patient's head to initiate endotracheal intubation in a traditional manner. The intubating laryngeal mask is a very efficient technique in this situation.

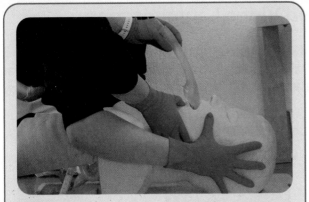

1 The first practitioner stabilizes the head from the front, while a second practitioner introduces the ILMA. The second practitioner checks the placement of the laryngeal mask with auscultation and inspection of the chest, and with ETCO$_2$, if available.

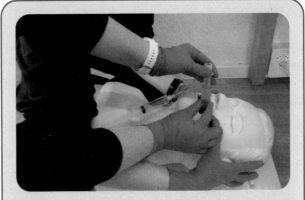

2 After making sure that the ILMA is in front of the laryngeal opening, the second practitioner introduces the endotracheal tube. Remember that the opening of the ILMA is at 4 to 5 cm from the teeth. It is therefore necessary to add this distance to the standard insertion depth of the ET tube (typically 4 cm with an i-gel Nr 5). The second practitioner carefully checks ET tube placement with auscultation, chest inspection, and ETCO$_2$ waveform assessment. Do not try to remove the ILMA before reaching the hospital: it provides excellent fixation for the ET tube and is an important backup should the ET tube become dislodged or obstructed.

Courtesy of J.C. Pitteloud MD, Switzerland.

Intubation With Airtraq Channeled Video Laryngoscope

Principle: The Airtraq device allows visualization of the glottis around the tongue and includes a channel to facilitate direction of the endotracheal tube through the vocal cords. (The King airway is another channeled video laryngoscope, which works in a very similar way.)

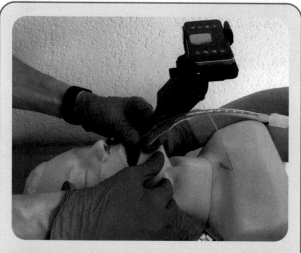

1 The second practitioner stabilizes the patient's head from the front while the first practitioner opens the cervical collar. The first practitioner turns on the light and slides the tube into the lateral channel of the Airtraq from the top, aligning the top with the end of the guiding channel. (*Warning:* Inserting the tube farther will obscure visualization, so keep the tip behind the light.) Suction the airway prior to laryngoscopy. This is particularly necessary when using video laryngoscopes. After suctioning the airway, leave the tip of the suction catheter in place below the vocal cords and sweep it to the left corner of the mouth to make space for the laryngoscope. While opening the mouth with the thumb of the nondominant hand, the first practitioner uses the dominant hand to facilitate insertion of the device into the patient's mouth. The Airtraq is held with the fingers and not with the palm of the hand, and it is not held from the top, so as to protect the patient's teeth.

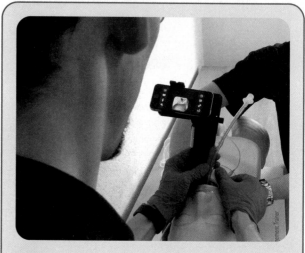

2 The first practitioner inserts the Airtraq into the midline of the patient's mouth, avoiding putting pressure on the upper teeth, until the tip has reached the back of the tongue. Once the Airtraq is inserted into the posterior oropharynx, the epiglottis, the arytenoids, and the vocal cords are identified.

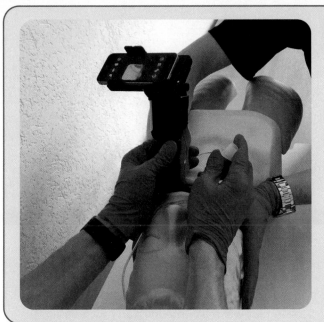

3 The first practitioner then advances the tube between the vocal cords by pushing it forward while keeping it inside the guiding channel. If the tip of the ET tube moves behind the vocal cords, pulling the laryngoscope 1 or 2 cm back will usually solve the problem. The first practitioner detaches the tube from the Airtraq by pulling the Airtraq laterally while holding the tube in position. The first practitioner confirms the correct position of the tube by auscultation and assessment of waveform capnography.

Photograph provided courtesy of J.C. Pitteloud M.D., Switzerland.

Surgical Cricothyroidotomy

Principle: A method of securing an airway in a patient with an airway obstruction that cannot be relieved by simple means.

Although there are many devices on the market, the technique described here utilizes simple and inexpensive materials stored in the ambulance. The equipment includes a scalpel, a curved hemostat, and a commercial tracheostomy tube (alternatively, a 5.0- to 7.0-mm endotracheal tube). Standard endotracheal tubes are a second choice because they are too long and carry the risk of mainstem bronchus intubation. This technique is not recommended in children younger than 12 years, because the very soft cartilage makes incision difficult and the thick mucosa under the glottis makes it very difficult to find the lumen.

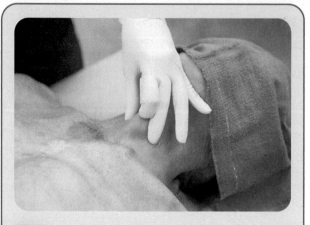

1 The left hand executes the "laryngeal handshake," with both the thumb and middle finger stabilizing the larynx while the index finger locates the cricothyroid membrane. The palm of the hand will help to keep the chin out of the way.

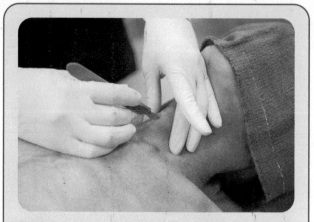

2 A 2- to 3-cm vertical incision is made over the cricothyroid cartilage down to the cricoid, and the membrane is located by palpation with the index finger. Using the thumb and the middle finger of the left hand to hold the skin taut will make the incision much easier. The scalpel is grasped in the right hand, with the heel of the hand firmly resting on the sternum. Remember that the carotid artery and jugular veins are nearby, so care should be taken in handling the sharp blade. Once located, the cricothyroid membrane is perforated with the scalpel blade and then enlarged horizontally. Keep the blade in place briefly until the next step to avoid losing access should the patient swallow or cough, a common occurrence in live patients. If this happens, getting the hole back can be very difficult.

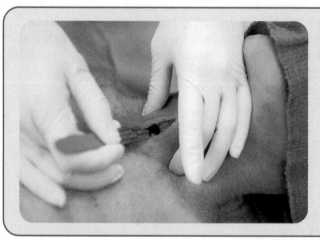

3 A hook is introduced into the incision and is lifted upward, providing an opening directed toward the trachea. The tube is introduced into the trachea, and the cuff is inflated. Check placement with auscultation and waveform capnography assessment. A word of caution if you use a standard ET tube for a surgical airway: because the standard ET tube is much longer than a cricothyrotomy cannula, it is very easy to end up in a mainstem bronchus.

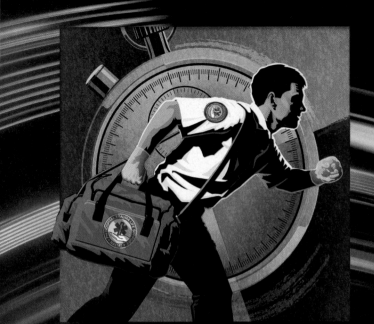

DIVISION **3**

Specific Injuries

© Ralf Hiemisch/Getty Images

CHAPTER **8**

Head and Neck Trauma

Lead Editors
Christine Ramirez, MD
Angela Lumba-Brown, MD
Deborah M. Stein, MD, MPH

CHAPTER OBJECTIVES

At the completion of this chapter, you will be able to do the following:

- Relate the physics of head trauma to the potential for traumatic brain injury (TBI).
- Recognize pathophysiologic manifestations of TBI in association with historical data to support the assessment of patients with head trauma and formulate a field impression.
- Discuss the importance of serial neurologic assessment, including Glasgow Coma Scale score, in prehospital settings with communication to receiving facilities.
- Formulate a plan of field intervention for both short and prolonged transport times for patients with suspected TBI.

- Compare and contrast the pathophysiology, management, and potential consequences of specific types of primary and secondary brain injuries.
- Recognize the importance of active airway management of patients with known or suspected TBIs.
- Identify criteria for patient care decisions with regard to transport, level of prehospital care, and hospital resources needed for the appropriate management of patients with head and neck injuries.

SCENARIO

On an 85°F (29°C) summer day, you and your partner are dispatched to a marathon race to assess a 30-year-old man who fell 14 feet (ft; 4.3 meters [m]) off a ladder while attempting to secure the finish line banner. Upon your arrival, the patient is supine and unresponsive. A bystander is holding the patient's head and neck in-line.

Upon initial assessment, you note an irregular breathing pattern that varies in depth of respirations and rate. There is blood-tinged fluid coming from both ear canals and nostrils of the patient. The patient's eyes are closed, and he is not responding to you talking to him.

You note an absence of gag reflex on your initial assessment and insert an oropharyngeal airway. Your partner ventilates the patient with a bag-valve mask at a rate of 12 breaths/minute. You note that the patient's right pupil is dilated. The radial pulse is 54 and regular. Oxygen saturation (SpO_2) is 96%. The patient's skin is cool, dry, and pale. His Glasgow Coma Scale (GCS) score is calculated to be 7, with eyes = 2, verbal = 1, and motor = 4 (E2V1M4).

(continues)

INTRODUCTION

Traumatic brain injury (TBI) is a public health problem that is a leading cause of injury-related deaths and disability.[1] Over 55 million people live with TBI-related disabilities worldwide, and the prevalence of TBI continues to increase. There are at least 3.5 million new cases of TBI per year in the United States alone.[2] According to the Centers for Disease Control and Prevention (CDC), there were approximately 61,000 TBI-related deaths in the United States in 2019, which is approximately 166 TBI deaths per day, and there are approximately 288,000 hospitalizations annually.[3] TBI is also the most frequent cause of death and disability among children, with more than 3 million children sustaining brain injuries yearly worldwide.[4] Mortality rates for moderate and severe brain injuries are about 10% and 30%, respectively. Of those who survive moderate or severe brain injuries, 50% to 99% have some degree of permanent neurologic disability.[3,5] Although patients with moderate and severe TBI have significant rates of morbidity and mortality, 80% of all TBIs are mild; most of these patients are discharged home from the emergency department (ED) or after primary care evaluations.[3]

Common causes of TBIs include motor vehicle crashes (MVCs), unintentional falls, penetrating injury (e.g., firearm), or assaults.[3] Unintentional falls account for the highest age-adjusted rate and proportion (52.3%) of all TBI-related hospitalizations and are most frequent among older adults at least age 75 years. MVCs are the second most common cause of TBI-related hospitalizations (20.4%), especially between ages 15 and 54 years. Falls and MVCs are also the most common principal mechanisms of injury in the pediatric population.[3]

The care of patients with suspected TBI in the prehospital setting is challenging for a variety of reasons. Mental status may be altered secondary to injury, posttraumatic seizure, comorbidities, hypoperfusion from concomitant shock, or coingestions. Symptoms of TBI, such as protracted vomiting, may make airway management a challenge. Coexisting injuries may impact hemodynamic stability and increase the risk of worsening brain injury and poor outcomes.

The prehospital care practitioner's goal is to rapidly identify likely TBI and stabilize the patient to minimize the risk of secondary injury during transport to a receiving facility. Prehospital treatments for TBI are aimed at optimizing respiratory and hemodynamic stability.

Anatomy

Knowledge of anatomy is important to understanding and identifying the complex pathophysiology of TBI. The scalp covers the head and offers some protection to the skull and brain. The scalp is composed of several layers, including skin, connective tissue, the aponeurosis (or **galea aponeurotica**), and the periosteum of the skull bones. The galea is a layer of tough, thick fibrous tissue that provides structural support to the scalp, while the periosteum provides nutrition to the bone. The scalp is highly vascular and may bleed profusely when injured.

The skull, or cranium, is composed of several bones that fuse into a single structure during childhood (see Figure 6-9). Several small openings (**foramina**) through the base of the skull provide pathways for blood vessels and cranial nerves. One large opening, the **foramen magnum**, is located at the base of the skull and serves as a passageway for the brain stem to the spinal cord (**Figure 8-1**). In infants, "soft spots" known as **fontanelles**, can be identified between the bones. The infant has no bony protection over these portions of the brain until the bones fuse, typically by 2 years of age. Because an infant's skull is not completely fused, hemorrhage within the skull can cause the bones to spread farther apart, allowing more blood to accumulate within the cranium.

The cranium provides significant protection to the brain. It is made of two layers of compact cortical tissue,

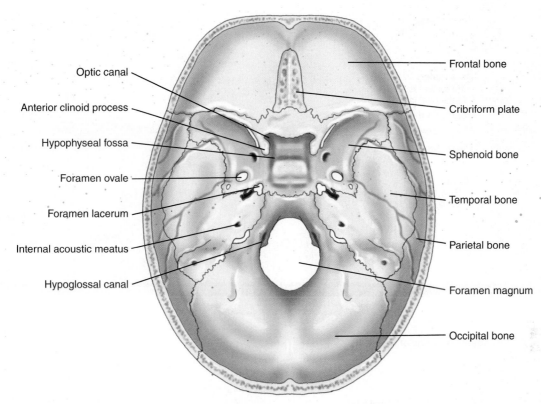

Figure 8-1 Internal view of the base of the skull.
© National Association of Emergency Medical Technicians (NAEMT)

known as the outer and inner tables, which encase a layer of spongy cancellous bone. Most of the bones forming the cranium, such as the frontal bone, are thick and strong. However, the skull is especially thin in the temporal and ethmoid regions and is therefore more prone to fracture in these regions. In addition, the interior surface of the skull base is rough and irregular (see Figure 8-1). When exposed to a blunt force, the brain may slide across these irregularities, producing cerebral contusions or lacerations.

The brain is covered by three separate membranes known as the **meninges**: the dura mater, arachnoid mater, and pia mater (**Figure 8-2**). The outermost layer, the **dura mater**, is composed of tough fibrous tissue and lines the inner table of the skull. Under normal circumstances, there is no space between the dura and the skull. However, this juncture is a potential space known as the **epidural space**, which may expand if the dura is stripped away from the skull. For example, the middle meningeal arteries are located in grooves in the temporal bones bilaterally, between the dura and the inner table. A temporal bone fracture may tear the middle meningeal artery, resulting in an **epidural hematoma**.

The **arachnoid mater** is deep to the dura mater and covers the brain and its blood vessels in a spiderweb appearance. The space between the dura mater and arachnoid mater is known as the subdural space. Unlike the epidural space, the subdural space is an actual space located beneath the dura mater. This space encompasses bridging veins—part of the vascular communications between the skull and the brain. The traumatic rupture of these veins often creates **subdural hematomas**, which may be associated with additional injury to brain tissue. Injury to these bridging veins accounts for the morbidity of subdural hematomas.

The deepest membrane is the **pia mater**. It is the final brain covering that is adherent to the brain. The space between the arachnoid mater and pia mater is known as the subarachnoid space, and it contains cerebral blood vessels that emerge from the base of the brain and cover the brain. Their rupture (usually from trauma or a ruptured cerebral aneurysm) will result in bleeding into the subarachnoid space, causing a **subarachnoid hematoma**. Subarachnoid hematomas can be indicators of other serious concomitant brain injuries.

The brain occupies about 80% of the **cranial vault** and is divided into three main regions: the **cerebrum**, **cerebellum**, and **brain stem** (**Figure 8-3**). The cerebrum consists of right and left hemispheres that can be subdivided into several lobes. The dominant hemisphere contains the language center and is the left side in the majority of right-handed individuals and 85% of left-handed individuals. The cerebrum is separated from the cerebellum by an extension of the dura mater called the **tentorium cerebelli**. The cerebellum is located in the posterior fossa of the cranium, behind the brain stem

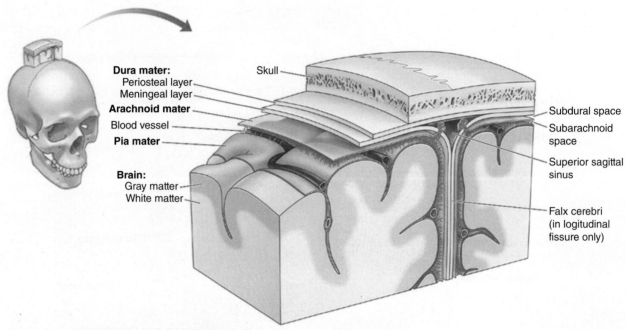

Figure 8-2 Meningeal coverings of the brain.
Courtesy of the American College of Surgeons.

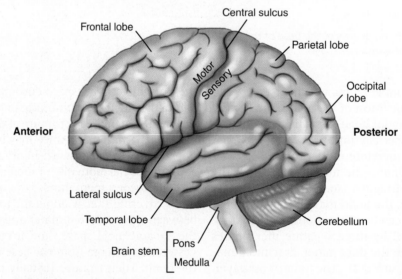

Figure 8-3 Regions of the brain.
© National Association of Emergency Medical Technicians (NAEMT)

and beneath the cerebrum. The brain stem sits inferior to the cerebrum and anterior to the cerebellum. **Table 8-1** lists the major regions of the brain and their functions. Much of the **reticular activating system**, the portion of the brain responsible for arousal and alertness, is also found in the brain stem. Blunt trauma can impair the reticular activating system, leading to a transient loss of consciousness.

The brain receives its arterial blood supply from the internal carotid arteries (anteriorly) and the vertebral arteries (posteriorly). Venous drainage occurs through a network of superficial and deep cerebral veins, which drain primarily into dural venous sinuses and the great cerebral vein of Galen, and eventually into the jugular veins and then the superior vena cava. At any time, the intracranial blood volume is 15% arterial and 40% venous, with the remaining 45% within the microcirculation.[6]

Cerebrospinal fluid (CSF) is produced in the ventricular system of the brain and travels within the subarachnoid space to surround the brain and spinal cord. Its primary role is to deliver and remove nutrients, hormones, and neurotransmitters to and from the brain. CSF production is approximately 500 milliliters (mL) per day and is constantly being produced and reabsorbed such

Table 8-1 The Brain	
Region	**Function**
Cerebrum	Sensory function, motor function, intelligence, memory
Frontal	Emotions, motor function, and expression of speech on the dominant side
Parietal	Sensory function, spatial orientation
Temporal	Regulation of certain memory functions; speech reception and integration in all right-handed and the majority of left-handed individuals
Occipital	Vision
Cerebellum	Movement
Brain stem	Signal relay between brain and spinal cord
Midbrain	Arousal and alertness via the reticular activating system
Pons	Respiratory apnea centers, conveyance of signals from cerebrum to medulla and cerebellum
Medulla	Cardiopulmonary centers (breathing, heart rate)

© National Association of Emergency Medical Technicians (NAEMT)

that the total CSF volume is approximately 150 mL. This volume is small compared to the volume of brain parenchyma and cerebral blood flow.[7]

There are 12 cranial nerves that originate from the brain and brain stem (**Figure 8-4**). Cranial nerve (CN) III (**oculomotor nerve**) controls pupillary constriction. CN III is important in assessing patients with suspected brain injury because it crosses the surface of the tentorium cerebelli and any hemorrhage or edema that causes downward herniation of the brain will compress the nerve, impairing its function and leading to pupil dilation.[7]

Physiology

Cerebral Blood Flow

The brain's neurons require continuous blood flow in order to provide oxygen and glucose for cell activity and survival. Cerebral blood flow occurs at rate of about 700 mL per minute, which is approximately 15% of the cardiac output. The cardiac output is the amount of blood the heart pumps in 1 minute, which normally ranges from 4 to 8 liters per minute. This constant cerebral blood flow is maintained by (1) an adequate pressure (cerebral perfusion pressure) to force blood through the brain and (2) a regulatory mechanism (autoregulation) that varies the resistance to blood flow as the perfusion pressure changes. Cerebral metabolic rate also affects cerebral blood flow, such that increased neuronal activity increases cerebral blood flow. This is important in the treatment of TBI, which will be discussed in a later section.[6]

Cerebral Perfusion Pressure

Cerebral perfusion pressure (CPP) is the amount of pressure available to propel blood through the cerebral circulation and maintain cerebral blood flow. Cerebral perfusion pressure relates directly to the patient's mean arterial pressure (MAP) and **intracranial pressure (ICP)**. The MAP is the average pressure in the arteries during one cardiac cycle and is an indicator of perfusion to vital organs. ICP is the combined pressure of brain tissue, blood, and CSF within the skull cavity.

Cerebral perfusion pressure is expressed by the following formula:

Cerebral perfusion pressure = Mean arterial pressure – Intracranial pressure

or

$$CPP = MAP - ICP$$

Normal MAP ranges from about 85 to 95 mm Hg. In adults, ICP is normally below 15 mm Hg. It is usually 3 to 7 mm Hg in children and 1.5 to 6 mm Hg in infants.[5] Therefore, CPP is normally about 70 to 80 mm Hg. Sudden increases or decreases in blood pressure and ICP, which can occur following TBI, may affect cerebral perfusion.

Autoregulation of Cerebral Blood Flow

The brain works very hard at keeping its cerebral blood flow constant over a wide range of changing conditions. This process is known as **autoregulation**. Autoregulation is crucial to the brain's normal function and is dependent on cerebral blood flow (CBF) and cerebral vascular resistance (CVR).

Cerebral perfusion pressure = Cerebral blood flow × Cerebral vascular resistance

or

$$CPP = CBF \times CVR$$

Because the brain's principal concern is cerebral blood flow, it is useful to rewrite this equation as:

$$CBF = CPP/CVR$$

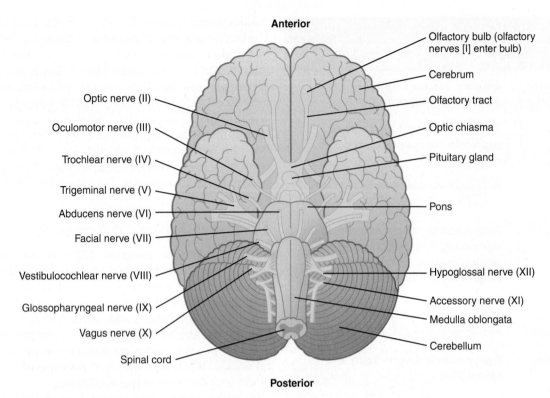

Figure 8-4 Inferior surface of the brain showing the origins of the cranial nerves.
© National Association of Emergency Medical Technicians (NAEMT)

Autoregulation is accomplished by adjusting CVR through either vasodilation or vasoconstriction. If CPP decreases, cerebral arterial vasodilation will decrease CVR to maintain CBF. Similarly, increased CPP will induce arterial vasoconstriction, subsequently increasing CVR. Typically, autoregulation can compensate for CPP between 50 and 150 mm Hg. Outside of this range, CBF will vary linearly with CPP. Hence, cerebral blood flow will begin to decrease once cerebral perfusion pressure is below 50 mm Hg.

Another way to compensate for reduced cerebral blood flow is by extracting more oxygen from the blood that is passing through the brain. The clinical signs and symptoms of ischemia (dizziness and altered mental status) will not be noticed until the diminished perfusion has exceeded the ability of increased oxygen extraction to meet the brain's metabolic needs.[6] As cerebral blood flow begins to fall, cerebral function will decline, and the risk of permanent cerebral injury from ischemia increases. Injured brains may require higher-than-normal cerebral perfusion pressures to activate autoregulation and keep cerebral blood flow adequate.

Cerebral perfusion pressure is used to estimate the adequacy of cerebral blood flow. The relationship between CPP, ICP, and MAP is important in trauma. Acute intracranial bleeding causes compression to surrounding tissues and an increased ICP. This is termed *mass effect*.

As the ICP increases, the amount of pressure needed to propel blood through the brain also increases. The MAP will subsequently increase to maintain CPP. If the MAP cannot keep up with the increase in ICP or if treatment to decrease the ICP is not rapidly instituted, the amount of blood flowing through the brain will start to decrease, leading to ischemic brain damage and impaired brain function. Therefore, in the absence of an ICP monitor, the best practice is to maintain a high-normal MAP.[8-15]

Cerebral Venous Drainage

Cerebral venous drainage is an often overlooked but significant contributor of ICP and autoregulation. Venous sinuses are susceptible to dilation and compression. For example, when cerebral blood inflow rises, venous drainage increases as an autoregulatory mechanism. However, there is a point at which the limits of compliance increase, and inadequate venous drainage can result in venous and intracranial hypertension. Acute compression, such as depressed skull fractures, expanding intracranial hematomas, and sinus thrombosis can also impair venous drainage, increasing ICP. Obstruction of the dominant sinus has more effects than obstruction of the nondominant sinus. Extracranial causes, such as jugular venous compression from head flexion or tight cervical collars, can also impair venous drainage by almost 10 mm Hg.[16-18]

Oxygen and Cerebral Blood Flow

The brain is a highly metabolic organ and therefore has high oxygen requirements. Decreased levels of oxygen (hypoxia) cause significant vasodilation in an effort to dramatically increase cerebral blood flow. This response typically does not occur until the arterial oxygen partial pressure (PaO_2) falls below 50 mm Hg. At times, cerebral blood flow can increase by up to 400% of resting levels.[6]

Carbon Dioxide and Cerebral Blood Flow

The cerebral blood vessels respond to changes in arterial carbon dioxide levels by constricting or dilating. Decreased levels of carbon dioxide (hypocapnia) result in vasoconstriction, whereas elevated levels (hypercapnia) cause vasodilation. Hyperventilation reduces the arterial carbon dioxide partial pressure ($PaCO_2$) by increasing the rate at which carbon dioxide is exhaled by the lungs. The resulting hypocapnia changes the acid–base balance in the brain, resulting in vasoconstriction. This cerebral vasoconstriction reduces the intravascular volume of the brain, reducing cerebral blood volume and, therefore, often ICP.[19-20]

Hyperventilation-induced cerebral vasoconstriction also increases CVR, regardless of whether CPP is adequate to maintain cerebral blood flow. As a result, hyperventilation can reduce CBF, placing the injured brain at greater risk for ischemic injury. A $PaCO_2$ of less than 35 mm Hg increases the risk of cerebral ischemia. As such, prophylactic hyperventilation is not recommended in the management of TBI.[15, 21-23]

Conversely, a $PaCO_2$ greater than the normal range of 35 to 45 mm Hg (hypercapnia) leads to dilation of cerebral arterioles, thus increasing cerebral blood flow while at the same time increasing intravascular volume and potentially increasing ICP.[15] Management of TBI using hyperventilation is discussed later in this chapter.

Pathophysiology of Traumatic Brain Injury

TBI can be divided into two categories: primary and secondary.

Primary Brain Injury

Primary brain injury is any mechanical injury that occurs at the time of the original trauma. This includes injury to the brain, its coverings, and associated vascular structures. Primary brain injuries include brain contusions, hemorrhages, and damage to nerves and brain vessels. Because neural tissue does not regenerate well and because little possibility exists for repair, there is minimal expectation of recovery of the structure and function lost with primary injury.

Mild TBI

Mild TBI, inclusive of concussion, is defined by the CDC as "a type of traumatic brain injury—or TBI—caused by a bump, blow, or jolt to the head or by a hit to the body that causes the head and brain to move rapidly back and forth. This sudden movement can cause the brain to bounce around or twist in the skull, creating chemical changes in the brain and sometimes stretching and damaging brain cells."[24] A neurometabolic cascade of injury occurs in mild TBI, often in the absence of macroscopic neural damage. However, with the advent of highly advanced neuroimaging, microhemorrhage and contusion may be visualized resulting in "complicated mild TBI," which may present with postconcussive symptoms (**Table 8-2**) lasting longer than the traditional recovery period of 2 to 4 weeks.[3]

Headache, dizziness, and nausea frequently occur acutely following mild TBI but also may be early symptoms of a more severe injury. Patients with these symptoms should be transported immediately for further evaluation. The formal diagnosis of a mild TBI will be made in the hospital once the patient has been clinically evaluated, observed, and/or when neuroimaging demonstrates an absence of clinically significant intracranial pathology. Up to 30% of patients with mild TBI experience persistent postconcussive symptoms for longer than 4 weeks. These symptoms include headaches, balance problems, oculomotor impairment, anxiety and mood disruption, and cognitive impairments such as difficulty concentrating.[25-29]

Intracranial Hemorrhage

Intracranial hemorrhages are divided into four general types: epidural, subdural, subarachnoid, and

Table 8-2 Common Postconcussive Symptoms

Categories	Symptoms
Vestibular	Imbalance, nausea, dizziness
Sensory	Blurry vision, migraines, tinnitus, photo/phonophobia
Cognitive	Difficulty focusing, forgetfulness
Emotional	Fatigue, insomnia, irritability, depression

Data from Quinn DK, Mayer AR, Master CL, Fann JR. Prolonged postconcussive symptoms. *Am J Psychiatry.* 2018;175(2):103-111. doi:10.1176/appi.ajp.2017.17020235

intracerebral. Because the signs and symptoms of each of these have significant overlap, specific diagnosis in the prehospital setting (as well as the ED) is almost impossible, although the prehospital care practitioner may suspect a particular type of hemorrhage based on the characteristic clinical presentation. Even so, a definitive diagnosis can be made only after a computed tomography (CT) scan is performed at the receiving facility. Because these hemorrhages often occupy space inside the rigid skull, they may produce rapid increases in ICP, especially if they are of a sizable volume.

Epidural Hematoma

Epidural hematomas often result from a relatively low-velocity blow to the temporal bone, such as the impact from a punch or baseball. A fracture of this thin bone damages the middle meningeal artery, which results in arterial bleeding that collects between the skull and dura mater (**Figure 8-5**). This high-pressure arterial blood can start to dissect, or peel, the dura off the inner table of the skull, creating an epidural space full of blood. Such an epidural hematoma has a characteristic lens shape, as seen on the CT scan, created by the dura holding the hematoma against the inner table of the skull. The principal threat to the brain is from the expanding mass of blood displacing the brain and threatening herniation.

The classic history for an epidural hematoma is a patient experiencing a brief loss of consciousness, then regaining consciousness, and then experiencing a rapid decline in consciousness. During the period of consciousness, or "lucid interval," the patient may be oriented, or lethargic and confused, or may complain of a headache. However, the majority of patients with epidural hematomas do not experience this lucid interval, and it may also occur with other types of intracranial hemorrhages, making it nonspecific for epidural hematoma. Nonetheless, a patient who experiences a lucid interval, followed by a neurologic decline, is at risk for a progressive intracranial process and needs emergency evaluation.

As a patient's consciousness worsens, the physical examination may reveal a dilated and sluggish or nonreactive pupil, most commonly on the ipsilateral side of the herniation. Because motor nerves cross over to the other side above the spinal cord, hemiparesis or hemiplegia typically occurs on the contralateral side. The mortality rate for an epidural hematoma is about 20%. However, with rapid recognition and hematoma evacuation, the mortality rate can be as low as 2%. This improved rate of outcome is because an epidural hematoma is usually an isolated space-occupying lesion, with little associated injury to the brain beneath. If the hematoma is quickly recognized and removed, the pathologic mass effect is corrected, and the patient can make an excellent recovery. Rapid removal reduces mortality as well as neurologic morbidity.

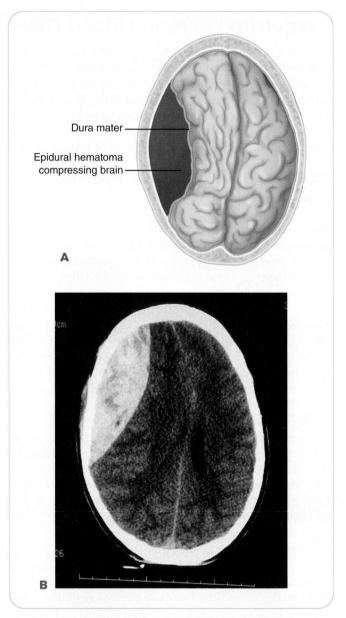

Figure 8-5 **A.** Epidural hematoma. **B.** CT scan of epidural hematoma.

Subdural Hematoma

Subdural hematomas are seen in between 5% and 25% of severe brain injuries, depending on the study, with a male-to-female ratio of 3:1.[30] In young adults, subdural hematomas are associated with high-energy trauma (e.g., MVCs) and in the elderly, subdural hematomas are associated with minor trauma (e.g., falls), with those older adults more likely to be on anticoagulant or antiplatelet therapy.[31] Older data indicate that 56% of subdural hematomas are due to MVCs and 12% are due to falls, whereas in older adults, 22% are due to MVCs and 56% are due to falls.[32]

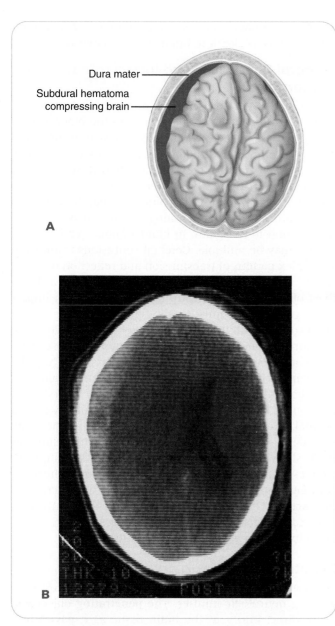

Figure 8-6 **A.** Subdural hematoma. **B.** CT scan of subdural hematoma.

A. © National Association of Emergency Medical Technicians (NAEMT); **B.** Courtesy of Peter T. Pons, MD, FACEP.

In addition to being more common than epidural hematomas, subdural hematomas also differ in etiology, location, and prognosis. Unlike the epidural hematoma, which is caused by arterial hemorrhage, a subdural hematoma generally results from a venous bleed. In this case, bridging veins are torn during an injury to the head. Blood collects in the subdural space, between the dura mater and the underlying arachnoid membrane (**Figure 8-6**).

Subdural hematomas present in two different ways. In patients who have experienced significant trauma, the disruption of the bridging veins results in relatively rapid accumulation of blood in the subdural space, with rapid onset of mass effect. Direct injury to the brain parenchyma beneath the subdural hematoma occurs concomitantly with venous disruption. As a result, the mass effect of subdural hematomas is often caused by both blood accumulation and cerebral edema of the underlying injured brain. Patients presenting with this type of acute mass effect will have an acutely depressed mental status and will need rapid identification of the emergency in the field with emergent transport to an appropriate receiving facility for CT scan, ICP monitoring and management, and possibly surgery.

However, clinically occult subdural hematomas can occur in other patients. In older adults or debilitated patients, such as those with chronic disease, the subdural space is enlarged secondary to brain atrophy. In such patients, blood may accumulate in the subdural space without exerting mass effect and is therefore asymptomatic. Such subdural hematomas can occur during falls in older adults or during minor trauma. Older patients receiving anticoagulants such as warfarin or the direct oral anticoagulants such as apixaban or rivaroxaban are at higher risk. Because these falls are minor, patients often do not present for evaluation and the bleeds are not identified. Many patients in whom chronic subdural hematoma is eventually identified do not even recall the traumatic event that caused the bleed because it seemed so minor.

In some patients with an occult subdural hematoma, the subdural blood liquefies but is retained within the subdural space. Over time, through a mechanism that includes repeated small bleeds into the liquid hematoma, the now-chronic subdural hematoma can expand and slowly start to exert mass effect on the brain. Because the onset of the mass effect is gradual, the patient will not have the dramatic presentation associated with an acute subdural hematoma. Instead, the patient is more likely to present with headache, visual disturbances, personality changes, difficulty speaking (**dysarthria**), and hemiparesis or hemiplegia of a slowly progressive nature. Only when some of these symptoms become pronounced enough to prompt the patient or caregiver to seek help is the chronic subdural hematoma discovered. On CT scan, a chronic subdural hematoma has a distinct appearance compared with the more emergent, acute subdural hematoma. Often the event precipitating transport for evaluation and care is the most recent of the small, repetitive subdural bleeds that create chronic subdural hematomas, and a small amount of acute blood may be found in a larger collection of chronic blood. The need for and the urgency of surgery are determined by the patient's symptoms, the amount of mass effect, and the patient's overall medical condition.

Prehospital care personnel frequently encounter these patients when called to facilities that care for chronically ill populations. Because the symptoms are nonspecific, diagnosing a chronic subdural hematoma in the field is rarely possible, and the symptoms may be confused with those of a stroke, infection, dementia, or even a generalized decline in the patient.

Although many subdural hematomas in these patients will be chronic, patients taking anticoagulants, after an apparently insignificant trauma, may have a subdural hematoma that expands over several hours and progresses to herniation resulting from the patient's inability to clot. These patients can have a benign presentation and then deteriorate several hours after their injury. Older adults, especially patients receiving anticoagulants who have experienced apparently minor falls, should be managed with a heightened sense of urgency and care.

Subarachnoid Hemorrhage

Subarachnoid hemorrhage (SAH) is bleeding that occurs beneath the arachnoid membrane, which lies under the subdural space covering the brain. Blood in the subarachnoid space cannot enter the subdural space. Many of the brain's blood vessels are located in the subarachnoid space, so injury to these vessels will cause subarachnoid bleeding, a layering of blood beneath the arachnoid membrane on the surface of the brain. This layering of blood is typically thin and rarely causes mass effect.

SAH is often associated with spontaneous rupture of cerebral aneurysms and causing the sudden onset of the worst headache of the patient's life; however, trauma is actually the most common cause of subarachnoid bleeding. A patient with an SAH will usually complain of a headache, which may be severe in nature, as well as nausea, vomiting, and dizziness. In addition, the presence of blood in the subarachnoid space may cause meningeal signs such as pain and stiffness of the neck, visual complaints, and photophobia (aversion to bright light). Bleeding from the posterior communicating artery can cause oculomotor nerve abnormalities or loss of movement on the ipsilateral side; the affected eye will look down and outward, and patients will not be able to lift their eyelids. These patients may also develop seizures, although seizure development is more common in cerebral aneurysm rupture or arteriovenous malformations than from trauma.

Because subarachnoid bleeding rarely causes mass effect, it does not require surgery for decompression. In fact, patients with SAH and mild neurologic deficits generally do extremely well.[33] However, traumatic SAH can be a marker for potentially severe brain injury whose presence increases the risk for other space-occupying lesions, elevated ICP, and intraventricular hemorrhage. Patients with traumatic SAH have a 63% to 73% increased risk of a cerebral contusion and a 44% risk of developing subdural hematomas. Those with greater than 1 centimeter (cm) of blood thickness or blood in the suprasellar or ambient cisterns have a positive predictive value of 72%

to 78% for a poor outcome, and traumatic SAH doubles the incidence of death in brain-injured patients.[34,35]

Cerebral Contusions and Intracerebral Hemorrhage

Damage to the brain itself may produce cerebral contusions. If this damage includes injury to the blood vessels within the brain, there will be bleeding within the brain, known as intracerebral hemorrhage. Cerebral contusions are relatively common both in patients with severe brain injuries and in those with moderate injuries. Although they are typically the result of blunt trauma, these injuries may also occur from penetrating trauma, such as a gunshot wound to the brain. In blunt trauma, cerebral contusions may be multiple. Cerebral contusions result from a complex pattern of transmission and reflection of forces within the skull. For example, when the head strikes a fixed object, it causes a coup injury at the site of impact and a contrecoup injury on the opposite site, where the brain collides with the opposite side of the skull. This type of injury is known as a **coup-contrecoup injury**. As a result, contusions often occur in locations remote from the site of impact, often on the opposite side of the brain.

Cerebral contusions often take 12 to 24 hours to appear on CT scans, and these patients may initially have a normal head CT scan. The only clue to its presence may be a depressed neurologic examination, with many patients showing moderate brain injuries. As the contusion evolves after injury, it becomes apparent on the head CT scan and can cause increased mass effect and increasing headaches. Of particular concern, cerebral contusions may cause moderate injuries to deteriorate to severe brain injuries in about 10% of patients.[36]

Penetrating Cranial Injury

Penetrating trauma of the brain is one of the most devastating neurologic injuries. The penetrating object will cause direct injury to the brain tissue as it passes into and, in some cases, through the brain parenchyma. The nature of the neurologic injury produced depends on the area of the brain injured. Gunshot wounds are particularly destructive because of the energy associated with the missile. (This type of injury is described further in Chapter 4, *The Physics of Trauma*.) Not only does a bullet cause direct injury as it passes through tissue, the associated shock wave damages tissue along the cavitation pathway. In particular, gunshot wounds that cross the midline and pass from one side of the brain to the other, thus involving both sides of the brain, are associated with a dismal outcome. In rare instances, such as when the bullet traverses only the frontal lobes, the patient may survive, albeit with significant impairment. The potential for survival is also better if the bullet passes from front to back on one side of the brain. Again, however, the patient will have persistent, significant neurologic deficit.

All penetrating brain injury results in open fracture of the skull. The potential for subsequent infection, if the patient survives, is high. In addition, penetrating injuries of the skull may damage other important structures such as the eyes, ears, and face, leading to impaired function.

Secondary Brain Injury

Secondary brain injury refers to further injury to structures after the initial inciting event. Following initial injury, pathophysiologic processes may occur that result in further injury to the brain for hours to weeks after the initial insult. The primary focus in the prehospital (and hospital) management of TBI is to identify and halt or limit these secondary injury mechanisms. The secondary effects are insidious in nature, and there can often be significant, ongoing damage that is not immediately apparent or appreciated. These effects play a significant role in death and disability after TBIs. By understanding the causes of secondary injury and anticipating the development of such injuries, prehospital care practitioners can prepare for, prevent, and intervene to correct these complications.

Pathologic mechanisms related to intracranial mass effect, elevated ICP, and mechanical shifting of the brain can lead to herniation, morbidity, and mortality. In adjunct to clinical exam, head CT and other advanced imaging modalities, as well as ICP monitoring, support

lifesaving interventions such as immediate neurosurgery. In the prehospital setting, rapid assessment and transport to a hospital with trauma and neurosurgical capabilities is a critical step in the treatment of patients with severe TBI and risk of herniation.

Two other important causes of secondary injury, discussed in further depth in dedicated sections, are hypoxia and hypotension. Unrecognized and untreated hypoxia and hypotension may be just as damaging to the injured brain as elevated ICP. In addition, impaired delivery of oxygen or glucose to an injured brain may be more devastating than it is in the normal brain. Therefore, hypoxia and hypotension must be prevented, identified, and treated immediately.[11,12,37-39]

Intracranial Causes of Secondary Brain Injury

Herniation

The **Monro-Kellie doctrine** states that the sum of the volume of brain tissue, blood, and CSF must remain constant in patients with an intact skull. Therefore, an increase in one component (such as from a hematoma, cerebral swelling, or tumor) must cause a decrease in one or two of the other components or the ICP will increase (**Figure 8-7**).[16]

In response to intracranial hemorrhage (ICH), the initial compensatory mechanism is to decrease the volume of intracranial CSF. The CSF naturally circulates

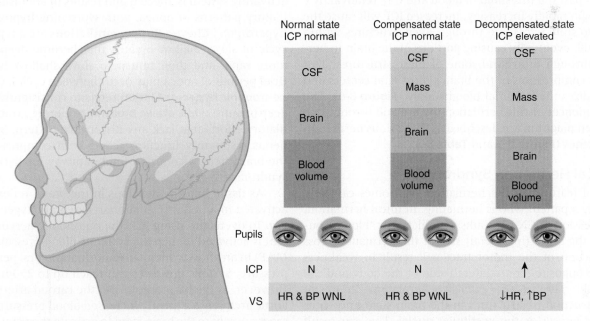

Figure 8-7 Monro-Kellie doctrine: The volume of intracranial contents must remain constant. If the addition of a mass such as a hematoma results in the decrease of an equal volume of CSF and blood, the ICP remains normal. However, when this compensatory mechanism is exhausted, an exponential increase in ICP occurs for minute increases in the volume of the hematoma.

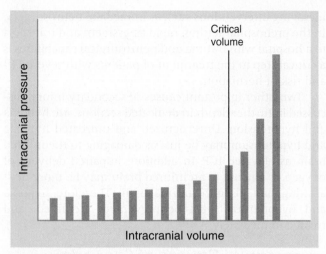

Figure 8-8 This graph demonstrates the relationship between intracranial volume and ICP. As the volume increases, the pressure remains relatively constant as CSF and blood are forced out. Eventually, a point is reached when no additional compensation can occur and ICP rises dramatically.

© National Association of Emergency Medical Technicians (NAEMT)

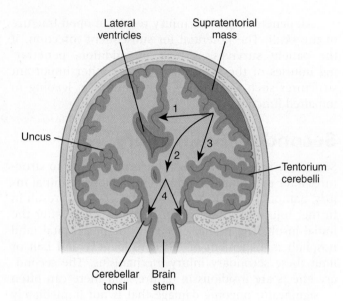

Figure 8-9 The various herniation syndromes that can result from mass effect and increased ICP: (1) cingulate herniation, (2) central herniation, (3) uncal herniation, (4) cerebellotonsillar herniation. These syndromes can occur in combination with each other.

© Jones & Bartlett Learning

within and around the brain, brain stem, and spinal cord. However, as ICH increases, CSF will be forced out of the head. Venous drainage will also increase to help reduce intravascular blood volume within the cranial vault. These two mechanisms prevent ICP from rising during the early phase of intracranial bleeding. As such, the patient can appear asymptomatic. However, as ICH increases past the threshold of blood and CSF removal, ICP will begin rapidly increasing. Increased ICP will cause the brain to shift across and through fixed structures within the skull, eventually causing portions of the brain to herniate through or around some of these structures. This causes compression of the brain's most vital centers and jeopardizes their arterial blood supply (**Figure 8-8**). The consequences of this herniation toward and through the foramen magnum are described as the various herniation syndromes (**Figure 8-9** and **Table 8-3**).

Clinical Herniation Syndromes

Clinical features of the herniation syndromes can help identify a patient who is herniating. In uncal herniation, compression of CN III results in a dilated or "blown" pupil on the same (ipsilateral) side of the herniation. Loss of function of the motor tract will result in weakness on the opposite (contralateral) side of the body and the Babinski reflex. More extensive herniation can result in destruction of structures in the brain stem known as the *red nucleus* or the **vestibular nuclei**. This can result in **decorticate posturing**, which involves abnormal flexion of the upper extremities and rigidity and extension of the lower extremities. A more ominous finding is **decerebrate posturing**, in which all extremities extend

and arching of the spine may occur. Decerebrate posturing occurs with injury and damage to the brain stem (**Figure 8-10**). As herniation progresses, the extremities become flaccid and motor activity becomes absent.[41,42]

With central and tonsillar herniation, the reticular activating system is affected and results in abnormal ventilatory patterns or apnea, with worsening hypoxia and hypercapnia. **Cheyne-Stokes ventilations** are a repeating cycle of slow, shallow breaths that become deeper and more rapid and then return to slow, shallow breaths. Brief periods of apnea may occur between cycles. **Central neurogenic hyperventilation** refers to consistently rapid, deep breaths, while **ataxic breathing** refers to erratic ventilatory efforts that lack any discernible pattern. Spontaneous respiratory function ceases with compression of the brain stem, a common final pathway for herniation syndromes.[40]

As tissue hypoxia develops in the brain, reflexes are activated in an effort to maintain cerebral oxygen delivery. To overcome rising ICP, the autonomic nervous system is activated to increase systemic blood pressure (and MAP) in an effort to maintain a normal cerebral perfusion pressure. Systolic pressures can reach up to 250 mm Hg. However, as the baroreceptors in the carotid arteries and aortic arch sense a greatly increased blood pressure, messages are sent to the brain stem to activate the parasympathetic nervous system. A signal then travels via the 10th cranial nerve, the vagus nerve, to slow the heart rate. The **Cushing reflex** results in the triad of findings that occur with increased ICP: (1) bradycardia, (2) increased

Table 8-3 Description of the Various Herniation Syndromes

Herniation Type	Movement
Uncal (transtentorial herniation)	The medial portion of the temporal lobe (uncus) is pushed toward the tentorium, putting pressure on the brain stem. Progressive herniation will compress CN III, the motor tract, and the reticular activating system on the same side (ipsilateral), resulting in an ipsilateral dilated or "blown" pupil, motor weakness on the opposite (contralateral) side, and respiratory dysfunction progressing to coma.
Central (downward herniation)	Parts of the temporal lobes of both cerebral hemispheres are squeezed through a notch in the tentorium (transtentorial). Downward herniation causes tearing of the basilar artery branches, resulting in small hemorrhages. The disrupted brain stem will result in decorticate posturing, respiratory center depression, and death.
Cingulate (subfalcine or transfalcine herniation)	Most commonly, the innermost part of the frontal lobe is drawn under the falx cerebri; the dura mater that separates the two hemispheres of the brain. This can cause injury to the medial cerebral hemispheres and the midbrain. It usually occurs in addition to uncal herniation and can present with abnormal posturing and coma.
Cerebellar (upward transtentorial herniation)	The midbrain is pushed upward through the tentorium. This movement can also occur in conjunction with uncal herniation.
Tonsillar (downward cerebellar herniation)	Cerebellar tonsils move downward through the foramen magnum, causing compression of the cerebellum and medulla and upper cervical spinal cord. Injury to the lower medulla results in cardiac and respiratory arrest, a common final event for patients with herniation. Tonsillar herniation is also referred to as "coning."[40]

© Jones & Bartlett Learning

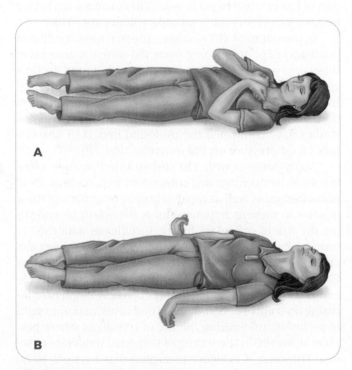

Figure 8-10 A. Decorticate posturing. **B.** Decerebrate posturing.
© Jones & Bartlett Learning

systolic blood pressure associated with a widened pulse pressure, and (3) irregular respirations such as Cheyne-Stokes breathing.[43]

Ischemia and Herniation

The herniation syndromes describe how increased ICP can result in compression and further brain injury. However, elevated ICP from cerebral swelling can also cause injury to the brain through decreased oxygen delivery and subsequent cerebral ischemia. Based on the cerebral perfusion pressure formula (CPP = MAP – ICP), an increase in ICP will result in a decrease in cerebral perfusion pressure and threatens cerebral perfusion. This is compounded by the ischemic insults sustained from other causes, such as systemic hypotension. These mechanical and ischemic insults bring about an endless cascade, resulting in more cerebral swelling that causes further mechanical and ischemic damage. This process will ultimately lead to herniation and death without intervention. Limiting secondary injury and breaking this cycle of injury are the principal goals of TBI management.

Cerebral Edema

Direct injury to the neuronal cell membranes allows intracellular fluid to collect within damaged neurons, leading to cerebral edema (brain swelling). In addition, injury can activate inflammatory responses that further injure neurons and the cerebral capillaries, leading to fluid collection within the neurons and interstitial spaces, leading to further cerebral edema. As the edema develops, the mechanical and ischemic injury previously described occurs, which aggravates these processes in an endless cycle of increasing edema and injury.

Cerebral edema often occurs at the site of a primary brain injury such as in association with intracranial hematomas or as a result of direct injury to the brain parenchyma such as in association with cerebral contusion. Cerebral edema may also be the result of diffuse brain injury from hypoxia or hypotension.

Mass Effect

In trauma, mass effect results from the accumulation of blood in the intracranial space. Intracranial hematomas, such as epidural, subdural, or intracerebral hematomas, are major sources of mass effect. Because mass effect is due to the hematoma size, rapid removal of these hematomas can break the cycle of edema and injury previously described. Unfortunately, hematomas often have associated cerebral edema, and other interventions, in addition to hematoma evacuation, are required to stop the cycle of injury and edema.

Venous Obstruction

Venous obstruction may occur secondary to external compression on the intracranial venous system or focal internal thrombosis. The walls of dural venous sinuses are thin and prone to external compression, most commonly due to depressed skull fractures or expanding masses. With external compression, the thin walls of the dural venous sinuses can be focally compressed, preventing venous outflow. Compression can also lead to venous thrombosis, which will further exacerbate venous obstruction.[16] Both external venous compression and venous thrombosis can begin an endless cycle of venous hypertension, further cerebral swelling, and further venous compression, all resulting in intracranial hypertension.

The most worrisome injuries are occipital skull fractures over the right transverse sinus because the right transverse sinus is the dominant sinus in most people. Focal internal obstructions such as dural sinus thromboses are rare but associated with high mortality. Treatment usually requires urgent surgical intervention.

In addition to intracranial venous obstruction, there are also extracranial causes of venous obstruction that can indirectly raise ICP. The venous tracts drain into the jugular veins, so any compression of the jugular veins can cause an upstream effect of intracranial venous obstruction. Poor head position, such as flexion or flexion with rotation, can cause significant increases in ICP (from a mean ICP of 8.8 to 16.2 mm Hg). This is even higher in children

who have larger occiputs and floppier necks.[7] Cervical collars can increase the ICP from 4 mm Hg to 14.5 mm Hg.[18] Increased intrathoracic and intra-abdominal pressure can also cause increased jugular venous pressure, affecting cerebral venous outflow. As a result, efforts should be made to keep the head in a neutral position and to avoid tight-fitting cervical collars.

Intracranial Hypertension

Additive factors related to cerebral edema, brain ischemia, venous obstruction, and mass effect exacerbate intracranial hypertension. ICP is measured as a way to quantify and assess the degree of cerebral edema. ICP monitors are placed in the hospital to allow healthcare practitioners to quantify cerebral edema, assess the risk of herniation, and monitor the effectiveness of therapies for cerebral edema. Elevated ICP may be a biomarker for cerebral edema. Although ICP monitoring is not routinely available in the prehospital environment, understanding the pathophysiology enables prehospital care practitioners target best management practices.

Extracranial Causes of Secondary Brain Injury

Hypotension

Brain ischemia is extremely common in severe brain injury. Studies have identified brain ischemia in 90% of patients who die of TBI and in many survivors.[44] Therefore, the impact of low cerebral blood flow on TBI outcomes has been a primary focus for limiting secondary injury after TBI.

In the national TBI database, the two most significant predictors of poor outcome from TBI were the amount of time spent with an ICP greater than 20 mm Hg and the time spent with a systolic blood pressure less than 90 mm Hg.[11] In fact, a single episode of systolic blood pressure less than 90 mm Hg can lead to a poorer outcome.[11] Several studies have confirmed the profound impact of low systolic blood pressure on the outcome after TBI.[12-14]

Many patients with TBI sustain other injuries, often involving hemorrhage and subsequent hypotension. Fluid resuscitation, as well as rapid definitive treatment of these injuries to prevent hypotension, is important in mitigating the risk of secondary injury. Insufficient data exist to recommend *specific* blood pressure *resuscitation* targets *that can be generalizable to all patients* in either the prehospital or ED setting. Both Prehospital Trauma Life Support (PHTLS) and Advanced Trauma Life Support (ATLS) emphasize focusing on control of hemorrhage and resuscitation to signs of perfusion, minimizing the use of crystalloid where possible. However, in the setting of suspected moderate or severe TBI, there is evidence to suggest that a systolic blood pressure of 110 mm Hg is an appropriate target.

In addition to hemorrhage, dysfunction in brain blood flow autoregulation may result in secondary injury.

Normal cortical cerebral blood flow is 50 mL per 100 grams (g) of brain tissue per minute (or 50 mL/100 g/minute [min]). After severe TBI, this value can drop to 30 mL or even as low as 20 mL/100 g/min. The cause of this decline in cerebral blood flow is unclear but may be due to a loss of autoregulation or a protective mechanism to downregulate the brain in response to injury. Decreased cerebral blood flow, compounded with hemorrhagic shock, further increases the ischemic threat to the brain.[11,20,45]

As previously discussed, injury to the brain also impairs the autoregulation mechanisms, and higher cerebral perfusion pressures are required to maintain adequate cerebral blood flow. Severely injured areas of the brain can lose almost all ability to autoregulate. In these areas, the blood vessels become dilated, causing hyperemia and shunting of blood toward the most severely injured brain areas and away from areas that could still be saved by adequate perfusion.[46,47] Finally, aggressive hyperventilation can further threaten cerebral blood flow and compound the ischemic threat by constricting blood vessels to compromised and unaffected areas of the brain.

This combination of physiologic downregulation, shunting, and hemorrhagic shock creates multiple ischemic threats to the salvageable areas of the brain and makes the aggressive management of hypotension an essential part of the management of TBI. For this reason, an aggressive approach in the prehospital environment, with prehospital fluid resuscitation aimed at keeping the systolic blood pressure above 110 mm Hg, is essential to limiting secondary injury in the brain-injured patient.

Hypoxia and Hyperoxia

One of the most critical substrates delivered to the injured brain by the circulation is oxygen. Irreversible brain damage can occur after only 4 to 6 minutes of cerebral anoxia. Studies have also demonstrated a profound impact of an oxygen saturation of hemoglobin (SpO_2) less than 90% in TBI patients.[8,11,23] A significant number of TBI patients present with low or inadequate SpO_2, which may be easily missed without the use of pulse oximetry.[38] The emphasis on prehospital airway management and oxygen delivery for brain-injured patients has been partly the result of these studies. Adequate ventilation and blood flow are critical in maintaining adequate oxygen delivery to the brain. One study of patients with severe TBI demonstrated a mortality rate of 26.9% if neither hypoxemia nor hypotension occurred, 28% with hypoxemia alone, and 57.2% if both were noted.[48] Therefore, prehospital care practitioners ensure adequate circulation by minimizing blood loss and provide adequate oxygenation by maintaining a patent airway and adequate ventilation.

It is important to note that too much concentrated oxygen delivery, or hyperoxia, has also been associated with worse outcomes. The administration of 100% oxygen may cause cerebral vasoconstriction, which may subsequently alter cerebral metabolism. The few available studies evaluating the effects of high levels of FiO_2 and high PaO_2 have demonstrated poor functional outcomes and higher mortality rates.[49-51] These studies suggest that there is likely an ideal therapeutic window for PaO_2 levels after TBI between 100 and 200 mm Hg. However, although both hyperoxia and hypoxia outside of normal ranges can be detrimental, hypoxia is considered to be more dangerous on even a transient basis and should be prevented whenever possible.

Anemia

The oxygen-carrying capacity of the blood is determined by the amount of hemoglobin it contains; hence, anemia results in lower hemoglobin levels, which impacts oxygen delivery to the brain. A 50% drop in hemoglobin has a much more profound effect on oxygen delivery to the brain than a 50% drop in the partial pressure of oxygen (PaO_2). For this reason, anemia from blood loss directly impacts TBI.[52]

Coagulopathy

Trauma, and TBI itself, has been associated with the induction of coagulopathy, including platelet dysfunction and alterations in fibrinogen and coagulation factors, which results in impaired clot formation. These hemostatic alterations contribute to hemorrhagic progression in TBI and are associated with higher morbidity and mortality compared to noncoagulopathic TBI patients.[53,54]

A major risk factor for worsening coagulopathy includes the use of preinjury anticoagulant and/or antiplatelet therapy, which is increasingly being prescribed for several indications in the elderly population. The highest incidence of TBI occurs in this population due to falls, and older patients who are currently taking anticoagulants have a threefold higher mortality and higher frequency of unfavorable 6-month outcomes compared to those without preinjury anticoagulant or antiplatelet therapy. One study demonstrated a mortality rate of 35.2% in anticoagulated patients versus 11.6% in nonanticoagulated patients.[54] It is therefore extremely important to ascertain whether patients are on preinjury anticoagulant or antiplatelet therapy so that the coagulopathy can be addressed as soon as possible to limit the progression of hemorrhage (**Table 8-4**). Prothrombin complex concentrate is most commonly used to rapidly reverse anticoagulants, and desmopressin to reverse antiplatelet medications.[55]

Studies have evaluated the effects of tranexamic acid (TXA) in patients with TBI. Tranexamic acid prevents fibrin clot breakdown and is often used to reduce bleeding. It is given as a loading dose of 1 gram over 10 minutes, followed by an infusion of 1 gram over 8 hours. The CRASH-2 trial demonstrated that early administration of TXA to bleeding trauma patients significantly reduced death due to bleeding by about 30% and all-cause mortality by about 20%.[56] Subgroup analysis of the CRASH-2

Table 8-4 Common Anticoagulant Medications

Drug Class	Examples	Reversal Agents
Vitamin K antagonist	Warfarin	Vitamin K Prothrombin complex concentrate (PCC)
Indirect thrombin inhibitor	Heparin Low molecular weight heparins (LMWH)	Protamine sulfate
Indirect factor Xa inhibitor	Fondaparinux	N/A
Direct-acting oral anticoagulant (DOAC)		PCC
Direct thrombin inhibitor	Argatroban Bivalirudin Dabigatran	Idarucizumab
Factor Xa inhibitor	Apixaban Rivaroxaban	Andexanet
Antiplatelet agent	Aspirin Clopidogrel Prasugrel	Desmopressin

Data from Yee J, Kaide CG. Emergency reversal of anticoagulation. *West J Emerg Med.* 2019;20(5):770-783. doi:10.5811/westjem.2018.5.38235

trial showed less intracranial hematoma expansion, fewer new intracranial hemorrhages, fewer new focal ischemic lesions, and trended toward improved mortality with TXA administration in bleeding patients with TBI, although the latter was not statistically significant.[57]

The follow-up 2019 CRASH-3 trial specifically looked at patients with TBI and found that rapid TXA treatment in the hospital (within 3 hours of injury) reduced head injury deaths in those with mild to moderate TBI. There was no effect in severe TBI.[58,59] A more recent multicenter cohort study (nonrandomized) evaluated outcomes in patients receiving prehospital TXA and found a substantially and statistically significantly higher 30-day mortality among those who received prehospital TXA.[60] Due to the controversial and limited data regarding the use of TXA in the prehospital setting, TXA is not currently recommended for use in the prehospital setting *except* in long prehospital transport times when definitive care will not be available for an extended period of time.

Hypocapnia and Hypercapnia

As discussed earlier in this chapter, both hypocapnia (decreased $PaCO_2$) and hypercapnia (increased $PaCO_2$) can worsen brain injury. When cerebral blood vessels constrict from significant hypocapnia, cerebral blood flow is compromised, leading to a decrease in oxygen delivery to the brain. Hypercapnia can result from hypoventilation from many causes, including drug or alcohol intoxication and abnormal ventilation patterns seen in patients with seizure and increased ICP. Hypercapnia causes cerebral vasodilation, which can further increase ICP.

Hypocapnia occurs as a result of hyperventilation, typically in patients who are mechanically ventilated. Hypocapnia causes cerebral vasoconstriction, which decreases cerebral blood volume and ICP. However, it also increases cerebral vascular resistance, which reduces cerebral blood flow and can cause further ischemia of the brain. Brain Trauma Foundation guidelines do not recommend prophylactic hyperventilation (with $PaCO_2$ of 25 mm Hg or less).[15,21-23] Ideally, normocapnia should be maintained to prevent the detrimental effects of both hypocapnia and hypercapnia.

Hypoglycemia and Hyperglycemia

When cerebral blood flow decreases, there is a decrease in oxygen delivery, as well as a decrease in the delivery of glucose and other necessary brain metabolites. Glucose is the primary fuel source of the adult brain, and changes in cerebral glucose metabolism are a hallmark response to TBI. Imaging studies have demonstrated a rapid transient increase in glucose uptake shortly after injury, followed by a prolonged period of depressed glucose metabolism. Glucose metabolism depression is greater in severely injured TBI patients, and the duration of this depression increases with age. The location of depressed metabolism is important, as higher metabolic rates in the thalamus, brain stem, and cerebellum have a significant positive correlation with levels of consciousness.[61-64]

Both elevations (hyperglycemia) and decreases (hypoglycemia) in blood glucose can jeopardize ischemic brain tissue. The disastrous impact of significant hypoglycemia on the nervous system, during injury and at other times, is well known. Because neurons are unable to store glucose, they require a continual supply of glucose to carry out cellular metabolism. In the absence of glucose, ischemic neurons can be permanently damaged. However, it is also true that a prolonged serum glucose level greater than 150 milligrams/deciliter (mg/dL), and probably greater than 200 mg/dL, may be harmful to the injured brain. Elevated blood glucose levels have been associated with poorer neurologic outcomes and should therefore be avoided.[65,66]

In the prehospital environment, hypoglycemia must be immediately assessed for and treated because the physiologic threat from low glucose is much more immediate than the danger from elevated serum glucose. Blood glucose measurement should be performed in the field in all patients with altered mentation and, if found to be below normal values, treated with intravenous (IV) or intramuscular glucose administration. In addition, any induced hyperglycemia is likely to be transient, and the tight glucose control required to manage these patients properly will be established upon admission to the hospital.

Seizures

A patient with acute TBI is at risk for seizures. Generalized seizure activity may be induced in the TBI patient due to hypoxia secondary to impaired ventilation, hypoglycemia, and electrolyte abnormalities. Additionally, ischemic or damaged brain tissue can serve as an irritable focus to produce partial or generalized seizures and/or **status epilepticus**. Seizures may aggravate preexisting hypoxia caused by impairment of respiratory function. The massive neuronal activity associated with generalized seizures rapidly depletes oxygen and glucose levels, further worsening cerebral ischemia.

Assessment and Management

A quick survey of the physics of trauma that caused the injury, combined with a rapid primary survey and subsequent secondary survey, will help identify potential life-threatening problems in a patient with suspected TBI. It is also critical to continually reassess these patients, perhaps more often than usual, because the pathophysiology of TBI is a dynamic process. Examination findings may fluctuate significantly as the condition of the patient changes over time.

Physics of Trauma

Knowledge of injury mechanisms is critical with all trauma patients, as it can aid in identifying specific injury patterns, especially in TBI. Key data about the physics of trauma will frequently come from observation of the scene or from bystanders. The windshield of the patient's vehicle may have a "spiderweb" pattern, suggesting an impact with the patient's head, or a bloody object may be present that was used as a weapon during an assault. A lateral impact on the side of the head can cause fracture

of the temporal bone of the skull with injury to the underlying middle meningeal artery, leading to epidural hematoma. High-impact injuries or rapid acceleration–deceleration injuries, such as high-speed MVCs, can result in a coup-contrecoup injuries. This important information should be reported to personnel at the receiving facility because it may be essential for proper diagnosis and management of the patient, not only as it relates to possible brain injury but also for other injuries.

Primary Survey

Effective management of a patient with TBI begins with orderly interventions focused on treating any life-threatening problems identified in the primary survey. Airway, breathing, and circulation are the very first assessments in the primary survey. Once these problems are addressed, the patient should be rapidly packaged and transported to the nearest facility capable of caring for TBI (**Box 8-1**).

Box 8-1 Alcohol Use and TBI

Alcohol use is a known risk factor for TBI, particularly subdural hematoma.[67,68] Multiple factors contribute to this known increase in risk. Physical shrinkage of the brain (cerebral atrophy) is commonly seen in patients who chronically ingest moderate to heavy volumes of alcohol over long periods. As the volume of the brain decreases, increasing tension is placed on the bridging veins, similar to how the cables on a suspension bridge hold the roadway in place. As this tension increases, it takes less shearing force to cause damage. Heavy alcohol consumption is also known to reduce clotting ability due to interference with the liver's ability to effectively produce clotting factors.[69]

Patients with a history of alcohol abuse or those who are acutely intoxicated may lack the ability to fully articulate the perceived extent of their injuries. This can confound physical assessment findings and make them less reliable—possibly obscuring the manifestations of a serious head injury.

The combined influence of these factors in individuals with a history of alcohol abuse or acute alcohol intoxication should lead to a lower threshold of suspicion for serious TBI in these patients. The forces necessary to cause serious injury in these patients may be significantly lower than those necessary to cause injury in individuals without a known history of alcohol abuse. Even patients who have suffered relatively minor head trauma should be evaluated fully, and transport to the hospital for in-depth medical evaluation should be strongly encouraged.

Exsanguinating Hemorrhage

The primary survey is the first assessment of any trauma patient, including a patient with TBI. The orderly, structured approach is the same for all trauma patients and begins with identification and control of exsanguinating hemorrhage. Airway and breathing are addressed either next or concurrently if sufficient resources are available on scene to address them without delaying the primary goal of achieving control of exsanguinating hemorrhage.

Direct pressure or pressure dressings should be applied to any external hemorrhage. Complex scalp wounds can produce significant external blood loss. Several gauze pads held in place by an elastic roller bandage create an effective pressure dressing to control bleeding. If this approach fails to control bleeding, the bleeding can often be controlled by applying direct pressure along the wound edges, thereby compressing the scalp vasculature between the skin and soft tissues and the galea. A pressure dressing should not be applied to a depressed or open skull fracture unless significant hemorrhage is present, because it may aggravate brain injury and lead to an increase in ICP. Direct gentle pressure may also limit the size of extracranial (scalp) hematomas.

Airway

The patency of the patient's airway is immediately examined and ensured. Patients with a depressed level of consciousness may be unable to protect their airway. Adequate oxygenation of the injured brain is critical to preventing secondary injury. Manual and simple airway skills, such as the jaw-thrust maneuver, are appropriate initial airway interventions. (See Chapter 7, *Airway and Ventilation*.) In unconscious individuals, the tongue may completely occlude the airway. Noisy ventilations indicate partial obstruction by either the tongue or foreign material. Emesis, hemorrhage, hematomas, and swelling from facial trauma are common causes of airway compromise in patients with TBI, and intermittent suctioning may be necessary.

Patients with facial fractures and laryngeal or other neck injuries will typically assume positions that maintain their airways. Attempts to force a patient to lie supine or wear a cervical collar may be met with extreme combativeness if the patient becomes hypoxic as a result of positional airway impairment. In these situations, airway patency takes precedence over spinal motion restriction, and patients may be transported in a partially upright position.[70] Cervical collars may also be deferred if thought to compromise the airway, although manual stabilization of the spine should still be provided. Conscious patients can often assist in managing their own airways by suctioning themselves when they feel it is needed. Facial trauma, including those injuries caused by gunshot wounds, is not a contraindication to endotracheal intubation; however, in some cases these patients may need to be managed using cricothyroidotomy.

Managing the airway is considered to be the first treatment priority after control of exsanguinating hemorrhage, and prehospital endotracheal intubation is traditionally advocated for patients who cannot protect their airway due to a severely depressed mental status. However, this prehospital intervention is controversial. Some studies support improved functional outcomes for those intubated in the field. However, other studies have suggested that prehospital endotracheal intubation may be associated with increased mortality.[71-77] A 2015 meta-analysis demonstrated that prehospital intubation by practitioners with limited experience was associated with a twofold increase in the odds of mortality, whereas intubation by experienced practitioners demonstrated no difference in mortality.[78] Several factors likely contribute to the higher mortality rates associated with inexperienced practitioners, including unrecognized episodes of hypoxia and/or hypotension. Prolonged or failed intubation attempts result in hypoxia, and medications used to facilitate intubation have hemodynamic effects, including hypotension. After successful intubation, inappropriate ventilation, including unintentional hyperventilation, can induce cerebral vasoconstriction and further complicate the patient's course.[73] Poorly performed intubation or poorly managed ventilation after intubation both appear to be more harmful than no intubation at all.

Furthermore, any delays in reaching the hospital and receiving definitive surgical intervention are associated with poorer outcomes. In urban settings, short transport times allow patients to be managed using alternate techniques and delivered fairly urgently to the ED, where the airway can be definitively managed in a more controlled setting. Conversely, in systems with longer transport times, intubation may be more beneficial than no intubation at all, even when done by a less experienced prehospital care practitioner. It is important to note that all studies have demonstrated the importance of practitioner experience in overall outcomes. Intubations by experienced practitioners do not increase scene time or total prehospital time and are associated with significantly lower mortality.[78,79] As such, the decision to intubate a patient depends on both the length of transport and prehospital care practitioner experience.

With these qualifiers in mind, prehospital care practitioners should consider active airway management for all patients who cannot protect their airway due to a severely depressed mental status. Such management can be extremely challenging due to patient combativeness, clenched jaw muscles (trismus), vomiting, and the need to maintain in-line cervical spine stabilization. As a result, intubation, if that is the method of airway management chosen, should be performed by the most skilled practitioner available. It is essential that the patient's SpO_2 be monitored continuously, and hypoxia (SpO_2 less than 90%) be avoided. Blind nasotracheal intubation can serve as an alternative technique, but the presence of midface trauma is a relative contraindication due to the possibility of inadvertent cranial and cerebral penetration with the nasotracheal tube in these patients. However, this complication is rare and has been reported only twice in head trauma patients.[80,81]

The use of neuromuscular blocking agents as part of a rapid-sequence intubation (RSI) protocol may facilitate successful intubation.[82] However, the safety and efficacy of RSI in the prehospital setting is undetermined. RSI with the use of lidocaine, fentanyl, and/or esmolol as premedication has not been demonstrated to decrease morbidity or mortality. However, some studies demonstrate that even though RSI improves intubation success, it can contribute to worse outcomes. Consequently, the routine use of paralytics in patients who are spontaneously breathing and maintaining SpO_2 greater than 90% on supplemental oxygen is not recommended.[48]

There is no single ideal airway management technique that is preferred over any other. Instead, manual and simple airway skills should be used as initial interventions, and complex airway interventions should be performed only if the airway cannot be maintained by less invasive means. In many cases, bag-mask ventilation with a nasal or oral airway is sufficient to oxygenate and ventilate the patient. Suction equipment should always be readily available. Airway management interventions and TBI will often precipitate episodes of vomiting. Prolonged attempts at complex airway interventions should be avoided, especially with a short transport time.

Breathing

Evaluation of respiratory function includes an assessment of the rate, depth, and adequacy of breathing. As noted previously, several different breathing patterns can result from severe brain injury, including disordered control of breathing secondary to seizure. In multisystem trauma patients, thoracic injuries can further impair both oxygenation and ventilation. Cervical spine fractures occur in about 2% to 5% of patients with TBI and may result in spinal cord injuries that significantly interfere with ventilation. Adjuncts described previously in the "Airway" section may be used to help obtain a definitive airway to assist with breathing, as with intubation and ventilation, or by using a bag-valve mask to support respiration and air exchange as needed.

Adequate oxygen delivery to the injured brain is essential to minimize secondary brain injury. Maintaining SpO_2 above 90% is critical; failure to do so results in poorer outcomes for brain-injured patients. All patients should be monitored with continuous pulse oximetry because hypoxia is often difficult to clinically detect otherwise. Oxygen concentration can be titrated by pulse oximetry for a goal SpO_2 of at least 90%, although 94% or higher is optimal. If hypoxia persists despite oxygen therapy, the prehospital care practitioner should attempt to identify and treat all likely etiologies, including aspiration and tension pneumothoraces. Use of positive end-expiratory pressure (PEEP), if available, may be considered to improve oxygenation. However, levels of PEEP greater than 15 centimeters of water (cm H_2O) may increase ICP.[83,84]

Because both hypocapnia and hypercapnia can aggravate TBI, controlling the ventilation rate is important.[48,85,86] In the hospital, arterial blood gases (ABGs) are available to directly measure and maintain $PaCO_2$ in a normal range of 35 to 40 mm Hg. However, ABGs and $PaCO_2$ are not routinely available in the prehospital environment. **Capnometry** is a useful alternative that can be used in the prehospital setting when ABGs are unavailable. It measures end-tidal carbon dioxide ($ETCO_2$), which is the maximum partial pressure of CO_2 obtained at the end of an exhaled breath. Studies have shown that $ETCO_2$ correlates well with $PaCO_2$, especially in healthy, hemodynamically stable patients. There is a potential discrepancy between $ETCO_2$ and $PaCO_2$ in severely traumatized patients due to potential instability in pulmonary perfusion, cardiac output, and patient temperature, which can result in lower $ETCO_2$ compared to $PaCO_2$. However, studies evaluating the use of $ETCO_2$ in TBI have demonstrated that $ETCO_2$ is still a reliable reflection of $PaCO_2$ and should be used in the prehospital setting to guide ventilation and prevent both hypocapnia and hypercapnia, especially when ABGs are not available.[87-97]

Normal ventilatory rates should be used when assisting ventilation in patients with TBI: 10 breaths/minute for adults, 20 breaths/minute for children, and 25 breaths/minute for infants. Excessively fast ventilatory rates and subsequent hypocapnia produce cerebral vasoconstriction, which, in turn, leads to a decrease in cerebral oxygen delivery. Routine prophylactic hyperventilation has been shown to worsen neurologic outcomes and should not be used. Both hyperventilation and severe hypoxia in the prehospital setting were associated with an increase in mortality. For adult patients, ventilating with a tidal volume of 350 to 500 mL at a rate of 10 breaths/minute should be sufficient to maintain adequate oxygenation without inducing hypocarbia.[48]

Hyperventilation of a patient in a controlled fashion may be considered in the specific circumstance of signs of herniation as discussed previously. These signs include asymmetric pupils, dilated and nonreactive pupils, extensor posturing or no response on motor examination, progressive neurologic deterioration, and the development of a Cushing reflex. In such cases, mild, controlled hyperventilation in the field may be performed during the prehospital phase of care. Mild hyperventilation is defined as an $ETCO_2$ of 30 to 35 mm Hg as measured by capnography or by careful control of the ventilatory rate (20 breaths/minute for adults, 25 breaths/minute for children, and 30 breaths/minute for infants younger than 1 year of age).[48]

Circulation

Blood loss resulting in hypotension is an important cause of secondary brain injury, so efforts should be made to prevent or treat these conditions. Maintaining a systolic blood pressure of at least 110 mm Hg is critical to preventing secondary brain injury. Understanding local protocols is critical in this situation because maintaining an SBP of greater than 110 mm Hg is preferred, but must be weighed

against the risk of excessive crystalloid administration and increased hemorrhage from noncompressible sources. In isolated TBI, maintaining SBP greater than 110 mm Hg in adults has been associated with improved outcomes.

Historically, SBP thresholds for pediatric patients were calculated using the formula: SBP = 70 + (2 × age in years).[98] However, these calculated thresholds are lower than the 75th percentile, and SBP less than 75th percentile has been associated with higher risk of in-hospital mortality in isolated severe TBI. **Table 8-5** compares the SBP thresholds based on calculated formulas.[99] As such, in the case of isolated TBI in the pediatric population, SBP should be maintained at greater than the 75th percentile for age.

Any external hemorrhage should be immediately controlled to prevent and/or minimize hypotension.

Table 8-5 Pediatric Systolic Blood Pressure Thresholds by Age

Age (years)	ATLS Definition: 70 +(2 × Age in Years) (mm Hg)	Systolic Blood Pressure 75th Percentile (mm Hg)	
		Boys	Girls
0	70	92	84
1	72	92	85
2	74	95	86
3	76	98	89
4	78	100	90
5	80	102	92
6	82	103	94
7	84	104	96
8	86	106	97
9	88	107	99
10	90	109	101
11	90	111	103
12	90	113	105
13	90	115	107
14	90	118	108
15	90	120	109
16	90	123	109
17	90	125	109

Age Group	Systolic Blood Pressure 75th Percentile (mm Hg)	
	Boys	Girls
Infant (0–12 months)	92	84
Toddler (1–2 years)	92–95	85–86
Preschool (3–5 years)	98–102	89–92
School age (6–12 years)	103–113	94–105
Adolescent (≥ 13 years)	115–125	107–109

© National Association of Emergency Medical Technicians (NAEMT)

Uncontrolled bleeding from a scalp injury can be an unrecognized cause of hemorrhagic shock and should be treated with application of direct pressure or a pressure dressing. If possible, the prehospital care practitioner should note and quantify evidence of external bleeding, and this information should be provided in the report to the receiving facility. In the absence of significant external blood loss, a weak, rapid pulse in a victim of blunt trauma suggests life-threatening internal hemorrhage in the pleural spaces, peritoneum, retroperitoneum, or soft tissues surrounding long-bone fractures. In an infant with open fontanelles, sufficient blood loss can occur inside the cranium to produce hypovolemic shock.

Because hypotension further worsens brain ischemia, standard measures should be employed to combat shock. In patients with TBI, the combination of hypoxia and hypotension is associated with a high mortality rate. If shock is present and major internal hemorrhage is suspected, prompt transport to a trauma center takes priority over other interventions. To preserve cerebral perfusion, adequate fluid should be given to maintain a systolic blood pressure of at least 110 mm Hg.[98] However, transport should not be delayed to establish IV access.

A randomized trial of patients with severe TBI showed that those who received prehospital resuscitation with hypertonic saline had almost identical neurologic functioning 6 months after injury compared to those treated with crystalloid.[100] Because of its increased cost and lack of benefit compared to normal saline or lactated Ringer solution, hypertonic saline is not recommended for routine prehospital volume replacement.

Autoregulation mechanisms to maintain cerebral perfusion pressure in the setting of increased ICP can lead to a recognized series of cardiovascular changes, mainly manifested as increased blood pressure. Attempts to treat hypertension should be avoided, because this will result in decreased cerebral perfusion pressure in the setting of high ICP, causing secondary brain injury. As discussed earlier, the Cushing phenomenon may be seen in severe intracranial hypertension, which is the combination of bradycardia, increased blood pressure associated with a widened pulse pressure, and irregular respirations, such as Cheyne-Stokes breathing.[39] These findings may indicate impending herniation. In a patient with potentially life-threatening injuries, transport should not be delayed for blood pressure measurements; it should be performed en route, as time permits.

Disability

After the initiation of appropriate measures to treat problems identified during the primary survey, a rapid neurologic examination should be performed. This includes obtaining a baseline GCS score and pupillary assessment. The GCS score is calculated by using the best response noted when evaluating the patient's eyes, verbal response, and motor response status. Each component of the score should be recorded individually, rather than just providing a total, so that specific changes can be noted over time (**Table 8-6**).[98,101,102] How to determine a patient's GCS score is covered in detail in Chapter 6, *Patient Assessment and Management*.

The GCS score is helpful to evaluate the patient's status and may impact transport and triage decisions. It can help to classify the severity of TBI and whether the patient's airway is patent and stable in the setting of a TBI. The lowest total GCS score is 3 and maximum total score is 15. A total GCS score of 13 to 15 likely indicates a mild TBI, whereas a score of 9 to 12 is indicative of moderate TBI. A GCS score of 3 to 8 suggests severe TBI. Standard guidelines recommend intubation for GCS scores equal to or less than 8.[48,103] Many other factors can also affect the GCS score, including the presence of intoxicants or other drugs.

The most critical portion of the GCS score is the motor score. Studies have demonstrated equal sensitivity and specificity between both motor and total GCS scores for neurologic assessment and prognostication. Obtaining

Table 8-6 Glasgow Coma Scale

Subcategory	Classification	Points
Eye opening	Spontaneous	4
	To sound	3
	To pressure	2
	None	1
Verbal response	Oriented	5
	Confused	4
	Words	3
	Sounds	2
	None	1
Motor response	Obey commands	6
	Localizing	5
	Normal flexion	4
	Abnormal flexion	3
	Extension	2
	None	1

© National Association of Emergency Medical Technicians (NAEMT)

the motor score in the prehospital setting is especially important because it is a dynamic score that often deteriorates from the field to the hospital. Admission values are often different than field values due to intubation, paralysis, and/or sedation, making the full GCS score less reliable. Studies have demonstrated that the field GCS motor score predicts 6-month mortality better than admission motor scores. Given these findings and the simplicity of determining the motor score, use of the motor score alone has been advocated in the prehospital triage setting.[103,104]

In addition to determining the GCS score, the pupils are examined quickly for symmetry and response to light. In adults, the resting pupil diameter is generally between 3 and 5 mm.[105] A difference of greater than 1 mm in pupil size is considered abnormal. A fixed pupil is defined as a response to bright light of less than 1 mm.[48] The combination of motor GCS score and admission pupillary reactivity has been demonstrated to accurately assess and predict TBI outcomes (**Box 8-2**). Acute pupillary dilation indicates a neurologic emergency and can suggest brain stem ischemia and/or uncal herniation. Uncal herniation from brain edema or mass effect can cause compression of the oculomotor

nerve (CN III), resulting in pupil dilation. Decreased blood flow to the brain stem and brain stem ischemia also cause pupillary dilation. Of note, a portion of the population has **anisocoria**, or unequal pupils, which is either congenital or acquired as the result of ophthalmic trauma. However, it is not always possible in the field to distinguish between pupillary inequality caused by trauma and congenital or preexisting posttraumatic anisocoria. Therefore, pupillary inequality should always be treated as secondary to the acute trauma until the appropriate workup has ruled out cerebral edema or motor or ophthalmic nerve injury.[106]

Because of the significant incidence of cervical spine fractures, spinal motion restriction should be applied for patients with suspected TBI as a result of blunt trauma. Some degree of caution must be exercised when applying a cervical collar to a patient with TBI, because a tightly fitted cervical collar can impede venous drainage of the head, thereby increasing ICP. *Application of a cervical collar is not mandatory as long as motion of the head and neck are sufficiently restricted.* Spinal immobilization is not recommended for victims of gunshot wounds to the head.

Expose/Environment

Patients who have sustained a TBI frequently have other injuries that threaten life and limb as well as the brain. All such injuries must be identified. The entire body should be examined for other potentially life-threatening problems.

Secondary Survey

Once life-threatening injuries have been identified and managed, a thorough secondary survey should be completed if time permits. The patient's head and face should be palpated carefully for wounds, depressions, and **crepitus**. The pupillary size and response should be rechecked at this time. Because of the incidence of associated cervical spine fractures in patients with TBI, as noted previously, the neck should be examined for tenderness and bony deformities. Any drainage of clear fluid from the nose or ear canals may be CSF. In most cases, however, the CSF will be mixed with blood, making formal recognition of this finding difficult. Specific head and neck injuries are discussed next.

In a cooperative patient, a more thorough neurologic examination may also be performed. This will include assessing the cranial nerves, sensation, and motor function in all extremities. Looking for complete or partial deficits as well as asymmetry in function may reveal important clues to a possible neurologic injury. Findings such as **hemiparesis** (weakness) or **hemiplegia** (paralysis) present on only one side of the body are considered "lateralizing signs" and usually are indicative of TBI.

Box 8-2 Refusal of Treatment

Patients who refuse medical treatment and/or transport are encountered frequently by emergency medical services (EMS) professionals. These encounters become more complicated when EMS professionals believe that it is in the patient's best interest to be transported and assessed at a hospital, yet the patient refuses and demonstrates no signs of neurologic impairment or deficit at the time of assessment. Often, TBI patients with severe mechanisms of injury may not experience the full severity of their injuries until hours or days later. Consider patients with an epidural bleed, where there is often a lucid interval, during which the patient feels well, before suffering the potentially fatal effects of hemorrhage hours later.

Patients who have suffered a possible head injury should be evaluated fully, with particular attention being paid to their decision-making capacity. In addition, the following signs and symptoms indicate the need for further medical attention, and this should be communicated to the patient:

- Unequal pupils
- Worsening headache
- Nausea and vomiting
- Drowsiness or difficulty wakening
- Slurring of speech
- Confusion or change in behavior
- Loss of consciousness
- Seizures
- Numbness
- Decreased coordination
- Trouble recognizing people or locations

© National Association of Emergency Medical Technicians (NAEMT)

When the EMS practitioner feels that it is in the best interest of the patient to be transported to the hospital for further assessment and a patient with full decision-making capacity refuses transport, every attempt should be made to clearly articulate the risks of refusal and benefits of care. This includes very direct warnings about the possibility of death and permanent disability that can result from delayed medical care if appropriate. Contacting medical direction sooner rather than later in these situations can be helpful, as patients may be more willing to listen to the advice of a physician in some cases. In the event that patients still refuse transport and further treatment, it should be made clear that they can change their minds at any time and EMS will be available to return and evaluate them.

When patients do not clearly possess full decision-making capacity, medical direction and law enforcement should be involved to the extent necessary to help facilitate what is in the patient's best interests—transporting them to the hospital for further evaluation.

Protocols, medical direction instructions, and local legal statutes should always be followed when making treatment decisions. Discussions regarding the proper course of action to take in scenarios similar to those discussed here are best had before the incident takes place and should be routinely incorporated into continuing education and initial employee training. The dictum of "first do no harm" should be foundational in the approach to care for all patients encountered by EMS professionals. Patients with questionable capacity are certainly no exception.

Specific Head and Neck Injuries

Scalp Injuries

As noted in the anatomy section, the scalp is composed of multiple layers of tissue and is highly vascular. Injuries can vary from simple small lacerations to complex injuries such as a degloving injury, in which a large area of the scalp is torn back from the skull. It is important to take note of how much blood loss occurred on scene from scalp injuries. Uncontrolled hemorrhage from these injuries can result in hypovolemic shock and even **exsanguination (Figure 8-11)**. This type of injury often occurs in an unrestrained front-seat occupant of a vehicle whose head impacts the windshield, as well as in workers

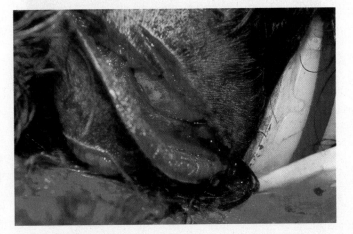

Figure 8-11 Extensive scalp injuries may result in massive external hemorrhage.
Courtesy of Peter T. Pons, MD, FACEP.

whose long hair becomes caught in machinery. A serious blow to the head may result in the formation of a scalp hematoma, which may be confused with a depressed skull fracture while palpating the scalp. Scalp hematomas may signify the concomitant presence of underlying intracranial injury.

Skull Fractures

Skull fractures can result from either blunt or penetrating trauma. Linear fractures are usually from blunt trauma. However, a powerful impact may produce a depressed skull fracture, in which fragments of bone are driven toward or into the underlying brain tissue (**Figure 8-12**). Although simple linear fractures can only be diagnosed with a radiographic study, depressed skull fractures can be palpated during a careful physical examination. A closed, nondepressed skull fracture by itself is of little clinical significance, but its presence increases the risk of an intracranial hematoma. Closed depressed skull fractures may require neurosurgical intervention because the decrease in intracranial space caused by the encroaching fracture results in increased ICP. As discussed earlier, skull fractures may cause extrinsic compression of dural venous sinuses, resulting in venous obstruction and subsequently increased ICP. Open skull fractures can result from a particularly forceful impact or a gunshot wound and serve as an entry site for bacteria, predisposing the patient to meningitis. If the dura mater is torn, brain tissue or CSF may leak from an open skull fracture. Because of the risk

of meningitis, these wounds require immediate neurosurgical evaluation.

Basilar skull fractures are fractures of the base of the skull that most commonly involve temporal bone fractures. These fractures can cause tears in membranes, resulting in leakage of CSF. In approximately 12% to 30% of basilar skull fractures, CSF can leak from the ears through a perforated eardrum (otorrhea) or from the nostrils (rhinorrhea).[107] Periorbital ecchymosis ("raccoon eyes") and Battle sign, in which ecchymosis is noted over the mastoid area behind the ears, can also occur with basilar skull fractures, although they may take several hours after the injury to become apparent. If permitted, examination of the tympanic membrane with an otoscope may reveal blood behind the eardrum, suggesting a basilar skull fracture.

Facial Injuries

Injuries to the face range from minor soft-tissue trauma to severe injuries associated with airway compromise or hypovolemic shock. The airway may be compromised by (1) structural damage, (2) extrinsic anatomic distortion from displaced and/or swollen tissue, or (3) obstruction by fluid or other objects within the airway. It is also important to note that the airway includes anything from the face to the carina of the tracheobronchial tree, and compromise can occur anywhere along this tract.[70] Structural changes may include deformities of fractured facial bones or hematomas that develop in the tissues. Because the head has a high concentration of blood vessels, injuries to this region frequently result in significant hemorrhage. Significant facial fractures are often associated with pooling of blood and secretions in the pharynx due to painful and less effective swallowing. The most common obstructing materials within the airway are blood and vomit. Facial trauma is often associated with alterations in consciousness and potentially severe trauma to the brain. Trauma to the face may result in fractures or displacement of teeth into the airway lumen. TBIs and swallowed blood from facial injuries may lead to vomiting, which may also lead to airway obstruction.

Trauma to the Eye and Orbit

Injury to the structures of the orbit and eye are common and often result from direct trauma to the face. Although injury of the globe (eyeball) itself is not often encountered, it must be considered whenever trauma to the face and orbit is noted, as proper management of a globe injury increases the salvage rate of the patient's vision.

Eyelid lacerations are treated by covering the eye with a protective rigid shield (*not* a pressure patch) that is placed over the bony orbit. No patching material should be placed under the shield. Eyelid lacerations can be associated with underlying globe injury. As such, the primary

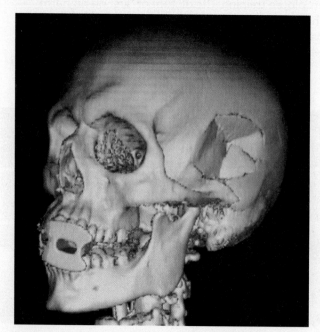

Figure 8-12 A three-dimensional reconstruction of a depressed skull fracture after an assault.
Courtesy of Peter T. Pons, MD, FACEP.

consideration is to avoid any pressure on the eye that might do further harm by forcing intraocular contents out through a corneal or scleral laceration.

A **corneal abrasion** is disruption of the protective epithelial covering of the cornea. This abrasion results in intense pain, tearing, light sensitivity (photophobia), and increased susceptibility to infection until the defect has healed (usually in 2 to 3 days). There is typically a history of antecedent trauma or contact lens use. Prehospital management for this disorder is to cover the eye with a patch, shield, or sunglasses to reduce the discomfort caused by light sensitivity.

Subconjunctival hemorrhage over the sclera of the eye results from bleeding between the **conjunctiva** and the **sclera** (**Figure 8-13**). It is easily visible without the use of diagnostic equipment. This injury is innocuous and resolves over a period of several days to several weeks without treatment. In the presence of antecedent trauma, one should be alert for another, more serious injury. For example, an occult globe rupture should be suspected if hemorrhage results in massive swelling of the conjunctiva, known as **chemosis**. Prehospital management of this disorder consists solely of transporting the patient to the hospital so that the diagnosis can be confirmed and other associated disorders ruled out.

Hyphema refers to blood in the anterior chamber of the globe between the **iris** and the **cornea**. This condition is usually seen in the setting of acute trauma from a direct blow to the eye. The eye should be examined with the patient sitting upright. If enough blood is present, the blood collects at the bottom of the anterior chamber and is visible as a layered hyphema (**Figure 8-14**). This blood may not be appreciated if the victim is examined while in a supine position or if the amount of blood is very small. A protective shield should be placed over the eye and the patient should be transported to the hospital in a sitting position (if there is no other contraindication) so that the blood can migrate to the inferior aspect of the anterior chamber and allow for a better examination of the anterior chamber and posterior segment of the eye when that is performed.

An **open globe** injury is a wound that goes through the cornea or sclera into the interior of the eyeball. If this is identified, the remainder of the eye examination should be discontinued and a protective shield immediately placed onto the bony orbit over the eye to protect it from further injury. Do *not* apply a pressure patch or instill any topical medication.

There are two primary concerns in the management of this condition. The first is to minimize manipulation of or additional trauma to the eye that might raise intraocular pressure and result in expulsion of intraocular contents through the corneal or scleral defect. The second is to prevent the development of **posttraumatic endophthalmitis**, an infection of the interior portion of the eye. This typically has devastating visual results. Expeditious transport to the hospital is warranted for ophthalmologic evaluation and surgical repair.

A penetrating injury to the eye or a ruptured globe may not always be obvious. Clues to occult rupture include the mechanism of injury (such as metal-on-metal hammering or eye injuries from weed-trimming tools) as well as clinical findings of large subconjunctival hemorrhage with chemosis, dark uveal tissue (the colored iris) present at or protruding through the junction of the cornea and the sclera, a distorted pupil (teardrop shaped), a leak from a lacerated or punctured corneal wound, or a decrease in vision. If an occult globe rupture is suspected, the patient should be treated as described previously for an obvious open globe. The relatively less severe appearance of the injury does not eliminate the threat of further injury to the eye from pressure (if subjected to

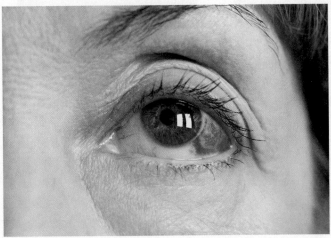

Figure 8-13 Subconjunctival hemorrhage.

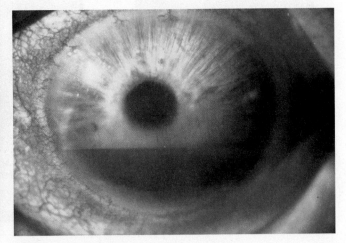

Figure 8-14 Hyphema.

external pressure) or endophthalmitis, so immediate shielding of the eye and rapid transport to the hospital are still essential.

Nasal Fractures

Fracture of the nasal bones is the most common fracture in the face. Indications that a nasal fracture is present include **ecchymosis**, **edema**, nasal deformity, swelling, and epistaxis (nosebleed). On palpation, bony crepitus may be noted.

High-force midface traumas may cause nasal bone fractures as well as fractures of the cribriform plate (the thin, horizontal bone in the skull through which the olfactory [CN I] nerve passes). Any clear rhinorrhea (CSF leak from the nose) occurring after significant force to the midface is significant for possible cribriform plate fracture.

Midface Fractures

Midface fractures can be categorized according to the Le Fort classification, shown in **Figure 8-15**.

- *Le Fort I fracture* involves a horizontal detachment of the maxilla from the nasal floor. Although air passage through the nares (nostrils) may not be affected, the oropharynx may be compromised by a blood clot or edema in the soft palate.
- *Le Fort II fracture*, also known as a pyramidal fracture, includes the right and left maxillae, the medial portion of the orbital floor(s), and the nasal bones. The sinuses are well vascularized, so this fracture may be associated with airway compromise from significant hemorrhage.
- *Le Fort III fracture* involves fractures that completely separate the facial bones from the skull (craniofacial disjunction). Because of the forces involved, this injury may be associated with airway compromise, presence of TBI, injuries to the tear ducts, malocclusion (misalignment) of teeth, and CSF leakage from the nares.

Patients with a midface fracture generally have loss of normal facial symmetry. The face may appear flattened, and the patient may be unable to close the jaws or teeth. If conscious, the patient may complain of facial pain and numbness. On palpation, crepitus may be noted over fracture sites. Displaced midface fractures can occasionally cause airway obstruction. High energy impacts to the fragile middle third of the facial skeleton can result in fragmented fractures that can collapse backwards and downwards, impacting posterior structures including the soft palate. This can result in swelling into the pharynx, potentially causing airway obstruction. Combined mandibular and middle third facial fractures are indicative of significant underlying injury, including associated brain injury and cervical spine injury.

Mandibular Fractures

Following fractures of the nasal bones, mandibular fractures are the second most common type of facial fracture. Often, the mandible (jawbone) is broken in more than one location. The most common complaint of a patient with a mandibular fracture, in addition to pain, is malocclusion of the teeth where the upper and lower teeth no longer meet in their usual alignment. Visual examination

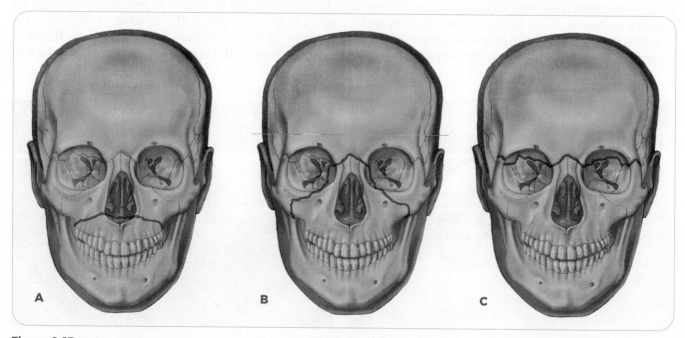

Figure 8-15 Types of Le Fort fractures of the midface. **A.** Le Fort I fracture. **B.** Le Fort II fracture. **C.** Le Fort III fracture.

may reveal a step-off or misalignment of the teeth. On palpation, a step-off type of deformity and crepitus may be noted. In a supine patient with a mandibular fracture, the tongue may occlude the airway as the bony support structure of the tongue is no longer intact.

Laryngeal Injuries

Fractures of the larynx typically result from a blunt blow to the anterior neck, such as when a motorcycle or bicycle rider's anterior neck is struck by an object. The patient may complain of a change in voice (usually lower in tone). On inspection, the prehospital care practitioner may note a neck contusion or loss of the prominence of the thyroid cartilage (Adam's apple). A fracture of the larynx may result in the patient coughing up blood (hemoptysis) or the development of subcutaneous emphysema in the neck, which may be detected on palpation. Endotracheal intubation is generally contraindicated in the presence of a laryngeal fracture because this procedure may dislodge fracture segments. If a patient with a suspected laryngeal fracture has a compromised airway, a surgical cricothyrotomy may be lifesaving.

Injuries to Cervical Vessels

A carotid artery and internal jugular vein traverse the anterior neck on either side of the trachea. The carotid arteries supply blood to the majority of the brain, and the internal jugular veins drain this region. Open injury to one of these vessels can produce profound hemorrhage. An added danger from internal jugular vein injuries is air embolism. If a patient is sitting up or the head is elevated, venous pressure may fall below atmospheric pressure during inspiration, permitting air to enter the venous system. A large air embolus can be fatal because it can interfere with both cardiac function and cerebral perfusion. An additional concern of trauma to the cervical vasculature is the development of an expanding hematoma that may lead to airway compromise as the hematoma expands and impinges on and distorts the normal airway anatomy. It may also cause jugular venous compression, occluding cerebral venous outflow and indirectly increasing ICP.

Blunt injury to the neck may also result in blunt cerebrovascular injury. These injuries can occur to the internal or common carotid artery or vertebral artery. Vertebral artery injuries are almost always associated with cervical spinal column injuries. Carotid injuries are associated with a number of other injuries including severe TBI, major facial fractures, basilar skull fractures, and major thoracic injury, among others. High-speed MVCs, direct blows to the neck, "clothesline" type injuries, and hangings place patients at risk of these injuries. These injuries can be highly morbid due to the risk of stroke.

Often these patients may manifest signs of stroke in the field and any unexplained neurologic deficit should prompt an evaluation for these injuries.[108]

History

A SAMPLER history (**S**ymptoms, **A**llergies, **M**edications, **P**ast medical history, **L**ast meal, **E**vents preceding the injury, **R**isk factors) should be obtained from the patient, family members, or bystanders if time and circumstances allow. Diabetes mellitus, seizure disorders, and drug or alcohol intoxication can mimic TBI or confound the evaluation of TBI. Any evidence of drug use or overdose should be noted, but the possibility of TBI should not be overlooked in the presence of intoxication. The use of antiplatelet and anticoagulation medications is also important to note, as it may change the management of TBI. The patient may have a history of prior head injury and may complain of persistent or recurring headache, visual disturbances, nausea and vomiting, or difficulty speaking.[96]

As previously discussed, it is important to take note of the events surrounding the trauma. This includes the mechanism of injury, any loss of consciousness, duration of unresponsiveness, any witnessed seizure activity and the subsequent level of alertness (postictal state). If the patient cannot recall the events, it can be helpful to determine the duration of amnesia of the events preceding (retrograde) or following (antegrade) the trauma.[98]

Serial Examinations

It is important to reevaluate the GCS score and determine what changes are occurring over time. The patient who initially presented with a GCS score that is now decreasing is of much greater concern for serious TBI than a patient who has an improving GCS score. A small number of patients with apparently mild brain injury (GCS score 14 or 15) may experience an unexpected deterioration in their mentation. During transport, both the primary survey and assessment of the GCS score should be repeated at frequent intervals. Patients whose GCS score deteriorates by more than two points during transport are at particularly high risk for an ongoing pathologic process.[106,109,110] These patients need rapid transport to an appropriate facility. The receiving facility will use GCS score trends during transport in the patient's early management. Trends in the GCS score or vital signs should be reported to the receiving facility and documented on the patient care report. Responses to management should also be recorded.[98,111]

Transport

To achieve the best possible outcome, patients with moderate and severe TBI should be transported directly to a trauma center that can perform CT imaging and provide prompt neurosurgical consultation and intervention (including ICP monitoring if indicated). If such a facility is not available, air medical transport from the scene to an appropriate trauma center should be considered.[111]

The patient's pulse rate, blood pressure, SpO_2, $ETCO_2$ when available, and GCS score should be reassessed and documented every 5 to 10 minutes during transport. PEEP valves may be used cautiously if persistent hypoxia exists up to levels of 15 cm of H_2O; PEEP greater than 15 cm H_2O may increase ICP. Normothermia should be maintained during transport. In general, patients with TBI should be transported in a supine position because of the presence of other injuries.[112] Although elevating the head on the ambulance stretcher or long backboard (reverse Trendelenburg position) may decrease ICP, cerebral perfusion pressure may also be jeopardized, especially if the head is elevated higher than 30 degrees.

The receiving facility should be notified as early as possible so that appropriate preparations can be made before the patient's arrival. The radio report should include information regarding the mechanism of injury, initial GCS score and any changes en route, focal signs (e.g., motor examination asymmetry, unilaterally or bilaterally dilated pupils) and vital signs, other serious injuries, and response to management.[113]

Prolonged Transport

Prolonged transport times may lower the threshold for performing advanced airway management. RSI may be used in this setting, especially if air medical transport is considered, because a combative patient in the confines of a helicopter represents a safety threat to everyone onboard. Efforts to control the airway should be performed while cervical spine stabilization is being applied. Oxygen should be administered to maintain an appropriate SpO_2 level. Because of the risk of developing pressure ulcers from lying on a hard backboard, appropriate padding should be used if a long backboard is employed for SMR, especially if the anticipated transport time is lengthy. Patients should be attached to continuous pulse oximetry, and serial vital signs, including ventilations, pulse, blood pressure, and GCS score, should be measured. Pupils should be periodically checked for response to light and symmetry.

When there is a delay in transport or a prolonged transport time to an appropriate facility, additional management options can be considered. For patients with an abnormal GCS score, the blood glucose level should be checked. If the patient is hypoglycemic, a 50% dextrose solution can be administered intravenously until the blood glucose is restored to a normal level. Benzodiazepines may be titrated intravenously if recurrent or prolonged seizures occur.

External hemorrhage should be controlled, and crystalloid fluids administered if signs of shock are apparent. Fluids should be titrated to maintain the systolic blood pressure greater than 110 mm Hg in the patient with suspected TBI. Associated injuries should be managed en route to the receiving facility. Fractures should be appropriately splinted to control both internal hemorrhage and pain. TXA can be considered in the setting of hemorrhage and suspected TBI only if there are prolonged transport times.

Appropriate management of increased ICP in the prehospital setting is extremely challenging because the ICP is not monitored in the field unless the patient is undergoing interfacility transfer and already has an ICP monitor or ventriculostomy in place. Although a declining GCS score may represent increasing ICP, it may also be the result of worsening cerebral perfusion from hypovolemic shock. Warning signs of possible increased ICP and herniation include the following:

- Decline in GCS score of two points or more
- Development of a sluggish or nonreactive pupil
- Development of hemiplegia or hemiparesis
- Cushing reflex

The decision to intervene and manage increased ICP is based on written protocol or made in consultation with medical oversight or online medical direction at the receiving facility. Possible temporizing management options include sedation, chemical paralysis, the use of osmotically active agents such as mannitol, and controlled hyperventilation (**Figure 8-16**). Small doses of benzodiazepine sedatives should be titrated cautiously because of the potential side effects of hypotension and ventilatory depression. Use of a long-acting neuromuscular blocking agent, such as vecuronium, may be considered if the patient is intubated. If the cervical collar is too tight, it may be loosened slightly or removed, provided that the head and neck are adequately immobilized with other measures. If feasible, the patient should be placed in reverse Trendelenburg, where the head is on a higher incline than the rest of the body to help facilitate cerebral venous drainage.

Hyperosmolar therapy, such as the use of hypertonic (3%) saline or mannitol (0.25 to 1.0 g/kg) can be used to lower ICP. Both medications are given intravenously. There is currently no good evidence to support its routine use in the prehospital setting.[114] Mannitol is a highly effective osmotic diuretic that may cause hypovolemia in patients who have not been systemically resuscitated; this may result in hypotension and thereby worsen cerebral perfusion. As such, it should not be used in patients with systolic blood pressures less than 90 mm Hg. Mannitol should be restricted to patients with signs of herniation and should be used with extreme caution.[15] In addition, a

Management of Suspected Traumatic Brain Injury

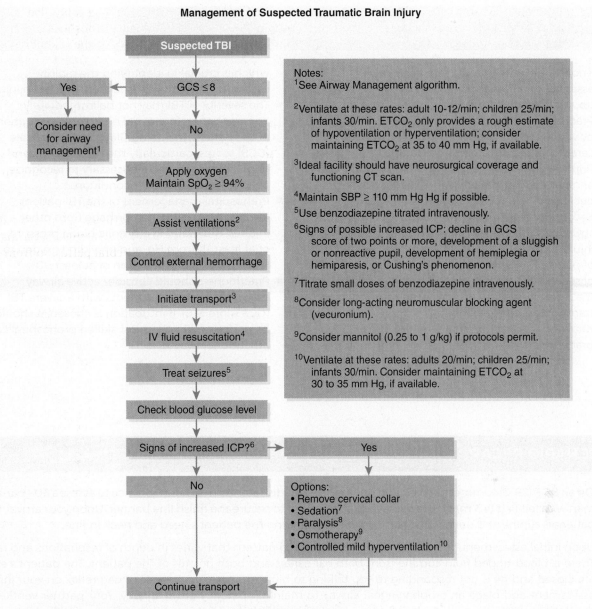

Figure 8-16 Management of suspected traumatic brain injury.
© National Association of Emergency Medical Technicians (NAEMT)

Foley catheter should be placed to monitor urine output if transport will be extremely prolonged.

An increased rate of ventilation (controlled, mild therapeutic hyperventilation) aimed at maintaining the $ETCO_2$ at 30 to 35 mm Hg may be considered for obvious signs of herniation. The following ventilatory rates should be used: 20 breaths/minute for adults, 25 breaths/minute for children, and 30 breaths/minute for infants. As stated previously, *prophylactic hyperventilation has no role in TBI, and therapeutic hyperventilation, if instituted, should be stopped if signs of intracranial hypertension resolve.* Steroids

have not been shown to improve the outcome of patients with TBI and should not be administered.[48]

Suspected seizures, especially if witnessed to be prolonged or multiple, can be treated with IV administration of a benzodiazepine, such as diazepam, lorazepam, or midazolam. However, these drugs should be cautiously titrated because hypotension and ventilatory depression may occur.

The primary focus for the TBI patient during prolonged transport or in austere environments is the best possible maintenance of cerebral oxygenation and perfusion and the best efforts possible to control cerebral edema.

SUMMARY

- Knowledge of head and brain anatomy is essential to understanding the pathophysiology of traumatic brain injury (TBI).
- Practitioners must understand the mechanisms by which the brain compensates for reduced cerebral blood flow following trauma.
- Primary brain injury occurs at the time of the original insult and is any injury that occurs because of the initial trauma.
- Secondary brain injury refers to further injury to structures that were unharmed by the primary injury. In the prehospital environment, recognition of pathophysiologic processes representative of secondary injury, including herniation from mass effect, hypoxia, and hypotension, and rapid transport are the key priorities.
- Knowing the mechanism of injury allows practitioners to anticipate certain injury patterns,

which is crucial in identifying the rapidly escalating conditions associated with brain injury.
- The severity of TBI may not be immediately apparent; therefore, serial neurologic evaluations of the patient, including Glasgow Coma Scale (GCS) scores, particularly the motor score, and pupillary response, are necessary to recognize changes in the patient's condition.
- Prehospital management of the TBI patient involves controlling hemorrhage from other injuries, maintaining a systolic blood pressure of at least 110 mm Hg, and providing oxygen to maintain oxygen saturation of at least 90%.
- Practitioners should consider active airway management for all patients with a severe TBI (GCS score ≤ 8). If intubation is chosen, it should be performed by the most skilled prehospital care practitioner available.

SCENARIO RECAP

On an 85°F (29°C) summer day, you and your partner are dispatched to a marathon race to assess a 30-year-old man who fell 14 ft (4.3 m) off a ladder while attempting to secure the finish line banner. Upon your arrival, the patient is supine and unresponsive. A bystander is holding the patient's head and neck in-line.

Upon initial assessment, you note an irregular breathing pattern that varies in depth of respirations and rate. There is blood-tinged fluid coming from both ear canals and both nostrils of the patient. The patient's eyes are closed and he is not responding to you talking to him. You note an absence of gag reflex on your initial assessment and place an oropharyngeal airway to maintain patency of the airway. Your partner ventilates the patient with a bag-mask device at a rate of 12 breaths/minute. You note that the patient's right pupil is dilated. The radial pulse is 54 and regular. Oxygen saturation (SpO$_2$) is 96%. The patient's skin is cool, dry, and pale. His Glasgow Coma Scale (GCS) score is calculated to be 7, with eyes = 2, verbal = 1, and motor = 4 (E2V1M4).

You rapidly prepare the patient for transport; you place him into your ambulance to perform the secondary survey while continuing to maintain c-spine precautions en route to the hospital. Palpation of the occiput generates a painful moan from the patient. You cover the patient with a warm blanket and measure his blood pressure, which is 184/102 millimeters of mercury (mm Hg). An electrocardiogram reveals sinus bradycardia with infrequent premature ventricular beats noted. The right pupil remains widely dilated.

- What injury is most likely present given the patient's presenting signs?
- What are your management priorities at this point?
- What actions may you need to take to address increased intracranial pressure and maintain cerebral perfusion during a prolonged transport?

SCENARIO SOLUTION

En route to the hospital, the patient begins to show palmar flexion of both hands. With this sign of impending herniation, you raise the head of the bed to support venous drainage and transiently increase the ventilation rate to 16 to 20 breaths/minute to temporarily target an $ETCO_2$ of 30 to 35 mm Hg. The patient remains unconscious. You consider insertion of a complex airway; however, because the SpO_2 is at 96% and transport time to the trauma center is only a few minutes, you decide to maintain him with the oral airway and bag-mask device with 100% oxygen.

References

1. Global Burden of Disease 2016 Traumatic Brain Injury and Spinal Cord Injury Collaborators. Global, regional, and national burden of traumatic brain injury and spinal cord injury, 1990-2016: a systematic analysis for the Global Burden of Disease Study 2016. *Lancet Neurol*. 2019;18(1):56-87.

2. Maas AIR, Menon DK, Adelson PD, Andelic N, Bell MJ, Belli A. Traumatic brain injury: integrated approaches to improve prevention, clinical care and research. *Lancet Neurol*. 2017;16(12):987-1048.

3. Centers for Disease Control and Prevention. Traumatic Brain Injury and Concussion. Accessed July 15, 2021. https://www.cdc.gov/traumaticbraininjury/

4. Dewan MC, Mummareddy N, Wellons III JC, Bonfield CM. Epidemiology of global pediatric traumatic brain injury: qualitative review. *World Neurosurg*. 2016;91:497-509.

5. Hyder AA, Wunderlich CA, Puvanachandra P, et al. The impact of traumatic brain injuries: a global perspective. *Neuro Rehabilitation*. 2007;22:341-353.

6. Cipolla MJ. *The Cerebral Circulation*. Morgan & Claypool Life Sciences; 2009.

7. Mtui E, Gruener G, Dockery P. *Fitzgerald's Clinical Neuroanatomy and Neuroscience*. 8th ed. Elsevier Saunders; 2021.

8. Chesnut RM, Marshall LF, Klauber MR, et al. The role of secondary brain injury in determining outcome from severe head injury. *J Trauma*. 1993;34:216-222.

9. Fearnside MR, Cook RJ, McDougall P, et al. The Westmead Head Injury Project outcome in severe head injury: a comparative analysis of prehospital, clinical, and CT variables. *Br J Neurosurg*. 1993;7:267-279.

10. Gentleman D. Causes and effects of systemic complications among severely head-injured patients transferred to a neurosurgical unit. *Int Surg*. 1992;77:297-302.

11. Marmarou A, Anderson RL, Ward JL, et al. Impact of ICP instability and hypotension on outcome in patients with severe head trauma. *J Neurosurg*. 1991;75:S59-S64.

12. Miller JD, Becker DP. Secondary insults to the injured brain. *J R Coll Surg Edinb*. 1982;27:292-298.

13. Berry C, Ley EJ, Bukur M, et al. Redefining hypotension in traumatic brain injury. *Injury*. 2012;43(11):1833-1837.

14. Brenner M, Stein DM, Hu PF, Aarabi B, Sheth K, Scalea TM. Traditional systolic blood pressure targets underestimate hypotension-induced secondary brain injury. *J Trauma Acute Care Surg*. 2012;72(5):1135-1139.

15. Carney N, Totten AM, O'Reilly C, et al. Guidelines for the management of severe traumatic brain injury, fourth edition. *Neurosurgery*. 2017;80(1):6-15.

16. Wilson MH. Monro-Kellie 2.0: the dynamic vascular and venous pathophysiological components of intracranial pressure. *J Cereb Blood Flow Metab*. 2016;36(8):1338-1350.

17. Mavrocordatos P, Bissonnette B, Ravussin P. Effects of neck position and head elevation on intracranial pressure in anaesthetized neurosurgical patients: preliminary results. *J Neurosurg Anesthesiol*. 2000;12:10-14.

18. Sundstrøm T, Asbjørnsen H, Habiba S, et al. Prehospital use of cervical collars in trauma patients: a critical review. *J Neurotrauma*. 2014;31:531-540.

19. Obrist WD, Gennarelli TA, Segawa H, et al. Relation of cerebral blood flow to neurological status and outcome in head injured patients. *J Neurosurg*. 1979;51:292-300.

20. Obrist WD, Langfitt TW, Jaggi JL, et al. Cerebral blood flow and metabolism in comatose patients with acute head injury. *J Neurosurg*. 1984;61:241-253.

21. Coles JP, Minhas PS, Fryer TD, et al. Effect of hyperventilation on cerebral blood flow in traumatic head injury: clinical relevance and monitoring correlates. *Crit Care Med*. 2002;30(9):1950-1959.

22. Imberti R, Bellinzona G, Langer M. Cerebral tissue PO_2 and $SjvO_2$ changes during moderate hyperventilation in patients with severe traumatic brain injury. *J Neurosurg*. 2002;96(1):97-102.

23. Stocchetti N, Maas AI, Chieregato A, van der Plas AA. Hyperventilation in head injury: a review. *Chest*. 2005;127(5):1812-1827.

24. Centers for Disease Control and Prevention. What is a concussion? n.d. https://www.cdc.gov/headsup/basics/concussion_whatis.html

25. Quinn DK, Mayer AR, Master CL, Fann JR. Prolonged postconcussive symptoms. *Am J Psychiatry*. 2018;175(2):103-111.

26. Babcock L, Byczkowski T, Wade SL, et al. Predicting postconcussion syndrome after mild traumatic brain injury in

children and adolescents who present to the emergency department. *JAMA Pediatr*. 2013;167(2):156-161.

27. Barlow M, Schlabach D, Peiffer J, Cook C. Differences in change scores and the predictive validity of three commonly used measures following concussion in the middle school and high school aged population. *Int J Sports Phys Ther*. 2011;6(3):150-157.

28. Broglio SP, McAllister T, Katz BP, et al. The natural history of sport-related concussion in collegiate athletes: findings from the NCAA-DoD CARE Consortium. *Sports Med*. 2021;52:403-415. doi: 10.1007/s40279-021-01541-7

29. Hume CH, Wright BJ, Kinsella GJ. Systematic review and meta-analysis of outcome after mild traumatic brain injury in older people. *Int Neuropsychol Soc*. 2021;1-20.

30. Meagher RL, Young WF. Subdural hematoma. eMedicine, Medscape. Updated July 26, 2018. Accessed January 3, 2022. http://emedicine.medscape.com/article/1137207-overview

31. Lucke-Wold BP, Turner RC, Josiah D, Knotts C, Bhatia S. Do age and anticoagulants affect the natural history of acute subdural hematomas? *Arch Emerg Med Crit Care*. 2016;1(2):1010.

32. Coughlin RF, Moser RP. Subdural hematoma. In: Domino FJ, ed. *The 5-Minute Clinical Consult 2013*. 21st ed. Wolters Kluwer Health/Lippincott Williams & Wilkins; 2013:1246-1247.

33. Quigley MR, Chew BG, Swartz CE, Wilberger JE. The clinical significance of isolated traumatic subarachnoid hemorrhage. *J Trauma Acute Care Surg*. 2013;74:581-584.

34. Brain Trauma Foundation. CT scan features. In: Bullock MR, Chesnut RM, Clifton GL, et al. *Management and Prognosis of Severe Traumatic Brain Injury*. 2nd ed. Brain Trauma Foundation; 2000.

35. Kihtir T, Ivatury RR, Simon RJ, et al. Early management of civilian gunshot wounds to the face. *J Trauma*. 1993;35:569-575.

36. Rimel RW, Giordani B, Barth JT. Moderate head injury: completing the clinical spectrum of brain trauma. *Neurosurgery*. 1982;11:344-351.

37. Miller JD, Sweet RC, Narayan RK, et al. Early insults to the injured brain. *JAMA*. 1978;240:439-442.

38. Silverston P. Pulse oximetry at the roadside: a study of pulse oximetry in immediate care. *BMJ*. 1989;298:711-713.

39. Stochetti N, Furlan A, Volta F. Hypoxemia and arterial hypotension at the accident scene in head injury. *J Trauma*. 1996;40:764-767.

40. Plum F. *The Diagnosis of Stupor and Coma*. 3rd ed. Oxford University Press; 1982.

41. Langfitt TW, Weinstein JD, Kassell NF, et al. Transmission of increased intracranial pressure. I. Within the craniospinal axis. *J Neurosurg*. 1964;21:989-997.

42. Langfitt TW. Increased intracranial pressure. *Clin Neurosurg*. 1969;16:436-471.

43. Ayling J. Managing head injuries. *Emerg Med Serv*. 2002; 31(8):42.

44. Graham DI, Ford I, Adams JH, et al. Ischaemic brain damage is still common in fatal non-missile head injury. *J Neurol Neurosurg Psychiatry*. 1989;52:346-350.

45. Obrist WD, Wilkinson WE. Regional cerebral blood flow measurement in humans by xenon-133 clearance. *Cerebrovasc Brain Metab Rev*. 1990;2:283-327.

46. Darby JM, Yonas H, Marion DW, et al. Local "inverse steal" induced by hyperventilation in head injury. *Neurosurgery*. 1988;23:84-88.

47. Marion DW, Darby J, Yonas H. Acute regional cerebral blood flow changes caused by severe head injuries. *J Neurosurg*. 1991;74:407-414.

48. Badjatia N, Carney N, Crocco TJ, et al. Guidelines for prehospital management of traumatic brain injury: 2nd edition. *Prehosp Emerg Care*. 2007;12(1):S1-S52.

49. Bostek CC. Oxygen toxicity: an introduction. *AANA J*. 1989;57(3):231-237.

50. Brenner M, Stein D, Hu P, et al. Association between early hyperoxia and worse outcomes after traumatic brain injury. *Arch Surg*. 2012;147(11):1042-1046.

51. Tolias CM, Reinert M, Seiler R, Gilman C, Scharf A, Bullock MR. Normobaric hyperoxia-induced improvement in cerebral metabolism and reduction in intracranial pressure in patients with severe head injury: a prospective historical cohort matched study. *J Neurosurg*. 2004;101(3):435-444.

52. Hare GMT, Mazer CD, Hutchison JS, et al. Severe hemodilutional anemia increases cerebral tissue injury following acute neurotrauma. *J Appl Physiol*. 2007;103:1021-1029.

53. Cucher D, Harmon D, Myer B, et al. Critical traumatic brain injury is associated with worse coagulopathy. *J Trauma*. 2021;91(2):331-335.

54. Bohm JK, Guting H, Thorn S, et al. Global characterization of coagulopathy in isolated traumatic brain injury (iTBI): a CENTER-TBI analysis. *Neurocrit Care*. 2021;35:184-196.

55. Yee J, Kaide CG. Emergency reversal of anticoagulation. *West J Emerg Med*. 2019;20(5):770-783.

56. CRASH-2 trial collaborators. Effects of tranexamic acid on death, vascular occlusive events, and blood transfusion in trauma patients with significant hemorrhage (CRASH-2): a randomized, placebo-controlled trial. *Lancet*. 2010;376(9734):23-32.

57. Perel P, Al-Shahi Salman R, Kawahara T, et al. CRASH-2 (Clinical randomization of an antifibrinolytic in significant haemorrhage) intracranial bleeding study: the effect of tranexamic acid in traumatic brain injury—a nested randomized, placebo-controlled trial. *Health Technol Assess*. 2012;16(13):iii-xii;1-54.

58. CRASH-3 trial collaborators. Effects of tranexamic acid on death, disability, vascular occlusive events and other morbidities in patients with acute traumatic brain injury (CRASH-3): a randomized, placebo-controlled trial. *Lancet*. 2019;394(10210):1713-1723.

59. CRASH-3 Intracranial Bleeding Mechanistic Study Collaborators. Tranexamic acid in traumatic brain injury: an explanatory study nested within the CRASH-3 trial. *Eur J Trauma Emerg Surg*. 2021;47:261-268.

60. Bossers SM, Loer SA, Bloemers FW, et al. Association between prehospital tranexamic acid administration and outcomes of severe traumatic brain injury. *JAMA Neurol*. 2021;78(3):338-345.

61. Caron MJ, Hovda DA, Mazziotta JC, et al. The structural and metabolic anatomy of traumatic brain injury in humans: a computerized tomography and positron emission tomography analysis. *J Neurotrauma*. 1993;10(suppl 1):S58.

62. Caron MJ, Mazziotta JC, Hovda DA, et al. Quantification of cerebral glucose metabolism in brain-injured humans utilizing positron emission tomography. *J Cereb Blood Flow Metab.* 1993;13(suppl 1):S379.

63. Caron MJ. PET/SPECT imaging in head injury. In: Narayan RK, Wilberger JE, Povlishock JT, eds. *Neurotrauma.* McGraw-Hill; 1996.

64. Jalloh I, Carpenter KLH, Helmy A, et al. Glucose metabolism following human traumatic brain injury: methods of assessment and pathophysiologic findings. *Metab Brain Dis.* 2015;30:615-632.

65. Lam AM, Winn HR, Cullen BF, et al. Hyperglycemia and neurological outcome in patients with head injury. *J Neurosurg.* 1991;75:545-551.

66. Young B, Ott L, Dempsey R, et al. Relationship between admission hyperglycemia and neurologic outcome of severely brain-injured patients. *Ann Surg.* 1989;210:466-472.

67. Mechtcheriakov S, Brenneis C, Egger K, Koppelstaetter F, Schocke M, Marksteiner J. A widespread distinct pattern of cerebral atrophy in patients with alcohol addiction revealed by voxel-based morphometry. *J Neurol Neurosurg Psychiatry.* 2007;78(6):610-614.

68. Mayer S, Rowland L. Head injury. In: Rowland L, ed. *Merritt's Neurology.* Lippincott Williams & Wilkins; 2000:401.

69. Dimmitt SB, Rakic V, Puddey IB, et al. The effects of alcohol on coagulation and fibrinolytic factors: a controlled trial. *Blood Coagul Fibrinolysis.* 1998;9(1):39-45.

70. Perry M, Dancey A, Mireskandari K, Oakley P, Davies S, Cameron M. Emergency care in facial trauma—a maxillofacial and ophthalmic perspective. *Injury.* 2005;36(8):875-896.

71. Davis DP, Hoyt DB, Ochs M, et al. The effect of paramedic rapid sequence intubation on outcome in patients with severe traumatic brain injury. *J Trauma Injury Infect Crit Care.* 2003;54:444-453.

72. Bochicchio GV, Ilahi O, Joshi M, et al. Endotracheal intubation in the field does not improve outcome in trauma patients who present without an acutely lethal traumatic brain injury. *J Trauma Injury Infect Crit Care.* 2003;54:307-311.

73. Davis DP, Peay J, Sise MJ, et al. The impact of prehospital endotracheal intubation in moderate to severe traumatic brain injury. *J Trauma.* 2005;58:933-939.

74. Bulger EM, Copass MK, Sabath DR, et al. The use of neuromuscular blocking agents to facilitate prehospital intubation does not impair outcome after traumatic brain injury. *J Trauma.* 2005;58:718-723.

75. Wang HE, Peitzman AB, Cassidy LD, et al. Out-of-hospital endotracheal intubation and outcome after traumatic brain injury. *Ann Emerg Med.* 2004;44:439-450.

76. Chi JH, Knudson MM, Vassar MJ, et al. Prehospital hypoxia affects outcome in patients with traumatic brain injury: a prospective multi-center study. *J Trauma.* 2006;61:1134-1141.

77. Mayglothling J, Duane TM, Gibbs M, et al. Emergency tracheal intubation immediately following traumatic injury: an Eastern Association for the Surgery of Trauma practice management guideline. *J Trauma Acute Care Surg.* 2012;73:5(S4).

78. Bossers SM, Schwarte LA, Loer SA, et al. Experience in prehospital endotracheal intubation significantly influences mortality of patients with severe traumatic brain injury: a systematic review and meta-analysis. *PLoS One.* 2015;10(10):1-26.

79. Meizoso JP, Valle EJ, Allen CJ, et al. Decreased mortality after prehospital interventions in severely injured trauma patients. *J Trauma Acute Care Surg.* 2015;79:227-231.

80. Marlow TJ, Goltra DD, Schabel SI. Intracranial placement of a nasotracheal tube after facial fracture: a rare complication. *J Emerg Med.* 1997;15:187-191.

81. Horellou MD, Mathe D, Feiss P. A hazard of nasotracheal intubation. *Anaesthesia.* 1978;22:78.

82. Davis DP, Ochs M, Hoyt DB, et al. Paramedic-administered neuromuscular blockade improves prehospital intubation success in severely head-injured patients. *J Trauma Injury Infect Crit Care.* 2003;55:713-719.

83. Cooper KR, Boswell PA, Choi SC. Safe use of PEEP in patients with severe brain injury. *J Neurosurg.* 1985;63:552-555.

84. McGuire G, Crossley D, Richards J, et al. Effects of varying levels of positive end-expiratory pressure on intracranial pressure and cerebral perfusion pressure. *Crit Care Med.* 1997;25:1059-1062.

85. Warner KJ, Cuschieri J, Copass MK, et al. The impact of prehospital ventilation on outcome after severe traumatic brain injury. *J Trauma.* 2007;62:1330-1336.

86. Godoy DA, Badenes R, Robba C, Cabezas FM. Hyperventilation in severe traumatic brain injury has something changed in the last decade or uncertainty continues? A brief review. *Front. Neurol.* 2021;12:573237.

87. Christensen MA, Bloom J, Sutton KR. Comparing arterial and end-tidal carbon dioxide values in hyperventilated neurosurgical patients. *Am J Crit Care.* 1995;4:116-121.

88. Grenier B, Dubreuil M. Noninvasive monitoring of carbon dioxide: end-tidal versus transcutaneous carbon dioxide. *Anesth Analg.* 1998;86:675-676.

89. Isert P. Control of carbon dioxide levels during neuroanaesthesia: current practice and an appraisal of our reliance upon capnography. *Anaesth Intensive Care.* 1994;22:435-441.

90. Kerr ME, Zempsky J, Sereika S, et al. Relationship between arterial carbon dioxide and end-tidal carbon dioxide in mechanically ventilated adults with severe head trauma. *Crit Care Med.* 1996;24:785-790.

91. Mackersie RC, Karagianes TG. Use of end-tidal carbon dioxide tension for monitoring induced hypocapnia in head-injured patients. *Crit Care Med.* 1990;18:764-765.

92. Russell GB, Graybeal JM. Reliability of the arterial to end-tidal carbon dioxide gradient in mechanically ventilated patients with multisystem trauma. *J Trauma Injury Infect Crit Care.* 1994;36:317-322.

93. Warner KJ, Cuschieri J, Garland B, et al. The utility of early end-tidal capnography in monitoring ventilation status after severe trauma. *J Trauma.* 2009;66:26-31.

94. Davis DP, Dunford JV, Poste JC, et al. The impact of hypoxia and hyperventilation on outcome after paramedic rapid sequence intubation of severely head injured patients. *J Trauma.* 2004;57:1-10.

95. Nagler J, Krauss B. Capnography: a valuable tool for airway management. *Emerg Med Clin N Am.* 2008;26(4):881-897.

96. Childress K, Arnold K, Hunter C, Ralls G, Papa L, Silvestri S. Prehospital end-tidal carbon dioxide predicts mortality in trauma patients. *Prehosp Emerg Care.* 2017;22(2):170-174.

97. Howard MB, McCollum N, Alberto EC, et al. Association of ventilation during initial trauma resuscitation for traumatic brain injury and post-traumatic outcomes: a systematic review. *Prehosp Disaster Med.* 2021;36(4):460-465.

98. American College of Surgeons Committee on Trauma. Head trauma. In: *Advanced Trauma Life Support for Doctors, Student Course Manual.* 10th ed. American College of Surgeons; 2017.

99. Suttipongkaset P, Chaikittisilpa N, Vavilala MS, et al. Blood pressure thresholds and mortality in pediatric traumatic brain injury. *Pediatrics.* 2018;142(2):e20180594. doi: 10.1542/peds.2018-0594

100. Cooper DJ, Myles PS, McDermott FT, et al. Prehospital hypertonic saline resuscitation of patients with hypotension and severe traumatic brain injury: a randomized controlled trial. *JAMA.* 2004;291:1350-1357.

101. The Glasgow structured approach to assessment of the Glasgow Coma Scale. Accessed February 8, 2022. http://www.glasgowcomascale.org

102. Teasdale G, Allen D, Brennan P, et al. The Glasgow Coma Scale: an update after 40 years. *Nurs Times.* 2014;110:12-16.

103. Majdan M, Steyerberg EW, Nieboer D, et al. Glasgow Coma Scale motor score and pupillary reaction to predict six-month mortality in patients with traumatic brain injury: comparison of field and admission assessment. *J Neurotrauma.* 2015;32(2):101-108.

104. Ross SE, Leipold C, Terregino C, et al. Efficacy of the motor component of the Glasgow Coma Scale in trauma triage. *J Trauma.* 1998;45(1):42-44.

105. Jarvis C, ed. Physical Examination and Health Assessment. 6th ed. Elsevier Publishers; 2012:71.

106. Brain Trauma Foundation. Glasgow coma score. In: Gabriel EJ, Ghajar J, Jagoda A, et al. Guidelines for Prehospital Management *of Traumatic Brain Injury.* Brain Trauma Foundation; 2000.

107. Prosser JD, Vender JR, Solares CA. Traumatic cerebrospinal fluid leaks. *Otolaryngol Clin N Am.* 2011;44:857-873.

108. Biffl WL, Cothren CC, Moore EE, et al. Western Trauma Association critical decisions in trauma: screening for and treatment of blunt cerebrovascular injuries. *J Trauma Acute Care Surg.* 2009;67(6):1150-1153.

109. Servadei F, Nasi MT, Cremonini AM. Importance of a reliable admission Glasgow Coma Scale score for determining the need for evacuation of posttraumatic subdural hematomas: a prospective study of 65 patients. *J Trauma.* 1998;44:868-873.

110. Winkler JV, Rosen P, Alfrey EJ. Prehospital use of the Glasgow Coma Scale in severe head injury. *J Emerg Med.* 1984;2:1-6.

111. Brain Trauma Foundation. Hospital transport decisions. In: Gabriel EJ, Ghajar J, Jagoda A, et al. *Guidelines for Prehospital Management of Traumatic Brain Injury.* Brain Trauma Foundation; 2000.

112. Feldman Z, Kanter MJ, Robertson CS. Effect of head elevation on intracranial pressure, cerebral perfusion pressure and cerebral blood flow in head-injured patients. *J Neurosurg.* 1992;76:207-211.

113. Schott JM, Rossor MN. The grasp and other primitive reflexes. *J Neurol Neurosurg Psychiatry.* 2003;74:558-560.

114. Lumba-Brown A, Totten A, Kochanek PM. Emergency department implementation of the Brain Trauma Foundation's Pediatric Severe Brain Injury Guideline Recommendations. *Pediatr Emerg Care.* 2020;36(4):e239-e241.

Suggested Reading

American College of Surgeons Committee on Trauma. Head trauma. In: *Advanced Trauma Life Support, Student Course Manual.* 10th ed. American College of Surgeons; 2017.

Badjatia N, Carney N, Crocco TJ, et al. Guidelines for prehospital management of traumatic brain injury: 2nd edition. *Prehosp Emerg Care.* 2007;12(1):S1-S52.

Carney N, Totten AM, O'Reilly C, et al. Guidelines for the management of severe traumatic brain injury: fourth edition. *Neurosurgery.* 2017;80(1):6-15.

CHAPTER **9**

Spinal Trauma

Lead Editors
Steven C. Ludwig, MD
Alexandra E. Thomson, MD, MPH
Ivan Ye, BA

CHAPTER OBJECTIVES   At the completion of this chapter, you will be able to do the following:

- Describe the epidemiology of spinal injuries.
- Compare and contrast the most common mechanisms that produce spinal injury in adults with those in children.
- Recognize patients with the potential for spinal trauma.
- Relate the signs and symptoms of spinal injury and neurogenic shock with their underlying pathophysiology.
- Integrate principles of anatomy and pathophysiology with assessment data and principles of trauma management to formulate a treatment plan for the patient with obvious or potential spinal injury.

- Describe the multifaceted decision-making process required to determine if spinal motion restriction is appropriate for a given patient.
- Discuss factors associated with prehospital findings and interventions that may affect spinal injury morbidity and mortality.
- Understand the principles of selective spinal immobilization and how the application of these principles may change, depending on the patient and the situation.
- Understand the controversy surrounding steroid administration for spinal cord injury, and understand novel treatments currently under investigation.

SCENARIO

You have been dispatched to the scene of a bicyclist who is reported down alongside a roadway. On arrival, the scene is safe, with traffic being controlled by law enforcement. The patient, a young woman, is lying supine on the side of the road away from traffic. A law enforcement officer is kneeling beside her and trying to talk to her, but she is not responding.

As you begin your primary survey, you are unable to ascertain the specific cause of the fall. It appears the woman fell from her bike while riding along the roadway, but you do not know whether she was struck by a motor vehicle. The law enforcement officers tell you there were no witnesses. The patient is wearing full cycling gear, including helmet and gloves. She has abrasions on her forehead and an obvious deformity of the right wrist. Her airway is open, and she is breathing regularly. She shows no obvious signs of external blood

(continues)

INTRODUCTION

Traumatic spine injury (TSI) is potentially life threatening, with severity largely dependent on the region of the spine injured and whether damage includes nearby structures, such as the spinal cord. The injury most often results from high-energy forces but may occur with a lower energy mechanism of injury in vulnerable populations such as older adults. Injury to the skeletal components of the spine may not result in damage to the spinal cord, and, in some cases, the spinal cord, blood vessels, and nerves may be damaged without fracture or dislocation of the vertebrae. Damaged bony structures and supportive ligaments may result in structural instability of the vertebral column, making the spinal cord and other nearby structures susceptible to injury unless spinal motion is appropriately restricted. Severe injuries may irreparably damage the spinal cord and leave the patient with a lifelong neurologic disability. Immediate spinal cord damage occurs as a result of the trauma event, or primary injury. Secondary injury may follow the initial injury and result in worsened neurologic deficit. This secondary injury can be provoked or exacerbated by pathologic motion from an injured spinal column. Failure to suspect, properly assess, and stabilize a patient with a potential spine injury may produce a poor outcome. Prompt recognition and prehospital management of these injuries are important for timely stabilization in the critically injured patient, may guide future diagnostic and management decisions, and will reduce the risk of secondary injury.

Sudden violent forces acting on the body can stress the osseous and ligamentous structures in the spine beyond their normal limits of motion. The following four concepts help clarify the possible effect of energy on the spine when evaluating the potential for injury:

1. Objects in motion tend to stay in motion, and objects at rest tend to stay at rest (Newton's first law).
2. The head is similar to a bowling ball perched on top of the neck, and its mass often moves in a different direction from the torso, resulting in strong forces being applied to the neck (cervical spine, spinal cord).
3. Sudden or violent movement of the upper legs displaces the pelvis, resulting in forceful movement of the lower spine. Because of the weight and inertia of the head and torso, force in an opposite (contra) direction is applied to the upper spine.
4. Lack of neurologic deficit does not rule out bone or ligament injury to the spinal column or conditions that have stressed the spinal cord to the limit of its tolerance.

About 54 people per 1 million of the population in the United States (approximately 17,900 people) will sustain some type of spinal cord injury (SCI) annually, with an estimated 252,000 to 373,000 people living with the ensuing disability. SCI can occur at any age; however, with aging trends in the United States the incidence of SCI is increasing in the population age 65 years and older. There has been a significant increase in the proportion of SCI resulting from falls between 1997 and 2012. In 2012 unintentional falls accounted for 40% of acute traumatic SCIs in the United States. These trends are predictable given the increasing average age of the U.S. population.[1] Men overwhelmingly outnumber women and account for over 78% of SCIs. Common causes are motor vehicle crashes (39%), falls (32%), penetrating injuries (14%), sports injuries (8%), and other injuries (7%).[2] In the older adult population, falls outnumber motor vehicle crashes as the primary cause of SCI.[3]

SCI can have profound effects on physical function, lifestyle, and financial circumstances. In addition, when compared to the general population, those who survive the initial SCI generally have a shorter life expectancy.[3] The spinal cord may be injured at any level, and the two main categories of SCI include complete and incomplete injury. Complete SCI affects both sides of the body and results in total loss of all function, including movement and sensation, below the level of the injury. Incomplete injury describes any SCI without complete loss of neurologic function. Movement, sensation, or both are preserved but may be asymmetric in a patient with an incomplete SCI. In general, physiologic dysfunction and long-term impairment are most devastating when injury occurs in the upper cervical spine and decrease progressively as injury level descends. Complete injury at the highest level in the cervical spine is catastrophic and often fatal before emergency personnel arrive on scene. The loss of motor and sensory function after SCI can range from mild weakness to requiring a wheelchair or even a ventilator.

Patients with severe injuries may experience profound changes to daily activity levels and independence. SCI also impacts the financial circumstances of the patient as well as the population in general.[4] A patient with this injury requires both acute and long-term care. The lifetime cost of this care is estimated to be between $1.2 and $5.2 million per patient who sustains a permanent SCI, with cost rising with injury severity and age at time of injury.[4]

Neurologic deficits may result from trauma to a number of different central and peripheral nervous system structures or may be the result of inadequate oxygenation or perfusion to the brain or spinal cord. Patients may have injuries to multiple organ systems in addition to peripheral nerve injuries, which can manifest as a deficit. For example, a patient with multiple different injuries may have sustained a direct blow to the head resulting in direct neurologic injury, a significant vascular injury resulting in shock and inadequate perfusion and thus an anoxic injury to neurologic structures, and an extremity injury that directly injures a peripheral nerve. Recovery from such injuries is variable, and although permanent in some cases, the potential for recovery is possible and must be assumed during the initial care of a patient. Although the presentation of these patients may be complex, spinal injury should be a considered in any of the following mechanisms[5,6]:

- Any blunt mechanism that produced a violent impact on the head, neck, torso, or pelvis
- Incidents that produce sudden acceleration, deceleration, or lateral bending forces to the neck or torso
- Any fall from a height, especially in older adults
- Ejection or a fall from any motorized or otherwise powered transportation device
- Any shallow-water diving incident

The practice of prehospital spinal immobilization using the traditional rigid long backboard has evolved significantly since first gaining support in the 1960s. The decision to perform spinal motion restriction is made after careful consideration of the mechanism of injury, comorbidities and unique risk factors, and physical examination of the patient. Understanding the limitations and potential complications of this intervention is equally important in clinical decision making.

More recently, the safety and efficacy of immobilization using the rigid long backboard has been challenged by researchers and has resulted in a paradigm shift away from traditional immobilization practices. The evolution in prehospital management of spine trauma has generated widespread adoption of evidence-based protocols for spinal motion restriction and management of acute SCI that reduce widely recognized complications associated with immobilization using a rigid backboard, while effectively limiting spinal motion in patients with an injured spine. The patient with a suspected spinal injury should be manually stabilized in a neutral in-line position until the need for continued spinal motion restriction has been assessed. The initial management of a patient with suspected spinal trauma must include aggressive resuscitation to ensure uninterrupted perfusion of neurologic tissue and spinal motion restriction to prevent secondary injury and worsened neurologic decline.

Anatomy and Physiology

Vertebral Anatomy

The spine is a complex structure that primarily functions to facilitate movement in all three planes and disperse the forces from loads of the head and trunk to the pelvis, while simultaneously shielding the tenuous neurologic tissue of the spinal cord. The spinal column comprises 33 bones called vertebrae, which are stacked on top of one another. Except for the first (C1) and second (C2) vertebrae at the top of the cervical spine and the fused sacral and coccygeal vertebrae at the lower spine, all of the vertebrae are similar in form, structure, and motion (**Figure 9-1**). The *body* is situated anteriorly and represents the largest part of each vertebra. Each vertebral body bears most of the weight of the vertebral column and torso superior to it. Two curved sides called the **neural arches** are formed by the pedicle and posteriorly by the lamina projecting back from the body. The spinous process is a midline bony protuberance from the posterior aspect of the lamina that serves as an attachment for muscles and ligaments. In the lower five cervical vertebrae, this **spinous process** points directly posterior; in the thoracic and lumbar vertebrae, it points slightly downward in a caudal direction (toward the feet). Each vertebra has a pair of facet joints on the posterior aspect. These joints are covered in cartilage, allowing the vertebrae to articulate with one another.

Arising laterally from the junction of the pedicles and the vertebral bodies are additional bony structures called **transverse processes** that serve as additional points for attachment of the paraspinal muscles. Several neural and vascular structures, including the root of each spinal nerve, spinal artery, and dorsal root ganglion, pass through an opening called the **intervertebral foramen** (also called neural foramen) present between every pair of vertebrae. The neural arches and the posterior part of each vertebral body form a near-circular shape with an opening in the center called the **vertebral foramen** (spinal canal). The spinal cord, surrounded by the thecal sac that contains cerebrospinal fluid, passes through this

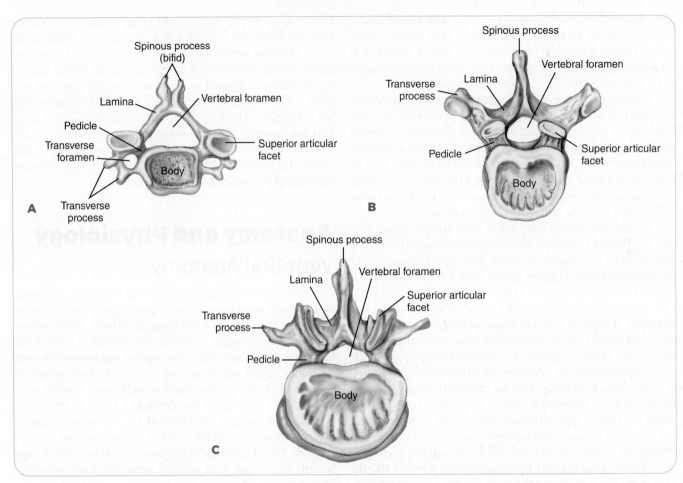

Figure 9-1 The body (anterior portion) of each vertebra becomes larger and stronger in the lower spine because it must support increasing mass as it approaches the pelvis. **A.** Fifth cervical vertebra. **B.** Thoracic vertebra. **C.** Lumbar vertebra.
© National Association of Emergency Medical Technicians (NAEMT)

space. The spinal cord is protected somewhat from injury by the bony vertebrae surrounding it, but it remains vulnerable to direct penetrating injury through the interlaminar space. Each vertebral foramen lines up with that of the vertebrae above and the vertebrae below to form the hollow spinal canal through which the spinal cord passes. Variability in the size of the foramen can result from pathologic processes (e.g., arthritic change, tumor, and spinal disc herniation), spinal loading, and posture. The risk of damaging the neurovascular structures that pass through these openings may increase if the foramen becomes narrowed.

Vertebral Column

The individual vertebrae are stacked in an S-shaped column (**Figure 9-2**). This organization allows extensive multidirectional movement while imparting maximum strength. The spinal column is divided into five individual regions for reference. Beginning at the top of the spinal column and descending downward, these regions are the cervical, thoracic, lumbar, sacral, and coccygeal regions. Vertebrae are identified by the first letter of the region in

which they are found and their sequence from the top of that region. The first cervical vertebra is called *C1*, the third thoracic vertebra *T3*, the fifth lumbar vertebra *L5*, and so on throughout the entire spinal column. Each vertebra supports increasing body weight as the vertebrae progress down the spinal column. Appropriately, the vertebrae from C3 to L5 become progressively larger to accommodate the increased weight and workload (see Figure 9-1).

Located at the cranial aspect of the spinal column are the seven *cervical* vertebrae that support the head and form the skeletal component of the neck. The cervical region is flexible to allow for total movement of the head. It is important to note that the vertebral arteries that supply the posterior aspect of the brain run through separate foramina in the cervical vertebra, usually entering at C6. In the case of significant displacement or fracture, this artery can become compromised, resulting in decreased perfusion to the brain, and the patient may present with stroke-like symptoms. Compared with lower regions of the spine, the cervical spine has relatively unrestricted mobility and is the region most commonly injured.[7,8] Next are 12 *thoracic* vertebrae. Each pair of ribs connects posteriorly to one of the thoracic vertebrae at the

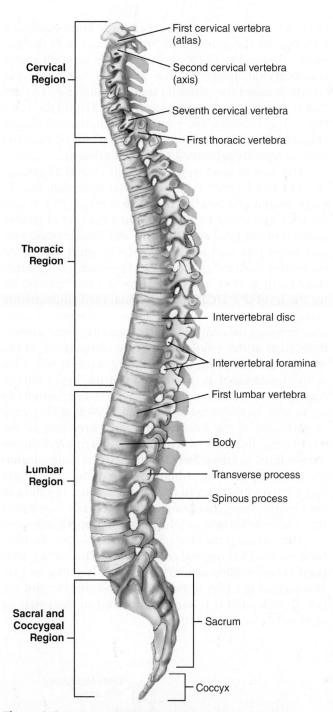

Figure 9-2 The vertebral column is not a straight rod but a series of blocks that are stacked to allow for several bends or curves. At each of the curves, the spine is more vulnerable to fractures; hence the origin of the phrase "breaking the S in a fall."
© National Association of Emergency Medical Technicians (NAEMT)

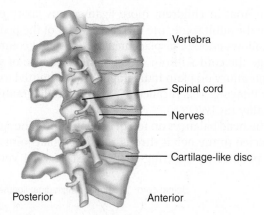

Figure 9-3 The cartilage between adjacent vertebral bodies is called the intervertebral disc.
© National Association of Emergency Medical Technicians (NAEMT)

costovertebral joints. The thoracic spine is more rigid and allows less movement than the cervical spine. The increased stability provided by the ribs extending between the thoracic vertebrae and sternum is a major reason why injury of the thoracic spine in a healthy adult patient typically requires the significant physical forces of high-energy mechanisms. However, the incidence of thoracic spine injury is higher in the older adult population and in those with factors that reduce the relative strength of the thoracic spine. Below the thoracic vertebrae are the five *lumbar* vertebrae. The lumbar spine is flexible, allowing for movement in several directions. The five *sacral* vertebrae fuse by adulthood to form a single bony structure called the **sacrum**. Similarly, the four *coccygeal* vertebrae fuse and form the *coccyx* (tailbone). The incidence of traumatic vertebral fracture is highest in the thoracic and lumbar spine (75–90%), with most localized to the thoracolumbar junction.[9-11] Conversely, SCI and the overall incidence of TSI (including injuries without fracture) occur most frequently in the cervical region.[7,8]

Each vertebra is separated from the one above and below it by the intervertebral disc (**Figure 9-3**). This disc consists of a fibrous annulus that is filled with a gelatinous interior called the nucleus pulposus. The discs serve as soft cushions that allow the spine to bend in multiple directions. They also act as shock absorbers by attenuating the gravitational and mechanistic axial load of the spine. If damaged, the intervertebral disc may protrude into the spinal canal, compressing the cord or the nerves that come through the intervertebral foramina.

Ligaments and muscles tether the spine from the base of the skull to the pelvis. These ligaments and muscles form a web that sheathes the entire bony part of the spinal column, holding it in normal alignment, providing stability, and allowing for movement. The anterior and posterior longitudinal ligaments connect the vertebral bodies anteriorly and inside the canal. Ligaments between the spinous processes provide support for flexion–extension (forward and backward) movement, and those between the lamina provide support during lateral flexion (side bending) (**Figure 9-4**). If the soft-tissue structures that stabilize the spine are torn, excessive movement of one vertebra in relation to another can occur. This excessive movement may result in dislocation of the vertebrae and could potentially narrow the space occupied by the spinal cord, called the spinal canal, severely enough to cause SCI. It is important to note that in children, more ligamentous laxity exists. Unlike the adult spine, the increased laxity of the pediatric spine allows enough displacement of the spinal column to damage the cord without radiographic evidence of spinal column injury on plain radiographs and computed tomography imaging. This is called SCI without radiographic abnormality (SCIWORA).

The head balances on top of the spine, and the spine is connected to the pelvis through the sacroiliac joints. The skull perches on the ring-shaped first cervical vertebra

(C1), referred to as the **atlas**. Very little bony stability is imparted by the joints of C1 and the skull, and the primary stabilization of this articulation is through strong craniocervical ligaments. The **axis**, C2, has a peg-like structure called the odontoid process (similar to a tooth) that protrudes upward. It is located just behind the anterior arch of the atlas, and it forms a rotational articulation (**Figure 9-5**). The articulation between C1 and C2 imparts 50% of the cervical spine's rotational motion.

The human head weighs between 16 and 22 pounds (lb; 7 to 10 kilograms [kg]), somewhat more than the average weight of a bowling ball. The cervical spine is particularly susceptible to injury due to a number of factors: position of the head atop the thin and flexible neck, normal forces that act upon the head, the small size of the supporting muscles, and the lack of protective bony structures (such as ribs). The cervical spinal canal narrows after the level of C1/C2, and the spinal cord consequently occupies 95% of the available space with minimal clearance between the cord and wall of the canal. Even a minor dislocation at this point can produce compression of the spinal cord. In contrast, the spinal cord occupies only 65% of the spinal canal as it terminates in the upper lumbar region. The posterior neck muscles are strong, permitting up to 60% of the range of flexion and 70% of the range of extension of the head without any stretching of the spinal cord. However, when sudden violent acceleration, deceleration, or lateral force is applied to the body, the momentum surpasses the stabilizing force of the osseous and ligamentous structures of the cervical spine, resulting in cord compromise. An example of this scenario would be a rear-end collision without the headrest properly adjusted.

The sacrum is the base of the spinal column, the platform on which the spinal column rests. The sacrum supports between 70% and 80% of the body's total weight. The sacrum is a part of both the spinal column and the pelvic girdle, and it is joined to the rest of the pelvis by immovable sacroiliac joints.

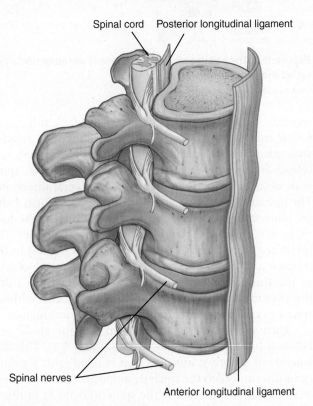

Figure 9-4 Anterior and posterior longitudinal ligaments of the vertebral column.
© National Association of Emergency Medical Technicians (NAEMT)

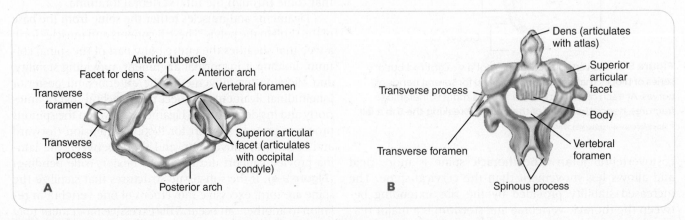

Figure 9-5 The first and second cervical vertebrae are uniquely shaped. **A.** Atlas (C1). **B.** Axis (C2).
© National Association of Emergency Medical Technicians (NAEMT)

Spinal Cord Anatomy

The spinal cord is a collection of neurons that carries outgoing and incoming signals between the brain and the rest of the body. It is continuous with the brain, beginning at the termination of the medulla oblongata, passing through the foramen magnum (the hole at the base of the skull) and respective vertebrae via the spinal canal to the level of the second lumbar (L2) vertebra. Blood is supplied to the spinal cord by the anterior and posterior spinal arteries.

The spinal cord is covered by three membranes, known as meninges: the pia, arachnoid, and dura mater, from innermost to outermost membrane, respectively. This meningeal covering continues to the second sacral vertebrae, where it terminates in a sac-like reservoir. The space between the pia mater and arachnoid mater contains cerebrospinal fluid (CSF), which is produced by the brain and encases the brain and spinal cord. In addition to removal of waste products from the brain, CSF protects against injury during rapid changes in acceleration that cause the brain to be pushed against the skull.

The spinal cord itself consists of gray matter and white matter. The gray matter consists primarily of the neuronal cell bodies. The white matter contains the long myelinated axons that make up the anatomic spinal tracts and serve as the communication pathways for nerve impulses. Spinal tracts are divided into two types: ascending and descending (**Figure 9-6**).

Ascending nerve tracts carry sensory impulses from distal body parts through the spinal cord up to the brain. Ascending nerve tracts can be further divided into those that carry different sensations: pain and temperature; touch and pressure; and sensory impulses of motion, vibration, position, and light touch. The tracts that carry pain and temperature sensation decussate or "cross over" in the spinal cord itself, meaning that the neuronal tract with the information from the right side of the body crosses over to the left side of the spinal cord and then travels up to the brain. In contrast, the nerve tract that carries the sensory information for position,

vibration, and light touch does not cross over in the spinal cord, but more cranially at the level of the medulla. Thus, this sensory information is carried up to the brain on the same side of the spinal cord as the nerve roots.

Descending nerve tracts are responsible for carrying motor impulses from the brain through the spinal cord down to the body, and they control all muscle movement and muscle tone. These descending tracts do not cross over in the spinal cord. Therefore, the motor tract on the right side of the spinal cord controls motor function on the right side of the body. These motor tracts do cross over in the brain stem, however, so the left side of the brain controls motor function on the right side of the body, and vice versa.

As the spinal cord continues to descend, pairs of nerves branch off from the spinal cord at each vertebra and extend to the various parts of the body (**Figure 9-7**). The spinal cord has 31 pairs of spinal nerves, named

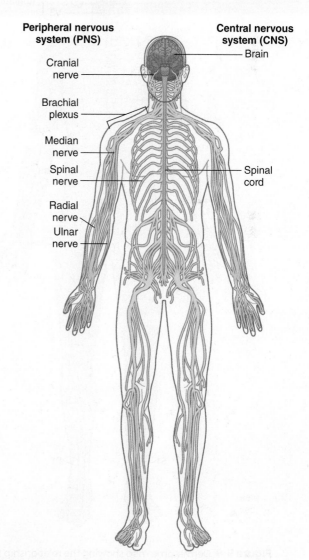

Peripheral nervous system (PNS)

- Cranial nerve
- Brachial plexus
- Median nerve
- Spinal nerve
- Radial nerve
- Ulnar nerve

Central nervous system (CNS)

- Brain
- Spinal cord

Figure 9-7 Nerves of the central nervous system (CNS) and peripheral nervous system (PNS).

Pyramidal tract (descending)
Motor function on the same side

Posterior columns (ascending)
Position and vibration sensation on the same side

Spinothalamic tract (ascending)
Pain and temperature sensation on the opposite side

Figure 9-6 Spinal cord tracts.

according to the level from which they arise. Each nerve has two roots (one dorsal and one ventral) on each side.

The **dorsal root** carries information for sensory impulses, and the ventral root carries motor impulse information. Neurologic stimuli pass between the brain and each part of the body through the spinal cord and respective pairs of these nerves. As they branch from the spinal cord, these nerves pass through a notch in the inferior lateral side of the vertebra, posterior to the vertebral body, called the intervertebral foramen.

A **dermatome** is the sensory area on the skin surface of the body innervated by a single dorsal root. Collectively,

dermatomes allow the body areas to be mapped out for each spinal level (**Figure 9-8**). Dermatomes help determine the level of an SCI. Three landmarks to keep in mind are the clavicles, which are the C4–C5 dermatome; the nipple level, which is the T4 dermatome; and the umbilicus level, which is the T10 dermatome. Remembering these three levels can help to quickly locate an SCI.

The process of inhalation and exhalation requires both chest excursion and proper changes in the shape of the diaphragm. The intercostal muscles as well as accessory respiratory muscles such as the trapezius also contribute to breathing. The diaphragm is innervated by the

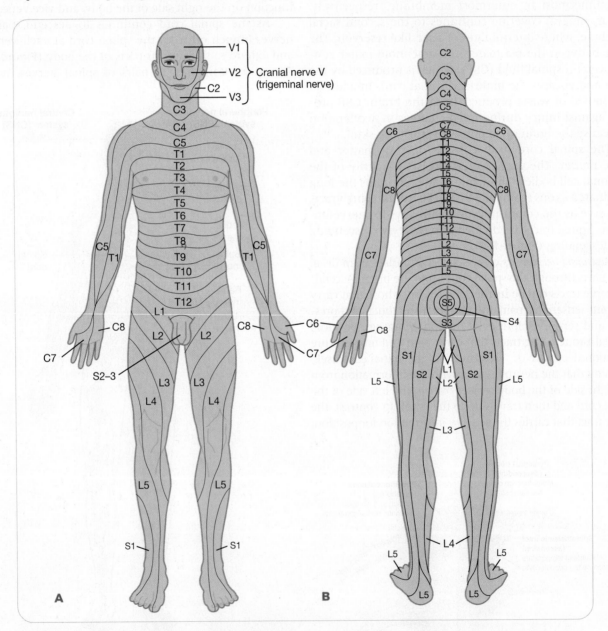

Figure 9-8 Dermatome map showing the relationship between areas of touch sensation on the skin and the spinal nerves that correspond to these areas. Loss of sensation in a specific area may indicate injury to the corresponding spinal nerve or level of injury of the spinal cord. **A.** Frontal view. **B.** Posterior view.

left and right phrenic nerves, which originate from the nerves arising from the spinal cord between levels C3 and C5. If the spinal cord is injured above the level of C3 or the phrenic nerves are cut, a patient will lose the ability to breathe spontaneously. A patient with this injury may asphyxiate before the arrival of practitioners unless bystanders initiate rescue breathing. Therefore, it is critical to maintain control of the airway in a patient with suspected SCI. Positive-pressure ventilation may need to be continued during transport.

Pathophysiology

The bony spine can normally withstand forces of up to 1,000 foot-pounds (1,360 joules) of energy. High-speed travel and contact sports can routinely exert forces on the spine well in excess of this amount. Even in a low- to moderate-speed vehicle crash, the body of an unrestrained 150-lb (68-kg) person can easily place 3,000 to 4,000 foot-pounds (4,080 to 5,440 joules) of force against the spine if the head is suddenly stopped by the windshield or roof. Similar force can occur when a motorcyclist is thrown over the front of the motorcycle or when a high-speed skier collides with a tree. Compression strength of the vertebral column increases caudally, likely reflecting the differences in vertebral size, shape, and bone mineral density (BMD) at various spine levels.[12-15] The large forces needed to cause TSI often result in associated injuries to visceral, vascular, and pulmonary structures, which further complicate patient management. Cervical injury has the highest risk of associated injury to structures other than the spine (65%), followed by injury to the lumbar (52%) and thoracic (50%) levels. Thoracic spine trauma should raise a particularly high index of suspicion for associated injury to the lung, diaphragm, ribs, and sternum. In addition to the region of spine injured, the risk of associated injury increases with increasing number of spine fractures or injured spine segments.[16]

Skeletal Injuries

Various types of injuries can occur to the spine, including the following[17]:

- Compression fractures, which produce wedge compression or total flattening of the body of the vertebra
- Burst fractures, which can violate the posterior vertebral wall and may produce small fragments of bone that may lie in the spinal canal near the cord
- Subluxation, which is a partial dislocation of a vertebra from its normal alignment in the spinal column
- Discoligamentous injury, which results from overstretching or tearing of the ligaments and muscles, producing instability between the vertebrae with or without bony injury

Although simple compression fractures are usually stable injuries, any of these injuries may immediately result in severe compression or (less commonly) transection of the spinal cord, resulting in irreversible injury. In some patients, however, damage to the vertebrae or ligaments results in an *unstable* spinal column injury but does not produce an immediate SCI. Should the fragments in an unstable spine shift position, they may then damage the spinal cord secondarily. In addition, patients who have one spine fracture have a 10% to 20% chance of having another, noncontiguous spinal column injury. Therefore, the entire spine should be considered when determining the need for spinal immobilization in a patient with a suspected injury to a particular spine segment.

A lack of neurologic deficit does not rule out a bony fracture or an unstable spine. Although the presence of good motor and sensory responses in the extremities indicates that the spinal cord is currently intact, it does not exclude a damaged vertebra or associated bony, ligamentous, or soft-tissue injury. The majority of patients with spine fractures have no neurologic deficit. A full assessment is required to determine the need for immobilization.

Specific Mechanisms of Injury That Cause Spinal Trauma

Axial loading of the spine can occur in several ways. Most often, this compression of the spine occurs when the head strikes an object and the weight of the still-moving body bears against the stopped head, such as when the head of an unrestrained occupant strikes the windshield or when the head strikes an object in a shallow-water diving incident. Compression and axial loading also occur when a patient sustains a fall from a substantial height and lands in a standing position. This type of injury drives the weight of the head and thorax down against the lumbar spine while the sacral spine remains stationary. About 20% of falls from a height greater than 15 feet (ft; 4.6 meters [m]) involve an associated lumbar spine fracture; however, it is important to recognize that certain patient populations, particularly older adults, have a significantly higher rate of spinal fracture after falling from much shorter distances than 15 ft (4.6 m).[18] During such an extreme energy exchange, the spinal column tends to exaggerate its normal curvature, and fractures and compressions occur at such areas. Many compression or burst fractures that result from axial loading occur at the apices of the lumbar lordosis or thoracic kyphosis.

Excessive flexion (**hyperflexion**), excessive extension (**hyperextension**), and excessive rotation (**hyper-rotation**) can cause osseous or ligamentous damage, resulting in impingement on or stretching of the spinal cord.

Sudden or excessive lateral bending requires much less movement than flexion or extension before tensile or compressive failure of the spinal column occurs, as motion in this direction is limited to begin with. During lateral impact, the torso and the thoracic spine are moved laterally. The head tends to remain in place until it is pulled along by the cervical attachments. The center of gravity of the head is above and anterior to its seat and attachment to the cervical spine; therefore, the head will tend to roll sideways. This movement often results in dislocations and bony fractures.

Distraction (over-elongation of the spine) occurs when one part of the spine is stable and the rest is in longitudinal motion. This pulling apart of the spine can easily cause stretching and tearing of the spinal cord. Distraction-type TSI is a common mechanism in pediatric playground injuries, hangings, and certain types of motor vehicle crashes.

There are many recognized mechanisms of SCI; however, most result from the following four major causes, listed in order of frequency[1,19]:

- Motor vehicle crashes
- Falls
- Acts of violence
- Sports/recreation-related activities, including shallow-water diving

Major causes of TSI and SCI in pediatric patients vary significantly by age and race. A significant proportion (17.5%) of spinal injuries in patients younger than 2 years result from violent physical abuse, while motor vehicle crashes and falls remain a common cause regardless of patient age.[20-23] The proportion of SCI related to falls has increased while those related to motor vehicle crashes has decreased since 2005.[1] Adolescents are more likely to sustain an injury during a sports-related activity than are younger children or adults.[24] Firearm-related injuries are responsible for nearly a quarter of all SCI in black adolescents in the United States.[25]

In practice, determining the exact mode of failure of the spinal column is difficult, as the injury mechanism can result in complex force patterns. One must always assume that an injury severe enough to cause fracture or neurologic injury has caused spinal instability until proven otherwise by further clinical and radiographic evaluation.

Spinal Cord Injuries

Primary injury occurs at the time of impact or force application and may cause spinal cord compression, direct SCI (usually from sharp, unstable bony fragments or projectiles), and interruption of spinal cord blood flow. Secondary injury occurs after the initial insult and can include swelling, ischemia, or movement of bony fragments.[26]

Cord concussion results from the temporary disruption of spinal cord functions distal to the injury. **Cord contusion** involves bruising or bleeding into the tissues of the spinal cord, which may also result in a temporary (and sometimes permanent) loss of spinal cord functions distal

to the injury (spinal "shock"). **Spinal shock** is a neurologic phenomenon that occurs for a variable amount of time after SCI (usually less than 48 hours), resulting in temporary loss of sensory and motor function, muscle flaccidity and paralysis, and loss of reflexes below the level of the SCI. Cord contusion is often caused by a penetrating type of injury or movement of bony fragments against the spinal cord. The severity of injury resulting from the contusion is related to the amount of bleeding into the spinal cord tissue. Damage to or disruption of the spinal blood supply can result in local cord tissue ischemia.

Cord compression is pressure on the spinal cord caused by swelling of local tissues but also may occur from traumatic disc rupture and bone fragments or development of a compressive hematoma. Cord compression may result in tissue ischemia and in some cases may require surgical decompression to prevent a permanent loss of function; thus prompt transport for imaging and definitive evaluation is important. **Cord laceration** occurs when spinal cord tissue is torn or cut. This type of injury usually results in irreversible neurologic injury.

Spinal cord transection can be categorized as complete or incomplete. In **complete cord transection**, all spinal tracts are interrupted, and all spinal cord functions distal to the site are lost. Because of the additional effects of swelling, determination of the extent of loss of function may not be accurate until 24 hours after the injury. Most complete spinal cord transections result in either paraplegia or quadriplegia, depending on the level of the injury. In **incomplete cord transection**, some tracts and motor/sensory functions remain intact. Prognosis for recovery is greater in these cases than with complete transection.

It is not possible in the prehospital environment to discern whether the resulting neurologic deficit is due to cord contusion, spinal shock, or a more severely damaged spinal cord. Therefore, all suspected SCI patients should be evaluated and managed without consideration of this distinction.

Types of incomplete cord injuries include the following:

- **Anterior cord syndrome** is typically a result of bony fragments or pressure on anterior spinal arteries resulting in infarction or damage to the anterior aspect of the spinal cord (**Figure 9-9**). Symptoms include loss of motor function and pain, temperature, and light touch sensations. However, some light touch, motion, position, and vibration sensations are spared through the intact posterior column.
- **Central cord syndrome** usually occurs with hyperextension of the cervical area, especially in patients who may have preexisting stenosis from degenerative or congenital etiologies (**Figure 9-10**). Symptoms include weakness or paresthesias in the upper extremities but less significant loss of strength and sensation in the lower extremities. This syndrome causes varying degrees of bladder dysfunction.

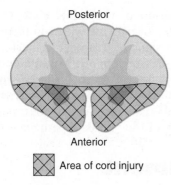

Posterior

Anterior

☒ Area of cord injury

Figure 9-9 Anterior cord syndrome.
© National Association of Emergency Medical Technicians (NAEMT)

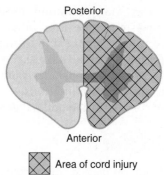

Posterior

Anterior

☒ Area of cord injury

Figure 9-11 Brown-Séquard syndrome.
© National Association of Emergency Medical Technicians (NAEMT)

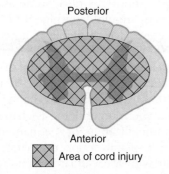

Posterior

Anterior

☒ Area of cord injury

Figure 9-10 Central cord syndrome.
© National Association of Emergency Medical Technicians (NAEMT)

- **Brown-Séquard syndrome** is caused by penetrating injury and involves hemi-transection of the spinal cord, involving only one side of the spinal cord (**Figure 9-11**). Symptoms include complete spinal cord damage and loss of function on the affected side (motor, vibration, motion, and position) with loss of pain and temperature sensation on the side opposite the injury.[27]

While *spinal shock* represents a loss of motor and sensory signal transmission in the spinal cord secondary to injury, this must be discriminated from *neurogenic shock*, a type of distributive shock with pathophysiologic signs caused by loss of sympathetic outflow to the heart and peripheral vessels. Without appropriate sympathetic stimulation, unopposed parasympathetic transmission results in bradycardia and dilation of peripheral arteries and veins. Dilation of arteries results in loss of peripheral systemic vascular resistance, and dilation of veins results in venous pooling. These findings reduce cardiac preload—the venous return to the right side of the heart. In combination with bradycardia, a serious decrease in cardiac output may occur. Recall that the hypovolemic shock patient presents with tachycardia in response to hypotension, and the skin is cool and clammy as the peripheral blood vessels constrict to shunt blood volume to vital organs in an attempt to maintain blood pressure. Conversely, the classic finding of the physiology associated with spinal shock is "hypotensive bradycardia" that may require treatment

with atropine (or other parasympathetic blocking agent) in addition to other methods of aggressive resuscitation. Other findings related to the unopposed parasympathetic tone include warm, flushed skin and priapism (abnormal, prolonged erection of the penis) as a result of vasodilation. In practice, patients with SCIs and spinal shock often have other injuries that may result in hypovolemic shock in addition to neurogenic shock, making assessment and management more challenging.

Spinal Cord Perfusion

Spinal cord blood flow is determined partially by the spinal cord perfusion pressure (SCPP):

Spinal cord perfusion pressure (SCPP) = Mean arterial pressure (MAP) – Extrinsic pressure

Several factors can affect spinal cord perfusion and oxygenation as well as extrinsic pressure on the cord:

1. *Mean arterial pressure (MAP).* The MAP primarily determines cord perfusion. Adequate resuscitation to a target MAP of 90 mm Hg with both fluid administration and medication is crucial to maintaining SCPP. Systemic hypotension (defined as a systolic blood pressure < 90 mm Hg) at any point acutely following SCI is associated with worsened neurologic outcome.[28]

2. *Spinal venous congestion.* This can be the effect of venous thrombosis or the result of extrinsic compression of the spinal veins resulting in inadequate blood outflow. On a microvascular level, the MAP must be higher in the setting of spinal venous congestion to push blood through the area of venous congestion in order to achieve adequate oxygen exchange.

3. *Hypoxia.* Trauma patients often have pulmonary issues that may result in decreased oxygen exchange in the lungs resulting in low partial pressure of arterial oxygen in the blood. Administering supplemental oxygen and maintaining control over the airway are crucial to maintaining adequate blood flow to the spinal cord.

4. *Medications.* Many common anesthetic agents, including morphine and other opioids, can reduce cardiac output due to negative inotropic effects on cardiac muscle.[29] Although pain control in a trauma patient is important, these agents must be used judiciously to allow for adequate cord perfusion and oxygenation.

Initial Resuscitation

Aggressive resuscitation plays a critical role in the prehospital management of SCI-related shock and in reducing neurologic deficit and preventing secondary neurologic damage. The pathogenesis of secondary neurologic injury stems from loss of autoregulation, leading to loss of spinal microcirculation, leading to further ischemic damage. Early, aggressive volume and blood pressure augmentation can improve this microcirculation and decrease the risk of secondary insults to the cord.[30] Additionally, up to 30% of SCI cases are associated with multitrauma and severe hemorrhage. This reflects the 20% mortality rate prior to hospital admission in SCI patients and the emphasis needed on adequate resuscitation efforts in the field.[31]

Ideally, initial resuscitation of the SCI patient should include measures to maintain a target MAP of 85 to 90 mm Hg for 7 days following the injury.[32,33] This is often accomplished using crystalloids, colloids, or blood products through appropriate venous access to restore as much neurologic blood flow as possible.[31] In the polytrauma SCI patient, it is important that prehospital practitioners weigh the potential risk and benefit of permissive hypotension. Given the risks of worsening SCI severity with transient low perfusion states, permissive hypotension should generally be avoided whenever SCI is suspected.[33-35] Volume-based resuscitation that includes glucose in the infusion fluids should be avoided for two reasons. First, glucose is metabolized quickly, leaving an excess of free water more likely to support the formation of edema. Second, too much glucose leads to hyperglycemia, which results in increased anaerobic cell metabolism, leading to increased lactate, decreased systemic pH, and a poorer outcome.[31]

It is also important to remember high SCIs (C5 or above) are more likely to require cardiovascular interventions such as vasopressors and pacemakers. Vasomotor sympathetic fibers exit the spinal cord between the levels of the first and fourth thoracic vertebrae and may be transected with higher cervical injuries while parasympathetic fibers travel in the vagus nerve outside of the spinal cord to the chest. This results in unabated parasympathetic flow and the paradox of bradycardia with hypotension.[36] Studies have shown that the average MAP of patients with complete cervical injuries is only 66 mm Hg when they arrived at the intensive care unit, far below the 90 mm Hg target MAP needed to maintain adequate perfusion of the spinal cord. One study revealed that 40% of patients with complete cervical SCI presented with signs of neurogenic shock and immediately required pressor support.[30] Although first responders must always be vigilant in their resuscitation efforts for all spinal injuries, it must be especially emphasized in cervical SCI patients to produce the best possible neurologic outcomes for this subset of patients.

Assessment

Spinal injury, as with other conditions, should be assessed in the context of other injuries and conditions present. After ensuring practitioner and scene safety, the primary survey is the first priority. A rapid scene assessment and history of the event should determine if the possibility of a spinal injury exists, which would require the need for protection of the spinal column with external immobilization. The head is brought into a neutral in-line position, unless contraindicated (see the section "Manual In-Line Stabilization of the Head" later in this chapter). The head is maintained in that position until the assessment reveals no indication for immobilization, or the manual stabilization is replaced with a spinal motion restriction device, such as cervical collar with a backboard, vacuum mattress, or vest-type device. If the mechanism of injury is unclear or the scene assessment cannot be adequately performed or is otherwise unreliable, one must assume the presence of spinal column injury and initiate external immobilization until a more thorough assessment can be performed.

Neurologic Examination

In the field, a rapid neurologic examination is performed to identify obvious deficits that are potentially related to an SCI. The patient is asked to move the arms, hands, and legs, and any inability to do so is noted. Then the patient is checked for the presence or absence of sensation, beginning at the shoulders and moving down the body to the feet. A complete neurologic examination does not need to be performed in the prehospital setting, as it will not provide additional information that will affect the decisions about needed prehospital care and serves only to expend precious time on scene and delay transport.

The rapid neurologic examination should be repeated after the patient has been immobilized, any time the patient is moved, and upon arrival to the receiving facility. This will help identify any changes in patient condition that may have occurred after the primary survey.

Using Mechanism of Injury to Assess SCI

Traditionally, prehospital care practitioners were taught that suspicion for a spinal injury is based solely on the mechanism of injury and that spinal immobilization is required for any patient with a suggestive mechanism of injury. Until recently, this generalization has caused a lack of clear clinical guidelines for assessment of SCIs. Mechanism of injury should never be the sole means of determining the need for spinal motion restriction, as it represents only one factor in a multifaceted decision-making process to determine whether spinal motion restriction is appropriate. Assessment of the neck and spine for spinal immobilization should also include assessment of motor and sensory function, presence of pain or tenderness, and patient reliability as predictors of spinal column injury. In addition, the patient may not complain of pain in the spinal column because of pain associated with a more distracting painful injury, such as a fractured femur.[36] The definition of what constitutes a distracting injury remains controversial; however, the prehospital practitioner should take associated injuries into consideration while assessing a patient for potential TSI and potentially lower the threshold for applying spinal motion restriction if a distracting injury may exist.[37-40] Alcohol or drugs that the patient may have ingested as well as traumatic brain injury (TBI) may also blunt the patient's perception of pain and mask serious injury. Spinal motion restriction is likely not indicated in conscious patients with a reliable examination, no neurologic deficit, no neck or back pain, and no significant distracting injury. In patients with any of these factors positive on examination or who are unable to provide a reliable examination, spinal motion restriction should be continued.

Blunt Trauma

Blunt trauma is a common mechanism for TSI and warrants careful evaluation by the prehospital practitioner. Motor vehicle crashes and falls are responsible for the more than half of all spine fractures related to blunt trauma.[19] Large meta-analyses that included over 500,000 patients have determined the rate of thoracolumbar fracture in all blunt trauma to be about 7%, with over a quarter severe enough to cause SCI.[19] Injuries of the cervical spine result in higher risk of SCI and resulting neurologic impairment compared with thoracic or lumbar spine injuries.[16] In studies evaluating similarly large numbers of patients, the cervical spine is injured in over 6% of cases of blunt trauma, with considerably higher numbers in those who are unconscious or have suffered a head injury.[41,42] Almost half of all cervical injuries from blunt trauma are unstable; thus, a critical opportunity exists for prehospital intervention to prevent secondary injury.[43]

As a general guideline, the presence of spinal injury and a potentially unstable spine should be presumed, manual stabilization of the cervical spine immediately performed, and an assessment of the spine conducted to

determine the need for immobilization with the following situations:

- Any blunt mechanism that produced a violent impact on the head, neck, torso, or pelvis (e.g., assault, entrapment in a structural collapse)
- Incidents that produced sudden acceleration, deceleration, or lateral bending forces to the neck or torso (e.g., moderate- or high-speed motor vehicle crashes, pedestrians struck by vehicle, involvement in explosion)
- Any fall, especially in older adults
- Ejection or fall from any motorized or otherwise powered transportation device (e.g., scooters, skateboards, bicycles, motor vehicles, motorcycles, recreational vehicles)
- Any shallow-water incident (e.g., diving, body surfing)

Other situations often associated with spinal damage include the following:

- Head injuries with any alteration in level of consciousness
- Significant helmet damage
- Significant blunt injury to the torso
- Impacted or other deceleration fractures of the legs or hips
- Significant localized injuries to the area of the spinal column

These mechanisms of injury should mandate a thorough and complete examination of the patient to determine whether indications are present that necessitate spinal motion restriction. If no indications are found, manual stabilization of the cervical spine can be discontinued.

Use of proper seat belt restraints has proven to save lives and reduce head, face, and thoracic injuries. However, the use of proper restraints does not completely rule out the possibility of spinal injury. In significant frontal-impact collisions when sudden severe deceleration occurs, the restrained torso stops suddenly as the seat and shoulder belts engage, but the unrestrained head can continue its forward movement. If the force of deceleration is strong enough, the head will move down until the chin strikes the chest wall, frequently rotating across the diagonal strap of the shoulder restraint. Such rapid, forceful hyperflexion and rotation of the neck can result in compression fractures of the cervical vertebrae, "jumped" facets (dislocation of the articular processes), and stretching of the spinal cord. Different mechanisms can also cause spinal trauma in restrained victims of rear or lateral collisions. The amount of damage to the vehicle and the patient's other injuries are the key factors in determining if a patient needs to be immobilized.

Penetrating Trauma

Penetrating injury represents a special consideration regarding the potential for spinal trauma.[44] In general, if a patient did not sustain definite neurologic injury at the moment that the penetrating trauma occurred, there is little concern for subsequent development of an SCI (**Box 9-1**). This is because of the mechanism of injury and the kinematics associated with the force involved. Penetrating objects generally do not produce unstable spinal fractures because penetrating trauma, unlike blunt injury, produces minimal risk of creating unstable ligamentous or bony injury. A penetrating object causes injury along the path of penetration. Gunshot wounds are common causes of cord contusion. While the bullet can transect the cord, causing irreversible injury, the ballistic shock of the bullet passing close to the cord more frequently results in a cord contusion that may recover. Knife injuries rarely result in SCI; however, injury is still possible. In addition to lacerating neurologic structures, knife injuries can cause local tissue swelling, resulting in cord contusion.

Indications for Spinal Motion Restriction

The mechanism of injury can be used as an aid to determine the need to restrict spinal motion (**Figure 9-12**) but it is not the sole determinant. The key point is that a complete physical assessment coupled with good clinical judgment will guide decision making.

In 2018, the American College of Surgeons Committee on Trauma, the National Association of EMS Physicians, and the American College of Emergency Physicians updated recommendations regarding the use of spinal motion restriction. Based on these recommendations and current literature, spinal motion restriction should be considered when a blunt mechanism of injury exists with any of the indications listed in **Box 9-2**.

Several important signs and symptoms are concerning for serious spinal trauma (**Box 9-3**). However, the absence of these signs does not definitively rule out spinal injury.

In an effort to reduce the unnecessary use of spinal motion restriction, particularly with a rigid long backboard, these professional bodies also recommend that immobilization on a backboard is not necessary if the patient meets all of the criteria listed in **Box 9-4**.[46]

Patients with a penetrating injury (e.g., gunshot or stab wound) to the head, neck, or torso and no evidence of spinal injury, such as neurologic signs or symptoms (e.g., numbness, tingling, and loss of motor or sensory function or actual loss of consciousness), should not be immobilized.[46-49] Numerous studies have shown that unstable spinal injuries rarely occur from penetrating trauma to the head, neck, or torso,[48,50-56] and isolated penetrating injuries by themselves are not indications for spinal motion restriction. Because of the very low risk of an unstable spinal injury and because the other injuries created by the penetrating trauma often require a higher priority in management, patients with penetrating trauma should *not* undergo spinal immobilization. In fact, a retrospective study using the National Trauma Data Bank documented that patients with penetrating trauma who received spinal immobilization in the field had a higher overall mortality rate than those who did not.[49]

Penetrating injuries by themselves are not indications for spinal motion restriction. Unless a secondary mechanism exists or there is evidence of spinal injury, spinal motion restriction should not routinely be performed in patients with penetrating injuries.

The primary focus of prehospital care is to recognize the indications for spinal motion restriction rather than to attempt to clear the spine.[57-64] Because many patients do not have a spinal injury, a selective approach to performing spinal motion restriction is appropriate, especially since spinal immobilization has been shown to produce adverse effects in healthy volunteers, including increases in respiratory effort, skin ischemia, and pain.[65] This selective approach to spinal motion restriction is even more important with older adult populations, who may be more susceptible to skin breakdown and have underlying pulmonary disease. Prehospital care practitioners should focus on appropriate indications for performing spinal motion restriction[47] but should perform the intervention only if indicated to prevent the associated complications.[45,46] If no indications are present after a careful and thorough examination, there may be no need for spinal motion restriction. The cornerstone to proper spinal care is the same as with all trauma care: superior assessment with appropriate and timely treatment.

When a patient has a concerning mechanism of injury in the absence of the conditions just listed, the reliability of the patient must be assessed. A reliable patient is calm and cooperative and has a completely normal mental status. An unreliable patient may exhibit any of the following:

- *Altered mental status.* Patients who have sustained a TBI resulting in an alteration in their levels of consciousness cannot be adequately evaluated and should be immobilized. Similarly, patients who are under the influence of drugs or alcohol are immobilized and managed as if they had spinal injury until they are calm, cooperative, and sober and physical examination is normal.
- *Distracting painful injuries.* Injuries that are severely painful may distract the patient from other, less painful injuries and interfere with giving reliable

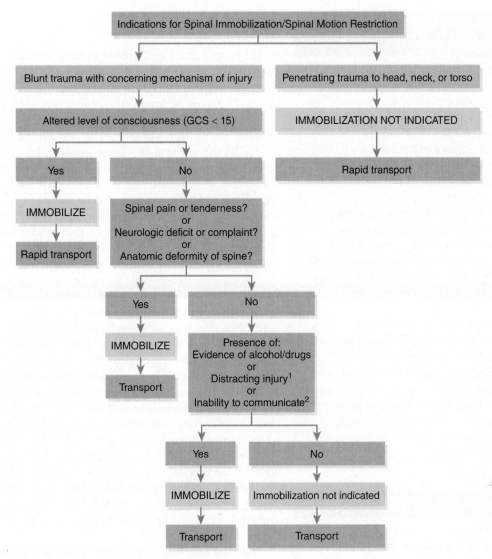

Figure 9-12 Indications for spinal immobilization.

Notes:
¹Distracting injury
   Any injury that may have the potential to impair the patient's ability to appreciate other injuries. Examples of distracting injuries include
   a) long bone fracture, b) a visceral injury requiring surgical consultation, c) a large laceration, degloving injury, or crush injury, d) large
   burns, or e) any other injury producing acute functional impairment.
   (Adapted from Hoffman JR, Wolfson AB, Todd K, Mower WR: Selective cervical spine radiography in blunt trauma: methodology of the
   National Emergency X-Radiography Utilization Study [NEXUS], *Ann Emerg Med*. 1998;461.)

²Inability to communicate.
   Any patients who, for reasons not specified above, cannot clearly communicate so as to actively participate in their
   assessment. Examples: speech or hearing impaired, those who only speak a foreign language, and small children.

responses during the assessment.³⁶ Examples include a fractured femur or a large burn (see Figure 9-12).

- *Communication barriers.* Communication problems may be encountered in patients who have language barriers, are hearing impaired, are preverbal or very young, or cannot communicate effectively for any reason.

The patient should be continually rechecked for reliability at all phases of an assessment. If at any time the patient exhibits these signs or symptoms or the reliability of the examination is in question, it should be assumed that the patient has a spinal injury, and full immobilization management techniques should be implemented.

In many situations, the mechanism of injury is not suggestive of neck injury (e.g., falling on an outstretched hand and producing a Colles' fracture [distal radius and ulna fracture]). In these patients, in the presence of a normal examination and proper assessment, spinal immobilization is not indicated.

Box 9-2 Indications for Immobilization/Spinal Motion Restriction

- *Midline neck or spinal pain and/or tenderness.*[45,46] This includes subjective pain or pain on movement, point tenderness, or guarding of the structures in the midline spinal area.
- *Altered level of consciousness or clinical intoxication* (e.g., TBI, Glasgow Coma Scale [GCS] score < 15, under the influence of alcohol or intoxicating substances).[45,46]
- *Paralysis or focal neurologic signs and/or symptoms* (e.g., numbness and/or motor weakness).[45,46] This includes bilateral paralysis, partial paralysis, paresis (weakness), numbness, prickling or tingling, and neurogenic spinal shock below the level of the injury. In men, a continuing erection of the penis (priapism) may be an additional indication of SCI.
- *Anatomic deformity of the spine.*[45,46] This includes any deformity of the spine noted on physical examination of the patient.
- *Presence of a distracting injury.*[45] This includes any associated injury of such severity that it may make the patient's report regarding the absence of pain in the spine otherwise unreliable (e.g., long-bone fracture, degloving injury).
- *Inability to communicate.*[46]

© National Association of Emergency Medical Technicians (NAEMT)

Box 9-3 Signs and Symptoms of Spinal Trauma

- Pain in the neck or back
- Pain on movement of the neck or back
- Pain on palpation of the posterior neck or midline of the back
- Deformity of the spinal column
- Guarding or splinting of the muscles of the neck or back
- Paralysis, paresis, numbness, or tingling in the legs or arms at any time after the incident
- Signs and symptoms of neurogenic shock
- Priapism

© National Association of Emergency Medical Technicians (NAEMT)

Box 9-4 Criteria to Determine When Spinal Motion Restriction Is Unnecessary

- Normal level of consciousness (GCS score of 15)
- No spine tenderness or anatomic abnormality
- No distracting injury
- No intoxication
- No neurologic findings or complaints

© National Association of Emergency Medical Technicians (NAEMT)

Management

If TSI is suspected and spinal motion restriction is appropriate, the prehospital practitioner should prepare the patient for transport by safely limiting motion of the spine. The goal of spinal immobilization is to limit spinal motion in patients who may have an unstable spinal column injury that could lead to secondary neurologic injury in the context of excess motion. It is controversial at this point, but some physicians believe that such limitation to motion can be accomplished by careful logrolling, using a sheet or sliding board to accomplish transfers, and keeping the patient flat on the ambulance stretcher or cot. Others believe that while such techniques represent the standard of care for protection of the spine within the hospital environment, using a device such as a backboard, scoop litter, or vacuum mattress to reduce the risk of displacement of an unstable spinal segment in the prehospital environment may be safer. Practitioners must understand that there is risk of secondary neurologic injury in some patients and that whatever means they employ to reduce those risks must be effective to avoid unnecessary neurologic disability. While there is a consensus regarding the general recommendations made within this text, there is acknowledgment that current scientific research and understanding of spinal motion restriction are incomplete and imperfect. As evidence grows and recommendations continue to evolve, clinical management is ultimately the responsibility of each practitioner based on specific protocols developed by the local medical director and in the context of utilization of equipment approved by the medical director.

Several methods of performing spinal motion restriction can be used. The rigid long backboard remains effective and appropriate for many short transports and short durations of application; however, this device should be avoided when possible for longer transports, as it is associated with complications such as increased discomfort, pressure ulcers, and restriction of breathing.[45-47,49,66-68] The scoop stretcher or vacuum mattress may be used as an alternative to a rigid long backboard, as these devices are often easier to apply and may be more comfortable (**Box 9-5**). The head, neck, torso, and pelvis should each be immobilized in a neutral in-line position to prevent any further movement of the unstable spine that could result in damage to the spinal cord. Spinal motion restriction follows the common principle of fracture management: immobilizing the joint above and the joint below an injury. Because of the anatomy of the spine, this principle of immobilization must be extended beyond just the joint above and below a suspected vertebral injury. The joint above the spine means the head, and the joint below means the pelvis.

Box 9-5 The Scoop Stretcher

The scoop stretcher (also known as clamshell stretcher, Robertson orthopedic stretcher, and scoop) was invented in 1943 by Wallace W. Robinson from Portland, Maine, and was patented in 1947.[69] It used just one opening joint at the foot end of the stretcher. The form we know today, with two opening joints, was patented by Ferno in 1970.

The scoop stretcher (**Figure 9-13**) has traditionally been made out of metal (aluminum or other lightweight metals), but modern plastics are now used more commonly. It is a two-part device, allowing the separated halves to be placed under each side of the patient without excessive manipulation. After fastening the two halves together, the patient can be lifted and transferred to an ambulance stretcher or vacuum mattress.

In its collapsed state, the scoop stretcher is roughly 5 ft, 5 inches (1.6 m) long and 16 inches (0.4 m) wide, but it can be extended to about 6 ft, 6 inches (2.0 m) to suit the size of the patient. The weight of a scoop is roughly the same as a long backboard. The acceptable patient weight limits vary according to the manufacturer's specifications (generally, 350 to 660 lb [160 to 300 kg]). The scoop stretcher can be used as a tool for transporting a patient over a long distance, provided the patient is properly secured with belts. There is some evidence that the scoop stretcher causes less discomfort than the rigid long backboard and may result in less spine movement during application of the device.[70]

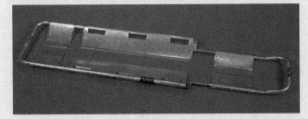

Figure 9-13 Scoop stretcher.
© Jones & Bartlett Learning. Courtesy of MIEMSS.

© National Association of Emergency Medical Technicians (NAEMT)

Box 9-6 The Vacuum Mattress Splint

The vacuum mattress (**Figure 9-14**) is a transport and immobilization tool that is used after the patient has been transferred to it with a scoop stretcher. The splint is an airtight polymer bag filled with small polystyrene balls and a valve. When the air inside the vacuum mattress is removed, the atmospheric pressure outside presses the balls together, forming a rigid "bed" for the patient that molds to the patient's body contours.

The vacuum mattress has evolved considerably in the past decade. It is now wider and longer than the original version, and it has an improved valve system to more easily remove the air from within the mattress. Removal of the air from the mattress involves using a vacuum pump (either an electric suction unit or a hand pump).

The mattress shown here has a V shape, enabling prehospital care practitioners to package the patient more securely. The belts for fixation and carrying are sewn onto the mattress, which makes it easy to use and handle.

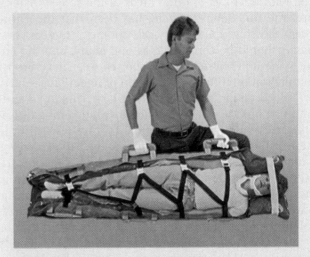

Figure 9-14 Vacuum mattress splint.
Courtesy of Hartwell Medical.

© National Association of Emergency Medical Technicians (NAEMT)

The vacuum mattress was invented by Loed and Haederlé in France (**Box 9-6**). Other sources give credit to Erik Runereldt, a Swede, who reportedly got the idea for it in the late 1960s after seeing a package of coffee beans being vacuum packed.

As with most medical tools, there are many different makes of vacuum mattresses; therefore, prehospital care practitioners must be familiar with their particular device and participate in frequent trainings.

Several studies have demonstrated that the vacuum mattress provides a much higher degree of comfort to the patient when compared to the long rigid backboard.[71-76] Of particular importance, the vacuum mattress is, similar to most backboards, x-ray penetrable, so the patient does not need to be removed from the immobilizing systems while being evaluated in the emergency department.

One important advantage of immobilizing a patient on a long backboard is ease of elevation of the head. Certain patients with TBI and evidence of increased intracranial pressure may benefit from elevation of the head. Some patients with airway difficulty, chest injury, or difficulty breathing may find that elevation of the head facilitates maintenance of the airway and allows the patient to continue to breathe independently better than would be possible while lying flat. In situations where the possibility of thoracolumbar spinal injury cannot be absolutely excluded, it is not generally possible to safely elevate the head of the patient who is not on a rigid device. Simply elevating the head of the stretcher for a patient in a supine position results in moving the patient to a semi-sitting position, which causes motion, malalignment, and potentially displacement in a patient with an unstable thoracolumbar spinal injury. Conversely, placing something under the board or rigid device to elevate the head in a patient who is on a long backboard results in elevation of the head without flexion deformity at the thoracolumbar spine. The same result can be accomplished using a vacuum mattress or scoop stretcher.

Fractures of one area of the spine are often associated with fractures of other areas of the spine.[56] Therefore, the traditional teaching has been that the entire weight-bearing spine (cervical, thoracic, lumbar, and sacral) should be considered as one entity, and the entire spine immobilized and supported to achieve proper immobilization if there is suspicion of underlying injury.

An exception to this general rule occurs in patients found ambulatory at the scene but complaining of isolated neck pain. Applying spinal motion restriction to these patients for thoracolumbar stabilization may be avoided if the patient is cognitively reliable (normal GCS and no evidence of drug or alcohol use), without back pain, has no back tenderness, and has normal distal neurologic function. A cervical collar alone for stabilization of the neck in the context of mild neck pain may be all that is indicated. Understand that there is variability in local protocols and that your medical director may recommend an alternative approach for these patients.

Patients usually present in one of four general postures: sitting, semi-prone, supine, or standing. If spinal column injury is suspected, the patient's spine needs to be protected and stabilized immediately and continuously from the time the patient is discovered until the patient is mechanically secured. Techniques and equipment, such as manual stabilization, half-spine boards, immobilization vests, scoop stretchers, proper logroll methods, and rapid extrication with full manual stabilization, are interim techniques used to protect a patient's spine. These techniques allow for safe movement from the position in which the patient was found until the patient arrives at a definitive care location.

In some instances, the patient may benefit from spinal precautions rather than complete spinal motion restriction using one of the previously mentioned devices. Spinal precautions can be performed by applying a rigid cervical collar and firmly securing the patient to the stretcher. This is likely more appropriate in the following situations[46]:

- Patients who are ambulatory on the scene
- Patients who have mild to moderate neck pain, are reliable, have no neurologic deficit or complaints, and have no back or other thoracolumbar pain
- Patients for whom a backboard or other spinal restricting device is not otherwise indicated based on the absence of a distracting injury, normal level of consciousness, and no evidence of intoxication

Often, too much focus is placed on particular immobilization devices without an understanding of the principles of spinal motion restriction and how to modify these principles to meet individual patient needs. Specific devices and immobilization methods can be safely used only with an understanding of the anatomic principles that are generic to all methods and equipment. Any inflexible, detailed method for using a device will not meet the varying conditions found in the field. Regardless of the specific equipment or method used, the management of any patient with an unstable spine should follow the general steps described in the next section.

General Method

When the decision is made to immobilize a trauma patient, follow these principles:

1. Move the patient's head into a proper neutral in-line position (unless contraindicated; see next section). Continue manual support and in-line stabilization without interruption.
2. Evaluate the patient by performing the primary survey, and provide any immediately required intervention.
3. Check the patient's motor ability, sensory response, and circulation in all four extremities, if the patient's condition allows.
4. Examine the patient's neck, and measure and apply a properly fitting, effective cervical collar.
5. Carefully, and without causing unnecessary motion of the spinal column, transfer the patient onto the appropriate immobilization device.
6. Stabilize the patient's torso to the device so that it cannot move up, down, left, or right.
7. Evaluate and pad behind the adult patient's head or pediatric patient's chest as needed.
8. Stabilize the patient's head to the device, maintaining a neutral in-line position.

9. Reevaluate the primary survey, and reassess the patient's motor ability, sensory response, and circulation in all four extremities, if the patient's condition allows.

Manual In-Line Stabilization of the Head

Once it has been determined from the mechanism of injury that an injured spine may exist, the first step is to provide manual in-line stabilization. The patient's head is grasped and carefully moved into a neutral in-line position unless contraindicated (see the following discussion). A proper neutral in-line position is maintained without any significant traction on the head and neck. The head should be constantly maintained in the manually stabilized neutral in-line position until mechanical immobilization of the torso and head is completed or the examination reveals no need for spinal stabilization. In this way, the patient's head and neck are immediately immobilized and remain so if indicated until after examination at the hospital. Moving the head into a neutral in-line position presents less risk than if the patient were carried and transported with the head left in an angulated position. In addition, both stabilization and transport of the patient are much simpler with the patient's head in a neutral position.

Contraindications

Movement of the patient's head into a neutral in-line position is contraindicated in a few cases. If careful movement of the head and neck into a neutral in-line position results in any of the following, the movement must be stopped:

- Resistance to movement
- Neck muscle spasm
- Increased pain
- Commencement or increase of a neurologic deficit, such as numbness, tingling, or loss of motor ability
- Compromise of the airway or ventilation

Neutral in-line movement should not be attempted if a patient's injuries are so severe that the head presents with such misalignment that it no longer appears to extend from the midline of the shoulders. In these situations, the patient's head must be immobilized in the position in which it was initially found. Fortunately, such cases are rare.

Rigid Cervical Collars

Rigid cervical collars alone do not provide complete stabilization; they simply aid in supporting the neck and promote a lack of movement. Stabilization of the body to a spinal motion restriction device or to the ambulance cot must be accomplished in order to effectively limit spinal motion during transfer and transport of patients.

Prehospital methods of spinal motion restriction necessarily still allow some movement of the patient and the spine because these devices only fasten to the patient externally, and the skin and muscle tissue move slightly on the skeletal frame even when the patient is extremely well secured. Most rescue situations involve some movement of the patient and spine when extricating, carrying, and loading the patient. This type of movement also occurs when an ambulance accelerates and decelerates in normal driving conditions.

An effective cervical collar sits on the chest, posterior thoracic spine and clavicle, and trapezius muscles, where the tissue movement is minimal. It still allows movement at C6, C7, and T1, but it helps limit compression of these vertebrae. The head is secured under the angle of the mandible and at the occiput of the skull. The rigid collar allows the unavoidable loading between the head and the torso to be transferred from the cervical spine to the collar, limiting the cervical compression that could otherwise result.

Even though it does not fully immobilize the spine and head, a cervical collar aids in limiting head movement. The rigid anterior portion of the collar also provides a safe pathway for the lower head strap across the anterior collar if the patient is further immobilized.

The collar must be the correct size for the patient. A collar that is too short will not be effective and will allow significant flexion or compression of the spine from axial loading; a collar that is too large will cause distraction of the spine, hyperextension, or full motion if the chin slips inside of it.[77] Also, a collar must be applied properly. A collar that is too loose will be ineffective in limiting head movement and can accidentally cover the anterior chin, mouth, and nose, obstructing the patient's airway; a collar that is too tight can compress the veins of the neck, causing increased intracranial pressure.

There are many different rigid cervical collars available. The method of determining the correct size and the application of the device should be done according to the manufacturer's recommendations. An ill-fitting, improperly sized cervical collar will not help the patient and may be detrimental if an unstable spinal column is present (**Box 9-7**).

The collar is applied after bringing the patient's head into a neutral in-line position. If the head cannot be returned to a neutral in-line position, use of any collar is difficult and should not be considered. In this case, the improvised use of a blanket or towel roll may assist in stabilization. A collar that does not allow the mandible to move down and the mouth to open without motion of the spine will produce aspiration of gastric contents into the lungs if the patient vomits and,

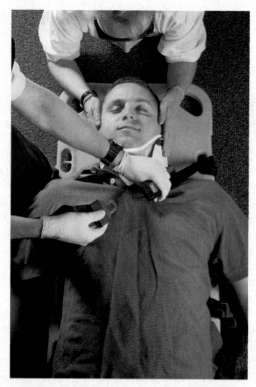

Figure 9-15 Cephalad movement of the upper torso is restricted by use of an oblique strap on each side.

© Jones & Bartlett Learning. Photographed by Darren Stahlman.

therefore, should not be used. Alternative methods to stabilize a patient when a collar cannot be used may include use of such items as blankets, towels, and tape. In the prehospital setting, the prehospital care practitioner may need to be creative when presented with these types of patients. Whatever method is used, the basic concepts of spinal motion restriction should be followed (Box 9-8).

There have been reports of increased intracranial pressure associated with cervical collar use in patients with TBI. If a patient with suspected TBI shows obvious signs of increasing intracranial pressure, loosening or opening the collar should be considered to provide some relief.[78,79]

Immobilization of Torso to the Board Device

Regardless of the specific device used, a patient with a suspected unstable spinal column injury must be stabilized so that the torso cannot move up, down, left, or right. The device is secured to the patient's torso so that the head and neck will be supported and immobilized when affixed to it. The patient's torso and pelvis are stabilized to the device so that the thoracic, lumbar, and sacral sections of the spine are supported and cannot move. The torso should be stabilized to the device before the head is secured. In this way, any movement of the device that may occur when fastening the torso straps is prevented from angulating the cervical spine.

There are many different methods for securing the device to the torso. Protection against movement in any direction—up, down, left, or right—should be achieved at both the upper torso (shoulders or chest) and the lower torso (pelvis) to avoid compression and lateral movement of the vertebrae of the torso. Limiting movement of the upper torso can be achieved with several specific methods; an understanding of the basic anatomic principles common to each method must be applied. Cephalad movement of the upper torso is restricted by use of a strap on each side, fastened to the board inferior to the upper margin of each shoulder, which then passes over the shoulder and is fastened at a lower point (Figure 9-15). Caudad movement of the torso can be restricted by use of straps that pass snugly around the pelvis and legs (Figure 9-16).

In one method, two straps are used to produce an X. A strap goes from each side of the board over the shoulder, then across the upper chest and through the opposite armpit, to fasten to the board on the armpit side. This approach limits any upward, downward, left, or right movement of the upper torso (Figure 9-17).

The same stabilization can be achieved by fastening one strap to the board and passing it through one armpit, then across the upper chest and through the opposite armpit, to fasten to the second side of the board. A strap, or cravat, is then added to each side and passed over the shoulder to fasten it to the armpit strap, similar to a pair of suspenders.

Stabilization of the upper torso of a patient with a fractured clavicle is accomplished by placing backpack-type loops around each shoulder through the armpit and fastening the ends of each loop in the same handhold. The straps remain near the lateral edges of the upper torso and do not cross the clavicles. With any of these methods, the straps are over the upper third of the chest and can be fastened tightly without producing the ventilatory compromise typically produced by tight straps placed lower on the thorax.

Stabilization of the lower torso can be achieved by use of a single strap fastened tightly over the pelvis at the iliac crests. If the long backboard will have to be upended or carried on stairs or over a distance, a pair of groin loops will provide stronger immobilization than the single strap across the iliac crests.

Lateral movement or anterior movement away from the rigid device at the midtorso can be limited by use of an additional strap around the midtorso. Any strap that surrounds the torso between the upper thorax and the iliac crests should be snug but not so tight that it inhibits chest excursion, impairing ventilatory function, or causes a significant increase in intra-abdominal pressure. Regardless of which strapping device or technique is used, the principle is to secure the torso and then the head to the board. The particular device and technique chosen depend on the judgment of the prehospital care practitioner and the given situation.

The Backboard Debate

Even though the backboard provides motion restriction of the entire spine, it is important to understand a number of facts about the backboard itself. Being placed onto a rigid board is an extremely uncomfortable experience for the patient. An unpadded board will lead to complaints of back discomfort after a relatively short time on the board. In addition, being strapped onto a rigid backboard leads to a significant amount of pressure being placed on bony prominences in contact with the board. Typically, the areas most affected include the occiput of the scalp, the scapulae (shoulder blades), the buttocks at the ischium and coccyx, and the heels. Over time (in most cases several hours), circulation to these areas can become compromised, leading to skin ischemia, necrosis, and decubitus ulcers. All these factors should prompt the prehospital care practitioner to place some padding under the patient and to minimize the amount of time a patient spends on the board.

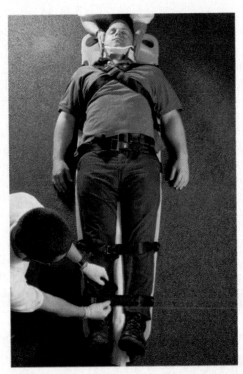

Figure 9-16 Caudad movement of the torso can be limited by use of straps that pass snugly around the pelvis and legs.

© Jones & Bartlett Learning. Photographed by Darren Stahlman.

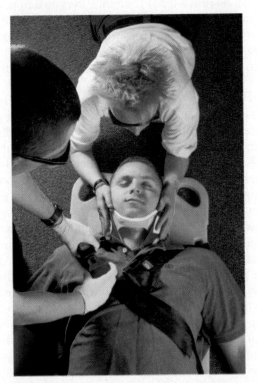

Figure 9-17 Use of two straps to produce an X across the upper chest helps to stop any upward, downward, left, or right movement of the upper torso.

© Jones & Bartlett Learning. Photographed by Darren Stahlman.

In addition, some patients, especially bariatric individuals, may experience respiratory compromise from being strapped supine onto a board.

All of these concerns have led to a growing move to decrease or completely cease the use of the backboard or to remove patients from the board once the patient has been placed on the stretcher. While it is clear that too many patients are unnecessarily immobilized based solely on the mechanism of injury, the conceptual framework surrounding the backboard cannot be disregarded. Like any intervention, the application of these management strategies must be carefully considered. In addition, while not the only method to achieve spinal motion restriction due to recognition of potential complications, the backboard is useful in select circumstances such as short transports.

It is certainly possible to maintain spinal alignment and limit motion by simply laying a patient on an ambulance cot in a supine position with a cervical collar in place. This is the technique used to immobilize patients in the hospital even after an unstable cervical or thoracolumbar injury has been formally diagnosed. If thoracolumbar injury cannot be excluded, however, it is not safe to allow such a patient to sit up by simply elevating the head portion of the stretcher, allowing the patient to flex at the hips and waist. If head elevation is desired to enhance airway protection, consider moving the stretcher to a reverse Trendelenburg position so that the spine remains in complete vertical alignment throughout. In the hospital, however, while patients can be safely moved by transfers using sheets and multiple personnel, and while they can be safely repositioned by logrolling to avoid pressure sore development, there is typically no need to move them vertically and potentially over uneven terrain as is often the case during operations in the field. There is also no need to transport them by vehicle over bumps and potholes and through traffic. Thus, the need for spinal column stabilization is not as profound in the hospital as it is in the field.

Furthermore, given that most EMS transport times in the United States are relatively short and that the length of time patients in the hospital need to maintain spinal motion restriction or immobilization is relatively long, the degree of discomfort associated with use of a longboard in the hospital is much greater than in the prehospital environment, and the risk of secondary spinal column displacement and resultant secondary neurologic injury is relatively small. This is the reason that patients should be (and routinely are) removed from backboards or immobilization devices soon after arrival at hospitals or trauma centers.

It is also possible to safely extricate patients from vehicles using temporary devices such as short backboards and sliding boards and to immediately position them onto ambulance cots without ever employing a long backboard. This technique requires increased attention to detail during patient transfers and a high degree of awareness of the need to maintain spinal precautions during all transfers by all personnel involved in such moves. Maintaining this level of control can be difficult, as it is not uncommon in the prehospital environment to employ the help of nonmedical first responders in executing such transfers. Nonetheless, this technique has the advantage of increased patient comfort and decreased scene time for physiologically unstable patients.

Elimination of the use of long backboards in the prehospital environment has occurred with increasing frequency in the United States and Europe without evidence in the literature to date of an increase in the incidence of catastrophic secondary neurologic injury. While some EMS agencies in the United States have eliminated the use of long backboards, others have chosen to modify their use of backboarding techniques to attempt to limit discomfort rather than expose patients to the potential risk of secondary catastrophic injury. EMS practitioners should be aware of the changes in their system and remain up to date on the latest evidence and protocol changes.

Maintenance of Neutral In-Line Position of the Head

In many patients, when the head is placed in a neutral in-line position, the posterior-most portion of the occipital region at the back of the head is between 0.5 and 3.5 inches (1.3 to 8.9 centimeters [cm]) anterior to the posterior thoracic wall (**Figure 9-18A**). Therefore, in most adults, a space exists between the back of the head and the board device when the head is in a neutral in-line position; thus, suitable padding should be added before securing the patient's head to the board device (**Figure 9-18B**). To be effective, this padding must be made of a material that does not readily compress. Firm, semirigid pads designed for this purpose or folded towels can be used. The amount of padding needed must be individualized for each patient; some individuals require none. If too little padding is inserted or if the padding is of an unsuitable spongy material, the head will be hyperextended when head straps are applied. If too much padding is inserted, the head will be moved into a flexed position. Both hyperextension and flexion of the head can increase spinal cord damage and should be avoided.

The same anatomic relationship between the head and back applies when most people are supine, whether on the ground or on a backboard. When most adults are supine, the head falls back into a hyperextended position. On arrival, the head should be moved into a neutral in-line position and manually maintained in that position, which in many adults will require holding the head up off the ground. If the patient is placed on a long backboard and the head is about to be fastened to the board, proper padding (as described) should be inserted between the back of the head and the board to maintain a neutral position. These principles should be used with all patients, including athletes with shoulder pads and

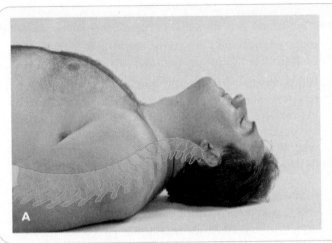
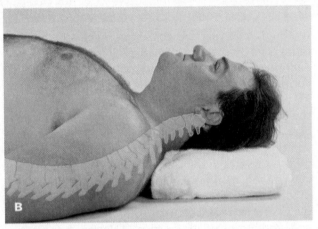

Figure 9-18 A. In some patients, allowing the skull to fall back to the level of the backboard can produce severe hyperextension of the spine. **B.** Padding is needed between the back of the head and the backboard in these patients to prevent hyperextension.
© National Association of Emergency Medical Technicians (NAEMT)

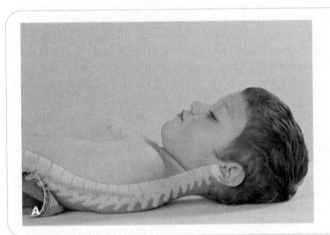
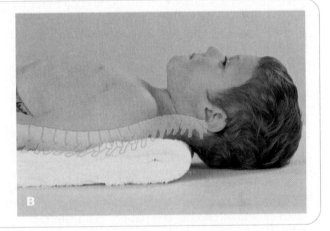

Figure 9-19 A. The larger size of a child's head relative to body size, combined with the reduced development of the posterior thoracic muscles, produces hyperflexion of the head when a child is placed on a backboard. **B.** Padding beneath the shoulders and torso will prevent this hyperflexion.
© National Association of Emergency Medical Technicians (NAEMT)

patients with abnormal curvature of the spine, such as those with severe kyphosis.

In small children, generally those with the body size of a 7-year-old or younger, the size of the head is much larger relative to the rest of the body than it is in adults, and the muscles of the back are less developed.[80] When a small child's head is in a neutral in-line position, the back of the head usually extends 1 to 2 inches (2.5 to 5 cm) beyond the posterior plane of the back. Therefore, if a small child is placed directly on a rigid surface, the head will be moved into a position of flexion (**Figure 9-19A**).

The placement of small children on a standard long backboard results in unwanted flexion of the head and neck. The long backboard needs to be modified either by creating a recess in the board for the occiput to fit into or by inserting padding under the torso to maintain the head in a neutral position (**Figure 9-19B**). The padding placed under the torso should be of the appropriate thickness so that the head lies on the board in a neutral position; too much will result in extension, too little in flexion. The padding under the torso must also be firm and evenly shaped. Use of irregularly shaped or insufficient padding or placing it only under the shoulders can result in movement and misalignment of the spine.

The challenge of undesirable deformity resulting from positioning on a board or other transport device is particularly pronounced in the situation where an athlete wearing protective equipment is injured. Spinal cord and spinal column trauma in high-energy athletes wearing protective equipment require careful consideration and potential modification of stabilization techniques to include additional padding (**Box 9-9**).

Box 9-9 Assessing Athletes and Athletic Equipment Removal

Although relatively rare, spinal trauma in athletes represents a potentially career-ending and life-altering event. Trauma during sporting activities comprises nearly 15% of all TSIs, 10% of all SCIs, and 2% to 3% of all sports-related hospital admissions in the United States.[81-83] The mechanism in which injury occurs varies based on the activity. Similarly, certain sporting activities carry higher risk of SCI than do others. Athletes in the United States who participate in wrestling, gymnastics, and football sustain a large proportion of cervical SCIs.[83] High school–age football players suffer severe cervical SCI more than any other age group involved in this sport.[84] Hockey, a sport that also carries a relatively higher risk of spine injury, will likely result in increased numbers of sports-related TSI if the popularity of the sport in the United States continues to rise.[83,85] It is important that prehospital practitioners are aware of the unique challenges faced while treating athletes (e.g., protective equipment such as helmets and face masks) to ensure that they can confidently and appropriately assess and manage these patients when a TSI is suspected. Similarly, EMS systems must collaborate with athletic trainers and recreational sporting programs in their community to ensure that all stakeholders are prepared with the equipment and training necessary for safe, effective prehospital management of an injured athlete.

The assessment and management of sports-related TSI must begin wherever the patient is encountered, with care taken before the patient is transferred from the field to a more controlled environment. Whenever an athlete is exposed to a traumatic mechanism of injury and complains of midline pain or tenderness of the spine, reduced range of motion, and/or neurologic signs or symptoms, manual stabilization of the spine should be performed with careful physical examination. If continued spinal motion restriction is appropriate (see criteria discussed previously in this chapter), practitioners should carefully prepare the patient for transfer to an appropriate hospital for further evaluation. In addition, any athlete found unconscious after a traumatic mechanism of injury should be treated as if a TSI has occurred until this can be ruled out by further diagnostic testing.[83] Although there is limited evidence to better guide this decision, it is currently recommended that whenever there are persistent neurologic complaints, pain, or reduced range of motion in the spine, the athlete should not be permitted to return to play.[86]

While special care for helmeted athletes is needed, the general principles of spinal immobilization taught in Prehospital Trauma Life Support (PHTLS) courses are appropriate and need to be followed. Patients who are not wearing any protective equipment, such as padding, helmet, or face mask, should be treated in the same fashion as any other patients undergoing spinal motion restriction. There have been recent changes in recommendations from professional organizations, such as the National Athletic Trainers' Association (NATA) and National Association of State EMS Officials (NASEMSO), regarding the removal of protective equipment.[85,87] If a helmet with a face mask is still in place when the athlete is encountered, careful removal of the face mask should be completed to ensure adequate access to effectively manage the airway.[83-85] The helmet can be removed on the field or in the emergency department, but should be removed only when enough trained personnel are available to assist.[83-85] Ideally, the helmet and shoulder pads should be removed as one unit. However, it is still possible to stabilize a player on a long backboard without causing hyperextension of the cervical spine when the helmet alone is removed. This is accomplished by the appropriate use of padding behind the head to maintain the head in neutral alignment with the rest of the spine if the shoulder pads are not removed.

Prehospital care practitioners must determine the specific medical needs for an injured athlete and take appropriate steps to meet those needs, which may often include immediate removal of the athletic equipment. Regardless of the decision, the methods of spinal motion restriction should be made with careful consideration of how protective athletic equipment may influence the ability to maintain neutral alignment of the spine, how excessive spinal motion can be prevented during transfer and transport, and whether the equipment will restrict the ability to assess or manage the patient in the prehospital environment. Athletic equipment should be removed by personnel trained and experienced in the removal of sports equipment. If the decision is made not to remove the equipment at the scene, someone knowledgeable in sports equipment removal should accompany the patient to the hospital.

Completing Stabilization

Head

Once the patient's torso has been stabilized to the rigid device selected and appropriate padding inserted behind the head as needed, the head should be secured to the device. Because of its rounded shape, the head cannot be stabilized on a flat surface with only straps or tape. Use of these alone allows the head to rotate and move laterally. Also, because of the angle of the forehead and the slippery nature of oily and moist skin and hair, a simple strap over the forehead is unreliable and can easily slide off. Although the human head weighs about the same as a bowling ball, it has a significantly different shape. The head is ovoid, longer than it is wide with almost completely flat lateral sides, resembling a bowling ball with about 2 inches (5 cm) cut off to form left and right sides. Adequate external stabilization of the head, regardless of method or device, can be achieved by placing pads or rolled blankets on these flat sides and securing them with straps or tape. In the case of vest-type devices, this is accomplished with hinged side flaps that are part of the vest.

The side supports, whether they are preshaped foam blocks or rolled blankets, are placed next to both sides of the head. The sidepieces should be at least as wide as the patient's ears, or larger, and be at least as high as the level of the patient's eyes with the patient supine. Two straps or pieces of tape surrounding these headpieces draw the sides together. When it is packaged between the blocks or blankets, the head now has a flat posterior surface that can be fixed to a flat device. The upper forehead strap is placed snugly across the front of the lower forehead (across the supraorbital ridge) to help prevent anterior movement of the head. If tape is used, avoid placing it directly onto the eyebrows. This strap should be pulled tightly enough to indent the blocks or blankets and rest firmly on the forehead.

The device, regardless of type, that holds the head also requires a lower strap to help keep the sidepieces firmly pressed against the lower sides of the head and to anchor the device further and prevent anterior movement of the lower head and neck. The lower strap passes around the sidepieces and across the anterior rigid portion of the cervical collar. This strap should not place too much pressure on the front of the collar, which could produce airway compression or a venous return problem at the neck.

Sandbags are not recommended for use as side supports because of the weight that may be placed on the head and neck when the stabilized patient is turned on the side.[88] The use of sandbags secured to the long backboard on the sides of the head and neck represents a dangerous practice. Regardless of how well the patient has been secured, these heavy objects can shift and move. Should the need arise to rotate the patient and board to the side, such as when the patient needs to vomit, the combined weight of the sandbags can produce localized lateral pressure against the head and cervical spine, forcing movement. Raising or lowering the head of the board when moving and loading the patient, or any sudden acceleration or deceleration of the ambulance can also produce shifting of the bags and movement of the head and neck.

The use of chin cups or straps encircling the chin prevents opening of the mouth to vomit, so these devices should not be used.

Whatever method of stabilization is chosen, it is essential that the practitioner recognize that rigid motion restriction of the cervical spine with these devices will impede the ability to manipulate the patient's mouth and gain access to the airway in a way that would allow for airway protection in the event of decreasing level of consciousness. It also potentially decreases the ability of patients to protect their airways in the event of vomiting or bleeding in the oropharynx. In addition, restrictive supine positioning that often results from spinal motion restriction has been shown to reduce airway patency in unconscious trauma patients when compared to lateral positioning.[89] This results in an increased risk of airway compromise.

The jaw-thrust maneuver results in less motion at unstable cervical injuries when compared with other airway maneuvers.[90] If airway management is required, it is recommended that the jaw-thrust maneuver be performed while a separate practitioner maintains neutral stabilization of the cervical spine. It is important to remember that the risk of secondary catastrophic neurologic injury in these patients, even with endotracheal intubation using direct laryngoscopy in the presence of an unstable cervical spine,[91] is small, regardless of the presenting signs, symptoms, and mechanism. It is also important to remember that the risk of airway compromise and aspiration in a patient with a decreased level of consciousness who is vomiting or bleeding into the oropharynx is real, substantial, and potentially devastating. Never allow the process of stabilization of the cervical spine to result in compromise of the ability to maintain and secure a patient's airway.

Legs

Tying the feet together can eliminate the significant outward rotation of the legs that can result from pelvic fractures or hip fractures. Placing a rolled blanket or piece of padding between the legs will increase comfort for the patient.

The patient's legs are secured to the stabilization device with two or more straps: one strap proximal to the knees at about midthigh and one strap distal to the knees. The average adult measures 14 to 20 inches (35 to

50 cm) from one side to the other at the hips and only 6 to 9 inches (15 to 23 cm) from one side to the other at the ankles. When the feet are placed together, a V shape is formed from the hips to the ankles. Because the ankles are considerably narrower than the device, a strap placed across the lower legs can prevent anterior movement but will not prevent the legs from moving laterally from one edge of the stabilization device to the other. If the device is angled or rotated, the legs will fall to the lower edge of the device, which can angulate the pelvis and produce movement of the spinal column.

One way to hold the patient's lower legs effectively in place is to encircle them several times with the strap before attaching it to the stabilization device. The legs can be kept in the middle of the device by placing blanket rolls between each leg and the edges of the device before strapping. It is important to ensure that the straps are not so tight that they impair distal circulation.

Arms

For safety, the patient's arms may be secured to the device or across the torso before moving the patient. One way to achieve this is with the arms placed at the sides on the device with the palms in, secured by a strap across the forearms and torso. This strap should be snug but not so tight as to compromise the circulation in the hands.

The patient's arms should not be included in the strap at the iliac crests or in the groin loops. If the straps are tight enough to provide adequate stabilization of the lower torso, they can compromise the circulation in the hands. If the straps are loose, they will not provide adequate stabilization of the torso or arms. Use of an additional strap exclusively to hold the arms allows the strap to be opened for taking a blood pressure measurement or starting an intravenous line once the patient is in the ambulance without compromising the stabilization. If the arm strap is also a torso strap, loosening it to free just an arm has the side effect of loosening the torso as well.

Most Common Spinal Stabilization Mistakes

The following are the most common spinal stabilization errors:

1. Failing to adequately provide spinal motion restriction such that the torso can move significantly up or down on the board device or the head can still move excessively.
2. Improperly sizing or improperly applying the cervical collar.
3. Immobilizing the patient with the head hyperextended. The most common cause is a lack of appropriate padding behind the head.
4. Securing the head before the torso or readjusting the torso straps after the head has been secured. This causes movement of the device relative to the torso, which results in movement of the head and cervical spine.
5. Using inadequate padding. Failure to fill the voids under a patient can allow for inadvertent movement of the spine, resulting in additional injury as well as increased discomfort for the patient.
6. Placing someone in spinal immobilization who does not meet immobilization criteria.
7. Taking excessive time to achieve immobilization in the context of a physiologically unstable or potentially unstable patient.
8. Using overly aggressive immobilization techniques that fail to prioritize maintaining and protecting airway integrity.

Complete spinal motion restriction is generally not a comfortable experience for the patient. As the degree and quality of the immobilization increase, the patient's comfort decreases. Spinal stabilization is a balance between the need to protect and immobilize the spine completely, the need to maintain and protect airway access, the need to expeditiously initiate transport, and the need to make it tolerable for the patient. This is why proper evaluation of the need for spinal stabilization is mandatory (**Box 9-10**).

Obese Patients

With the increasing epidemic of obesity, care of the *bariatric* (overweight, obese) patient is becoming necessary more frequently. Transport of a 400-lb (182-kg) patient is becoming an all-too-common occurrence, and special bariatric transport cots have been developed for this purpose. However, when using lifting and extrication devices that are not designed specifically to accommodate bariatric patients, special care is needed to ensure that the safe operating limits are not exceeded. Also, additional personnel must be present to help lift and extricate bariatric patients to avoid causing further injury to the patient or prehospital care practitioners. This subgroup of trauma patients presents the challenge of balancing safe packaging and moving procedures against the short scene times normally recommended for critically injured trauma patients.

Some obese patients may demonstrate an increased work of breathing to the point of respiratory failure if placed supine on a backboard. This phenomenon occurs secondary to the increased pressure being placed on the diaphragm by the adipose tissue of the abdomen. In these cases, the principles of spinal motion restriction should still be followed, but the practice may have to be changed. An obese patient's cervical spine may be manually maintained by the prehospital care practitioner's hands and a cervical collar, while the head of the stretcher is elevated in

Box 9-10 Criteria for Evaluating Spinal Stabilization Skills

Prehospital care practitioners must practice their stabilization skills in hands-on sessions using mock patients before use with real patients. When practicing or when evaluating new methods or equipment, the following criteria will serve as good tools for measuring how effective the intervention has been at restricting spinal motion:

1. Initiate manual in-line stabilization immediately, and maintain it until it is replaced mechanically.
2. Check neurologic function distally.
3. Apply an effective, properly sized cervical collar.
4. Secure the torso before the head.
5. Prevent movement of the torso up or down the device.
6. Prevent movement of the upper and lower torso left or right on the immobilization device.
7. Ensure ties crossing the chest do not inhibit chest excursion or result in ventilatory compromise.
8. Effectively stabilize the head so that it cannot move in any direction.
9. Provide padding behind the head, if necessary.
10. Maintain the head in a neutral in-line position.

11. Ensure that nothing inhibits or prevents the mouth from being opened and that sufficient access to the airway is present to effectively allow the practitioner to maintain and protect airway integrity.
12. Stabilize the legs so that they cannot move anteriorly, rotate, or move from side to side, even if the board and patient are rotated to the side.
13. Maintain the pelvis and legs in a neutral in-line position.
14. Ensure that the arms are appropriately secured to the device or torso.
15. Ensure that any ties or straps do not compromise distal circulation in any limb.
16. Reevaluate the patient if bumped, jostled, or in any way moved in a manner that could compromise an unstable spine while the device was being applied.
17. Complete the procedure within an appropriate time frame.
18. Recheck distal neurologic function.

Many methods and variations can meet these objectives. The selection of a specific method and specific equipment should be based on the situation, the patient's condition, and available resources.

© National Association of Emergency Medical Technicians (NAEMT)

a reverse Trendelenburg position. This approach will provide cervical and lumbosacral stabilization without causing increased respiratory distress.

Pregnant Patients

Occasionally a pregnant patient will require spinal immobilization. Depending on the gestational age, placing the patient in a fully supine position may cause compression of the inferior vena cava by the gravid uterus, leading to a decrease in venous blood return to the heart, thus decreasing the mother's blood pressure. In these circumstances, the patient should be secured to the backboard using standard techniques. Once secured, the backboard is tipped on an angle to place the patient in a relative left lateral position (left side down with blanket or padding under the right side of the patient sufficient to support this position). This position will move the uterus off of the vena cava, restoring blood pressure (**Figure 9-20**).

Use of Steroids

The use of steroids in the management of SCI remains controversial. The National Acute Spinal Cord Injury Studies (NASCIS) trials were multicenter, double-blinded,

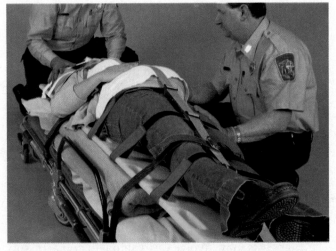

Figure 9-20 Tipping a pregnant patient onto her left side helps displace the uterus from the inferior vena cava and improves blood return to the heart, thus restoring blood pressure.
© Jones & Bartlett Learning. Courtesy of MIEMSS.

randomized control trials conducted in 1984, 1990, and 1997 to evaluate the benefit of steroids in acute SCI.[92-94] Although NASCIS I suggested that high doses of methylprednisolone started within 8 hours of the injury improved the neurologic outcome following acute SCIs from blunt trauma, NASCIS II and III did not find any benefit. The current national guidelines from the Congress of Neurological Surgeons in 2019 do not recommend routine use of methylprednisolone for acute SCI given insufficient evidence.[95] Steroids are also not indicated for SCI from penetrating trauma, even with neurologic deficits.

Steroid use has been associated with numerous adverse effects, including suppression of the adrenal gland and immune system. Therefore, the risk of complications associated with steroid administration may significantly outweigh the benefit, if any, they may confer. Numerous publications no longer recommend steroid use for spinal injury, either in the field or in the hospital.[96-100] In summary, the current medical literature does not support a role for the administration of steroids to the spinal cord–injured patient in the hospital or prehospital setting.[101,102]

Prolonged Transport

As with other injuries, the prolonged transport of patients with suspected or confirmed spine and spinal cord injuries presents special considerations. Although backboards may be valuable for transfers over short distances or duration, they should not be used as stabilization devices for periods exceeding 30 minutes. Such efforts should help reduce the risk for the development of pressure ulcers in a patient with SCI. Any areas where there could be pressure on the patient's body, especially over bony prominences, should be sufficiently padded. For transports that will exceed 30 minutes, consideration should be given to using a scoop stretcher to carefully lift the patient, removing the long backboard, and then placing the patient down onto the ambulance cot.

Patients who are immobilized in a supine position are at risk for aspiration should they regurgitate. In the event the patient begins to vomit, the device and patient should immediately be tipped onto the side. Suction should be kept near the head of the patient so it is readily accessible should vomiting occur. Insertion of a gastric tube (either nasogastric or orogastric), if allowed, and the judicious use of antiemetic medications may help reduce this risk.

High SCIs may involve the diaphragm and accessory respiratory muscles (i.e., intercostal muscles), predisposing patients to respiratory failure. Impending respiratory failure may be aggravated and hastened by straps placed across the trunk for spinal stabilization that further restrict respiration. Prior to initiating a prolonged transport, practitioners must double-check that the patient's torso is secured at the shoulder girdle and at the pelvis and that straps do not limit chest wall excursion.

As described earlier, patients with high SCIs may experience hypotension from loss of sympathetic tone (neurogenic shock). Although these patients rarely suffer from widespread hypoperfusion of their tissues, crystalloid boluses are generally sufficient to restore their blood pressure to normal. Vasopressors are rarely, if ever, necessary to treat neurogenic shock. Another hallmark of a high cervical spine injury is bradycardia. If associated with significant hypotension, bradycardia may be treated with intermittent doses of atropine, 1.0 mg administered intravenously.

The presence of tachycardia combined with hypotension should raise suspicion for the presence of hypovolemic (hemorrhagic), rather than neurogenic, shock. Careful assessment may pinpoint the source of hemorrhage, although intra-abdominal sources and pelvic fractures are most likely. Insertion of a urinary catheter will allow urine output to be used as another measure of tissue perfusion. In an adult, a urine output of greater than 30 to 50 milliliters per hour (mL/hour) generally indicates satisfactory end-organ perfusion. The loss of sensation that accompanies an SCI may prevent a conscious patient from perceiving peritonitis or other injuries below the level of the sensory deficit.

Patients with spinal injuries may have significant back pain or pain from associated fractures. Pain may be managed with small doses of intravenous narcotics titrated until pain is relieved. (See Chapter 12, *Musculoskeletal Trauma*, for further details.) Narcotics may exaggerate the neurogenic hypotension associated with SCI.

Patients with SCIs lose some ability to regulate body temperature, and this effect is more pronounced with injuries higher in the spinal cord. Thus, these patients are sensitive to the development of hypothermia, especially when they are in a cold environment.

Spine and spinal cord injuries are best managed at facilities that have excellent orthopedic or neurosurgical services and are experienced in the management of these injuries. All level I and II trauma centers should be capable of managing the SCI and any associated injuries. Some facilities that specialize in the management of spine and spinal cord injuries may directly accept a patient who has suffered only an SCI (e.g., a shallow-water diving injury with no evidence of aspiration).

SUMMARY

- The vertebral column comprises 24 separate vertebrae plus the sacrum and coccyx stacked on top of one another.
- The major functions of the spinal column are to support the weight of the body and allow movement.
- The spinal cord is enclosed within the vertebral column and is vulnerable to injury from abnormal movement and positioning. When support for the vertebral column has been lost as a result of injury to the vertebrae or to the muscles and ligaments that help hold the spinal column in place, injury to the spinal cord can occur.
- After ensuring practitioner and scene safety, the primary survey is the first priority. A rapid scene assessment and history of the event should determine if the possibility of a spinal injury exists.
- Mechanism of injury should never be the sole means of determining the need for spinal motion restriction, as it represents only one factor in a multifaceted decision-making process to determine if spinal motion restriction is appropriate. Assessment of the neck and spine for spinal motion restriction should also include assessment of motor and sensory function, presence of pain or

tenderness, and patient reliability as predictors of risk of spinal column injury.
- Prehospital care practitioners must be familiar with the devices (e.g., scoop stretchers, vacuum mattresses, rigid cervical collars) and the techniques (e.g., manual in-line stabilization, maintenance of in-line position of the head) used to restrict spinal motion. They must train frequently and stay up to date on local protocols.
- Special patient populations, including patients who are obese or pregnant, and prolonged transport times may require modifications to standard immobilization practices.
- The device selected should stabilize the head, chest, and pelvis areas in a neutral in-line position without causing or allowing movement.
- Depending on the patient, the severity of the patient's injuries, and the availability of equipment, the technique chosen should be based on the judgment of the prehospital care practitioner with the guidance of local emergency medical services medical direction.
- Properly fitting and applying equipment are paramount for the successful stabilization of trauma patients.

SCENARIO RECAP

You have been dispatched to the scene of a bicyclist who is reported down alongside a roadway. On arrival, the scene is safe, with traffic being controlled by law enforcement. The patient, a young woman, is lying supine on the side of the road away from traffic. A law enforcement officer is kneeling beside her and trying to talk to her, but she is not responding.

As you begin your primary survey, you are unable to ascertain the specific cause of the fall. It appears the woman fell from her bike while riding along the roadway, but you do not know whether she was struck by a motor vehicle. The law enforcement officers tell you there were no witnesses. The patient is wearing full cycling gear, including helmet and gloves. She has abrasions on her forehead and an obvious deformity of the right wrist. Her airway is open, and she is breathing regularly. She shows no obvious signs of external blood loss. Her skin appears dry and warm with normal color. As you are performing your primary survey, she begins to awaken but remains confused as to what happened.

- What pathologic processes explain the patient's presentation?
- What immediate interventions and further assessments are needed?
- What are the management goals for this patient?

SCENARIO SOLUTION

The patient's vital signs are as follows: pulse 66 beats/minute, ventilatory rate 14 breaths/minute, and blood pressure 86/70 mm Hg. As you continue your examination, you note that the patient is not moving her arms or legs. The physical findings, along with the vital signs, are suggestive of neurogenic hypotension. Interruption of the sympathetic nervous system and unopposed parasympathetic influence on the vascular system below the point of spinal injury result in an increased size of the vascular container and a relative hypovolemia. The patient's response to the spinal cord injury is a low blood pressure and bradycardia.

The first priorities of care are to continue to maintain a patent airway and oxygenation and assist ventilation as necessary to ensure an adequate minute volume while concurrently providing manual stabilization of the cervical spine. You stabilize the patient effectively and efficiently on a spinal motion restriction device and transport her to an appropriate facility 9 minutes away. You manage the neurogenic hypotension caused by the SCI with two separate 250-mL boluses of intravenous fluids. You splint the fractured arm while en route.

The goals of prehospital management for this patient are to prevent additional spinal cord trauma, maintain tissue perfusion, care for extremity trauma en route, and transport without delay to an appropriate facility for definitive care.

References

1. Jain NB, Ayers GD, Peterson EN, et al. Traumatic spinal cord injury in the United States, 1993–2012. *JAMA.* 2015;313(22):2236-2243. doi: 10.1001/jama.2015.6250

2. *Spinal Cord Injury: Facts and Figures at a Glance* [SCI data sheet]. National SCI Statistical Center; 2021.

3. Singh A, Tetreault L, Kalsi-Ryan S, Nouri A, Fehlings MG. Global prevalence and incidence of traumatic spinal cord injury. *Clin Epidemiol.* 2014;6:309-331.

4. DeVivo M, Chen Y, Mennemeyer S, Deutsch A. Costs of care following spinal cord injury. *Top Spinal Cord Inj Rehab.* 2011;16(4):1-9.

5. Meldon SW, Moettus LN. Thoracolumbar spine fractures: clinical presentation and the effect of altered sensorium and major injury. *J Trauma.* 1995;38:1110-1114.

6. Ross SE, O'Malley KF, DeLong WG, et al. Clinical predictors of unstable cervical spine injury in multiply-injured patients. *Injury.* 1992;23:317-319.

7. Greenbaum J, Walters N, Levy PD. An evidence-based approach to radiographic assessment of cervical spine injuries in the emergency department. *J Emerg Med.* 2009;36(1):64-71.

8. Stein DM, Knight WA IV. Emergency neurological life support: traumatic spine injury. *Neurocrit Care Soc.* 2017; 27:S170-S180.

9. Hu R, Mustard CA, Burns B. Epidemiology of incident spinal fracture in a complete population. *Spine.* 1996;21(4): 492-499.

10. Wood KB, Buttermann GR, Phukan R, et al. Operative compared with nonoperative treatment of a thoracolumbar burst fracture without neurological deficit: a prospective randomized study with follow-up at 16 and 22 years. *J Bone Joint Surg Am.* 2015;97:3-9.

11. Wood KB, Buttermann GR, Mehob A, Garvey T, Jhanjee R, Sechriest V. Operative compared with nonoperative treatment of a thoracolumbar burst fracture without neurological deficit: a prospective, randomized study. *J Bone Joint Surg Am.* 2003;85(5):773-781.

12. Adams MA, Dolan P. Spine biomechanics. *J Biomech.* 2005;38(10):1972-1983.

13. Izzo R, Guarnieri G, Guglielmi G, Muto M. Biomechanics of the spine. Part 1: spinal stability. *Eur J Radiol.* 2013;82:118-126.

14. Dreischarf M, Shirazi-Adl A, Arjmand N, Rohlmann A, Schmidt H. Estimation of loads on human lumbar spine: a review of *in vivo* and computational model studies. *J Biomech.* 2016;49:833-845.

15. Oxland TR. Fundamental biomechanics of the spine: what we have learned in the past 25 years and future directions. *J Biomechan.* 2016;49:817-832.

16. Leucht P, Fischer K, Muhr G, Mueller EJ. Epidemiology of traumatic spine fractures. *Injury.* 2009;40:166-172.

17. Lindsey RW, Gugala Z, Pneumaticos SG. Injury to the vertebrae and spinal cord. In: Feliciano DV, Mattox KL, Moore EE, eds. *Trauma.* McGraw Hill; 2008:479-510.

18. Jawa RS, Singer AJ, Rutigliano DN, et al. Spinal fractures in older adult patients admitted after low-level falls: 10-year incidence and outcomes. *J Am Geriatr Soc.* 2017;65(5):909-915.

19. Katsuura Y, Osborn JM, Cason GW. The epidemiology of thoracolumbar trauma: a meta-analysis. *J Orthop.* 2016;13:383-388.

20. Shin JI, Lee NJ, Cho SK. Pediatric cervical spine and spinal cord injury: a national database study. *Spine.* 2016;41(4):283-292.

21. Mohseni S, Talving P, Castelo Branco B, et al. Effect of age on cervical spine injury in pediatric population: a National Trauma Data Bank review. *J Pediatr Surg.* 2011;46:1771-1776.

22. Easter JS, Barkin R, Rosen CL, Ban K. Cervical spine injuries in children, part 1: mechanism of injury, clinical presentation, and imaging. *J Emerg Med.* 2011;41(2):142-150.

23. Patel JC, Tepas JJ III, Mollitt DL, Pieper P. Pediatric cervical spine injuries: defining the disease. *J Pediatr Surg*. 2001;36(2):373-376.

24. Parent S, Mac-Thiong J-M, Roy-Beaudry M, Sosa JF, Labelle H. Spinal cord injury in the pediatric population: a systematic review of the literature. *J Neurotrauma*. 2011;28:1515-1524.

25. Piatt JH Jr. Pediatric spinal injury in the US: epidemiology and disparities. *J Neurosurg Pediatr*. 2015;16:463-471.

26. Tator CH, Fehlings MG. Review of the secondary injury theory of acute spinal cord trauma with special emphasis on vascular mechanisms. *J Neurosurg*. 1991;75:15-26.

27. Tator CH. Spinal cord syndromes: physiologic and anatomic correlations. In: Menezes AH, Sonntag VKH, eds. *Principles of Spinal Surgery*. McGraw-Hill; 1995.

28. Ahuja CS, Martin AR, Fehlings M. Recent advances in managing a spinal cord injury secondary to trauma. *F1000Res*. 2016;5:ii.

29. Wu C, Fry CH, Henry J. The mode of action of several opioids on cardiac muscle. *Exp Physiol*. 1997;82:261-272.

30. Vale FL, Burns J, Jackson AB, Hadley MN. Combined medical and surgical treatment after acute spinal cord injury: results of a prospective pilot study to assess the merits of aggressive medical resuscitation and blood pressure management. *J Neurosurg*. 1997;87:239-246.

31. Bernhard M, Gries A, Kremer P, Bottiger BW. Spinal cord injury (SCI)—prehospital management. *Resuscitation*. 2005;66:127-139.

32. Dhall SS, Dailey AT, Anderson PA, et al. Congress of Neurological Surgeons systematic review and evidence-based guidelines on the evaluation and treatment of patients with thoracolumbar spine trauma: hemodynamic management. *Neurosurgery*. 2019;84(1):E43-E45.

33. Catapano JS, Hawryluk GWJ, Whetstone W, et al. Higher mean arterial pressure values correlate with neurologic improvement in patients with initially complete spinal cord injuries. *World Neurosurg*. 2016;96:72-79.

34. Carrick MM, Leonard J, Slone DS, Mains CW, Bar-Or D. Hypotensive resuscitation among trauma patients. *Biomed Res Int*. 2016;2016:8901938.

35. Ryken TC, Hurlbert RJ, Hadley MN, et al. The acute cardiopulmonary management of patients with cervical spinal cord injuries. *Neurosurgery*. 2013;72:84-92.

36. Bilello JP, Davis JW, Cunningham MA, et al. Cervical spinal cord injury and the need for cardiovascular intervention. *Arch Surg*. 2003;138:1127-1129.

37. Heffernan DS, Schermer CR, Lu SW. What defines a distracting injury in cervical spine assessment? *J Trauma Inj Infect Crit Care*. 2005;59(6):1396-1399.

38. Cason B, Rostas J, Simmons J, Frotan MA, Brevard SB, Gonzalez RP. Thoracolumbar spine clearance: clinical examination for patients with distracting injuries. *J Trauma Acute Care Surg*. 2015;80(1):125-130.

39. Konstantinidis A, Plurad D, Barmparas G, et al. The presence of nonthoracic distracting injuries does not affect the initial clinical examination of the cervical spine in evaluable blunt trauma patients: a prospective observational study. *J Trauma Inj Infect Crit Care*. 2011;71(3):528-532.

40. Lindborg R, Jambhekar A, Chan V, Laskey D, Rucinski A, Fahoum B. Distracting injury defined: does an isolated hip fracture constitute a distracting injury for clearance of the cervical spine? *Emerg Radiol*. 2018 Feb;25(1):35-39.

41. Young AJ, Wolfe L, Tinkoff G, Duane TM. Assessing incidence and risk factors of cervical spine injury in blunt trauma patients using the National Trauma Data Bank. *Am Surg*. 2015;81:879-883.

42. Hills MW, Deane SA. Head injury and facial injury: is there an increased risk of cervical spine injury. *J Trauma*. 1993;34(4):549-553.

43. Shekhar H, Kahn S. Cervical spine injuries. *Orthopaed Trauma*. 2016;30(5):390-401.

44. Connell RA, Graham CA, Munro PT. Is spinal immobilization necessary for all patients sustaining isolated penetrating trauma? *Injury*. 2003;34:912-914.

45. Fischer PE, Perina DG, Delbridge TR, et al. Spinal motion restriction in the trauma patient: a joint position statement. *Prehosp Emerg Care*. 2018;22(6):659-661. doi: 10.1080/10903127.2018.1481476

46. National Association of EMS Physicians and American College of Surgeons Committee on Trauma. EMS spinal precautions and the use of the long backboard. *Prehosp Emerg Care*. 2013;17(3):392-393.

47. Stuke LE, Pons PT, Guy JS, Chapleau WP, Butler FK, McSwain NE. Prehospital spine immobilization for penetrating trauma: review and recommendations from the Prehospital Trauma Life Support Executive Committee. *J Trauma Inj Infect Crit Care*. 2011;71(3):763-770.

48. Haut ER, Kalish BT, Efron DT, et al. Spine immobilization in penetrating trauma: more harm than good? *J Trauma Inj Infect Crit Care*. 2010;68(1):115-121.

49. Abram S, Bulstrode C. Routine spinal immobilization in trauma patients: what are the advantages and disadvantages? *Surgeon*. 2010;8:218-222.

50. Kennedy FR, Gonzales P, Beitler A, et al. Incidence of cervical spine injuries in patients with gunshot wounds to the head. *Southern Med J*. 1994;87:621-623.

51. Chong CL, Ware DN, Harris JH. Is cervical spine imaging indicated in gunshot wounds to the cranium? *J Trauma*. 1998;44:501-502.

52. Kaups KL, Davis JW. Patients with gunshot wounds to the head do not require cervical spine immobilization and evaluation. *J Trauma*. 1998;44:865-867.

53. Lanoix R, Gupta R, Leak L, Pierre J. C-spine injury associated with gunshot wounds to the head: retrospective study and literature review. *J Trauma*. 2000;49:860-863.

54. Barkana Y, Stein M, Scope A, et al. Prehospital stabilization of the cervical spine for penetrating injuries of the neck: is it necessary? *Injury*. 2003;34:912.

55. Cornwell EE, Chang, DC, Boner JP, et al. Thoracolumbar immobilization for trauma patients with torso gunshot wounds—is it necessary? *Arch Surg*. 2001;136:324-327.

56. American College of Surgeons Committee on Trauma. *Advanced Trauma Life Support for Doctors*. 9th ed. American College of Surgeons; 2012.

57. Ullrich A, Hendey GW, Geiderman J, et al. Distracting painful injuries associated with cervical spinal injuries in blunt trauma. *Acad Emerg Med*. 2001;8:25-29.

58. Domeier RM, Evans RW, Swor RA, et al. Prospective validation of out-of-hospital spinal clearance criteria: a preliminary report. *Acad Emerg Med*. 1997;4:643-646.

59. Domeier RM, Swor RA, Evans RW, et al. Multicenter prospective validation of prehospital clinical spinal clearance criteria. *J Trauma*. 2002;53:744-750.

60. Hankins DG, Rivera-Rivera EJ, Ornato JP, et al. Spinal immobilization in the field: clinical clearance criteria and implementation. *Prehosp Emerg Care*. 2001;5:88-93.

61. Stroh G, Braude D. Can an out-of-hospital cervical spine clearance protocol identify all patients with injuries? An argument for selective immobilization. *Ann Emerg Med*. 2001;37:609-615.

62. Dunn TM, Dalton A, Dorfman T, et al. Are emergency medical technician-basics able to use a selective immobilization of the cervical spine protocol? A preliminary report. *Prehosp Emerg Care*. 2004;8:207-211.

63. Domeier RM, Frederiksen SM, Welch K. Prospective performance assessment of an out-of-hospital protocol for selective spine immobilization using clinical spine clearance criteria. *Ann Emerg Med*. 2005;46:123-131.

64. Domeier RM, National Association of EMS Physicians Standards and Practice Committee. Indications for prehospital spinal immobilization. *Prehosp Emerg Care*. 1997;3:251-253.

65. Kwan I, Bunn F. Effects of prehospital spinal immobilization: a systematic review of randomized trials on healthy subjects. *Prehosp Disast Med*. 2005;20:47-53.

66. Akkuş Ş, Çorbacıoğlu ŞK, Çevik Y, Akıncı E, Uzunosmanoğlu H. Effects of spinal immobilization at 20° on respiratory functions. *Am J Emerg Med*. 2016;34:1959-1962.

67. Ham WHW, Shoonhoven L, Schuurmans MJ, Leenen LPH. Pressure ulcer development in trauma patients with suspected spinal injury: the influence of risk factors present in the emergency department. *Int Emerg Nurs*. 2017;30:13-19.

68. Ham WHW, Shoonhoven L, Schuurmans MJ, Leenen LPH. Pressure ulcers, indentation marks and pain from cervical spine immobilization with extrication collars and headblocks: an observational study. *Injury*. 2016;47:1924-1931.

69. Robinson WW, inventor. Scoop stretcher. U.S. patent 2417378. December 28, 1943.

70. Krell JM, McCoy MS, Sparto PJ, Fisher GL, Stoy WA, Hostler DP. Comparison of the Ferno scoop stretcher with the long backboard for spinal immobilization. *Prehosp Emerg Care*. 2006;10(1):46-51.

71. Lovell ME, Evans JH. A comparison of the spinal board and the vacuum stretcher, spinal stability and interface pressure. *Injury*. 1994;25(3):179-180.

72. Chan D, Goldberg RM, Mason J, Chan L. Backboard versus mattress splint immobilization: a comparison of symptoms generated. *J Emerg Med*. 1996;14(3):293-298.

73. Johnson DR, Hauswald M, Stockhoff C. Comparison of a vacuum splint device to a rigid backboard for spinal immobilization. *Am J Emerg Med*. 1996;14(4):369-372.

74. Hamilton RS, Pons PT. The efficacy and comfort of full-body vacuum splints for cervical-spine immobilization. *J Emerg Med*. 1996;14(5):553-559.

75. Cross DA, Baskerville J. Comparison of perceived pain with different immobilization techniques. *Prehosp Emerg Care*. 2001;5(3):270-274.

76. Luscombe MD, Williams JL. Comparison of a long spinal board and vacuum mattress for spinal immobilisation. *Emerg Med J*. 2003;20(5):476-478.

77. Ben-Galim P, Dreiangel N, Mattox KL, Reitman CA, Kalantar SB, Hipp JA. Extrication collars can result in abnormal separation between vertebrae in the presence of a dissociative injury. *J Trauma*. 2010;69(2):447-450.

78. Ho AMH, Fung KY, Joynt GM, Karmakar KM, Peng Z. Rigid cervical collar and intracranial pressure of patients with severe head injury. *J Trauma*. 2002;53:1185-1188.

79. Mobbs RJ, Stoodley MA, Fuller JF. Effect of cervical hard collar on intracranial pressure after head injury. *Anz J Surg*. 2002;72:389-391.

80. DeBoer SL, Seaver M. Big head, little body syndrome: what EMS providers need to know. *Emerg Med Serv*. 2004;33:47-52.

81. Nalliah RP, Anderson IM, Lee MK, Rampa S, Allareddy V, Allareddy V. Epidemiology of hospital-based emergency department visits due to sports injuries. *Pediatr Emerg Care*. 2014;30(8):511-515.

82. UAB Spinal Cord Injury Model System Information Network. The UAB-SCIMS information network. University of Alabama School of Medicine website. Accessed February 4, 2018. www.spinalcord.uab.edu

83. Puvanesurajah V, Qureshi R, Cancienne JM, Hassanzadeh H. Traumatic sports-related cervical spine injuries. *Trauma Spine Inj*. 2017;30(2):50-56.

84. Banerjee R, Palumbo MA, Fadale PD. Catastrophic cervical spine injuries in the collision sport athlete, part 1: epidemiology, functional anatomy, and diagnosis. *Am J Sports Med*. 2004;32(4):1077-1087.

85. Appropriate Care of the Spine Injured Athlete. National Athletic Trainers' Association. Updated August 5, 2015. Accessed February 4, 2018. https://www.nata.org /sites/default/files/Executive-Summary-Spine-Injury -updated.pdf

86. Schroeder GD, Vaccaro AR. Cervical spine injuries in the athlete. *J Am Acad Orthop Surg*. 2016;24(9):e122-e133.

87. Response to the National Athletic Trainers Association: appropriate care of the spine injured athlete; inter-association consensus statement. National Association of State EMS Officials. Published October 27, 2015. Accessed March 4, 2018. https://www.nasemso.org/Councils/MedicalDirectors /documents/NASEMSO-Response-to-NATA-Care-of-Spine -Injured-Athlete.pdf

88. Nesathurai S. Steroids and spinal cord injury: revisiting the NASCIS 2 and NASCIS 3 trials. *J Trauma*. 1998; 45:1088-1093.

89. Hyldmo PK, Vist GE, Feyling AC, et al. Is the supine position associated with loss of airway patency in unconscious trauma patients? A systematic review and meta-analysis. *Scan J Trauma Resusc Emerg Med*. 2013;23:50.

90. Prasarn ML, Horodyski EB, Scott NE, Konopka G, Conrad B, Rechtine GR. Motion generated in the unstable upper cervical spine during head tilt–chin lift and jaw thrust maneuvers. *Spine J*. 2014;14:609-614.

91. Hindman BJ, From RP, Fontes RB, et al. Intubation biomechanics: laryngoscope force and cervical spine motion during intubation in cadavers—cadavers vs. patients, the effect of repeated intubations, and the effect of type II odontoid fracture on C1-C2 motion. *Anesthesiology*. 2015;123(5):1042-1058.

92. Bracken MB, Collins WF, Freeman DF, et al. Efficacy of methylprednisolone in acute spinal cord injury. *JAMA*. 1984;251(1):45-52.

93. Bracken MB, Shepard MJ, Collins WF, et al. A randomized, controlled trial of methylprednisolone or naloxone in the treatment of acute spinal-cord injury: results of the Second National Acute Spinal Cord Injury Study. *N Engl J Med*. 1990;322(20):1405-1411. doi: 10.1056/NEJM199005173222001

94. Bracken MB, Shepard MJ, Holford TR, et al. Administration of methylprednisolone for 24 or 48 hours or tirilazad mesylate for 48 hours in the treatment of acute spinal cord injury: results of the Third National Acute Spinal Cord Injury Randomized Controlled Trial National Acute Spinal Cord Injury Study. *JAMA*. 1997;277(20):1597-1604.

95. Arnold PM, Anderson PA, Chi JH, et al. Congress of Neurological Surgeons systematic review and evidence-based guidelines on the evaluation and treatment of patients with thoracolumbar spine trauma: pharmacological treatment. *Neurosurgery*. 2019;84(1):E36-E38. doi: 10.1093/neuros/nyy371

96. Bledsoe BE, Wesley AK, Salomone JP. High-dose steroids for acute spinal cord injury in emergency medical services. *Prehosp Emerg Care*. 2004;8:313-316.

97. American College of Surgeons Committee on Trauma. Spine and spinal cord trauma. In: *Advanced Trauma Life Support for Doctors*. 8th ed. Chicago, IL: American College of Surgeons; 2008.

98. Short DJ, El Masry WS, Jones PW. High dose methylprednisolone in the management of acute spinal cord injury: a systematic review from the clinical perspective. *Spinal Cord*. 2000;38:273-286.

99. Coleman WP, Benzel D, Cahill DW, et al. A critical appraisal of the reporting of the National Acute Spinal Cord Injury Studies (II and III) of methylprednisolone in acute spinal cord injury. *J Spinal Disord*. 2000;13:185-199.

100. Hurlbert RJ. The role of steroids in acute spinal cord injury: an evidence-based analysis. *Spine*. 2001;26:S39-S46.

101. Bracken MB. Steroids for acute spinal cord injury (review). *Cochrane Database Syst Rev*. 2012 Jan 18;1(1):CD001046.

102. Evaniew N, Noonan VK, Fallah N, et al. Methylprednisolone for the treatment of patients with acute spinal cord injuries: a propensity score-matched cohort study from a Canadian multi-center spinal cord injury registry. *J Neurotrauma*. 2015;32(21):1674-1683.

Suggested Reading

American College of Surgeons Committee on Trauma. *Advanced Trauma Life Support for Doctors, Student Course Manual*. 9th ed. American College of Surgeons; 2012.

Pennardt AM, Zehner WJ. Paramedic documentation of indicators for cervical spine injury. *Prehosp Disaster Med*. 1994; 9:40-43.

White CC, Domeier RM, Millin MG; Standards and Clinical Practice Committee, National Association of EMS Physicians. EMS spinal precautions and the use of long backboard—resource document to the position statement of the National Association of EMS Physicians and the American College of Surgeons Committee on Trauma. *Prehosp Emerg Care*. 2014;18(2):306-314.

SPECIFIC SKILLS

Spine Management

These skills are meant to demonstrate the principles of spinal immobilization. The specific preference as to the particular device used will be determined by each agency, jurisdictional medical oversight, and local protocols.

Cervical Collar Sizing and Application

Principle: To select and apply an appropriate-sized cervical collar to assist in providing neutral alignment and stabilization of the patient's head and neck.

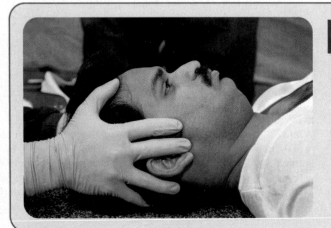

1 The first prehospital care practitioner provides manual neutral in-line stabilization of the patient's head and neck.

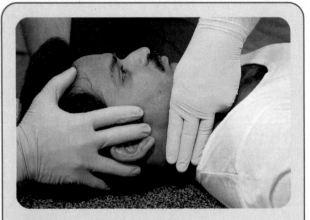

2 The second prehospital care practitioner uses their fingers to measure the patient's neck between the patient's lower jaw and shoulder.

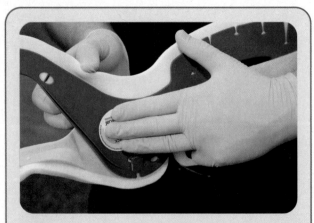

3 The second prehospital care practitioner uses this measurement to select the proper size collar or adjust an adjustable collar to the correct size.

Spine Management (continued)

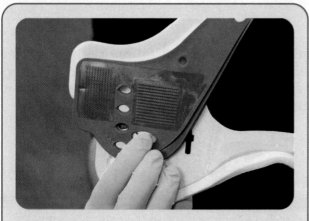

4 If an adjustable collar is utilized, make sure the collar is locked into the proper size.

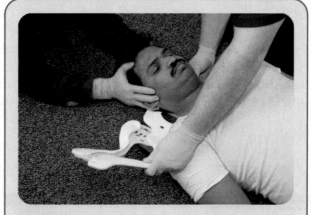

5 The second prehospital care practitioner applies the collar, while the first prehospital care practitioner continues to maintain the neutral in-line head and neck stabilization.

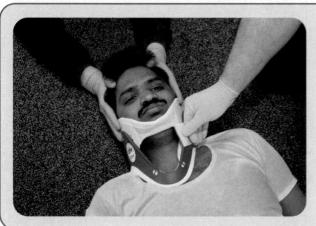

6 After applying and securing the cervical collar, manual in-line stabilization of the head and neck is maintained until the patient is secured to an appropriate device.

(continues)

Spine Management (continued)

Logroll

Principle: To turn a patient while maintaining manual stabilization with minimal movement of the spine. The logroll is indicated for (1) positioning a patient onto a long backboard or other device to facilitate movement of the patient and (2) turning a patient with suspected spinal trauma to examine the back.

A. Supine Patient

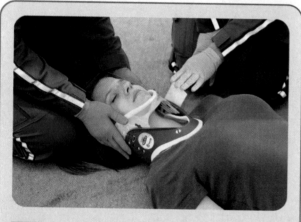

1 While one prehospital care practitioner maintains neutral in-line stabilization at the patient's head, a second prehospital care practitioner applies a properly sized cervical collar.

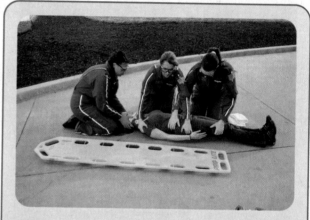

2 While one prehospital care practitioner maintains neutral in-line stabilization, a second prehospital care practitioner kneels at the patient's midthorax, and a third prehospital care practitioner kneels at the level of the patient's knees. The patient's arms are straightened and placed palms-in next to the torso while the patient's legs are brought into neutral alignment. The patient is grasped at the shoulder and hips in such a fashion as to maintain a neutral in-line position of the lower extremities. The patient is "logrolled" slightly onto the side.

Spine Management (continued)

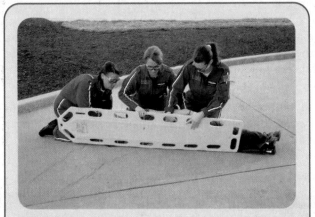

3 The backboard or other device is placed with the foot end of the board positioned between the patient's knees and ankles (the head of the backboard will extend beyond the patient's head). The backboard is held against the patient's back, the patient is logrolled back onto the long backboard, and the board is lowered to the ground with the patient.

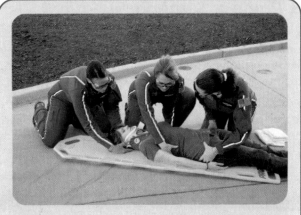

4 Once on the ground, the patient is grasped firmly by the shoulders, the pelvis, and the lower extremities.

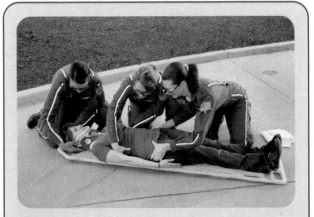

5 The patient is moved upward and laterally onto the long backboard. Neutral in-line stabilization is maintained without pulling on the patient's head and neck.

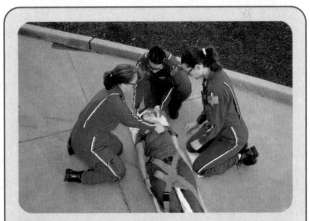

6 The patient is positioned onto the long backboard with the head at the top of the board and the body centered and secured to the device. If there is significant discomfort or if the transport will be prolonged, the backboard can be removed by log rolling the patient off the board once the patient has been safely transferred to the stretcher in a supine position.

(continues)

Spine Management (continued)

B. Prone or Semi-prone Patient

When a patient presents in a prone or semi-prone position, a stabilization method similar to that used for the supine patient can be used. The method incorporates the same initial alignment of the patient's limbs, the same positioning and hand placement of the prehospital care practitioners, and the same responsibilities for maintaining alignment.

The patient's arms are positioned in anticipation of the full rotation that will occur. When using the semi-prone logroll method, a cervical collar can be safely applied only after the patient is in an in-line position and supine on the backboard or other immobilization device, not before.

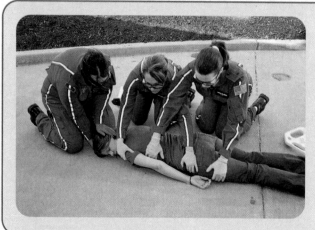

1 Whenever possible, the patient should be rolled away from the direction in which the patient's face initially points. One prehospital care practitioner establishes in-line manual stabilization of the patient's head and neck. Another prehospital care practitioner kneels at the patient's thorax and grasps the patient's opposite shoulder and wrist and pelvis area. A third prehospital care practitioner kneels at the patient's knees and grasps the patient's wrist and pelvis area and lower extremities.

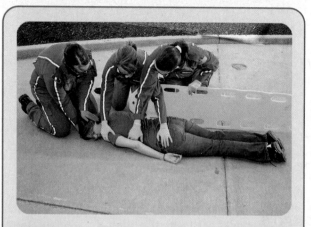

2 The backboard or other immobilization device is placed on the lateral edge and brought into position between the patient and the prehospital care practitioners.

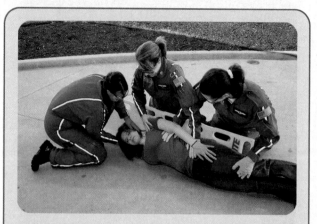

3 The board is placed with the foot of the board between the patient's knees and ankles, and the patient is logrolled onto the side. The patient's head rotates less than the torso, so by the time the patient is on the side (perpendicular to the ground), the head and torso have come into proper alignment.

Spine Management (continued)

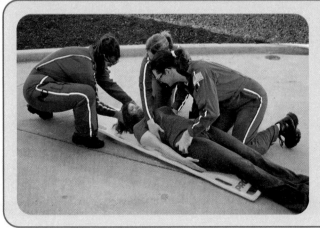

4 Once the patient is supine on the board, the patient is moved upward and toward the center of the board. The prehospital care practitioners should take care not to pull the patient but to maintain neutral in-line stabilization. Once the patient is positioned properly on the board, a properly sized cervical collar can be applied, and the patient can be secured to the board. If there is significant discomfort or if the transport will be prolonged, the board can be removed by log rolling the patient off once the patient has been safely transferred to the stretcher in a supine position.

© National Association of Emergency Medical Technicians (NAEMT)

Establishing Spinal Motion Restriction in a Patient Found in the Sitting Position

Principle: To manually stabilize a patient before and during movement from a sitting position.

A. Three or More Prehospital Care Practitioners

Sitting patients with indications for spinal motion restriction (see Figure 9-12) can be safely extricated.

Rapid extrication is indicated in the following situations:

- When the patient has life-threatening conditions identified during the primary survey that cannot be corrected where the patient is found
- When the scene is unsafe and clear danger to the prehospital care practitioner and patient exists, necessitating rapid removal to a safe location
- When the patient needs to be moved quickly to access other, more seriously injured patients

(continues)

Spine Management (continued)

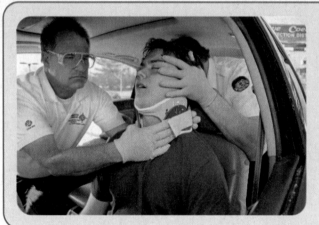

1 Once the decision is made to employ spinal motion restriction prior to extricating a patient, manual in-line stabilization of the patient's head and neck in a neutral position is initiated. This is best accomplished from behind the patient. If a prehospital care practitioner is unable to get behind the patient, manual stabilization can be accomplished from the side. Whether from behind the patient or the side, the patient's head and neck are brought into a neutral alignment, a rapid assessment of the patient is performed, and a properly sized cervical collar is applied.

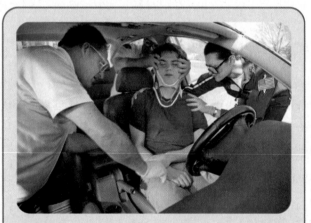

2 While manual stabilization is maintained, the patient's upper torso and lower torso and legs are controlled. The patient is rotated in a series of short, controlled movements.

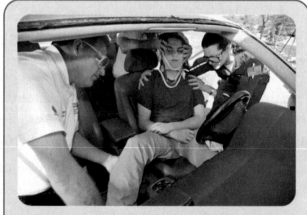

3 If the vehicle has a center console, the patient's legs should be moved one at a time over the console.

Spine Management (continued)

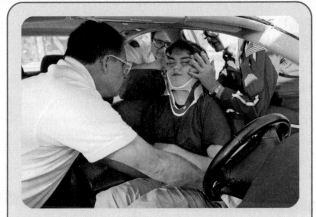

4 The prehospital care practitioner continues to rotate the patient in short, controlled movements until control of manual stabilization can no longer be maintained from behind and inside the vehicle. A second prehospital care practitioner assumes manual stabilization from the first prehospital care practitioner while standing outside of the vehicle.

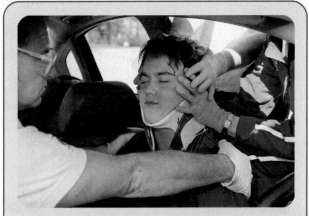

5 The first prehospital care practitioner can now move outside the vehicle and reassume manual stabilization from the second prehospital care practitioner.

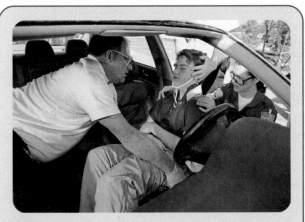

6 The rotation of the patient is continued until the patient can be lowered out of the vehicle door opening and onto the long backboard.

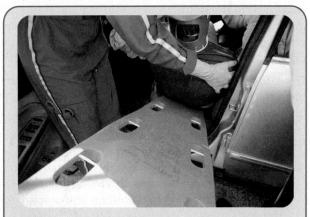

7 The long backboard or other spinal stabilization device is placed with the foot end of the board on the vehicle seat and the head end on the ambulance cot. If the cot cannot be placed next to the vehicle, other prehospital care practitioners can hold the long backboard while the patient is lowered onto it.

(continues)

Spine Management *(continued)*

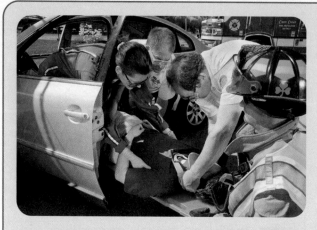

8 Once the patient's torso is down on the board, the weight of the patient's chest is controlled while the patient's pelvis and lower legs are controlled. The patient is moved upward onto the device. The prehospital care practitioner who is maintaining manual stabilization must be careful not to pull the patient and should continue to support the patient's head and neck.

After the patient is positioned onto the device, the prehospital care practitioners can secure the patient to the board and the board to the ambulance cot. The patient's upper torso is secured first, then the lower torso and pelvis area, then the head. The patient's legs are secured last. If the scene is unsafe, the patient should be moved to a safe area before being secured to the board or cot.

Note: This procedure represents only one example of extrication of a patient found in a sitting position. Because few field situations are ideal, prehospital care practitioners may need to modify the steps for extrication for the particular patient and situation. The principle of extrication should remain the same regardless of the situation: Maintain manual stabilization throughout the extrication process without interruption, and maintain the entire spine in an in-line position without unwarranted movement. Any positioning of the prehospital care practitioners that works can be successful. However, numerous position changes and hand position takeovers should be avoided because they invite a lapse in manual stabilization.

The extrication technique can effectively provide manual in-line stabilization of the patient's head, neck, and torso throughout a patient's removal from a vehicle. The following are three key points of extrication:

1. One prehospital care practitioner maintains stabilization of the patient's head and neck at all times, another rotates and stabilizes the patient's upper torso, and a third moves and controls the patient's lower torso, pelvis, and lower extremities.
2. Maintaining manual in-line stabilization of the patient's head and neck is impossible if attempting to move the patient in one continuous motion. The prehospital care practitioners need to limit each movement, stopping to reposition and prepare for the next move. Undue haste will result in movement of the spine.
3. Each situation and patient may require adaptation of the principles of extrication. This can only work effectively if the maneuvers are practiced. Each prehospital care practitioner needs to know the actions and movements of the other prehospital care practitioners.

Spine Management *(continued)*

B. Two Prehospital Care Practitioners

In some situations, an adequate number of prehospital care practitioners may not be available to extricate a critical patient rapidly. In these situations, a two-practitioner technique is useful.

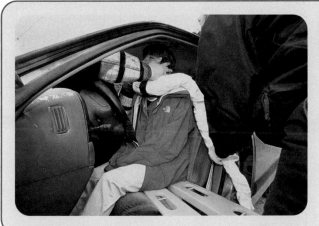

1 One prehospital care practitioner initiates and maintains manual in-line stabilization of the patient's head and neck. A second prehospital care practitioner places a properly sized cervical collar on the patient and places a prerolled blanket around the patient. The center of the blanket roll is placed at the patient's midline on the rigid cervical collar. The ends of the blanket roll are wrapped around the cervical collar and placed under the patient's arms.

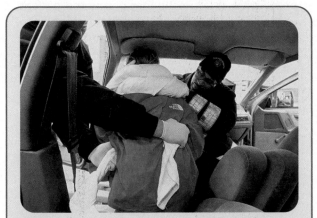

2 The patient is turned using the ends of the blanket roll and until the patient's back is centered on the door opening.

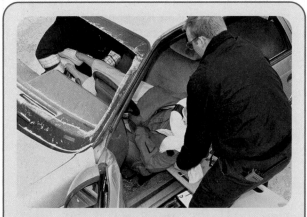

3 The first prehospital care practitioner takes control of the blanket ends, moving them under the patient's shoulders, and moves the patient by using the blanket, while the second prehospital care practitioner moves and controls the patient's lower torso, pelvis, and legs.

(continues)

Child Immobilization Device

Principle: To provide spinal motion restriction to a child with a suspected spinal injury.

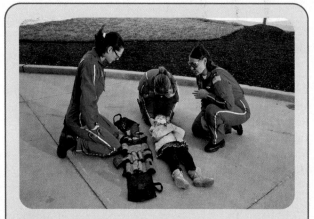

1 The first prehospital care practitioner kneels above the patient's head and provides manual in-line stabilization of the patient's head and neck. The second prehospital care practitioner sizes and applies a cervical collar while the first prehospital care practitioner maintains neutral in-line stabilization. The second prehospital care practitioner straightens the patient's arms and legs, if needed.

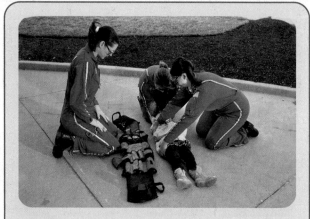

2 The second prehospital care practitioner now kneels at the patient's side between the shoulders and knees. The second prehospital care practitioner grasps the patient at the shoulder and hips in such a fashion as to maintain a neutral in-line position of the lower extremities. On command from the first prehospital care practitioner, the patient is logrolled slightly onto the side.

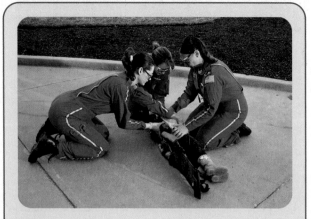

3 A third prehospital care practitioner positions the immobilization device behind the patient and holds it in place.

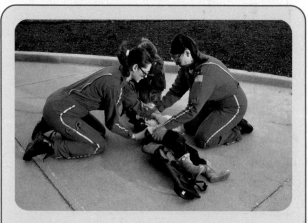

4 The device is held against the patient's back, the patient is logrolled onto the device, and the device is lowered to the ground with the patient.

Spine Management *(continued)*

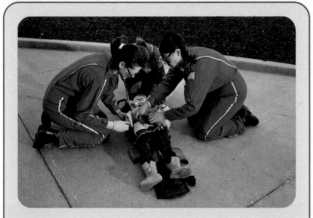

5 The patient is now secured to the immobilization device by the second and third prehospital care practitioner while the first prehospital care practitioner maintains head and neck stabilization.

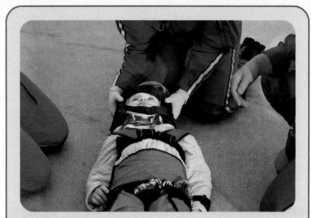

6 After securing the patient's torso and lower extremities to the device, the patient's head is secured to the device.

© National Association of Emergency Medical Technicians (NAEMT)

Helmet Removal

Principle: To remove a safety helmet while minimizing the risk of additional injury.

Patients who are wearing full-face helmets must have the helmet removed early in the assessment process. This provides immediate access for the prehospital care practitioner to assess and manage a patient's airway and ventilatory status. Helmet removal ensures that hidden bleeding is not occurring into the posterior helmet and allows the prehospital care practitioner to move the head (from the flexed position caused by large helmets) into neutral alignment. It also permits complete assessment of the head and neck in the secondary survey and facilitates spinal immobilization when indicated (see Figure 9-12). The prehospital care practitioner explains to the patient what will occur. If the patient verbalizes that the prehospital care practitioner should not remove the helmet, the prehospital care practitioner will explain that properly trained personnel can remove it by protecting the patient's spine. Two prehospital care practitioners are required for this maneuver.

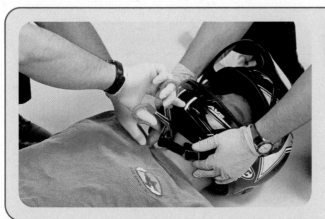

1 One prehospital care practitioner takes a position above the patient's head. With palms pressed on the sides of the helmet and fingertips curled over the lower margin, the first prehospital care practitioner stabilizes the helmet, head, and neck in as close to a neutral in-line position as the helmet allows. A second prehospital care practitioner kneels at the side of the patient, opens or removes the face shield if needed, removes eyeglasses if present, and unfastens or cuts the chin strap.

(continues)

Spine Management *(continued)*

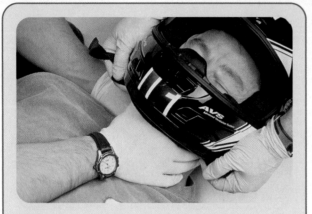

2 The patient's mandible is grasped between the thumb and the first two fingers at the angle of the mandible. The other hand is placed under the patient's neck on the occiput of the skull to take control of manual stabilization. The prehospital care practitioner's forearms should be resting on the floor or ground or on their own thighs for additional support.

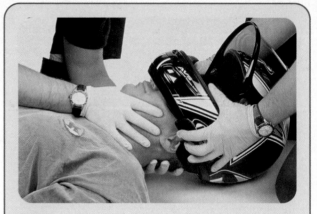

3 The first prehospital care practitioner pulls the sides of the helmet slightly apart, away from the patient's head, and rotates the helmet with up-and-down rocking motions while pulling it off of the patient's head. Movement of the helmet is slow and deliberate. The prehospital care practitioner takes care as the helmet clears the patient's nose.

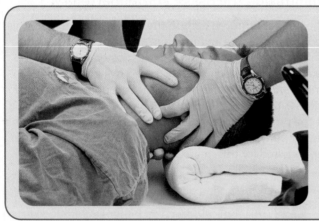

4 Once the helmet is removed, padding should be placed behind the patient's head to maintain a neutral in-line position. Manual stabilization is maintained, and a properly sized cervical collar is placed on the patient.

Note: Two key elements are involved in helmet removal, as follows:

1. While one prehospital care practitioner maintains manual stabilization of the patient's head and neck, the other prehospital care practitioner moves. At no time should both prehospital care practitioners be moving their hands.
2. The prehospital care practitioner rotates the helmet in different directions, first to clear the patient's nose and then to clear the back of the patient's head.

Vacuum Mattress Application

It is important to take proper care when using a vacuum mattress. Any sharp object on the ground or in the patient's clothes may pierce the mattress, rendering it useless.

The steps involved in applying a vacuum mattress may vary from the following steps, depending upon the particular vacuum mattress available. Prehospital care practitioners should become familiar with the steps specific to the particular device used in their agency.

The prehospital care practitioner places the vacuum mattress on the lowered stretcher, partially deflated. The valve of the vacuum mattress should be at the head. The plastic balls inside the vacuum mattress should be evenly spread out to form a relatively flat surface.

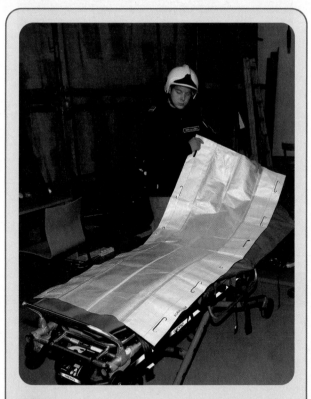

1 One prehospital care practitioner places a vacuum mattress on a lowered stretcher. The mattress should be deflated partially with the valve of the mattress at the head. The plastic balls inside the mattress should be spread out evenly to form a relatively flat surface. The prehospital care practitioner then places a sheet on the vacuum mattress.

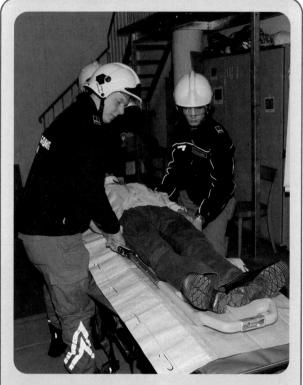

2 A scoop stretcher is used to transfer the patient onto the vacuum mattress.

(continues)

Spine Management *(continued)*

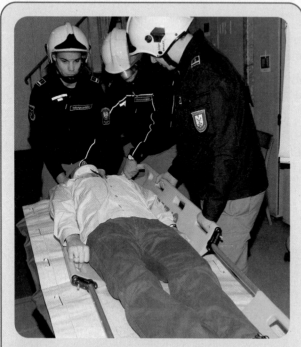

3 The scoop stretcher is removed carefully from beneath the patient.

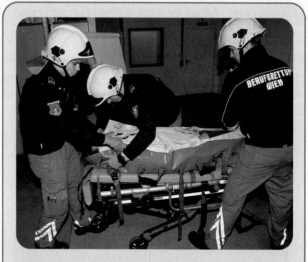

4 The vacuum mattress is molded to the body contours of the patient while one prehospital care practitioner maintains manual in-line stabilization of the patient's head. Once the mattress is molded to the patient, the valve of the vacuum mattress is opened and suction is applied to deflate the mattress.

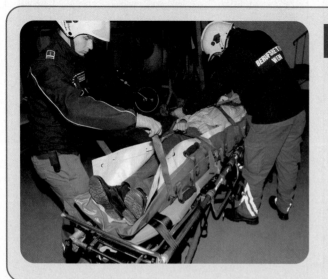

5 The valve is then closed and the patient secured with belts. A sheet or blanket should be placed over the patient.

CHAPTER **10**

Thoracic Trauma

Lead Editors
Anthony Loria, MD
Mark Gestring, MD, FACS

CHAPTER OBJECTIVES

At the completion of this chapter, you will be able to do the following:

- Discuss the anatomy and physiology of the thoracic organs.
- Explain the alterations in anatomy and physiology that result from thoracic injury.
- Discuss the relationships among the mechanism of thoracic trauma, anatomy and physiology, and various assessment findings consistent with the injuries listed here.
- Differentiate between patients in need of rapid stabilization and transport and those in whom further on-scene assessment and management are appropriate.

- Relate the signs, symptoms, pathophysiology, and management of the following injuries:
  - Rib fractures
  - Flail chest
  - Pulmonary contusion
  - Pneumothorax (simple, open, tension)
  - Hemothorax
  - Blunt cardiac injury
  - Cardiac tamponade
  - Commotio cordis
  - Traumatic aortic disruption
  - Tracheobronchial disruption
  - Traumatic asphyxia
  - Diaphragmatic rupture

SCENARIO

You and your partner are dispatched to an industrial construction site for a worker who was struck by a piece of metal. Upon arrival, you are led to an area where a safety officer explains that the patient was helping install metal studs. As he turned to grab another stud, he ran into the end of a stud that his partner had just trimmed, cutting through his shirt and puncturing his chest.

You find an approximately 35-year-old man sitting upright, leaning forward and holding a rag to the right side of his chest. You ask him what happened, and he tries to tell you but has to stop after every five to six words to catch his breath. You move the rag and notice a 2 inch (5 centimeter [cm]) long laceration with a

(continued)

INTRODUCTION

As with other forms of injury, thoracic trauma can result from blunt, penetrating, or blast mechanisms. Blunt force applied to the thoracic cavity can disrupt the normal anatomy and physiology of the thoracic organs. Similarly, penetrating wounds from firearms, knives, or other forms of impalement can injure the thorax and its contents. Blast injuries to the chest result from an intense over-pressurization, which may cause pulmonary barotrauma (contusions, hemorrhage, lacerations, pneumothorax, or air embolism). Most thoracic injuries do not require a *thoracotomy* (operative opening of the thoracic cavity). In fact, less than 10% of blunt chest injuries and 15% to 30% of penetrating chest injuries require operative intervention. The remaining injuries are well managed with relatively simple interventions, such as supplemental oxygen, analgesia, ventilatory support, or tube *thoracostomy* (chest tube placement) when necessary.[1-3]

The thoracic organs are intimately involved in the maintenance of oxygenation, ventilation, perfusion, and oxygen delivery. Consequently, an injury to the chest, especially if not promptly recognized and appropriately managed, can lead to morbidity and mortality. Inadequate or untimely management of a thoracic injury can contribute to **hypoxemia** (insufficient oxygen in the blood), **hypoxia** (insufficient oxygen in body tissues), **hypercarbia** (excessive carbon dioxide in the blood), *acidosis* (excessive acid in the blood), and *shock* (an abnormality of the circulatory system that results in inadequate organ perfusion and tissue oxygenation). These physiologic abnormalities resulting from thoracic injuries can also contribute to late complications, such as multisystem organ failure, which accounts for the 25% of trauma deaths that result from thoracic trauma.[1-3]

Anatomy

Simplistically, the thoracic or chest cavity is a hollow cylinder formed by bony and muscular structures. Of the 12 pairs of ribs, the upper 10 attach to the spinal column posteriorly and to the sternum or the rib above anteriorly. The lower two pairs of ribs attach only posteriorly to the spine and are thus referred to as "floating ribs." This bony architecture provides a great deal of protection to the internal organs of the thoracic cavity and upper abdomen (most notably the spleen and liver). This scaffolding of ribs is reinforced by the **intercostal muscles**, which lie between and connect the ribs to one another.

A number of muscle groups move the upper extremity and are part of the chest wall, including the major and minor *pectoral muscles*, anterior and posterior *serratus muscles*, and *latissimus dorsi muscle*, along with the various muscles of the back (**Figure 10-1**). All this "padding" means it takes a considerable amount of force to injure the internal organs.

The thorax also contains the muscles involved in breathing (ventilation), including the intercostal muscles; the *diaphragm*, a dome-shaped muscle attached around the lower aspect of the chest; and muscles in the neck that attach to the upper ribs. A nerve, artery, and vein course along the lower edge of each rib and provide blood and stimulation to the intercostal muscles.

Lining the interior of the cavity formed by these structures is a thin membrane called the **parietal pleura**. A corresponding membrane covers the two lungs within the chest cavity, called the **visceral pleura**. A small amount of fluid holds these two membranes together similar to how a layer of water will hold two sheets of glass together. This pleural fluid creates a surface tension, which opposes the elastic nature of the lungs, preventing their natural tendency to collapse. There is normally no space between these two membranes.

The lungs occupy the right and left sides of the chest cavity (**Figure 10-2**). The two sides are connected by a space called the **mediastinum**, which contains the trachea, the main bronchi, the heart, the major arteries and veins to and from the heart, and the esophagus.

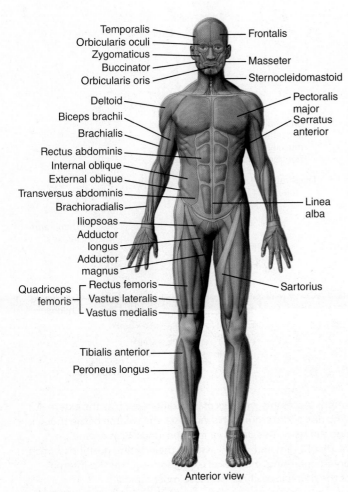

Figure 10-1 The muscular system.

© National Association of Emergency Medical Technicians (NAEMT)

Physiology

Breathing and *circulation* are the two components of chest physiology that are most likely to be impacted by injury.[1-3] Both processes need to be working properly, and in conjunction with one another, for oxygen to reach the organs and for carbon dioxide to be expelled. Understanding these processes helps clarify how an injury alters the body's physiology and clarifies the steps needed to manage these injuries.

Ventilation

The lay terms *breathing* and *respiration* refer to the physiologic process of ventilation. *Ventilation* is the mechanical act of drawing air through the mouth and nose into the upper airway and then into the lungs, where it arrives in small air sacs known as *alveoli*. **Respiration** is ventilation plus the delivery of oxygen to the cells. The process of drawing air in is called **inhalation**. Oxygen in the inhaled air is transported across the lining membrane of the alveoli, into adjacent small blood vessels known as **capillaries**. There, in a process called **oxygenation**, oxygen attaches to hemoglobin in the red blood cells for transport to the rest of the body. Simultaneously, the carbon dioxide that is dissolved in the blood diffuses out into the air within the alveoli for expulsion in the process of exhalation (**Figure 10-3**). **Cellular respiration** is the use of oxygen by the cells to produce energy. (See Chapter 3, *Shock: Pathophysiology of Life and Death*, and Chapter 7, *Airway and Ventilation*.)

    Inhalation occurs due to the contraction of the muscles of respiration (primarily the intercostal muscles and the diaphragm). The contraction of these muscles causes

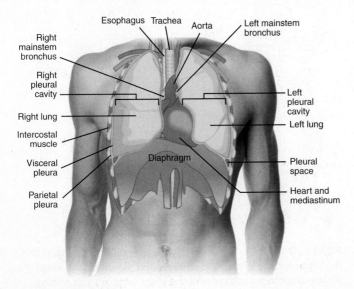

Figure 10-2 The thoracic cavity, including the ribs, intercostal muscles, diaphragm, mediastinum, lungs, heart, great vessels, bronchi, trachea, and esophagus.

© MariyaL/Shutterstock

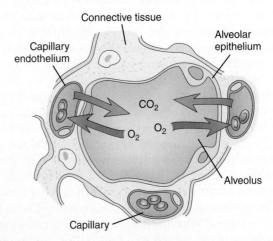

Figure 10-3 The capillaries and alveoli lie in close proximity; therefore, oxygen (O_2) in the alveoli can easily diffuse through the alveolar, capillary and red blood cell walls. Carbon dioxide (CO_2) can diffuse in the opposite direction.

© National Association of Emergency Medical Technicians (NAEMT)

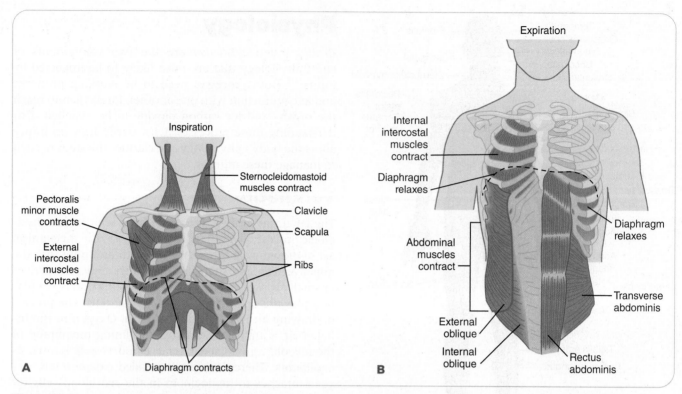

Figure 10-4 **A.** During inspiration, the diaphragm contracts and flattens. Accessory muscles of inspiration—such as the external intercostal, pectoralis minor, and sternocleidomastoid muscles—lift the ribs and sternum. This increases the volume of the thoracic cavity, which decreases the pressure in the chest compared to outside the body. This drives air into the lungs. **B.** In expiration during quiet breathing, the elasticity of the thoracic cavity causes the diaphragm and ribs to assume their resting positions, which decreases the volume of the thoracic cavity. In expiration during labored breathing, muscles of expiration—such as the internal intercostal and abdominal muscles—contract, causing the volume of the thoracic cavity to decrease more rapidly.

© National Association of Emergency Medical Technicians (NAEMT)

the ribs to lift and separate as the diaphragm moves downward. This increases the size of the thoracic cavity creating a negative pressure within the chest compared with the air pressure outside the body. As a result, air flows into the lungs (**Figure 10-4** and **Figure 10-5**). *Expiration* is achieved by relaxing the intercostal muscles and diaphragm, returning the ribs and diaphragm to their resting positions. This causes the pressure within the chest to exceed the pressure outside the body, forcing air from the lungs to be exhaled.

Ventilation is primarily controlled by the respiratory center in the brain stem, which monitors the partial pressure of arterial carbon dioxide ($PaCO_2$) and partial pressure of arterial oxygen (PaO_2) by specialized cells known as **central chemoreceptors**. If the central chemoreceptors detect increased $PaCO_2$, they stimulate the respiratory center to increase the depth and frequency of breaths, eliminating more carbon dioxide and returning $PaCO_2$ to normal (**Figure 10-6**). This process can increase the volume of air moved into and out of the lungs per minute by a factor of 10. Mechanoreceptors, found in the airways, lungs, and chest wall, measure the degree of stretch in these structures and provide feedback to the brain stem about lung volume.

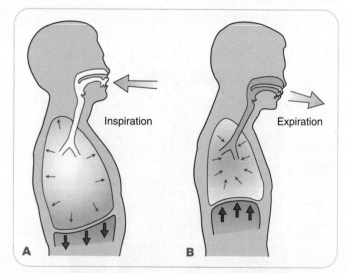

Figure 10-5 When the chest cavity expands during inspiration, the intrathoracic pressure decreases and air enters the lungs. As the diaphragm relaxes and the chest returns to its resting position, the intrathoracic pressure increases, and air is expelled. When the diaphragm is relaxed and the glottis is open, the pressure inside and outside the lungs is equal. **A.** Inspiration. **B.** Expiration.

© National Association of Emergency Medical Technicians (NAEMT)

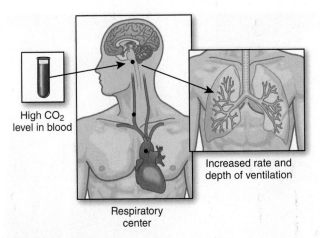

Figure 10-6 An increased level of carbon dioxide is detected by nerve cells sensitive to this change, stimulating the lung to increase both depth and rate of ventilation.

© National Association of Emergency Medical Technicians (NAEMT)

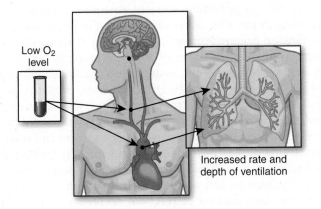

Figure 10-7 Receptors located in the aorta and carotid arteries are sensitive to the blood's oxygen level, stimulating the lungs to increase air movement into and out of the alveolar sacs.

© National Association of Emergency Medical Technicians (NAEMT)

In patients with chronic obstructive pulmonary disease (COPD), the lungs cannot efficiently eliminate carbon dioxide. This results in chronically elevated $PaCO_2$ levels causing the central chemoreceptors to become insensitive to changes in $PaCO_2$. As a result, **peripheral chemoreceptors** (in the aorta and carotid arteries) stimulate breathing in response to decreasing PaO_2. Analogous to when the central chemoreceptors detect an increase in $PaCO_2$ and stimulate increased respirations to lower the carbon dioxide level, the peripheral chemoreceptors sense changing PaO_2, sending feedback to the respiratory center that stimulate the respiratory muscles to be more active, increasing the ventilatory rate and depth to raise the PaO_2 to more normal values (**Figure 10-7**). This mechanism is often referred to as "hypoxic drive," as it is related to falling levels of oxygen in the blood.

Box 10-1 Important Definitions

- *Dead space.* Volume of air in the parts of the airway that are not involved in gas exchange (e.g., air in trachea and mainstem bronchi).
- **Minute ventilation (V°).** Total volume of air moved into and out of the lungs in 1 minute.
- **Tidal volume (V_t).** Amount of air that is inhaled and then exhaled during a normal breath (Normal = 0.5 liter or 7 milliliters/kilogram [mL/kg]).
- **Total lung capacity (*TLC*).** Total volume of air the lungs contain when maximally inflated. This volume declines with age from 6 liters in young adults to approximately 4 liters in elderly persons.
- **Work of breathing.** Physical effort performed in moving the chest wall and diaphragm to breathe. This work increases with rapid breathing, increasing minute ventilation, and when the lungs or chest wall are abnormally stiff.

© National Association of Emergency Medical Technicians (NAEMT)

The concept of the hypoxic drive has led to recommendations to limit the amount of oxygen given to patients with COPD for fear of suppressing their impetus to breathe. However, *trauma patients who are hypoxic should never be deprived of supplemental oxygen* in the prehospital setting.[4] The true existence of the hypoxic drive remains controversial. If it exists, it will not manifest itself in the acute setting, and the potential adverse consequences of inadequate oxygenation in a patient with a thoracic injury are far worse than the potential adverse consequences of temporarily suppressing hypoxic drive in a patient who is actively being monitored.

See **Box 10-1** for a list of important terms for understanding pulmonary physiology.[5]

Circulation

The other major physiologic process that may be affected following thoracic injury is circulation. The following discussion sets the stage for the pathophysiology of chest injury. Chapter 3, *Shock: Pathophysiology of Life and Death*, covers this topic more extensively.

The heart, which lies in the center of the chest within the mediastinum, functions as a biologic pump. For a pump to work, it must be primed with fluid and that fluid level must be maintained. For the heart, the return of blood occurs through two large veins, the **superior vena cava** and the **inferior vena cava**. The heart normally contracts 70 to 80 times per minute on average (normal range 60 to 100 beats/minute), ejecting approximately 70 mL of blood with each contraction to the body via the aorta.

Processes that interfere with the return of blood to the heart (e.g., loss of blood through hemorrhage, increased pressure in the chest cavity from tension pneumothorax) cause a decrease in the output of the heart and thus the blood pressure decreases. Similarly, processes that injure the heart itself (e.g., blunt cardiac injury) may make the heart a less efficient pump, causing the same physiologic abnormalities. Just as chemoreceptors recognize changes in carbon dioxide or oxygen levels, **baroreceptors** located in the arch of the aorta and the carotid sinuses of the carotid arteries recognize changes in blood pressure and direct the heart to change the rate and forcefulness of its beating to return the blood pressure to normal.

Pathophysiology

As mentioned earlier, blunt, penetrating, and blast mechanisms may disrupt the physiologic processes just described. The disturbances created by these mechanisms have several common elements.

Penetrating Injury

In penetrating injuries, objects of varying sizes and types traverse the chest wall, enter the thoracic cavity, and possibly injure the organs within the thorax. Normally, no space exists between the pleural membranes. However, when a penetrating wound creates a communication between the chest cavity and the outside world, air can enter into the pleural space. During inspiration, when the pressure in the chest is lower than outside the chest, air enters through the wound, disrupting the apposition of the pleural membranes and resulting in a **pneumothorax**. Air may be further encouraged to enter the pleural space if the resistance to airflow through the wound is less than that through the airways. Together, these processes cause the lung to collapse, preventing effective ventilation. Penetrating wounds result in an open pneumothorax only when the size of the chest wall defect is large enough that the surrounding tissues do not effectively close the wound during inspiration and/or expiration. Wounds to the airways or lung tissue caused by a penetrating object may also allow air to escape from the lung into the pleural space and result in collapse of the lung.

In either case, the patient becomes short of breath. To make up for the lost ventilation capacity, the respiratory center will stimulate more rapid breathing, increasing the work of breathing. The patient may be able to tolerate the increased workload for a time, but if not recognized and treated, the patient is at risk for ventilatory failure, which will be manifested by increasing respiratory distress as the carbon dioxide levels in the blood rise and the oxygen levels fall.

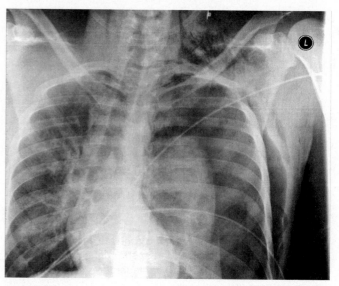

Figure 10-8 An x-ray showing a left tension pneumothorax.
Courtesy of Dr. Mark Gestring, MD, FACS.

If there is persistent entry of air into the chest cavity without any exit, pressure will begin to build, leading to **tension pneumothorax** (**Figure 10-8**). This condition further impedes the patient's ability to properly ventilate as venous return to the heart is progressively reduced by the persistently increasing intrathoracic pressure, potentially causing shock. In extreme cases, the *mediastinal structures* (organs and vessels located in the middle of the chest between the two lungs) displace toward the unaffected side of the chest, causing mechanical compromise of venous return. This causes decreased blood pressure but increased jugular venous distension, and the classic, but very late, finding of **tracheal deviation** away from the midline toward the uninvolved side of the chest.

Penetrating wounds to the chest may result in bleeding into the pleural space (**hemothorax**) from the chest wall muscles, the intercostal vessels, and the lung tissue (**Figure 10-9**). Penetrating wounds to the major vessels in the chest result in catastrophic bleeding as each pleural space can accommodate 2,500 to 3,000 mL of blood. Notably, bleeding into the pleural space may not be readily apparent externally, but it may be of sufficient magnitude to create a shock state. The presence of large volumes of blood in the pleural space will impede the patient's ability to breathe as the blood in the pleural space prevents expansion of the lung on that side. It is not uncommon for an injury to the lung to result in both a hemothorax and a pneumothorax, termed a *hemopneumothorax*. A hemopneumothorax results in collapse of the lung and impaired ventilation from both the air in the pleural space and the accumulation of blood in the thoracic cavity.

Wounds of the lung may also result in bleeding into the lung tissue itself. This blood floods the alveoli, preventing them from filling with air. Alveoli filled with blood cannot participate in gas exchange. The more

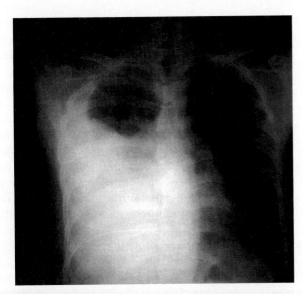

Figure 10-9 An x-ray showing a right massive hemothorax.
© Medicshots/Alamy Stock Photo

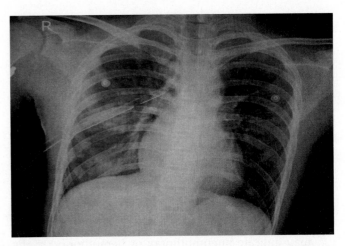

Figure 10-10 An x-ray showing a right pulmonary contusion.
© Richman Photo/Shutterstock

alveoli that are flooded, the more the patient's ventilation and oxygenation may be compromised.

Wounds of the lungs or airways may also result in an air embolism. These are uncommon but can be catastrophic. An air embolism results from a direct communication between a source of air (usually a larger airway injury) and the vasculature (usually a venous injury). Positive-pressure ventilation (bagging or mechanical ventilation) may increase the possibility of this phenomenon. Air emboli may result in hemodynamic instability, neurologic deficits (when arterial), or even cardiac arrest.

Blunt Force Injury

Blunt force applied to the chest wall is transmitted to the thoracic organs. This wave of energy can tear lung tissue, which may result in bleeding into the alveoli. In this context, the injury is called a **pulmonary contusion** (**Figure 10-10**). A pulmonary contusion is essentially a bruise of the lung that can be exacerbated by aggressive fluid resuscitation. The impact on oxygenation and ventilation is the same as with penetrating injury. If the force applied to the lung tissue also tears the visceral pleura, air may escape from the lung into the pleural space, creating a pneumothorax and the potential for a tension pneumothorax, as previously described.

Blunt force trauma can also break ribs, which can lacerate the lung, resulting in pneumothorax as well as hemothorax (both caused by bleeding from the broken ribs and from the torn lung and intercostal muscles). Blunt force injury typically associated with sudden deceleration incidents may cause shearing or rupture of the major blood vessels in the chest, particularly the aorta, leading to catastrophic hemorrhage. Finally, in some cases, blunt force can disrupt the chest wall, leading to instability of the chest wall and compromise of the changes in intrathoracic pressure, leading to impaired ventilation.

Assessment

As in all aspects of medical care, assessment involves taking a history and performing a physical examination. In trauma situations, we speak of a **SAMPLER history**, in which the patient's **S**ymptoms, **A**llergies, **M**edications, **P**ast medical history, time of the **L**ast meal, **E**vents surrounding the injury, and **R**isk factors are determined.[6] (See Chapter 6, *Patient Assessment and Management*.)

Patients with chest trauma will likely be experiencing chest pain, which may be sharp, stabbing, or constricting. Frequently, the pain is worse with respiratory efforts or movement. The patient may report a sense of being short of breath or being unable to take in an adequate breath. The patient may feel apprehensive or lightheaded if shock is developing. It is important to remember that the absence of symptoms does not equal the absence of injury.

The next step in assessment is the performance of a physical examination directed to thoracic injuries. There are four components to the physical examination: observation, auscultation, palpation, and percussion.

- *Observation.* The patient is observed for pallor of the skin and sweating, which may indicate the presence of shock. The patient may also appear apprehensive. The presence of **cyanosis** (bluish discoloration of skin, especially around the mouth and lips) is a late finding and may be evident in advanced hypoxia. The frequency of respirations and whether the patient appears to be having trouble breathing (gasping, contractions of the accessory muscles of respiration in the neck, nasal flaring) should be noted. Is the trachea in the midline, or deviated to one side or the other? Are the jugular veins distended? The chest is examined for contusions, abrasions, lacerations, and whether the chest wall expands symmetrically with breathing. Does any portion of the chest wall move paradoxically with respiration? (That is, instead of moving out during inspiration, does it collapse inward, and vice versa during exhalation?) If any wounds are identified, they are carefully examined to see if they are bubbling air as the patient breathes in and out.

- *Auscultation.* The entire chest is evaluated. Decreased breath sounds on one side compared to the other may indicate pneumothorax or hemothorax on the examined side. Pulmonary contusions may result in abnormal breath sounds (crackles). Although often difficult to discern in the field, muffled heart sounds from blood collecting around the heart and murmurs from valvular damage may also be noted on auscultation of the heart.
- *Palpation.* By gently pressing the chest wall, assessment for the presence of tenderness, crepitus (either bony or **subcutaneous emphysema**), and bony instability of the chest wall is performed.
- *Percussion.* This examination technique is difficult to perform in the field because the environment is often noisy, making evaluation of the percussion note difficult. In addition, there is little additional information to be obtained from percussion that will change the prehospital management.

The assessment should also include a determination of vital signs. Placement of a pulse oximeter to assess arterial oxygen saturation is a useful adjunct in the assessment of the injured patient.[6,7]

- *Pulse oximetry.* The level of oxygen bound to hemoglobin should be assessed and monitored to the extent possible to detect changes in the patient's condition and responses to therapy. The oxygen saturation should be maintained at 94% or greater. Because of difficulties in obtaining reliable pulse oximetry readings in the context of acute trauma and in the context of potential shock, hypoxia should be generally assumed to be present and oxygen administered by default unless overwhelming evidence of adequate oxygenation is present.
- *Waveform capnography.* Whether by sidestream assessment (with a nasal probe or mask) or by in-line assessment (in an intubated patient), capnography (measurement of end-tidal carbon dioxide) may be used to assess the level of carbon dioxide in expired air and is monitored to detect changes in the patient's condition and responses to therapy. In-line sampling measures the end-tidal carbon dioxide directly at the point of sampling, whereas sidestream assessment takes a sample of expired air and performs the carbon dioxide determination at the monitor location, which is remote from the sampling site.

- *Extended Focused Assessment with Sonography in Trauma (eFAST).* Point-of-care ultrasound (POCUS) is an emerging technology that is being actively studied in the prehospital setting. Although it requires additional training and experience, it is feasible during air or ground transport and might be a helpful adjunct to physical examination. In the context of thoracic trauma, the main role for POCUS is the identification of pneumothoraces and pericardial effusion (**Box 10-2**).[8,9] There is growing evidence that with appropriate education, prehospital practitioners can accurately identify traumatic thoracic pathology and retain this skill over time.[10-12] There is no evidence yet that use of such technology in the prehospital environment improves patient survival. One important concern is that introducing such technology to the field could increase scene times and delay transport, thus potentially increasing patient mortality.

Repeat determinations of the ventilatory rate during patient reassessment may be the most important assessment tool in recognizing that a patient is deteriorating. As patients become hypoxic and compromised, an early clue to this change is a gradual increase in the ventilatory rate.

Assessment and Management of Specific Injuries

Rib Fractures

Rib fractures are common and present in approximately 10% of blunt trauma patients.[15] Several factors contribute to the morbidity and mortality of patients with rib fractures, including the total number of ribs fractured, the presence of bilateral fractures, and age 65 years or older.[16] Regardless of age, mortality increases as more ribs are fractured. The mortality rate for a single rib fracture is 5.8%, increasing to 10% in those with five fractured ribs, to as high as 34% in those with eight rib fractures.[17,18] The elderly are especially susceptible to rib fractures, likely due to loss of cortical bone mass (osteoporosis), which allows the ribs to fracture after sustaining less force.[19]

The upper ribs are broad, thick, and well protected by the shoulder girdle and muscles.[1-3] Because it requires great energy to fracture the upper ribs, patients with upper rib fractures are at risk for other major injuries, such

Box 10-2 The Role of Extended Focused Assessment With Sonography in Trauma (eFAST) in Thoracic Trauma

- **Lung sliding sign.** During respiration, the visceral and parietal pleura slide across each other. On eFAST, the junction of these membranes appears as a "shimmering" (hyperechoic) white line. During normal respiration, the shimmering to and fro movement of the pleura define lung sliding. In the presence of a pneumothorax, air disrupts the pleural space, and this shimmering line is disrupted and cannot be identified. This sign must be combined with clinical features to diagnose a pneumothorax as other conditions can disrupt the lung sliding sign. This sign cannot be adequately demonstrated without a moving image. Prehospital practitioners with training in eFAST should continue their education and practice to maintain operator skills.
- The negative predictive value of lung sliding is nearly 100%. This means that if lung sliding is identified, a pneumothorax is essentially excluded. In fact, there is evidence that ultrasound can prevent harm from unnecessary needle decompression in patients with clinical suspicion for a pneumothorax.[13,14] However, these data have not yet been validated in prehospital settings.
- The positive predictive value of lung sliding exceeds 90%. This means that if no lung sliding is observed, then there is likely a pneumothorax. However, the positive predictive value is lower because other factors (such as operator experience, mode setting on the device, very low tidal volumes, severe consolidation, and prior pneumonectomy) can make identification of a pneumothorax more challenging. Again, the degree to which the positive predictive value in the prehospital setting matches that of the in-hospital setting is unknown.
- **Pericardial Effusion.** A pericardial effusion is a collection of fluid, usually blood in traumatic circumstances, that accumulates in the pericardial sac. Ultrasound examination using a subxiphoid cardiac view can identify a pericardial effusion. This blood can accumulate, resulting in hemodynamic instability (see the section "Cardiac Tamponade" later in this chapter).

as traumatic disruption of the aorta. The broken ends of the ribs may tear muscle, lung, and blood vessels, with the possibility of an associated pulmonary contusion, pneumothorax, or hemothorax.[1,3,20] Underlying pulmonary contusion is the most commonly associated injury seen with multiple rib fractures. In addition, compression of the lung may rupture the alveoli and lead to pneumothorax, as discussed previously. Fracture of the lower ribs[20-22] may be associated with injuries of the spleen and liver and may indicate the potential for other intra-abdominal injuries. These injuries may present with signs of blood loss or shock.[1,3,20]

Assessment

Patients with simple rib fractures will most often complain of difficulty breathing and chest pain with inspiration or with movement. They may have labored respirations. Careful palpation of the chest wall will usually reveal point tenderness directly over the site of the rib fracture, and crepitus may be felt as the broken ends of the rib grind against each other. The prehospital care practitioner assesses vital signs, paying particular attention to the ventilatory rate and depth of breathing. Monitoring should include pulse oximetry with supplemental oxygen administration if necessary or if the status of the patient's oxygenation is in any way uncertain.[1,23,24]

Management

The initial management of patients with rib fractures is ensuring adequate oxygenation, ventilation, and analgesia. Administering supplemental oxygen and assisting ventilations may be necessary to ensure adequate oxygenation. Achieving adequate analgesia (pain control) may involve reassurance to decrease anxiety and positioning of the patient's arms in a position of comfort. It is important to reassure and continuously reassess the patient, keeping in mind the potential for deterioration in ventilation and the development of shock. Establishing intravenous (IV) access should be considered, depending on the patient's condition and anticipated transport time. Administration of IV analgesics may be appropriate in some situations for advanced units with appropriate protocols and medical control and in situations where the pain from the rib fractures is impeding the patient's ability to breathe effectively. The patient is encouraged to take deep breaths and cough to prevent the collapse of the alveoli (**atelectasis**) and the potential for pneumonia and other complications. Rigid immobilization of the rib cage with tape or straps should be avoided because these interventions predispose to the development of atelectasis and pneumonia.[1,3]

Flail Chest

Flail chest occurs when two or more adjacent ribs are fractured in more than one place along their length. Consequently, a segment of the chest wall is in discontinuity, allowing the affected ribs to have paradoxical inward

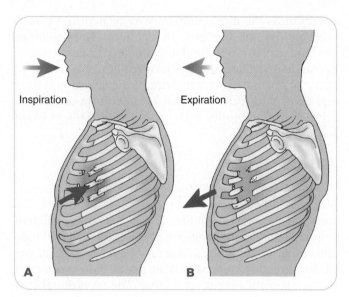

Figure 10-11 Paradoxical motion. **A.** If stability of the chest wall has been lost by ribs fractured in two or more places, as intrathoracic pressure decreases during inspiration, the external air pressure forces the chest wall inward. **B.** When intrathoracic pressure increases during expiration, the chest wall is forced outward.

© National Association of Emergency Medical Technicians (NAEMT)

movement during inspiration when the ribs should move out and upward (**Figure 10-11**). Similarly, during expiration, the segment may move outward as pressure inside the chest increases. This paradoxical motion of the flail segment makes ventilation less efficient. The degree of inefficiency is directly related to the size of the flail segment.

The significant force necessary to produce such an injury is generally transmitted to the underlying lung, resulting in a pulmonary contusion. Thus, the patient's ventilation and gas exchange is compromised by the flail segment and the underlying pulmonary contusion (which is the bigger problem when it comes to compromising ventilation). As described earlier, the pulmonary contusion does not allow for gas exchange in the contused portion of the lung because of alveolar flooding with blood.

Assessment

As with a simple rib fracture, assessment of flail chest will reveal a patient in pain. The pain is typically more severe, however, and the patient usually appears to be in distress. The ventilatory rate is elevated, and the patient does not take deep breaths because of the pain. Hypoxia may be present, as demonstrated by pulse oximetry or cyanosis. Paradoxical motion may or may not be evident or easily recognized. Initially, the intercostal muscles will be in spasm and tend to stabilize the flail segment. As

these muscles fatigue over time, the paradoxical motion becomes increasingly evident. The patient will have tenderness and potentially bony crepitus over the injured segment. The instability of the segment may also be appreciated on palpation.

Management

Management of flail chest is directed toward pain relief, ventilatory support, and monitoring for deterioration. The ventilatory rate and tidal volume may be the most important parameters to follow. Patients who are developing underlying pulmonary contusion and respiratory compromise will demonstrate an increase in their ventilatory rate over time. Pulse oximetry, if available, is also useful to detect hypoxia.[7] Oxygen should be administered to ensure an oxygen saturation of at least 94%.

IV access may be obtained, except in cases of extremely short transport times. Narcotic analgesics may be carefully titrated to provide pain relief.

Support of ventilation with bag-mask device assistance, continuous positive airway pressure (CPAP), or endotracheal intubation and positive-pressure ventilation may be necessary (particularly with prolonged transport times) for those patients who are having difficulty maintaining adequate oxygenation.[23] Efforts to stabilize the flail segment with sandbags or other means are contraindicated as they may further compromise chest wall motion and, thus, impair ventilations.[1]

Pulmonary Contusion

When lung tissue is lacerated or torn by blunt or penetrating mechanisms, bleeding into the alveolar air spaces can result in *pulmonary contusion*. As the alveoli fill with blood, gas exchange is impaired because air cannot enter these alveoli from the terminal airways. In addition, blood and tissue edema between the alveoli further impede gas exchange in the alveoli that are ventilated. Pulmonary contusion is almost always present in patients with a flail segment and is a common—and potentially lethal—complication of thoracic trauma.[3,20] Deterioration to the point of respiratory failure may occur over the first 24 hours after injury.

Assessment

Assessment findings are variable depending on the severity of the contusion (percentage of involved lung). Early assessment typically reveals no respiratory compromise. As the contusion progresses, the ventilatory rate will increase and crackles may be heard on auscultation. In fact, a rising ventilatory rate is often the earliest clue that a patient is deteriorating from a pulmonary contusion. A high index of suspicion is necessary, particularly in the presence of a flail segment.

Management

Management is directed toward support of ventilation. Prehospital care practitioners should repeatedly reassess the ventilatory rate and any signs of respiratory distress. Pulse oximetry should be utilized. Supplemental oxygen should be provided to all patients with suspected pulmonary contusion, with a goal of maintaining oxygen saturation in the normal range (≥ 94%). CPAP can be used to improve oxygenation in patients in whom supplemental oxygen alone proves to be inadequate for maintaining acceptable oxygen saturation levels.[25] Support of ventilation with a bag-mask device or positive-pressure ventilation via a supraglottic airway or endotracheal intubation may be necessary.[24]

Aggressive IV fluid administration may further increase edema and compromise ventilation and oxygenation and thus should be avoided. Instead, IV fluids should be administered judiciously and only as necessary to maintain blood pressure between 80 and 90 mm Hg. Pulmonary contusion is an important example of an injury in which fluid resuscitation may worsen outcome and therefore must be balanced with the patient's need to maintain a blood pressure of at least 80 mm Hg. (See Chapter 3, *Shock: Pathophysiology of Life and Death*.)

Pneumothorax

Pneumothorax is present in up to 20% of severe chest injuries.[17] The three types of pneumothoraces represent increasing levels of severity: simple, open, and tension.

Simple pneumothorax is the presence of air within the pleural space. As the amount of air in the pleural space increases, the lung on that side collapses (**Figure 10-12**). **Open pneumothorax** ("sucking chest wound") involves a pneumothorax associated with a defect in the chest wall that allows air to enter and exit the pleural space from the outside with ventilatory effort. *Tension pneumothorax* occurs when air continues to enter and is trapped in the pleural space with gradual increase in intrathoracic pressure. This leads to a shift of the mediastinum and results in decreased venous blood return to the heart and compromised circulatory function.

Simple Pneumothorax

Assessment

Assessment in simple pneumothorax is likely to demonstrate findings similar to those in patients with rib fractures. The patient frequently complains of pleuritic chest pain (pain that is exacerbated with breathing) and shortness of breath that may vary from mild to severe. The classic findings are decreased breath sounds on the side of injury. Any patient with respiratory distress and diminished breath sounds should be assumed to have a pneumothorax.

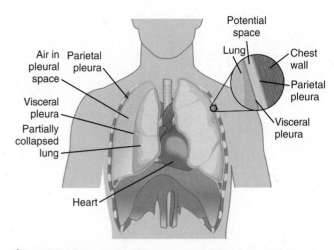

Figure 10-12 Air in the pleural space forces the lung inward, decreasing the amount of lung tissue that can be ventilated and, therefore, decreasing the oxygenation level of the blood leaving the lung.

© National Association of Emergency Medical Technicians (NAEMT)

Management

The prehospital care practitioner should administer supplemental oxygen, obtain IV access, and prepare to treat shock if it develops. Monitoring of pulse oximetry and waveform capnography, if available, is essential to detect early signs of respiratory deterioration.[17-22,26,27] If spinal motion restriction is not necessary, the patient may be more comfortable in a semi-recumbent position. Rapid transport is essential.[22,24,26] If the prehospital crew is functioning at the basic level and transport time will be prolonged, rendezvous with an advanced life support (ALS) unit should be considered.

A key point in management is the recognition that a simple pneumothorax may quickly evolve into a tension pneumothorax. The patient needs to be continuously monitored for the development of tension pneumothorax so that timely intervention can occur before there is a serious compromise of circulation.

Open Pneumothorax

Open pneumothorax, as with simple pneumothorax, involves air entering the pleural space, causing the lung to collapse. A defect in the chest wall that results in a communication between the outside air and the pleural space is the hallmark of an open pneumothorax. Mechanisms leading to open pneumothorax include gunshot wounds, shotgun blasts, stabbings, impalements, and (rarely) blunt trauma. When the patient attempts to inhale, air crosses the open wound and enters the pleural space because of the negative pressure created in the thoracic cavity as the muscles of respiration contract. In larger wounds, there may be free flow of air into and out of the pleural space with the different phases of respiration (**Figure 10-13**).

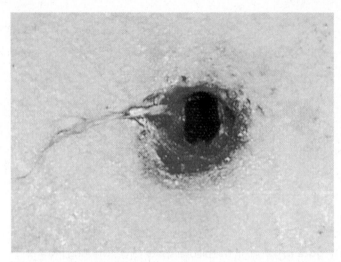

Figure 10-13 A gunshot or stab wound to the chest produces a hole in the chest wall through which air can flow both into and out of the pleural cavity.

Courtesy of Norman McSwain, MD, FACS, NREMT-P.

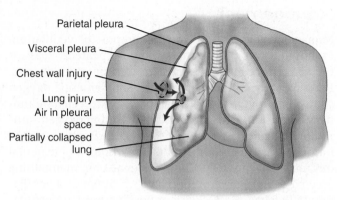

Parietal pleura
Visceral pleura
Chest wall injury
Lung injury
Air in pleural space
Partially collapsed lung

Figure 10-14 Because of the proximity of the chest wall to the lung, it would be extremely difficult for the chest wall to be injured by penetrating trauma and the lung not to be injured. Occluding the hole in the chest wall does not prevent air leakage into the pleural space from the lung.

© National Association of Emergency Medical Technicians (NAEMT)

Audible noise is often created as air travels into and out of the hole in the chest wall; thus, this wound has been referred to as a "sucking chest wound."

Because airflow follows the path of least resistance, this abnormal airflow through the chest wall may occur preferentially to the normal flow through the upper airway and trachea into the lung, especially if the open defect is similar or larger in size than the glottic opening to the lower airway. Resistance to the flow of air through a wound decreases as the defect size increases. Effective ventilation is then inhibited both by the collapse of the lung on the injured side and with the preferential flow of air into the pleural space through the wound rather than via the trachea into the alveoli of the lung. Although the patient is breathing, oxygen is prevented from entering the circulatory system.

Assessment

Assessment of the patient with open pneumothorax generally reveals obvious respiratory distress. The patient will typically be anxious and tachypneic (breathing rapidly). The pulse rate will be elevated and potentially thready (difficult to palpate). Examination of the chest wall will reveal the wound, which may make audible sucking sounds during inspiration, with bubbling during expiration.

Management

Initial management of an open pneumothorax involves sealing the defect in the chest wall and administering supplemental oxygen. Airflow through the wound into the pleural cavity is prevented by applying an occlusive dressing; using a commercially available chest seal; or using improvised methods, such as application of aluminum

foil or plastic wrap (unlike plain gauze, these materials do not allow airflow through them). Petroleum gauze or a defibrillator pad are both viable options if a commercial device is not available.

A patient with an open pneumothorax virtually always has an injury to the underlying lung, allowing for two sources of air leak, the first being the hole in the chest wall and the second being the hole in the lung. Even if an injury to the chest wall is sealed with an occlusive dressing, air leakage into the pleural space can continue from the injured lung, setting the stage for the development of a tension pneumothorax (**Figure 10-14**).

When treating an open pneumothorax, the occlusive dressing is secured on three sides.[1] This prevents airflow into the chest cavity during inspiration while allowing air to escape through the loose side of the dressing during exhalation and, hopefully, preventing the development of a tension pneumothorax. In contrast, taping the occlusive dressing on all four sides risks allowing a tension pneumothorax to develop. If there is an underlying leak in the lung tissue that allows air to continue to migrate into the pleural space with inspiration after sealing the open wound, the increasing size of the pneumothorax can cause it to transform into a tension pneumothorax. Sealing the wound on three sides should be effective, while simultaneously allowing for air to be released from the pleural space with time, thus avoiding the complications of tension pneumothorax.

A study in animals evaluated the physiologic response of an open pneumothorax model by comparing animals with a vented chest seal against those with an unvented chest seal.[28] This study showed that both seals improved the respiratory physiology associated with an open pneumothorax; however, the vented seal prevented the development of tension pneumothorax, whereas the

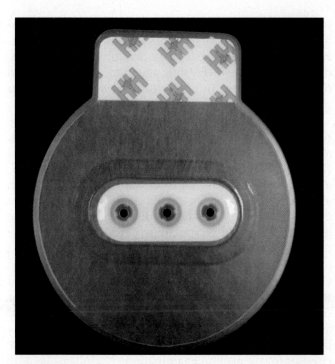

Figure 10-15 Vented chest seals have been shown in animal studies to prevent the development of tension pneumothorax after sealing of an open chest wound.[28]

Courtesy of H & H Medical Corporation.

unvented seal did not (**Figure 10-15**). This finding has led the military's Committee on Tactical Combat Casualty Care to recommend that, if available, a vented chest seal is preferred over an unvented chest seal.[29] An unvented chest seal is an acceptable alternative if the vented type is not available; however, the patient must be carefully observed for the subsequent development of a tension pneumothorax.[30]

In view of the research, Prehospital Trauma Life Support (PHTLS) now recommends the following approach to the management of an open pneumothorax:

- Place a vented chest seal over the open chest wound.
- If a vented seal is not available, place a plastic or foil square over the wound and tape on three sides.
- If none of these is available, an unvented chest seal or a material such as petroleum gauze that prevents ingress and egress of air may be used; however, this approach may allow the development of tension pneumothorax, so the patient must be observed carefully for signs of deterioration.
- If the patient develops tachycardia, tachypnea, or other indications of respiratory distress, elevate a corner of the dressing for a few seconds and allow any air under pressure to be released, and assist ventilations as necessary.
- If respiratory distress continues, assume the development of a tension pneumothorax, and perform a needle thoracostomy using a large-bore (10- to

16-gauge) needle that is 3.5 inches (8 cm) in length in the fifth intercostal space along the anterior axillary line.

If these measures fail to support the patient adequately, endotracheal intubation and positive-pressure ventilation may be necessary.[23] If positive pressure is utilized and a dressing has been applied to seal the open wound, the prehospital care practitioner needs to monitor the patient carefully for the development of tension pneumothorax. If signs of increasing respiratory distress develop, the dressing over the wound should be vented or removed to allow for decompression of any accumulating tension. If this is ineffective, needle decompression should be considered.[31]

In cases in which positive-pressure ventilation is being performed, sealing the wound is much less important from the perspective of restoring functional ventilation, although a sterile dressing is still valuable from the standpoint of limiting further wound contamination. The positive-pressure ventilation effectively manages the pathophysiology usually associated with the open pneumothorax by ventilating the lung directly.

Tension Pneumothorax

Tension pneumothorax is a life-threatening emergency. As air continues to enter the pleural space without any exit or release, intrathoracic pressure builds up. As intrathoracic pressure rises, ventilatory compromise increases and venous return to the heart decreases. The decreasing cardiac output coupled with worsening gas exchange results in profound shock (**Figure 10-16**). The increasing

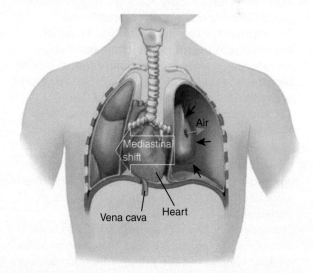

Figure 10-16 Tension pneumothorax. If the amount of air trapped in the pleural space continues to increase, not only is the lung on the affected side collapsed, but the mediastinum is shifted to the opposite side. The lung on the opposite side is then compressed and intrathoracic pressure increases, which kinks the vena cava and decreases blood return to the heart.

© National Association of Emergency Medical Technicians (NAEMT)

pressure on the injured side of the chest may eventually push the structures in the mediastinum toward the other side of the chest. This distortion of anatomy may further impede venous return to the heart through the kinking of the inferior vena cava as it passes through the diaphragm. Additionally, inflation of the lung on the uninjured side is increasingly restricted, and further respiratory compromise results.

Any patient with a thoracic injury is at risk for developing tension pneumothorax. Patients at particular risk are those who likely have a pneumothorax (e.g., patient with signs of rib fracture), those who have a known pneumothorax (e.g., patient with a penetrating wound to the chest), and those with chest injury who are undergoing positive-pressure ventilation. Such patients must be continuously monitored for signs of increasing respiratory distress associated with circulatory impairment and rapidly transported to an appropriate trauma facility.

Assessment

The findings during assessment depend on how much pressure has accumulated in the pleural space (**Box 10-3**).

Initially, patients will exhibit apprehension and discomfort. They will generally complain of chest pain and difficulty breathing. As the tension pneumothorax worsens, they will exhibit increasing agitation, tachypnea, and respiratory distress. In severe cases, cyanosis and apnea may occur.

The classic findings are absent breath sounds on the side of injury, a tympanitic percussion note (drum-like), and tracheal deviation away from the side of injury (a very late finding) all occurring in the context of progressive hemodynamic collapse. Constant practice with auscultation of all patients will hone this skill and make detection of absent or diminished breath sounds more likely. Detection of a tympanitic percussion note in the field is often not possible, but the finding is mentioned for the sake of completeness. If available, an ultrasound examination, usually performed between the second and third rib spaces with the patient supine, examining for signs of pneumothorax can be performed and repeated as needed. Transport and treatment should never be delayed for the purposes of performing percussion of the chest or for ultrasound examination.

Box 10-3 Signs of Tension Pneumothorax

Although the following signs are frequently discussed with a tension pneumothorax, many may not be present or are difficult to identify in the field.

Ultrasound

- *Absence of lung sliding.* Ideally, a pneumothorax can be identified and treated prior to the development of tension physiology. However, any change in respiratory status (regardless of any prior assessment of respiratory status) should prompt repeat clinical, and if available ultrasound, evaluation for a pneumothorax. See Box 10-2 and the section "Needle Decompression (Needle Thoracostomy)."

Observation

- *Cyanosis* may be difficult to see in the field. Poor lighting, variation in skin color, and dirt and blood associated with trauma often render this sign unreliable.
- *Distended neck veins* are described as a classic sign of tension pneumothorax. However, because a patient with a tension pneumothorax may also have lost a considerable amount of blood, distended neck veins may not be prominent.

Palpation

- *Subcutaneous emphysema* is a common finding. As the pressure builds up within the chest cavity,

air dissects through the tissues of the chest wall. Because tension pneumothorax involves significantly elevated intrathoracic pressure, the subcutaneous emphysema can often be palpated across the entire chest wall and neck and sometimes can involve the abdominal wall and face as well.

- *Tracheal deviation* is usually a late sign. Even when it is present, it can be difficult to diagnose by physical examination. In the neck, the trachea is bound to the cervical spine by fascial and other supporting structures; thus, the deviation of the trachea is more of an intrathoracic phenomenon, although deviation may be palpated in the jugular notch if it is severe. Tracheal deviation is not often noted in the prehospital environment.

Auscultation

- *Decreased breath sounds on the injured side.* The most helpful part of the physical examination is checking for decreased breath sounds on the side of the injury. However, to use this sign, the prehospital care practitioner must be able to distinguish between normal and decreased sounds. Such differentiation requires a great deal of practice. Listening to breath sounds during every patient contact will help.

Other physical findings that may be evident are jugular venous distension, chest wall crepitus, and cyanosis. Tachycardia and tachypnea become increasingly prominent as the intrathoracic pressure builds and the pulse pressure narrows, culminating in hypotension and uncompensated shock.

Management

The priority in management involves decompressing the tension pneumothorax.[23] Decompression should be performed when all of the following three findings are present:

1. Worsening respiratory distress or difficulty ventilating with a bag-mask device
2. Unilateral decreased or absent breath sounds
3. Decompensated shock (systolic blood pressure less than 90 mm Hg with a narrowed pulse pressure)[23-27,31]

Depending on the clinical setting and the training level of the prehospital care practitioner, several options for pleural decompression exist. If decompression is not an option (i.e., only basic life support [BLS] is available and there is no occlusive dressing to remove), rapid assessment and safe, expeditious transport to an appropriate facility while administering high-concentration oxygen (fraction of inspired oxygen [FiO_2] ≥ 94%) is imperative. Positive-pressure ventilatory assistance should be used only if the patient is hypoxic and fails to respond to supplemental oxygen, as this situation may rapidly worsen the tension pneumothorax. Assisting ventilations may result in air accumulating more rapidly in the pleural space. If ALS intercept is an option, it should be accomplished, but only if the intercept will be faster than delivery to an appropriate facility.

Suspected Tension Pneumothorax With an Occlusive Dressing

In the patient with an open pneumothorax, if an occluding dressing has been applied, it should be briefly opened or removed. This should allow the tension pneumothorax to decompress through the wound with a rush of air. This procedure may need to be repeated periodically during transport if symptoms of tension pneumothorax recur. If removing the dressing for several seconds is ineffective or if there is no open wound, an ALS practitioner should proceed with a needle thoracostomy.

Suspected Tension Pneumothorax in the Intubated Patient

In an intubated patient, a malpositioned endotracheal tube can be mistaken for a tension pneumothorax. If the endotracheal tube has slipped farther down from the trachea into one of the main bronchi (usually the right), the opposite lung will not be ventilated, and breath sounds and chest wall expansion may be markedly diminished. In these cases, the position of the endotracheal tube should be assessed and confirmed prior to any attempt at chest decompression.

Needle Decompression (Needle Thoracostomy)

Insertion of a needle (angiocatheter) into the pleural space on the affected side permits the accumulated air, under pressure, to escape. Successful decompression converts a tension pneumothorax into an open pneumothorax and reverses the hemodynamic compromise associated with decreased venous return caused by the shift of mediastinal contents away from the collapsed lung.[32] This, along with the immediate improvement in ability to oxygenate and ventilate, can be lifesaving.

Needle decompression has historically been performed through the second intercostal space in the midclavicular line on the affected side of the chest (lateral to the nipple). Recent evidence, however, supports using the fifth intercostal space along the anterior axillary line (lateral approach) as the preferred location for needle decompression (**Figure 10-17**).[1,33] Each location has advantages and disadvantages. Decompression in the midclavicular line has the advantage of ease of access in the prehospital environment, but chest wall thickness at this location can result in the inability of the catheter to reach the thoracic cavity or kinking of the catheter during patient movement. In addition, there is a small risk of inducing major hemorrhage from inadvertent placement of

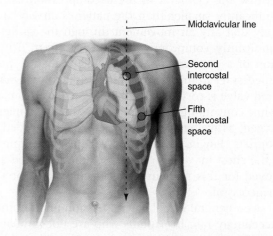

Figure 10-17 Needle decompression of the thoracic cavity for treatment of suspected tension pneumothorax. The procedure is performed using a large-bore (10- to 16-gauge) IV needle that is at least 3.5 inches (8 cm) in length. The needle should be placed at the fifth intercostal space along the anterior axillary line.

© MariyaL/Shutterstock

the catheter into the subclavian vessels (superiorly) or internal mammary artery, heart, or pulmonary vessels (medially).[34,35] For these reasons, the lateral approach is now recommended as the first-line technique for prehospital tension pneumothorax decompression.

Advantages of the anterior axillary line placement of the catheter include its relative safety and efficacy. The chest wall is thinner in this location across all body mass index (BMI) quartiles in both men and women. In addition, higher success rates have been reported using this location,[36,37] and evidence suggests that catheters placed at the fifth intercostal space at the anterior axillary line are more stable during transport and less likely to become dislodged,[38] although kinking may be an issue.[39]

Regardless of the location chosen, decompression should be performed with a large-bore (10- to 16-gauge) IV needle that is at least 3.5 inches (8 cm) in length. The needle and catheter should be advanced until a rush of air is encountered, but not beyond that point. The lung on the affected side is collapsed and shifted toward the contralateral side; therefore, it is unlikely to be injured during the procedure. Once the decompression is achieved, the needle is removed and the catheter is taped to the chest to prevent dislodgment. Careful monitoring of the patient following the procedure is mandatory. One study noted a 26% mechanical failure rate due to kinking, obstruction, or dislodgment of the angiocatheter, with 43% of decompression attempts ultimately failing to relieve the tension pneumothorax.[40]

This procedure, when successfully performed, converts the tension pneumothorax into a simple, open pneumothorax. The relief to respiratory effort far outweighs the negative effect of the open pneumothorax. Because the diameter of the decompression catheter is significantly smaller than the patient's airway, it is unlikely that any air movement through the catheter will significantly compromise ventilatory effort. Thus, creation of a one-way valve (Heimlich valve) is probably unnecessary from a clinical standpoint. Using a manufactured valve is costly, and fashioning a valve from a glove is time consuming. Continued provision of supplemental oxygen, as well as ventilatory support as needed, is appropriate. Finger thoracostomy or finger decompression of the chest may be an option for those trained and approved for this maneuver if a needle decompression is unsuccessful.

As a general rule, bilateral tension pneumothorax is exceedingly rare in patients who are not intubated and ventilated with positive pressure. The first step in reassessing the patient is to confirm the location of the endotracheal tube, ensuring that it has no kinks or bends causing compression of the tube, and determining if the tube has not inadvertently moved down into a main bronchus. Extreme caution should be exercised with bilateral needle decompression in patients who are not being ventilated with positive-pressure ventilation. If the prehospital care practitioner's assessment is in error, the creation of bilateral pneumothoraces can cause severe respiratory distress.

The patient should be rapidly transported to an appropriate facility. Intravenous access should be obtained during transport unless transport time is particularly short. The patient must be closely observed for deterioration. Repeat decompression and endotracheal intubation may become necessary.

Tube Thoracostomy (Chest Tube Insertion)

In general, the insertion of a chest tube (tube thoracostomy) is not performed in the prehospital setting because of concerns of time, procedural complications, and training issues. Needle decompression can be accomplished more rapidly than tube thoracostomy because fewer steps are necessary and less equipment is used. Published complication rates with tube thoracostomy range from 2.8% to 21%[41,42] and include infection potentially resulting in an empyema (collection of pus in the pleural space), damage to the heart or lungs, and malposition in the subcutaneous tissues of the chest wall or in the peritoneal cavity. Significant training is required to develop this skill, and ongoing practice is required to maintain skill proficiency.

Patients being transported with a chest tube in place are still at risk for the development of a tension pneumothorax, particularly if they are undergoing positive-pressure ventilatory assistance. If signs of a tension pneumothorax begin to manifest, first ensure that there are no kinks in the chest tube or connecting tubing. Next, ensure that the connecting tubing is correctly connected to a water seal and drainage device. Even with no identified problems, the patient with signs of an increasing tension pneumothorax may require needle decompression. Do not delay just because there is already a chest tube in place (**Box 10-4**).

Hemothorax

Hemothorax occurs when blood enters the pleural space. Because this space can accommodate a large volume of blood (2,500 to 3,000 mL), hemothorax can represent a source of significant blood loss. In fact, high-volume blood loss into the chest results in shock, and this can be of greater physiologic consequence than the actual collapse of the impacted lung (**Figure 10-19**). It is rare that enough blood accumulates to create a "tension hemothorax." The mechanisms resulting in hemothorax are the same as those causing the various types of pneumothoraces. The bleeding may come from the chest wall musculature, intercostal vessels, lung parenchyma, pulmonary vessels, or great vessels of the chest.

Box 10-4 Troubleshooting Tube Thoracostomy

Three Basic Components of Chest Tube Drainage Systems

1. *Seal*. Allows air to escape the pleural space but not return. The seal is generally a water seal that bubbles as air escapes the pleural space and rises with inspiratory negative pressure.
2. *Collecting system*. Collects and measures output. Observe for changes in volume of output and nature.
3. *Suction*. Provides negative pressure to assist drainage and expansion. Ensure that suction is appropriately attached and functioning. Review the basic operation of any drainage system with the patient's healthcare team prior to transfer of the patient (**Figure 10-18**).

Changes in Respiratory Status in Patients With Chest Tubes

■ *Assess vital signs, including pulse oximetry*. If the chest tube is not working properly, the patient may become tachycardic, tachypneic, and hypoxic. If tension pneumothorax is developing, subcutaneous emphysema, increasing respiratory distress, narrowing pulse pressure, and hypotension may result.
■ *Assess lung sounds*. The lung sounds may become diminished in the involved side if the chest tube is no longer functioning and instead is allowing air to reaccumulate within the chest.
■ *Assess ventilatory effort*. Ventilatory effort will increase when the chest tube is not functioning.
■ *Assess circulation*. If the chest tube is not working properly and is allowing air to accumulate within the chest, the patient may become tachycardic. If tension pneumothorax is developing, narrowing pulse pressure and hypotension may result.
■ *Assess level of consciousness*. If hypoxia or signs of shock develop, the patient may become agitated and anxious. As these complications progress, the patient's level of consciousness will decrease.

Troubleshooting Steps

■ Assess the dressing and tube site to ensure that the chest tube has not been dislodged during transfers.

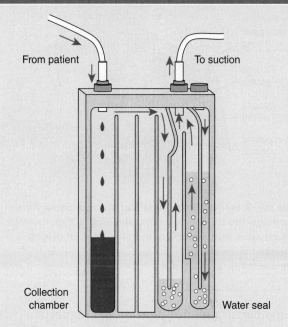

Figure 10-18 A chest drainage system provides negative pressure to assist drainage and expansion of the patient's chest.

© National Association of Emergency Medical Technicians (NAEMT)

■ Check that the chest tubing is tightly connected and unobstructed, with no kinks, blood clots, or clamps.
■ Check that the chest seal is intact and functioning. Is there any bubbling and/or variation with ventilations?
■ Assess whether the chest tube is fogging and/or drainage is continuing.
■ Ensure that the suction is functioning. Is there continuous bubbling or a negative pressure indicator throughout the ventilation cycle?
■ If the patient's ventilatory status continues to deteriorate, assess closely for signs of developing tension pneumothorax. If indicated, disconnect the chest tube from the drainage system; this should allow release of tension if the chest tube is properly placed and unobstructed. If this step does not relieve the condition, consider needle decompression, and contact online medical control.

© National Association of Emergency Medical Technicians (NAEMT)

Assessment

Assessment reveals a patient in some distress, depending on the amount of blood lost into the chest and the resultant compression of the lung on the involved side. Chest pain and shortness of breath are again prominent features, generally with signs of significant shock. The prehospital care practitioner monitors the patient for signs of shock: tachycardia, tachypnea, confusion, pallor, and hypotension. Breath sounds on the side of the injury are diminished or absent, but the percussion note is dull (compared to tympanitic for a pneumothorax).

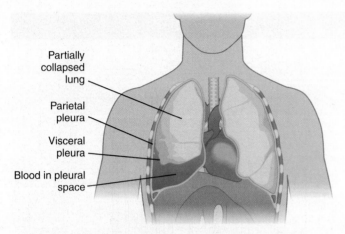

Partially collapsed lung

Parietal pleura

Visceral pleura

Blood in pleural space

Figure 10-19 Hemothorax. The blood loss associated with hemorrhage into the thoracic cavity (leading to hypovolemia) is a much more severe problem than the amount of lung compressed by this blood.

© National Association of Emergency Medical Technicians (NAEMT)

Pneumothorax may be present in conjunction with hemothorax, increasing the likelihood for cardiorespiratory compromise. Because of loss of circulating blood volume, distended neck veins often are not present.

Management

Management includes constant observation to detect physiologic deterioration while providing appropriate support. High-concentration oxygen should be administered and ventilation supported if necessary with a bag-mask device or endotracheal intubation, if available and indicated. Hemodynamic status is closely monitored. IV access should be obtained and appropriate fluid therapy provided, with a goal of maintaining adequate perfusion without indiscriminately administering large volumes of crystalloid. Blood product resuscitation may be appropriate if available. Rapid transport to an appropriate facility that is capable of immediate blood transfusion and surgical intervention completes the management algorithm for hemothorax. Needle decompression of the chest for hemothorax alone is not effective and not indicated.

Blunt Cardiac Injury

Cardiac injury most often results from application of force to the anterior chest, especially in a deceleration event such as a motor vehicle crash with violent frontal impact.[1,2,43] The heart is then compressed between the sternum anteriorly and the spinal column posteriorly (**Figure 10-20**). This compression of the heart causes an abrupt increase in the pressure within the ventricles to several times greater than normal, which results in cardiac contusion, sometimes valvular injury, and (rarely) cardiac rupture, as follows:

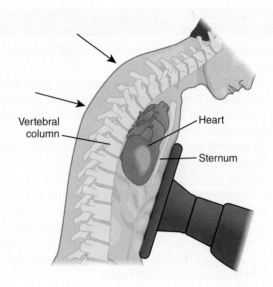

Vertebral column

Heart

Sternum

Figure 10-20 The heart can be compressed between the sternum (as the sternum stops against the steering column or dashboard) and the posterior thoracic wall (as the wall continues its forward motion). This compression can contuse the myocardium.

© National Association of Emergency Medical Technicians (NAEMT)

- *Cardiac contusion.* The most common result of cardiac compression is cardiac contusion. The heart muscle is bruised, with varying amounts of injury to the myocardial cells. This injury most often results in arrythmias, such as sinus tachycardia.[43] Of greater concern, but less common, are premature ventricular contractions or nonperfusing rhythms such as ventricular tachycardia and ventricular fibrillation. If the septal region of the heart is injured, the electrocardiogram (ECG) may demonstrate intraventricular conduction abnormalities, such as right bundle branch block. If a sufficient volume of myocardium is injured, the contractility of the heart may be impaired, and cardiac output falls, resulting in cardiogenic shock. Unlike the other forms of shock usually encountered in the trauma setting, this type of shock does not improve with fluid administration and may actually worsen.
- *Valvular rupture.* Rupture of the supporting structures of the heart valves or the valves themselves typically renders the valves incompetent. The patient will present in varying degrees of shock with symptoms and signs of acute congestive heart failure (CHF), such as *tachypnea*, crackles, and new-onset heart murmur.
- *Blunt pericardial rupture with cardiac herniation.* A rare event, blunt pericardial rupture occurs in less than 0.4% of patients with blunt chest trauma.[44] These patients may exhibit hemodynamic instability, especially upon laying the patient supine, where the heart can herniate through the pericardial defect and then compromise cardiac return.[45,46]

- *Blunt cardiac rupture.* A rare event, blunt cardiac rupture occurs in less than 1% of patients with blunt chest trauma.[43-48] Most of these patients will die at the scene from *exsanguination* into the chest or fatal cardiac tamponade. Surviving patients will typically present with cardiac tamponade.

Assessment

Assessment of the patient with the potential for blunt cardiac injury reveals a mechanism that imparted a frontal impact to the center of the patient's chest. A bent steering column accompanied by bruising over the sternum implies such a mechanism. As with other chest injuries, the patient is likely to complain of chest pain and/or shortness of breath. If a dysrhythmia is present, the patient may complain of palpitations. Physical findings of concern are bruising over the sternum, crepitus over the sternum, and sternal instability. With a floating sternum (**flail sternum**), the ribs on either side of the sternum are broken, allowing it to move paradoxically with respirations, similar to flail chest, as described earlier. If valvular disruption has occurred, a harsh murmur may be detectable over the precordium along with signs of acute CHF, such as hypotension, jugular venous distension, and abnormal breath sounds. ECG monitoring may demonstrate dysrhythmias (in descending order of frequency: sinus tachycardia, atrial fibrillation, premature ventricular contractions, and others).

Management

The key management strategy is correct assessment that blunt cardiac injury may have occurred and transmission of that concern along with the clinical findings to the receiving hospital. In the meantime, high-concentration oxygen is administered and IV access established for judicious fluid therapy. The patient should be placed on a cardiac monitor to detect dysrhythmias and ST-segment elevations, if present. If dysrhythmias are present and ALS practitioners are present, standard antiarrhythmic pharmacotherapy should be instituted. There are no data to support prophylactic antidysrhythmic therapy in blunt cardiac injury. Consider maintaining the patient sitting upright if immediate decompensation occurs upon placing supine. As always, ventilatory support measures should be implemented as indicated.

Cardiac Tamponade

Cardiac tamponade occurs when a wound of the heart or proximal great vessels allows fluid (usually blood) to acutely accumulate between the pericardial sac and the heart.[1,43] The pericardial sac is composed of a fibrous, inelastic tissue. Normally, there is a small amount of fluid in the pericardial sac, similar to the pleural space,

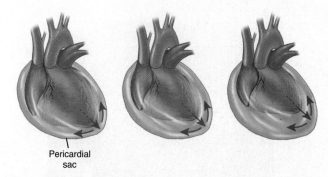

Pericardial sac

Figure 10-21 Cardiac tamponade. As blood courses from the cardiac lumen into the pericardial space, it limits expansion of the ventricle. Therefore, the ventricle cannot fill completely. As more blood accumulates in the pericardial space, less ventricular space is available to accumulate blood, and cardiac output is reduced.
© National Association of Emergency Medical Technicians (NAEMT)

as described earlier. Because the pericardium is inelastic, pressure begins to rise rapidly within the pericardial sac as fluid accumulates within it acutely. This rising pericardial pressure impedes venous return to the heart. This, in turn, leads to diminished cardiac output and blood pressure. With each contraction of the heart, additional blood may enter the pericardial sac, further impeding the heart's ability to fill in preparation for the next contraction (**Figure 10-21**). This condition can become profound enough to precipitate **pulseless electrical activity**, a life-threatening injury requiring coordinated response by prehospital care practitioners in all phases of care to achieve an optimal outcome. The normal adult pericardium may be able to accommodate as much as 300 mL of fluid before pulselessness occurs, but as little as 50 mL is usually enough to impede cardiac return and, thus, cardiac output.[1]

Most often, cardiac tamponade is caused by a stab wound to the heart. This mechanism of injury may result in penetration into one of the cardiac chambers or just a laceration of the myocardium. The right ventricle is the most anterior chamber in the heart and is therefore the most commonly injured chamber in penetrating trauma. Regardless of the anatomic location of injury, bleeding into the pericardial sac occurs. The rising pressure within the pericardium results in the cardiac tamponade physiology. At the same time, the increased pressure within the pericardium may temporarily impede further bleeding from the cardiac wound, allowing the patient to survive long enough to reach definitive medical care. In the case of gunshot wounds to the heart, the damage to the heart and pericardium is usually so severe that the pericardium cannot contain the hemorrhage, resulting in rapid exsanguination into the chest cavity. The same is true in the case of impalements. Blunt rupture of a cardiac chamber can result in cardiac tamponade but more often causes exsanguinating hemorrhage.

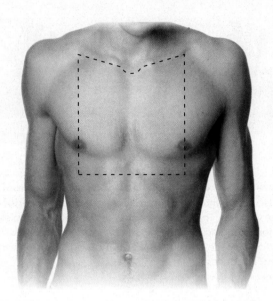

Figure 10-22 The index of suspicion for penetrating cardiac injury should be high if the penetrating wound occurs within the "cardiac box."

© MariyaL/Shutterstock

Cardiac tamponade should be kept in mind as a possibility when evaluating any patient with a thoracic penetration. This index of suspicion should be raised to the level of "present until proven otherwise" when the penetrating injury is within a rectangle (the cardiac box) formed by drawing a horizontal line along the clavicles, vertical lines from the nipples to the costal margins, and a second horizontal line connecting the points of intersection between the vertical lines and the costal margin (**Figure 10-22**). The presence of such a wound should be communicated to the receiving institution as soon as it is recognized to allow for appropriate preparation to manage the patient.

Assessment

Assessment involves quickly recognizing the presence of at-risk wounds, as previously described, in combination with an appreciation for the physical and ultrasound findings of pericardial tamponade (see Box 10-2). Beck triad is a constellation of findings indicative of cardiac tamponade: (1) distant or muffled heart sounds (the fluid around the heart makes it difficult to hear the sounds of the valves closing), (2) jugular venous distension (caused by the increasing pressure in the pericardial sac backing blood up into the neck veins), and (3) low blood pressure. Another physical finding described in cardiac tamponade is paradoxical pulse (**Box 10-5**).

Detection of some of these physical exam signs is difficult in the field, especially muffled heart tones and paradoxical pulse. Additionally, the components of Beck triad are present in only 22% to 77% of cases of

---

Box 10-5 Paradoxical Pulse

The **paradoxical pulse**, also known as pulsus paradoxus, is actually an accentuation of the normal, slight drop in systolic blood pressure (SBP) that occurs during inspiration. As the lungs expand, there is preferential filling and ejection of blood from the right side of the heart at the expense of the left side. Thus, peripheral blood pressure falls. This decrease in SBP is usually less than 10 to 15 mm Hg. A greater decrease in SBP constitutes the so-called paradoxical pulse.

© National Association of Emergency Medical Technicians (NAEMT)

---

tamponade.[49,50] Thus, the prehospital care practitioner needs to maintain a high index of suspicion, based on the location of the wounds and hypotension, and implement therapy accordingly and expeditiously.

Management

Management requires rapid, monitored transport to a facility that can perform immediate surgical repair.[22,25,51-55] The prehospital care practitioner first needs to recognize that cardiac tamponade likely exists and to inform the receiving facility so that preparations can be made for emergent surgical intervention. Oxygen in high concentration should be administered. IV access should be obtained and judicious fluid therapy initiated, because this can augment central venous pressure and thus improve cardiac filling for a time. Positive-pressure ventilation should be avoided if at all possible as this will decrease venous return and exacerbate the hemodynamic challenge.[56,57]

Definitive therapy requires release of the tamponade and repair of the cardiac injury. A patient with a suspected cardiac tamponade should be transported directly to a facility capable of immediate surgical intervention, if available. Draining some of the pericardial fluid by **pericardiocentesis** (insertion of a needle into the pericardial space) is often an effective temporizing maneuver (**Figure 10-23**). Risks of pericardiocentesis include injury to the heart and coronary arteries, resulting in increased tamponade and injury to the lung, great vessels, and liver. In very rare cases, resuscitative thoracotomy (opening the chest to control bleeding and repair internal wounds) has been performed in the field by physicians in systems in which they respond to field emergencies.[58,59]

Commotio Cordis

The term **commotio cordis** refers to sudden cardiac death following a nonpenetrating chest injury.[60,61] Data on over 220 cases from the National Commotio Cordis Registry, which has existed since the 1990s in the United States,

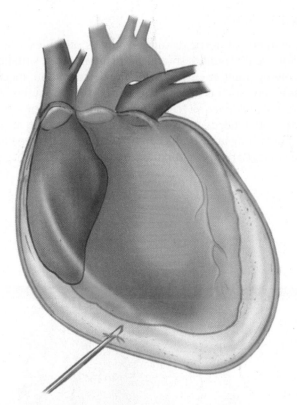

Figure 10-23 Draining some of the pericardial fluid by pericardiocentesis is often an effective temporizing maneuver for cardiac tamponade.

© National Association of Emergency Medical Technicians (NAEMT)

demonstrate that the average age of presentation is 15 years, 95% of cases are among males, and 75% of cases occur during athletic competition.[62] Most experts hypothesize that commotio cordis results from a relatively minor, nonpenetrating blow to the precordium during an electrically vulnerable portion of the cardiac cycle, while others believe that coronary artery vasospasm may play a role in its development. Regardless of the mechanism, the result is a cardiac dysrhythmia resulting in ventricular fibrillation and sudden cardiac arrest.

This condition most frequently occurs during amateur sporting events in which the patient is struck in the mid-anterior chest by a projectile or object, such as a baseball (most common), ice hockey puck, lacrosse ball, or softball. However, commotio cordis has also been reported after bodily impacts (e.g., karate blows), a low-velocity motor vehicle crash, and the collision of two outfielders trying to catch a baseball. After the impact, victims have been known to walk a step or two and then suddenly drop to the ground in cardiac arrest. Typically, no injury is noted to the ribs, sternum, or heart at autopsy. Most victims have no known history of heart disease. The use of chest wall protectors during sports play has not demonstrated a decrease in commotio cordis incidence. The American Heart Association and American Cardiology Association recommend preventive efforts focus instead on increased bystander and athletic staff training on recognition and management of commotio cordis including prompt notification of local EMS service.[63]

Assessment

Patients who have sustained commotio cordis are found in cardiopulmonary arrest. In some victims, a minor bruise is noted over the sternum. Ventricular fibrillation is the most common rhythm, although complete heart block and left bundle branch block with ST-segment elevations have also been seen.

Management

Once cardiac arrest is confirmed, cardiopulmonary resuscitation (CPR) is initiated. Commotio cordis is managed in a manner similar to cardiac arrests resulting from myocardial infarction rather than those resulting from trauma and blood loss. The cardiac rhythm should be determined as expeditiously as possible, with rapid defibrillation administered if ventricular fibrillation is identified. Prognosis is poor, with the chance of survival at 15% or less.[61] Virtually all survivors of this condition received both rapid bystander-initiated CPR and immediate defibrillation, often with an automated external defibrillator. Precordial thumps have not been shown to consistently terminate ventricular fibrillation; however, they may be attempted if a defibrillator is not immediately available. The initiation of CPR and electrical defibrillation should not be delayed to perform a precordial thump.[64] If immediate attempts at defibrillation are unsuccessful, the airway is secured and IV access initiated. Epinephrine and antidysrhythmic pharmacologic agents may be administered as outlined in medical cardiac arrest protocols.

Traumatic Aortic Disruption

Traumatic aortic disruption results from a deceleration/acceleration mechanism of significant force.[65] Examples include high-speed frontal-impact motor vehicle crashes and high falls.

The aorta arises from the upper portion of the heart in the mediastinum. The heart, ascending aorta, and aortic arch are relatively mobile within the chest cavity. As the arch of the aorta transitions to the descending aorta, it is "wrapped" with an investing layer of tissue and becomes adherent to the vertebral column. Thus, the descending aorta is relatively immobile. When there is a sudden deceleration of the body, such as occurs in a high-speed frontal impact, the heart and the aortic arch continue to move forward relative to the fixed (immobile) descending aorta. This contrast in velocity produces shear forces in the aortic wall at the junction between these two segments of the aorta.[54] Thus, the typical location for a traumatic aortic injury is just distal to the takeoff of the left subclavian artery. This shear force can disrupt the wall of the aorta in varying degrees (**Figure 10-24**). When the tear extends through the full thickness of the aortic wall, the patient rapidly exsanguinates into the pleural cavity. However, if the tear is only partially through the wall, leaving the outer layer (adventitia) intact, the patient may survive for a variable length of time. Rapid identification and treatment are essential for a successful outcome.[65]

Assessment

Assessment of aortic disruption hinges on index of suspicion. A high index should be maintained in situations involving high-energy deceleration/acceleration mechanisms. For such a devastating injury, there may be little external evidence of chest injury. The prehospital care practitioner needs to assess the adequacy of the airway and breathing and should carefully auscultate and palpate the chest. Careful examination may demonstrate that the

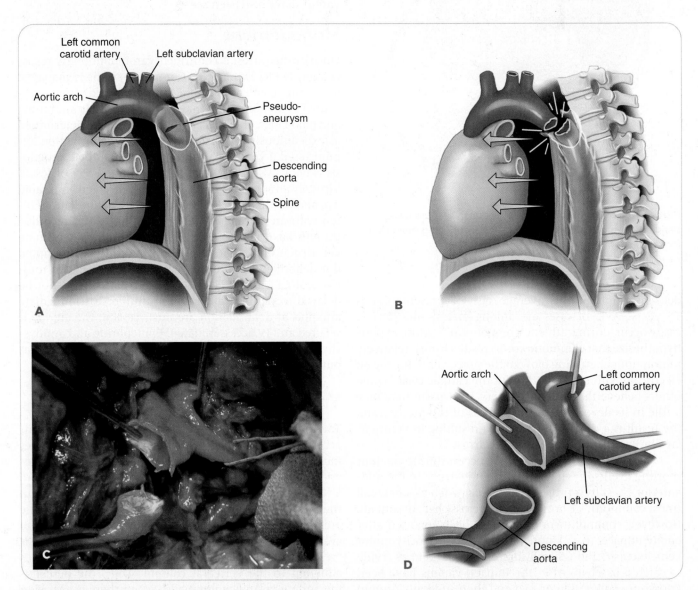

Figure 10-24   A. The descending aorta is a fixed structure that moves with the thoracic spine. The arch, aorta, and heart are freely movable. Acceleration of the torso in a lateral-impact collision or rapid deceleration of the torso in a frontal-impact collision produces a different rate of motion between the arch–heart complex and the descending aorta. This motion may result in a tear of the inner lining of the aorta that is contained within the outermost layer, producing a pseudo-aneurysm. **B.** Tears at the junction of the arch and descending aorta may also result in a complete rupture, leading to immediate exsanguination in the chest. **C.** and **D.** Operative photograph and drawing of a traumatic aortic tear.

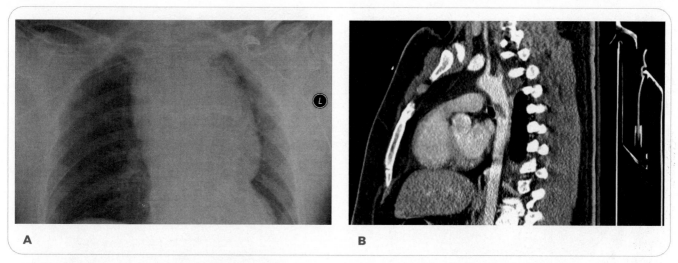

Figure 10-25 Chest x-ray and chest CT demonstrating aortic disruption. **A.** Widened mediastinum on chest x-ray suggestive of aortic injury. **B.** Chest CT demonstrating aortic dissection flap and aortic injury.

Courtesy of Dr. Mark Gestring, MD, FACS.

pulse quality may be different between the two upper extremities (pulse stronger in the right arm than the left) or between the upper (brachial artery) and lower extremities (femoral artery). Blood pressures, if measured, may be higher in the upper extremities than in the lower extremities, comprising the signs of a pseudo-coarctation (narrowing) of the aorta.

Definitive diagnosis of aortic disruption requires radiographic imaging in the hospital. Plain chest radiographs may demonstrate a variety of signs suggesting the injury is present. The most reliable of these is widening of the mediastinum (**Figure 10-25**). The injury is usually identified via a chest computed tomography (CT) angiography or **transesophageal echocardiography**.[65]

Management

Management of traumatic aortic disruption in the field is supportive. A high index of suspicion for its presence is maintained when the appropriate mechanism exists. High-concentration supplemental oxygen is administered and IV access is obtained en route, except in cases of extremely short transport times. Communication with the receiving facility about the mechanism and suspicion for aortic disruption should occur at the earliest opportunity. Strict blood pressure control is imperative to the successful outcome of these injuries (**Box 10-6**). Traumatic aortic disruption represents another situation in which balanced resuscitation is clinically important. Fluid resuscitation that results in normal or elevated blood pressure may result in rupture of the remaining tissue of the aorta and rapid exsanguination. If transport times are longer, blood pressure management should be guided by the highest blood pressure obtained, typically in the right arm. Control of both blood pressure and contractile force may be accomplished with the administration of beta blockers.[60]

Box 10-6 Blood Pressure Maintenance

Caution: When performing interhospital transfer of patients with suspected aortic disruption, it is important not to raise the patient's blood pressure aggressively because this may lead to exsanguinating hemorrhage (see Chapter 3, *Shock: Pathophysiology of Life and Death*). Many of these patients may be given infusions of medications, such as beta blockers (e.g., esmolol, metoprolol), to maintain the blood pressure at a lower level, typically a systolic blood pressure ≤ 100 mm Hg. Such therapy typically requires invasive monitoring, such as insertion of an arterial line, so that blood pressure can be monitored much more carefully.

© National Association of Emergency Medical Technicians (NAEMT)

Tracheobronchial Disruption

Tracheobronchial disruption is an uncommon, but potentially lethal, condition.[66] All lacerations of the lung involve disruption of airways to some degree; however, in these cases, the intrathoracic portion of the trachea itself or one of the main or secondary bronchi is disrupted. This disruption results in high flow of air through the injury into the mediastinum or pleural space (**Figure 10-26**). Pressure rapidly accumulates, resulting in tension pneumothorax or even tension pneumomediastinum, which is similar to cardiac tamponade except that it results from the presence of air and not blood or fluid. Unlike the usual situation in tension pneumothorax, needle thoracostomy may result in the continuous flow of air through the catheter and may fail to relieve the tension. This is caused by the ongoing high flow of air across these major airways into the

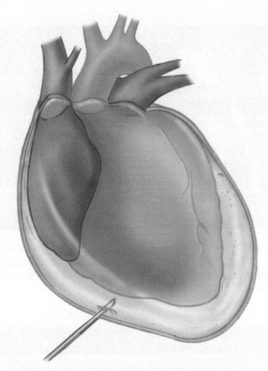

Figure 10-26 Tracheal or bronchial rupture. Positive-pressure ventilation can directly force large amounts of air through the trachea or bronchus, rapidly producing a tension pneumothorax.

© National Association of Emergency Medical Technicians (NAEMT)

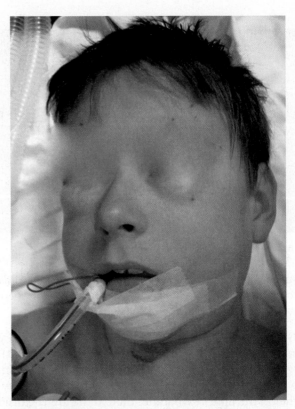

Figure 10-27 Patient with trauma to the anterior neck causing a tracheal disruption and subcutaneous emphysema of the face (eyelids) and neck.

Photograph provided courtesy of J.C. Pitteloud M.D., Switzerland

pleural space. Respiratory function may be significantly impaired because of preferential airflow across the lesion as well as the pressure. Positive-pressure ventilation efforts may worsen the tension. Penetrating trauma is more likely to cause this injury than blunt trauma. However, blunt injury of high energy may also cause tracheobronchial disruption.[67]

Assessment

Assessment of the patient with tracheobronchial disruption demonstrates an individual in obvious distress. The patient may be pale and diaphoretic and will demonstrate signs of respiratory distress, such as use of accessory muscles of respiration, grunting, and nasal flaring. Extensive subcutaneous emphysema, especially in the upper chest and neck, may be identified (**Figure 10-27**). Although traditionally taught as important findings, jugular venous distension may be obscured by subcutaneous emphysema, and deviation of the trachea may only be noted upon palpation of the trachea in the jugular notch. Ventilatory rate will be elevated, and oxygen saturation may be diminished. The patient may or may not be hypotensive and may cough up blood (hemoptysis). The hemorrhage associated with penetrating trauma may not be present in the blunt cases, but hemothorax is a possibility in both penetrating and blunt trauma.

Management

Successful management of tracheobronchial disruption requires administration of supplemental oxygen and judicious use of ventilatory assistance. If assisted ventilation makes the patient more uncomfortable, only oxygen is administered and the patient is rapidly transported to an appropriate facility. Continuous monitoring for signs of progression toward a tension pneumothorax is imperative, and rapid needle decompression should be attempted if these signs present. Complex advanced airway management, such as selective main bronchus intubation, is generally not possible in the field and attempts are associated with the potential for worsening a major bronchial injury.

Traumatic Asphyxia

Traumatic asphyxia is so named because the victims physically resemble strangulation patients. They exhibit the same bluish discoloration of the face and neck (and in the case of traumatic asphyxia, upper chest) as patients who have been strangled. Unlike strangled patients, however, traumatic asphyxia patients do not suffer from true asphyxia (cessation of air and gas exchange). The similarity in appearance to strangulation patients results from the impaired venous return from the head and neck that is present in both groups of patients.

The mechanism for traumatic asphyxia is an abrupt, significant increase in thoracic pressure resulting from a crush to the torso (e.g., car falling off a jack onto the patient's chest). This pressure results in blood being forced back out of the heart and into the veins in a retrograde direction. Because the veins of the arms and lower extremities contain valves, backward flow into the extremities is limited. However, the veins of the neck and head lack such valves, and blood is preferentially forced into these areas. Subcutaneous venules and small capillaries rupture and blood leaks out, resulting in the purplish discoloration of the skin. Rupture of small vessels in the brain and retina may result in brain and eye dysfunction. Traumatic asphyxia is reported to be a marker for blunt cardiac rupture.[68]

Assessment

The hallmark of traumatic asphyxia is plethora, a condition characterized by an excess of blood and turgescence (i.e., swelling and distension of blood vessels), with a reddish coloration of the skin. This appearance is most prominent above the level of the crush (**Figure 10-28**). The skin below the level of injury is normal. Because of the force

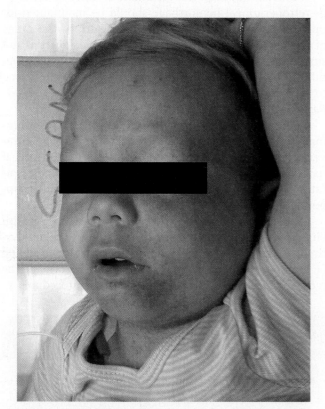

Figure 10-28 Child with traumatic asphyxia. Note the purple discoloration, particularly on the chin, and the multiple petechiae on the face and forehead.

Photograph provided courtesy of J.C. Pitteloud M.D., Switzerland

applied to the chest necessary to cause this injury, many of the injuries already discussed in this chapter may be present, as well as injuries to the spine and spinal cord.

Management

Management is supportive. High-concentration oxygen is administered, IV access obtained, and judicious ventilatory support provided, if indicated. The reddish-purple discoloration typically fades within 1 to 2 weeks in survivors.

Diaphragmatic Rupture

Small lacerations of the diaphragm may occur in penetrating injuries to the thoracoabdominal region.[1] Because the diaphragm rises and falls with respiration, any penetration that is below the level of the nipples anteriorly or the level of the scapular tip posteriorly is at risk for having traversed the diaphragm. Generally, these lesions do not present any acute problems on their own, but they usually require surgical repair because of the risk in the future for herniation and strangulation of abdominal contents through the defect. Significant injuries to thoracic or abdominal organs may accompany these otherwise apparently innocuous injuries.

Blunt diaphragmatic rupture results from the application of sufficient force to the abdomen to increase abdominal pressure acutely, abruptly, and sufficiently to disrupt the diaphragm. Unlike the small tears that usually accompany penetrating injury, the tears resulting from blunt mechanisms are frequently large and allow acute herniation of the abdominal viscera into the chest cavity[1] (**Figure 10-29**). Respiratory distress results from the pressure of the herniated organs on the lungs, preventing effective ventilation, as well as from contusion of the lungs. This impairment of ventilation may be life threatening. In addition to the ventilatory dysfunction, rib fractures, hemothorax, and pneumothorax may occur. Injury of intra-abdominal organs may also accompany the injury to the diaphragm, including injuries to the liver, spleen, stomach, or intestines, as these organs are forced through the tear in the diaphragm into the pleural cavity. These patients are frequently in acute distress and require rapid intervention to recover.

Assessment

Assessment frequently reveals a patient in acute respiratory distress who appears anxious, tachypneic, and pale. The patient may have contusions of the chest wall, bony crepitus, or subcutaneous emphysema. Breath sounds on the affected side may be diminished, or bowel sounds may be auscultated over the chest. The abdomen may be scaphoid if enough of the abdominal contents have herniated into the chest.

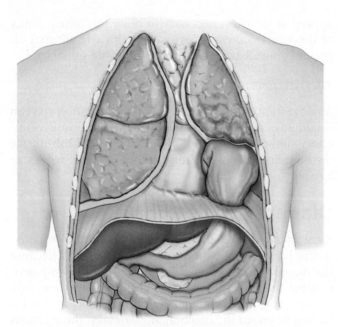

Figure 10-29 Diaphragmatic rupture may cause the bowel or other structures to herniate through the tear, causing partial compression of the lung and respiratory distress.
© National Association of Emergency Medical Technicians (NAEMT)

Management

Prompt recognition that diaphragmatic rupture may be present is necessary. Supplemental oxygen in high concentration should be administered and ventilation supported as necessary. Placement of a needle decompression catheter or chest tube is unlikely to provide benefit and may be dangerous due to the intra-abdominal organs displaced upward into the chest. The patient should be rapidly assessed and transported to an appropriate facility with surgical capability.

Prolonged Transport

Priorities for managing patients with known or suspected thoracic injuries during prolonged transport remain fundamental, including managing the airway, supporting ventilation and oxygenation, controlling hemorrhage, and providing appropriate volume resuscitation. When faced with a prolonged transport, prehospital care practitioners

may have a lower threshold for securing the airway with endotracheal intubation. Indications for performing endotracheal intubation include increasing respiratory distress or impending respiratory failure (after exclusion or treatment of a tension pneumothorax), a flail chest, open pneumothorax, or multiple rib fractures. Oxygen should be provided to maintain oxygen saturation ≥ 94%.

Ventilations should be assisted as necessary. Pulmonary contusions worsen over time, and the use of CPAP, positive end-expiratory pressure (PEEP) with a transport ventilator, or PEEP valves with bag-mask device may facilitate oxygenation. Any patient with significant thoracic trauma may have or develop a tension pneumothorax, and ongoing assessment should look for the hallmark signs. In the presence of decreased or absent breath sounds, worsening respiratory distress, difficulty squeezing the bag-mask device, increasing peak inspiratory pressures in patients on a ventilator, and hypotension, pleural decompression should be performed. A tube thoracostomy (insertion of a chest tube) may be performed by authorized and appropriately qualified personnel, typically air medical flight crews, if the patient requires needle decompression or is found to have an open pneumothorax. IV access should be secured and IV fluids administered judiciously.

Patients with suspected intrathoracic, intra-abdominal, or retroperitoneal hemorrhage should be maintained for up to 2 hours with systolic blood pressure in the range of 80 to 90 mm Hg when significant head injury is not suspected. Overaggressive volume resuscitation may significantly worsen pulmonary contusions, as well as lead to recurrent internal hemorrhage (see Chapter 3, *Shock: Pathophysiology of Life and Death*).

Patients with severe pain from multiple rib fractures may benefit from small doses of narcotics titrated intravenously or ketamine if trained and locally approved. If narcotic administration results in hypotension and respiratory failure, volume resuscitation and ventilatory support should be provided.

Patients with cardiac dysrhythmias associated with blunt cardiac injury may benefit from the use of antidysrhythmic medications. Any interventions performed should be carefully documented on the patient care report, and the receiving facility must be made aware of the procedures.

SUMMARY

- Patients with chest injury must be managed expeditiously and transported quickly for definitive care because they are frequently associated with multisystem trauma and patients are at risk for respiratory and circulatory compromise.

- When responding to penetrating injuries to the chest, prehospital care practitioners should be prepared to manage a hemothorax or a pneumothorax, or both, which is termed a *hemopneumothorax*.

SUMMARY (CONTINUED)

- When responding to blunt force trauma to the chest, injuries that prehospital care practitioners should be on the lookout for include pulmonary contusion, tears of the visceral pleura, broken ribs, shearing or rupture of the major blood vessels in the chest, and disruption of the chest wall. Associated conditions include hemothorax, pneumothorax, blunt cardiac or pericardial injury, commotio cordis, and catastrophic hemorrhage. Pulse oximetry and waveform capnography can be useful adjuncts for assessing ventilatory status and responses to therapy.
- Prehospital care practitioners must be prepared to recognize and manage the three types of pneumothoraces:
  - Simple pneumothorax is the presence of air within the pleural space.
  - Open pneumothorax ("sucking chest wound") involves a defect in the chest wall that allows air to enter and exit the pleural space from the outside with ventilatory effort.
  - Tension pneumothorax occurs when air continues to enter and is trapped in the pleural space with gradual increase in intrathoracic pressure. Signs of tension pneumothorax should be carefully sought because treatment in the field with needle decompression may correct this possible, and rapidly fatal problem.
- Because of the high risk of multisystem trauma in patients with blunt thoracic injury, spinal motion restriction should be employed when transporting these patients.
- Electrocardiographic monitoring may suggest blunt cardiac injury.
- Particular attention should be paid to the administration of supplemental high-concentration oxygen and the need for ventilatory support in any patient suspected of having chest trauma.
- Intravenous access should be obtained en route to the medical facility and fluid therapy administered with appropriate fluids and goals in mind.
- Although many thoracic injuries can be managed without surgical intervention, the patient with a chest injury must still be evaluated and managed at an appropriate medical facility.

SCENARIO RECAP

You and your partner are dispatched to an industrial construction site for a worker who was struck by a piece of metal. Upon arrival, you are led to an area where a safety officer explains that the patient was helping in-stall metal studs. As he turned to grab another stud, he ran into the end of a stud that his partner had just trimmed, cutting through his shirt and puncturing his chest.

You find an approximately 35-year-old man sitting upright, leaning forward and holding a rag to the right side of his chest. You ask him what happened, and he tries to tell you but has to stop after every five to six words to catch his breath. You move the rag and notice a 2 inch (5 cm) long laceration with a small amount of "bubbling" blood-tinged fluid. He is diaphoretic, has a rapid radial pulse, and decreased breath sounds on the right side. No other abnormal physical findings are noted.

- Is this patient in respiratory distress?
- Does the patient have life-threatening injuries?
- What interventions should you undertake in the field?
- What modality should be used to transport this patient?
- How would a different location (e.g., rural) impact your management and plans during prolonged transport?
- What other injuries do you suspect?

SCENARIO SOLUTION

The scene report, patient complaints, and physical examination lead you to suspect that this patient may have serious and potentially life-threatening injuries. He is awake and speaking coherently, indicating that he has a stable airway. He is experiencing severe respiratory distress as he is unable to speak in full sentences. He is experiencing hemodynamic instability as he is diaphoretic and tachycardic. The location of the wound, bubbling fluid, and decreased breath sounds indicate a sucking chest wound with an open pneumothorax that may have a tension component.

You move quickly to apply an occlusive dressing that is sealed on three sides, provide the patient with supplemental oxygen, and consider ventilatory assistance with a bag-mask device as necessary. The first priorities in this scenario are to recognize the seriousness of the injuries, stabilize the patient, and initiate transfer to an appropriate facility. Given this patient's respiratory distress and findings, he is at significant risk for complications. Transport to the closest trauma center is appropriate. IV access should be obtained en route.

There is risk for respiratory deterioration, and the patient's ventilatory status needs to be monitored closely. Signs of progressing circulatory compromise and respiratory distress would prompt you to first remove the occlusive dressing and, if there is no improvement, to perform needle decompression of the right chest. If transport time will be extended, air transport should be considered.

References

1. American College of Surgeons Committee on Trauma. Thoracic trauma. In: *Advanced Trauma Life Support, Student Course Manual*. 10th ed. American College of Surgeons; 2018.

2. Ghanta RK, Wall MJ, Mattox KL. Trauma thoracotomy: principles and techniques. In: Feliciano DV, Mattox KL, Moore EE, eds. *Trauma*. 9th ed. McGraw-Hill; 2020.

3. Livingston DH, Hauser CJ. Trauma to the chest wall and lung. In: Mattox KL, Feliciano DV, Moore EE, eds. *Trauma*. 5th ed. McGraw-Hill; 2004.

4. Howes DS, Bellazzini MA. Chronic obstructive pulmonary disease. In: Wolfson AB, Hendey GW, Ling LJ, et al., eds. *Harwood-Nuss' Clinical Practice of Emergency Medicine*. 5th ed. Wolters Kluwer/Lippincott Williams & Wilkins; 2010.

5. Wilson RF. Pulmonary physiology. In: Wilson RF. *Critical Care Manual: Applied Physiology and Principles of Therapy*. 2nd ed. Davis; 1992.

6. National Association of Emergency Medical Technicians. Advanced medical life support assessment for the medical patient. In: *Advanced Medical Life Support*, 3rd ed. Jones & Bartlett Learning; 2021:1-53.

7. Silverston P. Pulse oximetry at the roadside: a study of pulse oximetry in immediate care. *BMJ*. 1989;298:711.

8. Garrett PD, Boyd SY, Bauch TD, Rubal BJ, Bulgrin JR, Kinkler ES Jr. Feasibility of real-time echocardiographic evaluation during patient transport. *J Am Soc Echocardiogr*. 2003 Mar;16(3):197-201. doi: 10.1067/mje.2003.16

9. Roline CE, Heegaard WG, Moore JC, et al. Feasibility of bedside thoracic ultrasound in the helicopter emergency medical services setting. *Air Med J*. 2013;32(3):153-7. doi: 10.1016/j.amj.2012.10.013

10. Quick JA, Uhlich RM, Ahmad S, Barnes SL, Coughenour JP. In-flight ultrasound identification of pneumothorax. *Emerg Radiol*. 2016 Feb;23(1):3-7. doi: 10.1007/s10140-015-1348-z

11. Yates JG, Baylous D. Aeromedical ultrasound: the evaluation of point-of-care ultrasound during helicopter transport. *Air Med J*. 2017;36(3):110-115. doi: 10.1016/j.amj.2017.02.001

12. Pietersen PI, Mikkelsen S, Lassen AT, et al. Quality of focused thoracic ultrasound performed by emergency medical technicians and paramedics in a prehospital setting: a feasibility study. *Scand J Trauma Resusc Emerg Med*. 2021;29(1):40. doi: 10.1186/s13049-021-00856-8

13. Brun PM, Bessereau J, Levy D, Billeres X, Fournier N, Kerbaul F. Prehospital ultrasound thoracic examination to improve decision making, triage, and care in blunt trauma. *Am J Emerg Med*. 2014;32(7):817.e1-2. doi: 10.1016/j.ajem.2013.12.063

14. Kirkpatrick AW, Brown DR, Crickmer S, et al. Handheld portable sonography for the on-mountain exclusion of a pneumothorax. *Wilderness Environ Med*. 2001;12(4):270-272. doi: 10.1580/1080-6032(2001)012[0270:hhpsft]2.0.co;2

15. Ziegler DW, Agarwal NN. The morbidity and mortality of rib fractures. *J Trauma Acute Care Surg*. 1994;37(6):975-979.

16. Pressley CM, Fry WR, Philip AS, et al. Predicting outcome of patients with chest wall injury. *Am J Surg*. 2012;204(6):900-904.

17. Flagel BT, Luchette FA, Reed RL, et al. Half-a-dozen ribs: the breakpoint for mortality. *Surgery*. 2005;138:717-725.

18. Jones KM, Reed RL, Luchette FA. The ribs or not the ribs: which influences mortality? *Am J Surg*. 2011;202(5):598-604.

19. Bulger EM, Arneson MA, Mock CN, Jurkovich GJ. Rib fractures in the elderly. *J Trauma*. 2000;48(6):1040-1046;

discussion 1046-1047. doi: 10.1097/00005373-200006000-00007

20. Richardson JD, Adams L, Flint LM. Selective management of flail chest and pulmonary contusion. *Ann Surg.* 1982;196:481-487.

21. Di Bartolomeo S, Sanson G, Nardi G, et al. A population-based study on pneumothorax in severely traumatized patients. *J Trauma.* 2001;51(4):677-682.

22. Regel G, Stalp M, Lehmann U, et al. Prehospital care: importance of early intervention outcome. *Acta Anaesthesiol Scand Suppl.* 1997;110:71-76.

23. Barone JE, Pizzi WF, Nealon TF, et al. Indications for intubation in blunt chest trauma. *J Trauma.* 1986;26:334-337.

24. Mattox KL. Prehospital care of the patient with an injured chest. *Surg Clin North Am.* 1989;69(1):21-29.

25. Simon B, Ebert J, Bokhari F, et al. Management of pulmonary contusion and flail chest: an Eastern Association for the Surgery of Trauma practice management guideline. *J Trauma Acute Care Surg.* 2012 Nov;73(5 suppl 4):S351-S361.

26. Cooper C, Militello P. The multi-injured patient: the Maryland Shock Trauma Protocol approach. *Semin Thorac Cardiovasc Surg.* 1992;4(3):163-167.

27. Barton ED, Epperson M, Hoyt DB, et al. Prehospital needle aspiration and tube thoracostomy in trauma victims: a six-year experience with aeromedical crews. *J Emerg Med.* 1995;13:155-163.

28. Kheirabadi BS, Terrazas IB, Koller A, et al. Vented vs. unvented chest seals for treatment of pneumothorax (PTx) and prevention of tension PTx in a swine model. *J Trauma Acute Care Surg.* 2013;75:150-156.

29. Butler FK, Dubose JJ, Otten EJ, et al. Management of open pneumothorax in tactical combat casualty care: TCCC guidelines change 13-02. *J Special Ops Med.* 2013;13(3):81-86.

30. Kuhlwilm V. The use of chest seals in treating sucking chest wounds: a comparison of existing evidence and guideline recommendations. *J Spec Oper Med.* 2021;21(1):94-101.

31. Eckstein M, Suyehara DL. Needle thoracostomy in the pre-hospital setting. *Prehosp Emerg Care.* 1998;2:132.

32. Holcomb JB, McManus JG, Kerr ST, Pusateri AE. Needle versus tube thoracostomy in a swine model of traumatic tension hemopneumothorax. *Prehosp Emerg Care.* 2009;13(1):18-27.

33. American College of Surgeons Committee on Trauma. Thoracic trauma. In: *Advanced Trauma Life Support, Student Course Manual.* 10th ed. American College of Surgeons; 2018:66.

34. Netto FA, Shulman H, Rizoli SB, et al. Are needle decompressions for tension pneumothoraces being performed appropriately for appropriate indications? *Am J Em Med.* 2008;26;597-602.

35. Riwoe D, Poncia H. Subclavian artery laceration: a serious complication of needle decompression. *Em Med Aust.* 2011;23:651-653.

36. Inaba K, Branco BC Exkstein M, et al. Optimal positioning for emergent needle thoracostomy: a cadaver-based study. *J Trauma.* 2011;71:1099-1103.

37. Inaba K, Karamanos E, Skiada D, et al. Cadaveric comparison of the optimal site for needle decompression of tension pneumothorax by prehospital care providers. *J Trauma.* 2015;79(6):1044-1048.

38. Leatherman ML, Held JM, Fluke LM, et al. Relative device stability of anterior versus axillary needle decompression for tension pneumothorax during casualty movement: preliminary analysis of a human cadaver model. *J Trauma.* 2017;83(1):S136-S141.

39. Beckett A, Savage E, Pannell D, et al. Needle decompression for tension pneumothorax in tactical combat casualty care: do catheters placed in the midaxillary line kink more often than those in the midclavicular line? *J Trauma.* 2011;71:S408-S412.

40. Martin M, Satterly S, Inaba K, Blair K. Does needle thoracostomy provide adequate and effective decompression of tension pneumothorax? *J Trauma.* 2012;73(6): 1410-1415.

41. Davis DP, Pettit K, Rum CD, et al. The safety and efficacy of prehospital needle and tube thoracostomy by aeromedical personnel. *Prehosp Emerg Care.* 2005;9:191-197.

42. Etoch SW, Bar-Natan MF, Miller FB, et al. Tube thoracostomy: factors related to complications. *Arch Surg.* 1995; 130:521-525.

43. Newman PG, Feliciano DV. Blunt cardiac injury. *New Horizons.* 1999;7(1):26-34.

44. Sherren PB, Galloway R, Healy M. Blunt traumatic pericardial rupture and cardiac herniation with a penetrating twist: two case reports. *Scand J Trauma Resusc Emerg Med.* 2009;17:64.

45. Lindenmann J, Matzi V, Neuboeck N, Porubsky C, Ratzenhofer B, Maier A. Traumatic pericardial rupture with cardiac herniation. *Ann Thorac Surg.* 2010;89:2028-2030.

46. LeBlanc N, Tan L. Pericardial rupture with cardiac herniation following blunt thoracic trauma. *JTCVS Tech.* 2020 Dec;4:375–377. doi: 10.1016/j.xjtc.2020.08.011

47. Ivatury RR. The injured heart. In: Mattox KL, Feliciano DV, Moore EE, eds. *Trauma.* 5th ed. McGraw-Hill; 2004:555.

48. Symbas NP, Bongiorno PF, Symbas PN. Blunt cardiac rupture: the utility of emergency department ultrasound. *Ann Thorac Surg.* 1999;67(5):1274-1276.

49. Demetriades D. Cardiac wounds. *Ann Surg.* 1986;203(3): 315-317.

50. Jacob S, Sebastian JC, Cherian PK, et al. Pericardial effusion impending tamponade: a look beyond Beck's triad. *Am J Em Med.* 2009;27:216-219.

51. Ivatury RR, Nallathambi MN, Roberge RJ, et al. Penetrating thoracic injuries: in-field stabilization versus prompt transport. *J Trauma.* 1987;27:1066.

52. Bleetman A, Kasem H, Crawford R. Review of emergency thoracotomy for chest injuries in patients attending a UK accident and emergency department. *Injury.* 1996;27(2):129-132.

53. Durham LA III, Richardson RJ, Wall MJ Jr, et al. Emergency center thoracotomy: impact of prehospital resuscitation. *J Trauma.* 1992;32(6):775-779.

54. Honigman B, Rohweder K, Moore EE, et al. Prehospital advanced trauma life support for penetrating cardiac wounds. *Ann Emerg Med.* 1990;19(2):145-150.

55. Lerer LB, Knottenbelt JD. Preventable mortality following sharp penetrating chest trauma. *J Trauma.* 1994;37(1): 9-12.

56. Ho AM, Graham CA, Ng CS, et al. Timing of tracheal intubation in traumatic cardiac tamponade: a word of caution. *Resuscitation*. 2009;80(2):272-274. doi: 10.1016/j.resuscitation.2008.09.021

57. Möller CT, Schoonbee CG, Rosendorff C. Haemodynamics of cardiac tamponade during various modes of ventilation. *Br J Anaesth*. 1979;51(5):409-415. doi: 10.1093/bja/51.5.409

58. Wall MJ Jr, Pepe PE, Mattox KL. Successful roadside resuscitative thoracotomy: case report and literature review. *J Trauma*. 1994;36(1):131-135.

59. Coats TJ, Keogh S, Clark H, et al. Prehospital resuscitative thoracotomy for cardiac arrest after penetrating trauma: rationale and case series. *J Trauma*. 2001;50(4):670-673.

60. Zangwill SD, Strasburger JF. Commotio cordis. *Pediatr Clin North Am*. 2004;51(5):1347-1354.

61. Perron AD, Brady WJ, Erling BF. Commodio cordis: an underappreciated cause of sudden cardiac death in young patients: assessment and management in the ED. *Am J Emerg Med*. 2001;19(5):406-409.

62. Maron BJ, Estes NA 3rd. Commotio cordis. *N Engl J Med*. 2010;362(10):917-927.

63. Tainter CR, Hughes PG. Commotio cordis. In: StatPearls [Internet]. StatPearls Publishing. Updated September 28, 2021. Accessed February 10, 2022. https://www.ncbi.nlm.nih.gov/books/NBK526014/

64. 2010 American Heart Association Guidelines for Cardiopulmonary Resuscitation and Emergency Cardiovascular Care Science. *Circulation*. 2010;122:S745-S746.

65. Wall MJ, Ghanta RK, Mattox KL. Heart and thoracic vessels. In: Feliciano DV, Mattox KL, Moore EE, eds. *Trauma*. 9th ed. McGraw-Hill; 2020.

66. Fabian TC, Roger T. Sherman lecture: advances in the management of blunt thoracic aortic injury: Parmley to the present. *Am Surg*. 2009;75(4):273-278.

67. DuBose JJ, Scalea TM, O'Connor JV. Trachea, bronchi, and esophagus. In: Feliciano DV, Mattox KL, Moore EE, eds. *Trauma*. 9th ed. McGraw-Hill; 2020.

68. Rogers FB, Leavitt BJ. Upper torso cyanosis: a marker for blunt cardiac rupture. *Am J Emerg Med*. 1997;15(3):275-276.

Suggested Reading

Bowley DM, Boffard KD. Penetrating trauma of the trunk. *Unfallchirurg*. 2001;104(11):1032-1042.

Brathwaite CE, Rodriguez A, Turney SZ, et al. Blunt traumatic cardiac rupture: a 5-year experience. *Ann Surg*. 1990;212(6):701-704.

Helm M, Schuster R, Hauke J. Tight control of prehospital ventilation by capnography in major trauma victims. *Br J Anaesth*. 2003;90(3):327-332.

Lateef F. Commotio cordis: an underappreciated cause of sudden death in athletes. *Sports Med*. 2000;30:301-308.

Papadopoulos IN, Bukis D, Karalas E, et al. Preventable prehospital trauma deaths in a Hellenic urban health region: an audit of prehospital trauma care. *J Trauma*. 1996;41(5):864-869.

Rozycki GS, Feliciano DV, Oschner MG, et al. The role of ultrasound in patients with possible penetrating cardiac wounds: a prospective multicenter study. *J Trauma*. 1999;46:542-552.

Ruchholtz S, Waydhas C, Ose C, et al. Prehospital intubation in severe thoracic trauma without respiratory insufficiency: a matched-pair analysis based on the Trauma Registry of the German Trauma Society. *J Trauma*. 2002;52(5):879-886.

Streng M, Tikka S, Leppaniemi A. Assessing the severity of truncal gunshot wounds: a nation-wide analysis from Finland. *Ann Chir Gynaecol*. 2001;90(4):246-251.

SPECIFIC SKILLS

Thoracic Trauma Skills

Needle Decompression

Principle: To decrease intrathoracic pressure from a tension pneumothorax affecting the patient's breathing, ventilation, and circulation.

In patients with increasing intrathoracic pressure from a developing tension pneumothorax, the side of the thoracic cavity that has the increased pressure should be decompressed. If this pressure is not relieved, it will progressively limit the patient's ventilatory capacity and compromise venous return, producing inadequate cardiac output and death.

For patients in whom an open pneumothorax has been treated by the use of an occlusive dressing and a tension pneumothorax develops, decompression can usually be achieved through the wound, which provides an existing opening into the thorax. Opening the occlusive dressing over the wound for a few seconds should initiate a rush of air out of the wound as increased pressure in the thorax is relieved.

Once this pressure has been released, the wound is resealed with the occlusive dressing to allow for proper alveolar ventilation and to stop air from "sucking" into the wound. The patient should be monitored carefully, and, if any signs of tension recur, the dressing should be "burped" again to release the intrathoracic pressure.

Decompression in a closed tension pneumothorax is achieved by providing an opening—a thoracostomy—in the affected side of the chest. Different methods for performing a thoracostomy exist. Because needle thoracostomy is the most rapid method and does not require special equipment, it is the preferred method for use in the field.

Needle decompression carries minimal risk and can greatly benefit the patient by improving oxygenation and circulation. Needle decompression should be performed only when the following three criteria are met:

1. Evidence of worsening respiratory distress or difficulty with a bag-mask device
2. Decreased or absent breath sounds
3. Decompensated shock (systolic blood pressure less than 90 mm Hg)

Necessary equipment for needle chest decompression includes a needle, a syringe, ½-inch adhesive tape, and alcohol swabs. The needle used should be a large-bore, over-the-needle IV catheter between 10 and 14 gauge, at least 3.5 inches (8 cm) in length. A 16-gauge catheter can be used if a larger bore is not available.

One prehospital care practitioner attaches the needle to the syringe while a second prehospital care practitioner auscultates the patient's chest to confirm which side has the tension pneumothorax, which is indicated by absent or diminished breath sounds.

Thoracic Trauma Skills *(continued)*

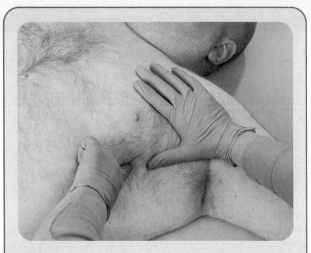

1 After confirmation of a tension pneumothorax, the anatomic landmarks are located on the affected side (second intercostal space along the midclavicular line *or* fifth intercostal space along the anterior axillary line).

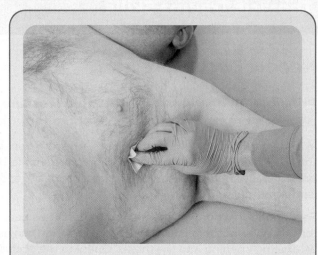

2 The site is swabbed with an antiseptic wipe.

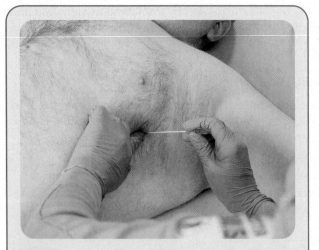

3 The skin over the site is stretched between the fingers of the nondominant hand. The needle and syringe are positioned over the top of the rib.

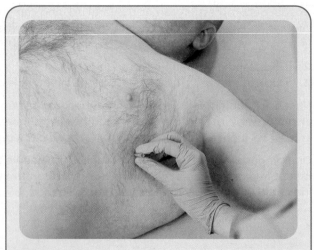

4 Once the needle enters into the thoracic cavity, air will escape into the syringe, and the needle should not be advanced further.

(continued)

Thoracic Trauma Skills (continued)

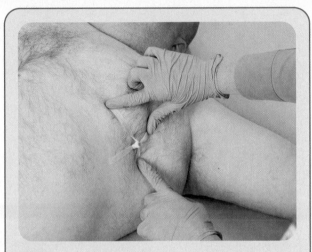

5 The catheter should be left in place and the needle removed, with care not to kink the catheter. As the needle is removed, a rush of air from the hub of the catheter should be heard. If no air escapes, the catheter should be left in place to indicate that needle decompression of the chest was attempted.

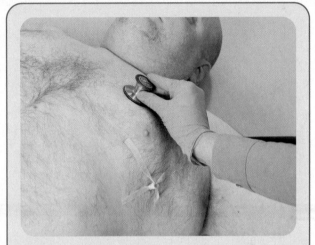

6 After the needle is removed, the catheter is taped in place with adhesive tape. After securing the catheter, the chest is auscultated to check for increased breath sounds. The patient is monitored and transported to an appropriate facility. The prehospital care practitioner need not waste time applying a one-way valve. Needle decompression may need to be repeated if the catheter becomes occluded with a blood clot and tension pneumothorax reoccurs.

CHAPTER 11

Abdominal Trauma

Lead Editors
Thomas Scalea, MD
Emily Esposito, DO

CHAPTER OBJECTIVES

At the completion of this chapter, you will be able to do the following:

- Analyze scene assessment data and mechanism of injury to determine the level of suspicion for abdominal or pelvic trauma.
- Understand the anatomy of the abdomen and pelvis to aid in the recognition and triage of patients with abdominal injury.
- Anticipate the pathophysiologic effects of a blunt or penetrating injury to the abdomen.
- Recognize the physical examination findings indicative of intra-abdominal injury.
- Correlate external signs of abdominal injury to the potential for specific abdominal organ injuries.
- Identify the indications for rapid intervention and transport in the context of abdominal or pelvic trauma.
- Understand appropriate field management decisions for patients with suspected abdominal trauma, including those with impaled objects, evisceration, and external genital trauma.
- Correlate the anatomic and physiologic changes associated with pregnancy to the pathophysiology and management of trauma.
- Discuss the effects of maternal trauma on the fetus and the priorities of management.

SCENARIO

You are called to a construction site for a male patient in his mid-20s who fell 3 hours earlier and is now complaining of increasing abdominal pain. He states that he tripped on a piece of wood at the site and fell, striking his left lower chest and abdomen on some stacked wood. The patient notes moderate pain over his lower left rib cage when he takes deep breaths and complains of mild difficulty breathing. His coworkers wanted to call for assistance when he fell, but he said the symptoms were not so bad and told them to hold off. He states that the discomfort has been increasing in intensity and that he is now feeling lightheaded and weak.

You find the patient sitting on the ground in visible discomfort. He is holding the left side of his lower chest and upper abdomen. He has a patent airway, a respiratory rate of 28 breaths/minute, a heart rate of 124 beats/minute, and a blood pressure of 94/58 millimeters of mercury (mm Hg). The patient's skin is pale and diaphoretic. You lay him down, and on physical examination, he has tenderness on palpation of the left lower ribs without

(continues)

SCENARIO (CONTINUED)

obvious bony crepitus. His abdomen is nondistended and soft to palpation, but he has tenderness and voluntary guarding in the left upper quadrant. No external ecchymosis or subcutaneous emphysema is present.

· What are the patient's possible injuries?
· What are the priorities in the care of this patient?
· Are signs of peritonitis present?

INTRODUCTION

The abdomen is the third most commonly injured body region in trauma.[1] Because physical signs of blunt abdominal trauma are often less obvious than penetrating injuries, abdominal injuries can be easily missed.[2] Unrecognized abdominal injury is one of the major causes of preventable death in trauma patients. Because of the limitations of prehospital assessment, patients with suspected abdominal injuries are best managed by prompt transport to the closest appropriate facility.[3,4]

Early death from severe abdominal trauma typically results from massive hemorrhage caused by either penetrating or blunt injuries. Any patient with unexplained shock after sustaining a traumatic injury to the trunk of the body should be assumed to have an intra-abdominal hemorrhage until proven otherwise. The absence of localized signs and symptoms does not rule out the possibility of abdominal trauma; signs and symptoms often take time to develop and are especially difficult to identify in the patient whose level of consciousness is altered by alcohol, drugs, or traumatic brain injury (TBI). Complications and death may occur from liver, spleen, colon, small intestine, stomach, or pancreatic injuries that were not initially detected. Consideration of the kinematics can raise the index of suspicion and alert the prehospital care practitioner to possible abdominal trauma and intra-abdominal hemorrhage. It is not necessary to be concerned with pinpointing the exact location or extent of abdominal trauma but rather to recognize the likelihood of injury, treat the clinical findings, and triage to the appropriate facility.

Anatomy

The abdomen contains the major organs of the digestive, endocrine, and urogenital systems and major vessels of the circulatory system. The abdominal cavity is located below the diaphragm; its boundaries include the anterior abdominal wall, the pelvic bones, the vertebral column, and the muscles of the abdomen and flanks. The abdominal cavity is divided into two regions based upon the relationship to the *peritoneum*, which covers many of the organs of the abdomen. The **peritoneal cavity** (the "true" abdominal cavity) contains the spleen, liver, gallbladder, stomach, portions of the large intestine (transverse and sigmoid colon), most of the small intestines (primarily the jejunum and ileum), and female reproductive organs (uterus and ovaries; **Figure 11-1**). The **retroperitoneal space** is the area in the abdominal cavity that is located behind the peritoneum and contains the kidneys, ureters, inferior vena cava, abdominal aorta, pancreas, much of the duodenum, ascending and descending colon, and rectum (**Figure 11-2**). The urinary bladder and male reproductive organs (penis, testes, and prostate) lie inferior to the peritoneal cavity.

A portion of the abdomen lies in the lower thorax. This is because the dome shape of the diaphragm allows the upper abdominal organs to rise up into the lower chest, particularly on expiration. This superior portion of the abdomen, sometimes referred to as the thoracoabdomen, is protected in front and along the flanks by the ribs and in back by the vertebral column. The thoracoabdomen contains the liver, gallbladder, spleen, and parts of the stomach anteriorly and the lower lobes of the lungs posteriorly, separated by the diaphragm. Additionally, the esophagus and large vessels such as the inferior vena cava extend between the thorax and abdomen through small openings in the diaphragm. Because of their location, the same forces that fracture ribs may injure the underlying abdominal organs.

The relationship of these abdominal organs to the lower portion of the thoracic cavity changes with the respiratory cycle. At peak expiration, the diaphragm extends to the fourth intercostal space anteriorly (nipple level in the male), the sixth intercostal space laterally, and the eighth intercostal space posteriorly, providing greater protection to abdominal organs from the rib cage (see **Figure 11-3**). Conversely, at peak inspiration, the dome of the contracted diaphragm lies at the level of the sixth intercostal space; the inflated lungs almost fill the thorax and largely push these abdominal organs out from under the rib cage. Patients who sustain a penetrating injury to the thorax below these anatomic locations may also have sustained an abdominal injury. Thus, the organs injured

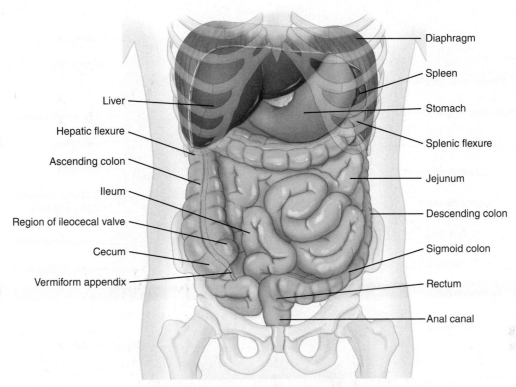

Figure 11-1 Organs in the peritoneal cavity include solid organs (spleen and liver), hollow organs of the gastrointestinal tract (stomach, small intestine, and colon), and reproductive organs.

© National Association of Emergency Medical Technicians (NAEMT)

by penetrating trauma to the thoracoabdomen may differ depending on which phase of respiration the patient was in when injured (Figure 11-3).

The most inferior portion of the abdomen is protected on all sides by the pelvis. This area contains the rectum, a portion of the small intestine (especially when the patient is upright), the urinary bladder, and the female reproductive organs. Retroperitoneal hemorrhage associated with a fractured pelvis is a major concern in this portion of the abdominal cavity.

The abdomen between the rib cage and the pelvis is protected only by the abdominal muscles and other soft tissues anteriorly and laterally. Posteriorly, the lumbar vertebrae and the thick, strong *paraspinal* muscles located along the length of the spine provide more protection (**Figure 11-4**).

For purposes of patient assessment, the surface of the abdomen is divided into four quadrants. These quadrants are formed by drawing two lines: one in the middle from the tip of the xiphoid to the symphysis pubis and one perpendicular to this midline at the level of the umbilicus (**Figure 11-5**). Knowledge of anatomic landmarks is important because of the high correlation of organ location to pain response. The right upper quadrant includes the liver and gallbladder, the left upper quadrant contains the spleen and stomach, and the right and left lower quadrants contain primarily the intestines, the distal ureters, and, in women, the ovaries. A portion of the intestinal tract exists in all four quadrants. The urinary bladder and the uterus in women are midline between the lower quadrants.

Pathophysiology

Dividing the abdominal organs into hollow, solid, and vascular (blood vessel) groups helps explain manifestations of injury to these structures. When injured, solid organs (liver, spleen) and blood vessels (aorta, vena cava) bleed, whereas hollow organs (intestine, gallbladder, urinary bladder) primarily spill their contents into the peritoneal cavity or retroperitoneal space (they too bleed but often not as briskly as do solid organs). Loss of blood into the abdominal cavity, regardless of its source, can contribute to or can be the primary cause of the development of hemorrhagic shock. The release of acids, digestive enzymes, and/or bacteria from the gastrointestinal tract into the peritoneal cavity results in **peritonitis**

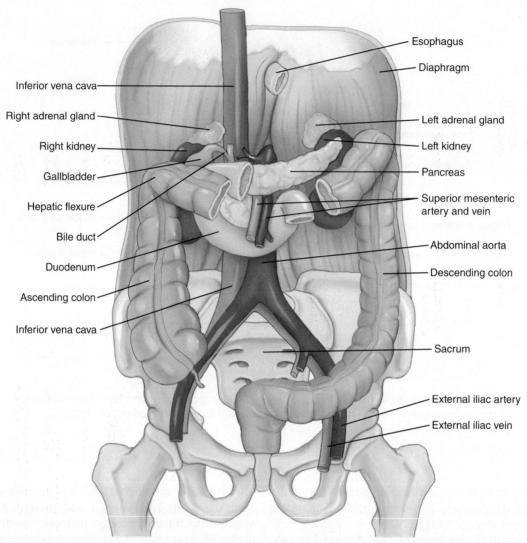

Figure 11-2 The abdomen is divided into two spaces: the peritoneal cavity and the retroperitoneal space. The retroperitoneal space includes the portion of the abdomen behind the peritoneum. Because the retroperitoneal organs are not within the peritoneal cavity, injury to these structures generally does not produce peritonitis; however, injury to the large blood vessels and solid organs may produce rapid and massive hemorrhage.

© National Association of Emergency Medical Technicians (NAEMT)

(inflammation of the peritoneum, or the lining of the abdominal cavity) and **sepsis** (systemic infection) if not recognized and promptly treated by surgical intervention. Because urine and bile are generally sterile (do not contain bacteria) and do not contain digestive enzymes, perforation of the gallbladder or urinary bladder does not produce peritonitis as quickly as material spilled from the intestine. Similarly, because it lacks acids, digestive enzymes, and bacteria, blood in the peritoneal cavity can take several hours to cause peritonitis. Bleeding from intestinal injury is typically minor, unless the larger blood vessels in the *mesentery* (the folds of peritoneal tissue that attach the bowel to the posterior wall of the abdominal cavity) are damaged.

Injuries to the abdomen can be caused by either penetrating, blunt, or blast trauma. Penetrating trauma, such as a gunshot or stab wound, is more readily visible than blunt trauma. Multiple organs may be damaged as a result of penetrating trauma, more commonly with gunshot wounds versus stab wounds given the high energy associated with the projectile-type injury and the relatively low energy of most objects used to stab a patient. A mental visualization of the potential trajectory of the penetrating object, such as a bullet or the path of a knife blade, can help identify possible injured internal organs. Penetrating wounds of the flanks and buttocks may involve organs in the abdominal cavity as well. These penetrating injuries may cause bleeding from a major vessel or

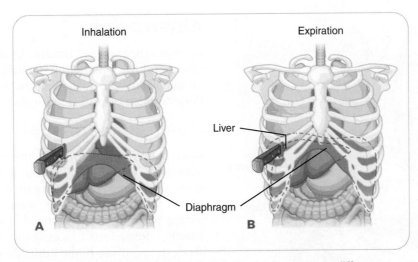

Inhalation

Expiration

Liver

Diaphragm

A

B

Figure 11-3 Relationship of abdominal organs to the thorax in different phases of respiration in a patient with a stab wound. **A.** Inhalation. **B.** Exhalation.

© National Association of Emergency Medical Technicians (NAEMT)

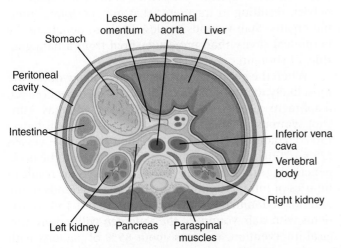

Stomach

Lesser omentum   Abdominal aorta   Liver

Peritoneal cavity

Intestine

Inferior vena cava

Vertebral body

Right kidney

Left kidney   Pancreas   Paraspinal muscles

Figure 11-4 This transverse section of the abdominal cavity provides an appreciation of the positions of the organs in the anteroposterior direction and the relatively limited protection, particularly anteriorly and laterally.

© National Association of Emergency Medical Technicians (NAEMT)

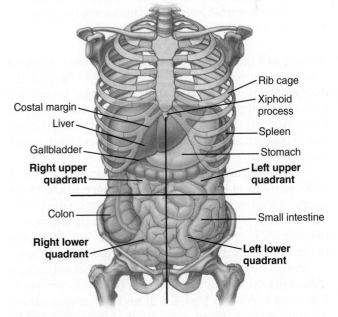

Rib cage

Xiphoid process

Costal margin

Liver

Spleen

Gallbladder

Stomach

Right upper quadrant

Left upper quadrant

Colon

Small intestine

Right lower quadrant

Left lower quadrant

Figure 11-5 As with any part of the body, the better the description of pain, tenderness, guarding, and other signs, the more accurate the diagnosis. The most common system of identification divides the abdomen into four quadrants: left upper, right upper, left lower, and right lower.

© National Association of Emergency Medical Technicians (NAEMT)

solid organ and perforation of a segment of the intestine, the most frequently injured organ in penetrating trauma.

Blunt trauma injuries are often more challenging to recognize than those caused by penetrating trauma. These injuries to abdominal organs result from either compression or shear forces. In **compression injuries**, the organs of the abdomen are crushed between solid objects, such as between the steering wheel and spinal column. **Shear forces** create rupture of the solid organs or rupture of blood vessels in the cavity as a result of the tearing forces exerted against their supporting ligaments. The liver and spleen can shear and bleed easily, and blood loss can occur at a rapid rate. Increased

intra-abdominal pressure produced by compression can rupture the diaphragm, causing the abdominal organs to move upward into the thoracic cavity (**Figure 11-6**). (See Chapter 4, *The Physics of Trauma*, and Chapter 10, *Thoracic Trauma*.) The intra-abdominal contents forced into the chest cavity can compromise lung expansion and affect both respiratory and cardiac function. Although rupture

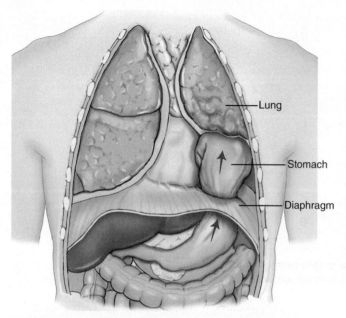

Figure 11-6 With increased pressure inside the abdomen, the diaphragm can rupture, allowing intra-abdominal organs such as the stomach or small intestine to herniate into the chest.
© National Association of Emergency Medical Technicians (NAEMT)

of each half of the diaphragm is now believed to occur equally, rupture of the left *hemidiaphragm* (half of the diaphragm) is diagnosed more often, as the underlying liver and its attachments on the right side often prevents herniation of abdominal contents into the right chest and makes the diagnosis of a right-side diaphragm injury more difficult.

Pelvic fractures may be associated with the loss of large volumes of blood caused by damage to the many smaller blood vessels adjacent to the pelvis. Other injuries associated with pelvic fractures include damage to the urinary bladder and the rectum, as well as injuries to the urethra in the male and the vagina in the female.

Primary blast injury to the abdomen primarily affects hollow organs such as the intestine. These may present in a delayed fashion as bowel wall necrosis or perforation. Secondary blast injury may occur due to penetrating fragments or debris striking the abdomen, and tertiary blast injury is similar to blunt trauma and occurs when the patient is thrown against another object.

Assessment

The assessment of abdominal injury can be difficult, especially with the limited diagnostic capabilities available in the prehospital setting. A high index of suspicion for abdominal injury should develop from a variety of sources of information, including mechanism of injury, the findings from the physical examination, and input from the patient or bystanders.

Kinematics

As with other types of trauma, knowledge of the mechanism of injury, whether blast, blunt, or penetrating, plays an important role in shaping the prehospital care practitioner's index of suspicion for abdominal trauma.

Penetrating Trauma

Most penetrating trauma in the civilian setting results from stab wounds and gunshot wounds from handguns. Occasionally, impalement with or onto an object occurs when, for example, someone falls onto a projecting piece of wood or metal. These low to moderate kinetic energy forces lacerate or cut abdominal organs along the pathway of the knife, projectile, or penetrating object. High-velocity injuries, such as those created by high-powered rifles and assault weapons, tend to create more serious injuries because of the larger temporary cavities created as the projectile moves through the peritoneal cavity. Projectiles may strike bones (ribs, spine, or pelvis), resulting in fragments that may perforate internal organs. Stab wounds are less likely to penetrate the peritoneal cavity than projectiles fired from a handgun, rifle, or shotgun.

When the peritoneum is penetrated, stab wounds are most likely to injure the liver (40%), small bowel (30%), diaphragm (20%), and colon (15%), whereas gunshot wounds most commonly damage the small bowel (50%), colon (40%), liver (30%), and abdominal vessels (25%).[5,1] Because of the thicker musculature of the back, penetrating trauma to the back is less likely to result in injuries of intraperitoneal structures than wounds to the anterior abdominal wall. Overall, only about 15% of patients with stab wounds to the abdomen will require surgical intervention, whereas about 85% of patients with gunshot wounds will need surgery for definitive management of their abdominal injuries. Tangential gunshot wounds may pass through subcutaneous tissues but never enter the peritoneal cavity. Explosive devices may also propel fragments that penetrate the peritoneum and injure internal organs.

Blunt Trauma

Numerous mechanisms lead to the compression and shear forces that may damage abdominal organs. A patient may experience considerable deceleration or compression forces when involved in motor vehicle and motorcycle crashes, when struck or run over by a vehicle, or after falling from a significant height. In a motor vehicle collision, location of impact should be considered in relationship to the passengers in the vehicle. For example, driver's side impact raises suspicion for splenic injury, as opposed to deceleration and compression injuries of a head-on collision. Although abdominal organs are most often injured in events associated with significant kinetic injury, such as those with rapid deceleration or severe compression, abdominal injuries may result from more innocuous-appearing mechanisms, such as assaults, falls down a flight of stairs, and sporting activities (e.g., being tackled in football). Any protective devices or gear used by the patient should be noted, including seat belts, airbags, or sports padding.

Compression of a solid organ may result in splitting of its structure (e.g., hepatic laceration), whereas similar forces applied to a hollow structure, such as a loop of bowel or the bladder, may cause the structure to burst open ("rupture"), spilling its contents into the abdomen. Shearing forces may result in tears of structures at sites of tethering to other structures, such as where the more mobile small bowel joins the ascending colon, which is fixed in the retroperitoneum. The organs most commonly injured following blunt trauma to the abdomen include the spleen, liver, and small bowel. Not all injuries to solid organs require surgical intervention (**Box 11-1**). Many of these types of solid organ injuries can be carefully observed in the hospital, as they often stop bleeding on their own.

Blast Injury

Explosions from any source (e.g., munitions, industrial, fuel), generate large amounts of energy in different forms. In a matter of milliseconds, an intense overpressure impulse, referred to as a "blast wave" passes through the environment (i.e., air, water). This impulse rapidly diminishes in air in inverse proportion to the third power of the radius.[7] People in close proximity to this overpressure impulse sustain what is called a *primary blast injury*. This is immediately followed by energized fragments, which will quickly decrease in number and in their kinetic energy depending on time and distance traveled.[8] Injury secondary to flying debris and fragments is termed *secondary blast injury*.[9] Next, the gaseous products of detonation and a physical movement generated by the "blast wind" can push the victim into surrounding structures generating a significant blunt force, causing injuries similar to those of motor vehicle collisions or decelerating injuries of falls. Injuries caused by these blunt mechanisms are termed *tertiary blast injury*. Finally, other problems related to the explosion, including related injuries (e.g., burns, crush) or illnesses (e.g., psychological effects or breathing problems from dust, smoke, or toxic fumes) are generated and can affect any part of the body. These related injuries are termed *quaternary blast injury*.

As mentioned earlier, the environment in which the blast occurs is important mechanistically.[10] An explosion in the air generates a blast wave that disburses energy, compressing the air as it travels. The energy of

> **Box 11-1** Nonoperative Management of Solid Organ Injuries
>
> Suspected injuries of the spleen, liver, or kidney no longer mandate surgical exploration in the modern trauma center. Experience has shown that many of these injuries stop bleeding prior to the development of shock and then heal without surgical repair. Research has shown that even significant solid organ injuries may be safely observed, provided the patient is not experiencing hypovolemic shock or peritonitis. Patients are admitted to the hospital for close monitoring of their vital signs, blood count, and abdominal exam, often initially in the intensive care unit. The advantage of this approach is that it prevents the patient from undergoing a potentially unnecessary operation. Because the spleen performs an important role in fighting infections, removal of the spleen (splenectomy) predisposes patients (especially children) to certain bacterial infections.
>
> Successful nonoperative management of these injuries was first reported for splenic injuries in children, but this approach is now often applied to adult patients, as well as to patients who sustain injuries to the liver or kidney. Following blunt trauma, data indicate that about 84% of splenic injuries can be managed in this manner, with reported success rates over 90% at high-volume trauma centers.[2] Similarly, many liver injuries are managed nonoperatively, with a success rate of over 90%.[6] Nonoperative management may include angiographic embolization of bleeding, not simply observation.
>
> The risk of failure of this technique (rebleeding, with the development of shock requiring surgical intervention) is greatest in the first several days following injury. Prehospital care practitioners should be aware of this approach, as they may respond to patients who are experiencing rebleeding after discharge from the hospital.
>
> © National Association of Emergency Medical Technicians (NAEMT)

the primary blast wave dissipates after traveling only a short distance. On the other hand, blasts in confined air spaces can generate additional blast wave injury because the wave reflects off of structures and then reengages with the victim with a second or more waves. A blast wave from an underwater explosion also behaves differently and can be more damaging. Water is, in essence, incompressible and the blast wave from an underwater explosion will dissipate its energy slowly and travel three times farther than it would in the air.

Specific to the abdominal cavity, a primary blast injury may lead to bowel wall injury, which can present in a delayed fashion as a perforation.[11] Secondary blast injuries result in penetrating injuries, which may or may not penetrate the peritoneal cavity but need further hospital evaluation. Tertiary blast injuries result in blunt abdominal injuries, which may include splenic, renal, and hepatic lacerations, as well as bowel injuries.

History

History may be obtained from the patient, family, or bystanders, and it should be documented on the patient care report and relayed to the receiving facility. Obtaining a photograph of the scene and sharing this with emergency department personnel may be valuable in communicating the mechanism of injury clearly. In addition to the components of the SAMPLER history (Symptoms, Allergies, Medications, Past medical history, Last meal, Events preceding the injury, Risk factors), questions should be tailored to the mechanism of injury and the presence of comorbid conditions that can potentially increase mortality or morbidity. For example, in the case of a motor vehicle collision, questions may be asked to determine the following:

- Type of collision, position of patient in the vehicle, or ejection from the vehicle
- Estimated vehicle speed at time of event
- Extent of vehicle damage, including intrusion into the passenger compartment, steering wheel deformity, windshield damage, and requirement for extrication
- Use of safety devices, including seat belts, deployment of airbags, and presence of child safety seats

In the case of penetrating injury, questions may be asked to determine the following:

- Type of weapon (handgun or rifle, caliber, length of knife)
- Number of times the patient was shot or stabbed
- Distance from which the patient was shot
- Amount of blood at the scene (although accurate estimation is often difficult)
- Previous history of penetrating injury (may have retained ballistic fragments)

Physical Examination

Primary Survey

Most severe abdominal injuries present as abnormalities identified in the primary survey, primarily in the evaluation of breathing and circulation. Unless there are associated injuries, patients with abdominal trauma generally present with a patent airway. The alterations found in the breathing, circulation, and disability assessments generally correspond to the degree of shock present. Patients with early, compensated shock may have a mild increase in their respiratory rate, whereas those with severe hemorrhagic shock demonstrate marked tachypnea. Rupture of a hemidiaphragm often compromises respiratory function when abdominal contents herniate into the chest on the affected side, and bowel sounds may be heard over the thorax when auscultating breath sounds. Similarly, shock from intra-abdominal hemorrhage may range from mild tachycardia with few other findings, to severe tachycardia, marked hypotension, and pale, cool, clammy skin.

The most reliable indicator of intra-abdominal bleeding is the presence of hypovolemic shock from an unexplained source. When assessing disability, the prehospital care practitioner may note only subtle signs, such as mild anxiety or agitation, in the patient with compensated shock from abdominal trauma, whereas patients with life-threatening hemorrhage may be barely arousable or have other serious depression in their mental status. When abnormalities are found in the assessment of these systems and while preparing for immediate transport, the abdomen should be exposed and examined for evidence of trauma, such as bruising or penetrating wounds.

Secondary Assessment

During the secondary assessment, the abdomen is examined in greater detail. This examination primarily involves inspection and palpation of the abdomen and should be approached systematically.

Inspection

The abdomen is examined for soft-tissue injuries and distension. Intra-abdominal injury may be suspected when soft-tissue trauma is noted over the abdomen, flanks, or back. Such findings may include contusions, abrasions, stab or gunshot wounds, obvious bleeding, and unusual findings such as evisceration, impaled objects, or tire marks. The "seat belt sign" (ecchymosis or abrasion across the abdomen resulting from compression of the abdominal wall against the shoulder harness or lap belt) indicates that significant force was applied to the abdomen as a result of sudden deceleration (**Figure 11-7**) and increases the likelihood of intra-abdominal injury eightfold.[12] The incidence of intra-abdominal injuries in pediatric patients with seat belt signs is greater than the incidence in adults. The injuries associated with restraints are typically to the bowel and its supporting mesentery, as they are compressed and crushed between the seat belt and anterior abdominal wall and the spinal

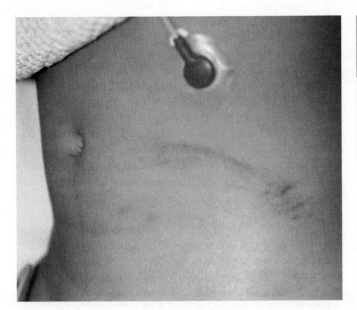

Figure 11-7 An abdominal "seat belt sign" resulting from the patient decelerating against a lap belt.

Courtesy of Peter T. Pons, MD, FACEP.

column posteriorly, and often present in a delayed fashion. Grey-Turner sign (ecchymosis involving the flanks) and Cullen sign (ecchymosis around the umbilicus) indicate retroperitoneal bleeding; however, these signs are often delayed and may not be seen in the first few hours after injury.

The contour of the abdomen should be noted, assessing if it is flat or distended. Distension of the abdomen may indicate significant internal hemorrhage; however, the adult peritoneal cavity can hold up to 1.5 liters of fluid before showing any obvious signs of distension. Abdominal distension may also be the result of a stomach filled with air, as can occur during artificial ventilation with a bag-mask device. Although these signs may indicate intra-abdominal injury, some patients with substantial internal injury may lack these findings.

Palpation

Palpation of the abdomen is undertaken to identify areas of tenderness. Ideally, palpation is begun in an area in which the patient does not complain of pain. Then, each of the abdominal quadrants is palpated. While palpating a tender area, the prehospital care practitioner may note that the patient "tenses up" the abdominal muscles in that area. This reaction, called **voluntary guarding**, protects the patient from the pain resulting from palpation. **Involuntary guarding** represents rigidity or spasm of the abdominal wall muscles in response to peritonitis. **Box 11-2** lists physical findings consistent with the presence of peritonitis. Unlike voluntary guarding, involuntary guarding remains when

the patient is distracted (e.g., with conversation) or the abdomen is surreptitiously palpated (e.g., with pressure on the stethoscope while appearing to auscultate bowel sounds). Although the presence of **rebound tenderness** has long been considered an important finding indicating peritonitis, many surgeons now believe that this maneuver—pressing deeply on the abdomen and then quickly releasing the pressure—causes excessive pain. If rebound tenderness is present, the patient will note more severe pain when the abdominal pressure is released.

Deep or aggressive palpation of an obviously injured abdomen should be avoided because, in addition to the pain it causes, palpation may theoretically aggravate bleeding or other injury. Great care during palpation should also be exercised if there is an impaled object in the abdomen. In fact, there is little additional useful information to be gained by palpating the abdomen in a patient with an impaled object.

Although tenderness is an important indicator of intra-abdominal injury, several factors may confound the assessment of tenderness. Patients with altered mental status, such as those with a TBI or those under the influence of drugs or alcohol, may have an *unreliable* examination; that is, the patient may not report tenderness or respond to palpation even when significant internal injuries are present. Pediatric and geriatric patients are more likely to have unreliable abdominal examinations because of impaired pain responses. Conversely, patients with lower rib fractures or a pelvic fracture may have an *equivocal* (ambiguous) examination, with tenderness resulting from either the fractures or associated internal injuries. If the patient has distracting pain from injuries, such as extremity or spinal fractures, abdominal pain may not be elicited on palpation.

Palpation of the pelvis in the prehospital setting provides little information that will alter the management of the patient. If time is taken to perform this examination, it is performed only once, because any clot that has formed at the site of an unstable fracture may be disrupted, thus exacerbating hemorrhage. During this examination, the pelvis is palpated gently to assess for instability and tenderness. This evaluation involves two steps as follows:

1. Pressing inward on the iliac crests
2. Pressing posteriorly on the pubic symphysis

If instability or pain is noted during any step of the examination, no further palpation of the pelvis should be performed and a pelvic binder should be applied.

Auscultation

Hemorrhage and spillage of intestinal contents in the peritoneal cavity may result in an *ileus*, a condition in which the peristalsis of the bowel ceases. This results in a "quiet" abdomen, as bowel sounds are diminished or absent. Auscultation of bowel sounds is generally not a helpful prehospital assessment tool. Time should not be wasted trying to determine their presence or absence because this diagnostic sign will not alter the prehospital management of the patient. If bowel sounds are heard over the thorax during auscultation of breath sounds, however, the presence of a diaphragmatic rupture may be considered.

Percussion

Although percussion of the abdomen may reveal tympanic or dull sounds, this information does not alter prehospital management of the trauma patient and only expends valuable time; therefore, it is not recommended as a prehospital assessment tool. Significant tenderness on percussion or pain when the patient is asked to cough represents a key finding of peritonitis. Peritoneal signs are summarized in Box 11-2.

Special Examinations and Key Indicators

Surgical evaluation and, in many cases, intervention remain key needs for most patients who have sustained abdominal injuries; time should not be wasted in attempts to determine the exact details of injury. In many patients, identification of specific organ injury will not be revealed until the abdomen is further evaluated by computed tomography (CT) scanning or surgical exploration.

In the emergency department, ultrasound has become the primary bedside modality used to assess a trauma patient for intra-abdominal hemorrhage.[5,13-16] The focused assessment with sonography for trauma (FAST) examination involves three views of the peritoneal cavity and a fourth view of the pericardium to assess for the presence of fluid, presumably blood, around the heart. The extended FAST (eFAST) adds additional views of the right and left hemithoraces to evaluate for pneumothorax[17] (**Figure 11-8** and **Box 11-3**). Because fluid does not reflect the ultrasound waves back to the device, all fluids appear anechoic (sonographically black). Presence of fluid in one or more areas is worrisome; however, ultrasonography cannot differentiate blood from other types of fluids (ascites, urine from a ruptured bladder, etc.).

Compared to other techniques used to evaluate the peritoneal cavity, FAST can be rapidly performed at the patient's bedside, does not interfere with resuscitation, is noninvasive, does not involve radiation exposure, and is much less costly than CT scanning. The primary disadvantage of FAST is that it does not definitively diagnose location of injury but only indicates the presence of fluid that may be blood. Other disadvantages of the FAST exam are that imaging is dependent on the operator's skill and experience, and its utility is compromised in patients who are obese, have subcutaneous air, or have had previous surgery. Perhaps most important, a negative FAST exam does not rule out the presence of an injury, including one that might require surgical intervention. A negative FAST exam only means that, at the moment when the exam was performed, fluid was not visualized in the abdomen. This result could be because no injury exists or because not enough blood had accumulated in the abdomen to be seen (which is a real possibility given a rapid response by emergency medical services [EMS] to the trauma incident scene).

Because of ease of use and improved ultrasound technology, some ground and air EMS systems and military teams have implemented FAST in the prehospital setting. The FAST exam has been shown to be feasible in the field and is being used to determine need for initiation of prehospital blood products or to activate a massive transfusion protocol more quickly.[25] Published prehospital studies demonstrating improved outcomes for patients with abdominal trauma, however, are limited.[18-21,26-28] An outcomes study of patients in the emergency department, has shown significantly decreased time to operative care, improved resource use, and lower hospital charges in patients with suspected torso trauma. FAST may also have utility in the austere environment or a mass-casualty situation. However, use of FAST is not recommended by Prehospital Trauma Life Support (PHTLS) for routine prehospital care, primarily because it may delay transport to the receiving facility or may provide false reassurance about the actual condition of the patient.

Despite all of these different components, the assessment of abdominal injury can be difficult. The following are key indicators for establishing the index of suspicion for abdominal injury:

- Obvious signs of trauma (i.e., soft-tissue injuries, gunshot wounds)
- Presence of hypovolemic shock without another obvious cause
- Degree of shock greater than what can be explained by other injuries (e.g., fractures, external hemorrhage)
- Presence of peritonitis

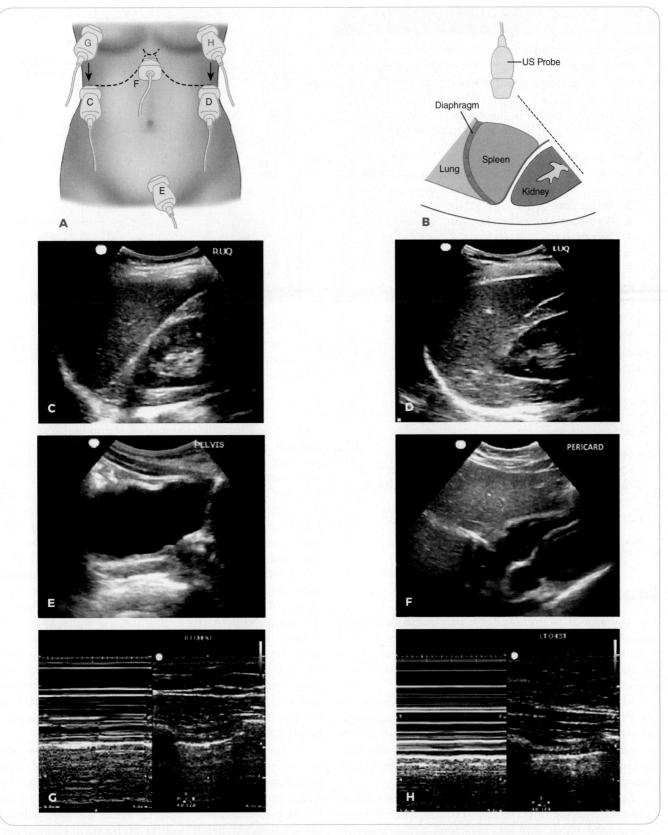

Figure 11-8 Extended focused assessment with sonography for trauma (eFAST). **A.** Probe placement for six views that constitute the eFAST examination. **B.** Orientation of lung, spleen, diaphragm, and kidney to ultrasound probe for splenorenal view. **C.** Normal view of the right upper quadrant. **D.** Normal view of the left upper quadrant. **E.** Normal view of the pelvis. **F.** Normal view of the pericardium. **G.** Normal view of the right chest. **H.** Normal view of the left chest.

A & B. © National Association of Emergency Medical Technicians (NAEMT). **C–H.** Reproduced from Cormack C, Lavender I, Coombs P, Ptasznik R. Sonographer credentialing in extended focussed assessment by sonography in trauma (eFAST). *Sonography*. 2019;6(2):50-55.

The eFAST examination has value in the trauma patient because most significant intra-abdominal injuries are associated with hemorrhage into the peritoneal cavity. Although ultrasound cannot differentiate the type of fluid present, any fluid in the trauma patient is presumed to be blood.

Technique

- Five acoustic windows (views) are imaged, three of which evaluate the peritoneal cavity:
  1. Pericardial
  2. Perihepatic (Morrison pouch)
  3. Perisplenic
  4. Pelvic
  5. Anterior thorax
- Accumulated fluid appears anechoic (sonographically black).
- Presence of fluid in one or more of the areas indicates a positive scan.

Advantages

- Can be rapidly performed
- Can be done at the bedside
- Does not interfere with resuscitation
- Is noninvasive
- Is less costly than CT

Disadvantages

- Results are compromised in patients who are obese, who have subcutaneous air, or who have had previous abdominal surgery.
- Skill at imaging is operator dependent.

*FAST and eFAST have been studied in several prehospital systems.[18-24]
© National Association of Emergency Medical Technicians (NAEMT)

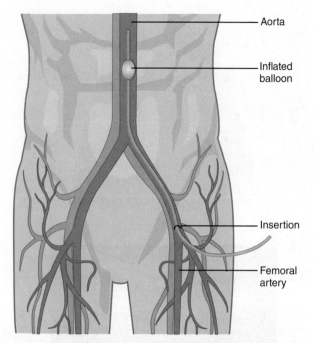

Figure 11-9 Resuscitative endovascular balloon occlusion of the aorta (REBOA) for uncontrolled hemorrhage in the torso.
© National Association of Emergency Medical Technicians (NAEMT)

Labels: Aorta; Inflated balloon; Insertion; Femoral artery

Management

The key aspects of prehospital management of patients with abdominal trauma are to recognize the presence of potential injury and initiate rapid transport, as appropriate, to the closest facility that is capable of managing the patient.

Abnormalities in vital functions identified in the primary survey are supported during transport. Supplemental oxygen is administered to maintain saturation at 94% or greater, an airway is obtained if necessary, and ventilations are assisted as needed. External hemorrhage is controlled with direct pressure or a tourniquet.

Patients with abdominal trauma often require transfusion and surgical intervention to control internal hemorrhage and repair injuries; therefore, patients should be transported to facilities that have immediate surgical capability, such as a trauma center, if available. Findings particularly indicative of the need for prompt surgical intervention include evidence of abdominal trauma associated with hypotension or peritoneal signs, and the presence of an evisceration or impaled object. Taking a patient with intra-abdominal injuries to a facility that does not have an available operating room and a surgical team defeats the purpose of rapid transport. In a rural setting where there is no hospital with general surgeons on staff, consideration should be given to direct transfer to a trauma center, either by ground or air, as early surgical intervention is the key to survival of the unstable patient with abdominal trauma. Case reports describe prehospital use of resuscitative endovascular balloon occlusion of the aorta (REBOA) by highly trained teams to control hemorrhage in thoracoabdominal trauma in order to allow time for transfer to definitive care[29] (**Figure 11-9**). Given the requirement for specialized training, the unclear benefit to outcomes, and potential for significant complications, this intervention is undergoing trials in the prehospital setting but is not currently recommended by PHTLS.

If the patient has sustained blunt trauma that also could have produced spinal or pelvic injury, stabilization is performed as appropriate. For proper instructions on spinal motion restriction, see Chapter 9, *Spinal Trauma*. In hemodynamically unstable blunt trauma patients with suspected pelvic injury, prehospital practitioners are advised to stabilize, or "close," the pelvis by securing it with a sheet or applying a commercial pelvic binder (**Figure 11-10**). Securing the pelvis in this fashion reduces

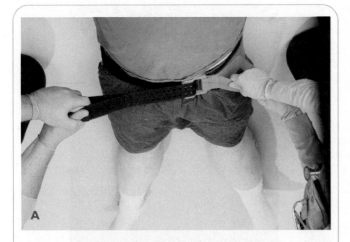

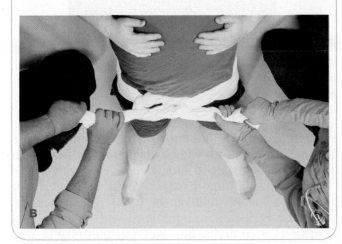

Figure 11-10 Examples of prehospital pelvic stabilization techniques. **A.** Commercially available pelvic binder. **B.** Sheet used for binding.

© Jones & Bartlett Learning. Photographed by Darren Stahlman.

pelvic volume and stabilizes fracture fragments, thus helping to reduce the risk of major hemorrhage during transport to definitive care. Guidance for recommended application of a pelvic binder is shown in **Box 11-4**.

During transport, intravenous (IV) access should be obtained. The decision to administer crystalloid fluid replacement en route depends on the patient's clinical presentation. Abdominal trauma represents one of the key situations in which a balanced resuscitation is indicated. Aggressive administration of IV fluid may elevate the patient's blood pressure to levels that will disrupt any clot that has formed and result in recurrence of bleeding that had ceased because of blood clotting and hypotension.[31] (Further discussion of IV fluid administration is provided in Chapter 3, *Shock: Pathophysiology of Life and Death*.) Although prehospital teams equipped with blood products and strict protocols to guide transfusion in hypotensive trauma patients have been established in some areas, with some data suggesting a 30-day mortality reduction,

Box 11-4 Pelvic Binder Indications

A pelvic binder should be applied for cases of suspected pelvic fracture in the following circumstances[30]:

- Severe blunt force (i.e., motorcycle crash) or blast injury with one or more of the following indications:
  · Pelvic pain
  · Physical exam findings suggestive of a pelvic fracture
  · Any major lower limb amputation or near amputation
  · Shock
  · Unconsciousness (complaints of pain or findings of tenderness will not be possible)

© National Association of Emergency Medical Technicians (NAEMT)

this remains a resource-limited intervention and is not yet a standard of care.[32-34] Whether crystalloid or blood products are available, prehospital care practitioners must achieve a delicate balance: maintain a blood pressure that provides perfusion to vital organs without restoring blood pressure to elevated or even normal ranges, which may reinitiate bleeding sites in the abdomen or pelvis. In the absence of TBI, the target systolic blood pressure is 80 to 90 mm Hg (mean arterial pressure of 60 to 65 mm Hg). For patients with suspected intra-abdominal bleeding and a TBI, the systolic blood pressure is maintained at a minimum of 110 mm Hg.

Tranexamic acid (TXA) is a clot-stabilizing medication that has been used for years to control bleeding and has started to make its way into the prehospital environment. TXA works by binding to plasminogen and preventing it from becoming plasmin, thereby preventing the breakdown of fibrin in a clot. Ongoing studies will assist in determining the appropriate prehospital role for TXA. Chapter 3, *Shock: Pathophysiology of Life and Death*, discusses TXA in greater detail.

Special Considerations
Impaled Objects

Because removal of an impaled object may cause additional trauma and because the object may be actively controlling the bleeding (*tamponade effect*), removal of an impaled object from the abdomen in the prehospital environment is contraindicated (**Figure 11-11**). The prehospital care practitioner should neither move nor remove an object impaled in a patient's abdomen. In the hospital, these objects are not removed until their shape and

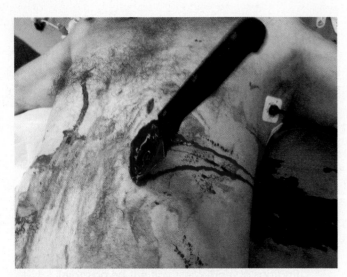

Figure 11-11 Removal of an impaled object from the abdomen is contraindicated in the prehospital environment.

Courtesy of Lance Stuke, MD, MPH.

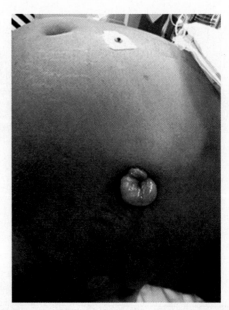

Figure 11-12 Bowel eviscerated through a wound in the abdominal wall.

Courtesy of Lance Stuke, MD, MPH.

location have been identified by radiographic evaluation (when stable) and until blood replacement and a surgical team are present and ready. Often these objects are removed in the operating room.

A prehospital care practitioner may stabilize the impaled object, either manually or mechanically, to prevent any further movement in the field and during transport. In some circumstances the impaled object may need to be cut in order to free the patient and permit transport to the trauma center. If bleeding occurs around it, direct pressure should be applied around the object to the wound with the practitioner's hand. Psychological support of the patient is important, especially if the impaled object is visible to the patient.

The abdomen should not be palpated or percussed in these patients because these actions may produce additional organ injury from the distal end of the object. Further examination is unnecessary because the presence of impaled objects indicates the need for management by a surgeon.

Evisceration

In an abdominal **evisceration**, a section of intestine, tissue, or other abdominal organ is displaced through an open wound and protrudes outside the abdominal cavity (**Figure 11-12**). The tissue most often visualized is the fatty **omentum** that lies over the intestines. Attempts should not be made to replace the protruding tissue into the abdominal cavity. The **viscera** should be left on the surface of the abdomen or protruding as found.

Treatment efforts should focus on protecting the protruding segment of intestine or other organ from further damage. Most of the abdominal contents require a moist

environment. If the intestine or other abdominal organs become dry, cell death will occur. Therefore, the eviscerated abdominal contents should be covered with a clean or sterile dressing that has been moistened with saline (normal saline IV fluid can be used). These dressings should be periodically remoistened with saline to prevent them from drying out. Wet dressings may be covered with a large, dry or occlusive dressing to keep the patient warm.[35]

Psychological support is extremely important for patients with an abdominal evisceration, and care should be taken to keep the patient calm. Any action that increases pressure within the abdomen, such as crying, screaming, or coughing, can force more of the organs outward. These patients should be expeditiously transported to a trauma center.

Trauma in the Obstetric Patient

Trauma in pregnancy can range from mild, such as a fall from standing, or major, including penetrating or a high-velocity blunt injury sustained in a motor vehicle collision. Trauma in pregnancy has increased over the last few decades and is now the leading cause of nonobstetric maternal death in the United States.[36] Motor vehicles account for half of all traumatic injuries during pregnancy and 82% of trauma related to fetal death. The improper use of seat belts is the main reason for many of these accidents. Pelvic fracture is the most common maternal injury that leads to fetal death. In a review of women with pelvic fractures, the rate of fetal mortality was 35%.[37] The causes of death included direct fetal injury (20%), placental abruption (32%), and maternal shock (36%). Dilated vasculature, as a part of maternal physiologic changes, puts the mother at increased risk for hemorrhage following pelvic fractures, and mortality in these mothers is as high as 9%. Injuries from direct blunt trauma may include placental abruption and uterine rupture. Abruption is thought to complicate 1% to 6% of minor injuries and up to half of major injuries. Uterine rupture occurs in less than 1% of pregnant trauma patients. Maternal mortality is more favorable following penetrating injury, as the gravid uterus serves as protection to the maternal internal organs. However, fetal mortality is up to 73% following penetrating trauma.[38] Appropriate knowledge the anatomic and physiologic changes that occur during pregnancy is essential to most effectively recognize injuries in a pregnant patient.

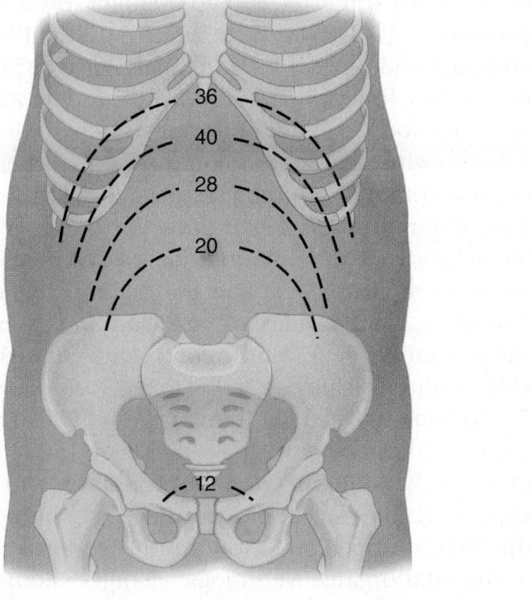

Anatomic and Physiologic Changes

Pregnancy causes both anatomic and physiologic changes to the body's systems. These changes can affect the patterns of injuries seen and make the assessment of an injured pregnant patient especially challenging. The prehospital care practitioner is dealing with two or more patients and must be aware of the changes that have occurred to the woman's anatomy and physiology throughout the pregnancy.

A human pregnancy typically lasts about 40 weeks from conception to birth, and this gestational period is divided into three sections, or trimesters. The first trimester ends at about the 12th week of gestation, and the second trimester is slightly longer than the other two, ending at about week 28.

Following conception and implantation of the fetus, the uterus continues to enlarge through the 38th week of pregnancy. Until about the 12th week, the growing uterus remains protected by the bony pelvis. By the 20th week of gestation, the top of the uterus (fundus) is at the umbilicus, and the fundus approaches the xiphoid process by the 38th week. This anatomic change makes the uterus and its contents more susceptible to both blunt and penetrating injury (**Figure 11-13**). Injury to the uterus can include rupture, penetration, *abruptio placentae* (when a portion of the placenta is pulled away from the uterine wall), and premature rupture of the membranes (**Figure 11-14**). The placenta and gravid uterus are

Figure 11-13 Fundal height. As pregnancy progresses, the uterus becomes more susceptible to injury.

© National Association of Emergency Medical Technicians (NAEMT)

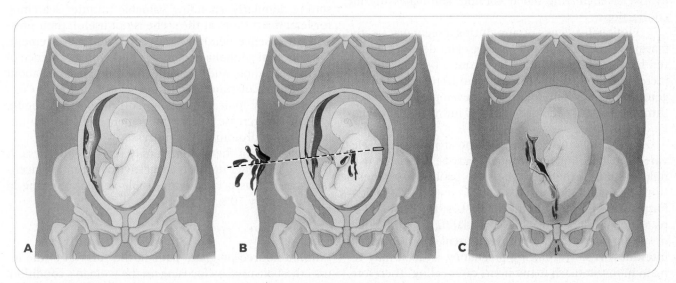

Figure 11-14 Diagram of uterine trauma. **A.** Abruptio placentae. **B.** Gunshot to the uterus. **C.** Ruptured uterus.

© National Association of Emergency Medical Technicians (NAEMT)

highly vascular; injuries to these structures can result in profound hemorrhage. Because the hemorrhage can be concealed inside the uterus or peritoneal cavity, it may not be externally visible.

Although a marked protuberance of the abdomen is obvious in late pregnancy, the rest of the abdominal organs remain essentially unchanged, with the exception of the uterus. The uterus stretches and eventually becomes the largest intra-abdominal organ. This thin-walled structure is susceptible to injury. Intestine that is displaced superiorly is shielded by the uterus in the last two trimesters of pregnancy. The increased size and weight of the uterus alter the patient's center of gravity and increase the risk of falls. Because of its prominence, the gravid abdomen is often injured in a fall. As is the case with nonpregnant blunt trauma patients, the spleen remains the most commonly injured organ.

In addition to these anatomic changes, physiologic changes occur during pregnancy. The woman's heart rate normally increases throughout pregnancy by 15 to 20 beats/minute above normal by the third trimester. This makes the interpretation of tachycardia more difficult. Systolic and diastolic blood pressures normally drop 5 to 15 mm Hg during the second trimester but often return to normal at term. By the 10th week of pregnancy, the woman's cardiac output increases by 1 to 1.5 liters/minute. By term, the woman's blood volume has increased by about 50%. Blood flow increases from a nonpregnant state of 60 milliliters per minute (mL/min) to 600 mL/min at term. *Because of these increases in cardiac output and blood volume, healthy pregnant patients may lose 1,200 to 1,500 mL of blood before exhibiting signs and symptoms of hypovolemia.*[39] Hypovolemic shock may induce premature labor in patients in the third trimester. Oxytocin, which is released along with antidiuretic hormone in response to loss of circulating blood volume, stimulates uterine contractions.

Dilutional anemia occurs during pregnancy, as the plasma volume increases to a far greater degree than the red blood cell mass. The liver becomes hypermetabolic, increasing production of coagulation factors and fibrinogen. The patient is more prone to developing a deep vein thrombosis (DVT) and disseminated intravascular coagulation (DIC).

During the third trimester, the diaphragm is elevated 2 to 4 centimeters (cm) and may be associated with mild dyspnea, especially when the patient is supine. If supine positioning causes dyspnea, reverse Trendelenburg positioning may be helpful. Chest tubes should be placed 2 cm higher to avoid potential injury to the liver or spleen. Peristalsis (propulsive, muscular movements of intestines) is slower during pregnancy, so food may remain in the stomach many hours after eating. Therefore, the pregnant patient is at greater risk for vomiting and subsequent aspiration, particularly with intubation.

Toxemia of pregnancy (also known as eclampsia) is a late complication of pregnancy. Whereas *preeclampsia* is characterized by edema and hypertension, **eclampsia** is characterized by mental status changes and seizures, thus mimicking TBI. A careful neurologic assessment and asking about potential complications of pregnancy and other medical conditions such as known diabetes, hypertension, or seizure history are important.

Assessment

Pregnancy typically does not alter the woman's airway, but significant respiratory distress may occur if a patient in her third trimester is placed supine on a board. The decrease in peristalsis of the gastrointestinal tract makes vomiting and aspiration more likely. Airway patency and pulmonary function are assessed, including auscultation of breath sounds and monitoring of pulse oximetry.

As with hemoperitoneum from other sources, intra-abdominal bleeding associated with uterine injury may not produce peritonitis for hours. More likely, blood loss from an injury may be masked by the pregnant woman's increased cardiac output and blood volume. Therefore, a high index of suspicion and assessment for subtle changes (e.g., skin color, mental status) may provide important clues.

In general, the condition of the fetus will depend on the condition of the woman; however, the fetus may be in jeopardy while the woman's condition and vital signs appear hemodynamically normal. This occurs because the body shunts blood away from the uterus (and fetus) to the vital organs. Neurologic changes should be noted and documented, although the exact etiology may not be identifiable in the prehospital setting.

As with the nonpregnant patient, auscultation of bowel sounds is generally not helpful in the prehospital setting. Similarly, spending valuable minutes searching for fetal heart tones at the scene is not useful; their presence or absence will not alter prehospital management. The external genitalia should be checked for evidence of vaginal bleeding, and the patient should be asked about the presence of contractions and fetal movement. Contractions may indicate that premature labor has begun, whereas a decrease in fetal movement may be an ominous sign of profound fetal distress.

Palpation of the abdomen may reveal tenderness. A firm, hard, tender uterus is suggestive of abruptio placentae, which is associated with visible vaginal bleeding in approximately 70% of cases.[39]

Management

With an injured pregnant patient, the survival of the fetus is best ensured by focusing on the woman's condition. In essence, for the fetus to survive, usually the woman needs to survive. Priority is given to ensuring an adequate

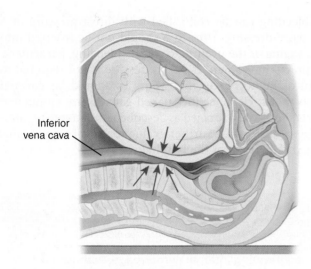

Figure 11-15 Full-term uterus compressing the vena cava.
© National Association of Emergency Medical Technicians (NAEMT)

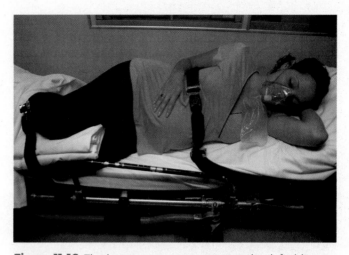

Figure 11-16 Tipping a pregnant woman onto her left side helps displace the uterus from the inferior vena cava and improves blood return to the heart, thus restoring blood pressure.
© Jones & Bartlett Learning. Courtesy of MIEMSS.

patent airway and supporting respiratory function. Sufficient oxygen should be administered to maintain a pulse oximetry reading of 95% or higher. Ventilations may need to be assisted, especially in the later stages of pregnancy. It is wise to anticipate vomiting and have suction nearby.

The goals of shock management are essentially the same as for any patient and include judicious IV fluid administration, especially if evidence of decompensated shock is present. Any evidence of vaginal bleeding or a rigid, board-like abdomen with external bleeding in the last trimester of pregnancy may indicate abruptio placentae or a ruptured uterus. These conditions threaten not only the life of the fetus but also that of the woman because exsanguination can occur rapidly. No good data exist to define the best target blood pressure for an injured pregnant patient. However, restoration of normal systolic and mean blood pressures will most likely result in better fetal perfusion, despite the risk of promoting additional internal hemorrhage in the woman.

Some women may have significant hypotension when supine. This supine hypotension of pregnancy typically occurs in the third trimester and is caused by the compression of the inferior vena cava by the enlarged uterus. This dramatically decreases venous return to the heart, and because there is less filling, cardiac output and blood pressure fall[39] (**Figure 11-15**).

The following maneuvers may be used to relieve supine hypotension (**Figure 11-16**):

1. The woman may be placed on her left side (left lateral decubitus position), or if spinal motion restriction is indicated, 4 to 6 inches (10 to 15 centimeters [cm]) of padding should be placed under the right side of the transport device.

2. If the patient cannot be rotated, her right leg should be elevated to displace the uterus to the left.

3. The uterus may be manually displaced toward the patient's left side.

These three maneuvers reduce compression on the vena cava, increasing venous return to the heart and improving cardiac output.

Transport of the pregnant trauma patient should not be delayed. Every pregnant trauma patient—even those who appear to have only minor injuries—should be rapidly transported to the closest appropriate facility. An ideal facility is a trauma center that has both surgical and obstetric capabilities immediately available. Adequate resuscitation of the woman is the key to survival of the woman and fetus.

Genitourinary Injuries

Injuries to the kidneys, ureters, and bladder most often present with *hematuria* (blood in the urine). This sign will generally not be noted unless the patient has a urinary catheter inserted. Because the kidneys receive a significant portion of cardiac output, blunt or penetrating injuries to these organs may result in life-threatening retroperitoneal hemorrhage.

Pelvic fractures may be associated with lacerations of the urinary bladder and the walls of the vagina or the rectum. Open pelvic fractures, such as those with deep groin or perineal lacerations, may result in severe external hemorrhage and lacerations to the vagina or the rectum may result in life-threatening infectious complications.

Trauma to the external genitalia may occur from multiple mechanisms, although injuries resulting from ejection from a motorcycle or motor vehicle, an industrial accident, straddle-type mechanisms, gunshot wounds, or sexual assault predominate. Because of the numerous nerve endings in these organs, these injuries are associated with significant pain and psychological concern. These organs contain numerous blood vessels, and copious amounts of blood may be seen. In general, this type of bleeding can be controlled with direct pressure or a pressure dressing. Dressings should not be inserted into the vagina or the urethra to control bleeding, particularly in pregnant women. If direct pressure is not required to control hemorrhage, these injuries should be covered with moist, clean, saline-soaked gauze. Any amputated parts should be managed as described in Chapter 12, *Musculoskeletal Trauma*. Further evaluation of all genital injuries should occur at the hospital.

SUMMARY

- Intra-abdominal injuries are often life threatening because of internal hemorrhage and spillage of gastrointestinal contents into the peritoneal cavity.
- The extent of internal injuries is not identifiable in the prehospital setting; therefore, mechanism of injury in combination with signs of abdominal or pelvic trauma should increase the prehospital care practitioner's index of suspicion.
- Management of patients with abdominal trauma includes oxygenation, hemorrhage control, and rapid packaging for transport. Spinal motion restriction should be used in blunt trauma patients with torso injury. The pelvis should be further stabilized with a binder if hemodynamically unstable.
- Balanced resuscitation permits perfusion of vital organs while potentially minimizing the risk of aggravating internal hemorrhage. Prehospital resuscitation with blood products has been shown in studies to reduce 30-day mortality, but programs are resource intensive and not yet widely available.
- Because emergent surgical intervention may be lifesaving, a patient with abdominal trauma should be transported to a trauma center with immediate surgical capability.
- The anatomic and physiologic changes of pregnancy have implications for the pattern of injury, presentation of signs and symptoms of trauma, and management of the pregnant trauma patient.
- Management of potential fetal compromise caused by trauma is accomplished through effective resuscitation of the woman.

SCENARIO RECAP

You are called to a construction site for a male patient in his mid-20s who fell 3 hours earlier and is now complaining of increasing abdominal pain. He states that he tripped on a piece of wood at the site and fell, striking his left lower chest and abdomen on some stacked wood. The patient notes moderate pain over his lower left rib cage when he takes deep breaths and complains of mild difficulty breathing. His coworkers wanted to call for assistance when he fell, but he said the symptoms were not so bad and told them to hold off. He states that the discomfort has been increasing in intensity and that he is now feeling lightheaded and weak.

You find the patient sitting on the ground in visible discomfort. He is holding the left side of his lower chest and upper abdomen. He has a patent airway, a respiratory rate of 28 breaths/minute, a heart rate of 124 beats/minute, and a blood pressure of 94/58 mm Hg. The patient's skin is pale and diaphoretic. You lay him down, and on physical examination, he has tenderness on palpation of the left lower ribs without obvious bony crepitus. His abdomen is nondistended and soft to palpation, but he has tenderness and voluntary guarding in the left upper quadrant. No external ecchymosis or subcutaneous emphysema is present.

- What are the patient's possible injuries?
- What are the priorities in the care of this patient?
- Are signs of peritonitis present?

SCENARIO SOLUTION

The patient is tender over his left lower ribs and left upper quadrant. These findings can represent injuries to the thorax, intra-abdominal organs, or both. His vital signs are consistent with compensated hypovolemic shock, and a hemothorax or intra-abdominal bleeding must be considered. More likely, the tenderness over the lower ribs may indicate fractured ribs with an associated laceration of the spleen, resulting in intraperitoneal hemorrhage.

Oxygen is administered, and the patient is packaged for transport. En route to the trauma center, intravenous access is obtained; however, given the patient's blood pressure, crystalloid fluid administration is avoided unless the blood pressure falls below 80 mm Hg, as aggressive fluid infusion may raise his blood pressure too much and lead to increased bleeding.

References

1. American College of Surgeons (ACS) Committee on Trauma. Abdominal trauma. In: *Advanced Trauma Life Support for Doctors, Student Course Manual*. 8th ed. ACS; 2008:111-126.

2. Banerjee A, Duane TM, Wilson SP, et al. Trauma center variation in splenic artery embolization and spleen salvage: a multicenter analysis. *J Trauma Acute Care Surg.* 2013;75(1):69-75.

3. Hemmila MR, Wahl WL. Management of the Injured Patient. In: Doherty GM, ed. *Current Surgical Diagnosis and Treatment.* McGraw-Hill Medical; 2008:227-228.

4. Aldemir M, Tacyildiz I, Girgin S. Predicting factors for mortality in the penetrating abdominal trauma. *Acta Chir Belg.* 2004;104:429-434.

5. American College of Surgeons (ACS) Committee on Trauma. Abdominal and pelvic trauma. In: *Advanced Trauma Life Support, Student Course Manual.* 10th ed. ACS; 2018:82-101.

6. Boese CK, Hackl M, Müller LP, et al. Nonoperative management of blunt hepatic trauma: a systematic review. *J Trauma Acute Care Surg.* 2015;79(4):654-660.

7. Centers for Disease Control and Prevention. Explosions and Blast Injuries: A Primer for Clinicians. Accessed February 28, 2022. https://www.cdc.gov/masstrauma/preparedness/primer.pdf

8. Ritenour AE, Blackbourne LH, Kelly JF, et al. Incidence of primary blast injury in US military overseas contingency operations: a retrospective study. *Ann Surg.* 2010;251(6):1140-1144.

9. U.S. Department of Defense, Blast Injury Research Coordinating Office. What Is Blast Injury. Last updated June 18, 2019. Accessed February 28, 2022. https://blastinjuryresearch.amedd.army.mil/index.cfm/blast_injury_101#:~:text=Tertiary%20blast%20injuries,Traumatic%20amputations

10. Champion HR, Holcomb JB, Young LA. Injuries from explosions: physics, biophysics, pathology, and required research focus. *J Trauma Acute Care Surg.* 2009 May 1;66(5):1468-1477.

11. Owers C, Morgan JL, Garner JP. Abdominal trauma in primary blast injury. *J British Surg.* 2011;98(2):168-179.

12. Velmahos GC, Tatevossian R, Demetriades D. The "seat belt mark" sign: a call for increased vigilance among physicians treating victims of motor vehicle accidents. *Am Surg.* 1999;65(2):181-185.

13. Rozycki GS, Ochsner MG, Schmidt JA, et al. A prospective study of surgeon-performed ultrasound as the primary adjuvant modality for injured patient assessment. *J Trauma Inj Infect Crit Care.* 1995;39(3):492-500.

14. Rozycki GS, Ochsner MG, Feliciano DV, et al. Early detection of hemoperitoneum by ultrasound examination of the right upper quadrant: a multicenter study. *J Trauma Inj Infect Crit Care.* 1998;45(5):878-883.

15. Rozycki GS, Ballard RB, Feliciano DV, et al. Surgeon-performed ultrasound for the assessment of truncal injuries: lessons learned from 1540 patients. *Ann Surg.* 1998;228(4):557-567.

16. Polk JD, Fallon WF Jr. The use of focused assessment with sonography for trauma (FAST) by a prehospital air medical team in the trauma arrest patient. *Prehosp Emerg Care.* 2000;4(1):82-84.

17. Bloom BA, Gibbons RC. Focused assessment with sonography for trauma. 2021 Jul 31. In: *StatPearls.* StatPearls Publishing; Published July 31, 2021. Accessed February 28, 2022. https://pubmed.ncbi.nlm.nih.gov/29261902/

18. Melanson SW, McCarthy J, Stromski CJ, et al. Aeromedical trauma sonography by flight crews with a miniature ultrasound unit. *Prehosp Emerg Care.* 2001;5(4):399-402.

19. Walcher F, Kortum S, Kirschning T, et al. Optimized management of polytraumatized patients by prehospital ultrasound. *Unfall-Chirurg.* 2002;105(11):986-994.

20. Strode CA, Rubal BJ, Gerhardt RT, et al. Wireless and satellite transmission of prehospital focused abdominal sonography for trauma. *Prehosp Emerg Care.* 2003;7(3):375-379.

21. Heegaard WG, Ho J, Hildebrandt DA. The prehospital ultrasound study: results of the first six months (abstract). *Prehosp Emerg Care.* 2009;13(1):139.

22. Partyka C, Coggins A, Bliss J, et al. A multicenter evaluation of the accuracy of prehospital eFAST by a physician-staffed helicopter emergency medical service. *Emerg Radiol.* 2021 Nov 24:1-8.

23. Partyka CL, Coggins A, Bliss J, et al. An evaluation of the accuracy of prehospital eFAST in the assessment of polytrauma by a physician-staffed helicopter emergency medical service. *medRxiv.* Jan 1, 2020. doi: 10.1101/2020.12.02.20242453

24. Press GM, Miller SK, Hassan IA, et al. Prospective evaluation of prehospital trauma ultrasound during aeromedical transport. *J Emerg Med.* 2014 Dec 1;47(6):638-645.

25. Yates JG, Baylous D. Aeromedical ultrasound: the evaluation of point-of-care ultrasound during helicopter transport. *Air Med J.* 2017 May 1;36(3):110-115.

26. Heegard WG, Hildebrandt D, Spear D, et al. Prehospital ultrasound by paramedics: results of field trial. *Acad Em Med.* 2010;17(6):624-630.

27. Jorgensen H, Jensen CH, Dirks J. Does prehospital ultrasound improve treatment of the trauma patient? A systematic review. *Eur J Emerg Med.* 2010;17(5):249-253.

28. Rooney KP, Lahham S, Lahham S, et al. Pre-hospital assessment with ultrasound in emergencies: implementation in the field. *World J Emerg Med.* 2016;7(2):117-123.

29. Sadek S, Lockey DJ, Lendrum RA, Perkins Z, Price J, Davies GE. Resuscitative endovascular balloon occlusion of the aorta (REBOA) in the pre-hospital setting: an additional resuscitation option for uncontrolled catastrophic haemorrhage. *Resuscitation.* 2016;107:135-138.

30. Shackelford S, Hammesfahr R, Morisette D. The use of pelvic binders in tactical combat casualty care. *J Spec Oper Med.* 2016 Nov 7:135-147.

31. Sondeen JL, Coppes VG, Holcomb JB. Blood pressure at which rebleeding occurs after resuscitation in swine with aortic injury. *J Trauma Acute Care Surg.* 2003;54(5):S110-S117.

32. Guyette FX, Sperry JL, Peitzman AB, et al. Prehospital blood product and crystalloid resuscitation in the severely injured patient: a secondary analysis of the Prehospital Air Medical Plasma Trial. *Ann Surg.* 2021;273(2):358-364. doi: 10.1097/SLA.0000000000003324

33. Pusateri AE, Moore EE, Moore HB, et al. Association of prehospital plasma transfusion with survival in trauma patients with hemorrhagic shock when transport times are longer than 20 minutes: a post hoc analysis of the PAMPer and COMBAT clinical trials. *JAMA Surg.* 2020;155(2):e195085. doi: 10.1001/jamasurg.2019.5085

34. Sperry JL, Guyette FX, Brown JB, et al; PAMPer Study Group. Prehospital plasma during air medical transport in trauma patients at risk for hemorrhagic shock. *N Engl J Med.* 2018 Jul 26;379(4):315-326. doi: 10.1056/NEJMoa1802345

35. Riesberg JC, Gurney JM, Morgan M, et al. The management of abdominal evisceration in tactical combat casualty care: TCCC guideline change 20-02. *J Spec Oper Med.* 2021 Jan 1;21(4):138-142.

36. Krywko DM, Toy FK, Mahan ME, Kiel J. Pregnancy trauma. In: *StatPearls.* StatPearls Publishing. Updated Jul 2, 2021. Accessed 10/12/2021. https://www.ncbi.nlm.nih.gov/books/NBK430926/

37. Leggon RE, Wood GC, Indeck MC. Pelvic fractures in pregnancy: factors influencing maternal and fetal outcomes. *J Trauma.* 2002;53(4):796-804.

38. Mason SM, Schnitzer PG, Danilack VA, Elston B, Savitz DA. Risk factors for maltreatment-related infant hospitalizations in New York City, 1995–2004. *Ann Epidemiol.* 2018;28(9):590-596.

39. American College of Surgeons (ACS) Committee on Trauma. Chapter 12, Trauma in pregnancy and intimate partner violence. In: *Advanced Trauma Life Support, Student Course Manual.* 10th ed. ACS; 2018:229.

Suggested Reading

Beldowicz GC, Leshikar D, Cocanour CS. Trauma in pregnancy. In: Moore EE, Feliciano DV, Mattox KL, eds. *Trauma.* 9th ed. McGraw-Hill; 2020:709.

Berry MJ, McMurray RG, Katz VL. Pulmonary and ventilatory responses to pregnancy, immersion and exercise. *J Appl Physiol.* 1989:66(2):857.

Jones LA. Abdominal trauma. In: Stone C, Humphries RL, eds. *Current Diagnosis and Treatment Emergency Medicine.* 8th ed. McGraw-Hill; 2017.

Kim FJ, Donalisio da Silva R. Genitourinary tract. In: Moore EE, Feliciano DV, Mattox KL, eds. *Trauma.* 9th ed. McGraw-Hill; 2020:669.

Raja AS, Zabbo CP. Trauma in pregnancy. *Emerg Med Clin North Am.* 2012;30:937-948.

CHAPTER 12

Musculoskeletal Trauma

Lead Editors
Gerard Slobogean, MD
Christopher Renninger, MD

© Ralf Hiemisch/Getty Images

CHAPTER OBJECTIVES

At the completion of this chapter, you will be able to do the following:

- List the three categories used to classify patients with extremity injuries, and relate this classification to priority of care.
- Describe the primary and secondary surveys as related to extremity trauma.
- Discuss the significance of hemorrhage in both open and closed fractures of the long bones and pelvis.
- List the five major pathophysiologic problems associated with extremity injuries that may require management in the prehospital setting.

- Explain the management of extremity trauma as an isolated injury and in the presence of multisystem trauma.
- Given a scenario involving an extremity injury, select an appropriate splint and splinting method.
- Describe the special considerations involved in femur fracture management.
- Discuss the management of amputations.

SCENARIO

It is a beautiful Saturday afternoon in June. You have been dispatched to a local motorcycle racetrack for a rider who has been injured. Upon arrival, you are escorted by track officials to an area on the track just in front of the grandstand where the track's medical crew (two-person, emergency medical responders, nontransport) is attending to a single patient lying supine on the track.

One of the emergency medical responders tells you that the patient was a rider in a 350-cc class race with 14 other motorcycles and that three of them collided in front of the grandstand. The other two riders were not injured, but the patient was unable to stand or move without significant pain in his right leg and pelvis. There was no loss of consciousness and no complaints other than leg pain. The medical crew has maintained the patient in a supine position with manual stabilization of the right lower extremity.

As you assess the patient, you find that he is a 19-year-old man, conscious and alert without past medical or trauma history. The patient's initial vital signs are as follows: blood pressure is 104/68 millimeters of mercury (mm Hg), pulse is 112 beats/minute, respirations are 24 breaths/minute, and skin is pale and diaphoretic.

(continues)

SCENARIO (CONTINUED)

The patient states that he collided with another rider when he came out of a corner and that the collision caused him to lose balance and slide across the track. He states his right leg was run over by at least one other bike. Visual inspection of his right leg reveals shortening of the leg and no open wounds when compared to the left side, tenderness, and bruising of the mid-anterior thigh area.

- What does the mechanism of injury from this event tell you about the potential injuries for this patient?
- What type of injury do you suspect, and what would your management priorities be?

INTRODUCTION

Musculoskeletal injury, although common in trauma patients, rarely poses an immediate life-threatening condition. Skeletal trauma can be life threatening, however, when it produces significant blood loss (hemorrhage), either externally or from internal bleeding into the extremity or into the pelvis.

When caring for a critical trauma patient, the prehospital care practitioner has three primary considerations with regard to extremity injuries:

1. Maintain assessment priorities. Do not be distracted by dramatic, non-life-threatening musculoskeletal injuries (**Figure 12-1**).
2. Recognize potentially life-threatening musculoskeletal injuries.
3. Recognize the mechanism of injury and the force that created the musculoskeletal injuries and the potential for other life-threatening injuries caused by that energy transfer.

If a life-threatening or potentially life-threatening condition is discovered during the primary survey, the secondary survey should not be started. Any problems found during the primary survey should be corrected before moving to the secondary survey (see later discussion). This may mean delaying the secondary survey until the patient is en route to the hospital or even, in some cases, waiting until arrival at the emergency department (ED).

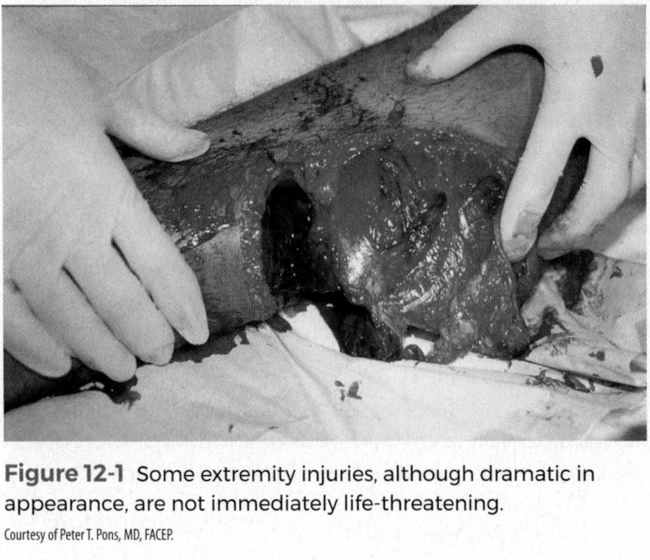

Figure 12-1 Some extremity injuries, although dramatic in appearance, are not immediately life-threatening.

Courtesy of Peter T. Pons, MD, FACEP.

Critical trauma patients may be secured to and transported on backboards or other equivalent devices to facilitate moving the patient and to allow for resuscitation and treatment of both critical and noncritical injuries. Use of such devices allow for stabilization of the entire patient and all injuries, when appropriate, on a single platform that makes it possible to move the victim without disturbing the splinting. Details of spinal motion restriction are discussed in Chapter 9, *Spinal Trauma*. The prehospital practitioner must consider the risk of delayed transport time versus the benefit of splinting extremities that have musculoskeletal pain without obvious deformity or crepitus. In general, any deformity in the extremities should be straightened, or otherwise generally realigned, and then immobilized for transport. The prehospital practitioner is unlikely to impart any more force or injury than what was sustained during the time of the trauma, and there are substantial downsides to leaving a limb in a severely deformed position for a prolonged time.

Anatomy and Physiology

Understanding the gross anatomy and physiology of the human body is an important piece of the prehospital care practitioner's fund of knowledge. Although this text does not discuss all of the anatomy and physiology of the musculoskeletal system, it reviews some of the basics.

The mature human body has approximately 206 bones (**Figure 12-2**). The skeleton is divided into two primary divisions: the axial skeleton and the **appendicular skeleton**. The axial skeleton comprises the bones of the central part of the body, including the skull, spine, sternum, and ribs. The appendicular skeleton is made up of

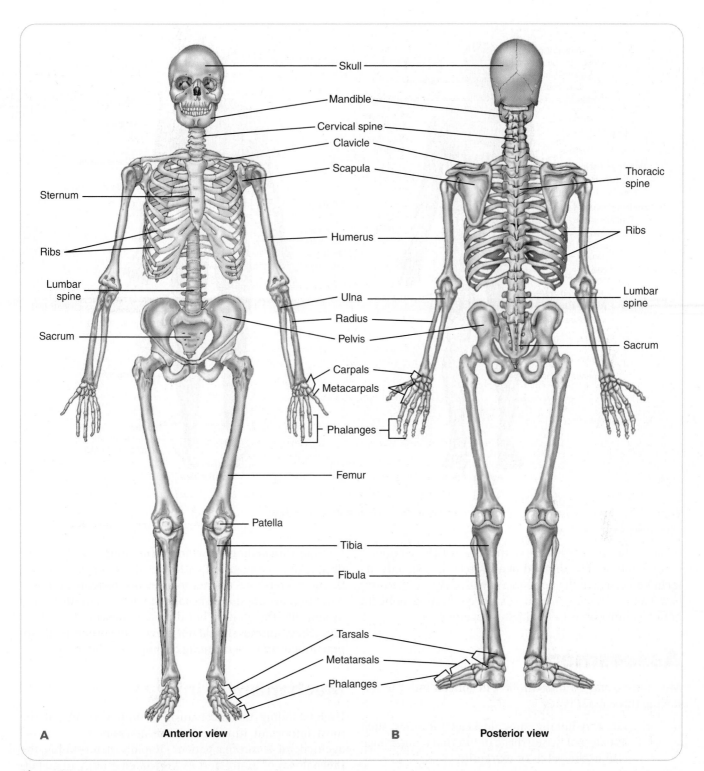

Figure 12-2 The human skeleton. **A.** Anterior view. **B.** Posterior view.
© National Association of Emergency Medical Technicians (NAEMT)

the bones of the upper and lower extremities, shoulder girdle, and pelvis (excluding the sacrum).

The human body has almost 650 individual muscles, which are categorized by their function. The muscles that are specific to this chapter are the voluntary, or skeletal,

muscles. These muscles are categorized as skeletal because they move the skeletal system. Muscles in this category voluntarily move the structures of the body (**Figure 12-3**).

Other important structures discussed in this chapter are tendons and ligaments. A **tendon** is a band of tough,

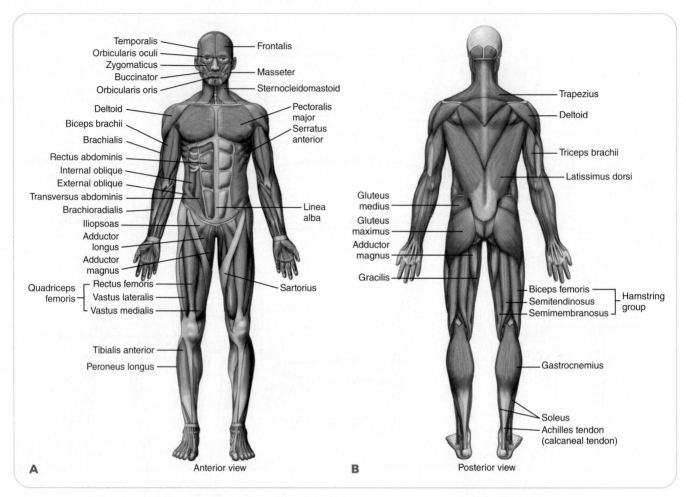

Figure 12-3 Major muscles of the human body. **A.** Anterior view. **B.** Posterior view.
© National Association of Emergency Medical Technicians (NAEMT)

inelastic, fibrous tissue that connects a muscle to bone. It is the white part at the end of a muscle that directly attaches a muscle to the bone that it will move. A **ligament** is a band of tough, fibrous tissue connecting bone to bone; its function is to hold joints together.

Assessment

Musculoskeletal trauma can be categorized into the following three main types:

1. Life-threatening musculoskeletal injuries, such as external hemorrhage or internal hemorrhage within the pelvis or extremity
2. Non-life-threatening musculoskeletal trauma associated with multisystem life-threatening trauma (life-threatening injuries plus limb fractures)
3. Isolated non-life-threatening musculoskeletal trauma (isolated limb fractures)

The purpose of the primary survey is to identify and treat life-threatening conditions. The presence of a non-life-threatening musculoskeletal injury can be an indicator of force involved with the injury and should alert the prehospital practitioner to assess for possible multisystem trauma. Care should be taken to not become distracted by non-life-threatening but dramatic musculoskeletal injury. These injuries should not prevent the prehospital care practitioner from performing a complete primary survey.

Mechanism of Injury

Understanding the mechanism of injury is one of the most important functions of the assessment and management of a trauma patient. Rapidly determining the mechanism of injury and its associated energy (e.g., falling from standing vs. being thrown from a motorcycle at high speed) will help the prehospital care practitioner to suspect and recognize the most critical injuries or conditions. The best source for determining the mechanism of injury is directly from the patient. If the patient is unresponsive, details of the injury can be obtained from witnesses. If none of these options is available, collect observations at the scene and the pattern of injuries found on physical examination, and present this information directly to the receiving facility. This information should also be documented on the patient care report (PCR).

Based on the mechanism of injury, the prehospital care practitioner may develop a high index of suspicion for the injuries that a patient might have sustained. This consideration and knowledge of various injury patterns may bring to mind additional injuries for which the patient should be assessed. Consider the following examples:

- If a patient jumps out of a window feetfirst, the primary injury suspicion would be fractures of the lower extremity, pelvis, and spine. Secondary injuries to consider would be abdominal injuries due to possible shearing mechanisms.
- If a patient is involved in a motorcycle collision with a telephone pole and the patient's head hits the pole, primary injuries will include head, cervical spine, and thoracic injury. A secondary injury might include a femur fracture from "striking" the femur on the handlebars of the motorcycle.
- If a passenger in a motor vehicle crash sustains a side-impact collision, consideration to musculoskeletal trauma would include upper and lower extremity fractures and pelvis injury. Associated injury patterns to consider include head injury, rib or lung injury, and abdominal injury.

Primary and Secondary Surveys

Primary Survey

The first steps of any patient assessment are to ensure scene safety and evaluate the situation. Once the scene is as safe as possible, the patient can be assessed. The primary survey is based on components necessary for sustaining life: airway, breathing, and circulation.

Although angulated fractures or partial amputations may draw the prehospital care practitioner's attention because of their visual impact, life-threatening conditions must take priority. Exsanguinating hemorrhage, airway, breathing, circulation, disability, and expose/environment (XABCDE) remain the most important parts of the primary survey. For a patient with life-threatening conditions identified in the primary survey, management of musculoskeletal trauma should be delayed until those problems are corrected. Exsanguinating external hemorrhage (X) is often due to musculoskeletal causes and should be addressed first in the primary survey, typically with direct pressure followed by immediate proximal tourniquet application. If the patient has life-threatening injuries, the prehospital care practitioner will next assess and address airway, breathing, and circulation. If the patient has no life-threatening injuries, the practitioner can proceed to the secondary survey.

Secondary Survey

With the exception of assessing and addressing exsanguinating extremity hemorrhage, which occurs during the primary survey, assessment of the extremities occurs during the secondary survey. To facilitate the physical examination, the prehospital care practitioner considers removing any clothing that was not removed during the primary survey, as allowed by the environment. If the mechanism of injury is not obvious, every effort should be made to safely expose the pelvis and both upper and lower extremities, including the hands and feet. Additionally, the patient or bystanders can be questioned about how the injuries occurred. The patient should also be queried about the presence of pain in the extremities. Most patients with significant musculoskeletal injuries have pain, unless a spinal cord injury is present.

Assessment of the extremities includes evaluating any pain, weakness, or abnormal sensations in the extremities. Specific attention is paid to the following:

- *Injury to the bones and joints*. This evaluation is accomplished by inspecting for deformities that may represent fractures or dislocations (**Table 12-1**) and palpating the extremity for tenderness and crepitus. The lack of these physical findings does not exclude the possibility of fracture or other musculoskeletal injury. Crepitus is the grinding feeling that bones make when the fractured ends rub against one another. Crepitus can be elicited by palpating the site of injury and by movement of the extremity. Crepitus sounds like a "snap, crackle, and pop" or the popping of plastic "bubble wrap" used for packing. This feeling of bones grating against one another during the assessment of a patient can produce further injury; therefore, once the crepitus is noted, no additional or repetitive steps should be taken to produce it. Crepitus is a distinct feeling that is not easily forgotten, and immediate immobilization is indicated once it has been identified.
- *Soft-tissue injuries*. The prehospital care practitioner visually inspects for swelling, lacerations, abrasions, hematomas, skin color, and wounds. Consider the possibility that a wound close to an apparent fracture is an open fracture. Firmness and tenseness of the soft tissues along with pain that appears out of proportion to the general findings may indicate the presence of a **compartment syndrome**. Compartment syndrome is a limb-threatening injury and should be communicated to the hospital practitioner (management of compartment syndrome is discussed later in this chapter).
- *Perfusion*. Perfusion should be evaluated by identifying the most distal palpable pulse (radial or ulnar in the upper extremity and dorsalis pedis or posterior tibial in the lower extremity) and noting capillary refill time in the fingers or toes. Absence of distal pulses

Table 12-1 Common Joint Dislocation Deformities

Joint	Direction	Deformity
Shoulder	Anterior	Abducted and externally rotated
	Posterior	Locked in internal rotation
Elbow	Posterior	Olecranon prominent posteriorly
Hip	Anterior	Extended, abducted, externally rotated
	Posterior	Flexed, adducted, internally rotated
Knee	Anteroposterior	Loss of normal contour, extended*
Ankle	Lateral is most common	Externally rotated, prominent medial malleolus
Subtalar joint	Lateral is most common	Laterally displaced os calcis (calcaneus)

*May spontaneously reduce prior to evaluation

Reproduced from American College of Surgeons Committee on Trauma. *Advanced Trauma Life Support*. 10th ed. Author; 2018:155.

Table 12-2 Peripheral Nerve Assessment of Upper Extremities

Nerve	Motor	Sensation	Anticipated Injury Location
Ulnar	Index and little finger abduction	Little finger	Elbow injury
Median distal	Thenar contraction with opposition	Distal tip of index finger	Wrist fracture or dislocation
Median, anterior interosseous	Index tip flexion	None	Supracondylar fracture of humerus (children)
Musculocutaneous	Elbow flexion	Radial forearm	Anterior shoulder dislocation
Radial	Thumb, finger metacarpophalangeal extension	First dorsal web space	Distal humeral shaft, anterior shoulder dislocation
Axillary	Deltoid	Lateral shoulder	Anterior shoulder dislocation, proximal humerus fracture

Reproduced from American College of Surgeons Committee on Trauma. *Advanced Trauma Life Support*. 10th ed. Author; 2018:161.

in the extremities can indicate disruption of an artery, compression of the vessel by a hematoma or bone fragment, or a compartment syndrome. Large or expanding hematomas may indicate the presence of an injury to a large vessel.

• *Neurologic function.* The prehospital care practitioner's neurologic assessment should include both motor and sensory function in both upper and lower extremities. For most situations in the prehospital setting, evaluating gross neurologic functioning is sufficient. **Table 12-2** shows large nerve motor and sensory distributions with the most common associated location of injury. Lack of injury at the anticipated site in the presence of nerve dysfunction should prompt practitioners to ask more questions and the need of further examination.

Table 12-3 Peripheral Nerve Assessment of Lower Extremities

Nerve	Motor	Sensation	Injury
Femoral	Knee extension	Anterior knee	Pubic rami fractures
Obturator	Hip adduction	Medial thigh	Obturator ring fractures
Posterior tibial	Toe flexion	Sole of foot	Knee dislocation
Superficial peroneal	Ankle eversion	Lateral dorsum of foot	Fibular neck fracture, knee dislocation
Deep peroneal	Ankle/toe dorsiflexion	Dorsal first to second web space	Fibular neck fracture, compartment syndrome
Sciatic nerve	Ankle dorsiflexion or plantar flexion	Foot	Posterior hip dislocation
Superior gluteal	Hip abduction	Upper buttocks	Acetabular fracture
Inferior gluteal	Gluteus maximus hip extension	Lower buttocks	Acetabular fracture

Reproduced from American College of Surgeons Committee on Trauma. *Advanced Trauma Life Support*. 10th ed. Author; 2018:161.

- *Motor function*. Motor function can be assessed by first asking the patient if any weakness is noted. Motor function in the upper extremity is evaluated by having the patient open and close a fist and by testing the patient's grip strength (the patient squeezes the prehospital care practitioner's fingers), while lower extremity motor function is tested by having the patient wiggle the toes and push-pull against the examiner's hands with the feet. A patient's ability to clench gluteal muscles and squeeze the buttock cheeks does not eliminate the need for a rectal examination during a full neurologic examination once the patient reaches the hospital.
- *Sensory function*. Sensory function is evaluated by asking about the presence of any deficits or changes in sensations. Sensory function should be tested at the most distal aspect of each extremity. Table 12-2 and **Table 12-3** provide information on performing more detailed evaluations of motor and sensory function of the extremities.

Repeat evaluation of extremity perfusion and neurologic functioning should be performed after any splinting procedure.

Associated Injuries

While performing the secondary survey, clues based on the mechanism of injury may help uncover particular commonly associated injury patterns. Such injury patterns can prompt the prehospital care practitioner to assess for occult injuries associated with specific fractures. **Table 12-4** provides some examples of associated injuries.

Specific Musculoskeletal Injuries

Injuries to the extremities result in two primary problems that require management in the prehospital setting: hemorrhage and pulselessness.

Hemorrhage

Bleeding can be dramatic or subtle. Regardless of the wound's appearance, it is the amount of blood lost and the rate of its loss that determines whether the patient will be able to compensate for the loss of blood volume or whether the patient will descend into shock. A good rule to remember is, "No bleeding is minor; every red blood cell counts." Even a small trickle of blood can add up to substantial blood loss if it is ignored for a long enough period.

External Hemorrhage

External arterial bleeding should be identified during the primary survey, as it can be life threatening. Generally, this type of bleeding is easily recognized, but assessment can be difficult when blood is hidden underneath a

Table 12-4 Injuries Commonly Associated With Musculoskeletal Trauma	
Musculoskeletal Injury	**Missed/Associated Injury**
Clavicular fracture Scapular fracture Fracture and/or dislocation of shoulder	Major thoracic injury, especially pulmonary contusion and rib fractures Scapulothoracic dissociation
Fracture/dislocation of elbow	Brachial artery injury Median, ulnar, and radial nerve injury
Femur fracture	Femoral neck fracture Ligamentous knee injury Posterior hip dislocation
Posterior knee dislocation	Femoral fracture Posterior hip dislocation
Knee dislocation Displaced tibial plateau	Popliteal artery and nerve injuries
Calcaneal fracture	Spine injury or fracture Fracture-dislocation of talus and calcaneus Tibial plateau fracture
Open fracture	High incidence of associated nonskeletal injury

Reproduced from American College of Surgeons Committee on Trauma. *Advanced Trauma Life Support.* 10th ed. Author; 2018:164.

patient or in heavy or dark clothing. Obvious hemorrhage requires immediate attention and should be assessed and controlled while or even before the patient's airway and breathing are being managed.

Estimation of external blood loss can be extremely difficult. Although less experienced individuals tend to overestimate the amount of external hemorrhage, underestimation is also possible, as overt signs of external blood loss are not always apparent. One study suggested that prehospital estimates of blood loss were inaccurate and not clinically beneficial.[1] The reasons for these inaccurate blood loss estimates are many and include that the patient may have been moved from the site of injury or that lost blood may have been absorbed by clothing or soil or washed away in water or by rain. Regardless of accuracy of estimated blood loss, prehospital control of external hemorrhage remains a crucial lifesaving intervention.

Internal Hemorrhage

Internal hemorrhage is common with musculoskeletal trauma, and it is often missed. It may result from damage to major blood vessels (many of which are located in close proximity to the long bones of the body), from disrupted muscle, and from fractured bones. Continued swelling of an extremity or a cold, pale, pulseless extremity could indicate internal hemorrhage from major

arteries or veins. Significant internal blood loss can be associated with fractures. Open fractures can be associated with a combination of internal and external hemorrhage that is substantial, but supporting data for the amount of blood lost for any given fracture are lacking. Nonetheless, the thigh and pelvis can hold enough volume to make the blood loss life threatening.

Both the potential internal and the external blood loss associated with extremity trauma must be considered when evaluating the patient. This will help the prehospital care practitioner anticipate the potential for the development of shock, prepare for the possibility of systemic deterioration, and intervene appropriately to minimize its occurrence.

Management

The initial management of external hemorrhage involves the application of direct pressure to the wound. Elevation of an extremity has not been shown to slow hemorrhage, and in musculoskeletal trauma, it may aggravate injuries that are present. (See discussion in Chapter 3, *Shock: Pathophysiology of Life and Death.*) If external hemorrhage is not immediately and completely controlled with direct pressure or a pressure dressing, a tourniquet should be applied. (Follow the principles described in Chapter 3, *Shock: Pathophysiology of Life and Death.*) A second tourniquet should be applied next to the first if hemorrhage control is not achieved with placement of the first tourniquet. A recommended topical hemostatic agent can be considered for hemorrhage that is not amenable to use of a tourniquet, such as in the groin or axilla. Such agents may also be considered for prolonged transport situations.

Tourniquet use is the standard of care in the prehospital management of exsanguinating extremity injuries. See Chapter 3, *Shock: Pathophysiology of Life and Death* for an in-depth discussion of prehospital tourniquet use.

Internal hemorrhage associated with extremity trauma can be substantial and can lead to shock in some situations. Like all other internal hemorrhage, management of internal extremity hemorrhage in the field is difficult and may be only marginally effective. Immobilization of fractures may help. In cases of pelvic fracture with instability, a pelvic binder or sheet wrapped around the pelvis may effectively reduce pelvic volume and thus indirectly reduce hemorrhage.

After controlling bleeding in patients with life-threatening hemorrhage from an extremity, prehospital care practitioners can repeat the primary survey and focus on airway, breathing, and circulation resuscitation and rapid transport to the facility that can best treat the patient's condition. During transport, administration of oxygen and initiation of intravenous (IV) fluid resuscitation for patients with shock can begin, keeping in mind that when internal hemorrhage is suspected, the target systolic blood pressure is 80 to 90 mm Hg (mean blood pressure is 60 to 65 mm Hg) and 110 mm Hg for patients with suspected traumatic brain injury. For patients with minor bleeding and no signs of shock or other life-threatening problems, bleeding can be controlled with direct pressure, and the secondary survey should be performed.

Pulseless Extremity

During your assessment of the patient, when trying to locate and identify distal pulses on each of the extremities, one thing to consider is that the fracture deformity may be the cause of decreased limb perfusion. In general, once the primary survey has been completed (XABCs), if there is a deformed limb that is noted to be without a pulse, attempt to realign the limb to the general appearance of an uninjured extremity. At that point, recheck pulses to see if the realignment helped restore blood flow. It is important to note that the purpose of this realignment is not to reduce an open fracture, restore function, or definitively treat the injury. The purpose is simply to provide a direct path for blood flow and remove any kink or compression of the vessels that may be caused by the deformity.

If pulses are restored or capillary refill is appropriate, this is the position in which the extremity should be splinted. This information should be communicated to the receiving facility.

The same mechanism of action that creates compartment syndrome can also cause distal occlusion from bleeding and associated swelling within isolated compartments proximally in the extremities. Assessing for a compartment syndrome (discussed later in this chapter) should be considered in evaluation of a pulseless extremity. Remember, a pulseless extremity is a limb-threatening injury, and transport to a hospital with immediate surgical capabilities is crucial.

Pelvic Fracture

Severe pelvic fractures or other severe disruptions of the pelvic ring present a number of challenging problems for prehospital care practitioners (**Figure 12-4**). The first is identification of a patient who is hemodynamically unstable from a pelvis fracture. In the field, consideration of the mechanism of injury, amount of energy imparted on the body during the injury, and the lower extremity deformity are additional ways to assess for pelvic injury. Potentially, an accurate assessment can mean the difference between life and death. Few injuries in orthopedics are truly life threatening, but pelvic ring disruptions can be.

The greatest immediate concern in pelvic fracture is internal hemorrhage, which can be very difficult to manage. Pelvic fractures can range from minor, relatively insignificant fractures to life-threatening injuries associated with massive internal and external hemorrhage (**Box 12-1**). Fractures of the **pelvic ring** are associated with overall mortality rates ranging from 9% to 20%. Furthermore, the presence of a pelvic ring fracture in blunt trauma is an independent risk factor for death

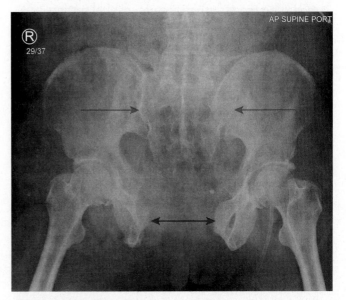

Figure 12-4 Severe pelvic ring disruption. The blue arrows show marked anterior symphyseal widening. The red arrows show bilateral sacroiliac injuries posteriorly.

Courtesy of Andrew Pollak, MD.

Box 12-1 Pelvic Binders

At least three pelvic binders are commercially available: PelvicBinder® (PelvicBinder, Inc.), SAM® Pelvic Sling II (SAM Medical Products), and Trauma Pelvic Orthotic Device (T-POD; Teleflex, Inc.).

Rationale

Some pelvic ring fractures are associated with an increase in the pelvic volume, permitting large amounts of intra-abdominal hemorrhage. Because the volume is increased, there is less tissue surrounding the pelvis to **tamponade** bleeding. Patients with hemodynamic instability often undergo surgical application of pelvic external fixation to help reduce the volume and assist with hemodynamic stability. This measure should be an afterthought to field application of a binder.

Binder Use

The concern for causing further injury during the application of a potential lifesaving pelvic binder should not prevent the application of a binder. The energy imparted on the body at the time of the initial trauma is far greater than that caused by a logroll or positioning while applying the binder. The literature has shown no detrimental effect to applying a binder early, even after full radiographic evaluation suggested it was not warranted.[3] Not applying one, however, in the context of major pelvic ring disruption with increased intrapelvic volume, could result in fatal exsanguination. Overall, the literature regarding binder use in the prehospital setting is relatively low quality regarding the magnitude of benefit, but there is unlikely to be any significant detrimental effect from placement in the prehospital setting.[4]

and doubles the chance of death.[2] Patients with pelvic fractures frequently have associated injuries, including traumatic brain injuries, long-bone fractures, thoracic injuries, urethral disruption in men, splenic trauma, and liver and kidney trauma.

To assess the pelvis, gentle manual pressure anterior to posterior and from the sides may identify crepitus or instability. Palpation over the mons pubis region may demonstrate a large gap between the left and right hemipelvis, indicating significant pelvic ring disruption. Once identified by physical exam, further examination to assess pelvic stability is contraindicated, as it could lead to worsening hemorrhage or clot disruption.

Open fractures of the pelvis may lacerate the rectum or vagina, and an obvious source of external blood loss may not be readily apparent. It is not the role of the prehospital care practitioner to identify and classify pelvic fracture patterns or to determine whether there is a hidden laceration making it an open fracture. The primary goal is to identify life-threatening pelvic fractures and provide appropriate treatment.

Some pelvic ring fractures are associated with an increase in pelvic volume due to the fracture pattern and degree of displacement, thus allowing large volumes of intrapelvic hemorrhage to occur that can be life threatening. Closed reduction of the pelvis by application of a binder requires simple, but specific, placement to ensure it does what it is supposed to do. A binder is designed for hemodynamic stabilization by limiting intrapelvic volume and therefore decreasing blood loss associated with pelvis fractures; it is not designed for fracture stabilization. In the prehospital environment, the ability to reliably ascertain stable versus unstable pelvic ring injuries has proven to be quite difficult.[5-7] There is limited evidence that pelvic binders applied prior to radiographic evaluation may decrease hospital and intensive care unit (ICU) lengths of stay and decrease initial transfusion requirements.[8] Therefore, in the setting of an appropriate mechanism of injury (high-energy) and clinical concern for pelvic ring injury (especially in the setting of hemodynamic instability), consensus recommendation is to apply a pelvic binder in the prehospital setting.[9-11]

The binder should be centered over the greater trochanters, not the pelvic brim. Commonly, binders are placed too superiorly, which can compress the abdomen and, in extreme cases, make it difficult to ventilate. Confirming the proper location allows for the transfer of compression from the binder to the pelvis regardless of body habitus. The result of proper placement is a reduction of pelvic volume, stabilization of the pelvis, and, ideally, a decrease in ongoing bleeding.

Femur Fracture

Femur fractures, like pelvis injuries, can be life threatening due to the large amount of associated hemorrhage into each thigh. An adult can lose enough blood from a femur fracture to develop hemodynamic instability and shock. In the absence of life-threatening conditions, a traction splint should be applied to stabilize suspected midshaft femoral fractures. The application of traction, both manually and by use of a mechanical device, can help decrease internal bleeding as well as decrease the patient's pain.

Splinting the femur represents a unique splinting situation because of the musculature of the thigh. The powerful thigh muscles often make reduction, realignment, and stabilization with splinting or traction difficult.

Contraindications to the use of a traction splint include the following:

- Avulsion or amputation of the ipsilateral ankle and foot
- Suspected fractures adjacent to the knee (A traction splint may be used as a rigid splint in this situation, but traction should not be applied.)

Instability (Fractures and Dislocations)

Tears of the supporting structures of a joint, fracture of a bone, and major muscle or tendon injury contribute to the instability of an injured extremity.

Fractures

If a bone is fractured, immobilizing it may decrease pain. The energy imparted at the time of injury to cause a fracture causes more damage and injury than anything a prehospital practitioner can do by realigning an extremity and immobilizing it with a splint or traction.

In general, fractures are classified as either closed or open. In a **closed fracture**, the skin is not open to bone, whereas in an **open fracture**, the integrity of the skin has been interrupted and bone is functionally or even potentially grossly exposed (**Figure 12-5A**). Orthopaedic surgeons may classify fractures by their patterns, but knowledge of the fracture pattern does not alter field management, whereas knowledge of the associated skin integrity might.

Closed Fractures

Closed fractures are fractures in which the bone has been broken but the patient has no associated loss of skin integrity (i.e., the skin is not broken in the region of the fracture; **Figure 12-5B**). Signs of a closed fracture include pain, tenderness, deformity, hematomas, swelling, and crepitus. In some patients, however, pain and tenderness may be the only findings. Pulses, skin color, and motor and sensory function should be assessed distal to the suspected fracture site. It is not always true that an extremity is not fractured because the patient can voluntarily move it or, in the case of a lower extremity, even walk on it; adrenalin from a traumatic event may motivate patients to endure pain they would not tolerate normally. Additionally, some patients have a remarkably high pain tolerance.

Open Fractures

Open fractures usually occur when a sharp bone end penetrates the skin from the inside out or, less commonly, when the trauma or an object lacerates the skin and muscle at a fracture site (from the outside in; **Figure 12-5C**). When a fracture is open to the outside environment, the

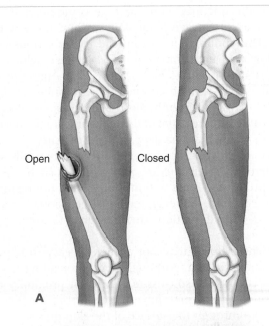

Open   Closed

A

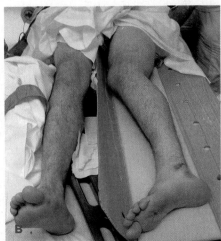

B

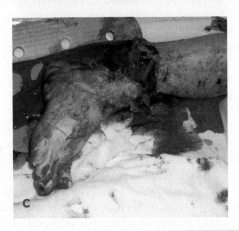

C

Figure 12-5 A. Open versus closed fracture. **B.** Closed fracture of the femur. Note the internal rotation and shortening of the left leg. **C.** Open fracture of the tibia.

A. © National Association of Emergency Medical Technicians (NAEMT); B. Courtesy of Norman McSwain, MD, FACS, NREMT-P; C. Courtesy of Peter T. Pons, MD, FACEP.

ends of the fractured bone become contaminated with bacteria from the overlying skin or from the environment. This contamination can lead to the serious complication of a bone infection (*osteomyelitis*), which can interfere with healing of the fracture. Although the skin wound associated with an open fracture often is not associated with significant hemorrhage, persistent bleeding may come from the canal of the bone or from the decompression of a hematoma deep inside the tissue.

Any open wound near a possible fracture needs to be considered an open fracture and treated as such. Generally, a protruding bone or bone end should not be intentionally replaced; however, the bones occasionally return to a near-normal position when realigned for splinting or immobilization.

Open fractures may not always be easy to identify in a trauma patient. Although bone protruding from a wound is obvious, soft-tissue injuries in proximity to a fracture/deformity may have resulted from a bone end that broke through the surface of the skin only to recede back into the tissue.

Management

The first consideration in managing fractures is to control hemorrhage and treat for shock. Direct pressure and pressure dressings will control virtually all external hemorrhage encountered in the field. Open wounds or exposed bone ends should be covered with a sterile dressing moistened with sterile normal saline or water. Consider realigning the deformed extremity at time of splinting for pain control, ease of splinting, fracture stabilization, and possibly, to improve perfusion by restoration of gross limb alignment. If the bone ends of an open fracture retract into the wound during reduction or splinting, this information must be documented on the PCR and reported to ED personnel. Some recent literature supports the administration of weight-based antibiotics, and some data show that earlier delivery of antibiotics may reduce infection rates. Antibiotic administration is controversial. There is, however, no evidence that field administration of antibiotics in urban or suburban environments decreases infection rates.[12]

Prior to splinting, an injured extremity should generally be returned to its normal anatomic position, including the use of gentle traction if necessary to realign an extremity to its normal length as best as possible and within reasonable clinical judgment. A "reduced fracture," one that is returned to normal anatomic alignment, is easier to splint. Second, restoring alignment may alleviate compression of arteries or nerves and result in improved perfusion and neurologic functioning. Realigning fractures also decreases hemorrhage and assists with pain control.

If the fracture is open and bone is exposed, the bone end should be gently rinsed with sterile water or normal saline (as time allows) to remove obvious contamination prior to an attempt to restore normal anatomic position. It is not of major concern if the bone ends retract back into the skin during this manipulation, as open fractures require irrigation and **debridement** in the operating room regardless. However, the fact that the bone was exposed prior to reduction is key information that should be passed on during the patient report at the receiving facility. No more than two attempts should be made to restore an extremity to normal position, and, if unsuccessful, the extremity should be splinted "as is."

The primary objective of splinting is to prevent movement of the fractured body part. Doing so will help decrease the patient's pain and stabilize the fragments. To immobilize any long bone in an extremity effectively, the entire limb should be immobilized. To do this, the injured site should be supported manually while the joint and bone above (proximal to) and the joint and bone below (distal to) the injury site are immobilized. Numerous types of splints are available, and most can be used with both open and closed fractures (**Box 12-2**). With virtually all splinting techniques, further inspection of the extremity is limited, and therefore a thorough assessment should be performed before splinting.

Four additional points are important to remember when applying any type of splint:

1. Pad splints to prevent movement of the extremity inside the splint, to help increase the patient's comfort, and to prevent pressure sores.

Box 12-2 Types of Splints

Various splints and splinting materials are available (**Figure 12-6**), including the following:

- *Rigid splints* cannot be changed in shape. They require that the body part be positioned to fit the splint's shape. Examples of rigid splints include board splints (wood, plastic, or metal) and backboards. Rigid splints are best used for long-bone injuries.
- *Formable splints* can be molded into various shapes and combinations to accommodate the shape of the injured extremity. Examples of formable splints include vacuum splints, air splints, pillows, blankets, cardboard splints, wire-ladder splints, and foam-covered moldable metal splints. Formable splints are best used for ankle, wrist, and long-bone injuries.
- *Traction splints* are designed to maintain mechanical in-line traction to help realign fractures. Traction splints are most often used to stabilize femur shaft fractures.

© National Association of Emergency Medical Technicians (NAEMT)

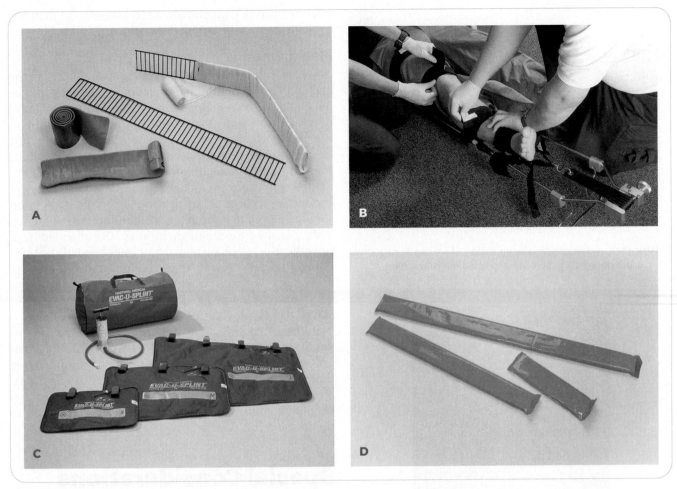

Figure 12-6 **A.** Formable splint. **B.** Traction splint. **C.** Vacuum splint. **D.** Board splint.

A & D. © National Association of Emergency Medical Technicians (NAEMT); **B.** © Jones & Bartlett Learning. Photographed by Darren Stahlman. **C.** Courtesy of Hartwell Medical.

2. Remove jewelry and watches so that these objects will not inhibit circulation as additional swelling occurs. Lubrication with soap, lotion, or a water-soluble jelly may facilitate removal of tight rings.

3. Assess neurovascular functions distal to the injury site before and after applying any splint and periodically thereafter. A pulseless extremity indicates either a vascular injury or a compartment syndrome, and rapid transport to an appropriate facility becomes even more of a priority.

4. After splinting, consider elevating the extremity, if possible, to decrease edema and throbbing. Ice or cold packs can also be used to decrease pain and swelling and may be placed on the splinted extremity near the suspected fracture site.

Dislocations

Joints are held together by ligaments. The bones that make up a joint are attached to their muscles by tendons.

Movement of an extremity is accomplished by the contraction (shortening) of muscles. This reduction of muscle length pulls the tendons that are attached to a bone and moves the extremity at a joint. A dislocation is a separation of two bones at the joint, resulting from significant disruption to the ligaments that normally provide supporting structure and stability at a joint (**Figure 12-7** and **Figure 12-8**). A dislocation, similar to a fracture, produces an area of instability that the prehospital care practitioner needs to secure. Dislocations can produce great pain. A dislocation can be difficult to distinguish clinically from a fracture without radiographic evaluation and may be associated with fractures as well (fracture-dislocation). Deformity of a joint provides a clue to the type and direction of dislocation.

The proper description to provide to the hospital practitioner should be based on the more distal segment when describing the dislocation. For example, a knee dislocation is based on the direction the tibia travels in relation to the femur. A posterior knee dislocation means the tibia is posterior to the femur.

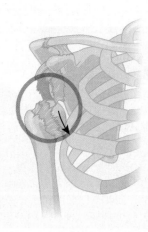

Figure 12-7 A dislocation is a separation of a bone from a joint; the picture depicts a typical anterior shoulder dislocation.

© Jones & Bartlett Learning

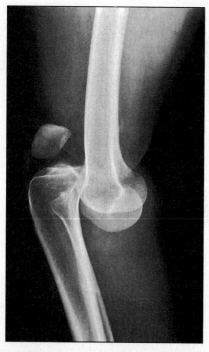

Figure 12-8 Right anterior knee dislocation with overriding tibia on the femur. Note the tibia (distal segment) has traveled anterior to the femur (proximal segment).

© Steven Needell/Science Source

Individuals who have had prior dislocations have ligaments that are more lax than normal and may be prone to more frequent dislocations unless the problem is corrected surgically. Unlike those sustaining a dislocation for the first time, these patients are often familiar with their injury and can help in assessment and stabilization. Chronic or frequent dislocators do not necessarily need a field reduction attempted. Taking these patients to the hospital with dislocated joints when they are unable to self-reduce them is often less dangerous and better tolerated from a pain and discomfort standpoint than it is for patients with first-time dislocations.

Management

As a rule, suspected dislocations should be splinted in the position found. Gentle manipulation of the joint can be done to try to return blood flow when the pulse is absent or weak. Realignment may improve the vascular status of the patient's limb. When faced with a brief transport time to the hospital, however, the better decision is to initiate transport rather than attempt manipulation. This manipulation will cause the patient great pain, so the patient should be prepared before moving the extremity. A splint should be used to immobilize most dislocations, whereas a sling is used for shoulder injuries. Documentation of how the injury was sustained and found and of the presence of pulses, movement, sensation, and color before and after splinting is important. During transport, ice or cold packs can be used to decrease pain and swelling. Analgesia can be provided as necessary to reduce pain.

Attempted reduction of a dislocation should be undertaken only when permitted by written protocols or online medical control and when the prehospital care practitioner has been properly trained in the appropriate techniques. All attempts at reduction of a dislocation should be properly documented and communicated to the hospital clinician.

Special Considerations

Critical Multisystem Trauma Patient

Adherence to the primary survey priorities in patients with multisystem trauma that includes injured extremities does not imply that extremity injuries should be ignored or that injured extremities should not be protected from further harm. Rather, it means that *life takes precedence over limb* when faced with a critically injured trauma patient with extremity injuries that are not life threatening. The focus should be on maintaining vital functions through resuscitation, and only limited measures should be taken to address the extremity injuries, regardless of how dramatic the injuries appear. By properly immobilizing a patient to a backboard or other full body immobilization device such as a vacuum mattress, all extremities and the entire skeleton are essentially splinted in an anatomic position and the patient is easily moved. A secondary survey can be omitted if the life-threatening problems identified in the primary survey require ongoing interventions and if transport time is short. If a secondary survey is deferred, the prehospital care practitioner can simply document the findings that precluded performing the secondary survey.

Compartment Syndrome

Compartment syndrome refers to a limb-threatening condition in which the blood supply to an extremity is compromised by increased pressure within that limb. The muscles of extremities are enveloped by dense connective tissue called **fascia**. This fascia forms numerous compartments in the extremities in which the muscles are contained. Muscle fascia has minimal stretch, and anything that increases the pressure inside the compartments may result in a compartment syndrome.

The two most common causes of compartment syndrome are hemorrhage within a compartment from a fracture or vascular injury and third-space edema that forms when ischemic muscle tissue is reperfused after a period of diminished or absent blood flow. However, a splint or cast that is applied too tightly may produce a compartment syndrome by external compression. As the pressure in the compartment increases beyond that of capillary pressure, blood flow is impaired through the capillaries. The tissue served by these vessels then becomes ischemic. The pressure may continue to build to the point that even arterial flow and nerve function are compromised by compression.

The two early signs of a developing compartment syndrome are (1) pain that is above the baseline pain appropriate to the trauma and that does not respond to pain-relieving measures and (2) altered sensation (abnormal sensations or reduced/absent sensation) of the involved extremity. Pain is often described as out of proportion to the injury. This pain may be dramatically increased on passive movement of a finger or toe in that extremity. Nerves are extremely sensitive to their blood supply, and any compromised blood flow will manifest as paresthesia. The fact that these symptoms are normally associated with a fracture underscores the need for baseline circulatory, motor, and sensory examinations followed by serial examinations so that the prehospital care practitioner can identify changes.

The other three classical signs of compartment syndrome—pulselessness, pallor, and paralysis—are late findings and indicate a clear compartment syndrome and a limb that is in jeopardy of necrosis (muscle death). Compartments may be extremely tense and firm to palpation, although it is difficult to judge the compartment pressures by physical examination alone.

Management

In the hospital, compartment pressures can be measured by hospital clinicians in extremities where compartment syndrome is suspected. Compartment syndrome must be definitively managed with emergent surgical intervention (*fasciotomy*), which involves an incision through the skin and fascia into the affected compartments to decompress the affected muscle tissue.

Only basic maneuvers can be attempted in the field. Any tightly applied splint or dressings should be removed and distal perfusion reassessed. Splinting the extremity provides stability. Elevation of the extremity is not recommended. Keeping the extremity level with the heart is ideal. Additionally, the ankle should be dorsiflexed when splinted to reduce anterior compartment pressure on the lower leg. Because compartment syndrome may develop during a long-distance transfer, serial examinations are essential for early identification of this problem.

Mangled Extremity

A "mangled extremity" refers to a complex injury resulting from high-energy transfer in which significant injury occurs to two or more of the following: (1) skin and muscle, (2) tendons, (3) bone, (4) blood vessels, and (5) nerves (**Figure 12-9**). Common mechanisms producing mangled extremities include motorcycle crash, ejection from a motor vehicle, and a pedestrian being struck by an automobile. When encountered, patients may be in shock from either external blood loss or hemorrhage from associated injuries, which are common because of the high-energy mechanism. Most mangled extremities involve severe open fractures, and amputation is frequently necessary. Limb salvage is possible in some patients, typically involving multiple surgical procedures, and substantial long-term disability is common.

Management

Even with a mangled extremity, the focus is still on the primary survey to rule out or address life-threatening conditions. Hemorrhage control, including the use of a tourniquet, may be required. The mangled extremity

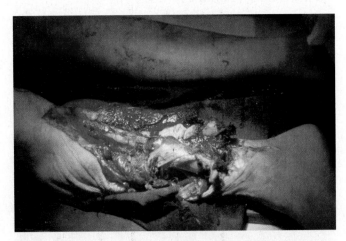

Figure 12-9 Mangled extremity resulting from crushing injury between two vehicles. The patient has fractures and extensive soft-tissue injury.
Courtesy of Peter T. Pons, MD, FACEP.

should be splinted, if the patient's condition allows. These patients are probably best cared for at high-volume level I trauma centers.

Amputations

When tissue has been totally separated from an extremity, the tissue is completely without nutrition and oxygenation. This type of injury is termed an amputation. An amputation is the loss of part or all of a limb. All amputations may be accompanied by significant bleeding, but it is more common with partial amputations. When vessels are completely transected, they retract and constrict, and blood clots may form, decreasing or stopping hemorrhage; however, when a vessel is only partially transected, the two ends cannot retract, and blood continues to pour out of the hole.

Amputations are often evident on the scene (**Figure 12-10**). This type of injury receives great attention from bystanders, and the patient may or may not know that the extremity is missing. Psychologically, the prehospital care practitioner needs to deal with this injury cautiously (**Box 12-3**).

The missing extremity should be located for possible reattachment. This is especially true for the upper extremity and thumb. Lower extremity amputations are generally not reattached in the setting of traumatic amputations because lower extremity prostheses are effective and the success of replantation in the lower extremity is poor.

The primary survey should be performed before looking for a missing extremity, unless adequate numbers of emergency response personnel are present to assist. The appearance of an amputation may be horrifying, but if the patient does not have a patent airway or is not breathing, the loss of the limb is secondary to the life-threatening priorities.

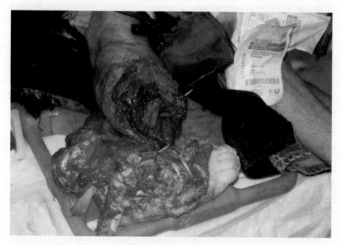

Figure 12-10 Complete amputation of the right leg after it became entangled in machinery.
Courtesy of Peter T. Pons, MD, FACEP..

Box 12-3 Phantom Pain

In some circumstances, the patient may complain of pain distal to the amputation. This "phantom pain" is the sensation that pain exists in a missing extremity. The reason for phantom pain is not understood completely, but the brain may not realize that the extremity is not present. This sensation usually is not present at the time of the injury.

© National Association of Emergency Medical Technicians (NAEMT)

Amputations can be very painful. Pain management should be employed as necessary once life-threatening problems have been excluded in the primary survey (**Figure 12-11**).

Management

Principles of managing an amputated part include the following:

1. Clean the amputated part by gentle rinsing with lactated Ringer (LR) solution.
2. Wrap the part in sterile gauze moistened with LR solution and place it in a plastic bag or container.
3. After labeling the bag or container, place it in an outer container filled with crushed ice.
4. Do not freeze the part by placing it directly on the ice or by adding another coolant such as dry ice.
5. Transport the part along with the patient to the closest appropriate facility.[13,14]

The longer the amputated portion is without oxygen, the less likely that it can be replaced successfully. Cooling the amputated body part, without freezing it, will reduce the metabolic rate and prolong this critical time. However, replantation is not a guarantee of successful attachment or ultimate function. Because lower extremity prostheses, particularly in the case of amputations below the knee, often allow the patient to resume a near-normal life, lower extremities are rarely considered for replantation. Furthermore, only cleanly separated amputations in otherwise healthy, younger individuals are usually considered for replantation. Smokers are less likely to have successful replantation because the nicotine in tobacco is a potent vasoconstrictor and may compromise blood flow to the replanted segment. Patients who are candidates for replantation of fingers (particularly the thumb) or a hand/forearm should be transported to a level I trauma center with specific replantation capabilities because level II and III facilities often lack replantation capability. Ultimately, it will be up to the surgical team to determine whether a replantation is possible.

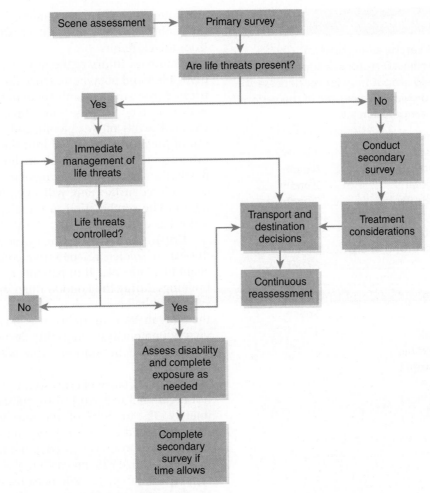

Figure 12-11 Primary survey algorithm.
© National Association of Emergency Medical Technicians (NAEMT)

Transport of a patient should not be delayed to locate a missing amputated part. If the amputated part is not readily found, law enforcement officials or other emergency responders should remain at the scene to search for it. When the amputated part is transported in a separate vehicle from the patient, the prehospital care practitioner must ensure that the transporters of the amputated part understand clearly where the patient is being transported and how to handle the part once it is located. The receiving facility should be notified as soon as the part is located, and transport of the part should be initiated as soon as possible.

Field Amputation

In general, many extremities that appear hopelessly entrapped can be released with additional extrication expertise. If the patient has an extremity entangled in a machine, an often-overlooked expert is the maintenance person who repairs the machine. This person usually has the technical knowledge to expeditiously disassemble and remove parts from a machine, allowing extrication. On rare occasions, however, a patient may

have an entrapped extremity for which a field amputation may be the only reasonable option. A regional trauma system should consider development of an appropriately equipped field amputation team (**Box 12-4**). While rarely used, such a team has been shown to save lives.[15] Although formal field amputation is not considered part of the scope of practice of prehospital care practitioners in the United States, some entrapped extremities may be connected by only a small strand of tissue. The decision to cut this tissue or wait for a physician to arrive at the scene must be made in consultation with medical oversight. If a substantial amputation is necessary, it should ideally be performed by a trained physician because of the anatomic knowledge and technical expertise required. Significant sedation may need to be administered for the procedure, including general anesthesia and intubation.

Crush Syndrome

An extremity that is crushed during a traumatic injury can cause a reaction called rhabdomyolysis. This condition is associated with death of the muscle in the affected extremity and release of **myoglobin**. Clinically, rhabdomyolysis is characterized by renal failure, end-organ injury, and potentially, death. The timing of the impact from this myoglobin release is after the crushing force is removed from the extremity.

Traumatic injury to the muscle causes release of both myoglobin and potassium. Once the patient has been extricated, the affected limb suddenly becomes reperfused with new blood; at the same time, the old blood with elevated levels of myoglobin and potassium is washed out of the injured area and into the rest of the body. Elevated potassium can result in life-threatening cardiac dysrhythmias, and free myoglobin will produce tea- or cola-colored urine and will eventually result in renal failure. The combination of these events is typically described as crush syndrome.

Crush syndrome was first described in World War I in German soldiers rescued from collapsed trenches, then again in World War II in patients rescued from collapsed buildings during the London Blitz. In World War II, crush syndrome had a mortality rate in excess of 90%. During the Korean War, mortality was 84%, but after the advent of hemodialysis, mortality decreased to 53%. In the Vietnam War, the mortality rate was approximately the same, at 50%.

The importance of crush syndrome, however, should not be limited to historical or military interest. Approximately 3% to 20% of the survivors of earthquakes have sustained a crush injury, and approximately 40% of survivors from collapsed buildings will have crush injuries.[16-19] In 1978, an earthquake near Beijing, China, injured more than 350,000 persons, with 242,769 deaths. More than 48,000 of these people died from crush syndrome. More commonly, mechanisms of crush syndrome include entrapment from a trench collapse, construction collapse, or motor vehicle collision.

Patients with crush syndrome are identified by the following:

- Prolonged entrapment
- Traumatic injury to muscle mass
- Compromised circulation to the injured area

Of note, traumatic rhabdomyolysis can also occur in patients, often the elderly, who fall, perhaps fracture a hip, and are unable to get up or in patients who fall in a bathroom and become wedged next to the bathtub and toilet. They are found hours or days later, having lain in the same position, often on a hard surface. The weight of their body on the muscles for a prolonged period leads to muscle breakdown and the findings of traumatic rhabdomyolysis.

Management

The key to improving outcomes in crush syndrome is early and aggressive fluid resuscitation. It is important for the prehospital care practitioner to remember that toxins are accumulating within the entrapped limb during the extrication process. Once the entrapped limb is freed, the accumulated toxins wash into the central circulation, similar to a bolus of poison. Therefore, success will depend on minimizing the toxic effects of accumulated myoglobin and potassium before release of the limb. Resuscitation needs to begin before extrication.[20] A delay in fluid resuscitation will result in renal failure in 50% of the patients, and a delay of 12 hours or more produces renal failure in almost 100% of the patients. Some authors have advocated that final extrication be delayed until the patient has been adequately resuscitated.[21] A poorly resuscitated patient may go into cardiac arrest during extrication because of the sudden release of metabolic acid and potassium into the bloodstream when the compression on the extremity is released.[22]

Fluid resuscitation should proceed with normal saline at a rate of up to 1,500 milliliters per hour (mL/hr) to ensure adequate renal output of 150 to 200 mL/hr. LR solution is avoided until urine output is adequate because of the presence of potassium in the IV fluid. The addition of 50 milliequivalents (mEq) of sodium bicarbonate and 10 grams of mannitol to each liter of fluid used during the extrication period may help decrease the incidence of renal failure. Once the patient has been extricated, the normal saline fluids can be slowed to 500 mL/hr, alternating with 5% dextrose in water (D_5W), with one ampule of sodium bicarbonate per liter.[23]

Once the blood pressure is stabilized and volume status restored, attention is turned toward prophylaxis against **hyperkalemia** and the toxic effects of serum myoglobin. Hyperkalemia in the field can be recognized by the development of peaked T waves on the cardiac monitor. Treatment of the increased potassium follows standard protocols for hyperkalemia, including IV sodium bicarbonate administration, inhaled beta-agonists (albuterol), administration of dextrose and insulin (if available), and, if life-threatening cardiac dysrhythmias occur, IV calcium chloride. Alkalinization of the urine will provide some degree of protection to the kidneys; however, the key is to maintain increased urine output (typically in the range of 50 to 100 mL/hr).

Sprains

A **sprain** is an injury in which ligaments are stretched or torn. Sprains are caused by a sudden twisting of the joint beyond its normal range of motion. They are characterized by significant pain, swelling, and possible hematoma. Externally, sprains may resemble a fracture or dislocation. Definitive differentiation between a sprain and a fracture is accomplished only through a radiographic study. In the prehospital setting, it is reasonable to splint a suspected sprain in case it turns out to be a fracture or dislocation. An ice or cold pack may help relieve pain. Use of narcotic pain medication is generally not necessary or desirable and should be reserved for cases with significant pain that is unresponsive to splinting, elevation, and ice.

Management

The general management for suspected sprain includes the following steps:

1. Identify and treat any and all life-threatening injuries found in the primary survey.
2. Stop any external bleeding and treat the patient for shock.
3. Evaluate for distal neurovascular function.
4. Support the area of injury.
5. Immobilize the injured extremity.
6. Apply ice or cold packs to control pain and swelling.
7. Reevaluate the injured extremity after immobilization for changes in distal neurovascular function.

Prolonged Transport

Patients with extremity trauma often have coexisting injuries. Ongoing internal blood loss may be from abdominal or thoracic injuries, and during a prolonged transport, the primary survey will need to be reassessed frequently to ensure that all life-threatening conditions are identified and no new ones have emerged. Vital signs should be obtained at regular intervals. Intravenous crystalloid solutions should be administered at a rate to maintain adequate perfusion, unless significant internal hemorrhage is suspected in the pelvis, abdomen, or thorax. In settings where compartment syndrome is suspected, pulses are diminished, or active hemorrhage has occurred, frequent checks are necessary.

During long transports, the prehospital care practitioner needs to focus greater attention on extremity perfusion. In limbs with compromised vascular supply, the practitioner can attempt to restore normal anatomic positioning to optimize the chance for improved blood flow. Similarly, in the face of prolonged transport times, consideration should be given to reduction of dislocations with impaired distal circulation prior to initiation of transport. Distal perfusion, including pulses, color, and temperature, as well as motor and sensory function, should be examined in a serial manner. Compartments should be monitored for the development of a potential compartment syndrome. These examinations, including any changes that develop, should be carefully recorded and communicated to the clinician at the receiving facility.

Measures to ensure patient comfort should be taken. Splinting devices should be comfortable and well padded.

The limbs should be assessed for any pressure points inside the splint where pressure could contribute to the creation of an ulcer, especially in an extremity with compromised perfusion. Parenteral narcotic analgesia should be given at regular intervals if necessary, with careful monitoring of ventilatory rate, blood pressure, pulse oximetry, and capnography.

Contaminated wounds should be flushed with normal saline irrigation so that gross particulate matter (e.g., soil, grass) is removed. Antibiotics may be administered for open fractures if there is a prolonged transport or a delay to receiving care from a hospital practitioner. Guidelines exist for antibiotic type, and gram-positive coverage is typical (cephalosporin; e.g., Ancef), with many authors advocating addition of gram-negative coverage for more severe and contaminated injuries (aminoglycosides). Penicillin is added for farm injuries. If a body part has been amputated, it should also be periodically assessed so that it remains cool but does not freeze or become macerated (softened) by soaking in water.

SUMMARY

- In patients with multisystem trauma, attention is directed toward the primary survey first and the identification and management of all life-threatening injuries, including internal or external hemorrhage in the extremities.
- Prehospital care practitioners must be careful not to be distracted from addressing life-threatening conditions by the gross, dramatic appearance of any noncritical injuries or by the patient's request for their management.
- Once the patient has been fully assessed and found to have only isolated injuries without systemic implication, then noncritical injuries should be addressed.
- Musculoskeletal injuries should be immobilized for stability and to provide comfort and some relief from pain.

- Rapidly determining the mechanism of injury and energy transferred will help the prehospital care practitioner suspect and recognize the most critical injuries or conditions.
- The first consideration in managing fractures is to control hemorrhage and treat for shock.
- As a rule, suspected dislocations should be splinted in the position found.
- Crush syndrome results from the reperfusion of areas of the body that have been trapped and ischemic for prolonged periods of time. Damaged muscle tissue releases myoglobin and potassium into the bloodstream, which can be toxic to the kidneys and heart.

SCENARIO RECAP

It is a beautiful Saturday afternoon in June. You have been dispatched to a local motorcycle racetrack for a rider who has been injured. Upon arrival, you are escorted by track officials to an area on the track just in front of the grandstand where the track's medical crew (two-person, emergency medical responders, nontransport) is attending to a single patient lying supine on the track.

One of the emergency medical responders tells you that the patient was a rider in a 350-cc class race with 14 other motorcycles and that three of them collided in front of the grandstand. The other two riders were not injured, but the patient was unable to stand or move without significant pain in his right leg and pelvis. There was no loss of consciousness and no complaints other than leg pain. The medical crew has maintained the patient in a supine position with manual stabilization of the right lower extremity.

As you assess the patient, you find that he is a 19-year-old man, conscious and alert without past medical or trauma history. The patient's initial vital signs are as follows: blood pressure is 104/68 mm Hg, pulse is 112 beats/minute, respirations are 24 breaths/minute, and skin is pale and diaphoretic. The patient states that he collided with another rider when he came out of a corner and that the collision caused him to lose balance and slide across the track. He states his right leg was run over by at least one other bike. Visual inspection of

SCENARIO RECAP (CONTINUED)

his right leg reveals shortening of the leg and no open wounds when compared to the left side, with tenderness, and bruising of the mid-anterior thigh area.

- What does the mechanism of injury of this event tell you about the potential injuries for this patient?
- What type of injury do you suspect, and what would your management priorities be?

SCENARIO SOLUTION

After completing the primary survey and ensuring that this was an isolated musculoskeletal injury, with your partner's help, you were able to apply a traction splint to the midshaft femur fracture of the right leg. After securing your patient to a long backboard, you were able to move the patient to the ambulance for transport to the hospital. Once in the ambulance, oxygen via mask was administered, and an IV was established. The patient stated that after the splint was applied, his pain improved significantly and that he did not need any analgesic at the moment. The patient's vital signs remained unchanged throughout the transport.

References

1. Williams B, Boyle M. Estimation of external blood loss by paramedics: is there any point? *Prehosp Disaster Med.* 2007;22(6):502-506.

2. Shulman JE, O'Toole RV, Castillo RC, et al. Pelvic ring fractures are an independent risk factor for death after blunt trauma. *J Trauma.* 2010;68:930-934.

3. Pierrie SN, Seymour RB, Wally MK, Studnek J, Infinger A, Hsu JR; Evidence-based Musculoskeletal Injury and Trauma Collaborative (EMIT). Pilot randomized trial of pre-hospital advanced therapies for the control of hemorrhage (PATCH) using pelvic binders. *Am J Emerg Med.* 2021 Apr;42:43-48. doi: 10.1016/j.ajem.2020.12.082

4. Pap R, McKeown R, Lockwood C, Stephenson M, Simpson P. Pelvic circumferential compression devices for prehospital management of suspected pelvic fractures: a rapid review and evidence summary for quality indicator evaluation. *Scand J Trauma Resusc Emerg Med.* 2020;28(1):65.

5. van Leent EAP, van Wageningen BV, Sir Ö, Hermans E, Biert J. Clinical examination of the pelvic ring in the pre-hospital phase. *Air Med J.* 2019;38(4):294-297.

6. Zingg T, Piaget-Rosssel R, Steppacher J, et al. Prehospital use of pelvic circumferential compression devices in a physician-based emergency medical service: a 6-year retrospective cohort study. *Sci Rep.* 2020;10(1):1-8.

7. Yong E, Vasireddy A, Pavitt A, Davies GE, Lockey DJ. Pre-hospital pelvic girdle injury: improving diagnostic accuracy in a physician-led trauma service. *Injury.* 2016; 47(2):383-388.

8. Hsu S-D, Chen C-J, Chou Y-C, Wang S-H, Chan D-C. Effect of early pelvic binder use in the emergency management of suspected pelvic trauma: a retrospective cohort study. *Int J Environ Res Public Health.* 2017;14(10):1217. doi: 10.3390/ijerph14101217

9. Coccolini F, Stahel PF, Montori G, et al. Pelvic trauma: WSES classification and guidelines. *World J Emerg Surg.* 2017;12:5.

10. Scott I, Porter K, Laird C, Greaves I. Bloch M. The pre-hospital management of pelvic fractures: initial consensus statement. *Emerg Med J.* 2013;30(12):1070-1072.

11. McCreary D, Cheng C, Lin ZC, Nehme Z, Fitzgerald M, Mitra B. Haemodynamics as a determinant of need for pre-hospital application of a pelvic circumferential compression device in adult trauma patients. *Injury.* 2020;51(1):4-9.

12. Garner MR, Sethuraman SA, Schade MA, Boateng H. Antibiotic prophylaxis in open fractures: evidence, evolving issues, and recommendations. *J Am Acad Orthop Surg.* 2020 Apr 15;28(8):309-315. doi: 10.5435/JAAOS-D-18-00193

13. Seyfer AE, American College of Surgeons Committee on Trauma. *Guidelines for Management of Amputated Parts.* ACS; 1996.

14. Harbour PW, Malphrus E, Zimmerman RM, Giladi AM. Delayed digit replantation: what is the evidence? *J Hand Surg Am.* 2021 Oct;46(10):908-916. doi: 10.1016/j.jhsa .2021.07.007

15. Sharp CF, Mangram AJ, Lorenzo M, Dunn EL. A major metropolitan "field amputation" team: a call to arms . . . and legs. *J Trauma.* 2009;67(6):1158-1161.

16. Pepe E, Mosesso VN, Falk JL. Prehospital fluid resuscitation of the patient with major trauma. *Prehosp Emerg Care.* 2002;6:81.

17. Better OS. Management of shock and acute renal failure in casualties suffering from crush syndrome. *Ren Fail.* 1997;19:647.

18. Vanholder R, Borniche D, Claus S, et al. When the earth trembles in the Americas: the experience of Haiti and

Chile 2010. *Nephron Clin Pract*. 2011;117(3):c184-c197. doi: 10.1159/000320200

19. Lameire N, Sever MS, Van Biesen W, Vanholder R. Role of the international and national renal organizations in natural disasters: strategies for renal rescue. *Semin Nephrol*. 2020 Jul;40(4):393-407. doi: 10.1016/j.semnephrol.2020.06.007

20. Michaelson M, Taitelman U, Bshouty Z, et al. Crush syndrome: experience from the Lebanon war, 1982. *Isr J Med Sci*. 1984;20:305-307.

21. Pretto EA, Angus D, Abrams J, et al. An analysis of prehospital mortality in an earthquake. *Prehosp Disaster Med*. 1994;9:107-117.

22. Collins AJ, Burzstein S. Renal failure in disasters. *Crit Care Clin*. 1991;7:421-435.

23. Sever MS, Vanholder R, Lameire N. Management of crush-related injuries after disasters. *N Engl J Med*. 2006; 354:1052-1063.

Suggested Reading

American College of Surgeons Committee on Trauma. Musculoskeletal trauma. In: ACS Committee on Trauma. *Advanced Trauma Life Support*. 10th ed. ACS; 2018:148-167.

Ashkenazi I, Isakovich B, Kluger Y, et al. Prehospital management of earthquake casualties buried under rubble. *Prehosp Disast Med*. 2005;20(2):122-133.

Coppola PT, Coppola M. Emergency department evaluation and treatment of pelvic fractures. *Emerg Med Clin North Am*. 2003;18(1):1-27.

SPECIFIC SKILLS

Traction Splint for Femur Fractures

Principle: To immobilize femur fractures to minimize ongoing internal thigh hemorrhage.

This type of immobilization is used for fractures of the shaft of the femur. The application of traction and immobilization helps to reduce muscle spasm and pain while at the same time decreasing the potential for the fractured ends of the bone to produce additional damage and increased bleeding. Traction splints should be applied only if the patient's condition is stable and time permits. Traction splints should not be used if there are associated fractures or injuries to the knee or tibia. The Hare traction splint is shown for illustrative purposes. Other traction splints, such as the Sager traction splint, may be used in accordance with local protocol and policy.

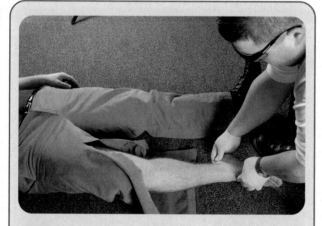

1 The prehospital care practitioner exposes the leg and assesses the patient's neurovascular status both before and after any manipulation. The practitioner explains to the patient what is going to happen and then performs the action.

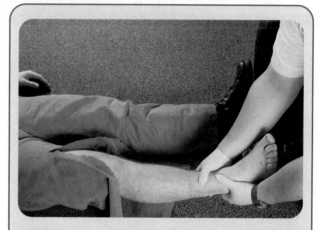

2 If the fractured extremity has marked deformity, the second prehospital care practitioner grasps the ankle and foot and applies gentle traction to straighten out the fracture and restore the patient's leg to length.

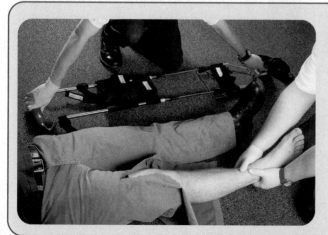

3 The splint is measured against the uninjured leg and adjusted to the appropriate length (approximately 8 to 10 inches [20 to 25 cm] beyond the heel of the leg).

(continues)

Traction Splint for Femur Fractures (continued)

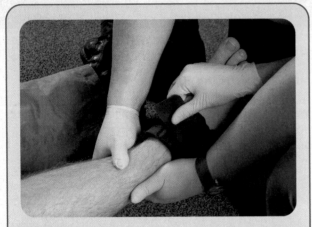

4 The ankle strap is applied to the injured leg. The strap may be used to maintain traction as necessary.

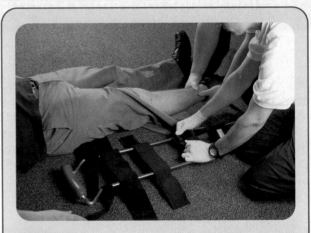

5 All Velcro securing straps are opened.

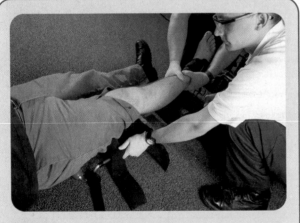

6 The patient's leg is elevated, and the proximal end of the traction splint is seated against the ischial tuberosity of the pelvis.

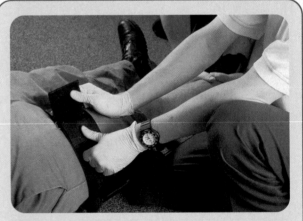

7 The prehospital care practitioner applies the proximal (pubic) strap around the proximal thigh to secure it in place.

Traction Splint for Femur Fractures (*continued*)

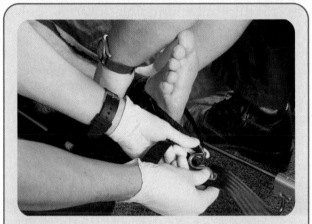

8 The ankle strap is attached to the traction hitch at the distal end of the splint.

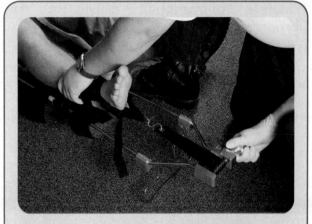

9 While maintaining manual traction, the prehospital care practitioner slowly turns the traction hitch mechanism to take over the traction function. Once the patient's leg has been restored to the same length as the uninjured leg, the practitioner stops turning the traction hitch mechanism.

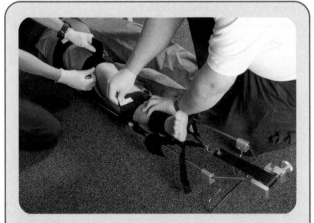

10 The prehospital care practitioner applies all remaining Velcro straps to secure the leg to the traction splint.

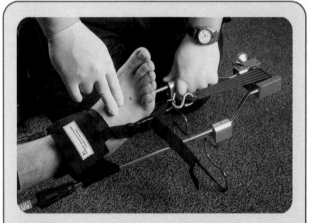

11 The prehospital care practitioner reassesses the patient's neurovascular status.

Pelvic Binder Placement for Pelvic Ring Fractures

Principle: To immobilize pelvic ring fractures to minimize ongoing internal pelvis hemorrhage.

This type of immobilization is used for fractures of the pelvic ring. The application of a pelvic binder immobilizes the pelvis, potentially improving pain, and decreases the pelvic volume, which may help prevent additional damage and increased bleeding. Pelvic binders may be safely placed in any patient suspected of sustaining an unstable pelvic ring injury. Any one of a number of commercially available binders or a well-placed sheet with clamps, may be used in accordance with local protocol and policy.

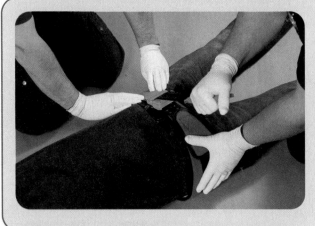

1 Assess the patient's neurovascular status both before and after placement. The binder is placed under the patient at the level of the greater trochanters using a standard log roll technique. The binder is then tightened and secured using the Velcro or ratcheted tightening mechanism depending on the model of binder employed. Reassess blood pressure and distal neurovascular status after application of the device. Be certain that the device is not positioned substantially above the level of the greater trochanters as it could easily impair the ability of the patient's chest to expand during inspiration.

CHAPTER 13

Burn Injuries

Lead Editors
Jennifer M. Gurney, MD, FACS
Spogmai Komak, MD
Brian H. Williams, MD, FACS

CHAPTER OBJECTIVES

At the completion of this chapter, you will be able to do the following:

- Describe the etiology, pathophysiology, systemic effects, and clinical consequences of burn injury.
- Describe the underlying fluid shifts in burn injury.
- Define the modern classification system for burn depth.
- Explain how ice can deepen the depth of burns.
- Estimate burn size using the rule of nines.
- Calculate fluid resuscitation and understand the different formulas.
- Calculate the initial rate for fluid resuscitation of an adult using the U.S. Army Institute of Surgical Research (USAISR) Rule of Ten.
- Describe the additional fluid needs in pediatric patients with burns.

- Describe the unique aspects of pediatric burns and child abuse.
- Describe appropriate burn dressings for prehospital care.
- Explain the unique concerns of electrical injuries and resuscitation implications.
- Describe the special considerations in radiation and chemical burns.
- Describe concerns in patients with circumferential burns and the management of these injuries.
- Describe the three elements of smoke inhalation.
- Describe prehospital management and management priorities in patients with severe burn injuries.
- Discuss the criteria for transfer of patients to burn centers.

SCENARIO

You are called to a residential structure fire. When your unit arrives, you witness a two-story house that is fully involved with fire and has thick black smoke pouring out of the roof and windows. You are directed to a victim who is being cared for by emergency medical responders (EMRs). They tell you that the patient reentered the burning building in an attempt to rescue his dog, and he was carried out unconscious by firefighters.

Your patient is a man who appears to be in his thirties. The majority of his clothes have been burned off. He has obvious burns to his face, and his hair has been singed. He is unconscious; he is breathing spontaneously, but with snoring respirations. The EMRs have placed the patient on high-flow oxygen with a nonrebreathing mask. On physical examination, his airway is patent with manual assistance (jaw thrust); he ventilates easily. The sleeves of his shirt have been burned off. His arms have circumferential burns, but his radial pulse is easily

(continues)

palpable. His heart rate is 118 beats/minute, blood pressure is 148/94 millimeters of mercury (mm Hg), ventilatory rate is 22 breaths/minute, and oxygen saturation (SpO_2), taken by pulse oximeter, is 92%. On physical examination, you determine that the patient is burned on his entire head and has blistering of the anterior chest and abdomen, along with full-thickness burns of his entire right and left arm and hand.

- What is the extent of burns for this patient?
- What are the initial steps for managing this patient?
- How does the prehospital care practitioner recognize an inhalation injury?

INTRODUCTION

Acute thermal injury continues to be a significant medical problem, claiming an estimated 180,000 lives worldwide annually.[1] Over 10 million people worldwide were treated for burn injuries in 2020.[1] Over 95% of fatal fire-related burns occur in low- and middle-income countries, with children and the elderly being the most vulnerable population with the highest mortality.[1] Major burns are serious traumatic injuries that require highly specialized care throughout the entire continuum to obtain good clinical outcomes. Burn trauma is unique in that it is frequently associated with significant disfigurement and deformity, in addition to prolonged intensive care unit (ICU) care, repeated episodes of sepsis, and multiorgan dysfunction.

Etiology of Burn Injury

The majority of burns are a result of thermal injury due to flame (55%), followed by scald (40%) injury. Fire is the most common cause of burn in adults, whereas scald burns from hot liquids are the most common burns to children and older adults. House fires are related to approximately 4% of burn admissions but have a 12% fatality rate (in patients hospitalized from house fires); this rate is much higher than the 3% fatality rate of patients with burns from other causes and is presumably associated with inhalation injury.[2] The cause of the increased risk of fire and burn fatalities in low-income populations is multifactorial and includes living in older buildings that were not built to meet current fire safety codes, crowded living conditions, and the absence of smoke detectors.

The elderly and young are the most susceptible populations to burn injury. Scald burns are the most common burns seen in children between the ages of 1 and 5 years. Child abuse accounts for a large proportion of immersion scald burns.[3] Intentional burn injuries can usually be distinguished from accidental burns based on the pattern and site of the burn. Nonaccidental burns often have clear-cut edges as found in a stocking or glove distribution, where a child's foot or hand has been held in scalding water. Accidental burns, such as those caused by a child spilling hot liquid, most often occur on the head, trunk, and palmar surface of the hands and feet. Other causes of burn injury include cold temperature, electricity, chemical agents, and radiation injury.

Pathophysiology of Burn Injury

Skin is a relatively poor conductor of heat; as such, it provides an extensive barrier to heat injury. Heat transfer within the skin is determined by thermal conductivity of the heated material, the area through which heat is transferred, and the temperature of the object. Acute transfer of heat to skin results in burn injury with rapid dysregulation of the barrier function of skin, impairing temperature regulation, protection against infection, and maintenance of fluid homeostasis. Burn injury causes a distributive form of shock secondary to an alteration in systemic circulation. Burn shock is complex and multifactorial but a loss of vascular wall integrity, with resultant loss of protein into the interstitium, is part of the pathophysiology that results in both hypovolemic and distributive forms of shock. Fluid translocation into the interstitial space increases due to increased capillary permeability, and an imbalance in hydrostatic and oncotic forces causes rapid fluid shifts from the intravascular compartment. With large burn injuries, the dramatic loss of fluids, electrolytes, and protein results in loss of effective circulating plasma volume, massive edema formation, decreased end-organ perfusion, and depressed cardiovascular function.[4]

Fluid Shifts in Burn Injury

Burn injury is characterized by the disruption of the integumentary system with impressive systematic physiologic changes. Thermal injury leads to disruption of homeostasis secondary to local and systemic inflammatory responses culminating in "burn shock," a unique combination of distributive and hypovolemic shock physiologies characterized by intravascular volume depletion, low pulmonary artery occlusion pressure, increased systemic vascular resistance, and depressed myocardial contractility. Direct thermal injury causes changes in microvascular circulation manifested by local hyperemia, edema, and resultant capillary leakage. Edema results because of the effects on the vascular endothelium and permeability, which is influenced by various mediators and cytokines (histamine, bradykinin, and interleukins), which are thought to drive the early phase of edema formation (12 to 24 hours) post burn. This edema formation can be profound and contributes to burn shock.

Fluid administration is the cornerstone of effective resuscitation, with the goal of restoring intravascular volume and perfusion. The type, quantity, duration, and endpoints of burn shock resuscitation have been debated over the last century; however, without fluid resuscitation, large burn wounds are uniformly fatal. Prior to the 1950s, hypovolemic shock or shock-induced renal failure was the leading cause of death after thermal injury.[5] Targeted fluid resuscitation should start in the prehospital environment. Overresuscitation is associated with morbidity as well, so understanding the timeliness and rate of prehospital fluid resuscitation is an important factor in the overall management of resuscitation during the first 24 hours after a burn injury. The aim of fluid resuscitation in burn injury is to restore intravascular volume and support the patient through the post-burn hypovolemia.

Several different resuscitation formulas may be used, with variability in the composition of resuscitation fluid. The consensus is to give the least amount of fluid necessary to maintain adequate end-organ perfusion and that the replacement of extracellular salt lost in the burned tissue is essential.[6-8]

Systemic Effects of Burn Injury

Burn injury results in a dramatic hypermetabolic response driven by multifold increases in circulating catecholamines after injury. Burns exceeding 30% of the total body surface area (TBSA) are characterized by massive release of cytokines and inflammatory mediators into the systemic circulation.

Early cardiovascular response to burn injury is a reduction in cardiac output accompanied by an elevation in peripheral vascular resistance. This response is seen immediately after burn injury, secondary to the intravascular volume depletion from movement of fluid into the interstitium. After initiation of fluid resuscitation and replacement of plasma volume, cardiac output increases, surpassing normal cardiac output due to a hyperdynamic state, driven by an attenuated hypermetabolic response.

Release of catecholamines, vasopressin, and angiotensin causes peripheral and splanchnic bed vasoconstriction, which can affect end-organ function. Glomerular filtration rate and renal blood flow are decreased initially because of a decrease in intravascular volume. Additionally, there is decreased mesenteric blood flow, decreased bowel mucosal integrity, and integumentary capillary leakage after burn injury. This leads to gastrointestinal (GI) dysfunction and translocation of bacteria into the portal circulation.

Pulmonary function is also altered in burn injury, as it is in other forms of traumatic injury. There is an increase in respiratory rate and tidal volume after resuscitation, resulting in increased minute ventilation. Circulating cytokines cause an increase in pulmonary vascular resistance, which results in deceased pulmonary capillary hydrostatic pressure and may contribute to pulmonary dysfunction during the initial resuscitation phase of injury.

Anatomy of the Skin

The skin is the largest organ in the human body. It serves multiple complex functions, including protection from the external environment, regulation of fluids, thermoregulation, sensation, and metabolic adaptation (**Figure 13-1**). The skin covers about 16.1 to 21.5 square feet (1.5 to 2.0 square meters [m]) in the average adult. It is made up of two layers: the **epidermis** and the **dermis**. The outer epidermis is about 0.05 millimeter (mm) thick in areas such as the eyelids and can be as thick as 1 mm on the sole of the foot. The epidermis is derived from ectoderm and

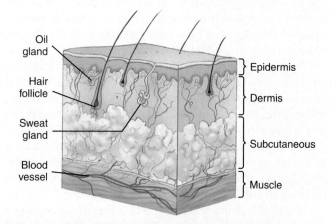

Figure 13-1 Normal skin. The skin is composed of two layers: epidermis and dermis. The subcutaneous layer and associated muscle are located below the skin. Some layers contain structures such as glands, hair follicles, blood vessels, and nerves. All of these structures are interrelated in the maintenance, loss, and gain of body temperature.

is capable of regenerative healing. The epidermis is connected to the dermis via the basement membrane zone, which contains epidermal projection (rete ridges) that interdigitate with dermal projections (papillae).

The dermis layer of skin is derived from mesoderm and is divided into the papillary dermis and the reticular dermis. The papillary dermis is extremely bioactive and is the reason that superficial partial-thickness burns generally heal faster than deeper partial-thickness burns (as the papillary component is lost in deeper burns).

The deeper dermis is on average 10 times thicker than the epidermis. The subcutaneous layer, or *hypodermis*, is made up of adipose (fat) and connective tissue that helps keep the outer layers of the skin attached to the underlying structures. The subcutaneous layer also contains some of the larger blood vessels and nerves.

The skin of males is thicker than the skin of females, and the skin of children and older adults is thinner than that of the average adult. These facts explain why one individual can sustain burns of varying depths from exposure to a singular burning agent, why a child might experience a deep burn while an adult with the same exposure has only a superficial injury, or why an elderly person will sustain a deeper burn than a younger adult.

Burn Characteristics

Burn injury is caused by applied heat with resultant damage to the skin, subcutaneous tissue, fat, muscle, and even bone. Changes at the cellular level following acute thermal injury cause denaturation of proteins and loss of plasma membrane integrity. Temperature and duration of contact are important determinants in the depth of burn injury.

Acute thermal injury causes tissue necrosis at the center of injury with progressively less damage at the periphery. The depth of heat injury depends on the degree of heat exposure and depth of heat penetration.

Injury to the skin can occur in two phases: immediate and delayed. Immediate injury is from acute thermal exposure resulting in immediate loss of plasma membrane integrity and protein denaturation. Delayed injury results from inadequate resuscitation, desiccation, edema, and wound infection. Skin is capable of tolerating temperatures of 104°F (40°C) for brief periods. However, once temperatures exceed this point, there is a *logarithmic* increase in the magnitude of tissue destruction.[9]

A full-thickness burn has three zones of tissue injury that essentially form circles (**Figure 13-2**).[10] The central zone is known as the **zone of coagulation**, and this is the region of greatest tissue destruction. The tissue in this zone is *necrotic* (dead) and is not capable of undergoing repair.

Adjacent to the zone of necrosis is a region of lesser injury. This zone, referred to as the **zone of stasis**, is

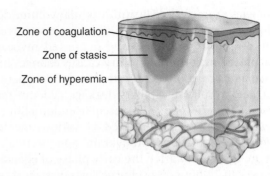

Figure 13-2 Three zones of burn injury.
© National Association of Emergency Medical Technicians (NAEMT)

characterized by the presence of both viable and nonviable cells. This zone often has tenuous blood flow immediately after injury with associated capillary vasoconstriction and ischemia. Timely and appropriate burn care, including systemic fluid resuscitation and avoidance of vasoconstriction, is critical in prevention of necrosis in this zone of injury. Local wound care, including nondesiccating dressings, topical antimicrobials, and frequent monitoring of the wound for infection, can further ensure that damaged cells do not progress to tissue necrosis. Failure to resuscitate the patient appropriately results in death of the cells in the injured tissue and in tissue necrosis.

A common error that results in damage to the zone of stasis is the application of ice by a bystander or prehospital care practitioner. While stopping the burning process is critical, ice applied to the skin will result in vasoconstriction, preventing reestablishment of the blood flow that is critically needed for the injured tissue. While ice application to a burn will result in reduction in pain, this will be at the expense of additional tissue destruction. For small burns, this is not significant; however, for larger burns ice should be withheld for local tissue reasons and also to prevent hypothermia. Analgesia should be provided with oral or parenteral (all other routes) medications.

The outermost zone of injury is known as the **zone of hyperemia**. This zone has minimal cellular injury and is characterized by increased blood flow secondary to an inflammatory reaction initiated by the burn injury. The zone of hyperemia is characterized by viable cells and usually recovers unless further injured as a result of hypoperfusion or wound infection. One of the goals of burn resuscitation is to preserve this area to decrease the amount of surgery and skin grafting the patient will need.

Burn Depth

Estimation of burn depth can be deceptively difficult for even the most experienced practitioners. Often, a burn that appears to be **partial thickness** can evolve to be

full thickness. Or, in other cases, the surface of a burn may appear to be partial thickness at first glance, but later, after **debridement** in the hospital, the superficial epidermis separates, revealing a white, full-thickness burn **eschar** underneath. In the prehospital environment, estimation of burn depth, with the exception of clear full-thickness injuries, is even more challenging because the wound can evolve with the resuscitation needs of the patient. Often it is best to simply tell patients that the injury is either superficial or deep and that further evaluation is required to determine ultimate burn depth. Furthermore, a treating practitioner should not attempt to estimate burn depth until attempts have been made to initially assess and debride the wound in the hospital.

Superficial Burns

Superficial burns involve only the epidermis and are characterized as red and painful (**Figure 13-3**). These burns extend into the papillary dermis and characteristically do not form blisters. These wounds blanch with pressure, and blood flow to this area is increased compared to adjacent normal skin. Superficial dermal wounds usually heal within 2 to 3 weeks without scar formation. These wounds do not require surgical excision and grafting. Burns of this depth are not included when calculating the percentage of TBSA that is burned or used for fluid administration.

Partial-Thickness Burns

Partial-thickness burns, once referred to as *second-degree burns*, are those that involve the epidermis and varying portions of the underlying dermis (**Figure 13-4**). They can be further classified as either *superficial* or *deep*. Partial-thickness burns will appear as blisters (**Box 13-1**) or as **denuded** burned areas with a glistening or wet-appearing base. Superficial dermal burns extend into the papillary dermis. These wounds blanch with pressure, and the blood flow to the dermis is increased over that

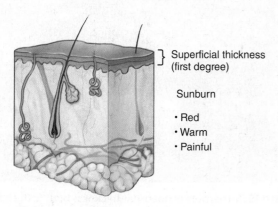

Figure 13-3 Superficial burn.
© National Association of Emergency Medical Technicians (NAEMT)

of normal skin due to vasodilation. These wounds are painful. Because remnants of the dermis survive, these burns can often heal but generally take approximately 3 weeks to do so. A deep partial-thickness burn involves destruction of most of the dermal layer, with few viable

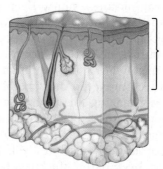

Figure 13-4 Partial-thickness burn.
© National Association of Emergency Medical Technicians (NAEMT)

Box 13-1 Blisters

Much discussion has been generated about blisters, including whether to open and debride them and how to approach the blister associated with partial-thickness burns. A blister occurs when the epidermis separates from the underlying dermis and fluid that is leaking from nearby vessels fills the space between the layers. The presence of *osmotically active* proteins in the blister fluid draws additional fluid into the blister space, causing the blister to continue to enlarge. If the blister continues to enlarge, it can create pressure on the injured tissue of the wound bed, which increases the patient's pain.

Many think that the skin of the blister acts as a sterile dressing and prevents contamination of the wound. However, the skin of the blister is not normal and frequently becomes violated, allowing bacteria to enter the space; when this happens, the blister does not serve as a protective barrier. Additionally, maintaining the blister intact prevents application of topical antibiotics directly on the injury. For these reasons, most burn specialists open and debride blisters after arrival of the patient to the hospital.[11]

In the prehospital setting, blisters should be left intact for transport. When blisters are debrided, the wounds are cleaned, and antimicrobial dressings are applied; this cannot be accomplished well either in the field or during transport. Blisters that have already ruptured should be covered with a clean, dry dressing.

epidermal cells. Blisters do not generally form because the nonviable tissue is thick and adheres to underlying viable dermis (eschar). Blood flow is compromised, and it is often difficult to distinguish between a deep partial-thickness and full-thickness burn wound; however, the presence of sensation to touch indicates that the burn is a deep partial-thickness injury. Deep partial-thickness wounds that have not healed in 3 weeks should undergo excision and grafting.

In partial-thickness burns, the zone of necrosis involves the entire epidermis and varying depths of the superficial dermis. If not well cared for, the zone of stasis can progress to necrosis, making these burns larger, potentially resulting in conversion to full-thickness injuries, and leading to a larger area requiring excision and grafting. A superficial partial-thickness burn will heal with vigilant wound care. Deep partial-thickness burns will often require surgery depending on their location, size, and patient factors; skin grafting can minimize scarring and limit functional deformities, particularly in areas such as the hands.

Full-Thickness Burns

Full-thickness burns are deep into the tissue and result in complete destruction of the epidermis and dermis, leaving no residual epidermal cells to repopulate the wound. They can result from prolonged contact with flame, liquid, or chemical elements. Full-thickness burns may have several appearances (**Figure 13-5**). Most often these wounds will appear as thick, dry, white, leathery burns, regardless of the patient's race or skin color (**Figure 13-6**). This thick, leathery damaged skin is referred to as an *eschar*. In severe cases, the skin will have a charred appearance with visible *thrombosis* (clotting) of blood vessels (**Figure 13-7**). Full-thickness burn eschar is insensate and will feel dry, thick, and leathery.

Even though full-thickness burn areas are insensate, they are typically surrounded by areas of partial-thickness burns. Additionally, it can be challenging to distinguish (prior to showering the patient and cleaning the wounds) between deep partial-thickness and full-thickness wounds. Any wound that is not full-thickness will cause the patient significant pain. Also, because full-thickness burns lose their tissue pliability, the patients can feel this constrictive effect, especially if the eschars (full-thickness burn wounds) are circumferential. Circumferential full-thickness burn wounds around the thorax can be life threatening because they impede chest movement and ventilation. Similarly, full-thickness burn wounds around an extremity can lead to edema and compartment syndrome. Extremities with full-thickness wounds should be elevated as much as possible during transport to prevent additional edema. Full-thickness burns can be disabling and life threatening; patients with full-thickness burns should be managed at a burn center. Prompt surgical excision and intensive rehabilitation at a specialized center are required.

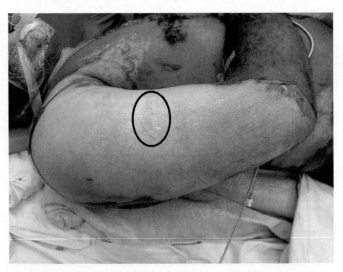

Figure 13-6 This patient has sustained partial-thickness burns and a full-thickness burn, characterized as white and leathery in appearance.
Courtesy of Dr. Jeffrey Guy.

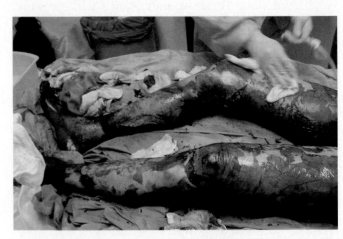

Figure 13-7 Example of deep, full-thickness burn with charring of the skin and visible thrombosis of blood vessels.
Courtesy of Dr. Jeffrey Guy.

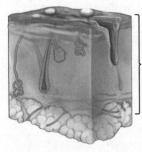

Full thickness
(third degree)
• Leathery
• White to charred
• Dead tissue
• Victims will have pain from burned areas adjacent to the full-thickness burn.

Figure 13-5 Full-thickness burn.
© National Association of Emergency Medical Technicians (NAEMT)

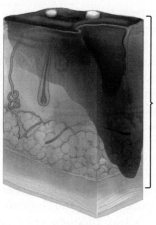

Fourth degree
(full thickness with
deep tissue damage)

Figure 13-8 Subdermal burn.
© National Association of Emergency Medical Technicians (NAEMT)

Subdermal Burns

Subdermal burns (previously referred to as fourth-degree burns) are those that not only burn all layers of the skin but also burn underlying fat, muscles, bone, or internal organs (**Figure 13-8** and **Figure 13-9**). These burns are, in fact, full-thickness burns that also result in deep tissue damage. These burns can be extremely debilitating and disfiguring as a result of the damage done to the skin and underlying tissues and structures. Significant debridement of dead and **devitalized** tissue may result in extensive soft-tissue defects.

Burn Assessment

Primary Survey and Resuscitation

The goal of the primary survey is to systematically evaluate and treat life-threatening disorders in order of importance to preserve life. The primary survey algorithm has to be acutely remembered in burn patients, given the distracting nature of major burn injuries. After stopping the burn process and ensuring the scene is safe, the management algorithm begins starting with assessment for hemorrhage. The XABCDE (eXsanguinating hemorrhage, Airway, Breathing, Circulation, Disability, and Expose/Environment) method of trauma care applies to the management of burn patients, although burn patients present unique challenges along every step of the assessment and resuscitation.

Major burns can be highly morbid, and while survivability and outcomes depend on the TBSA burned, the burn itself is rarely the injury that is immediately life threatening. The overall appearance of the burns can be dramatic, and their strong smell can be disturbing; this

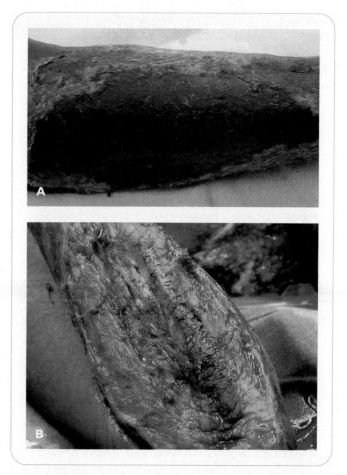

Figure 13-9 Subdermal burns are full-thickness burns with deep tissue damage. **A.** Skin. **B.** Subcutaneous fat, muscle, and bone.
Courtesy of Dr. Jeffrey Guy.

should not distract from prehospital management. Sophisticated prehospital care practitioners will be mindful that the patient may also have suffered from mechanical trauma in addition to the burn and have less apparent internal injuries that pose a more immediate life threat.

Control of Severe External Bleeding

Burn patients are trauma patients! Given the distracting nature of the burn injuries, this basic fact cannot be forgotten. Even in trauma and burn centers, practitioners can become distracted by burn injuries and fail to follow the trauma care management algorithms (**Box 13-2**). Burns are obvious and sometimes intimidating injuries, but it is vital to assess for other, less obvious internal injuries that may be imminently life threatening. For example, in attempts to escape being burned, patients may leap from the windows of buildings, elements of the burning structure may collapse and fall on the patient, or the patient may be trapped in the burning wreckage of a motor vehicle crash. In all of these cases, the patient may

- Becoming distracted by the burn injury and not recognizing and treating hemorrhage or other life-threatening injuries
- Overaggressive crystalloid resuscitation in patients with burns and hemorrhage
- Failing to recognize that the burn may not be the most life-threatening injury
- Failing to rule out hemorrhage in burn patients with hypotension
- Failing to prevent hypothermia
- Over- or underestimating burn size and over- or underresuscitating the patient

Box 13-3 Airway Management Pitfalls in Burn Patients

- Not recognizing signs of thermal injury to the airway. Concerning signs include: hoarseness, stridor, drooling, tissue hyperemia/blistering.
- Not securing the airway early. Once airway edema worsens, endotracheal intubation can be exceedingly difficult.
- Not being prepared for a surgical airway.
- Placing a laryngeal mask airway or temporizing airway device that is not a cuffed tube below the vocal cords. Burn patients must have definitive airways placed to bypass the problems associated with vocal cord edema.
- Using tape to secure the endotracheal tube or cricothyroidotomy. Tape does not stick to the skin of burn patients; never rely on tape to secure any important tube in a patient with burn injury.

have sustained both burns and associated traumatic injuries such as pelvic fractures, long-bone fractures, brain injuries, and thoracoabdominal injuries. The immediate life threat that needs to be excluded or treated is hemorrhage from an associated injury.

Airway

Burn injury is a subset of acute traumatic injury, and as in all trauma patients, attention to airway management priorities is paramount (**Box 13-3**). Thermal injury from acute exposure to flame can cause edema of the airway above the level of the vocal cords that can occlude the airway. Therefore, careful initial, as well as continuous, evaluation is required. Prehospital care practitioners who are likely to experience prolonged transport times need to be particularly vigilant about airway assessment. Airway management in burn patients is more challenging when there is a concern for smoke injury or when the initial thermal injury is from fire in an enclosed space. More than 30% of thermally injured patients admitted to burn centers in the United States have a concomitant smoke inhalation injury.[12] Direct thermal insult to the upper airways results in edema formation leading to progressive swelling of mucosa, which can increase resistance to the inflow of air during inhalation. Initially, 100% humidified oxygen should be given to all patients when no signs of obvious respiratory distress are present. The patient should be thoroughly inspected, paying particular attention to the presence of chest rise and circumferential torso burns, which may restrict adequate chest rise and ventilation.

Endotracheal intubation is necessary for patients in acute respiratory distress, those with increasing work of breathing, and those who have sustained burns to the face or neck, which may result in edema and airway obstruction. It is imperative to pay particular attention to the cervical spine, especially in patients who have sustained burn injury from an explosion or deceleration accident. Signs of impending airway obstruction are stridor, severe hoarseness, and drooling. Inhalation injury can result in soot in the airways as well, so a patient coughing up a large amount of black/carbonaceous sputum must be monitored closely for airway compromise.

If the patient is intubated, special precautions must be taken when securing the endotracheal (ET) tube to prevent inadvertent dislodgment or extubation. Following facial burns, the skin of the face will often peel or weep fluid, rendering adhesive tapes unsuitable for securing the ET tube. The ET tube can be secured using two umbilical tapes (**Figure 13-10A**) or pieces of intravenous (IV) tubing wrapped around the head. One piece should be draped over the ear and the second under the ear (**Figure 13-10B**). Commercially available cloth and Velcro devices are also suitable.

Breathing

As with any trauma patient, breathing can be adversely affected by such problems as fractured ribs, pneumothoraces, and other closed or open chest wounds. In the event of a circumferential chest wall burn, the chest wall compliance progressively decreases to such an extent that it inhibits the patient's ability to move air and ventilate. Prompt escharotomies of the chest wall should be performed in this case and the patient should be taken to the nearest hospital with surgical capability. Signs a patient needs an escharotomy are difficulty with bag ventilation or increased ventilatory pressure alarms on the ventilator. If a pneumothorax has already been excluded and the patient has circumferential full-thickness chest wall burn, then escharotomies may be necessary to ventilate circumferential injuries. Burned extremities should be elevated during transport to reduce the degree of swelling in the affected limb.

Establishment of two large-bore IV catheters capable of the rapid flow rate needed for large-volume resuscitation is a requirement for burns that involve more than 20% TBSA. Ideally, the IV catheters should not be placed through or adjacent to burned tissue; however, placement through the burn is appropriate if no alternative sites are available. When the catheter is placed in or near a burn, special measures must be taken to ensure that the catheter is not inadvertently dislodged. Adhesive tapes and dressings typically used to secure IV catheters will be ineffective when applied on or adjacent to burned tissue. Burn centers will frequently suture IV catheters in place because adhesives do not stick well to patients with burn injuries. Alternative means to secure the lines include wrapping the site with Kerlix or Coban rolls. In some patients, the prehospital care practitioner may not be able to obtain venous access. Intraosseous (IO) access is a reliable alternative method to administer IV fluids as well as narcotics.

Disability

A source of life-threatening neurologic disability that is unique to burn victims is the effect of inhaled toxins such as carbon monoxide and hydrogen cyanide gas. These toxins can produce asphyxiation (see the section on "Smoke Inhalation Injuries").

Evaluate the patient for neurologic and motor deficits as one would do for any other trauma patient. Identify and splint fractures of long bones after applying a clean sheet or dressing if the extremity is burned. Establish spinal motion restriction if you suspect a potential spinal injury.

Expose/Environment

The next priority is to expose the patient completely. All jewelry should be promptly removed because the gradually developing swelling of burned areas will cause jewelry to act as a constricting band and compromise distal circulation. In the event of mechanical trauma, all of the patient's clothes are removed in order to identify injuries that might be concealed by the clothing. In a burn victim, removal of the clothing can potentially have a therapeutic benefit. Clothing and jewelry can retain residual heat, which may continue to injure the patient. Following chemical burns, the clothing may be soaked with the agent that burned the patient. In the case of chemical burns, improper handling of the victim's clothing that has been saturated with a potentially hazardous material can result in injury to both the patient and the prehospital care practitioner. Any clothing that smells of chemicals should be handled with caution and prehospital

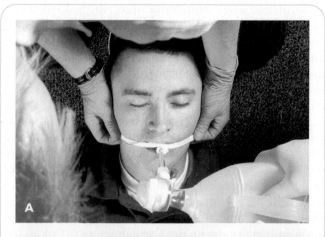
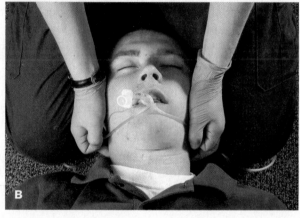

Figure 13-10 Prehospital care practitioners can use umbilical tape or IV tubing to secure an ET tube if the patient has burns to the face. **A.** Umbilical tape. **B.** IV tubing.

© Jones & Bartlett Learning. Photographed by Darren Stahlman.

the patient. An **escharotomy** is a surgical procedure that involves making an incision through the hardened burn eschar, allowing the chest wall to expand and move with the patient's respiratory movements. Partial-thickness burns do not cause these constrictive effects on the chest wall and do not require escharotomies.

Circulation

The process of evaluating and managing circulation includes the measurement of blood pressure, evaluation of circumferential burns (see the "Circumferential Burns" section in this chapter), and establishment of IV catheters. Accurate measurement of blood pressure becomes difficult or impossible with burns to the extremities, and if a blood pressure can be obtained, it may not correctly reflect systemic arterial blood pressure because of full-thickness burns and edema of the extremities. Even if the patient has adequate arterial blood pressure, distal limb perfusion may be critically reduced because of

practitioners must wear protective gear including eye protection.

Controlling the environmental temperature is critical when caring for patients with large burns. Patients with large surface area burns are unable to maintain their own body heat and are extremely susceptible to hypothermia. The burn leads to vasodilation in the skin, which, in turn, allows for increased heat loss. In addition, as open burn wounds weep and leak fluid, evaporation further exacerbates the patient's body heat loss. Make every effort to preserve the patient's body temperature. Apply several layers of blankets over the dry sheet that is placed over the patient. Keep the passenger compartment of the transporting ambulance or aircraft warm, regardless of the time of year. As a general rule, if the prehospital care practitioners are comfortable, then ambient temperature is too cold and the patient is at risk for hypothermia.

Secondary Survey

After completing the primary survey, the next objective is completion of the secondary survey as for any trauma patient. The secondary survey of a patient with a burn injury is no different from that of any other trauma patient. The prehospital care practitioner should conduct a complete head-to-toe evaluation. And, as stated, while the appearance of the burns can be dramatic, these wounds typically are not immediately life threatening. A thorough, methodical, and systematic secondary survey needs to be performed the same as would be done for any other trauma patient. IV access should be attempted, but there should not be a delay in transporting the patient to an emergency facility due to an inability to establish access. If the transport time to the nearest facility is less than 60 minutes, then transport should not be delayed for access. If IV access is established, then lactated Ringer's solution should be infused at a rate dependent on the burn size. The U.S. Army Institute of Surgical Research (USAISR) Rule of Ten can be used for this initial fluid rate (discussed later). In general, the burn size should be multiplied by 10 to get the initial fluid rate; so, in adult of average weight, a patient with a 30% TBSA should get 300 milliliters/hour (mL/hr), a patient with a 40% TBSA should get 400 mL/hr, and a patient with a 50% TBSA burn should get 500 mL/hr. Children over the age of 5 should get 100 to 250 mL/hr depending on the size of the burn and the size of the child.

Burn Size Estimation (Assessment)

A careful evaluation of burn wounds is conducted once the primary and secondary surveys are complete. The wounds are cleansed and assessed. Estimation of burn size is necessary to resuscitate the patient appropriately and prevent the complications associated with

hypovolemic shock from burn injury. Burn size determination is also used as a tool for stratifying injury severity and triage. The most widely applied method is the rule of nines, which applies the principle that major regions of the body in adults are considered to be 9% of the total body surface area (**Figure 13-11**). The perineum, or genital area, represents 1%.

Burns can also be assessed using the rule of palms (**Figure 13-12**). The use of the patient's palm has been a widely accepted and long-standing practice for estimating the size of smaller burns. However, there has not been uniform acceptance of what defines a palm and how large it is.[13] The average area of the palm alone (not including the extended fingers) is 0.5% TBSA in males and 0.4% in females. Including the palmar aspect of all five extended digits along with the palm increases the area to 0.8% TBSA for males and 0.7% TBSA for females.[13] Aside from gender differences of palm size, the size of the palm also varies with body weight of the patient. As the patient's body mass index (BMI) increases, the total skin surface area of the body increases, and the TBSA percentage of the palm decreases.[14] In most cases, the palm plus the fingers of the patient can be grossly estimated to be approximately 1% of the patient's TBSA.

Estimation of burn size in children is different from that for adults due to the relative increase of TBSA in the head. Additionally, the proportion of TBSA of children's heads and lower extremities differs with age. The *Lund-Browder chart* is a diagram that takes into account age-related changes in children. Using these charts, a prehospital care practitioner maps the burn and then determines burn size based on an accompanying reference table (**Figure 13-13**). This method requires drawing a map of the burns and then converting the map to a calculated burned surface area. The complexity of this method makes it difficult to use in a prehospital situation.

Dressings

Before transport, the wounds should be dressed. The goal of the dressings is to prevent ongoing contamination and to decrease airflow over the wounds, which will help with pain control.

Dressings in the form of a dry sterile sheet or towel are sufficient before transporting the patient. Several layers of blankets are then placed over the sterile burn sheets to help the patient maintain body heat. Topical antibiotic ointments and creams should not be applied until the patient has been evaluated by the burn center.

Transport

Patients who have multiple injuries in addition to their burns should first be transported to a trauma center, where hemorrhage and other life-threatening injuries

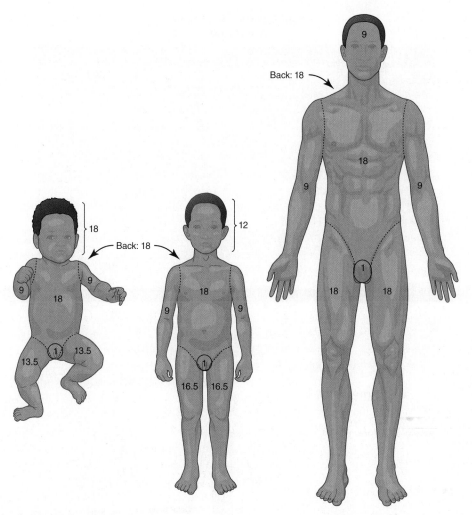

Figure 13-11 Rule of nines.

© Jones & Bartlett Learning

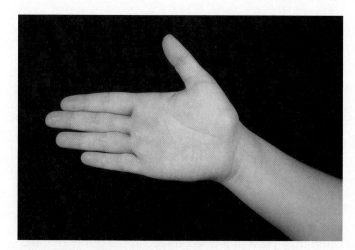

Figure 13-12 The rule of palms uses the patient's palm plus the fingers to estimate the size of smaller burns.

© Jones & Bartlett Learning. Photographed by Kimberly Potvin.

can be identified and surgically treated, if necessary. Once stabilized at a trauma center, the patient with burns can be transported to a burn center for definitive burn care and rehabilitation. The American Burn Association and the American College of Surgeons have identified criteria for transport or transfer of burn patients to a burn center, as outlined in **Figure 13-14**. In geographic areas with no easy access to a burn center, local medical direction will determine the preferred destination for such cases.

Management

Initial Burn Care

The initial step in the care of a burn patient is to stop the burning process. The most effective and appropriate method of terminating the burning is irrigation with

Burn Estimate and Diagram
Age vs Area

Area	Birth 1 yr.	1–4 years	6–9 years	10–14 years	15 years	Adult	2nd degree	3rd degree	Total	Donor Areas
Head	19	17	13	11	9	7	2			
Neck	2	2	2	2	2	2	2			
Ant. Trunk	13	13	13	13	13	13	7	5		
Post. Trunk	13	13	13	13	13	13	8			
R. Buttock	2½	2½	2½	2½	2½	2½				
L. Buttock	2½	2½	2½	2½	2½	2½	1.5			
Genitalia	1	1	1	1	1	1	1			
R. U. Arm	4	4	4	4	4	4				
L. U. Arm	4	4	4	4	4	4	1			
R. L. Arm	3	3	3	3	3	3	1			
L. L. Arm	3	3	3	3	3	3	2			
R. Hand	2½	2½	2½	2½	2½	2½	2			
L. Hand	2½	2½	2½	2½	2½	2½	2.5			
R. Thigh	5½	6½	8	8½	9	9½	4			
L. Thigh	5½	6½	8	8½	9	9½	4	2		
R. Leg	5	5	5½	6	6½	7				
L. Leg	5	5	5½	6	6½	7				
R. Foot	3½	3½	3½	3½	3½	3½				
L. Foot	3½	3½	3½	3½	3½	3½				
Total							38	7	45%	

Burn Diagram

Age   39
Sex   M
Weight   Pre Burn Wt. 59.6 kg

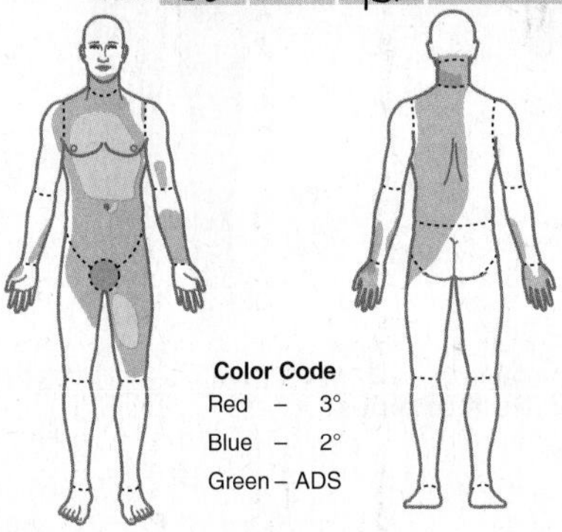

Color Code
Red – 3°
Blue – 2°
Green – ADS

Figure 13-13 An example of a filled-out Lund-Browder chart.
© National Association of Emergency Medical Technicians (NAEMT)

copious volumes of room-temperature water. The application of ice will stop the burning and provide analgesia, but it will also stimulate local vasoconstriction, which risks increasing the extent of tissue damage in the zone of stasis (**Box 13-4**). Remove all clothing and jewelry; these items maintain residual heat and will continue to burn the patient. In addition, jewelry may constrict digits or extremities as the tissues begin to swell. Clothing items that have burned and melted onto the skin should not be removed but should be cooled with room-temperature water.

To effectively dress a recent burn, sterile, nonadherent dressings are applied, and the area is covered with a clean, dry sheet. If a sheet is not readily available, substitute a sterile surgical gown, drapes, towels, or Mylar rescue blanket. The dressing will prevent ongoing environmental contamination while helping to prevent the patient from experiencing pain from air flowing over the exposed nerve endings. Airflow or any contact or movement of burned skin will cause a significant amount of pain for the patient. There has to be a balance with stopping the burning process and preventing air movement/contamination of the burn wound. Certain commercial dressings with sterile hydrogels can be used for both processes and may be beneficial in the prehospital environment.

Prehospital care practitioners have often been unsatisfied and frustrated with the simple application of sterile sheets to a burn. However, topical ointments and conventional topical antibiotics should not be applied because they prevent a direct inspection of the burn. Such topical ointments and antibiotics are removed on admission to the burn center to allow direct visualization of the burn and determination of burn severity. Also, some topical medications may complicate the application of tissue-engineered products used to aid wound healing.

Burn Center Referral Criteria

A burn center may treat adults, children, or both.

Burn injuries that should be referred to a burn center include:

1. Partial thickness burns greater than 10% total body surface area (TBSA).
2. Burns that involve the face, hands, feet, genitalia, perineum, or major joints.
3. Third degree burns in any age group.
4. Electrical burns, including lightning injury.
5. Chemical burns.
6. Inhalation injury.
7. Burn injury in patients with preexisting medical disorders that could complicate management, prolong recovery, or affect mortality.
8. Any patient with burns and concomitant trauma (such as fractures) in which the burn injury poses the greatest risk of morbidity or mortality. In such cases, if the trauma poses the greater immediate risk, the patient may be initially stabilized in a trauma center before being transferred to a burn unit. Physician judgment will be necessary in such situations and should be in concert with the regional medical control plan and triage protocols.
9. Burned children in hospitals without qualified personnel or equipment for the care of children.
10. Burn injury in patients who will require special social, emotional, or rehabilitative intervention.

Severity Determination

First Degree (*Partial Thickness*)
Superficial, red, sometimes painful.

Second Degree (*Partial Thickness*)
Skin may be red, blistered, swollen. Very painful.

Third Degree (*Full Thickness*)
Whitish, charred or translucent, no pin prick sensation in burned area.

Percentage Total Body Surface Area (TBSA)

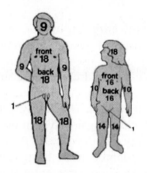

Figure 13-14 American Burn Association criteria for tranport or transfer of a burn patient to a burn center.

Courtesy of the American College of Surgeons.

Box 13-4 Burn Cooling

A potentially controversial topic is the practice of burn cooling. Several investigators have evaluated the effect of various cooling methods on the microscopic appearance of the burned tissue, as well as the impact on wound healing. In one study, the researchers concluded that burn cooling had a beneficial effect on the experimental burn wound.[15] Burns treated with cooling had less cellular damage than those that were not cooled.

Investigators have been able to directly measure the impact of cooling on the temperature of the burned dermis, the microscopic structure of the tissue, and wound healing. A study evaluated the outcomes of various cooling methods. These investigators compared burns cooled with tap water (59°F [15°C]) to application of a commercially available gel. Each of these methods was applied immediately after the burns as well as after a 30-minute delay. Immediate tap water cooling was almost twice as effective in reducing the temperature within the burned tissue. In this trial, wounds that were cooled had better microscopic appearance and wound healing at 3 weeks after injury.[16]

Overaggressive cooling with ice is harmful and will increase the injury to the tissue already damaged by the burn. This finding was demonstrated in an

animal model; cooling the burn immediately by the application of ice was more harmful than application of tap water or no treatment at all.[17] The application of ice water at a temperature of 34–46°F (1–8°C) resulted in more tissue destruction than was seen in burns that received no cooling treatment at all. In contrast, cooling with tap water at a temperature of 54–64°F (12–18°C) showed less tissue necrosis and a faster rate of healing than was observed in wounds not cooled.[18]

An important consideration is that the research on cooling was performed on experimental animals, and the burns were very limited in size. Ten percent TBSA was the largest burn size evaluated.

In summary, not all methods of burn cooling are equivalent. In the prehospital setting, cooling can be performed with room-temperature water to stop the acute burning process; however, it should not extend beyond this as cooling that is too aggressive may lead to additional tissue damage. Additionally, ongoing cooling (beyond that which stops the acute burning process) will contribute to hypothermia in patients with large burns. Another potential hazard of cooling a burn is that in the patient with both burns and mechanical trauma, systemic hypothermia has predictable and detrimental effects on the ability of blood to form a clot.

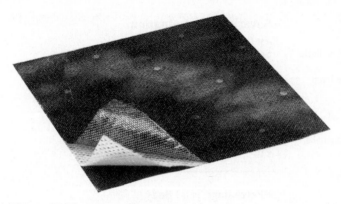

Figure 13-15 Acticoat dressing.
Courtesy of Smith & Nephew.

High-concentration antimicrobial-coated dressings have become the mainstay of wound care in burn centers (**Figure 13-15**). Dressings are used with a form of silver, sulfur, or even honey. Some dressings use impregnated silver, which is time-released over several days when applied to an open burn wound. The released silver has a strong antimicrobial effect against common organisms contaminating and infecting wounds. Recently, these dressings have been adapted from burn center use to prehospital applications. These large antimicrobial sheets can be rapidly applied to the burn and can eradicate contaminating organisms. This method of wound care allows prehospital care practitioners to apply a nonpharmaceutical device that greatly reduces burn wound contamination within 30 minutes of application.[19-21] An advantage of these dressings in wilderness and military applications is their compact size and light weight. An entire adult can be covered with antimicrobial dressings that can be stored in a container the size of a manila envelope with minimal weight.

Fluid Resuscitation

Burn injury results in direct disruption of cellular integrity and ongoing release of inflammatory mediators, causing vascular permeability and an increase in microvascular hydrostatic pressure. This drives the large efflux of fluid from the intravascular space into the interstitium. The underlying goal of early initial fluid resuscitation is to replace the intravascular volume and support the patient through the hypovolemia in the first 24 to 48 hours.

The resuscitation of a patient with a burn injury is aimed not only at the restoration of the loss of intravascular volume but also at the replacement of anticipated intravascular losses at a rate that mimics those losses as they occur (**Box 13-5**). In trauma patients, the prehospital care practitioner is replacing the volume that the patient has already lost from hemorrhage from an open fracture or bleeding viscera. In contrast, when treating the patient with a burn injury, the objective is to calculate

> **Box 13-5** Resuscitating a Patient With a Burn Injury
>
> Resuscitating a patient with a burn injury can be compared to filling a leaking bucket. The bucket is leaking water at a constant rate. The bucket has a line drawn inside near the top. The objective is to keep the water level at the line. Initially the water depth will be low. The longer the bucket has been unattended, the lower the water level will be and the greater the amount of fluid that needs to be replaced. The container will continue to leak, so once the bucket has been filled to an appropriate level, water will need to be continuously added at a constant rate to maintain the desired level.
>
> The longer the patient with a burn injury is not resuscitated or remains underresuscitated, the more hypovolemic the patient becomes. Therefore, greater amounts of fluids are required to establish a "level" of homeostasis. Once the patient has been resuscitated, the vascular space continues to leak in the same manner as the bucket. To maintain equilibrium with this homeostatic point, additional fluids need to be provided to replace the ongoing losses. It is important to keep track of the fluid that is being administered because overresuscitation can be as harmful as underresuscitation. In patients with transport times longer than 1 hour, communication with the receiving center should occur regarding the fluid resuscitation plan. Some centers are starting to use plasma for burn resuscitation, and as this practice gets adopted more widely it may migrate to the prehospital environment.

and replace the fluids that the patient has already lost as well as replace the patient's anticipated losses over the first 24 hours after the burn injury. Early fluid resuscitation is aimed at preventing progression of patients to burn shock. Maintaining urine output is essential in burn patients and is the primary indicator of adequate resuscitation. Patients with a > 20% burn should have their urine output monitored closely and all patients with > 40% TBSA burn should have a urinary catheter placed to monitory hourly urine output. Burn resuscitation can be guided by urine output, and the formulas presented in this chapter are aimed to restore intravascular volume, which can be monitored by average hourly urine output. Challenges to using urine output as a goal for fluid resuscitation are when large burn patients have sufficient shock to result in acute kidney injury and anuria; then other endpoints of resuscitation, such as lactate and base deficit, need to be closely monitored.

Adult Patient

The use of IV fluids, especially lactated Ringer's solution, is the best way to initially manage the fluid resuscitation of a burn patient. All the resuscitation formulas are initial guidance for fluid resuscitation volumes that are adjusted based on the physiologic response to resuscitation. Urine output is the best monitor of burn resuscitation with the goal output being 0.5 to 1.0 mL/kilogram (kg)/hr of ideal body weight. Overresuscitation can have just as many deleterious effects as underresuscitation and must be avoided. The fluid administered for resuscitation and the hourly urine output should be monitored for all patients with burns exceeding 40% TBSA. The amount of fluids administered in the first 24 hours after injury is typically 2 to 4 mL/kg/% TBSA burned (using only the total of the partial- and full-thickness burns). Current recommendations are to initiate fluid resuscitation at 2 mL/kg/% TBSA burned. This is a starting rate and the rate is subsequently adjusted based on the measured urine output. There are several formulas that guide fluid resuscitation in the burn patient. The most notable are the *Parkland Formula* and the *Brook Formula*. The *Parkland Formula*, which delivers 4 mL × body weight in kg × percentage of area burned. Half of this fluid needs to be administered within the first 8 hours of injury and the remaining half of the volume from hours 8 to 24.

Note, the first half of the fluid is administered within 8 hours from the time the patient sustained the burn injury, not from the time the prehospital care practitioner started to resuscitate the patient. This detail is especially important in wilderness or military settings, in which there may be an initial delay in treatment. For example, if the patient presents for emergency care 3 hours after the injury with no or little fluid administration, the first half of the calculated total needs to be administered over the next 5 hours. Thus, the patient will have received the target volume by hour 8 after the injury.

Lactated Ringer's solution is preferred to 0.9% normal saline for burn resuscitation. Burn patients typically require large volumes of IV fluids. Patients who receive large amounts of normal saline in the course of burn resuscitation will often develop a condition known as **hyperchloremic acidosis** because of the large amounts of chloride in the normal saline solution. Normal saline should be avoided in burn patients.

Calculation of Fluid Resuscitation Measures

The initial fluid rate for the resuscitation of burn patients is based on either the Brook formula (2 mL/kg/% TBSA) or the Parkland formula of 4 mL/kg/% TBSA.

For example, consider a 176-pound (lb; 80-kg) man who has sustained third-degree burns to 30% of his TBSA and who is managed on scene shortly after the injury.

The fluid resuscitation volume would be calculated as follows using the Parkland formula:

$$\text{24-hour fluid total} = \text{4 mL/kg} \times \text{weight in kg} \times \text{\% TBSA burned}$$
$$= \text{4 mL/kg} \times \text{80 kg} \times \text{30\% TBSA burned}$$
$$= \text{9,600 mL}$$

Note that in this formula, the units of kilograms and percent cancel out so that only mL is left, thus making the calculation 4 mL × 80 × 30 = 9,600 mL.

Once the 24-hour total is calculated, divide that number by 2:

$$\text{Amount of fluid to be given from time of injury to hour 8} = \text{9,600 mL/2} = \text{4,800 mL}$$

To determine the hourly rate for the first 8 hours, divide this total by 8:

$$\text{Fluid rate for the first 8 hours} = \text{4,800 mL/8 hours} = \text{600 mL/hr}$$

(The Brook formula would be half of this, or 300 mL/hr.)

The fluid requirement for the next period (hours 8 to 24) is calculated as follows:

$$\text{Amount of fluid to be given from hours 8 to 24} = \text{9,600 mL/2} = \text{4,800 mL}$$

To determine the hourly rate for the final 16 hours, divide this total by 16:

$$\text{Fluid rate for final 16 hours} = \text{4,800 mL/16 hours} = \text{300 mL/hr}$$

The USAISR Rule of Ten for Burn Resuscitation

In an effort to simplify the process of calculating fluid requirements for burn patients in the prehospital setting, researchers from the USAISR developed the Rule of Ten to help guide initial fluid resuscitation.[22] The percentage of body surface area burned is calculated and rounded to the nearest 10. For example, a burn of 37% would be rounded to 40%. The percentage is then multiplied by 10 to get the number of milliliters per hour of crystalloid. Thus, in the previous example, the calculation would be 40 × 10 = 400 mL/hr. This formula is used for adults weighing 88 to 154 lb (40 to 70 kg). If the patient exceeds this weight range, for each 10 kg in body weight over 70 kg, an additional 100 mL/hr is given.

If the Rule of Ten is compared to the Parkland formula, it will immediately become apparent that the fluid volumes calculated only differ to a small extent. Regardless of which method is used to calculate fluid requirements, the calculated volume is an estimate of the fluid needs, and the actual volume given to the patient must be adjusted based on the clinical response of the patient. The best indicators of the clinical response are urine output, normal blood pressure, and appropriate mental status in the absence of brain injury.

Pediatric Patient

Resuscitation in burned children is often initiated following a smaller TBSA burned (10% to 20%) compared to adults.[23,24] Pediatric patients require relatively larger volumes of IV fluids than adults with similar-sized burns (reported in some cases to range from 5.8 to 6.2 mL/kg/% TBSA burned).[23-25] Fluid losses are proportionally greater in children due to their small body weight to body surface ratio.[26] Additionally, children have less metabolic glycogen reserves in their livers to maintain adequate blood glucose during the periods of burn resuscitation. For these reasons, children should receive 5% dextrose-containing IV fluids (D_5LR) at a standard maintenance rate in addition to burn resuscitation fluids. Pediatric burn patients with longer than 1 hour transport time should have their glucose checked to ensure that they are not becoming hypoglycemic. Additionally, communication with the receiving burn center should occur to help guide the management of a pediatric patient with a large burn.

Smoke Inhalation: Fluid Management and Other Considerations

The patient with both thermal burns and inhalational injury may require larger volumes of fluid resuscitation. It is often difficult to judge the presence of inhalational injury in the prehospital environment as diagnosis is done with bronchoscopy at the burn center.[27] Resuscitation in this group has been reported to require significantly more fluid compared to similar burns without inhalational injury.[27,28] Patients who have sustained an inhalational injury will likely have other signs such as stridor and singed nasal hairs and will likely require prehospital airway and breathing management.

More about smoke inhalation and inhalational injury, as well as management considerations, will be discussed in subsequent sections.

Analgesia

Burns are extremely painful and, as such, warrant appropriate attention to pain relief, beginning in the prehospital setting. Narcotic analgesics such as fentanyl (1 microgram [mcg] per kg body weight) or morphine (0.1 milligram [mg] per kg body weight) in adequate dosages will be required to control pain. Ketamine 0.5 mg/kg can be used safely in burn patients every hour to augment pain control and decrease the risk of complications associated with use of narcotic analgesics.

Special Considerations

Electrical Injuries

Electrical injuries can be devastating injuries, with underlying tissue destruction and necrosis that may not be

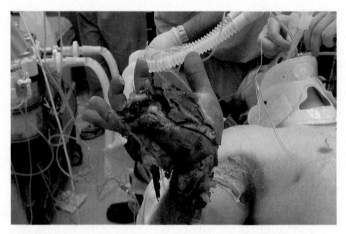

Figure 13-16 Patient after electrical injury from high-tension wires.
Courtesy of Dr. Jeffrey Guy.

apparent merely from the appearance of the overlying skin injury. The severity of electrical injury is determined by voltage, current, path of current flow, duration of contact, and resistance at the point of contact.

Electrical injury is the result of electric current, either alternating current (AC) or direct current (DC). Electrical injuries can be low voltage (< 1,000 volts [V]) or high voltage (> 1,000 V). Electric current generally follows the path of least resistance (through nerves and blood vessels), although high-voltage current may take a direct path between the point of entrance and the ground. Current is concentrated at its entrance point and then diverges and reconverges before exiting, causing the most severe tissue damage to occur at site of contact and the site of exit from the tissue (**Figure 13-16**). High-voltage electrical wounds are often charred, deep burns that leave a black metallic coating on the skin. Severity of damage to tissue is greatest around the contact sites, with damage to vital organs occurring in relation to the path of current.

In the treatment of electrical burns, prehospital care practitioners must keep in mind that the fluid resuscitation requirements usually cannot be estimated using TBSA measurements, as the damage to underlying tissues is easily underestimated. Underlying devitalized tissue is often extensive and involves muscular tissue damage. Often, fascia surrounding the affected muscle limits limb swelling, with resultant rising pressures in the affected compartment. This can lead to compartment syndrome within the affected limb.

Continued ischemia secondary to the initial electrical injury and ongoing increasing compartment pressures can result in irreversible muscle damage after 6 to 8 hours. Muscle necrosis within the compartment results in further release of cytokine mediators, increasing vascular permeability and extravasation of fluid into the injury site. Release of hemoglobin from necrotic muscle is circulated through the kidney. Release of myoglobin,

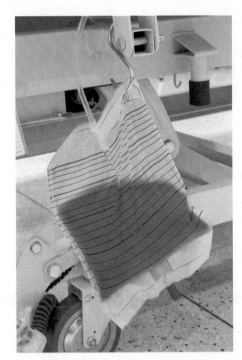

Figure 13-17 Urine of a patient who sustained electrical injury from high-tension wires. The patient has myoglobinuria after extensive muscle destruction.
© Suphatthra China/Shutterstock

another molecule found in the muscle, results in obstruction of the renal collecting tubules, leading to acute renal failure. This condition, myoglobinuria, is evidenced by tea- or cola-colored urine (**Figure 13-17**). There is limited management that can be done for compartment syndrome during transport of the patient with an electrical injury. Alerting the receiving team regarding concerns for compartment syndrome based on the current path is important.

Electrical and crush injuries share many similarities. In both injuries, there is massive destruction of large muscle groups with resultant release of both potassium and myoglobin. (See Chapter 12, *Musculoskeletal Trauma*.) The release of muscle potassium causes a significant increase in the serum level, which can result in cardiac dysrhythmias. Elevated potassium levels can make administration of the depolarizing muscle relaxant succinylcholine prohibitively dangerous.[29] If chemical paralysis of the patient is required, such as for rapid-sequence intubation, nondepolarizing agents such as vecuronium or rocuronium may be used. Succinylcholine should not be used in burn or crush patients secondary to the risk of severe hyperkalemia.

It is common for prehospital care practitioners to be called to provide interhospital transfers of patients with electrical injuries. Patients with electrical injury undergoing interfacility transport should have their electrolytes checked prior to transport and should be transported with a urinary catheter in place. Patients with myoglobinuria

require aggressive fluid administration to maintain a urine output of greater than 100 mL/hr in adults or 1 mL/kg/hr in children to avoid acute kidney injury. Sodium bicarbonate is administered in some cases to make the myoglobin more soluble in urine and reduce the likelihood of renal injury; however, its actual benefit in preventing acute kidney injury remains a topic of debate and it is exceptionally difficult to alkalize the urine to the appropriate pH to have the intended effect. Urine alkalization should not be attempted in the prehospital setting or during interhospital transport.

Patients with electrical burns may have associated mechanical injuries as well. Approximately 15% of patients with electrical injuries also have traumatic injuries. This rate is twice that seen in patients burned by other mechanisms.[30,31] Tympanic membranes may rupture, resulting in hearing difficulties. Intense and sustained muscle contraction (*tetany*) can result in shoulder dislocations and compression fractures of multiple levels of the spine as well as long bones, and for this reason, spinal motion restriction should be considered for patients with electrical injury. Long-bone fractures should be splinted when detected or suspected. Intracranial bleeds and cardiac dysrhythmias may also occur.

If the electric current crossed the thorax, the heart could have received some of the current. Cardiac arrest in the field is the most common cause of immediate death from electrical injury. If the patient has return of cardiac function, there may be continued myocardial instability. Low levels of calcium and magnesium can exacerbate this. Patients being transferred to a burn center from another hospital should have an electrocardiogram and electrolytes checked prior to transfer.

Circumferential Burns

Circumferential burns of the trunk or limbs are capable of producing a life- or limb-threatening condition as a result of the thick, inelastic eschar that is formed. Circumferential burns of the chest can constrict the chest wall to such a degree that the patient suffocates from the inability to inhale. Circumferential burns of the extremities create a tourniquet-like effect that can render an arm or leg pulseless. Therefore, all circumferential burns should be handled as emergencies and patients transported to a burn center, or to the local trauma center if a burn center is not immediately available. As discussed previously, escharotomies are surgical incisions made through the burn eschar to allow expansion of the deeper tissues and decompression of previously compressed and often occluded vascular structures (**Figure 13-18**).

Smoke Inhalation Injuries

The leading cause of death in fires is not thermal injury; it is the inhalation of toxic smoke. Any patient with a history of exposure to smoke in an enclosed space should

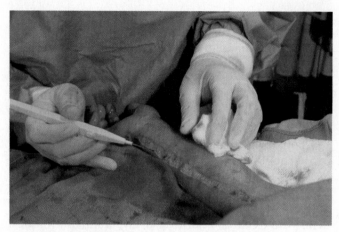

Figure 13-18 Escharotomies are performed to release the constricting effect of circumferential burns.

Courtesy of Dr. Jeffrey Guy.

Box 13-6 Clues Suggesting Smoke Inhalation/Inhalational Injury

- Burn occurred in a confined space
- Confusion or agitation
- Burns to face or chest
- Singeing of eyebrows or nasal hair
- Cardiac arrest (hypoxia or carbon monoxide)
- Soot in the sputum (carbonaceous sputum)
- Hoarseness, loss of voice, or stridor

---

be considered to be at risk of having an inhalational injury. Victims with burns to the face or soot in the sputum are at risk for a smoke inhalation injury; however, the absence of these signs does not exclude the diagnosis of a toxic inhalation (Box 13-6). Maintaining a high index of suspicion is vitally important because signs and symptoms may not manifest for days after the exposure.

Inhalational injury is caused by steam, hot air, gases, or toxic fumes. Inhalational injury can result in upper airway injury, lower airway injury, pulmonary parenchymal injury, and systemic toxicity. Depending on the setting of the fire, a wide variety of materials and chemicals may be part of the combustion process; many of these compounds may act together to increase injury and morbidity. The extent of injury is affected by the ignition source, temperature, concentration, and solubility of gases generated.

Edema formation in the oropharynx, bronchial areas, and lung parenchyma accounts for many of the effects of smoke inhalation injury. Ongoing edema contributes to the microvascular disruption, inhibiting gas exchange. The edema may also obstruct the oropharynx, making it difficult for the patient to breathe and also making intubation challenging. This is one of the reasons that early

intubation and control of the airway can be imperative. If there is any concern for airway or inhalational injury, intubation prior to aggressive fluid resuscitation and resultant edema formation is necessary.

Toxic Gas Inhalational Injury

Two gaseous products that are clinically important are *carbon monoxide* and *hydrogen cyanide*. Both molecules are classified as asphyxiants and, thus, cause cell death by cellular hypoxia. Patients with asphyxia from smoke containing one or both of these compounds will have inadequate delivery of oxygen to tissues despite an adequate blood pressure or pulse oximeter reading.

Carbon Monoxide

Carbon monoxide is an odorless, colorless gas that is produced by incomplete combustion of common products such as wood, paper, and cotton. It can also be produced by car exhaust. Carbon monoxide binds to hemoglobin with much greater affinity than oxygen does. This competitive binding to hemoglobin reduces delivery of oxygen to tissues, leading to severe hypoxia, especially in tissues with high oxygen extraction (i.e., the brain and heart). The symptoms of carbon monoxide inhalation depend on the duration or severity of exposure and the resultant serum levels. Symptoms can range from mild headache to confusion, unconsciousness, cardiac arrest, convulsions, and death (Box 13-7). Traditional teaching is that patients poisoned with carbon monoxide develop "classic" cherry-red skin coloration. Unfortunately, this is often a late sign and should not be relied on when considering the diagnosis. Diagnosis should be based on direct measurements of carboxyhemoglobin in arterial or venous blood. The inability to differentiate oxyhemoglobin from carboxyhemoglobin limits the use of pulse

---

Box 13-7 Symptoms of Carbon Monoxide Poisoning

- Mild
  - Headache
  - Fatigue
  - Nausea
- Moderate
  - Severe headache
  - Vomiting
  - Confusion
  - Drowsiness/sleepiness
  - Increased heart rate and respiratory rate
- Severe
  - Seizures
  - Coma
  - Cardiorespiratory arrest

oximetry. The pulse oximeter can read as normal in a patient with severe cellular hypoxia secondary to carbon monoxide poisoning. Pulse oximetry should not be relied upon to detect carbon monoxide poisoning, nor should it be used to determine that it is safe to withhold supplemental oxygen from a patient with suspected inhalation injury.

Portable pulse carbon monoxide monitors that noninvasively measure the amount of carbon monoxide in the bloodstream are available for use in the prehospital setting (**Figure 13-19**). These monitors look and operate like pulse oximeters. Patients will generally complain of mild symptoms with levels of 10% to 20% carboxyhemoglobin. As the level of carbon monoxide in the blood increases, symptoms progressively get worse. As levels exceed 50% to 60%, seizures, coma, and death result.

Treatment of carbon monoxide toxicity is removal of the patient from the source and administration of oxygen. When breathing room air (21% oxygen), the body will eliminate half the carbon monoxide in 250 minutes.[32] When the patient is placed on 100% oxygen, the half-life of the carbon monoxide–hemoglobin complex is reduced to 40 to 60 minutes.[33] All patients with suspected carbon monoxide poisoning should be placed on 100% oxygen regardless of pulse oximetry readings.

The use of hyperbaric oxygen therapy is controversial but should be considered if carbon monoxide elimination is not achieved as expected with the use of normobaric therapy (100% oxygen). Hyperbaric treatment is delivered in a hyperbaric chamber with a typical regimen consisting of several sessions at 2 to 3 atmospheres. Limited studies have shown an improvement in neurologic complications from carbon monoxide poisoning with the use of hyperbaric treatment.[34] If the decision to use hyperbaric therapy is made, then it should not be delayed. Rapid return to normoxia in these patients is associated with improved outcomes; the longer a patient remains with high carbon monoxide levels, the more damage occurs to the brain and heart. A review of seven randomized trials compared hyperbaric oxygen treatment to 100% oxygen therapy. It found mixed results regarding improvement of neurologic sequelae.[35-36] The role of hyperbaric treatment in inhalational injury at the present time remains controversial and should only be considered on a patient-specific basis if treatment with normobaric oxygen is not achieving adequate clearance of oxygen and if there is significant underlying neurologic compromise as a result of carbon monoxide exposure.

Hydrogen Cyanide

Cyanide gas is produced from the burning of plastics or polyurethane. Cyanide poisons the cellular processes of energy production and prevents the cells from using oxygen. Hydrogen cyanide inhibits cellular oxygenation with resultant tissue anoxia, which is caused by reversible inhibition of cytochrome *c* oxidase. The patient can die from asphyxia despite having adequate amounts of oxygen in the blood. Symptoms of cyanide toxicity include altered level of consciousness, dizziness, headache, and tachycardia or tachypnea. Patients with carbon monoxide toxicity from a structure fire should also be considered to be at risk for cyanide poisoning.

The treatment of cyanide poisoning is rapid administration of an antidote. The preferred antidote for cyanide poisoning is a medication that directly binds to the cyanide molecule, rendering it harmless. *Hydroxocobalamin* (Cyanokit) detoxifies the cyanide by directly binding to it and forming cyanocobalamin (vitamin B_{12}), which is nontoxic. Hydroxocobalamin is available for prehospital use in Europe and the United States. It should be liberally used if there is any suspicion of cyanide poisoning. A second chelating agent that has been used in Europe for cyanide poisoning is *dicobalt edetate*; however, if this medication is administered in the absence of cyanide poisoning, cobalt toxicity is a risk.

For historical purposes, the "Lilly kit" or "Pasadena kit" was the traditional cyanide antidote kit used in the United States and may still be utilized in some settings. Most prehospital systems should have the Cyanokit available; however, practitioners should be aware of the Lilly kit. This method of treating cyanide poisoning was developed in the 1930s and found to be effective in detoxifying animals poisoned with 21 times the lethal dose of cyanide.[37] The goal of this antidote therapy is to induce the formation of a second poison (methemoglobin) in the

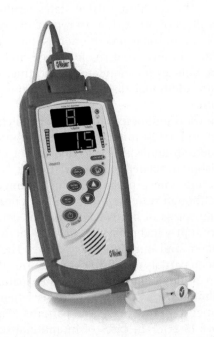

Figure 13-19 Masimo prehospital carbon monoxide monitor, Rad-57.

Courtesy of Masimo Corporation.

patient's blood. This therapeutically induced poison binds with the cyanide and allows the body to slowly detoxify and excrete the cyanide.

The Lilly kit contains three medications that are administered in a specified order. The first medication is a nitrate, either amyl nitrate or sodium nitrate (both of which are provided in the kit). Amyl nitrate comes in an ampule that is broken open, releasing fumes that the patient inhales; sodium nitrate, which is given IV, is the preferred method because it is more efficient and avoids exposure of healthcare practitioners to amyl nitrate fumes. The nitrate medications change some of the patient's hemoglobin into a form called methemoglobin, which attracts the cyanide away from the site of toxic action in the mitochondria of the cell. Once the cyanide binds with the methemoglobin, the mitochondria can once again begin to produce energy for the cell. Unfortunately, methemoglobin is toxic because it does not carry oxygen to cells as well as hemoglobin does. This decrease in oxygen delivery can exacerbate the tissue hypoxia associated with increased carbon monoxide levels that the victim may also have as a result of smoke inhalation.[38,39] The third medication in the kit is sodium thiosulfate, which is given IV after the nitrate to bind the methemoglobin. The thiosulfate and cyanide from the methemoglobin are metabolized to thiocyanate, which is safely excreted in the patient's urine. Because of the toxicity of methemoglobin and the time needed to administer the full Lilly kit, hydroxocobalamin (Cyanokit) has become the preferred antidote for the treatment of cyanide poisoning.

Toxin-Induced Lung Injury

In simplified terms, smoke is the product of incomplete combustion—that is, chemical dust. The chemicals in the smoke react with the lining of the trachea and lungs and damage the cells lining the airways and lungs.[40-42] Compounds such as ammonia, hydrogen chloride, and sulfur dioxide form corrosive acids and alkalis when they are inhaled and react with water.[43] These poisons cause necrosis of the cells lining the trachea and bronchioles. Normally, these cells have tiny hair-like structures called *cilia*. On these cilia is a blanket of mucus that captures and transports normally inhaled debris to the oropharynx, where the debris is swallowed into the GI tract. Several days after an inhalation injury, these cells die. The debris from these necrotic cells and the debris these cells typically capture accumulate instead of being removed. The result is an increase in secretions, plugging of the airways with mucus and cellular debris, and an increased rate of life-threatening pneumonia.

Prehospital Management

The initial and most important element of caring for a patient with smoke exposure is determining the need for endotracheal intubation. Continuous reevaluation of airway patency is required in order to recognize developing signs of airway obstruction. Change in the character of the voice, difficulty handling secretions, and drooling are signs of impending airway occlusion. Whenever patency of the patient's airway is in doubt, the prehospital care practitioner can proceed with securing the airway using endotracheal intubation.[44,45] In some cases, rapid-sequence intubation (avoiding the use of succinylcholine) may be necessary. In the event of long transport times, communication with the receiving facility as well as rendezvous with an agency capable of providing definitive airway management should be considered. These patients can be challenging to intubate even in very experienced hands; therefore, the capability to perform a surgical airway should be readily available.

Patients with smoke inhalation should be transported to burn centers even in the absence of cutaneous burns. Burn centers treat a greater volume of patients with smoke inhalation and offer unique modes of mechanical ventilation and occasionally hyperbaric oxygen therapy.

Child Abuse

Burn injuries are the third most common injury causing death in children.[46] Approximately 20% of all child abuse is the result of intentional burning. The majority of the children intentionally burned are 1 to 2 years of age.[46,47] Per the federal Child Abuse Prevention and Treatment Act, healthcare practitioners are mandatory reporters of suspected child maltreatment in 47 states and most U.S. territories. The remaining three states require any person, regardless of profession, to report suspected abuse. Therefore, prehospital practitioners should alert hospital providers of any concerns for abuse and be familiar with state policies for mandatory reporting, which may require an additional direct report by the prehospital practitioner.

The most common form of burn seen in child abuse is secondary to forcible immersion. These injuries typically occur when an adult places a child in hot water, often as a punishment related to toilet training.[47-49] Immersion scalds are often deep because of the prolonged skin exposure (although water temperature may not be as high as in other forms of burns). Factors that determine the severity of injury include age of the patient, temperature of the water, and duration of exposure. The child may sustain deep partial- or full-thickness burns of the hands or feet in a glove-like or stocking-like pattern. Practitioners should be especially suspicious when the burns are symmetric and lack splash patterns (**Figure 13-20** and **Figure 13-21**).[50] In cases of intentional scalding, the child will tightly flex the arms and legs into a defensive posture because of fear or pain. The resultant burn pattern will spare the flexion creases of the popliteal fossa

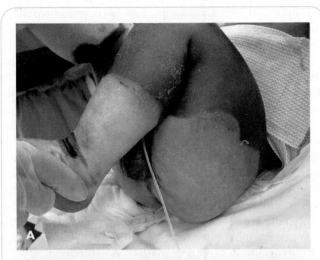

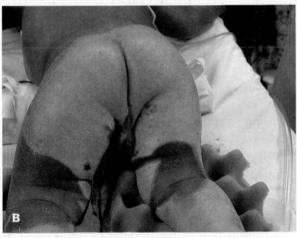

Figure 13-20 The straight lines of the burn pattern and absence of splash marks indicate that this burn is the result of abuse. **A.** Side view. **B.** Posterior view.

Courtesy of Dr. Jeffrey Guy.

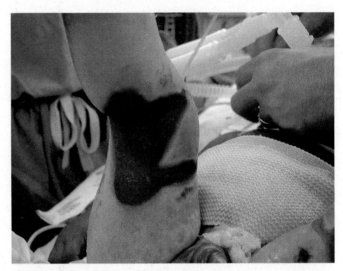

Figure 13-21 The sparing of the areas of flexion and the sharp lines of demarcation between burned and unburned skin indicate that this child was in a tightly flexed, defensive position before injury. Such a posture indicates that the scald is not accidental.

Courtesy of Dr. Jeffrey Guy.

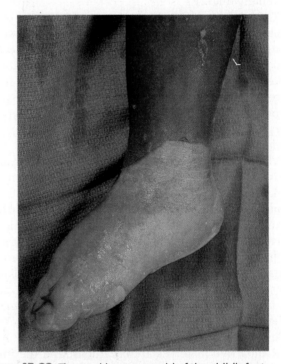

Figure 13-22 The stocking-type scald of the child's foot indicates intentional immersion burn injury consistent with child abuse.

Courtesy of Dr. Jeffrey Guy.

(knees), the antecubital fossa (elbows), and the groin. Sharp lines of demarcation will also be seen between burned and unburned tissue, essentially indicating a dip **(Figure 13-22)**.[51,52]

In accidental scald injuries, the burns will have variable burn depth, irregular margins, and smaller burns remote from the large burns, indicating splash.[53] A common mechanism of accidental scald injuries is from microwaved noodle soup.

Contact Burns

Contact burns are the second most common mechanism of burn injury in children, whether accidental or intentional. All body surfaces have some degree of curvature. When an accidental contact burn occurs, the burning agent makes contact with the curved body surface area. The burning instrument is deflected off the curved surface, or the victim withdraws from the hot object. The resultant injury has an irregular burn edge and depth. When a child receives an intentional contact burn, the inflicting implement is pressed onto the child's skin and there are sharp lines of demarcation with a uniform depth.[52] Common objects involved in contact burns include curling irons, steam irons, radiators, and hot pots and pans.

Radiation Burns

Radiation burn injuries can be difficult to diagnosis because the patient is not always aware that an exposure to radiation occurred. The severity of burns produced from the various forms of radiation is secondary to the amount of energy absorbed by the target tissue. The various forms of radiation include electromagnetic, x-ray, gamma ray, and particulate. These different forms of radiation transfer varying degrees of energy to tissue. While electromagnetic radiation is able to pass through tissue and not cause significant damage, other forms of radiation such as neutron exposure get absorbed by the tissue, resulting in significant damage. It is the absorption of the radiation that results in damage to the absorbing tissue. The absorption capacity of the radiation is more damaging than the actual dose of radiation. Equivalent doses of different forms of radiation will have dramatically different effects on an individual.

The current most common cause of radiation exposure is an industrial or occupational incident. However, with the increasing threat of global terrorism, the detonation of a radiation dispersal device (conventional explosive with radioactive material added) or a small, improvised nuclear device is a possibility, and all practitioners should have some awareness of this type of injury. (See Chapter 18, *Explosions and Weapons of Mass Destruction*, for more detail.)

The detonation of a nuclear weapon in a metropolitan area would be a catastrophic event that would injure and kill many. The mechanisms of injury from a nuclear detonation depend on proximity to the blast and include thermal burns from the initial firestorm; supersonic destructive blast causing blunt and penetrating trauma; and production of radiation, resulting in organ damage. Mortality from a combination of thermal and radiation burns is greater than that from either thermal or radiation burns alone of equal magnitude. The combination of thermal and radiation burns after a nuclear weapon explosion has a synergistic effect on mortality.[54]

Radioactive materials are hazardous, and the initial priorities are the same as for any patient exposed to a hazardous material: utilize appropriate personal protective equipment, remove the patient from the source of contamination, remove contaminated clothing, and initiate copious irrigation with water. Remember that any removed clothing should be considered contaminated and should be handled with caution. Irrigation is performed carefully to remove any radioactive debris or particles from contaminated areas without spreading the injury to uncontaminated body surfaces. Irrigation should continue until contamination has been minimized to a steady state, as determined by a full-body survey with a Geiger counter.[55]

The exception to this approach is the patient who has sustained major trauma in addition to radiation injury. In these cases, clothing should be removed immediately, obvious contaminants irrigated, and simultaneous stabilization of the traumatic injury provided. It is important that prehospital practitioners continue to take precautions to not expose themselves to radiation injury no matter how seriously the patient is injured. Acute radiation injury associated with vomiting and diarrhea is indicative of a large dose of radiation poisoning and is highly lethal. These patients will need supportive care with resuscitation fluids in the prehospital environment and transfer to a hospital with expertise in radiation toxicity management.

After a nuclear event, IV supplies, infusion pumps, and receiving medical facilities may be in short supply. If the prehospital care practitioner is unable to provide the patient with IV resuscitation, the patient can be resuscitated with oral fluids. In fact, oral resuscitation is considered for thermal injury as well, and some hospitals are assessing outcomes of using oral resuscitation in lieu of large volume of IV fluids, but this practice has not yet migrated into the prehospital environment. However, in any contingency with resource limitations, oral rehydration and resuscitation should absolutely be considered and current and future investigations will inform whether this therapy also improves outcomes. In the case of resource limitations, such as after a catastrophic event that generates large volumes of burn or radiation casualties, patients who are cooperative should be encouraged to drink a balanced salt solution to maintain urine output; alternatively, fluids can be delivered by nasogastric or nasoenteric tubes. Oral balanced salt solutions include Moyer's solution (4 grams [g] sodium chloride [0.5 teaspoon of salt] and 1.5 g sodium bicarbonate [0.5 teaspoon baking soda] in 1 liter of water) and World Health Organization oral rehydration solution (WHO ORS). Animal research has shown encouraging results with such resuscitation strategies in patients with burns as large as 40% TBSA. Administration of balanced salt solution to the GI tract at a rate of 20 mL/kg provided resuscitation equivalent to standard IV fluid resuscitation.[56]

Chemical Burns

All prehospital care practitioners need to be familiar with the basics of treating chemical injuries. Prehospital care practitioners in urban settings may be called to a chemical incident at an industrial setting, whereas a rural prehospital care practitioner may be summoned to an incident involving agents used in agriculture. Tons of hazardous materials are transported through urban and rural settings daily by both highways and rail systems. Military prehospital care practitioners may treat casualties of chemical burns caused by weapons or incendiary devices, chemicals used to fuel or maintain equipment, or chemical spills after damage to civilian installations.

Injuries from chemicals are often the result of prolonged exposure to the offending agent, in contrast to thermal injuries, which usually involve a very brief exposure duration. The severity of chemical injury is determined by four factors: nature of the chemical, concentration of the chemical, duration of contact, and mechanism of action of the chemical.

Chemical agents are classified as acid, base, organic, or inorganic. **Acids** are chemicals with a pH between 7 (neutral) and 0 (strong acid). **Bases** are agents with a pH between 7 and 14 (strong base) (**Figure 13-23**). Acids damage tissue by a process called **coagulative necrosis**; the damaged tissue coagulates and transforms into a barrier that prevents deeper penetration of the acid. In contrast, alkali burns destroy the tissue by **liquefaction necrosis**; the base liquefies the tissue, allowing the chemical to penetrate more deeply and cause increasingly deeper tissue damage. Alkali agents dissolve proteins of tissue and form alkaline proteins, which are soluble and allow further reaction deeper into affected tissues. Organic solutions will dissolve the liquid membranes of cell walls and cause disruption of cellular architecture, and cause damage predominantly through this mechanism. Inorganic solutions, in contrast, remain on the exterior of the cell. Chemical burns can be much deeper than what appears on the surface. Copious, and sometimes continuous, irrigation may be required. Ideally, the surface pH should be checked and should be < 8 for alkali injury. In patients with long transport times, continuous irrigation might be required for alkali injuries.

Prehospital Management

The greatest priority in the care of a patient exposed to chemical agents is personal and scene safety. As in any emergency, the prehospital care practitioner should always be protected first. If there is any possibility of exposure to a chemical hazard, ensure scene safety and determine if any special garment or breathing apparatus is required or if any specially trained personnel or equipment is necessary. Avoid contamination of equipment and emergency vehicles; a contaminated vehicle creates an exposure risk to all others in its path. Attempt to obtain identification of the chemical agent as soon as possible.

Remove all clothing from the patient, as it may be contaminated with the chemical agent in either liquid or powder form. The contaminated clothing needs to be discarded with care. If any particulate substance is on the skin, it should be brushed away. Next, wash (*lavage*) the patient with copious amounts of water. Lavage will dilute the concentration of the injurious agent and wash away any remaining reagent. The key to lavage is to use large amounts of water. A common error is to rinse 1 or 2 liters of water across the patient and then stop the lavage process once the water starts to pool and accumulate on the floor. When lavaged with only small amounts of fluid, the offending agent is spread across the patient's body surface area and not flushed away.[57,58]

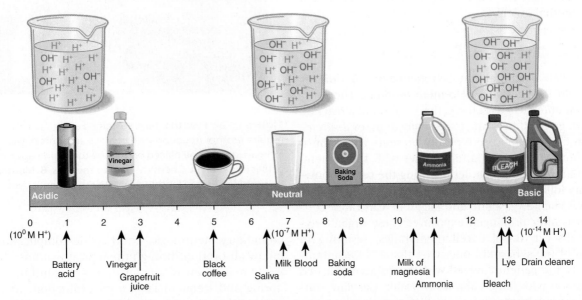

Figure 13-23 Chemical agents are classified as acid, neutral, or base, depending on the amount of hydrogen or hydroxide ions. Many household items are acids or bases and require care in handling.

Failure to provide adequate runoff and drainage of lavage fluid may cause injury to previously unexposed and uninjured areas of the patient's body as the contaminated lavage accumulates beneath the patient. One simple way of promoting runoff in a prehospital setting is to place the patient on a backboard and then tilt it with cribbing or other means to elevate the head. At the lower end of the board, tuck a large plastic garbage bag to capture the contaminated runoff.

Neutralizing agents for chemical burns should not be used or carried by prehospital practitioners. These neutralizing agents often give off heat in an exothermic reaction. Therefore, a well-meaning prehospital care practitioner may create a thermal burn in addition to the chemical burn. Most commercially available decontamination solutions are made for the purpose of decontaminating equipment, not people.

Chemical Burns to the Eye

Injuries to the eye caused by exposure to alkali may be encountered. A small exposure to the eye can threaten vision and ocular function. The eyes should be immediately irrigated with large amounts of irrigation fluid. If possible, ocular decontamination with continuous irrigation using a Morgan lens is performed (**Figure 13-24**). It can take more than 5 liters of continuous irrigation to treat a chemical burn to the eye. If a Morgan lens is not available, continuous irrigation may be accomplished manually with handheld IV tubing or, if both eyes are involved, a nasal cannula placed on the bridge of the nose and attached to IV tubing and an IV bag. Application of an ophthalmic local anesthetic such as proparacaine will simplify the patient's care for the prehospital care practitioner. These patients must be transferred to a center that has an ophthalmologist.

Specific Chemical Exposures

Cement is an alkali that may be retained on the clothing or fall into the footwear of cement workers. The powdered cement reacts with the patient's sweat in a reaction that both gives off heat and excessively dries, or *desiccates*, the skin.[59] This exposure typically presents with a burn injury hours or the day after contact with the cement. The initial treatment includes brushing the cement powder away followed by copious irrigation.

Fuels such as gasoline and kerosene can cause contact burns after prolonged exposure. These organic hydrocarbons can dissolve cell membranes, resulting in necrosis of the skin and underlying tissue.[60] Decontamination of the patient covered with fuel is accomplished by irrigation with large volumes of water. Gasoline contact exposure can lead to full-thickness tissue injury. An exposure of sufficient duration or severity may result in systemic toxicity. Severe cardiovascular, renal,

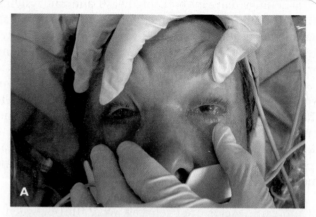
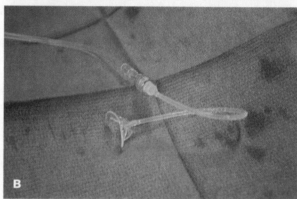
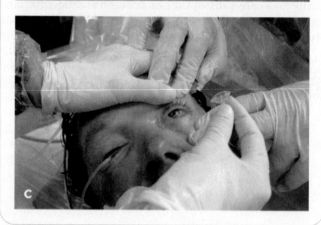

Figure 13-24 Eyes that have sustained a chemical injury require prompt irrigation with copious amounts of saline. A Morgan lens can be placed on the eye to provide appropriate ocular irrigation. **A.** Chemical burn to the eyes. **B.** Morgan lens. **C.** Inserting Morgan lenses to irrigate the patient's eyes.
Courtesy of Dr. Jeffrey Guy.

pulmonary, neurologic, and hepatic complications may follow absorption through the topical wounds; these patients require an ICU admission with continuous monitoring and frequent laboratory evaluation. In cases of suspected systemic toxicity, emergency surgical debridement may be warranted if there is concern for ongoing absorption of toxins from the wound.

Hydrofluoric acid is a dangerous substance widely used in domestic, industrial, and military settings. It is primarily found in the manufacturing of refrigerants but is also used when making herbicides, pharmaceuticals, high-octane gasoline, aluminum, plastics, electrical components, and fluorescent lightbulbs. In addition, it is used to etch glass and metal and is found in rust removers and automobile wheel cleaners. The real danger of this chemical is the fluoride ion, which produces profound alterations of electrolytes, especially calcium and magnesium.[61] The fluoride ion chelates positively charged ions like calcium and magnesium, causing an efflux of intracellular calcium with resultant cell death. The fluoride ion remains active until it is completely neutralized and can effectively penetrate to bone. Even small amounts of hydrofluoric acid can lead to profound, and potentially lethal, *hypocalcemia* (low serum calcium level). Hypocalcemia quickly results in cardiac arrhythmias. Left untreated, hydrofluoric acid will liquefy tissues, leach calcium from the patient's bones, and cause lethal cardiac arrhythmias. Initial treatment for hydrofluoric acid exposure is irrigation with water, followed by application of calcium gluconate gel at an emergency department. Patients with hydrofluoric acid burns should be promptly transferred to a burn center for additional treatment.

Injuries from phosphorus are often seen in military settings. **White phosphorus** (WP) is a powerful incendiary agent used in the production of munitions. It burns violently when exposed to air, producing brilliant flames and dense smoke. It will continue to burn until all of the agent has been consumed or is deprived of oxygen. When in contact with skin, WP will produce deep chemical and thermal burns. These burns require surgical excision or rapid treatment with a copper solution, which is rarely available, particularly in the prehospital environment.

The initial treatment is to deprive the WP of access to oxygen. All clothing needs to be rapidly removed because it may contain some retained phosphorus particles that could ignite the clothing. Keep the affected areas immersed in water or saline-soaked dressings, and re-moisten the dressings during transport. If the dressings dry out, any retained WP will reignite and could ignite the dressings and burn the patient.

Hypochlorite solutions are often used to produce household bleaches and industrial cleaners. These solutions are strong alkalis; the commonly available solutions are 4% to 6% and are not usually lethal unless large areas of the body are exposed to the chemical. **Sulfur mustard** and **nitrogen mustard** are compounds that are classified as **vesicants** or **blister agents**. These agents have been used as chemical weapons and are recognized as a threat in chemical terrorism. These chemicals will burn and blister skin on exposure. They are irritants to the skin and cause irritation to the lungs and the eyes. After exposure, patients will complain of a burning sensation in the throat and eyes. The skin involvement develops several hours later as redness and is followed by blistering in the exposed or contaminated areas. After intense exposure, victims will develop full-thickness necrosis and respiratory failure.[62-64] The principal treatment in the field is decontamination to prevent inadvertent cross-contamination.

In caring for victims of vesicant exposure, prehospital care practitioners must wear appropriate gloves, garments, and breathing equipment. The Scene Management chapter covers this topic in detail. The patients must be decontaminated and irrigated with water or saline. Other agents used to decontaminate victims, used by specially trained personnel, include dilute hypochlorite solution and fuller's earth powder, which is available commercially and functions as an absorbent agent. Additional specialized treatment is required when the patient arrives at a burn center.

Tear gas and similar chemicals are known as **riot control agents**. A riot control agent will rapidly and briefly disable those exposed to it by causing irritation to the skin, mucous membranes, lungs, and eyes. The extent of the injury is determined by the magnitude of exposure to the agent. The duration of the irritation typically lasts 30 to 60 minutes. Treatment consists of removing those exposed to the riot control agent from the source of the exposure, removing contaminated clothing, and irrigating the patients' skin and eyes.

SUMMARY

- All burns are serious, regardless of their size.
- Potentially life-threatening burns include large thermal burns, electrical injuries, and chemical burns.
- Unlike in mechanical trauma (e.g., penetrating, blunt), the body has little to no adaptive mechanisms to survive a burn injury and burn injuries that require hospitalization should be managed at specialty burn centers.
- Burn injuries are not isolated to the skin; these are systemic injuries of unparalleled magnitude. Patients with major burn injury will experience

(continues)

SUMMARY (CONTINUED)

dysfunction of the cardiovascular, pulmonary, gastrointestinal, renal, and immune systems.

- Failure to provide appropriate fluid resuscitation will lead to refractory shock, multiorgan dysfunction, and even deepening of the burns. The role of prehospital care practitioners is, therefore, crucial in optimizing survival after a burn injury.
- Although complicated and dangerous, burns are rarely rapidly fatal. A patient with severe smoke inhalation and large thermal burns may take several hours or days to die. Patients with burns also are likely to have other mechanical trauma. Trauma priorities stay the same for burn patients, and practitioners should not be distracted by the burn wounds.
- Dramatic burns may direct the prehospital care practitioner's attention away from other, potentially life-threatening injuries. Performing primary and secondary surveys will reduce the likelihood of missing these injuries (e.g., pneumothorax, pericardial tamponade, splenic rupture).

- The highest priority is personal and scene safety. Often the injuring agent still poses a risk for injuring the prehospital care practitioners.
- Even small burns in areas of high function (hands, face, joints, perineum) may result in long-term impairment from scar formation.
- Familiarity with burn center transport criteria will help to ensure that all patients can achieve maximum functional recovery after burn injury.
- The leading cause of death in patients with burns is complications from smoke inhalation: asphyxiation, thermal injury, and delayed toxin-induced lung injury. Patients often do not develop symptoms of respiratory failure for 48 hours or longer. Even without burns to the skin, victims of smoke inhalation should be transported to burn centers.
- Victims of burn injury from hazardous materials, such as chemicals or radioactive agents, should undergo decontamination to avoid inadvertent spread of the material to prehospital and healthcare practitioners.

SCENARIO RECAP

You are called to a residential structure fire. When your unit arrives, you witness a two-story house that is fully involved with fire and has thick black smoke pouring out of the roof and windows. You are directed to a victim who is being cared for by EMRs. They tell you that the patient reentered the burning building in an attempt to rescue his dog, and he was carried out unconscious by firefighters.

Your patient is a man who appears to be in his thirties. The majority of his clothes have been burned off. He has obvious burns to his face, and his hair has been singed. He is unconscious; he is breathing spontaneously, but with snoring respirations. The EMRs have placed the patient on high-flow oxygen with a nonrebreathing mask. On physical examination, his airway is patent with manual assistance (jaw thrust); he ventilates easily. The sleeves of his shirt have been burned off. His arms have circumferential burns, but his radial pulse is easily palpable. His heart rate is 118 beats/minute, blood pressure is 148/94 mm Hg, ventilatory rate is 22 breaths/minute, and oxygen saturation (SpO$_2$), taken by pulse oximeter, is 92%. On physical examination, you determine that the patient is burned on his entire head and has blistering of the anterior chest and abdomen, along with full-thickness burns of his entire right and left arm and hand.

- What is the extent of burns for this patient?
- What are the initial steps for managing this patient?
- How does the prehospital care practitioner recognize an inhalation injury?

SCENARIO SOLUTION

The patient has sustained critical injuries. Given that the patient was found collapsed in a burned building with burns to the face and labored respirations, you must be concerned that the patient has inhaled a large amount of smoke.

Evaluate and reevaluate for airway edema and an inhalational injury. Airway patency needs to be a concern; however, the patient currently is managing his own airway. Keeping in mind that often the best person to manage an airway is the patient, you need to balance the time required to transport the patient with the difficulties of airway management in a patient with an edematous airway. If transport will be prolonged or delayed, secure the airway by endotracheal intubation and use umbilical tape to secure the ET tube. The patient requires 100% oxygen given the exposure to smoke and concerns about asphyxiants. A portable carbon monoxide monitor placed on the patient reports a carboxyhemoglobin level of 16%, which is already being treated since the patient is on 100% oxygen. You consult the local protocol regarding management of smoke inhalation with potential cyanide poisoning.

Both upper extremities have deep, full-thickness burns. You are not able to identify any veins to establish an IV line. Neither leg is burned, nor is there evidence of any fractures. An IO line is started in the left tibia, and an infusion of lactated Ringer's solution is started.

The patient is burned on the entire head, both upper extremities, and the anterior trunk. Each limb is approximately 9% of TBSA, the anterior trunk is 18%, and the head is approximately 9%. Therefore, the estimated TBSA burned is approximately 45%. The patient weighs approximately 175 pounds, or 80 kg. Estimate the patient's initial fluid needs using the USAISR Rule of Ten:

45% TBSA burned × 10 mL/hr = 450 mL/hr as the initial fluid rate

If the patient requires a transport longer than 1 hour then fluid rate adjustments should be made depending on hemodynamics and urine output. Communication with the receiving burn center can help with en route resuscitation decision support for longer transports.

References

1. World Health Organization. Burns: Key facts. Published March 6, 2018. Accessed November 21, 2021. https://www.who.int/news-room/fact-sheets/detail/burns/

2. Vyrosek SB, Annest JL, Ryan GW. Surveillance for fatal and non-fatal injuries—United States, 2001. *MMWR Surveill Summ*. 2004;53(7):1-57.

3. Herndon DN. *Total Burn Care*. 5th ed. Elsevier; 2018:15-26.

4. Goodwin CW, Dorethy J, Lam V, Pruitt BA Jr. Randomized trial of efficacy of crystalloid and colloid resuscitation on hemodynamic response and lung water following thermal injury. *Ann Surg*. 1983 May;197(5):520-531.

5. Evans EI, Purnell OJ, Robinett PW, Batchelor A, Martin M. Fluid and electrolyte requirements in severe burns. *Ann Surg*. 1952;135:804-817.

6. Shires GT. Proceedings of the Second NIH Workshop on Burn Management. *J Trauma*. 1979;19(11 suppl):862-863.

7. Schwartz SL. Consensus summary on fluid resuscitation. *J Trauma*. 1979;19(11 suppl):876-877.

8. Moyer CA, Margrave HW, Monafo, WW. Burn shock and extravascular sodium deficiency: treatment with Ringer's solution with lactate. *Arch Surg*. 1965;90:799-811.

9. Mortiz AR, Henrique FC Jr. Studies of thermal injury: the relative importance of time and surface temperature in the causation of cutaneous burn injury. *Am J Pathol*. 1947;23:695-720.

10. Robinson MC, Del Becarro EJ. Increasing dermal perfusion after burning by decreasing thromboxane production. *J Trauma*. 1980;20:722-725.

11. Heggers JP, Ko F, Robson MC, et al. Evaluation of burn blister fluid. *Plast Reconstr Surg*. 1980;65:798-804.

12. Pruitt BA Jr, Goodwin CW, Mason AD Jr. Epidemiological, demographic and outcome characteristics of burn injury. In: Herndon DN, ed. *Total Burn Care*. 2nd ed. WB Saunders; 2002:16-32.

13. Rossiter ND, Chapman P, Haywood IA. How big is a hand? *Burns*. 1996;22(3):230-231.

14. Berry MG, Evison D, Roberts AH. The influence of body mass index on burn surface area estimated from the area of the hand. *Burns*. 2001;27(6):591-594.

15. de Camara DL, Robinson MC. Ultrastructure aspects of cooled thermal injury. *J Trauma*. 1981;21:911-919.

16. Jandera V, Hudson DA, de Wet PM, Innes PM, Rode H. Cooling the burn wound: evaluation of different modalities. *Burns*. 2000;26:265-270.

17. Sawada Y, Urushidate S, Yotsuyanagi T, Ishita K. Is prolonged and excessive cooling of a scalded wound effective? *Burns*. 1977;23(1):55-58.

18. Venter TH, Karpelowsky JS, Rode H. Cooling of the burn wound: the ideal temperature of the coolant. *Burns*. 2007;33:917-922.

19. Dunn K, Edwards-Jones VT. The role of Acticoat with nanocrystal-line silver in the management of burns. *Burns*. 2004;30(suppl):S1.

20. Wright JB, Lam K, Burrell RE. Wound management in an era of increasing bacterial antibiotic resistance: a role for topical silver treatments. *Am J Infect Control*. 1998;26:572-577.

21. Yin HQ, Langford R, Burrell RE. Comparative evaluation of the antimicrobial activity of Acticoat antimicrobial dressing. *J Burn Care Rehabil*. 1999;20:195-200.

22. Chung KK, Salinas J, Renz EM, et al. Simple derivation of the initial fluid rate for the resuscitation of severely burned adult combat casualties: in silico validation of the rule of 10. *J Trauma*. 2010;69:S49-S54.

23. Merrell SW, Saffle JR, Sullivan JJ, Navar PD, Kravitz M, Warden GD. Fluid resuscitation in thermally injured children. *Am J Surg*. 1986;152:664-669.

24. Graves TA, Cioffi WG, McManus WF, Mason AD Jr, Pruitt BA Jr. Fluid resuscitation of infants and children with massive thermal injury. *J Trauma*. 1988;28:1656-1659.

25. Carvajal HF. Fluid therapy for the acutely burned child. *Compr Ther*. 1977;3:17-24.

26. Herndon DN. *Total Burn Care*. 2nd ed. WB Saunders; 2002.

27. Navar PD, Saffle JR, Warden GD. Effect of inhalation injury on fluid resuscitation requirements after thermal injury. *Am J Surg*. 1985;150:716-720.

28. Lalonde C, Picard L, Youn YK, Demling RH. Increased early postburn fluid requirement and oxygen demands are predictive of the degree of airway injury by smoke inhalation. *J Trauma*. 1995;38(2):175-184.

29. RxList. Anectine: warnings. Reviewed January 31, 2011. Accessed September 1, 2013. http://www.rxlist.com/anectine-drug/warnings-precautions.htm

30. Dash S, Arumugam PK, Muthukumar V, Kumath M, Sharma S. Study of clinical pattern of limb loss in electrical burn injuries. *Injury*. 2021 Jul;52(7):1925-1933. doi: 10.1016/j.injury.2021.04.028

31. Herndon DN. *Total Burn Care*. 5th ed. Elsevier; 2018:398-400.

32. Forbes WH, Sargent F, Roughton FJW. The rate of carbon monoxide uptake by normal men. *Am J Physiol*. 1945;143:594-608.

33. Mellins RB, Park S. Respiratory complications of smoke inhalation in victims of fires. *J Pediatr*. 1975;87(1):1-7. doi: 10.1016/s0022-3476(75)80059-x

34. Weaver LK, Hopkins RO, Chan KJ, et al. Hyperbaric oxygen for acute carbon monoxide poisoning. *N Engl J Med*. 2002;347(14):1057-1067.

35. Juurlink DN, Buckley NA, Stanbrook MB, Isbister GK, Bennett M, McGuigan MA. Hyperbaric oxygen for carbon monoxide poisoning. *Cochrane Database Syst Rev*. 2005;(1):CD002041.

36. Han S, Cho YS. Hyperbaric oxygen therapy in carbon monoxide poisoning: still controversial. *J Emerg Med*. 2021 Nov;61(5):619-620.

37. Chen KK, Rose CL, Clowes GH. Comparative values of several antidotes in cyanide poisoning. *Am J Med Sci*. 1934;188:767-781.

38. Feldstein M, Klendshoj NJ. The determination of cyanide in biological fluids by microdiffusion analysis. *J Lab Clin Med*. 1954;44:166-170.

39. Vogel SN, Sultan TR. Cyanide poisoning. *Clin Toxicol*. 1981;18:367-383.

40. Herndon DN, Traber DL, Niehaus GD, et al. The pathophysiology of smoke inhalation in a sheep model. *J Trauma*. 1984;24:1044-1051.

41. Till GO, Johnson KJ, Kunkel R, et al. Intravascular activation of complement and acute lung injury. *J Clin Invest*. 1982;69:1126-1135.

42. Thommasen HV, Martin BA, Wiggs BR, Quiroga M, Baile EM, Hogg JC. Effect of pulmonary blood flow on leukocyte uptake and release by dog lung. *J Appl Physiol Respir Environ Exerc Physiol*. 1984;56:966-974. doi: 10.1152/jappl.1984.56.4.966

43. Trunkey DD. Inhalation injury. *Surg Clin North Am*. 1978;58:1133-1140.

44. Haponik E, Summer W. Respiratory complications in the burned patient: diagnosis and management of inhalation injury. *J Crit Care*. 1987;2:121-143.

45. Cahalane M, Demling R. Early respiratory abnormalities from smoke inhalation. *JAMA*. 1984;251:771-773.

46. Herndon DN. *Total Burn Care*. 5th ed. Elsevier; 2018: 16-19.

47. Hight DW, Bakalar HR, Lloyd JR. Inflicted burns in children: recognition and treatment. *JAMA*. 1979;242:517-520.

48. U.S. Department of Justice, Office of Justice Programs, Office of Juvenile Justice and Delinquency Prevention. Burn injuries in child abuse. Published May 1997. Reprinted June 2001. Accessed December 17, 2013. https://www.ojp.gov/pdffiles/91190-6.pdf

49. Başaran A, Narsat MA. Clinical outcome of pediatric hand burns and evaluation of neglect as a leading cause: a retrospective study. *Ulus Travma Acil Cerrahi Derg*. 2022 Jan;28(1):84-89.

50. Chadwick DL. The diagnosis of inflicted injury in infants and young children. *Pediatr Ann*. 1992;21:477-483.

51. Adronicus M, Oates RK, Peat J, et al. Nonaccidental burns in children. *Burns*. 1998;24:552-558.

52. Purdue GF, Hunt JL, Prescott PR. Child abuse by burning: an index of suspicion. *J Trauma*. 1988;28:221-224.

53. Lenoski EF, Hunter KA. Specific patterns of inflicted burn injuries. *J Trauma*. 1977;17:842-846.

54. Brooks JW, Evans EI, Ham WT, Reid JD. The influence of external body radiation on mortality from thermal burns. *Ann Surg*. 1953;136:533-545.

55. American Burn Association. Radiation injury. In: *Advanced Burn Life Support Course*. ABA; 1999:66.

56. Michell MW, Oliveira HM, Vaid SU, et al. Enteral resuscitation of burn shock using intestinal infusion of World

Health Organization oral rehydration solution (WHO ORS): a potential treatment for mass casualty care. *J Burn Care Rehabil*. 2004;25:S48.

57. Bromberg BF, Song IC, Walden RH. Hydrotherapy of chemical burns. *Plast Reconstr Surg*. 1965;35:85-95.

58. Leonard LG, Scheulen JJ, Munster AM. Chemical burns: effect of prompt first aid. *J Trauma*. 1982;22(5):420-423.

59. Alam M, Moynagh M, Orr DS, Lawlor C. Cement burns—the Dublin national burns experience. *J Burns Wounds*. 2007;7:33-38.

60. Mozingo DW, Smith AD, McManus WF, Mason AD. Chemical burns. *J Trauma*. 1988;28(5):642-647.

61. Mistry D, Wainwright D. Hydrofluoric acid burns. *Am Fam Physician*. 1992;45:1748-1754.

62. Willems JL. Clinical management of mustard gas casualties. *Ann Med Milit Belg*. 1989;3S:1-61.

63. Papirmeister B, Feister AJ, Robinson SI, et al. The sulfur mustard injury: description of lesions and resulting incapacitation. In: Papirmeister B, Feister A, Robinson S, Ford R, eds. *Medical Defense Against Mustard Gas*. CRC Press; 1990:13.

64. Sidell FR, Takafuji ET, Franz DR. *Medical Aspects of Chemical and Biological Warfare*. Washington, DC: Office of the Surgeon General; 1997.

CHAPTER 14

Pediatric Trauma

Lead Editors
Jessica Naiditch, MD, FACS, FAAP
Katherine Remick, MD, FAAP, FACEP, FAEMS
David Tuggle, MD, FACS, FAAP

© Ralf Hiemisch/Getty Images

CHAPTER OBJECTIVES

At the completion of this chapter, you will be able to do the following:

- Identify the anatomic and physiologic differences in children that account for unique pediatric injury patterns.
- Demonstrate an understanding of the special importance of managing the airway and restoring adequate tissue oxygenation in pediatric patients.

- Identify the quantitative vital signs for pediatric patients.
- Demonstrate an understanding of management techniques for the various injuries found in pediatric patients.
- Describe the signs of pediatric trauma suggestive of nonaccidental trauma.

SCENARIO

You are called to the scene of a motor vehicle crash on a heavily traveled highway. Two vehicles were involved in a frontal offset collision. One of the vehicle's occupants is a child who was improperly restrained in a child booster seat. No weather-related factors are present on this spring afternoon.

On arrival at the scene, you see that the police have secured and blocked traffic from the area around the crash. As your partner and the other arriving crew are assessing the other patients, you approach the child. You see a young boy, approximately 2 years of age, sitting in the booster seat, which is slightly turned at an angle; there is blood on the back of the headrest of the seat in front of him. Despite numerous abrasions and minor bleeding from the head, face, and neck, the child appears very calm.

Your primary and secondary surveys reveal a 2-year-old boy who weakly repeats "ma-ma, ma-ma." His pulse rate is 180 beats/minute, with the radial pulses weaker than the brachial; his blood pressure (BP) is 50 millimeters of mercury (mm Hg) by palpation. His ventilatory rate is 18 breaths/minute, slightly irregular, but without abnormal sounds. As you continue to assess him, you note that he has stopped saying "ma-ma" and seems to just stare into space. You also note that his pupils are slightly dilated, and his skin is pale and sweaty. A woman who identifies herself as the family's nanny tells you that the mother is en route and that you should wait for her.

- What are the management priorities for this patient?
- What are the most likely injuries in this child?
- Where is the most appropriate destination for this child?

INTRODUCTION

Annual data reporting from the Centers for Disease Control and Prevention (CDC) continue to show that injury is the most common cause of death for children in the United States.[1]

In 2019, more than 7,000 children under the age of 19 died as a result of unintentional injury according to the CDC.[2] The leading causes of these deaths were motor vehicle collisions, suffocation, drowning, poisoning, fires, and falls. Careful evaluation of available data regarding these deaths suggests that sadly, childhood injury is often preventable. Even more disturbing is the fact that there are important racial and ethnic disparities in the rate of unintentional injury deaths among different groups of children. For example, between 2010 and 2019, death rates due to injuries sustained as a result of motor vehicle collisions increased 9% among Black children while it fell 24% among White children. Poisoning death rates increased 50% in Hispanic children and 24% in Black children while they fell 9% among White children over the same time period[2] (**Figure 14-1**). Hopefully, these data can be used to target prevention strategies and interventions in ways that will most effectively decrease the risks to the most vulnerable populations.

As with all aspects of pediatric care, proper assessment and management of an injured child requires a thorough understanding of not only the unique characteristics of childhood growth and development (including immature anatomy and developing physiology) but also their unique mechanisms of injury.

The adage holds true that "children are not just little adults." Children have distinct, reproducible patterns of injury, different physiologic responses, and special treatment needs, based on their physical and psychosocial development at the time of injury.

This chapter begins by describing the special characteristics of pediatric trauma patients, then reviews optimal trauma management and its rationale. Although the unique characteristics of pediatric injury are important for prehospital care practitioners to understand, the fundamental basic and advanced life support treatment approach using the primary and secondary surveys is the same for every patient, regardless of age or size.

Children as Trauma Patients

Demographics of Pediatric Trauma

The unique needs and characteristics of pediatric patients require special attention when assessing an acutely injured child. The relative incidence of blunt (vs. penetrating) trauma is highest in the pediatric population, with penetrating trauma accounting for only 7.8% of injuries.[3] Penetrating trauma often results in injury to one body system, whereas blunt trauma mechanisms have a greater propensity for multisystem injury.

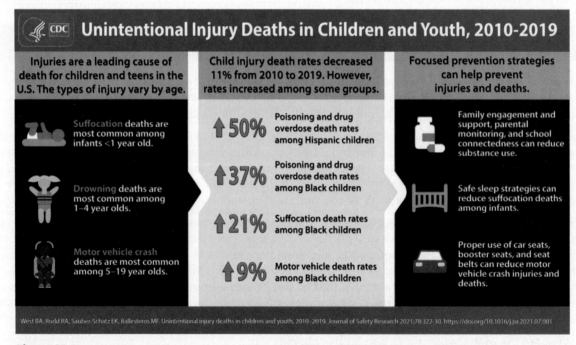

Unintentional Injury Deaths in Children and Youth, 2010-2019

Injuries are a leading cause of death for children and teens in the U.S. The types of injury vary by age.

Suffocation deaths are most common among infants <1 year old.

Drowning deaths are most common among 1–4 year olds.

Motor vehicle crash deaths are most common among 5–19 year olds.

Child injury death rates decreased 11% from 2010 to 2019. However, rates increased among some groups.

↑50% Poisoning and drug overdose death rates among Hispanic children

↑37% Poisoning and drug overdose death rates among Black children

↑21% Suffocation death rates among Black children

↑9% Motor vehicle death rates among Black children

Focused prevention strategies can help prevent injuries and deaths.

Family engagement and support, parental monitoring, and school connectedness can reduce substance use.

Safe sleep strategies can reduce suffocation deaths among infants.

Proper use of car seats, booster seats, and seat belts can reduce motor vehicle crash injuries and deaths.

West BA, Rudd RA, Sauber-Schatz EK, Ballesteros MF. Unintentional injury deaths in children and youth, 2010–2019. Journal of Safety Research 2021;78:322-30. https://doi.org/10.1016/j.jsr.2021.07.001

Figure 14-1 Unintentional injury deaths in children and youth, 2010–2019.

Falls, pedestrians struck by automobiles, and occupant injury as a result of motor vehicle crashes are the most common causes of pediatric injury in the United States, with falls alone accounting for more than 2.4 million injuries per year in children younger than age 15 years.[4] Worldwide, the World Health Organization estimates that approximately 830,000 children die from trauma each year and tens of millions are hospitalized with nonfatal injuries.[5] As in the United States, traffic-related accidents are the most common cause of pediatric death, with burns, homicide, and falls the next most common.

For a variety of reasons, which will be discussed throughout this chapter, multisystem involvement is the rule rather than the exception in major pediatric trauma. Although minimal external evidence of injury may be present, potentially life-threatening internal injury may still exist and must be evaluated at an appropriately equipped trauma center.

The Physics of Trauma and Pediatric Trauma

A child's size produces a smaller surface area to which forces from fenders, bumpers, and falls are applied. Minimal cushioning from body fat, increased elasticity of connective tissues, and proximity of the viscera to the surface of the body limit children's ability to dissipate these forces in the same manner as an adult; therefore, energy is more readily transmitted to underlying organs. Additionally, the skeleton of a child is incompletely calcified, contains multiple active growth centers, and is more resilient than that of an adult. As a result, there may be significant internal injuries without obvious evidence of external trauma.

Common Patterns of Injury

The unique anatomic and physiologic characteristics of children, combined with the age-specific common mechanisms of injury, produce distinct, but predictable, patterns of injury (**Table 14-1**). Improper seat belt usage or front seat placement in the vehicle with resulting airbag impact can lead to significant injury (**Box 14-1**). Trauma is frequently a time-critical illness, and familiarity with these patterns can assist prehospital care practitioners in optimizing management decisions for injured children in an expeditious manner. For example, blunt pediatric trauma involving closed head injury results in apnea, hypoventilation, and hypoxia much more commonly than hypovolemia and hypotension. Therefore, clinical care guidelines for pediatric trauma patients should include greater emphasis on focused management of the airway and breathing.

Table 14-1 Common Patterns of Injury Associated With Pediatric Trauma	
Type of Trauma	**Patterns of Injury**
Motor vehicle crash (child is passenger)	Unrestrained: Multisystem trauma (including chest and abdomen), head and neck injuries, scalp and facial lacerations
	Restrained: Chest and abdomen injuries, lower spine fractures
Motor vehicle crash (child is pedestrian)	Low speed: Lower extremity fractures
	High speed: Multisystem trauma (including chest and abdomen), head and neck injuries, lower extremity fractures
Fall from a height	Low: Upper extremity fractures
	Medium: Head and neck injuries, upper and lower extremity fractures
	High: Multisystem trauma (including chest and abdomen), head and neck injuries, upper and lower extremity fractures
Fall from bicycle	Without helmet: Head and neck lacerations, scalp and facial lacerations, upper extremity fractures
	With helmet: Upper extremity fractures
	Striking handlebar: Internal abdominal injuries

Modified from American College of Surgeons Committee on Trauma. Pediatric trauma. In: *ATLS® Advanced Trauma Life Support® Student Course Manual.* 10th ed. ACS; 2018:186-213.

Box 14-1 Pediatric Injuries Associated With Seat Belts and Airbags

Despite laws in all 50 states requiring the use of car safety seats or child restraint devices for young children, evidence suggests that child restraints are often installed improperly.[6] Furthermore, if a child is the front-seat occupant in a vehicle with a passenger-side airbag, the child is just as likely to sustain serious injury whether appropriately restrained or not.[7] A child exposed to a passenger-side airbag is twice as likely to sustain significant injury as a front-seat passenger without an airbag.[8]

Children with lap belts or inappropriate seat belt placement are at increased risk for bowel injury in motor vehicle crashes. These types of seat belt injuries can also cause pancreatic, aortic, and lumbar spine injuries, putting these children at risk for serious multisystem trauma. It is reasonable to assume that any child who was restrained by a lap belt and is found with abdominal wall bruising after a motor vehicle crash has an intra-abdominal injury until proven otherwise.

Approximately 1% of all motor vehicle crashes involving children result in exposure of the child to a deployed passenger airbag. Up to 14% of children who were involved in a motor vehicle collision with first-generation airbag deployment suffered serious injury.[9] With improvements in airbag technology, the risk of injury during deployment, while still significant, has decreased to 10%.[10,11] These injuries may include minor upper torso and facial burns and lacerations or major chest, neck, face, and upper extremity injury.[9]

Thermal Homeostasis

The ratio between a child's body surface area and body mass is highest at birth and diminishes throughout infancy and childhood. Consequently, more surface area exists through which heat can be quickly lost, not only providing additional stress to the child but also altering the child's physiologic responses to metabolic derangements and shock. Profound hypothermia can result in severe *coagulopathy* and potentially irreversible cardiovascular collapse. In addition, many of the clinical signs of hypothermia are similar to those of impending decompensated shock, thereby potentially muddying a prehospital care practitioner's clinical assessment.

Psychosocial Issues

The psychological ramifications for an injured child can present a major challenge. Particularly with a very young child, regressive psychological behavior may result when stress, pain, or other perceived threats impair the child's ability to process frightening events. Unfamiliar individuals in strange surroundings can limit a child's ability to fully cooperate with history taking, physical examination, and treatment. An understanding of these characteristics and a willingness to soothe and comfort an injured child are frequently the most effective means of achieving good rapport and obtaining a comprehensive assessment of the child's physiologic state.

The child's parents or caregivers also frequently require special attention and may be considered "parent patients." The treatment of all patients begins with effective communication, but communication becomes even more important when dealing with these parent patients. It may consist of simple words of compassion or great lengths of patience, but you cannot be an effective prehospital care practitioner for the pediatric patient if you are ignorant of the needs of the parents or caregivers.

Parents or primary caregivers may require information about their child's injuries and planned treatment or reassurance about their child's condition. If ignored, parents might become angry or aggressive and present significant obstacles to effective care. However, when you include them in the process, they can often act as functional members of their child's emergency care team.

The concept of family-centered care is a dynamic approach to building collaborative relationships between healthcare professionals and family, and using those relationships to assist in providing quality EMS care.[12] Family-centered care recognizes that the family's knowledge of one of their member's condition is an important tool to enhance quality of care and communication and inclusion of the family as a member of the team. Furthermore, parental or caregiver engagement signals to the child that you are endorsed as a "safe" person, increasing the likelihood of the child's cooperation. Practitioners must remember that whenever a child is sick or injured, the caregivers are also affected and should be considered patients as well.

Recovery and Rehabilitation

Unique to pediatric trauma patients is the effect that even minor injury may have on subsequent growth and development. Unlike an anatomically mature adult, a child must not only recover from the injury but also continue normal growth. The effect of injury on this process, especially in terms of permanent disability, growth deformity, or subsequent abnormal development, cannot be overestimated. Children sustaining even minor traumatic brain injury (TBI) may have prolonged disability in cerebral function, psychological adjustment, or other regulated organ systems. These disabilities can have a substantial effect on siblings and parents, resulting in a high incidence of family dysfunction, including divorce.

The effects of inadequate or suboptimal care in the acute injury phase may have far-reaching consequences, not only on the child's immediate survival but also, perhaps more important, on the long-term quality of the child's life. Therefore, it is extremely important to maintain a high index of suspicion for injury and to use clinical "common sense" when caring for and making transport decisions for an acutely injured child.

Pathophysiology

The final outcome for an injured child may be determined by the quality of care rendered in the first moments following an injury. During this critical period, a coordinated, systematic primary survey is the best strategy to avoid unnecessary morbidity and prevent overlooking a potentially fatal injury. As in an adult patient, the three most common causes of immediate death in a child are hypoxia, massive hemorrhage, and overwhelming central nervous system (CNS) trauma. These three common causes of immediate death are detailed in this section. Expedient triage, stabilizing emergency medical treatment, and transport to the most appropriate center for treatment can optimize the potential for a meaningful recovery.

Hypoxia

Confirming that a child has an open and functioning airway does not preclude the need for supplemental oxygen and assisted ventilation, especially when CNS injury, hypoventilation, or hypoperfusion is present. Well-appearing injured children can rapidly deteriorate from mild tachypnea to a state of total exhaustion and apnea. Once an airway is established, the rate and depth of ventilation should be carefully evaluated to confirm adequate ventilation. If ventilation is inadequate, merely providing an excessive concentration of oxygen will not prevent ongoing or worsening hypoxia.

The effects of even *transient* (brief) hypoxia on the traumatically injured brain deserve special attention. A child may have significant alteration in level of consciousness (LOC) yet retain an excellent potential for a complete functional recovery if cerebral hypoxia is avoided.

Pediatric patients who require aggressive airway management should be preoxygenated before attempting to place an advanced airway device. This oxygenation, or rather denitrogenation, attempts to replace alveolar nitrogen with oxygen to achieve an intrapulmonary oxygen reserve that will allow apnea to be as prolonged as possible with the least possible associated oxyhemoglobin desaturation. This improves the margin of safety when placement of an advanced airway is performed. A period of hypoxia during multiple or prolonged attempts at placing an advanced airway may be more detrimental

to the child than simply ventilating the child with a bag-mask device and transporting rapidly.[13-15] Attempting advanced airway management is unnecessary and potentially harmful if the child is adequately ventilated and oxygenated using good basic life support skills, such as bag-mask ventilation.

Hemorrhage

Most pediatric injuries do not cause immediate exsanguination. However, children who sustain injuries that result in major blood loss frequently die within moments of the injury or shortly after arrival at a receiving facility. These fatalities frequently result from multiple injured internal organs, with at least one significant injury causing acute blood loss. This bleeding may be minor, such as a simple laceration or contusion, or may be a life-threatening hemorrhage, such as a ruptured spleen, lacerated liver, or avulsed kidney.

Injured children compensate for hemorrhage by increasing systemic vascular resistance; however, this is at the expense of peripheral perfusion. Children are physiologically more adept at this response because pediatric vasoconstriction is not limited by preexisting peripheral vascular disease. Using blood pressure measurements alone is an inadequate strategy to identify the early signs of shock. Tachycardia, although it may be the result of fear or pain, should be considered to be secondary to hemorrhage or hypovolemia until proven otherwise. A narrowing pulse pressure and increasing tachycardia may be the first subtle signs of impending shock.

Furthermore, prehospital care practitioners must pay close attention to signs of ineffective organ perfusion as evidenced by alterations in respiratory efforts, decreased LOC, and diminished skin perfusion (decreased temperature, poor color, and prolonged capillary refill time). Unlike in adults, these early signs of hemorrhage in a child may be subtle and difficult to identify, leading to a delayed recognition of shock. If the practitioner misses these early signs, a child may lose enough circulating blood volume that compensatory mechanisms fail. When this happens, cardiac output plummets, organ perfusion decreases, and the child can rapidly decompensate, often leading to irreversible, fatal hypotension and shock. Therefore, every child who sustains blunt trauma should be carefully monitored to detect these subtle signs that might signal that there is ongoing hemorrhage, long before frank vital sign abnormalities.

A major reason for the rapid transition to decompensated shock is the loss of red blood cells (RBCs) and their corresponding oxygen-carrying capacity. Restoration of lost intravascular volume with crystalloid solutions will provide a transient increase in blood pressure, but circulating volume will dissipate quickly as the fluid shifts across capillary membranes. As blood is lost and intravascular volume is replaced with crystalloids, the remaining

RBCs are diluted in the bloodstream, reducing the blood's ability to carry oxygen to the tissues. Therefore, any child who requires more than one 20-milliliter/kilogram (mL/kg) bolus of crystalloid solution may be rapidly deteriorating and likely needs a transfusion of RBCs so that oxygen-delivery capacity is restored in parallel to intravascular volume resuscitation. Early administration of blood products should be considered in any pediatric patient with signs of ongoing hemorrhage. This may commence prior to administration of two fluid boluses.

However, once vascular access has been secured, there is a tendency to inadvertently overresuscitate an injured child who is not in frank shock. Normal saline is acidotic and, when given at room temperature, has the potential to cause both cooling and mild acidosis, which can compromise clotting and therefore worsen any ongoing hemorrhage. In a child with moderate bleeding, no evidence of end-organ hypoperfusion, and normal vital signs, fluid resuscitation should be limited to no more than one or two normal saline boluses of 20 mL/kg. The intravascular component of one bolus represents approximately 25% of a child's blood volume. Therefore, if more than two boluses are required, prehospital care practitioners must take care to reassess the child for sources of previously undetected ongoing bleeding.

In a child with TBI, fluid resuscitation should be given to prevent hypotension, a known and preventable contributor to secondary brain injury.[16,17] The cerebral perfusion pressure is the difference between the intracranial pressure (the pressure inside the skull) and the mean arterial pressure (the pressure driving blood into the skull). TBI can cause an increase in intracranial pressure. Therefore, even though blood may be adequately oxygenated, if the systemic blood pressure is low, oxygenated blood may not perfuse the brain; thus, hypoxic brain injury can still occur. Although overresuscitation should be avoided to prevent iatrogenic cerebral edema, hypotension must be prevented or quickly treated with fluid resuscitation, as a single episode of hypotension can increase mortality by as much as 150%.[18] Careful assessments of the child's vital signs and frequent reevaluation after therapeutic interventions should guide ongoing management decisions.

Isotonic crystalloid solutions should be the fluid of choice for resuscitation of a child with TBI, because hypotonic crystalloid solutions (e.g., dextrose in water) are known to increase cerebral edema. Furthermore, although hypertonic crystalloid solutions (e.g., hypertonic saline) may be useful for treatment of cerebral edema in the pediatric intensive care unit where there is extensive monitoring, evidence to date has not demonstrated improved outcomes of pediatric trauma patients when administered in the field. In the setting of impending herniation, evidence of blown pupil or markedly decreased Glasgow Coma Scale (GCS) score (as indicated by a drop of 2 or more points) and in the context of prolonged transport, hypertonic saline might be considered in the out-of-hospital environment.

Central Nervous System Injury

The pathophysiologic changes after severe CNS trauma begin within minutes. Early and adequate resuscitation is the key to maximizing potential survival of children with CNS trauma. Although some CNS injuries are overwhelmingly fatal, many children with the appearance of a devastating neurologic injury go on to a complete and functional recovery after deliberate, coordinated efforts to prevent secondary injury. These recoveries are achieved through the prevention of subsequent episodes of hypoperfusion, hypoventilation, hyperventilation, and ischemia. Adequate ventilation and oxygenation (while avoiding hyperventilation) are as critical in the management of TBIs as the avoidance of hypotension.[17]

For given degrees of CNS injury severity, children have lower mortality and a higher potential for survival than adults. However, the addition of injuries outside the brain lessens the child's chances of a favorable outcome, illustrating the potentially negative effect of shock from associated injuries.

Children with TBI frequently present with an alteration in consciousness, possibly sustaining a period of unconsciousness not witnessed during the initial evaluation. A history of loss of consciousness is one of the most important prognostic indicators of potential CNS injury and should be recorded for every case. In the event that the injury was not witnessed, amnesia to the event is commonly used as a surrogate for a loss of consciousness. Furthermore, complete documentation of baseline neurologic status is important, including the following:

1. GCS score (modified for pediatrics)
2. Pupillary reaction
3. Response to sensory stimulation
4. Motor function

These are essential steps in the initial pediatric trauma assessment for neurologic injury. The absence of an adequate baseline assessment makes ongoing follow-up and evaluation of interventions extremely difficult.

Attention to detail in history taking is especially important in pediatric patients with possible cervical spine injury. A child's skeleton is incompletely calcified with multiple active growth centers, often preventing radiographic diagnosis of injury from a mechanism causing a stretching, contusion, or blunt injury to the spinal cord. This condition is called spinal cord injury without radiographic abnormality, or SCIWORA. A transient neurologic deficit that resolves prior to facility arrival may be the only indicator of a significant spinal cord injury. Despite quick symptom resolution, children with

SCIWORA can develop spinal cord edema up to 4 days after the initial injury, with devastating neurologic disabilities if left untreated.

Assessment

Primary Survey

The small and variable sizes of pediatric patients (**Table 14-2**), the diminished caliber and size of the blood vessels and circulating volume, and the unique anatomic characteristics of the airway frequently make the standard procedures used in basic life support extremely challenging and technically difficult. Effective pediatric trauma resuscitation mandates the availability of appropriately sized airways, laryngoscope blades, endotracheal (ET) tubes, supraglottic airway devices, nasogastric tubes, blood pressure cuffs, oxygen masks, bag-mask devices, and associated equipment. Attempting to place an overly large intravenous (IV) catheter or an inappropriately sized airway can do more harm than good, not only because of the potential physical damage to the patient but also because it may delay transport to the appropriate facility. Color-coded, length-based resuscitation guides (discussed later in this chapter) provide practical medication and equipment references.[19]

Emergency assessment of children of all ages begins with an initial impression. In children, practitioners should use a rapid approach to quickly determine criticality (i.e., sick or not sick) based on understanding their developmental stage and their visual and auditory appearances. Using the **Pediatric Assessment Triangle (PAT)** at the point of first contact with the patient helps to establish a level of severity, determine urgency for treatment, and identify the general category of the physiologic problem (**Figure 14-2**).[4,20,21]

The three components of the PAT are appearance, work of breathing, and circulation to the skin. Typically, this is performed from a distance to create an initial impression as to how critical the patient is. The first step is to use the TICLS mnemonic to assess the child's overall general appearance:

- *Tone.* Strong truncal tone, sits or stands (age appropriate)
- *Interactiveness.* Appears alert, attentive to activities and people in the immediate environment, reaches for toys/objects (e.g., penlight)
- *Consolability.* Has differential response to caregiver
- *Look/gaze.* Makes eye contact with clinician, tracks visually
- *Speech/cry.* Has strong cry or uses age-appropriate speech

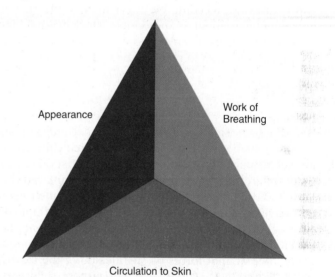

Figure 14-2 Pediatric Assessment Triangle (PAT).

Table 14-2 Height and Weight Range for Pediatric Patients			
		Range of Mean Norms	
Group	**Age**	**Average Height (cm)**	**Average Weight (kg)**
Neonate	0 to 1 month	51 to 63	4 to 5
Infant	1 month to 1 year	56 to 80	4 to 11
Toddler	1 to 2 years	77 to 91	11 to 14
Preschooler	3 to 5 years	91 to 122	14 to 25
School-age child	6 to 12 years	122 to 165	25 to 63
Adolescent	12 to 15 years	165 to 182	62 to 80

The second step is to assess the work of breathing. This step involves listening for abnormal airway sounds and looking for abnormal positioning, retractions, and flaring. Third, practitioners must assess the circulation to the skin by looking for pallor, mottling, or cyanosis. Combining these three PAT components allows for formation of a general primary impression. The general primary impression is the clinician's overall evaluation of the child's ability to compensate for the acute insult or injury—sick or not sick.

Stabilization Priorities

The survival rate from immediate exsanguinating injury is low in the pediatric population. Fortunately, the incidence of this type of injury is also low. The initial priority is to identify any exsanguinating external hemorrhage and control the bleeding by direct manual pressure or tourniquet placement as appropriate. Once exsanguinating hemorrhage has been addressed or if it is not present, the practitioner should manage the child's airway.

Airway

As in an injured adult, the next priority and focus after ensuring scene safety and addressing or excluding exsanguinating hemorrhage in an acutely injured child are on airway management. However, there are several anatomic differences that complicate the care of injured children. Children have a relatively large occiput and tongue and have an anteriorly positioned airway. Additionally, the smaller the child, the greater the size discrepancy between the cranium and the midface. Therefore, the relatively large occiput forces passive flexion of the cervical spine (**Figure 14-3**). These factors predispose children to a higher risk of anatomic airway obstruction than adults. In the absence of trauma, a pediatric patient's airway is best protected by a slightly superior–anterior position of the midface, known as the **sniffing position** (**Figure 14-4**). In the presence of trauma, however, the **neutral position** best protects the cervical spine by keeping it immobilized to prevent the flexion at the fifth and sixth cervical vertebrae (C5 to C6) and the extension at C1 to C2 that occurs with the sniffing position. In this position, a jaw-thrust maneuver can be used to facilitate airway opening if needed.

Manual stabilization of the cervical spine is performed during airway management and maintained until the child is immobilized with an appropriate cervical immobilization device, whether it is commercially purchased or a simple solution such as towel rolls. Additionally, placing a pad or blanket of about 1 inch (2 to 3 centimeters [cm]) in thickness under an infant's torso can lessen the acute flexion of the neck and help keep the airway patent. Bag-mask ventilation with high-flow (at least 15 liters/minute) 100% oxygen probably represents the best choice when

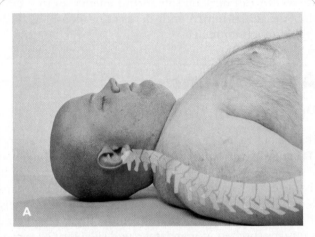
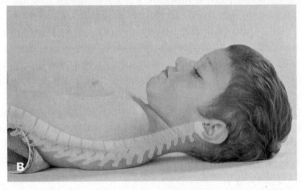

Figure 14-3 A. Compared to an adult, a child has a larger occiput and less shoulder musculature. **B.** When placed on a flat surface, these factors result in flexion of the neck.
© Jones & Bartlett Learning. Photographed by Darren Stahlman.

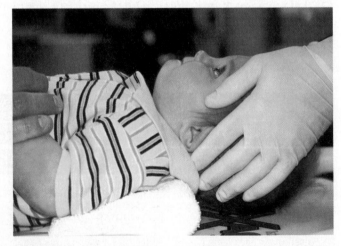

Figure 14-4 Sniffing position.
© American Academy of Orthopaedic Surgeons

an injured child requires assisted ventilation.[13] Use a properly fitted oxygen mask and the "squeeze-release-release" timing technique. Watch for rise and fall of the chest, and if end-tidal carbon dioxide ($ETCO_2$) monitoring is available, maintain levels between 35 and 40 mm Hg. Even in a young child, two-person bag-mask ventilation is preferred to one-person ventilation, when feasible. Intubation in the setting of uncorrected hypoxia can lead to worse outcomes in an injured child. Therefore, every effort should be made to correct hypoxia and optimize airway management prior to any intubation attempt.

If the child is unconscious, an oropharyngeal airway may be considered, but due to risk of vomiting, it should not be used in a child with an intact gag reflex. This is also true of the laryngeal mask and King LT airways, both of which are supraglottic airways; when sized appropriately, these devices can be considered for airway management in pediatric trauma patients when resources and personnel are limited, or when long transport times are anticipated, limiting the utility of two-person bag-mask ventilation. In very young children, especially those weighing less than 44 pounds (20 kg), these devices can cause iatrogenic upper airway obstruction by causing the relatively larger pediatric epiglottis to fold into the airway. Compared to endotracheal intubation, supraglottic airways have the benefit of being placed rapidly.

In comparison to that of the adult, the child's larynx is smaller in size and is slightly more anterior and *cephalad* (forward and toward the head), making it more difficult to visualize the vocal cords during intubation attempts (**Figure 14-5**). Endotracheal intubation, despite being the most reliable means of ventilation in the child with airway compromise, should be reserved for those situations in which airway management needs to be tightly controlled (e.g., severe head injury), impending airway obstruction, or insufficient resources to maintain effective bag-mask ventilation. Nasotracheal intubation is not recommended in children. This technique requires a spontaneously breathing patient, involves blind passage around the relatively acute posterior nasopharyngeal

angle, and can cause more severe bleeding in children. Additionally, in a patient with a basilar skull fracture, it can inadvertently penetrate the cranial vault.

Surgical cricothyroidotomy is usually not indicated in the care of pediatric trauma patients, though it may be considered in a larger child (usually at the age of 12 years).[22] The procedure should be reserved for those practitioners specifically trained in this technique and specifically credentialed to perform it.

Breathing

As in all trauma patients, a significantly traumatized child typically needs supplemental oxygen administration with an oxygen concentration of 85% to 100% (fraction of inspired oxygen [FiO_2] of 0.85 to 1.0). This concentration is maintained by the use of supplemental oxygen and an appropriately sized clear plastic pediatric mask. When hypoxia occurs in a small child, the body compensates by increasing the ventilatory rate (tachypnea) and by a strenuous increase in ventilatory effort, including increased thoracic excursion efforts and the use of accessory muscles in the neck and abdomen. This increased metabolic demand can produce severe fatigue and result in ventilatory failure, as an increasing percentage of the patient's cardiac output becomes devoted to maintaining this respiratory effort. Ventilatory distress can rapidly progress from a compensated ventilatory effort to ventilatory failure, then respiratory arrest, and ultimately a hypoxic cardiac arrest. Central (rather than peripheral) cyanosis is a fairly late and often inconsistent sign of respiratory failure. Prehospital care practitioners should not depend on this finding to identify impending respiratory failure.

Evaluation of the child's ventilatory status with early recognition of the signs of distress and the provision of

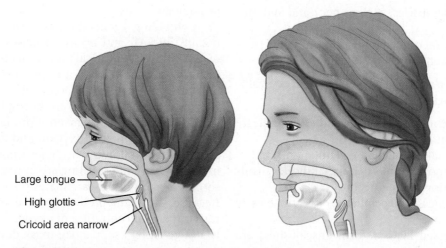

Large tongue
High glottis
Cricoid area narrow

Figure 14-5 Comparison of the adult and pediatric airways.

Table 14-3 Ventilatory Rates for Pediatric Patients

Group	Age	Ventilatory Rate (breaths/minute)	Ventilatory Rate That Indicates Possible Need for Ventilatory Assistance With Bag-Mask Device (breaths/minute)
Neonate	0 to 1 month	30 to 60	< 30 or > 60
Infant	1 month to 1 year	30 to 53	< 30 or > 53
Toddler	1 to 2 years	22 to 37	< 22 or > 37
Preschooler	3 to 5 years	20 to 28	< 20 or > 28
School-age child	6 to 12 years	18 to 25	< 18 or > 25
Adolescent	12 to 15 years	12 to 20	< 12 or > 20

Data from American Heart Association (AHA). Vital signs in children. *Pediatric Advanced Life Support*. AHA; 2020.

ventilatory assistance are key elements in the management of pediatric trauma patients. The normal ventilatory rate of infants and children younger than age 4 years is typically two to three times that of adults (**Table 14-3**).

Tachypnea with signs of increased effort or difficulty may be the first manifestations of respiratory distress and shock. As distress increases, additional signs and symptoms include shallow breathing or minimal chest movement. Breath sounds may be weak or infrequent, and air exchange at the nose or mouth may be reduced or minimal. Ventilatory effort becomes more labored and may include the following:

- Head bobbing with each breath
- Gasping or grunting
- Flared nostrils
- Stridor or snoring respirations
- Suprasternal, supraclavicular, subcostal, or intercostal retractions
- Use of accessory muscles, such as neck and abdominal wall muscles
- Distension of the abdomen when the chest falls (seesaw effect between the chest and abdomen)

The effectiveness of a child's ventilation should be evaluated using the following indicators:

- Rate and depth (minute volume) and effort indicate adequacy of ventilation.
- Pink skin may indicate adequate ventilation.
- Dusky, gray, cyanotic, or mottled skin indicates insufficient oxygenation and perfusion.
- Anxiety, restlessness, and combativeness can be early signs of hypoxia.
- Lethargy, depressed LOC, and unconsciousness are probably advanced signs of hypoxia.
- Breath sounds indicate the depth of exchange.

- Wheezing, rales (crackles), or rhonchi may indicate inefficient oxygenation.
- Declining pulse oximetry and/or declining capnography indicate respiratory failure.

A rapid evaluation of ventilation includes assessment of the patient's ventilatory rate (particularly tachypnea), ventilatory effort (degree of labor, nostril flaring, accessory muscle use, retraction, and seesaw movement), auscultation (air exchange, bilateral symmetry, and pathologic sounds), skin color, and mental status.

In a child who initially presents with tachypnea and increased ventilatory effort, normalization of the ventilatory rate and apparent lessening of the respiratory effort should not be immediately interpreted as a sign of improvement, as it may indicate exhaustion or impending respiratory failure. As with any change in the patient's clinical status, frequent reassessment is necessary to determine if this is an improvement or deterioration in physiologic status.

Combining a general impression of the child's status, use of the PAT, and an assessment of the child's work of breathing, prehospital care practitioners can quickly identify children in need of respiratory support. Children with a good appearance according to the PAT and increased work of breathing are in respiratory distress and require attention to airway positioning (with spinal stabilization), supplemental oxygen, and careful frequent reassessments. Children who have a poor appearance and increased work of breathing are in respiratory failure and should be considered candidates for ventilatory support. Because the main problem is one of inspired volume rather than concentration of oxygen, assisted ventilation is best given by use of a bag-mask device, supplemented with an oxygen reservoir attached to high-concentration oxygen (FiO_2 of 0.85 to 1.0). Because a child's airway is so small, it is prone to obstruction from increased secretions, blood, body fluids, and foreign materials; therefore, early and periodic suctioning may be necessary. In infants, who are obligate nose breathers, the nostrils should be suctioned.

When obtaining a mask seal in infants, caution should be exercised to avoid compressing the soft tissues underneath the chin because doing so pushes the tongue against the soft palate and increases the risk of occluding the airway. Pressure on the uncalcified, soft trachea should also be avoided. One or two hands can be used to obtain a mask seal, depending on the size and age of the child. Two hands are generally preferred across all age ranges.

Use of the correct-sized bag-mask device is essential for obtaining a proper mask seal, providing the proper tidal volume, and ensuring that the risks of hyperinflation and barotrauma are minimized. Ensure appropriate depth of ventilation by bagging only until chest rise is seen. Adequacy of ventilation can also be assessed by monitoring $ETCO_2$ with a goal level between 35 and 40 mm Hg. Ventilating a child too forcefully or with a tidal volume that is too great can lead to gastric distension. In turn, gastric distension can result in regurgitation, aspiration, or prevention of adequate ventilation by limiting diaphragmatic excursion. Aggressive ventilation can lead to a tension pneumothorax that can result in both severe respiratory distress and sudden cardiovascular collapse, as the mediastinum is more mobile in children. This mobility protects children from traumatic aortic injuries but increases the susceptibility to tension pneumothorax. The more mobile mediastinum compresses easily, allowing for earlier respiratory compromise and cardiovascular collapse than occurs in an adult.

Changes in a child's ventilatory status can be subtle, but ventilatory effort can rapidly deteriorate until ventilation is inadequate and hypoxia ensues. The patient's breathing should be evaluated as part of the primary survey and carefully and periodically reassessed to ensure its continued adequacy. Pulse oximetry should also be monitored, and efforts should be made to keep oxygen saturation (SpO_2) at greater than 94% (at sea level).

Whenever a child is manually ventilated, it is important to carefully control the rate at which ventilations are being administered. It is relatively easy to inadvertently hyperventilate patients, which will decrease the carbon dioxide level in the blood and cause cerebral vasoconstriction. This can lead to poorer outcomes in patients with TBI. Furthermore, excessive ventilation pressures can lead to gastric insufflation. A distended stomach can subsequently push up into the more pliable pediatric thorax and limit tidal volume capacity. Ensure chest rise when delivering tidal volumes while bagging to avoid underventilation and hypoxia.

Circulation

After stopping any exsanguinating hemorrhage, ensure adequate airway patency and breathing, then proceed to a circulatory assessment. The child's heart rate should be assessed and identified as tachycardic (heart beating too quickly), normal, or bradycardic (heart beating too slowly). If the child is bradycardic, go back and reassess the airway. For normal or fast heart rates, look for signs of hypoperfusion (pallor, mottling, poor capillary refill time).

A child with hemorrhagic injury can maintain adequate circulating volume by increasing peripheral vascular resistance to maintain mean arterial pressure. Clinical evidence of this compensatory mechanism includes prolonged capillary refill time, peripheral pallor or mottling, cool peripheral skin temperature, and decreased intensity of the peripheral pulses. In children, signs of significant hypotension develop with the loss of approximately 30% of the circulating volume. Hypotension is a late sign of hypovolemia. Because of their increased physiologic reserve, children with hemorrhagic injury frequently present with only slightly abnormal vital signs. Initial tachycardia may be from psychological stress, pain, or fear, but in a traumatized child it should always be assumed to be secondary to hypovolemia. If the child is tachycardic but has a normal blood pressure, the child may be in compensated shock. Look for signs of hypoperfusion, and complete frequent reassessments. If increased peripheral vascular resistance is not sufficient to compensate for loss of circulating volume, then the blood pressure will fall. The concept of evolving shock must be of paramount concern in the initial management of an injured child and is a major indication for transport to an appropriate trauma facility for expeditious evaluation and treatment.

A child who is tachycardic with hypotension is experiencing a critical life-threatening emergency (decompensated shock). Stop all external bleeding! If the bleeding is from an extremity injury, tourniquet placement may be lifesaving.[23,24] Fluid resuscitation should be initiated as soon as possible, but transport to a trauma center should not be delayed. Intravenous access and fluids may be initiated en route.

As in the assessment of the airway, a single measurement of heart rate or blood pressure does not equate with physiologic stability. Serial measurements and changing trends of vital signs and perfusion status are critical in gauging a child's evolving hemodynamic state in the acute injury phase. Close monitoring of vital signs is absolutely essential to recognizing the signs of impending shock, enabling the appropriate interventions to be performed to prevent clinical deterioration. **Table 14-4** and **Table 14-5** provide the normal ranges for pulse rate and blood pressure

Table 14-4 Pulse Rate for Pediatric Patients

Group	Age	Awake Rate (beats/minute)	Asleep Rate (beats/minute)	Pulse Rate That Indicates a Possible Serious Problem* (beats/minute)
Neonate	0 to 1 month	120 to 205	100 to 160	< 100 or > 160
Infant	1 month to 1 year	100 to 180	90 to 160	< 80 or > 150
Toddler	1 to 2 years	98 to 140	80 to 120	< 60 or > 140
Preschooler	3 to 5 years	80 to 120	65 to 100	< 60 or > 130
School-age child	6 to 12 years	75 to 118	60 to 90	< 50 or > 120
Adolescent	12 to 15 years	60 to 100	50 to 90	< 45 or > 100

*Bradycardia or tachycardia.

Data from American Heart Association (AHA). Vital signs in children. *Pediatric Advanced Life Support.* AHA; 2020.

Table 14-5 Blood Pressure for Pediatric Patients

Group	Age	Expected BP Range (mm Hg)	Lower Limit of Systolic BP (mm Hg)
Neonate	0 to 1 month	Systolic: 67 to 84 Diastolic: 35 to 53 Mean arterial pressure: 45 to 60	> 60
Infant	1 month to 1 year	Systolic: 72 to 104 Diastolic: 37 to 56 Mean arterial pressure: 50 to 62	> 70
Toddler	1 to 2 years	Systolic: 86 to 106 Diastolic: 42 to 63 Mean arterial pressure: 49 to 62	> 70
Preschooler	3 to 5 years	Systolic: 89 to 112 Diastolic: 46 to 72 Mean arterial pressure: 58 to 69	> 75
School-age child	6 to 12 years	Systolic: 97 to 120 Diastolic: 57 to 80 Mean arterial pressure: 66 to 79	> 80
Adolescent	12 to 15 years	Systolic: 110 to 131 Diastolic: 64 to 83 Mean arterial pressure: 73 to 84	> 90

Data from American Heart Association (AHA). Vital signs in children. *Pediatric Advanced Life Support.* AHA; 2020.

Box 14-2 Pediatric Vital Signs and Quantitative Norms

The term *pediatric*, or child, includes a vast range of physical development, emotional maturity, and body sizes. The approach to the patient and the implications of many injuries vary greatly between an infant and an adolescent.

In most anatomic and therapeutic dosage considerations, a child's weight (or specific height or length) serves as a more accurate indicator than exact chronologic age.[19] Table 14-2 lists the average height and weight for healthy children of varying ages.

The acceptable ranges of vital signs also vary for the different ages within the pediatric population. Adult norms cannot be used as guidelines in smaller children. An adult ventilatory rate of 30 breaths/minute is tachypneic, and an adult heart rate of 120 to 140 beats/minute is tachycardic. Both are considered alarmingly high in an adult and are significant pathologic findings. However, the same findings in an infant may be within the normal ranges.

Normal ranges of vital signs for different age groups may not be consistent across all pediatric references. In an injured child without a previous history of normal vital signs, borderline vital signs may be viewed as pathologic, even though the signs may

be physiologically acceptable in that specific child. The guidelines in Table 14-4 and Table 14-5 can aid in evaluating vital signs in pediatric patients. These tables present statistically common ranges into which most children in these age groups will fall.

Several commercially available items serve as rapid reference guides for pediatric vital signs and equipment size. These include length-based resuscitation tape, several slide-rule-type plastic scales, and mobile applications. The following guideline formulas can also be used to estimate the expected finding for ages 1 to 10 years:

**Lowest acceptable systolic BP (mm Hg)
= 70 + (2 × Child's age [years])**

**Total vascular blood volume (mL)
= 80 mL × Child's weight (kg)**

Quantitative vital signs in children, although important, are only one piece of information used in making an assessment. A child with a normal set of vital signs can rapidly deteriorate into either critical ventilatory difficulty or decompensated shock. Vital signs should be considered along with mechanism of injury and other clinical findings.

---

by pediatric age group. **Box 14-2** presents further discussion of pediatric vital signs and quantitative norms.

Disability

After assessment of exsanguinating hemorrhage, airway, breathing, and circulation, the primary survey must include an assessment of neurologic status. Although the AVPU scale (**A**lert, responds to **V**erbal stimulus, responds to **P**ainful stimulus, **U**nresponsive) is a simple, rapid assessment tool for the child's neurologic status, it is less informative than the Glasgow Coma Scale. The GCS should be combined with a careful examination of the pupils to determine whether they are equal, round, and reactive to light. As in adults, the GCS score provides a more thorough assessment of neurologic status and should be calculated for each pediatric trauma patient. There are modifications to the GCS for pediatric trauma patients, which allows for various developmental stages (**Table 14-6**).

The score of the motor component of the GCS may be as helpful as calculating the total GCS.[25,26] For further discussion of the importance of the motor component, see Chapter 6, *Patient Assessment and Management*.

The GCS score should be repeated frequently and used to document progression or improvement of

neurologic status during the postinjury period (refer to Chapter 6, *Patient Assessment and Management* for a review of the GCS). A more thorough assessment of motor and sensory function should be performed in the secondary survey, if time permits.

Expose/Environment

Children should be examined for other potentially life-threatening injuries; however, while exposure is critical and necessary to identify injuries, children may be frightened at attempts to remove their clothes. If the toddler or preschool child is not critically injured, a "toe-to-head" approach to the physical exam may be less frightening. Explain as you expose each area, and have a parent present whenever possible. In addition, because of children's high body surface area, they are more prone to developing hypothermia. Once the examination to identify other injuries is complete, the child should be covered to preserve body heat and prevent further heat loss.

Secondary Survey

The secondary survey of a pediatric patient should follow the primary survey only after life-threatening conditions

Table 14-6 Pediatric Glasgow Coma Scale

	Score	> 1 year	< 1 year	
Eye opening	4	Spontaneously	Spontaneously	
	3	To verbal command	To shout	
	2	To pain	To pain	
	1	No response	No response	
Motor response	6	Obeys	Spontaneous movements	
	5	Localized pain	Localizes pain	
	4	Flexion-withdrawal	Flexion-withdrawal	
	3	Abnormal flexion	Abnormal flexion	
	2	Abnormal extension	Abnormal extension	
	1	No response	No response	
		> 5 years	**2–5 years**	**0–23 months**
Verbal response	5	Oriented and converses	Appropriate works and phrases	Coos and smiles appropriately
	4	Disoriented and converses	Inappropriate words	Cries
	3	Inappropriate words	Cries and/or screams	Inappropriate crying and/or screaming
	2	Incomprehensible sounds	Grunts	Grunts
	1	No response	No response	No response

Modified from Low A, Hulme J. *ABC of Transfer and Retrieval Medicine*. John Wiley & Sons; 2014.

have been identified and managed. The head and neck should be examined for obvious deformities, contusions, abrasions, punctures, burns, tenderness, lacerations, or swellings. The thorax should be reexamined. Potential pulmonary contusions may become evident after volume resuscitation, manifested by respiratory distress or abnormal lung sounds. Trauma patients are infrequently *nil per os* (NPO [fasting]) at the time of their injuries. Insertion of a nasogastric or orogastric tube may be indicated, if local protocols allow, keeping in mind that the nasal route is contraindicated when there is significant facial and/or head trauma concerning for a possible skull base fracture. Gastric decompression is especially important for children who are **obtunded** or who have posttraumatic seizure activity.

Examination of the abdomen should focus on distension, tenderness, discoloration, ecchymosis, and presence of a mass. Careful palpation of the iliac crests may suggest an unstable pelvic fracture and increase the suspicion for possible retroperitoneal or urogenital injury as well as increased risk for hidden blood loss. An unstable pelvis should be noted, but repeated examinations of the pelvis should not be performed, as this may result in further injury and increased blood loss. Appropriate spinal motion restriction should be employed during patient movement and transport.

Each extremity should be inspected and palpated to rule out tenderness, deformity, diminished vascular supply, and neurologic deficit. A child's incompletely calcified skeleton, with its multiple growth centers, increases the possibility of physeal (growth plate) disruption. Accordingly, any area of edema, pain, tenderness, or diminished range of motion should be treated as if it were fractured until evaluated by radiographic examination. In children, as in adults, a missed orthopedic injury in an extremity may have little effect on mortality but may lead to long-term deformity and disability.

Management

The keys to pediatric patient survival from a traumatic injury are rapid cardiopulmonary assessment, age-appropriate aggressive management, and transport to a facility capable of managing pediatric trauma. A color-coded, length-based resuscitation tape was devised to serve as a guide that allows for rapid identification of a patient's height with a correlated estimation of weight, the size of equipment to be used, and appropriate dosages of potential resuscitative drugs. In addition, most prehospital systems have a guideline for selecting appropriate destination facilities for pediatric trauma patients. Not all trauma centers have the capabilities (i.e., pediatric readiness) to adequately manage the injured child. Pediatric-ready trauma centers are associated with a two-fold decrease in mortality for injured children.[27] Because trauma remains the leading cause of death in children, beginning in 2023, all ACS-verified trauma centers will be required to develop a plan to assess and address deficiencies in pediatric readiness. Be sure to review the destination protocol prior to arrival at the scene for expedited decisions in critical children.

Control of Severe External Hemorrhage

In the primary assessment of a trauma patient, external hemorrhage must be identified and controlled. If gross exsanguinating external hemorrhage is present, this bleeding must be controlled even before addressing the airway. Control of hemorrhage may be accomplished through direct pressure. This is accomplished by placing 4 × 4-in. (10 × 10-cm) gauze pads directly on the bleeding site and holding pressure. Pressure must be held during the entire transport. Tourniquet placement may be necessary for extremity bleeding when direct pressure does not adequately control the hemorrhage (or for extremity amputations). Some tourniquets may be too large or ineffective on smaller children or infants. If a ratchet or windlass style tourniquet is too large, an elastic-style tourniquet may be needed. Control of exsanguinating hemorrhage is imperative. If the patient is having ongoing hemorrhage, perfusion will not improve and the patient will progress to hemorrhagic shock.

Airway

Ventilation, oxygenation, and perfusion are as essential to an injured child as to an adult. Thus, the primary goal of the initial resuscitation of an injured child is restoration of adequate tissue oxygenation as quickly as possible. The first priority of assessment and resuscitation after establishing scene safety and addressing any exsanguinating external hemorrhage is the establishment of a patent airway.

A patent airway should be ensured and maintained with suctioning, manual maneuvers, and airway adjuncts. As in an adult, initial management in a pediatric patient includes in-line cervical spine stabilization. Unless a specialized pediatric spine board that has a depression at the head is used, adequate padding (about 1 inch [2 to 3 cm]) should be placed under the torso of the small child so that the cervical spine is maintained in a straight line rather than forced into slight flexion because of the disproportionately large occiput (**Figure 14-6**). When adjusting and maintaining airway positioning, compressing the soft tissues of the neck and trachea should be avoided.

Once manual control of the airway is achieved, an oropharyngeal airway can be placed if no gag reflex is present. The device should be inserted carefully and gently, parallel to the course of the tongue rather than turned 90 or 180 degrees in the posterior oropharynx as in the adult. Use of a tongue blade to depress the tongue can be helpful in pediatric patients.

Endotracheal intubation under direct visualization of the trachea may be indicated for long transports (**Box 14-3**). However, this procedure should be initiated only by experienced personnel and when adequate oxygenation cannot be maintained by a bag-mask device. Importantly, there are no data to show improved survival or neurologic outcome in pediatric trauma patients intubated early in the field versus those managed with bag-mask ventilation. In fact, there is some evidence suggesting equal or worse outcomes.[18] Multiple prehospital intubation attempts have been associated with significant complications (**Box 14-4**).[28,29]

Although several different supraglottic airway devices have been proven to be effective rescue airway devices for adult trauma victims,[37,38] in some cases, their large size and the lack of smaller sizes make them

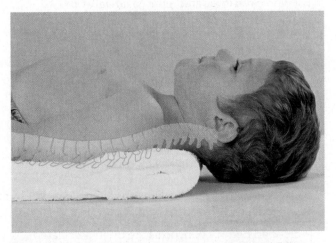

Figure 14-6 Provide adequate padding under the child's torso, or use a spine board with a cutout for the child's occiput.
© National Association of Emergency Medical Technicians (NAEMT)

Box 14-3 Pediatric Endotracheal Intubation

Endotracheal intubation of a pediatric patient should include careful attention to cervical spine stabilization. One prehospital care practitioner should maintain the child's spine in a neutral position while another practitioner intubates.

The narrowest portion of the pediatric airway is the cricoid ring, creating a "physiologic cuff." Although uncuffed ET tubes were previously used in children due to this difference, newer recommendations endorse the use of cuffed tubes for all ages. The cuffed tube allows prehospital care practitioners to inflate the cuff fully, partially, or not at all, depending on the strength of the seal and the child's oxygenation and ventilation. To prevent iatrogenic tracheal injury, cuff pressures should not exceed 25 centimeters of water (cm H_2O). The appropriate size for a cuffed ET tube can be estimated by using the diameter of the child's fifth finger or the external nares, or by using the following formula:

$$(Age \div 4) + 3.5$$

Although routine cricoid pressure is no longer recommended, a slight amount of cricoid pressure may be tried to bring the anterior structures of the child's larynx into better view. However, pediatric tracheal rings are relatively soft and pliable, and overzealous cricoid pressure may completely occlude the airway.

A common error that occurs during the intubation of pediatric patients under emergency circumstances is aggressive advancement of the ET tube, resulting in its placement into the right main bronchus. The ET tube should never be advanced more than three times the ET tube size (in centimeters). For example, a 3.0-cm ET tube should rest at the lips at a depth no greater than 9 cm.

The chest and epigastrium should always be auscultated after the ET tube is placed and capnometry used to monitor $ETCO_2$. ET tube placement should be frequently reassessed, especially after any movement of the patient. In addition to confirming ET tube placement, auscultation may rule out the possibility of other pulmonary injury. A child with a compromised airway and a pulmonary injury who has been successfully intubated may be in greater jeopardy for the development of a tension pneumothorax as a result of positive-pressure ventilation.

Box 14-4 Prehospital Pediatric Intubation: The Great Debate

It might seem intuitive that providing an ET tube as early as possible in the management of a child with TBI would be of benefit. A retrospective review showed improved survival in adult patients with TBI who were intubated prior to arrival at the receiving hospital.[30] Subsequent studies evaluated rapid-sequence intubation (RSI), demonstrating its improved efficiency and success rate in intubation of adults and children.[31,32] However, many retrospective and prospective case-control studies found that prehospital intubation compared with bag-mask ventilation did not improve survival or neurologic outcome and might have been detrimental.[14,33,34] A systematic review of pediatric airway management in the prehospital setting suggests that bag-mask ventilation is associated with improved survival and decreased complications compared to any form of advanced airway management.[35]

Prolonged periods of hypoxia are often associated with the intubation process, as well as periods of overaggressive ventilation following intubation in patients being transported to the trauma center.[15]

Data supporting prehospital pediatric endotracheal intubation are limited and ambiguous. In the spontaneously breathing child, endotracheal intubation with or without pharmacologic assistance is not recommended. Emergency medical services programs that perform pediatric prehospital intubation should include at least the following[36]:

1. Close medical direction and supervision
2. Training and continuing education, including hands-on operating room experience
3. Resources for patient monitoring, drug storage, and ET tube placement confirmation
4. Standardized RSI protocols
5. Availability of an alternate airway such as a laryngeal mask airway or King LT airway
6. Intensive continuing quality assurance/quality control and performance review program

inadequate as rescue devices for smaller children (under 4 feet [122 cm] in height). The laryngeal mask airway, iGels, and the smaller sizes of the King LT airways provide an alternate airway device choice in older children (> 8 years of age, when the airway is more similar to that of an adult). However, early studies demonstrate no improvement in outcomes among children with the use of supraglottic airways in place of endotracheal tube intubation.[39] Additionally, bag-mask ventilation is associated with improved outcomes relative to supraglottic airways in the pediatric population.[40]

For pediatric patients, the risks may outweigh the benefits of endotracheal intubation and must be carefully considered before attempting the procedure, especially in children for whom bag-mask ventilation is providing adequate ventilation and oxygenation. Consideration of the risks associated with endotracheal intubation is increasingly important as additional non-visualized advanced airway devices become available and are added into the prehospital care practitioner's practice.[33,34]

Breathing

A child's minute volume and ventilatory effort should be evaluated carefully. Because of the potential for rapid deterioration from mild hypoxia to ventilatory arrest, ventilation should be assisted if dyspnea and increased ventilatory effort are observed. A properly sized bag-mask device with a reservoir and high-flow oxygen to provide an oxygen concentration of between 85% and 100% (FiO_2 of 0.85 to 1.0) should be used. Continuous pulse oximetry serves as an adjunct for ongoing assessment of airway and breathing. The SpO_2 should be kept at greater than 94% (at sea level, with slightly lower expected oxygen saturations at higher altitudes).

In any intubated pediatric patient, ET tube placement should be confirmed using multiple methods, including directly visualizing the ET tube passing through the vocal folds, listening for the presence of equal bilateral breath sounds, and listening for the absence of sounds over the epigastrium when ventilated. Continuous $ETCO_2$ monitoring should be used to document continuing appropriate ET tube placement and to avoid extremes of hypercarbia and hypocarbia, both of which can be just as detrimental to recovery from a traumatic brain injury as hypoxia. $ETCO_2$ should be targeted at 35 to 40 mm Hg.[15]

Tension Pneumothorax

Children are more susceptible than adults to acute cardiovascular collapse from a tension pneumothorax. Most children with tension pneumothoraces will present with acute cardiac decompensation secondary to decreased venous return before any detectable changes in oxygenation and ventilation have occurred. Any child who acutely decompensates, especially after initiation of positive-pressure ventilation by bag-mask device or advanced airway placement, should be emergently assessed for tension pneumothorax.

Jugular venous distension may be difficult to determine because an extrication collar has been applied or because of the presence of hypovolemia from hemorrhage. Tracheal shift is a late sign of tension pneumothorax and may only be determined by palpating the trachea in the jugular notch. In these pediatric patients, unilateral absent breath sounds, in association with cardiovascular compromise, represent an indication for emergency needle decompression or finger thoracostomy. In an intubated pediatric patient, diminished sounds on the left may indicate a right main bronchus intubation, but when associated with acute cardiac decompensation, these sounds may represent tension pneumothorax. Careful reassessment of the patient's airway and respiratory status is needed to distinguish these subtle differences in the presentation.

The adult literature supports finger thoracostomy in the field for suspected tension pneumothorax, although systematic review has suggested that neither needle decompression nor finger thoracostomy has been shown definitively to have better outcomes. There is no literature comparing these two interventions for tension pneumothorax in pediatric patients. In a survey of experienced practitioners, there was a preference for needle decompression in younger pediatric patients and finger thoracostomy in older pediatric patients. Needle decompression of a tension pneumothorax in a pediatric patient should be performed in the second intercostal space at the midclavicular line. This approach is in contrast to a recent change in the adult recommendations for decompression at the midaxillary line at the fifth intercostal space.[41,42] For more on needle decompression and finger thoracostomy, see Chapter 10, *Thoracic Trauma*. Thoracic decompression is often more immediately effective in a child because the mediastinum rapidly shifts back to its normal position and venous return is quickly restored. The prehospital practitioner should be cautious of and watch closely for dislodgment after the angiocatheter is placed.

Circulation

Once a pediatric patient's external hemorrhage is controlled, perfusion should be evaluated. Controlling external hemorrhage involves applying direct manual pressure on the bleeding point, the use of advanced hemostatic dressings, and the use of tourniquets in cases of significant or problematic extremity hemorrhage. Managing external hemorrhage is not just a matter of covering the bleeding site with layer after layer of absorbent dressing. If the initial dressing becomes saturated in blood, it is better to add an additional dressing rather than to replace it, as the removal may dislodge any clot that has begun to form. At the same time, consider additional interventions to stop the ongoing hemorrhage such as wound packing or tourniquet application.

The pediatric vascular system is usually able to maintain a normal blood pressure until severe collapse occurs, at which point it is often unresponsive to resuscitation. Fluid resuscitation should be started whenever signs of compensated hypovolemic shock are present and must be started immediately in pediatric patients who present with decompensated shock. Normal saline solution in 20-mL/kg boluses should be used first. Early administration of blood and/or tranexamic acid (TXA) should be considered in any child felt to be in hemorrhagic shock. Specific guidelines for inclusion and exclusion are based on local protocols.

For pediatric trauma patients who display any signs of hemorrhagic shock or hypovolemia, key factors to survival are appropriate volume resuscitation and rapid initiation of transport to a suitable facility. Transport should never be delayed to obtain vascular access or administer IV fluid.

Vascular Access

Fluid replacement in a pediatric patient with severe hypotension or signs of shock must deliver adequate fluid volume to the right atrium to avoid further reduction in cardiac preload. The most appropriate initial sites for IV access are the *antecubital fossa* (anterior aspect of the forearm at the elbow) and the saphenous vein at the ankle. Access through the external jugular vein is another possibility, but airway management takes priority in such a small space and a cervical collar may make the neck poorly accessible.

In an unstable or potentially unstable pediatric patient, attempts at peripheral access should be limited to two in 90 seconds. If peripheral access is unsuccessful, IO access should be established (**Box 14-5**).

Placement of a subclavian or internal jugular catheter in a pediatric patient should be performed only under the most controlled circumstances within the hospital; this should not be attempted in the prehospital environment.

The determination of which pediatric patients should have intravascular access depends on the severity of injury, the experience of the involved prehospital care practitioners, and transport times, among other factors. If uncertainty exists regarding which pediatric patients

---

Box 14-5 Pediatric Intraosseous Infusion

Intraosseous (IO) infusion can provide an excellent alternative site for resuscitative volume replacement in injured children of all ages. This is an effective route for infusion of medications, blood, or high-volume fluid administration.

The most accessible site for IO infusion is the anterior tibia just inferior and medial to the tibial tuberosity. After preparing the skin antiseptically and securing the leg adequately, a site is chosen on the anterior medial portion of the tibia, 0.4 to 0.8 inch (1 to 2 cm) below and medial to the tibial tuberosity. Specially manufactured IO infusion needles are optimal for the procedure, but spinal or bone marrow needles may also be used. Spinal needles that are 18 to 20 gauge work well because they have a trocar to prevent the needle from being obstructed as it passes through the bony cortex into the marrow. Any 14- to 20-gauge needle can be used in an emergency.

A variety of commercially available devices are available that ease the difficulty of placing an IO needle, using various mechanical devices. For example, one device uses a high-speed drill to insert a specially designed IO needle, and another uses a spring-loaded mechanism. The needle is placed at a 90-degree angle to the bone and advanced firmly through the cortex into the marrow.

Evidence that the needle is adequately within the marrow includes the following:

1. A soft "pop" is heard and no resistance is felt after the needle has passed through the cortex.
2. Bone marrow aspirates into the needle.
3. Fluid flows freely into the marrow without evidence of subcutaneous infiltration.
4. The needle is secure and does not appear loose or wobbly.

IO infusion should be considered during initial resuscitation if percutaneous venous cannulation (venous IV insertion) has been unsuccessful. Because the flow rate is limited by the bone marrow cavity, the administration of fluids and medications should normally be done under pressure, and the IO route alone will seldom be sufficient after initial resuscitation.

Proper location of the insertion site is important, perhaps even more so in a pediatric patient. Failure to properly identify landmarks could lead to misplacement of the IO device and ineffective resuscitation or possibly compartment syndrome if fluid is inadvertently infused in large amounts into the soft tissues of the extremity as opposed to being introduced into the systemic circulation.

need intravascular access or if fluid replacement is needed during transport, online medical direction should be obtained.

Fluid Therapy

Isotonic crystalloid solution is the initial resuscitation fluid of choice for a hypovolemic pediatric patient. Fluid choices, when available, should take into account acidity, which may worsen coagulopathy and electrolyte concentrations (i.e., potassium) in the setting of massive tissue injury. The time that a crystalloid fluid remains in the intravascular space is relatively short, which is one reason why resuscitation with whole blood remains much more effective. This is discussed further in Chapter 3, *Shock: Pathophysiology of Life and Death.*

Historically, fluid resuscitation would begin with a 20-mL/kg fluid bolus, and a repeat crystalloid bolus if physiologically indicated prior to proceeding with blood product infusion. The current recommendation, however, is to start infusing blood products earlier if hemorrhagic shock is suspected. This can be with packed RBCs or whole blood, and may even be the first "fluid" given for these severely injured patients. A crystalloid bolus may temporarily restore cardiovascular stability as it transiently fills and then leaks from the circulatory system. However, until circulating RBCs are replaced and oxygen transport is restored, hypoxic injury can continue.

Pain Management

As with adults, pain management should be considered for children in the prehospital setting. Small doses of a narcotic analgesia that are appropriately titrated will not compromise the neurologic or abdominal examination. Both morphine and fentanyl are acceptable choices, but they should be administered only according to written prehospital care guidelines or with orders from online medical control. Because of the side effects of hypotension and hypoventilation, all pediatric patients receiving IV narcotics should be monitored with pulse oximetry and serial vital signs. In general, benzodiazepines should not be administered in combination with narcotics because of their synergistic effects on respiratory depression, possibly resulting in respiratory arrest. If local protocols for ketamine use are available, this may be a useful alternative in the prehospital setting as well.

Transport

Because timely arrival at the most appropriate facility may be the key element in a child's survival, triage is an important consideration in the management of a pediatric patient.

The tragedy of preventable pediatric traumatic death has been documented in multiple studies reported over the past three decades. It is estimated that the majority of pediatric trauma deaths can be classified as preventable or potentially preventable. These statistics have been one of the primary motivations for the development of regionalized pediatric trauma centers, where continuous, coordinated, high-quality, sophisticated care can be provided. Recent studies have demonstrated that adult trauma centers are not necessarily pediatric ready. Injured children evaluated at trauma centers that are not pediatric ready are associated with as much as a two-fold increase in mortality.[27] The American College of Surgeons Committee on Trauma supports the integration of pediatric readiness among all verified trauma centers. When feasible, EMS systems should preferentially transport severely injured children to pediatric-ready trauma centers and, ideally, pediatric trauma centers. Early identification of any physiologic abnormality (heart rate, ventilatory rate, or BP) should increase suspicion for multisystem injury and the need for a pediatric trauma center.

Many urban areas have both pediatric trauma centers and adult trauma centers. Ideally, a pediatric multisystem trauma patient will benefit from the initial resuscitation capability and definitive care available at a pediatric trauma center because of its specialization in treating traumatized children. It may be appropriate to bypass an adult trauma center in favor of transport to a pediatric-capable trauma center. For many communities, however, the nearest specialized pediatric trauma center may be hours away. In these cases, a seriously traumatized child should be transported to the nearest adult trauma center because early resuscitation and evaluation before transport to a pediatric facility may improve the child's chances of survival.[43-45]

In areas where there is no specialized pediatric trauma center nearby, personnel working in adult trauma centers should be experienced in the resuscitation and treatment of both adult and pediatric trauma patients. In areas where neither facility is close, a seriously injured child should be transported to the nearest appropriate hospital capable of caring for trauma victims, according to local prehospital triage guidelines.

Aeromedical transport may be considered in rural areas to expedite transport. There is little evidence that aeromedical transport provides any benefit in urban areas where ground transport to a pediatric trauma center is almost as fast.[46] It is becoming increasingly evident that using aeromedical transport exposes both the patient and the crew to a significant amount of risk.[47-49] These concerns must be carefully weighed when deciding whether to utilize this resource.

Many EMS and trauma systems use pediatric triage criteria, which may be dictated by state, regional, or local guidelines. All prehospital care practitioners need to be familiar with the triage protocols in place within their own systems.

Specific Injuries

Traumatic Brain Injury

Among children and youth aged 0 to 14 years in the United States, each year TBI results in an estimated 3,000 deaths and 29,000 hospitalizations.[50] Although many of the most severe brain injuries are treatable only by prevention, initial resuscitative measures may minimize secondary brain injury and, consequently, the severity of the child's injury. Adequate ventilation, oxygenation, and perfusion are needed to prevent secondary morbidity. While the recovery of pediatric patients sustaining severe TBI is typically considered to be better than in adults, growing evidence indicates that a wide variety of impairments persist, including functional, cognitive, and behavioral abnormalities.[51]

The results of the initial neurologic assessment are useful for prognosis. Even with a normal initial neurologic evaluation, however, any child who sustains a significant brain injury may be susceptible to cerebral edema, hypoperfusion, and secondary insults (**Box 14-6**). Furthermore, victims of nonaccidental trauma may have little external evidence of trauma, yet may have sustained considerable intracranial injury. A baseline GCS score should be recorded and frequently repeated during transport. Supplemental oxygen should be administered, and if possible, pulse oximetry should be monitored.

As with hypoxia, hypovolemia with resultant hypotension may dramatically worsen the outcome of the original TBI. External hemorrhage must be controlled and the child's fractured extremities immobilized to limit internal blood loss associated with these injuries. An attempt should be made to keep these pediatric patients in a *euvolemic* (normal volume) state with IV volume resuscitation. On rare occasions, infants younger than about age 6 months may become hypovolemic as a result of intracranial bleeding because they have open cranial sutures and fontanelles. An infant with an open fontanelle may better tolerate an expanding intracranial hematoma and thus not become symptomatic until rapid expansion occurs. An infant with a bulging fontanelle should be considered to have a more severe TBI.

For children with a GCS score of 8 or less, adequate oxygenation and ventilation should be the goal at all times, not the placement of an ET tube. Prolonged attempts at securing an endotracheal airway may increase periods of hypoxia and delay transport to an appropriate facility. The best airway for a pediatric patient is the one that is both safest and most effective. Ventilation with a bag-mask device while being prepared to suction emesis, should it occur, is often the best airway for the child with TBI.[13-15]

Box 14-6 Pediatric Concussion

The issue of concussion, or mild traumatic brain injury, in pediatric patients, particularly those engaged in sports activities, has become a topic of great importance.[52,53] Between 2006 and 2013, the Nationwide Emergency Department Sample database estimated there were 6.1 million (2.83%) pediatric patients evaluated in U.S. emergency departments with a TBI diagnosis, with the number of pediatric TBI patients increasing by 34.1% over the period of the study. In the distant past, when a pediatric athlete sustained a concussion, the child was kept out of the game for a short time and was allowed to return to play as soon as able. However, repeated blows to the head and brain lead to long-term difficulties with cognition, behavior, and function.[54] Any pediatric athlete who has sustained a concussion should be removed from play and not be permitted to participate for the duration of the event and until cleared for participation by a qualified physician.

The recognition of concussion is of key importance. Where it was once thought that concussion involved a brief loss of consciousness with a return to normal function, it is now understood that loss of consciousness is not necessary to make the diagnosis. Concussion may involve a variety of symptoms and complaints, including headache, nausea, balance problems, feeling dazed or stunned, confusion, and asking questions slowly or repetitively. It is recommended that medical personnel present at a sporting event have a formal method for assessing pediatric athletes for concussion using a standard sideline assessment tool as well as a neurologic examination.[55]

Full recovery from a concussion may take a week or longer—in some cases, months. Until the pediatric athlete has fully recovered from the concussion and is asymptomatic, the child should not be allowed to return to play. Once asymptomatic, the child may return to activity and play in a graded, structured format with repeat evaluations to assess for relapse of symptoms. Return of symptoms indicates incomplete recovery, and the pediatric athlete should refrain from participation in sports until improvement has occurred. Direction of return to play should be provided by a qualified physician. No child should return to play after a concussion without a thorough evaluation.

A pediatric patient with signs and symptoms of intracranial hypertension or increased intracranial pressure, such as a sluggishly reactive or nonreactive pupil, systemic hypertension, bradycardia, and abnormal breathing patterns, may benefit from temporary mild hyperventilation to lower intracranial pressure. However, this effect of hyperventilation is transient and also decreases overall oxygen delivery to the CNS, actually causing additional secondary brain injury.[56] It is strongly recommended that this strategy not be used unless the child is exhibiting signs of active herniation or *lateralizing* signs (distal neurologic abnormalities such as weakness on one side from injury to an area of the brain). $ETCO_2$ monitoring should guide management in an intubated pediatric patient, with the target range about 35 mm Hg. Hyperventilation to an $ETCO_2$ of less than 25 mm Hg has been associated with worse neurologic outcome.[15] If capnography is not available, a ventilation rate of 25 breaths/minute for children and 30 breaths/minute for infants should be used.[57]

During prolonged transports, small doses of mannitol (0.5 to 1 g/kg body weight), or hypertonic saline, may benefit children with evidence of intracranial hypertension, if local protocols permit. However, the use of mannitol in the setting of insufficient volume resuscitation may result in hypovolemia and worsening shock. Mannitol should not be given in the field without discussing this option with online medical control, unless permitted by standing orders or protocol, in which case the risks and benefits should be carefully weighed. Regardless, use of hypertonic saline or mannitol in the prehospital setting should be reserved for cases of impending herniation. Brief seizures may occur soon after a TBI and, aside from ensuring patient safety, oxygenation, and ventilation, often do not require specific treatment by prehospital care practitioners. However, recurrent seizure activity is worrisome and may require IV boluses of a benzodiazepine, such as midazolam (0.1 mg/kg/dose). All benzodiazepines should be used with extreme caution in these patients because of the potential side effects of ventilatory depression and hypotension, as well as their ability to cloud the neurologic examination.

Spinal Trauma

The indication for maintaining spinal motion restriction in a pediatric patient is based on the mechanism of injury and physical findings; the presence of other injuries that suggest violent or sudden movement of the head, neck, or torso; or the presence of specific signs of spine injury, such as deformity, pain, or a neurologic deficit. As with adult patients, the correct prehospital management of a suspected spine injury is in-line manual stabilization followed by the use of a properly fitting cervical collar and use of an appropriate device so that the head, neck, torso, pelvis, and legs are maintained in a neutral in-line

position. Pediatric patients with a neurologic deficit that quickly resolves may have SCIWORA and may be susceptible to delayed secondary sequelae. Spinal motion restriction should be employed in these patients even if their symptoms resolve prior to hospital arrival. This should be achieved without impairing the child's ventilation or ability to open the mouth or disrupting any other resuscitative efforts.

The threshold for performing spinal motion restriction is lower in young children because of their inability to communicate or otherwise participate in their own assessment. No studies have validated the safety of clinically clearing a child's spine in the field. The same immaturity discussed previously also contributes to children's fear and lack of cooperation with immobilization. A child who strongly fights attempts at spinal motion restriction may be at increased risk of worsening any existing spinal injuries. It may be valid to decide not to restrain such a pediatric patient if the child can be persuaded to lie quietly without restraints. However, any decision to stop stabilization attempts in the interest of patient safety must be supported by careful and thoroughly documented reasoning, as well as serial assessment of neurologic status during and immediately after transport. Ideally, this decision would be made in concert with online medical control.

When most small children are placed on a rigid surface, the relatively larger size of the child's occiput will result in passive neck flexion. Sufficient padding (about 1 inch [2 to 3 cm]) should be placed under the child's torso to elevate it and allow the head to be in a neutral position. The padding should be continuous and flat from the shoulders to the pelvis and extend to the lateral margins of the torso to ensure that the thoracic, lumbar, and sacral spine are on a flat, stable platform without the possibility of anterior–posterior movement. Padding should also be placed between the sides of the child and the edges of the board to ensure that no lateral movement occurs when the board is moved or if the patient and board need to be rotated to the side to avoid aspiration during vomiting episodes.

Various new pediatric stabilization devices are available. The prehospital care practitioner should practice regularly and be familiar with any specialized equipment used in the practitioner's system as well as the required adjustments necessary when immobilizing a child using adult-sized equipment. If a vest-type device is used on a pediatric patient, adequate stabilization while at the same time preventing respiratory compromise must be ensured. In the past, it was recommended that infants or young children be immobilized in a car safety seat if that is where they were found.[58,59] The National Highway Traffic Safety Administration now recommends that the pediatric patient be secured and transported in an appropriately sized pediatric stabilization device instead of the car seat. Keeping the injured child in an upright position in the car seat increases the axial load placed on the spine by the patient's head; therefore, standard spinal motion restriction techniques are preferred to the car seat.[60] A child who is not immobilized should not be transported on a caregiver's lap; rather, the child should be appropriately restrained in a car seat for transport.

Thoracic Injuries

The extremely resilient rib cage of a child often results in less injury to the bony structure of the thorax, but there is still risk for underlying pulmonary injury, such as pulmonary contusion, pneumothorax, or hemothorax. Although rib fractures are rare in childhood, they are associated with a high risk of intrathoracic injury when present. Crepitus may be appreciated on examination and may be a sign of pneumothorax. The risk of mortality increases with the number of ribs fractured. A high index of suspicion is the key to identifying these injuries. Every pediatric patient who sustains trauma to the chest and torso should be carefully monitored for signs of respiratory distress and shock. Abrasions or contusions over a pediatric patient's torso after blunt force trauma may be the only clues to the prehospital care practitioner that the child has suffered thoracic trauma.

Additionally, when transporting a pediatric patient who has sustained a high-impact blunt thoracic injury, the child's cardiac rhythm should be monitored en route to a medical facility. In all cases, the key items in managing thoracic trauma involve careful attention to ventilation, oxygenation, and timely transport to an appropriate facility.

Abdominal Injuries

The presence of blunt trauma to the abdomen, an unstable pelvis, posttraumatic abdominal distension, rigidity or tenderness, or otherwise unexplained shock can be associated with possible intra-abdominal hemorrhage. A "seat belt sign" (or mark) or a handlebar mark across the abdomen of a pediatric patient is often an indicator of serious internal injuries (**Figure 14-7**).

The key prehospital elements in management of abdominal injuries include targeted fluid resuscitation, supplemental high-concentration oxygen, and rapid transport to an appropriate facility with continued careful monitoring en route. There are really no definitive interventions that prehospital care practitioners can offer to pediatric patients with intra-abdominal injuries, and, as such, every effort should be made to transport pediatric patients rapidly to the closest, most appropriate facility.

Extremity Trauma

Compared with the adult skeleton, the child's skeleton is actively growing and consists of a large proportion of cartilaginous tissue and metabolically active growth plates. The ligamentous structures that hold the skeleton together are frequently stronger and better able to withstand mechanical disruption than the bones to which they are attached. As a result, children with skeletal trauma frequently sustain major traumatic forces before developing long-bone fractures, dislocations, or deformities. Incomplete ("greenstick") fractures are common and may be indicated only by bony tenderness and pain on use of the affected extremity.

Primary joint disruption from injury other than penetrating injury is uncommon compared with disruption of the *diaphyseal* (shaft) or *epiphyseal* (end) segments of bone. Fractures that involve the growth plate are unique in that they must be carefully identified and managed in the acute injury phase to not only ensure adequate healing but also prevent subsequent displacement or deformity as the child continues to develop. The association of neurovascular injuries with orthopedic injuries in children should always be considered, and the distal vascular and neurologic examination should be carefully evaluated. Often, the presence of a potentially debilitating injury can be determined only by radiologic study or, when the slightest suggestion of a decrease in distal perfusion exists, by *arteriography* (x-ray study of a blood vessel that has been injected with radiopaque contrast material).

The apparent gross deformity sometimes associated with extremity injury should not distract focus from potentially life-threatening injuries. Uncontrolled hemorrhage represents the most life-threatening consequence of extremity trauma. In multisystem pediatric and adult trauma patients alike, the initiation of transport to an appropriate facility without delay after completion of the primary survey, resuscitation, and rapid packaging remains paramount in reducing mortality. If basic splinting

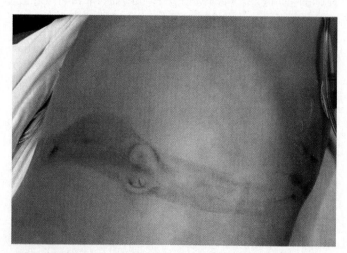

Figure 14-7 "Seat belt sign" in a 6-year-old patient who was found to have a ruptured spleen. Seat belt signs are often associated with serious intra-abdominal injuries.
Courtesy of Dr. Jeffrey Guy.

can be provided en route without detracting from the child's resuscitation, it will help to minimize bleeding and pain from long-bone fractures, but attention to life-threatening injuries should always remain the primary focus.

Burn Injuries

Following motor vehicle crashes and drowning, burns rate third as a cause of pediatric trauma deaths.[2] Caring for an injured child always poses significant physical and emotional challenges to the prehospital care practitioner, and these difficulties are amplified when caring for a pediatric patient with burns. A child with burns may have an *edematous* (swollen) airway, IV access may be complicated by burns of the extremity, and the child may be hysterical from pain.

The primary survey should be followed as in other causes of pediatric trauma, but every step of the primary survey may be more complicated than in a child without thermal injuries. Most deaths related to structure fires are not directly related to soft-tissue burns but are secondary to smoke inhalation. When children are trapped in a structure fire, they often hide from the fire under beds or in closets. These children frequently die, and their recovered bodies often have no burns; they die from carbon monoxide or hydrogen cyanide toxicity and hypoxia.

Thermally induced edema of the airway is always a concern in patients with burns, but especially in children. The smaller diameter of the pediatric trachea means that 1 mm of edema will produce a greater magnitude of airway obstruction than in an adult with a larger diameter airway. A pediatric patient with an edematous airway may be sitting forward and drooling or complaining of hoarseness or voice changes. These symptoms should prompt rapid preparations for and initiation of transport to the hospital. While en route, supplemental oxygen is administered and preparations made for airway intervention should the symptoms progress or the child develop respiratory or cardiac arrest.

If an ET tube is placed, it needs to be protected against inadvertent dislodgment or removal. If a pediatric burn patient accidentally becomes extubated, the prehospital care practitioner may not be able to intubate the child again due to progressive edema, and the results could be disastrous. Securing an ET tube in a pediatric patient who has peeling facial skin and moist wounds is also difficult. Securing the ET tube to the face with adhesive tape should not be attempted in a child with facial burns. The ET tube should be secured with two pieces of umbilical tape, with one piece draped above the ear and the second piece placed below the ear. An effective alternative to umbilical tape is IV tubing. If these supplies are not available but extra hands are, designate a practitioner to be solely responsible for holding the airway in place.

Fluid Resuscitation

Rapid establishment of intravascular access is vital to prevent the development of shock in pediatric burn patients. Delayed fluid resuscitation in pediatric patients has been associated with significantly worse clinical outcomes and an increased mortality rate, especially in burned infants.[61-63]

After securing an airway and providing adequate ventilation and oxygenation, it is critical that venous access be obtained quickly. Children have a relatively small intravascular volume, and a delay in fluid resuscitation may lead to the rapid development of hypovolemic shock. To provide the large volumes of IV fluids required in critical burns, such pediatric patients usually require two peripheral IV catheters to achieve the required IV flow rates. The insertion of a single large-bore IV catheter is often challenging, so two IV catheters is all the more so. Burns on the extremities may make it difficult to impossible to establish enough access for an appropriate fluid resuscitation.

In children with burns, as in adult patients with burns, fluid needs are calculated from the time of the injury, so a delay of even 30 minutes to the beginning of fluid resuscitation can result in hypovolemic shock. Excessive fluids can result in respiratory complications as well as excessive edema, which can complicate burn care.

At the beginning of a fluid resuscitation, the amount of fluids typically given to a patient with burns is calculated based on the estimated percentage of total body surface area (TBSA) burned, with later resuscitation guided by perfusion and urine output. TBSA is used with the "rule of nines," a rapid and imprecise method of estimating resuscitative fluid needs based on adult battlefield burn casualties. The premise of this method of burn size estimation is that major regions of the adult body (e.g., head, arm, anterior torso) each comprise 9% of the total body surface area. Children's anatomic regions are proportionally different from those in adults; children have larger heads and smaller limbs. There is a tendency to overestimate TBSA of burn in children. Remember that superficial burns (intact erythematous skin) are not included in the TBSA estimation. Estimation of pediatric burn size should use diagrams that are age specific, such as the Lund-Browder chart, and not the rule of nines. Using this chart, each leg can be estimated at 13.5%, arms are 9%, the chest and back are 18% each, and the head is 18%. If charts and diagrams are not available, the "rule of palms" may be used. Using this method, the size of the pediatric patient's palm plus fingers represents approximately 1% of the body surface area. This is useful when estimating burn area for scattered areas that do not involve an entire body part. (See Chapter 13, *Burn Injuries*, for further discussion of these burn estimation methods.)

The volume of IV fluids needed for resuscitation is determined based on the percentage of TBSA burned (see Chapter 13, *Burn Injuries*). Two important pediatric considerations merit mention. First, small children have a limited reserve of glycogen. Glycogen is essentially glucose molecules strung together, and it is used for carbohydrate storage. Stored glycogen is mobilized in times of stress. If these limited glycogen stores become depleted, the child may rapidly develop hypoglycemia. Second, children have a large volume-to-surface area ratio; the general shape of an adult is a cylinder, whereas children resemble a sphere (**Figure 14-8**). The clinical implication is that a child will require more IV fluids for a given TBSA burned. For the initial prehospital resuscitation, glucose should be checked on any child with an altered mental status. If the child is tachycardic with poor perfusion, a 20-mL/kg fluid bolus should be administered. Total fluids administered should be reported to the hospital upon arrival.

Once peripheral IV access has been obtained, provisions must be made to ensure that the IV line is not inadvertently removed or dislodged. The usual techniques used to secure IV lines are often ineffective when a line is placed in or adjacent to a burn because adhesive tape and dressings may not adhere to burned tissue. If possible, the IV line is secured with a Kerlix dressing, although circumferential dressings must be frequently monitored as edema develops, to prevent the dressing from becoming a constricting band.

When peripheral venous access cannot be obtained, IO catheters should be used for an unstable and/or unconscious pediatric patient. Although previously advocated only for pediatric patients younger than 3 years of age, IO infusions are now used in older children as well as adults.

Abuse

Approximately 10% of pediatric burns are nonaccidental.[64] Up to 50% of these children may experience recurrent abuse, and 30% of this group eventually die from abuse.[65,66] An increased awareness of this problem among prehospital care practitioners can improve detection of this cause of pediatric trauma. Careful documentation of the situation surrounding the injury, as well as of the injury patterns themselves, may aid officials in the prosecution of the offenders.[67]

The two most common mechanisms by which these children receive burns are scalds and contact burns. Scalds are the most common source of nonaccidental burns. Scalding injuries typically are inflicted on children of toilet-training age. The usual scenario is that the child urinates or defecates other than on the toilet and is subsequently immersed in a tub of scalding water. These scald burns are characterized by a pattern of sharp demarcation between burned and unburned tissue and sparing of flexion creases, as the child will frequently draw the legs up to avoid the scalding water (see Chapter 13, *Burn Injuries*).

Contact burns are the second most common mechanism of abuse burns. Common items used to inflict contact burns are curling irons, clothing irons, lighters, and cigarettes. Cigarette burns appear as circular, uniform wounds measuring slightly over 0.4 inches (1 cm) in diameter (typically 0.5 inches [1.3 cm]). To conceal these injuries, the abuser may place the burns in areas usually covered by clothing (e.g., the back, feet), above the hairline in the scalp, or even in the axillae.

All of the surfaces of the human body have some degree of curvature; thus, a hot item that accidentally falls onto the body surface will have an initial point of contact and will then deflect from the point of contact. The resultant burns will have irregular borders and uneven depths. In contrast, when a hot item is deliberately used to burn someone, the item is pressed onto the region of the body. The burn will have a pattern with a sharp, regular outline and uniform burn depth (see Chapter 13, *Burn Injuries*).

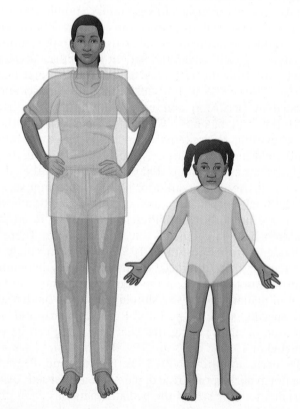

Figure 14-8 Children have a large volume-to-surface area ratio; the general shape of an adult is a cylinder, whereas children resemble a sphere.

© National Association of Emergency Medical Technicians (NAEMT)

A high index of suspicion for abuse is important, and all cases of suspected abuse should be reported. Make meticulous observations of the surroundings, such as the position of various pieces of furniture, presence of curling irons, and depth of bath water. Record the names of the individuals present at the scene. Any pediatric patient suspected of being abused by burns, regardless of the size of the burns, needs to be cared for at a center experienced in pediatric burn care.

Child abuse and neglect are further discussed later in this chapter.

Motor Vehicle Injury Prevention

The American Academy of Pediatrics (AAP) has defined optimal restraint for children in motor vehicles (**Table 14-7**). The AAP recommends that children should always ride in the rear seat and face the rear of the seat until 2 years of age. Children who have outgrown the rear-facing weight or height limit for their convertible seat should use a forward-facing seat with a harness for as long as possible, based on the highest weight and height allowed by the car safety seat manufacturer.

Children then graduate into a belt-positioning booster seat until they are age 8 to 12 years. At that time, the standard three-point (seat belt–shoulder harness combination) adult restraint can be used. The lap belt alone should never be used. All children should remain in the back seat until they are age 13 years.

Suboptimal restraint is defined as the lack of use of a child safety seat or booster seat for anyone younger than age 8 years and lack of a three-point restraint for a child older than age 8 years (see Box 14-1).[68] In a review study, when these guidelines were observed, the risk of abdominal injury in children who were appropriately restrained was 3.5 times less than in the suboptimally restrained pediatric population.[69] The protective benefit of the rear-seat position is such that risk of death is decreased by at least 30%, even if restrained with a lap belt only in the rear seat versus three-point restraint in the front seat.[70] For more information on injury prevention, see Chapter 16, *Injury Prevention*.

Child Abuse and Neglect

Child abuse (maltreatment or nonaccidental trauma) is a significant cause of childhood injury. In 2018, there were approximately 678,000 substantiated cases of child

Table 14-7 Types of Car Seats		
Age Group	**Type of Seat**	**General Guidelines**
Infants and toddlers	■ Rear-facing only ■ Rear-facing convertible	All infants and toddlers should ride in a **rear-facing seat** until they are at least **2 years of age** or reach the highest weight or height allowed by their car seat manufacturer.
Toddlers and preschoolers	■ Convertible ■ Forward-facing with harness	Children who have outgrown the rear-facing weight or height limit for their convertible seat should use a **forward-facing seat** with a harness for as long as possible, up to the highest weight or height allowed by their car safety seat manufacturer.
School-age children	■ Booster seats	All children whose weight or height exceeds the forward-facing limit for their car safety seat should use a **belt-positioning booster seat** until the vehicle seat belt fits properly, typically when they have reached 4 feet 9 inches in height and are ages 8 to 12 years. All children younger than age 13 years should ride in the back seat.
Older children	■ Seat belts	When children are old enough and large enough for the vehicle seat belt to fit them correctly, they should always use **lap and shoulder seat belts** for the best protection. All children younger than age 13 years should ride in the back seat.

Reproduced from American Academy of Pediatrics (AAP). Car seats: information for families. Updated March 6, 2018. Accessed April 2, 2018. https://www.healthychildren.org/English/safety-prevention/on-the-go/Pages/Car-Safety-Seats-Information-for-Families.aspx

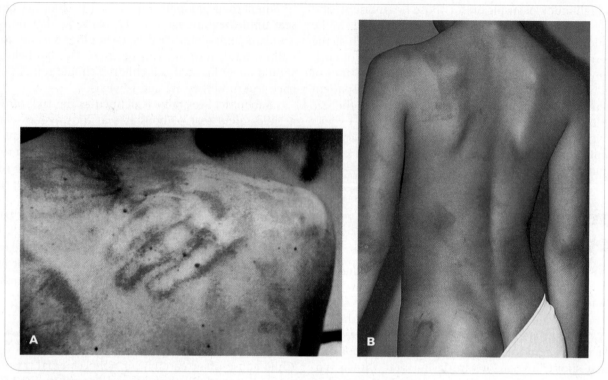

Figure 14-9 Indicators of possible nonaccidental trauma. **A.** Bruises that resemble hand prints. **B.** Bruises that are in multiple stages of healing.

A: Courtesy of Moose Jaw Police Service; **B:** Courtesy of Ronald Dieckmann, MD.

abuse in the United States and 1,738 fatalities due to abuse. Prehospital care practitioners must always consider the possibility of child abuse when circumstances warrant.

Prehospital care practitioners should suspect abuse or neglect if they note any of the following scenarios:

- Discrepancy between the history and the degree of physical injury or frequent changes in the reported history.
- Inappropriate response from the family.
- Prolonged interval between time of injury and call for medical care.
- History of the injury inconsistent with the developmental level of the child. For example, a history indicating that a neonate rolled off a bed would be suspect because neonates are developmentally unable to roll over.

Certain types of injuries also suggest abuse, such as the following (**Figure 14-9**):

- Multiple fractures or bruises in varying stages of resolution (excluding the palms, forearms, tibial areas, and the forehead in ambulatory children, who are frequently injured in normal falls). Accidental bruises usually occur over bony prominences; bruises

from intentional harm may appear on the buttocks, abdomen, or back.
- Unusual injuries such as bite marks, cigarette burns, rope marks, imprint of a hand, or any pattern injury.
- Sharply demarcated burns or scald injuries in unusual areas (see Chapter 13, *Burn Injuries*).

The TEN-4-FACESp Bruising Clinical Decision Rule is a highly sensitive and specific tool in identifying bruising that is concerning for abuse (**Figure 14-10**).[71]

- TEN: Bruising on Torso (chest, abdomen, back, buttocks, GU region, hip), Ears, or Neck
- FACES: Bruising on Frenulum, Angle of jaw, Cheek (fatty portion), Eyelids, Subconjunctivae
- 4: "TEN 4 FACES" Bruising in a child younger than age 4 years or any bruising in an infant age 4 months or younger
- p: Patterned bruising

In many jurisdictions, prehospital care practitioners are legally mandated reporters if they identify potential child abuse. Generally, practitioners who act in good faith and in the best interests of the child are protected from legal action. Reporting procedures vary, so practitioners should be familiar with the appropriate agencies that handle child abuse cases in their location.

TEN-4 Bruising Rule

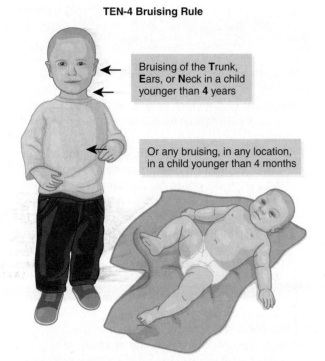

Bruising of the **T**runk, **E**ars, or **N**eck in a child younger than **4** years

Or any bruising, in any location, in a child younger than 4 months

Figure 14-10 The TEN-4-FACESp Bruising Clinical Decision Rule is a highly sensitive and specific tool in identifying bruising that is concerning for abuse.

© National Association of Emergency Medical Technicians (NAEMT)

Prolonged Transport

Occasionally a situation arises as a result of patient location, triage decisions, or environmental considerations in which transport will be prolonged or delayed and prehospital personnel need to manage the ongoing resuscitation of a pediatric patient. Even though this may be suboptimal because of the lack of field resources (e.g., blood) and the inability to perform diagnostic and therapeutic interventions, by applying the principles discussed in this chapter in an organized fashion, many children can be safely managed until arrival at a trauma center. If radio or cell phone contact with the receiving facility is possible, constant communication and feedback are crucial for both prehospital and hospital-based members of the trauma team.

Management consists of continued serial evaluation of the components of the primary survey. Spinal motion restriction should be maintained throughout. Removal from a hard board and maintenance of spinal motion restriction on a cot is preferred for significantly prolonged transports to avoid significant pressure discomfort and for patients with altered levels of consciousness, and potentially, pressure ulcerations. In these cases, great care must be taken during transfers from the ambulance cot to maintain strict spinal motion restriction and limit the risk of secondary spinal cord injury. If the airway is tenuous and the crew is well trained in pediatric airway management, including endotracheal intubation, then definitive airway stabilization should be performed if the child's condition warrants. Otherwise, conscientious bag-mask ventilation is an acceptable management strategy, assuming it provides adequate oxygenation and ventilation.

Pulse oximetry should be monitored and preferably $ETCO_2$ as well, especially in a child with a head injury. If signs of shock exist, 20-mL/kg boluses of lactated Ringer's or normal saline solution are administered until the child improves or is transferred to definitive care.

The GCS score should be calculated early and followed serially. Assessment for other injuries should continue, and all efforts to keep the child normothermic should be standard practice. Fractures should be splinted and stabilized with serial neurovascular assessments. This cycle of continued reassessment of the primary survey should be repeated until the child can be safely transported or transferred to definitive care.

Any change or decompensation in the pediatric patient's condition requires immediate reassessment of the primary survey. For example, if SpO_2 begins to decline, is the ET tube still secure and in the airway? If so, has the child developed a tension pneumothorax? Is the ET tube now in the right main bronchus? If the pediatric patient has received what was thought to be sufficient fluid and is still in shock, is there now cardiac tamponade, severe cardiac contusion, or perhaps an occult source of bleeding, such as intra-abdominal injury or missed scalp laceration? Has the GCS score changed? Are there now lateralizing signs suggesting progressive brain injury and requiring more aggressive treatments? Is the circulation and neurologic function of the extremities still intact? Is the child normothermic? If radio contact is available, continued advice and guidance should be sought throughout the resuscitation and transport.

By paying attention to the basics and continually reassessing your pediatric patient, adequate resuscitation can be performed until the child can be transferred to definitive care.

SUMMARY

- The primary survey and management of the pediatric patient in the prehospital setting require application of standard trauma life support principles modified to account for the unique characteristics of pediatric patients.
- Traumatic brain injury is the leading cause of death from trauma, as well as the most common injury for which pediatric patients require airway management.
- Children should not be thought of as "little adults." They present unique anatomic and developmental considerations, and both they and their caregivers may require psychological support.
- The pediatric assessment triangle (PAT) helps practitioners to form a general impression—sick or not sick. The three components of the PAT are appearance, work of breathing, and circulation to the skin.
- Children have the ability to compensate for volume loss longer than adults, but when they decompensate, they deteriorate suddenly and severely.
- Significant underlying organ and vascular injury can occur with few or no obvious signs of external injury.
- Pediatric patients with the following signs are unstable and should be transported without delay to an appropriate facility, ideally a pediatric trauma center:
  - Respiratory compromise
  - Signs of shock or circulatory instability
  - Any alteration to mental status
  - Significant blunt trauma to the head, thorax, or abdomen
  - Any evidence of multiple fractures or significant fractures (ribs or pelvis)
  - Any concern for nonaccidental trauma
- Always consider the possibility of abuse or nonaccidental trauma when the history of the injury does not match the presentation of the patient.

SCENARIO RECAP

You are called to the scene of a motor vehicle crash on a heavily traveled highway. Two vehicles were involved in a frontal offset collision. One of the vehicle's occupants is a child who was improperly restrained in a child booster seat. No weather-related factors are involved on this spring afternoon.

On arrival at the scene, you see that the police have secured and blocked traffic from the area around the crash. As your partner and the other arriving crew are assessing the other patients, you approach the child. You see a young boy, approximately 2 years of age, sitting in the booster seat, which is slightly turned at an angle; there is blood on the back of the headrest of the seat in front of him. Despite numerous abrasions and minor bleeding from the head, face, and neck, the child appears very calm.

Your primary and secondary surveys reveal a 2-year-old boy who weakly repeats "ma-ma, ma-ma." His pulse rate is 180 beats/minute, with the radial pulses weaker than the carotid; his blood pressure is 50 mm Hg by palpation. His ventilatory rate is 18 breaths/minute, slightly irregular, but without abnormal sounds. As you continue to assess him, you note that he has stopped saying "ma-ma" and seems to just stare into space. You also note that his pupils are slightly dilated, and his skin is pale and sweaty. A woman who identifies herself as the family's nanny tells you that the mother is en route and that you should wait for her.

- What are the management priorities for this patient?
- What are the most likely injuries in this child?
- Where is the most appropriate destination for this child?

SCENARIO SOLUTION

You correctly identify this child as a victim of multisystem trauma who is critically injured. His ventilatory rate is low. The first priority is manual cervical spine control and supplemental oxygen with bag-valve mask. You are also acutely aware of the tachycardia and weak peripheral pulses. You quickly search for any obvious signs of bleeding and note there are no obvious sources. You correctly assume the patient is in hypovolemic shock, probably the result of an unrecognized intra-abdominal injury. This child has major multisystem trauma and requires aggressive care to give him a chance to survive.

Because of the nature of the child's injuries, you consult with online medical control, who agrees that helicopter transport to the closest pediatric trauma center is more appropriate than ground transport to a nearby community hospital that has no pediatric critical care, neurosurgical, or orthopedic resources. Brief efforts at peripheral venous access are successful. You begin a crystalloid bolus of 20 mL/kg. The child's mother arrives just as you are transferring care to the helicopter crew.

References

1. National Center for Injury Prevention and Control, Centers for Disease Control and Prevention. 10 leading causes of death reports, 2005–2018. Updated September 22, 2021. Accessed March 4, 2022. https://www.cdc.gov/injury/wisqars/LeadingCauses.html

2. Centers for Disease Control and Prevention. Injuries among children and teens. Last reviewed September 22, 2021. Accessed February 23, 2022. https://www.cdc.gov/injury/features/child-injury/index.html

3. American College of Surgeons. National Trauma Data Bank 2013: Pediatric Report. American College of Surgeons; 2016. Accessed March 12, 2018. https://www.facs.org/~/media/files/quality%20programs/trauma/ntdb/ntdb%20pediatric%20annual%20report%202016.ashx

4. National Center for Injury Prevention and Control, Centers for Disease Control and Prevention. Updated November 20, 2020. Accessed March 4, 2022. https://wisqars.cdc.gov/nonfatal-leading

5. Peden M, Oyegbite K, Ozanne-Smith J, et al., eds. *World Report on Child Injury Prevention*. World Health Organization; 2008.

6. Bachman SL, Salzman GA, Burke RV, Arbogast H, Ruiz P, Upperman JS. Observed child restraint misuse in a large, urban community: results from three years of inspection events. *J Safety Res*. 2016 Feb;56:17-22.

7. Grisoni ER, Pillai SB, Volsko TA, et al. Pediatric airbag injuries: the Ohio experience. *J Pediatr Surg*. 2000;35(2):160-162.

8. Durbin DR, Kallan M, Elliott M, et al. Risk of injury to restrained children from passenger air bags. *Traffic Injury Prev*. 2003;4(1):58-63.

9. Durbin DR, Kallan M, Elliott M, et al. Risk of injury to restrained children from passenger air bags. *Annu Proc Assoc Adv Auto Med*. 2002;46:15-25.

10. Ferguson SA, Schneider LW. An overview of frontal air bag performance with changes in frontal crash-test requirements: findings of the Blue Ribbon Panel for the evaluation of advanced technology air bags. *Traffic Inj Prev*. 2008;9(5):421-431.

11. Arbogast KB, Kallan MJ. The exposure of children to deploying side air bags: an initial field assessment. *Ann Proc Assoc Adv Automot Med*. 2007;51:245-259.

12. EMSC-Partnership for Children, National Association of Emergency Medical Technicians. Guidelines for Providing Family-Centered Care. Published July 2000. Accessed March 22, 2022. https://www.nh.gov/safety/divisions/fstems/ems/documents/emscguidelines.pdf

13. Gausche M, Lewis RJ, Stratton SJ, et al. Effect of out-of-hospital pediatric endotracheal intubation on survival and neurological outcome: a controlled clinical trial. *JAMA*. 2000;283(6):783-790.

14. Davis DP, Hoyt DB, Ochs M, et al. The effect of paramedic rapid sequence intubation on outcome in patients with severe traumatic brain injury. *J Trauma Injury Infec Crit Care*. 2003;54(3):444-453.

15. Davis DP, Dunford JV, Poste JC, et al. The impact of hypoxia and hyperventilation on outcome after paramedic rapid sequence intubation of severely head-injured patients. *J Trauma Injury Infect Crit Care*. 2004;57(1):1-8.

16. York J, Arrillaga A, Graham R, Miller R. Fluid resuscitation of patients with multiple injuries and severe closed-head injury: experience with an aggressive fluid resuscitation strategy. *J Trauma Injury Infect Crit Care*. 2000;48(3):376-380.

17. Manley G, Knudson MM, Morabito D, et al. Hypotension, hypoxia, and head injury: frequency, duration, and consequences. *Arch Surg*. 2001;136(10):1118-1123.

18. Chesnut RM, Marshall LF, Klauber MR, et al. The role of secondary brain injury in determining outcome from severe head injury. *J Trauma*. 1993;34(2):216-222.

19. Luten R. Error and time delay in pediatric trauma resuscitation: addressing the problem with color-coded resuscitation aids. *Surg Clin North Am*. 2002;82(2):303-314.

20. Fernández A, Ares MI, Garcia S, Martinez-Indart L, Mintegi S, Benito J. The validity of the pediatric assessment triangle as the first step in the triage process in a pediatric emergency department. *Pediatr Emerg Care*. 2017 Apr;33(4):234-238.

21. Gausche-Hill M, Eckstein M, Horeczko T, et al. Paramedics accurately apply the pediatric assessment triangle to drive management. *Prehosp Emerg Care*. 2014;18(4):520-530.

22. American College of Surgeons Committee on Trauma. Pediatric trauma. In: ACS Committee on Trauma. *Advanced Trauma Life Support for Doctors, Student Course Manual*. 8th ed. ACS; 2008:225-245.

23. Sokol KK, Black GE, Azarow KS, Long W, Martin MJ, Eckert MJ. Prehospital interventions in severely injured pediatric patients: rethinking the ABCs. *J Trauma Acute Care Surg*. 2015;79(6):983-989.

24. Kragh JF Jr, Cooper A, Aden JK, et al. Survey of trauma registry data on tourniquet use in pediatric war casualties. *Pediatr Emerg Care*. 2012 Dec;28(12):1361-1365.

25. Chou R, Totten AM, Pappas M, et al., eds. *Glasgow Coma Scale for Field Triage of Trauma: A Systematic Review* [Report No.: 16(17)-EHC041-EF]. Agency for Healthcare Research and Quality; 2017.

26. Van de Voorde P, Sabbe M, Rizopoulos D, et al.; PENTA study group. Assessing the level of consciousness in children: a plea for the Glasgow Coma Motor subscore. *Resuscitation*. 2008;76(2):175-179.

27. Newgard C, Lin A, Olson L, et al. Evaluation of emergency department pediatric readiness and outcomes among US trauma centers. *JAMA Pediatr*. 2021;175(9):947-956. doi: 10.1001/jamapediatrics.2021.1319

28. National Vital Statistics System, Centers for Disease Control and Prevention. Deaths: final data for 1997. *Morb Mortal Wkly Rep*. 1999;47(19):1.

29. Ehrlich PF, Seidman PS, Atallah D, et al. Endotracheal intubation in rural pediatric trauma patients. *J Pediatr Surg*. 2004;39:1376-1380.

30. Winchell RJ, Hoyt DB. Endotracheal intubation in the field improves survival in patients with severe head injury. *Arch Surg*. 1997;132(6):592-597.

31. Davis DP, Ochs M, Hoyt DB, et al. Paramedic-administered neuromuscular blockade improves prehospital intubation success in severely head-injured patients. *J Trauma Injury Infect Crit Care*. 2003;55(4):713-719.

32. Pearson S. Comparison of intubation attempts and completion times before and after the initiation of a rapid sequence intubation protocol in an air medical transport program. *Air Med J*. 2003;22(6):28-33.

33. Hansen ML, Lin A, Eriksson C, et al. A comparison of pediatric airway management techniques during out-of-hospital cardiac arrest using the CARES database. *Resuscitation*. 2017;120:51-56.

34. Gerritse BM, Draaisma JM, Schalkwijk A, van Grunsven PM, Scheffer GJ. Should EMS-paramedics perform paediatric tracheal intubation in the field? *Resuscitation*. 2008;79(2):225-229.

35. Weihing VK, Crowe EH, Wang HE, Ugalde IT. Prehospital airway management in the pediatric patient: a systematic review. *Acad Emerg Med*. 2021. doi: 10.1111/acem.14410

36. Davis BD, Fowler R, Kupas DF, Roppolo LP. Role of rapid sequence induction for intubation in the prehospital setting: helpful or harmful? *Curr Opin Crit Care*. 2002;8(6):571-577.

37. Heins M. The "battered child" revisited. *JAMA*. 1984;251(24):3295-3300. doi: 10.1001/jama.251.24.3295

38. Davis DP, Valentine C, Ochs M, et al. The Combitube as a salvage airway device for paramedic rapid sequence intubation. *Ann Emerg Med*. 2003;42(5):697-704.

39. Fukuda T, Sekiguchi H, Taira T, et al. Type of advanced airway and survival after pediatric out-of-hospital cardiac arrest. *Resuscitation*. 2020;150:145-153.

40. Hernandez MC, Antiel RM, Balakrishnan K, Zielinski MD, Klinkner DB. Definitive airway management after prehospital supraglottic rescue airway in pediatric trauma. *J Pediatr Surg*. 2018;53(2):352-356.

41. Inaba K, Karamanos E, Skiada D, et al. Cadaveric comparison of the optimal site for needle decompression of tension pneumothorax by prehospital care providers. *J Trauma*. 2015;79(6):1044-1048.

42. Leatherman ML, Held JM, Fluke LM, et al. Relative device stability of anterior versus axillary needle decompression for tension pneumothorax during casualty movement: preliminary analysis of a human cadaver model. *J Trauma*. 2017;83(1):S136-S141.

43. McCarthy A, Curtis K, Holland AJ. Paediatric trauma systems and their impact on the health outcomes of severely injured children: an integrative review. *Injury*. 2016;47(3):574-585.

44. Lerner EB, Drendel AL, Cushman JT, et al. Ability of the physiologic criteria of the field triage guidelines to identify children who need the resources of a trauma center. *Prehosp Emerg Care*. 2017;21(2):180-184.

45. Larson JT, Dietrich AM, Abdessalam SF, Werman HA. Effective use of the air ambulance for pediatric trauma. *J Trauma Injury Infect Crit Care*. 2004;56(1):89-93.

46. Eckstein M, Jantos T, Kelly N, Cardillo A. Helicopter transport of pediatric trauma patients in an urban emergency medical services system: a critical analysis. *J Trauma Injury Infect Crit Care*. 2002;53(2):340-344.

47. Englum BR, Rialon KL, Kim J, et al. Current use and outcomes of helicopter transport in pediatric trauma: a review of 18,291 transports. *J Pediatr Surg*. 2017;52(1):140-144.

48. Polites SF, Zielinski MD, Fahy AS, et al. Mortality following helicopter versus ground transport of injured children. *Injury*. 2017;48(5):1000-1005.

49. Brown JB, Leeper CM, Sperry JL, et al. Helicopters and injured kids: improved survival with scene air medical transport in the pediatric trauma population. *J Trauma Acute Care Surg*. 2016;80(5):702-710.

50. National Center for Injury Prevention and Control, Centers for Disease Control and Prevention. Injuries among Children and Teens. https://www.cdc.gov/traumaticbraininjury/data/index.html#:~:text=Children%20(birth%20to%2017%20years,related%20deaths1%20in%202019

51. Goh MS, Looi D, Goh J, et al. The impact of traumatic brain injury on neurocognitive outcomes in children: a systematic review and meta-analysis. *J Neurol Neurosurg Psychiatry*. 2021. doi: 10.1136/jnnp-2020-325066

52. Halstead ME, Walter KD, Council on Sports Medicine and Fitness. Clinical report—sport-related concussion in children and adolescents. *Pediatrics*. 2010;126:597-615.

53. McCrory P, Meeuwisse W, Aubry M, et al. Consensus statement on concussion in sport: the 4th International Conference on Concussion in Sport held in Zurich, November 2012. *J Sci Med Sport*. 2013;16(3):178-189.

54. Centers for Disease Control and Prevention (CDC). Sports-related recurrent brain injuries—United States. *Morb Mortal Wkly Rep*. 1997;46(10):224-227.

55. Halstead ME, Walter KD, Moffatt K; Council on Sports Medicine and Fitness. Sport-related concussion in children and adolescents. *Pediatrics*. 2018;142(6):e20183074. doi: 10.1542/peds.2018-3074

56. Carmona Suazo JA, Maas AI, van den Brink WA, et al. CO_2 reactivity and brain oxygen pressure monitoring in severe head injury. *Crit Care Med*. 2000;28(9):3268-3274.

57. Adelson PD, Bratton SL, Carney NA, et al. Guidelines for the acute medical management of severe traumatic brain injury in infants, children, and adolescents. Chapter 4. Resuscitation of blood pressure and oxygenation and prehospital brain-specific therapies for the severe pediatric traumatic brain injury patient. *Pediatr Crit Care Med*. 2003;4(suppl 3):S12-S18.

58. De Lorenzo RA. A review of spinal immobilization techniques. *J Emerg Med*. 1996;14(5):603-613.

59. Valadie LL. Child safety seats and the emergency responder. *Emerg Med Serv*. 2004;33(7):68-69.

60. U.S. Department of Transportation, National Highway Traffic Safety Administration. Working group best-practice recommendations for the safe transportation of children in emergency ground ambulances. DOT HS 811 677. September 2012. Accessed March 22, 2022. https://www.nhtsa.gov/staticfiles/nti/pdf/811677.pdf

61. Williams FN, Herndon DN, Hawkins HK, et al. The leading causes of death after burn injury in a single pediatric burn center. *Crit Care*. 2009;13(6):183.

62. Hollén L, Coy K, Day A, Young A. Resuscitation using less fluid has no negative impact on hydration status in children with moderate sized scalds: a prospective single-centre UK study. *Burns*. 2017;43(7):1499-1505.

63. Müller Dittrich MH, Brunow de Carvalho W, Lopes Lavado E. Evaluation of the "early" use of albumin in children with extensive burns: a randomized controlled trial. *Pediatr Crit Care Med*. 2016;17(6):e280-e286.

64. Loos MHJ, Almekinders CAM, Heymans MW, de Vries A, Bakx R. Incidence and characteristics of non-accidental burns in children: a systematic review. *Burns*. 2020;46(6):1243-1253. doi: 10.1016/j.burns.2020.01.008

65. Peck MD, Priolo-Kapel D. Child abuse by burning: a review of the literature and an algorithm for medical investigations. *J Trauma*. 2002;53(5):1013-1022.

66. Hettiaratchy S, Dziewulski P. ABC of burns: pathophysiology and types of burns. *BMJ*. 2004;328(7453):1427-1429.

67. Hight DW, Bakalar HR, Lloyd JR. Inflicted burns in children: recognition and treatment. *JAMA*. 1979;242:517.

68. American Academy of Pediatrics Committee on Injury and Poison Prevention. Selecting and using the most appropriate car safety seats for growing children: guidelines for counseling parents. *Pediatrics*. 2002;109(3):550.

69. Nance ML, Lutz N, Arbogast KB, et al. Optimal restraint reduces the risk of abdominal injury in children involved in motor vehicle crashes. *Ann Surg*. 2004;239(1):127-131.

70. Bauer M, Hines L, Pawlowski E, et al. Using Crash Outcome Data Evaluation System (CODES) to examine injury in front vs. rear-seated infants and children involved in a motor vehicle crash in New York State. *Inj Epidemiol*. 2021;8(1):32. doi: 10.1186/s40621-021-00328-8

71. Pierce MC, Kaczor K, Aldridge S, et al. Bruising characteristics discriminating physical child abuse from accidental trauma. *Pediatrics*. 2010;125:67-74.

Suggested Reading

EMSC Partnership for Children, National Association of EMS Physicians. Model pediatric protocols: 2003 revision [no authors listed]. *Prehosp Emerg Care*. 2004;8(4):343.

CHAPTER 15

Geriatric Trauma

Lead Editors
Danielle Hashmi, DO
Angel Ramon Lopez, MD
Robert D. Barraco, MD, MPH, FACS, FCCP

© Ralf Hiemisch/Getty Images

CHAPTER OBJECTIVES

At the completion of this chapter, you will be able to do the following:

- Discuss the epidemiology of trauma in the older adult population.
- Describe the anatomic and physiologic effects of aging as factors in causes of geriatric trauma and as factors in the pathophysiology of trauma.
- Explain the interaction of preexisting medical problems with traumatic injuries in geriatric patients and how these interactions produce differences in the pathophysiology and manifestations of trauma.
- Discuss the physiologic effects of specific common classes of medications on the pathophysiology and manifestations of geriatric trauma.

- Compare and contrast the assessment techniques and considerations used in the older adult population with those used in younger populations.
- Demonstrate modifications in spinal immobilization techniques for safe and effective spinal immobilization of the older adult patient with the highest degree of comfort possible.
- Compare and contrast the management of the older adult trauma patient with that of the younger trauma patient.
- Assess the scene and older patient for signs and symptoms of abuse and neglect.

SCENARIO

Your unit is dispatched to the home of a 78-year-old woman who has fallen down a flight of stairs. Her daughter states that they had spoken on the telephone just 15 minutes earlier and that she was coming to her mother's house to take her to do some shopping. When she got to the house, she found her mother on the floor and called for an ambulance.

Upon initial contact, you find the patient lying at the bottom of a flight of stairs. You note that the patient is an older woman whose appearance matches her reported age. While maintaining in-line stabilization of the spine, you note that the patient is unresponsive to your commands. She has a visible laceration of the forehead and an obvious deformity of the left wrist. There is no obvious major external hemorrhage. She is wearing a Medic Alert bracelet that indicates that she has diabetes.

- Did the fall cause the change in mental status, or was there an antecedent event?
- How do the patient's age, medical history, and medications interact with the injuries received to make the pathophysiology and manifestations different from those in younger patients?
- Should advanced age alone be used as an additional criterion for transport to a trauma center?

INTRODUCTION

The older adult population represents the fastest growing age group in the United States. As of 2019, over 54 million Americans (16% of the U.S. population) are 65 years or older, and this number is expected to reach 94.7 million by 2060, with the population of those older than 80 years expected to triple in that same time frame.[1,2] Similarly, the worldwide number of people older than 60 years was just over 900 million in 2015 (12% of the world population) and will increase to just over 2 billion by 2050 (22% of the world population).[3]

Injuries in older adults present unique challenges in prehospital (and hospital) care management. Some of the earliest data that examine the effect of age on outcome are from a retrospective study published in 1990, the Major Trauma Outcome Study by the American College of Surgeons Committee on Trauma.[4] Outcome data from patients age 65 years and older were compared to those of younger patients. Mortality increased in ages 45 to 55 years and doubled by age 75 years. This age-adjusted risk of death occurred across the spectrum of injury severity. Studies have continued to demonstrate an increased mortality rate for geriatric trauma patients, as compared with younger patients.[5] Despite the increased mortality and morbidity, older adults are historically less likely to receive medical care at a trauma center than younger patients with similar injuries.[6]

With an ever-growing population of older adults, an increasing number of geriatric patients suffer traumatic injuries. Trauma is the third leading cause of death in persons ages 55 to 64 years and is the seventh leading cause of death in those age 65 years and older.[7] Trauma-related deaths in this age group account for 35% of all trauma deaths nationwide.[8] By 2050, an estimated 40% of all trauma patients will be older adults.[9] Specific mechanisms and patterns of injury are also unique to the older adult population.[10] Although motor vehicle crashes are the overall leading cause of trauma deaths, falls are the predominant mechanism of death in patients older than 75 years.

This chapter aims to highlight the unique needs and increased level of risk among older adult trauma patients. Specifically, the aging process and the effects of coexisting medical problems on an older patient's response to trauma and trauma management must be understood. The special considerations outlined in this chapter should be included in the assessment and management of any trauma patient who is 65 years or older, physically appears older, or is middle-aged with any medical problems typically associated with the older adult population. Early recognition of traumatic injuries and rapid treatment are paramount for the care of the older trauma patient.

Anatomy and Physiology of Aging

The aging process causes changes in physical structure, body composition, and organ function, which can create unique problems during prehospital care. The aging process influences mortality and morbidity rates.

Aging, or **senescence**, is a natural biologic process that begins during the years of early adulthood. By this time, organ systems have achieved maturation, and a turning point in physiologic growth has been reached. The body gradually loses its ability to maintain **homeostasis** (the state of relative constancy of the body's internal environment), and viability declines over a period of years until death occurs.

The process of aging occurs at the cellular level and is reflected in both anatomic structure and physiologic function. The period of "old age" is generally characterized by frailty, slower cognitive processes, impairment of psychological functions, diminished energy, the appearance of chronic and degenerative diseases, and a decline in sensory acuity. Functional abilities are reduced, and the well-known external signs and symptoms of older age appear, such as skin wrinkling, changes in hair color and quantity, osteoarthritis, and slowness in reaction time and reflexes (**Figure 15-1**). It is important to note, however, that quality of life does not necessarily decrease with the aging process.

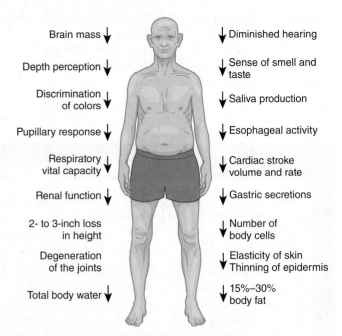

Figure 15-1 Changes caused by aging.
© National Association of Emergency Medical Technicians (NAEMT)

Influence of Chronic Medical Problems

Although some individuals can reach an advanced age without any serious medical problems, older people are significantly more likely to have health conditions that limit their ability to work and to live normal lives (**Table 15-1**). Historically, older adults consume healthcare resources, including the emergency department (ED), at a higher rate than other age groups in the United States.[11,12] Older adult patients also use emergency medical services (EMS) at a higher frequency than younger patients, as older age has been found to be an independent risk factor for EMS transport to the ED.[13]

As a person ages, additional medical problems can occur, often with cumulative negative consequences. The total influence on the body usually is greater than the sum of each individual effect. As each condition progresses and reduces the quality of the body's vital functions, the ability to withstand even modest anatomic or physiologic insults is greatly diminished (**Box 15-1**).

Table 15-1 Percentage of Patients With Chronic Conditions

Number of Chronic Conditions	Age 55 to 64 years	Age 65 years and over
1+ chronic conditions	69.5%	85.6%
2+ chronic conditions	37.1%	56.0%
3+ chronic conditions	14.4%	23.1%

Note: Chronic conditions include arthritis, current asthma, cancer, cardiovascular disease, chronic obstructive pulmonary disease, and diabetes.

Data from Centers for Disease Control and Prevention. Percent of U.S. adults 55 and over with chronic conditions. Accessed May 23, 2022. https://www.cdc.gov/nchs/health_policy/adult_chronic_conditions.htm

Box 15-1 Preventive Care

Preventive care is key to maintaining optimum health, especially in older adults. Unfortunately, some older adults may not receive preventive care because of a lack of financial resources.

Regardless of whether the patient is pediatric, middle-aged, or geriatric, the priorities, intervention needs, and life-threatening conditions that usually result from serious trauma are the same. However, because of these preexisting physical conditions, older adult patients often die from less severe injuries and die sooner than younger patients. Data show that preexisting conditions impact the mortality of an older trauma patient, and the more conditions a trauma patient has, the higher the mortality rate (**Table 15-2**). Several conditions increase mortality because they interfere with the physiologic ability to respond to trauma (**Table 15-3**).

Ears, Nose, and Throat

Tooth decay, gum disease, and dental trauma result in the need for various prostheses. The brittle nature of capped teeth, dentures, and fixed or removable bridges poses a special problem; these foreign bodies can be easily broken and aspirated and can subsequently obstruct the airway.

Older adults are more likely to experience dry mouth. There is a small decrease in number of acinar cells of the salivary glands, which can cause a reduction of up to 50% in maximal saliva production.[14] This can have various effects on chewing and swallowing and will not accurately demonstrate evidence or absence of hypovolemia. In addition, certain medications have been demonstrated to be associated with dry mouth.

Changes in the contours of the face result from resorption of the mandible, in part because of the absence of teeth (**edentulism**). This resorption causes a characteristic look of an infolding and shrinking mouth and can adversely affect the ability to create a seal with a bag-mask device or to sufficiently visualize the airway during endotracheal intubation.

The nasopharyngeal tissues become increasingly fragile with age. In addition to the risk this change poses

Table 15-2 Number of Preexisting Diseases (PEDs) and Patient Outcome After Trauma

Number of PEDs	Survived	Died	Mortality Rate (%)
0	6,341	211	3.2
1	868	56	6.1
2	197	36	15.5
3 or more	67	22	24.7

Data from Milzman DP, Boulanger BR, Rodriguez A, Soderstrom CA, Mitchell KA, Magnant CM. Pre-existing disease in trauma patients: a predictor of fate independent of age and injury severity score. *J Trauma.* 1992;32:236–244.

Table 15-3 Prevalence of Preexisting Diseases (PEDs) and Associated Mortality Rates After Trauma

PED	Number of Patients	PED Present (%)	Total (%)	Mortality Rate (%)
Hypertension	597	47.9	7.7	10.2
Pulmonary disease	286	23	3.7	8.4
Cardiac disease	223	17.9	2.9	18.4
Diabetes	198	15.9	2.5	12.1
Obesity	167	13.4	2.1	4.8
Malignancy	80	6.4	1	20
Neurologic disorder	45	3.6	0.6	13.3
Renal disease	40	3.2	0.5	37.5
Hepatic disease	41	3.3	0.5	12.2

Data from Milzman DP, Boulanger BR, Rodriguez A, Soderstrom CA, Mitchell KA, Magnant CM. Pre-existing disease in trauma patients: a predictor of fate independent of age and injury severity score. *J Trauma*. 1992;32:236–244.

during the initial trauma, interventions such as nasopharyngeal airway insertion may induce profuse bleeding if not performed with care.

Respiratory System

Ventilatory function declines in the older person partly from decreased chest wall elasticity and partly from stiffening of the airway. Chest wall and lung compliance declines with age and may result in increased work of breathing. This is associated with higher risk of respiratory failure with chest trauma.[15] Blunted cardiac response to hypoxia can also make identifying respiratory failure more difficult.[15] With declines in the efficiency of the respiratory system, the older person uses more effort to breathe, and carrying out daily activities requires greater exertion.

The alveolar surface area in the lungs decreases with age. A 70-year-old person, for example, would have a 16% reduction in alveolar surface area. Any alteration of the already-reduced alveolar surface further decreases oxygen uptake. Additionally, as the body ages, its ability to saturate hemoglobin with oxygen decreases, leading to lower baseline oxygen saturation and less available oxygen reserve.[16] Because of impaired mechanical ventilation and diminished surface for gas exchange, the older trauma patient is less capable of compensating for physiologic losses associated with trauma.

Changes in the airway and lungs of older adults may not always be related to senescence alone. Cumulative chronic exposure to environmental toxins over the course of their lives may be caused by occupational hazards or tobacco smoke. This can lead to chronic obstructive pulmonary disease (COPD). Impaired cough and gag

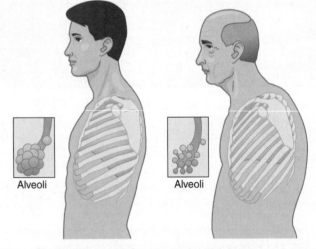

Figure 15-2 Spinal curvature can lead to an anteroposterior hump, which can cause ventilatory difficulties. Reduction in the alveolar surface area can also reduce the amount of oxygen that is exchanged in the lungs.
© National Association of Emergency Medical Technicians (NAEMT)

reflexes, along with poor cough strength and diminished esophageal sphincter tone, result in an increased risk of **aspiration pneumonitis**. A reduction in the number of **cilia** (hairlike projections of the cells in the respiratory tract that propel foreign particles and mucus from the bronchi) predisposes the older person to problems caused by inhaled particulate matter.

Another factor that affects the respiratory system is a physical change in the spinal curvature. Curvature changes, primarily increasing **kyphosis**, accompanied by an anteroposterior hump, often lead to impaired biomechanics and additional ventilatory compromise (**Figure 15-2**).

Changes that affect the diaphragm can also contribute to ventilatory problems. Stiffening of the rib cage can cause more reliance on the activity of the diaphragm to achieve negative inspiration pressure. This increased reliance on the diaphragm makes an older person especially sensitive to changes in intra-abdominal pressure. Thus, a supine position or a full stomach from a large meal can provoke ventilatory insufficiency.

Injuries to the chest wall may compound these underlying respiratory changes in older patients. In fact, older trauma patients with rib fractures have a significantly increased mortality and risk of complications such as pneumonia, compared with younger patients.[17] The combination of underlying lung disease and physiologic changes of aging may predispose older patients to respiratory compromise after trauma.

Cardiovascular System

In 2019, heart disease was the leading cause of death in people age 65 years and older in the United States.[7] In fact, heart disease accounted for so many deaths in this age group that it was the leading cause of death for all age groups combined, despite not being the leading cause of death in any other age group.[7]

Age-related decreases in arterial elasticity lead to increased peripheral vascular resistance. The myocardium and blood vessels rely on their elastic, contractile, and *distensible* (stretchable) properties to function properly. The compliance of the walls of the heart decreases, resulting in a decrease in cardiac index of about 1% per year. Simultaneously, vascular resistance increases by 1% per year.[18] With advancing age, the cardiovascular system becomes less efficient at moving fluids around the body.

Atherosclerosis is a narrowing of the blood vessels, a condition in which the inner layer of the arterial wall thickens as fatty deposits build up within the artery. These deposits, called plaques, decrease the inner diameter of the vessel, increasing resistance and making it more difficult to move blood forward. This same luminal narrowing occurs in the coronary vessels. Almost 50% of the U.S. population has coronary artery stenosis by age 65 years.[5]

One result of this narrowing is **hypertension**, a condition that commonly affects adults in the United States. Calcification of the arterial wall reduces compliance and the ability to respond to endocrine and central nervous system stimuli. The decrease in circulation can adversely affect any of the vital organs and is a common cause of heart disease. This is significant because the baseline blood pressure of the older trauma patient may be higher than in younger patients. A common pitfall in the assessment and management of geriatric trauma patients is failure to recognize a "normal"-appearing blood pressure as a sign of shock.

With age, the heart itself shows an increase in fibrous tissue and size (**myocardial hypertrophy**). Atrophy of the cells of the conduction system results in the increased incidence of cardiac dysrhythmias. The normal reflexes in the heart that respond to hypotension diminish with age, reducing the ability of older patients to increase their heart rate and stroke volume to compensate for a low blood pressure. Patients with pacemakers and patients on beta blocker medications have a decreased ability to adjust heart rate and cardiac output to meet the increased demands for oxygen consumption accompanying the stress of trauma.

In an older trauma patient, this reduced circulation contributes to cellular hypoxia. Cellular hypoxia may result in cardiac dysrhythmia, acute heart failure, and even sudden death. The body's ability to compensate for blood loss or other causes of shock is significantly lowered in older people because of a diminished *inotropic* (cardiac contraction) response to **catecholamines**. In addition, total circulating blood volume decreases, creating less physiologic reserve for blood loss from trauma. Diastolic dysfunction makes the patient more dependent on atrial filling to augment cardiac output, which is diminished in hypovolemic states.

The reduced circulation and circulatory-defense responses, coupled with increasing cardiac failure, produce a significant problem in managing shock in older trauma patients. Fluid resuscitation needs to be carefully monitored because of the reduced compliance of the cardiovascular system. Care must be taken when treating hypotension and shock to avoid causing volume overload with aggressive fluid resuscitation.[19]

Nervous System

As individuals age, brain weight and the number of neurons (nerve cells) decrease. The weight of the brain reaches its peak (3 pounds [1.4 kilograms]) at approximately 20 years of age. By 80 years of age, the brain has lost about 10% of its weight, with progressive cerebral atrophy.[20] Additionally, the dural bridging veins become more stretched and thus susceptible to tearing. This results in a lower frequency of epidural hemorrhage and a higher frequency of subdural hemorrhage. The body compensates for the loss of size with increased cerebrospinal fluid. Although this additional space around the brain can protect it from contusion, it also allows for more brain movement in response to acceleration/deceleration injuries. The increased space in the cranial vault also allows significant volumes of blood to accumulate around the brain in older patients with minimal or no symptoms.

The speed with which nerve impulses are conducted along certain nerves also decreases. These decreases result in only small effects on behavior and thinking. Reflexes are slower, but not to a significant degree. Compensatory functions can be impaired, particularly in patients with diseases such as Parkinson disease, resulting in an increased incidence of falls. The peripheral nervous system is also affected by the slowing of nerve impulses, resulting in tremors and an unsteady gait.

General information and vocabulary abilities increase or are maintained, whereas skills requiring mental and muscular activity (psychomotor ability) may decline. The intellectual functions that involve verbal comprehension, arithmetic ability, fluency of ideas, experiential evaluation, and general knowledge tend to increase after age 60 years in those who continue learning activities. Exceptions are those who develop dementia and related disorders such as Alzheimer disease.

Dementia is a general term for a decrease in cognitive capabilities that causes an interference with daily life. Alzheimer disease is the most common form of dementia. Most commonly, memory, attention, communication skills, and judgment may be impaired; however, symptoms may vary. Dementia affects 1 in 10 people over the age of 65 in the United States. It is the fifth leading cause of death for older adults and a major cause of disability.[21] Cognitive effects from dementia are usually gradual in onset.

Delirium differs from dementia. Delirium is an abrupt and acute change in mental status characterized by inattention, cognitive dysfunction, and a fluctuating course associated with a medical cause. It is generally reversible once the underlying acute process is corrected. However, delirium has been linked with increased mortality and morbidity. A study from Yale University found a 1-year increase in mortality associated with delirium that presented during intensive care unit (ICU) admission.[22] A recent meta-analysis demonstrates persistent findings that delirium may be associated with increase odds of mortality, especially in ICU patients.[23]

Older adults also have significant mental health burdens. Depression is common in older people. While depression, dementia, and organic brain disease may be considerations, it is critical that traumatic brain injury, hypoxia, and shock take priority when assessing an older trauma patient. (See Chapter 8, *Head and Neck Trauma*.)

Sensory Changes

Vision and Hearing

Overall, men tend to be more likely to have hearing difficulties, whereas both sexes have a similar incidence of sight-related impairment (**Box 15-2**).

Box 15-2 Impact of Sensory Changes With Age

Vision and hearing changes may be so subtle and may occur over such a long period of time that the patient may not realize that changes have occurred. Preventive check-ups with primary care practitioners should include screenings to evaluate for any subtle sensory changes.

Poor vision is challenging at any age, but it may be even more problematic for older people. Poor vision may have detrimental effects on reading prescription labels and safe driving abilities. In addition, older people have progressive decreases in visual acuity, ability to differentiate colors, and night vision. The cells of the lens of the eye are incapable of restoration to their original molecular structure. Eventually, the lens loses its capability to increase in thickness and curvature. The result is almost universal farsightedness (*presbyopia*) in those older than 40 years that requires glasses for reading.

Because of changes to the various structures of the eye, older people have more difficulty seeing in dimly lit environments. With age, the lens of the eye begins to become cloudy and impenetrable to light. This gradual process results in a **cataract**, or a milky lens that blocks and distorts light that enters the eye and blurs vision. Over half of people over age 80 are affected by cataracts.[24] This deterioration of vision increases the risk of a motor vehicle crash, particularly when driving at night.

A gradual decline in hearing (*presbycusis*) is also characteristic of aging. **Presbycusis** is usually caused by loss of conduction of sound into the inner ear; the use of hearing aids can compensate for this loss to some degree. This hearing loss is most pronounced when attempting to discriminate complex sounds, such as when many people are speaking at once, or with loud, ambient noise present, such as the wailing of sirens.

Pain Perception

Because of the aging process and the presence of diseases such as diabetes, older adults may not perceive pain normally, placing them at increased risk of injury from excesses in heat and cold exposure. Many older adults have conditions such as arthritis that result in chronic pain. Living with daily pain can cause an increased tolerance to pain, which may result in a patient's failure to identify areas of injury. When evaluating patients, especially those who usually have pain at baseline, prehospital care practitioners should locate areas in which the pain has increased or in which the painful area has enlarged. It is also important to note the pain characteristics or exacerbating factors since the trauma occurred.

Renal System

Changes common with aging include reduced levels of filtration by the kidneys and a reduced excretory capacity. Renal mass is lost rapidly after age 50 years, followed by a fall in glomerular filtration rate (GFR) after age 60 years due to loss of nephrons.[18] These changes should be considered when administering medications normally cleared by the kidneys. Creatinine clearance becomes a more reliable predictor of renal function rather than serum creatinine, as this value declines with declining muscle mass.[18] In addition, atherosclerotic vascular changes related to age can result in decreased percentage of renal blood flow, further affecting GFR.[18] Chronic renal insufficiency typically affects older people and contributes to a reduction in a patient's overall health status and ability to withstand trauma. For example, renal dysfunction may be one cause of chronic anemia, which would lower a patient's **physiologic reserve**.

Musculoskeletal System

Bone loses minerals as it ages. The loss of bone (**osteoporosis**) is unequal between the sexes. During young adulthood, bone mass is greater in women than in men. However, bone loss is more rapid in women and accelerates after menopause. With this higher incidence of osteoporosis, older women have a greater probability of fractures, particularly of the neck of the femur (hip). Causes of osteoporosis include decreased estrogen levels, increased periods of inactivity, and inadequate intake and inefficient use of calcium.

Osteoporosis contributes significantly to hip fractures and spontaneous compression fractures of the vertebral bodies. The incidence approaches 1% per year for men and 2% for women over age 85 years.[25]

Older persons are sometimes shorter than they were in young adulthood due to a decrease in height of the vertebral discs. As the discs flatten, a loss of approximately 2 inches (5 centimeters) in height occurs between ages 20 and 70 years. Kyphosis (curvature of the spine) in the thoracic region can also contribute to height loss and is often caused by osteoporosis (**Figure 15-3**). As the bones become more porous and fragile, erosion occurs anteriorly, and compression fractures of the vertebrae may develop. As the thoracic spine becomes more curved, the head and shoulders appear to be pushed forward. If COPD, particularly emphysema, is present, the kyphosis may be more pronounced because of the increased development of the accessory muscles of breathing.

Arthritis is also common in older adults. **Osteoarthritis (OA)** is a degenerative condition that affects the joints, which leads to damage of the cartilage that normally provides smooth surfaces for joint movement. **Rheumatoid arthritis (RA)** is an inflammatory disorder caused by an autoimmune response, which can lead to joint swelling and deformity. These chronic conditions can cause decreased mobility and chronic pain. These limitations need to be considered during assessment and transport of older patients.

Absolute levels of growth hormones decrease with aging, in conjunction with a decline in responsiveness to anabolic hormones. The combined effect is a reduction in muscle mass of older adults. Muscle loss is measured microscopically by both absolute number of muscle cells and reduction in cell size.

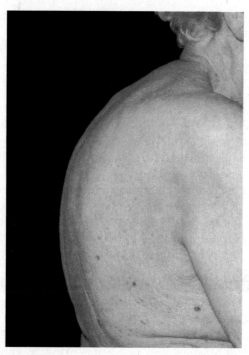

Figure 15-3 Kyphosis, typically caused by osteoporosis.
© Dr. P. Marazzi/Science Source

Deficits that relate to the musculoskeletal system (e.g., inability to flex the hip or knee adequately with changes in terrain) predispose older adults to falls. Muscle fatigue can cause many problems that affect movement, especially falls. Changes in the body's normal posture are common, and changes in the spine make the curvature become more acute with aging. Some degree of osteoporosis is universal with aging. Because of this progressive bone resorption, the bones become less pliant, more brittle, and more easily broken. The decrease in bone strength, coupled with reduced muscle strength caused by less active exercise, can result in multiple fractures with only mild or moderate force. The most common sites of fractures in older persons include the proximal femur (hip), humerus, and wrist. The increased incidence of falls as a mechanism of injury frequently results in Colles fractures of the distal radius, as the dorsiflexed hand is outstretched to anticipate the fall.

The entire vertebral column changes with age, primarily because of the effects of osteoporosis, **osteophytosis** (bone spurs), and calcification of the supporting ligaments. This calcification results in decreased range of motion and narrowing of the spinal canal. The narrowed canal and progressive osteophytic disease put these patients at high risk for spinal cord or nerve root injury with even minor trauma. The narrowing of the spinal canal is called **spinal stenosis**, and it increases the likelihood of cord or nerve compression without any actual break in the bony spine. The combined forces of osteoporosis and posture changes lead to increased falls. Even ground-level falls can cause fractures in older patients.[26]

Skin

Significant changes in the skin and connective tissues are associated with aging, and they result in difficulties with response to trauma as well as direct wound healing. Cell numbers decrease, tissue strength is lost, and the skin has impaired functional status. As the skin ages, sweat and sebaceous glands are lost. Loss of sweat glands reduces the body's ability to regulate temperature. Loss of sebaceous glands, which produce oil, makes the skin dry and flaky. Production of melanin, the pigment that gives color to skin and hair, declines, causing an aging pallor. The skin thins and appears translucent, primarily because of changes in underlying connective tissue, and therefore is more prone to sustaining damage from relatively minor trauma. The thinning and drying of the skin also reduce its resistance to minor injury and microorganisms, resulting in an increased infection rate from open wounds. As elasticity is lost, the skin stretches and falls into wrinkles and folds, especially in areas of heavy use, such as those overlying the facial muscles of expression. Thinning of the skin also results in the potential for significant tissue loss and injury in response to relatively low-energy transfers.

Loss of fatty tissue can predispose older adults to hypothermia. The loss of dermal thickness with advanced age and an associated loss in vascularity are also responsible for impaired thermoregulatory function. However, hypothermia should also suggest the possibility of occult sepsis, hypothyroidism, or phenothiazine overdose in the older population. This loss of fatty tissue also leads to less padding over bony prominences, such as the head, shoulders, spine, buttocks, hips, and heels. Prolonged immobilization without additional padding can result in tissue necrosis and ulceration in these areas as well as increased pain and discomfort during treatment and transport. Therefore, complications from skin breakdown must be considered during the transport and immobilization of older patients.

Nutrition and the Immune System

With aging, a reduction in lean body mass and decreases in metabolic rate cause a reduction in caloric needs. However, because of inefficient utilization, protein requirements may in fact increase. These competing changes often result in preexisting malnutrition in older trauma patients. The financial status of retired individuals may also affect their choices of and access to quality nutrition.

The ability of the immune system to function decreases as it ages. Grossly, organs associated with the immune response (thymus, liver, and spleen) all decrease in size. A decrease in cell-mediated and humoral responses to infection also results. Coupled with any preexisting nutritional problems common in the older adult population, there is an increased susceptibility to infection. *Sepsis* is a common cause of late death after severe or even insignificant trauma in older patients.

Assessment

In 2019, 26% of people 65 years and older had an ED visit within the prior year.[27] Although the basic prehospital assessment is the same for all patients, there are specific considerations to keep in mind when assessing an elderly patient. This section will discuss those considerations as well as the most common injury mechanism and patterns for this patient population.

Physics of Trauma

Falls

Falls are the leading cause of traumatic death and disability in older adults. Approximately one in four people older than 65 years falls each year, leading to 3 million ED visits and approximately 30,000 deaths.[28,29] Although men and women fall with equal frequency, women are more than twice as likely to sustain a serious injury because of more pronounced osteoporosis. Falls, even those that occur from a standing position, can result in serious injury and life-threatening trauma, with up to 20% to 30% of those who fall sustaining a moderate to severe injury.[28]

The cause of falls is multifactorial. They result from changes in posture and gait. Declining visual acuity from cataracts, glaucoma, and loss of night vision contribute to the loss of visual cues used to navigate safely. Diseases of the central and peripheral nervous systems and the vascular instability of cardiovascular disease further precipitate falls. Compounding these preexisting conditions that predispose older adults to falls are the medications used, such as benzodiazepines, beta blockers, and antidepressants.[24] The latter can be particularly important after the COVID-19 pandemic, where rising rates of anxiety and depression were noted in the older population, notably due to social isolation, among other factors.[30] Finally, environmental factors are also important contributors to falls. Physical barriers in the environment, such as slippery floors, throw rugs, stairs, poorly fitting shoes, and poor lighting, create additional hazards.

Long-bone fractures account for the majority of injuries, with fractures of the hip region resulting in the greatest mortality and morbidity rates. The mortality rate from hip fractures is 20% at 1 year after the injury and rises to 33% at 2 years. Mortality is due to multiple causes but is postulated to be related to the effects of decreased mobility. Prehospital care practitioners must have a high level of suspicion for serious injury given the increased incidence of falls, rate of injury, and severity of complications from falls among older patients. Preventive programs like the Centers for Disease Control and Prevention's Stopping Elderly Accidents, Deaths & Injuries (STEADI) can be effective in decreasing the incidence of these injuries. In addition, many EMS agencies perform home visits to help achieve fall prevention.[30] It should be noted, however, that a multicenter randomized trial did not find a statistically significant difference in outcomes with the implementation of multifactorial prevention strategies targeting decreased falls in the elderly, and falls continue to have a large impact on the healthcare industry.[28]

Vehicular Trauma

From 2000 to 2018, the number of older adult drivers increased by more than 60%.[31] Vehicle fatalities in this age group have increased 31%, while pedestrian fatalities increased over 55% from 2010 to 2019.[32] Unfortunately, as age increases, so too does the risk of being injured in a vehicle crash. When comparing fatalities per mile driven, an increase in fatality rates is seen in drivers starting at ages 70 to 74 years, with the highest rates being among drivers 85 years and older (**Box 15-3**).[32]

These high fatality rates have been attributed to certain physiologic changes. In particular, subtle changes in memory and judgment, together with impaired visual and auditory acuity can result in delayed reaction time. Alcohol use is reported less frequently than in other patient populations, however not all patients are tested for alcohol use and these statistics are therefore inferred.[31]

Older pedestrians represent 10% of all pedestrian injuries and 20% of all pedestrian fatalities.[31] Because of slower walking speeds, the time allowed by traffic signals may be too short for an older person to traverse the crosswalk safely.

Box 15-3 Older Drivers

The American Medical Association (AMA), with support from the National Highway Traffic Safety Administration (NHTSA), has produced a program called Physician's Guide to Assessing and Counseling Older Drivers.[33] This program is available online at the NHTSA website: https://one.nhtsa.gov /people/injury/olddrive/olderdriversbook/pages /contents.html.

Elder Abuse

Global data indicate that 15% of people age 60 years and older have experienced abuse.[34] This includes neglect; physical, sexual, and emotional abuse; and financial exploitation. Despite the vulnerability of the older population, cases are under-reported.[35] See the "Elder Maltreatment" section for more details.

Burns

Patients age 60 years and older have higher mortality rates for every category of burn severity. Older patients are also more likely to face complications related to burn injuries and subsequent hospitalizations. The top complications include pneumonia, urinary tract infection, and respiratory failure. Unlike in younger patient populations, those age 60 years and older have a greater mortality rate with significantly smaller burn size. In patients ages 60 to 69 years, mortality exceeds 50% at 40% total body surface area (TBSA); for those ages 70 to 79 years, mortality exceeds 50% at 30% TBSA; and for patients 80 years and older, mortality exceeds 50% at 20% TBSA. The mechanisms of injury are most commonly flame injury, scald, or contact with hot objects.[36]

Traumatic Brain Injury

The incidence of traumatic brain injury (TBI) among older patients is high, leading to an estimated 12,000 deaths in the United States each year.[37] There is an increased mortality rate from TBI for older patients compared to younger patients and also an increased need for long-term care facilities and rehabilitation care following injury.

Because of brain atrophy, a fairly large subdural hemorrhage can exist with minimal clinical findings. The combination of head trauma and hypovolemic shock yields a greater fatality rate. Preexisting medical conditions or their treatment may be a cause of altered mentation in older patients. When in doubt regarding whether confusion represents an acute or a chronic process, it is safest to assume that injured patients have sustained a TBI, and they should be preferentially transported to a trauma center for evaluation when possible. The use of anticoagulants is another important factor to consider, as seemingly minor injuries can result in significant TBI with their use. Addressing whether or not a patient is on an anticoagulant or blood thinner is an integral component of the initial assessment.

Primary Survey

Exsanguinating Hemorrhage

Look for correctable causes of life-threatening hemorrhage in trauma patients. External sites of severe bleeding should be recognized early.

Airway

After establishing scene safety and controlling any exsanguinating hemorrhage, evaluation of an older patient proceeds with assessment of the airway. Changes in mentation may be secondary to hypoxia from partial airway occlusion or obstruction. Examine the oral cavity for foreign objects, such as dentures or teeth that have become fractured or dislodged.

Breathing

As in any other adult, older patients who breathe at a rate of less than 10 or greater than 30 breaths/minute will not have an adequate minute volume and will require appropriate airway support. In most adults, a ventilatory rate between 12 and 20 breaths/minute is normal and confirms that an adequate minute volume is present. However, in an older patient, reduced tidal volume may result in an inadequate minute volume, even at rates of 12 to 20 breaths/minute. Because of these changes, breath sounds should be immediately assessed even if the ventilatory rate is normal. Keep in mind, these sounds may be harder to hear because of smaller tidal volumes.

An older patient's vital capacity is often diminished by as much as 50%. Kyphotic changes of the spine (anteroposterior) result in a ventilation–perfusion mismatch at rest. Hypoxia is much more likely to be a consequence of shock than in younger patients. Older patients also have decreased chest excursion. Reductions in capillary oxygen and carbon dioxide exchange are significant. Hypoxemia tends to be progressive.

Circulation

Some findings can only be interpreted properly by knowing the individual patient's pre-event, or baseline, status. Expected ranges of vital signs and other findings usually accepted as normal are not "normal" in every individual, and deviation is much more common in the older patient. Although the typical ranges are broad enough to include most individual adult differences, an individual of any age may vary beyond these norms; therefore, such variation in older patients should be expected.

Medication may contribute to these changes. For example, in the average adult, a systolic blood pressure of 120 millimeters of mercury (mm Hg) is considered normal and generally unimpressive. However, in a chronically hypertensive patient who normally has a systolic blood pressure of 150 mm Hg or higher, a pressure of 120 mm Hg would be a concern, suggestive of occult bleeding (or some other mechanism causing hypotension) of such a degree that decompensation has occurred. Likewise, heart rate is a poor indicator of trauma in older patients because of the effects of medications such as beta blockers

and the heart's dampened response to circulating catecholamines (epinephrine). Quantitative information or objective signs should not be used in isolation from other findings. Failing to recognize that such a change occurred or that it is a serious pathologic finding can lead to a poor outcome for the patient.

Delayed capillary refill time is common in older patients because of less efficient circulation from peripheral arterial disease and may be a less reliable indicator of acute circulatory changes. Mildly reduced motor, sensory, and circulatory function in the extremities may represent a normal finding in older patients.

Disability

All findings should be viewed collectively to maintain an increased level of suspicion for neurologic injury in an older patient. Orientation to time and place should be assessed by careful and complete questioning in older patients. Wide differences in mentation, memory, and orientation (to the past and present) can exist in older persons. Unless someone on the scene can describe the baseline mental status of an older patient (or any patient for that matter), it should be assumed that any deficits present are indicative of an acute neurologic injury, hypoxia, hypotension, or a combination of the three. Establishing the baseline mental status for an older patient is crucial and may involve obtaining information from the patient, family members, and/or caretakers.

Expose/Environment

Older persons are more susceptible to ambient environmental changes. They have a reduced ability to respond to environmental temperature changes with impairments of both heat production and heat dissipation. Thermoregulation may be related to an imbalance of electrolytes, lower basal metabolic rate, decreased ability to shiver, arteriosclerosis, and the effects of drugs or alcohol. Hyperthermia may result from cerebrovascular accidents (strokes) or medications such as diuretics, antihistamines, and antiparkinsonian drugs. Hypothermia is often associated with decreased metabolism, reduced body fat, less efficient peripheral vasoconstriction, and poor nutrition.

Secondary Survey

The secondary survey in an older trauma patient is performed in the same manner as for younger patients and only after urgent life-threatening conditions have been addressed. However, many factors can complicate the assessment of an older patient, and prehospital care practitioners should consider how changes of aging may impact presentation when assessing older patients.

Communication Challenges

Many factors come into play when communicating with geriatric patients, from the normal biologic effects of the aging process to generational expectations of the practitioner–patient relationship. Understanding how best to communicate with older individuals will help prehospital care practitioners deliver prompt, efficient care.

- *Additional patience may be needed because of an older patient's hearing or visual impairments.* Empathy and compassion are essential. A patient's intelligence should not be underestimated merely because communication may be difficult or absent.

- *A significant other or caregiver may need to be involved.* With the patient's permission, involving the caregiver, spouse, or partner may be necessary to gather valuable information if the patient is unable to reliably provide a detailed history. Remember to still involve the patient in any discussions as appropriate. Some older patients may be reluctant to give information without the assistance of a relative or support person. Others may not want any others present, and this should be recognized and respected.

- *Be mindful of how impaired hearing, sight, comprehension, and mobility impact your history and physical examination.* Noise, distractions, and interruptions may impact your interaction with the patient. For example, the patient might be unable to hear or understand verbal instructions during an assessment and examination, making it difficult to truly assess acute deficits.

- *Be respectful and avoid language that may be interpreted as condescending.* Patients should be addressed by their last name, unless otherwise instructed by the patient. Words that may be considered condescending or dismissive should be avoided, such as "honey" or "dear." It may take the patient a few additional seconds to process questions, especially during the stress of an emergency. Ask the patient one question at a time, and wait for the patient to respond before asking another question.

Physiologic Changes

Prehospital care practitioners must be prepared for the physiologic distinctions that are often encountered in the geriatric age group.

- *Changes in physiology lead to altered pathophysiology compared to younger patients.* Typical findings of serious illness such as fever, pain, or tenderness may take longer to develop in an older patient and can confuse the presenting signs and symptoms. In addition, many medications can adversely affect the physiologic response to illness and injury. Often a prehospital care practitioner will have to depend on the patient's history alone.

- *Altered comprehension or neurologic disorders are a significant problem for many older patients.* These impairments can range from delirium to a dementia, such as Alzheimer disease. Not only may these patients have difficulty in expressing themselves, they also may have difficulty with receiving information or helping in the assessment. They may be restless and sometimes combative.

- *Older patients may not be properly nourished or hydrated.* Shake the patient's hand to feel for grip strength, skin turgor, and body temperature. Look at the patient's state of nourishment. Does the patient appear to be well, thin, or emaciated? Older patients have a decreased thirst response, a drop in the amount of body fat (15% to 30%) as well as total body water.

- *Older patients have a decrease in skeletal muscle weight, widening and weakening of bones, degeneration of joints, and osteoporosis.* They have an increased probability of fractures with comparatively minor injuries and a higher risk of fractures to the vertebrae, hips, and ribs. The ease of rising or sitting should be observed, as it provides clues about muscle strength.

- *Older patients have degeneration of heart muscle cells and fewer pacemaker cells.* Older persons are prone to dysrhythmia as a result of a loss of elasticity of the heart and major arteries. Widespread use of beta blockers, calcium channel blockers, and diuretics further complicates this problem. Often after injury, older patients present with low cardiac output with hypoxia despite the absence of lung injury. Heart rate, stroke volume, and cardiac reserve all decrease, resulting in increased morbidity and mortality after trauma. Consider baseline vital signs when assessing for signs of early decompensation. A blood pressure that would be "normal" for a healthy person may represent significant hypotension for an older patient with comorbid conditions.

Environmental Factors

The environment in which the patient is found can tell you a lot about the patient's well-being. Chronic underlying illness may be exacerbated by environmental factors and poor living conditions. Weather-related illness should also be considered in an older patient. Heat- and cold-related death rates increase with age, particularly for those older than 75 years.[38]

- *Look for behavioral problems or manifestations that do not fit the scene.* Look at the patient's physical appearance and grooming. Are the attire and grooming appropriate for where and how the patient was found? Does the patient appear capable of accomplishing normal activities of daily living? Is the living space clean and well kept? Is there a potential for elder abuse or neglect? Is the appropriate temperature control and clothing in the living environment consistent with the regional climate?

Detailed History

Medications

Knowledge of a patient's medications can provide key information in determining prehospital care. Preexisting disease in an older trauma patient is a significant finding. The following classes of drugs are of particular interest because of their frequent use by older persons and their potential to impact the physical examination and management of an older trauma patient:

- Beta blockers (e.g., propranolol, metoprolol) may account for a patient's absolute or relative bradycardia. In this situation, an increasing tachycardia as a sign of developing shock may not occur. The drug's inhibition of the body's normal sympathetic compensatory mechanisms can mask the true level of the patient's circulatory deterioration. Such patients can rapidly decompensate, seemingly without warning.
- Calcium channel blockers (e.g., diltiazem) may prevent peripheral vasoconstriction and accelerate hypovolemic shock.
- Nonsteroidal anti-inflammatory agents (e.g., ibuprofen) may contribute to platelet dysfunction and increase bleeding.
- Anticoagulants and antiplatelet agents (e.g., clopidogrel, aspirin, warfarin, dabigatran, apixaban, rivaroxaban) may increase bleeding and blood loss. Any bleeding from trauma will be more brisk and difficult to control when a patient is taking an anticoagulant. More important, internal bleeding can progress rapidly, leading to shock and death.
- Hypoglycemic agents (e.g., insulin, metformin, rosiglitazone) may be causally related to the events that led to injury, affect mentation, and make blood glucose stabilization difficult if their use is unrecognized.
- Over-the-counter medications, including herbal preparations and supplements, are frequently used. Their inclusion in the list of medications is often omitted by patients, who often do not consider over-the-counter supplements as "medicine." Thus, patients should be specifically questioned about their use. These preparations may be unregulated and have unpredictable effects and medication interactions. Complications of these agents include bleeding (garlic) and myocardial infarction (ephedrine/ma huang).

Assessing an older trauma patient's medication list can prove challenging when the patient has impaired awareness or an extensive list of medications with difficult names. In some communities, EMS agencies have promoted programs such as the File of Life Project (www.folife.org). These programs advocate for standardizing the location of detailed medical history to intuitive locations such as the refrigerator door. The patient completes a medical history form that is then placed into a magnetic holder that is applied to the refrigerator, alerting prehospital care practitioners to the File of Life (**Figure 15-4**). Additionally, many electronic medical records systems used by hospitals and physicians include the most recent medication lists in their discharge instructions, providing another location to find such information.

Older patients also have a higher rate of **polypharmacy**, a term used to describe the administration of more than five medications. In fact, nearly half of older patients fit the definition of polypharmacy.[39] This can be a significant cause of morbidity in these patients. One in six older adults experiences adverse events due to medications. In an effort to address polypharmacy and its complications, the American Geriatrics Society has established the Beers criteria for identifying potentially inappropriate medication use among older patients.[40] Prehospital care practitioners should recognize the impact of home medications, especially among older patients with traumatic injuries.

Because older patients often are taking numerous medications, the possibility of medication interactions or inadvertent overdose must be considered as a possible cause of the patient's trauma, altered mental status, or changes in vital signs.

Medical Conditions as a Precursor to Traumatic Injury

A number of medical conditions may predispose individuals to traumatic events, especially those that result in an alteration in the level of consciousness or neurologic deficit. Common examples include seizure disorders, hypoglycemia due to improper medication dosing, syncope from antihypertensive medication, cardiac dysrhythmia from an acute coronary syndrome, and cerebrovascular accidents. Because the incidence of chronic medical conditions increases with age, geriatric patients are more likely to suffer trauma as a consequence of a medical problem when compared to younger victims. The astute prehospital care practitioner should note clues from the primary and secondary surveys that may point to a medical problem that precipitated the traumatic event, such as the following:

- Bystander reports that a victim appeared unconscious prior to a crash
- A Medic Alert bracelet that indicates an underlying condition such as diabetes
- An irregular heartbeat or cardiac dysrhythmia seen during electrocardiogram monitoring

Prehospital care practitioners may be the only source of this information, all of which is highly pertinent to the receiving facility.

FILE OF LIFE

KEEP INFORMATION UP TO DATE !!
Review At Least Every Six Months !
MEDICAL DATA REVIEWED AS OF ___ MO.___ YR.

Name: _____ Sex: M F

Address: _____

Doctor: _____ Phone #: _____

Doctor: _____ Phone #: _____

EMERGENCY CONTACTS

Name: _____ Phone #: _____

Address: _____

Name: _____ Phone #: _____

Address: _____

KEEP INFORMATION UP TO DATE !!
Review At Least Every Six Months !
MEDICAL DATA REVIEWED AS OF ___ MO.___ YR.

Name: _____ Sex: M F

Address: _____

Doctor: _____ Phone #: _____

Preferred Hospital: _____

EMERGENCY CONTACTS

Name: _____ Phone #: _____

Address: _____

Name: _____ Phone #: _____

Address: _____

MEDICAL DATA
Use pencil for ease in making changes.

Special Conditions/Remarks:

_____

Medication	Dosage	Frequency

Pharmacy: _____ Phone: _____

Date of Birth: _____

Blood Type: _____ Religion: _____

Health Care Proxy on file at: _____

Living Will on file at: _____

® **FILE OF LIFE**   SEE BACK OF CARD FOR ADDITIONAL INFORMATION

Use Pencil for ease in making changes

Recent Surgery: _____ Date: _____

_____

Do you have an EMS-NO CPR Directive or a DNR form ?
YES ☐   NO ☐   Where is it located ?

MEDICAL CONDITIONS
Check all that exist

☐ No known medical conditions
☐ Abnormal EKG
☐ Adrenal Insufficiency
☐ Angina
☐ Asthma
☐ Bleeding Disorder
☐ Cancer
☐ Cardiac Dysrhythmia
☐ Cataracts
☐ Clotting Disorder
☐ Coronary Bypass Graft
☐ Dementia ☐ Alzheimer's
☐ Diabetes/Insulin Dependent
☐ Eye Surgery
☐ Glaucoma
☐ Hearing Impaired
☐ Heart Valve Prosthesis
☐ Other:

☐ Hemodialysis
☐ Hemolytic Anemia
☐ Hepatitis-Type [   ]
☐ Hypertension
☐ Hypoglycemia
☐ Laryngectomy
☐ Leukemia
☐ Lymphomas
☐ Memory Impaired
☐ Myasthenia Gravis
☐ Pacemaker
☐ Renal Failure
☐ Seizure Disorder
☐ Sickle Cell Anemia
☐ Stroke
☐ Tuberculosis
☐ Vision Impaired

ALLERGIES

☐ Aspirin   ☐ Insect Stings   ☐ Penicillin
☐ Barbiturate ☐ Latex   ☐ Sulfa
☐ Codeine   ☐ Lidocaine   ☐ Tetracycline
☐ Demerol   ☐ Morphine   ☐ X-Rays Dyes
☐ Horse Serum ☐ Novocaine   ☐ No Known Allergies
☐ Environmental:

☐ Other: _____

MEDICAL INSURANCE

Med Ins Co: _____

Policy #: _____

Other Med Ins Co: _____

Policy #: _____

Medicaid #: _____ Medicare #: _____

Figure 15-4 File of Life.

Courtesy of the File of Life Foundation.

Management

Exsanguinating Hemorrhage

Severe external bleeding may lead to rapid exsanguination. This life-threatening bleeding needs to be recognized and addressed rapidly. Direct pressure should be applied to any area of hemorrhage. If severe bleeding involves an extremity site, a tourniquet should be applied to control hemorrhage if direct pressure is unsuccessful.

Airway

The presence of dentures, common among older adults, may affect airway management. Ordinarily, dentures should be left in place to maintain a better seal around the mouth with a mask. However, partial dentures may become dislodged during an emergency and may completely or partially block the airway; these should be removed.

Fragile nasopharyngeal mucosal tissues and the possible use of anticoagulants put older trauma patients at increased risk of bleeding from placement of a nasopharyngeal airway. This hemorrhage may further compromise the patient's airway and result in aspiration.

Arthritis may affect the temporomandibular joints and cervical spine. The decreased flexibility of these areas may make airway management techniques such as endotracheal intubation more difficult.

The objective of airway management is primarily to ensure a patent airway for the delivery of adequate tissue oxygenation. Early mechanical ventilation by either bag-mask device or advanced airway interventions should be considered in older trauma patients because of their greatly limited physiologic reserve.

Breathing

In all trauma patients, supplemental oxygen should be administered as soon as possible. Oxygen saturation should generally be kept at greater than or equal to 94%. The older population has a high prevalence of COPD. Even if a patient has severe COPD, it is unlikely that high-flow oxygen administration will be detrimental to the respiratory drive during routine urban or suburban transports. However, if the prehospital care practitioner notes *somnolence* (a state of drowsiness) or a slowing respiratory rate, ventilations can be assisted with a bag-mask device with consideration for advanced airway management.

Older persons experience increased stiffness of the chest wall. In addition, reduced chest wall muscle power and decreased flexibility of the cartilage make the chest cage less flexible. These and other changes are responsible for reductions in lung volumes. An older patient may need ventilatory support by assisted ventilations with a bag-mask device earlier than younger trauma patients. The mechanical force applied to the resuscitation bag may need to be increased slightly to overcome the increased chest wall resistance. However, as indicated by lower lung volumes at baseline, large tidal volumes are often not needed when providing assisted bag-mask ventilations as this may lead to unintended consequences such as gastric distension or pneumothorax.

Capnography, a measure of end-tidal carbon dioxide ($ETCO_2$), may be another tool used to help assess respiratory status. Capnography measurements for severely injured older trauma patients should be correlated with all other clinical information available.

Circulation

Older persons may have poor cardiovascular reserve. Reduced circulating blood volume, possible chronic anemia, and preexisting myocardial and coronary disease leave the patient with little tolerance for even modest amounts of blood loss.

Because of the laxity of skin or use of anticoagulant and antiplatelet agents, geriatric patients are prone to the development of larger hematomas and potentially more significant internal hemorrhage. Early control of hemorrhage through direct pressure on open wounds, stabilization or immobilization of fractures, and rapid transport to a trauma center are essential. Fluid resuscitation should be guided by the index of suspicion for serious bleeding based on the mechanism of injury and an overall appearance of shock. At the same time, overadministration of intravenous fluids must be avoided, as older patients are less able to tolerate excessive fluid loads. Urine output is a poor measure of perfusion in older persons, especially in the prehospital setting.

Spinal Motion Restriction

Protection of the cervical, thoracic, and lumbar spine in trauma patients who have sustained multisystem blunt injury is the standard of care. For patients with normal mentation and no distracting injuries, such traditional spinal stabilization is not necessary in the absence of specific evidence of spinal injury. In the older population, these standards must apply not only in trauma situations but also during acute medical problems in which attempts to maintain airway patency are a priority. Degenerative arthritis of the cervical spine may subject the older patient to spinal cord injury from positioning and manipulating the neck to manage the airway, even without injury to the bony spine. EMS practitioners must know their local protocols, in addition to understanding the potential value of immobilizing the spine.

Prehospital practitioners should be careful to ensure that if a cervical collar applied to an older patient with

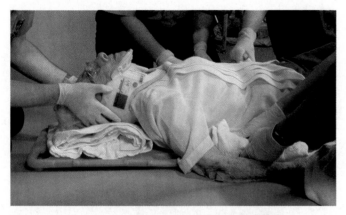

Figure 15-5 Correct technique for achieving spinal motion restriction in a kyphotic patient when using a backboard. Padding is placed behind the head to fill the space that is formed as a result of the thoracic kyphotic deformity.

© Jones & Bartlett Learning

severe kyphosis, it does not inadvertently compress the airway or carotid arteries. Less traditional means of immobilization, such as a rolled towel and head block, may be preferable if standard collars are inappropriate for a specific patient.

Padding may need to be placed under the patient's head and between the shoulders when stabilizing a kyphotic supine older patient (**Figure 15-5**). In systems that have access to one, a vacuum mattress can mold to the patient's anatomy to reduce pressure points and to provide appropriate support and greater comfort. Because of the thin skin and lack of *adipose tissue* (fat) in frail, older patients, they are more likely to develop pressure (*decubitus*) ulcers from lying on their backs. Additional padding may be necessary if the patient is immobilized on a long backboard. It is always a good idea to check for pressure points when the patient is resting on the board and pad appropriately. When applying leg straps, older patients may not be able to straighten their legs fully because of decreased range of motion of the hips and knees. This may require the placement of padding under the legs for comfort and security during transport.[41]

Temperature Control

Older patients should be monitored closely for hypothermia and hyperthermia during treatment and transport. Although it is appropriate to expose the patient to facilitate a thorough examination, older persons are especially prone to heat loss. Once the physical examination is complete, the patient should be covered with a blanket or other available covering to preserve body heat.

The effects of various medications, such as those used to treat Parkinson disease, depression, psychosis, and nausea, may make a patient more prone to overheating. Cooling measures should be considered if the patient cannot be moved quickly to a controlled environment.

(See Chapter 19, *Environmental Trauma I: Heat and Cold*, for a detailed discussion of management of hyperthermia.)

Prolonged extrication in the extremes of heat and cold may place an older patient at risk and should be rapidly addressed. External methods of heating or cooling older trauma patients should be considered and the risks balanced by the possibility of direct thermal injury to the site of application with the patient's attenuated skin structure. Therefore, a sheet or some of the patient's clothing should be placed between the heat or cooling source and the patient's skin.

Legal Considerations

Several legal considerations can become issues when providing care to older trauma patients. In most states, spouses, siblings, children, spouses of children, and parents have no automatic legal standing in making medical decisions for an adult. Persons with power of attorney or court-appointed conservators may have authority over an individual's financial affairs, but they do not necessarily have control over that individual's personal medical decisions. Court-appointed custodians or guardians may or may not have the power to make medical decisions, depending on the local laws and the specific charge of their appointments. Such powers are considered to exist only when a guardianship of person or a durable power of attorney for health care is specified and clear documentation of such third-party powers is present.

While providing care on a trauma scene, it may be difficult to make such a fine legal distinction. Because the ambulance was summoned and a "call for help" was made, the concept of *implied consent* to care for the patient applies in cases of patients who are unconscious or have reduced mental capacity. If relatives of the patient object to the actions of the prehospital care practitioners or attempt to interfere with care of the patient, law enforcement should be summoned to the scene to assist. In addition, the practitioners can contact their medical direction and have their online supervising physician speak directly with the relatives. Documentation within the patient's medical record should clearly reflect the decisions made by the practitioners on scene.

Reporting Elder Abuse

As of 2019, healthcare workers, including prehospital care practitioners, in all states are legally bound to report cases of suspected elder maltreatment to the authorities.[42] Should further clarification be necessary or anyone attempt to interfere with prehospital care, law enforcement should be called to the scene (if not already present) and the problem presented to the police officer in charge. The law generally provides a protocol for a law enforcement officer to make a timely decision at the scene, with clarification to occur later at the hospital when time allows. Such events should be documented carefully and completely as a part of the EMS medical record.

Elder Maltreatment

There is no universal definition of elder abuse. However, the National Center for Elder Abuse, as well as the Centers for Disease Control and Prevention (CDC), use the term to include an act or failure to act that results in the harm of an older person. This includes physical, emotional, and sexual abuse as well as financial exploitation and neglect.[35]

Elder abuse is not uncommon, but it remains underreported. According to the CDC, 1 in 10 people age 60 years and older experiences some form of abuse each year. Men experience higher rates of nonfatal assault and homicide than women, and unfortunately, rates of homicide in the older patient population have been increasing.[43] Underreporting has been attributed to several factors, including lack of a clear, universal definition of abuse; reluctance on the part of the abused to report due to dependence on the abuser or for other reasons; and regulations that vary by state for mandated reporters.

The U.S. Preventive Services Task Force did not find sufficient evidence to recommend screening for elder abuse.[44] However, there are signs of abuse that prehospital practitioners should be aware of, as your ability to recognize these signs and subsequently report suspected abuse may be instrumental in breaking the cycle of abuse. These include emotional signs, such as anxiety and depression, and physical signs, including the following[35]:

- Broken bones
- Bruises
- Poor living conditions
- Untreated decubitus ulcers
- Wounds
- Torn or stained clothing

Categories of Maltreatment

Abuse can be categorized in several ways as follows:

- *Physical abuse* includes assault, physical force, or physical coercion that results in bodily injury, as well as force feeding and chemical means of restraint. The signs of physical abuse may be obvious, such as the imprint left by an item (e.g., fireplace poker), or may be subtle. The signs of elder abuse are similar to those of child abuse (**Figure 15-6**). (See Chapter 14, *Pediatric Trauma*.)
- *Emotional abuse* can take the forms of verbal abuse, infantilizing, intimidation, threats, or deprivation of sensory stimulation.

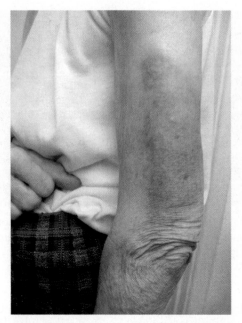

Figure 15-6 Bruises in varying stages of healing are highly suggestive of physical abuse. For example, if a 70-year-old man were brought from his caregiver's home to the ED with bruises such as the ones depicted here, prehospital care practitioners would need to consider the possibility of abuse.
© Libby Welch/Alamy Stock Photo

- *Financial* exploitation can include theft of valuables or embezzlement as well as improper use of guardianship or power of attorney.
- *Sexual assault and/or abuse* includes nonconsensual sexual contact and any sexual interaction with an elderly person who lacks the capacity to give consent.
- *Neglect* refers to not fulfilling the duties of care for an older person, such as nutrition, maintenance of the living environment, and personal care.

COVID-19 Impact on Elder Abuse

Older adults are not only more susceptible to serious illness due to COVID-19, but they are also subject to negative consequences from measures enacted to reduce the spread of the virus. Social distancing has led to several downstream effects that put the elder population at greater risk of abuse. Closing of businesses deemed "nonessential" creates access issues for health care, finances, and personal needs. This can worsen underlying conditions such as dementia in addition to putting additional strain on caregivers who may or may not be equipped or prepared to care for an elderly family member, friend, or neighbor during a pandemic. Stock market drops may lead to loss of retirement funds, leading to financial distress and putting older persons at risk of financial exploitation. These factors create an increased risk of people facing elder abuse and also put them in a situation in which the abuse may be less likely to be reported.[45]

Important Points

Many abused patients are terrorized into making false statements for fear of retribution or because they wish to protect the individual. In the case of elder abuse by family members, fear of removal from the home environment can cause an older patient to lie about the origin of the abuse. In other cases of elder abuse, sensory deprivation or dementia may impair adequate explanation. Prehospital care practitioners should identify abuse and uncover any pathology reported by the patient. Any history of maltreatment or findings consistent with abuse should be documented on the patient care report.

Further trauma to a patient may be reduced by identifying and reporting an abusive situation. A high index of suspicion for abuse can allow for referral to protective services from social services and public safety agencies (Box 15-4).

Disposition

One of the greatest challenges with prehospital care of injured patients is defining which patients are most likely to benefit from specialized trauma care and advanced

---

Box 15-4 Reporting Elder Abuse and Neglect

In most states, EMS personnel are legally mandated reporters of suspected elder (or adult) abuse, neglect, and exploitation. Mandated reporters must report directly to the social services agency responsible for investigating adult abuse rather than relying on intermediaries such as hospital personnel. If the individual is in immediate danger or has been sexually assaulted, law enforcement must be notified as well. In the event of a death that appears to be the result of abuse or neglect, mandatory reporters must notify the office of the medical examiner or coroner and law enforcement.

Mandatory reporters are liable for failing to report suspected abuse, neglect, and exploitation. They are protected against civil and criminal liability associated with reporting and may be able to keep their identities confidential. Reporting individuals are allowed to share medical information that is pertinent to the case, even though this information would otherwise be protected under the Health Insurance Portability and Accountability Act (HIPAA). Laws governing the mandatory reporting of elder abuse are enacted at the state level. All prehospital care practitioners must be aware of the laws in the state in which they work.

---

treatment options available at a trauma center. For many of the reasons mentioned previously, traditional triage criteria may be less reliable in older patients because of physiologic changes or effects of medications. The CDC's *Guidelines for Field Triage of Injured Patients* recommends that trauma patients older than 55 years be considered for transport to a trauma facility.[46]

Because of the differences between injured older and younger patients, and the differences in outcomes, much work is being done to determine if unique criteria are needed to identify older adults who need to be transported to a trauma center. Although some studies have shown that using geriatric-specific triage criteria increased the number of older adults meeting criteria for transport to a trauma center, others have failed to demonstrate any increase.[47,48]

Prolonged Transport

The majority of care for older trauma patients follows the general guidelines for prehospital care of any injured patient. However, several special circumstances exist in prolonged transport scenarios. For example, geriatric patients with less significant anatomic injuries should be triaged directly to trauma centers.

Treatment of shock in the prehospital environment over an extended period requires careful reassessment of vital signs during transport. After control of hemorrhage with local measures, fluid resuscitation should be titrated to physiologic response to optimize resuscitation of intravascular volume status while avoiding potential volume overload in patients with impaired cardiac function.

Immobilization on a long backboard places a geriatric patient at increased risk for pressure-related skin breakdown over extended transports. Weakened skin structure and impaired vascular supply may lead to earlier complications than in younger trauma patients. Prior to a long transport, consideration should be given to logrolling a patient onto an appropriately padded long backboard, vacuum mattress, or ambulance cot to protect the patient's skin. Agencies in remote regions should consider purchasing a specially designed, low-pressure backboard or vacuum mattress that immobilizes the patient while limiting the potential for skin breakdown.

Environmental control is essential for geriatric patients with a lengthy transport. Limiting body exposure and controlling the ambient temperature of the vehicle are important to limit hypothermia and prevent its complications.

Finally, transport of geriatric trauma patients from remote regions may be a valid use of aeromedical assets. Transport via helicopter may limit the duration of environmental exposure, reduce the duration of shock, and ensure earlier access to trauma center care, including early surgery and blood transfusion.

Prevention

Given the emergence of mobile integrated health care and community paramedicine programs, prehospital practitioners may have an increased role in trauma prevention efforts. Many current community paramedicine programs have a specific focus on patients with chronic medical conditions, many of whom are older patients. These programs may represent a unique opportunity to identify safety hazards, such as fall risks, for older patients and allow for education and/or interventions to help prevent injury. EMS systems and practitioners should consider these types of programs to improve the health of their communities.

SUMMARY

- The older adult population is growing rapidly.
- Although general guidelines for care of injured patients remain the same, several specific approaches are unique to care of injured geriatric patients.
- Anatomic and physiologic changes associated with aging, chronic disease, and medications can make certain types of trauma more likely, complicate traumatic injuries, and cause a decreased ability to compensate for shock. Older patients have less physiologic reserve and tolerate physical insult poorly.
- Knowledge of an older trauma patient's medical history and medications is essential to being able to provide excellent care.

- Many factors in geriatric trauma patients can mask early signs of deterioration, increasing the possibility of sudden, rapid decompensation without apparent warning.
- With an older trauma patient, more serious injury may have occurred than indicated by the initial presentation.
- Prehospital care practitioners should recognize the signs of elder abuse and report any suspicions to the proper authority.
- A lower threshold for direct triage of geriatric trauma patients to trauma centers is important.

SCENARIO RECAP

Your unit is dispatched to the home of a 78-year-old woman who has fallen down a flight of stairs. Her daughter states that they had spoken on the telephone just 15 minutes earlier and that she was coming to her mother's house to take her to do some shopping. When she got to the house, she found her mother on the floor and called for an ambulance.

Upon initial contact, you find the patient lying at the bottom of a flight of stairs. You note that the patient is an older woman whose appearance matches her reported age. While maintaining in-line stabilization of the spine, you note that the patient is unresponsive to your commands. She has a visible laceration of the forehead and an obvious deformity of the left wrist. There is no obvious major external hemorrhage. She is wearing a Medic Alert bracelet that indicates that she has diabetes.

- Did the fall cause the change in mental status, or was there an antecedent event?
- How do the patient's age, medical history, and medications interact with the injuries received to make the pathophysiology and manifestations different from those in younger patients?
- Should advanced age alone be used as an additional criterion for transport to a trauma center?

SCENARIO SOLUTION

When assessing trauma in older patients, it is not always immediately possible to determine if the trauma was the primary event or was secondary to a medical event, such as a stroke, myocardial infarction, or syncopal episode. Prehospital practitioners should look for signs of a preceding medical event that may have led to a traumatic injury.

Your primary survey reveals that this patient is maintaining a patent airway and is breathing at a rate of 16 breaths/minute. There is no major external hemorrhage, and the bleeding from the forehead laceration is easily controlled with light direct pressure. The patient's heart rate is 84 beats/minute, and blood pressure is 154/82 mm Hg. You manually control the head and spine and immobilize the patient to a vacuum mattress using appropriate padding underneath the patient. Because the patient is known to have diabetes, you check her blood glucose level to see if there is a correctable cause for her altered mentation. Given her age, the apparent traumatic brain injury, and the magnitude of the fall, you transport her emergently to the closest trauma center.

References

1. U.S. Census Bureau. State and county quick facts. Updated July 1, 2021. Accessed January 25, 2022. https://www.census.gov/quickfacts/fact/table/US#viewtop

2. Mather M, Jacobsen L, Pollard K, Population Reference Bureau. Aging in the United States. *Popul Bull.* 2015;70(2):2-17. Accessed January 25, 2022. https://www.prb.org/resources/population-bulletin-vol-70-no-2-aging-in-the-united-states/

3. United Nations, Department of Economic and Social Affairs, Population Division. *World Population Prospects: The 2015 Revision; Key Findings and Advance Tables.* United Nations; 2015.

4. Champion H, Copes WS, Sacco WJ, et al. The Major Trauma Outcome Study: establishing national norms for trauma care. *J Trauma.* 1990;30(11):1356-1365.

5. Hashmi A, Ibrahim-Zada I, Rhee P, et al. Predictors of mortality in geriatric trauma patients: a systematic review and meta-analysis. *J Trauma Acute Care Surg.* 2014;76(3):894-901.

6. Lane P, Sorondo B, Kelly JJ. Geriatric trauma patients: are they receiving trauma center care? *Ann Emerg Med.* 2003;10(3):244-250.

7. Centers for Disease Control and Prevention, National Center for Injury Prevention and Control, Web-Based Injury Statistics Query and Reporting System (WISQARS). Ten leading causes of death by age group, United States—2018. Accessed January 25, 2022. https://www.cdc.gov/injury/images/lc-charts/leading_causes_of_death_by_age_group_2018_1100w850h.jpg

8. American College of Surgeons Committee on Trauma. *Advanced Trauma Life Support, Student Course Manual.* 9th ed. American College of Surgeons; 2012:272-284.

9. Caterino J, Brown N, Hamilton M, et al. Effect of geriatric-specific trauma triage criteria on outcomes in injured older adults: a statewide retrospective cohort study. *J Am Geriatr Soc.* 2016;64(10):1944-1951.

10. Jacobs D. Special considerations in geriatric injury. *Curr Opin Crit Care.* 2003;9(6):535-539.

11. U.S. Department of Health and Human Services, Centers for Disease Control and Prevention, National Center for Health Services. Hospitalizations for patients aged 85 and over in the United States, 2000–2010. Published 2015. Accessed January 25, 2022. https://www.cdc.gov/nchs/data/databriefs/db182.pdf

12. Roberts D, McKay M, Shaffer A. Increasing rates of emergency department visits for elderly patients in the United States, 1993 to 2003. *Ann Emerg Med.* 2008;51(6):769-774.

13. Jones C, Wasserman E, Li T, et al. The effect of older age on EMS use for transportation to an emergency department. *Prehosp Disaster Med.* 2017;13:1-8.

14. Smith CH, Boland B, Daureeawoo Y, Donaldson E, Small K, Tuomainen J. Effect of aging on stimulated salivary flow in adults. *J Am Geriatr Soc.* 2013;61(5):805-808. doi: 10.1111/jgs.12219

15. American College of Surgeons Committee on Trauma. *Advanced Trauma Life Support, Student Course Manual.* 10th ed. American College of Surgeons; 2018:214-224.

16. Smith T. Respiratory system: aging, adversity, and anesthesia. In: McCleskey CH, ed. *Geriatric Anesthesiology.* Williams & Wilkins; 1997.

17. Bergeon E, Lavoie A, Clas D, et al. Elderly trauma patients with rib fractures are at greater risk of death and pneumonia. *J Trauma.* 2003;54(3):478-485.

18. Jacobs D, Plaisier BR, Barie PS, et al. Practice management guidelines for geriatric trauma: the EAST Practice Management Guidelines Work Group. *J Trauma.* 2003;54(2):391-416. doi: 10.1097/01.TA.0000042015.54022.BE

19. Deiner S, Silverstein JH, Abrams K. Management of trauma in the geriatric patient. *Curr Opin Anaesthesiol.* 2004;17(2):165-170.

20. Carey J. *Brain Facts: A Primer on the Brain and Nervous System.* Society for Neuroscience; 2002.

21. Alzheimer's Association. 2017 Alzheimer's disease facts and figures. *Alzheimer's Dement.* 2017;13:325-373.

22. Pisani M, Kong S, Kasl S, et al. Days of delirium are associated with 1 year mortality in an older intensive care unit population. *Am J Crit Care Med.* 2009;180:1092-1097.

23. Aung Thein M, Pereira J, Nitchingham A, Caplan G. A call to action for delirium research: meta-analysis and regression of delirium associated mortality. *BMC Geriatrics.* 2020;20(325):1-12.

24. U.S. Department of Health and Human Services, National Institutes of Health, National Eye Institute. Facts about cataracts. Updated August 3, 2019. Accessed January 25, 2022. https://www.nei.nih.gov/learn-about-eye-health/eye-conditions-and-diseases/cataracts

25. EPOS Group. Incidence of vertebral fracture in Europe: results from the European Prospective Osteoporosis Study (EPOS). *J Bone Miner Res*. 2002;17:716-724.

26. Blackmore C. Cervical spine injury in patients 65 years old and older: epidemiologic analysis regarding the effects of age and injury mechanism on distribution, type, and stability of injuries. *Am J Roentgenol*. 2002;178:573-577.

27. Administration for Community Living. 2020 profile of older Americans. Published May 2021. Accessed January 25, 2022. https://acl.gov/sites/default/files/Aging%20and%20Disability%20in%20America/2020ProfileOlderAmericans.Final_.pdf

28. Bhasin S, Gill TM, Reuben DB, et al. A randomized trial of a multifactorial strategy to prevent serious fall injuries. *N Engl J Med*. 2020;393(2):129-140.

29. Centers for Disease Control and Prevention. Facts about falls. Last reviewed August 6, 2021. Accessed January 25, 2022. https://www.cdc.gov/falls/facts.html

30. Centers for Disease Control and Prevention. STEADI: Stopping Elderly Accidents, Deaths & Injuries. Accessed January 25, 2022. https://www.cdc.gov/steadi/materials.html

31. Centers for Disease Control and Prevention, National Center for Injury Prevention and Control, Division of Unintentional Injury Prevention. Older adult drivers. Updated December 7, 2020. Accessed August 29, 2021. https://www.cdc.gov/transportationsafety/older_adult_drivers/index.html

32. National Highway Traffic Safety Administration. Traffic safety facts: 2019 data: pedestrians. Published May 2021. Accessed August 30, 2021. https://crashstats.nhtsa.dot.gov/Api/Public/ViewPublication/813121

33. Joseph CB. Physician's guide to assessing and counseling older drivers: second edition. *J Med Libr Assoc*. 2013;101(3):230-231. doi: 10.3163/1536-5050.101.3.017

34. Yon Y, Mikton CR, Gassoumis ZD, Wilber KH. Elder abuse prevalence in community settings: a systematic review and meta-analysis. *Lancet Glob Health*. 2017 Feb;5(2):e147-e156.

35. National Center for Elder Abuse. Welcome to the National Center on Elder Abuse. Accessed August 30, 2021. https://ncea.acl.gov/

36. American Burn Association. 2016 National Burn Repository. Accessed January 25, 2022. https://ameriburn.org/wp-content/uploads/2017/05/2016abanbr_final_42816.pdf

37. Richmond R, Aldaghlas TA, Burke C, et al. Age: is it all in the head? Factors influencing mortality in elderly patients with head injuries. *J Trauma*. 2011;71(1):E8-E11.

38. Berko J, Ingram D, Saha S, et al. Deaths attributed to heat, cold, and other weather events in the United States, 2006–2010. *Natl Health Stat Rep*. 2014;76.

39. Maher R, Hanlon J, Hajjar E. Clinical consequences of polypharmacy in elderly. *Expert Opin Drug Saf*. 2014;13(1):57-65.

40. American Geriatrics Society. 2019 updated AGS Beers criteria for potentially inappropriate medication use in older adults. *J Am Geriatr Soc*. 2019;67:674-694. doi: 10.1111/jgs.15767

41. National Association of Emergency Medical Technicians, American Geriatrics Society, Snyder, DR. *Geriatric Education for Emergency Medical Services*. 2nd ed. Jones & Bartlett Learning; 2015.

42. American Bar Association. Adult Protective Services reporting chart. Published December 2019. Accessed January 25, 2022. https://www.americanbar.org/content/dam/aba/administrative/law_aging/2020-elder-abuse-reporting-chart.pdf

43. Centers for Disease Control and Prevention. Preventing Elder Abuse. Updated June 2, 2021. Accessed September 1, 2021. https://www.cdc.gov/violenceprevention/elderabuse/fastfact.html

44. U.S. Preventive Services Task Force. Intimate Partner Violence, Elder Abuse, and Abuse of Vulnerable Adults: Screening. Published October 23, 2018. Accessed September 1, 2021. https://www.uspreventiveservicestaskforce.org/uspstf/recommendation/intimate-partner-violence-and-abuse-of-elderly-and-vulnerable-adults-screening

45. Makaroun LK, Bachrach RL, Rosland AM. Elder abuse in the time of COVID-19: increased risks for older adults and their caregivers. *Am J Geriatr Psychiatry*. 2020;28(8):876-880. doi: 10.1016/j.jagp.2020.05.017

46. Sasser SM, Hunt RC, Faul M. Guidelines for field triage of injured patients: recommendations of the National Expert Panel on Field Triage 2011. *Morb Mortal Wkly Rep*. 2012;61(1):1-20.

47. Ichwan N, Darbha S, Shah M, et al. Geriatric-specific triage criteria are more sensitive than standard adult criteria in identifying need for trauma center care in injured older adults. *Ann Emerg Med*. 2015;65(1):92-100.

48. Phillips S, Rond P, Kelly S, et al. The failure of triage criteria to identify geriatric patients with trauma: results from the Florida Trauma Triage Study. *J Trauma*. 1996;40(2):278-283.

Suggested Reading

American College of Surgeons Committee on Trauma. Geriatric trauma. In: *Advanced Trauma Life Support, Student Course Manual*. 10th ed. American College of Surgeons; 2018:214-225.

American Geriatrics Society, Snyder DR. *Geriatric Education for Emergency Medical Services*. 2nd ed. Jones & Bartlett Learning; 2015.

Reske-Nielsen C, Medzon R. Geriatric trauma. *Emer Med Clin North Am*. 2016;34(3):483-500.

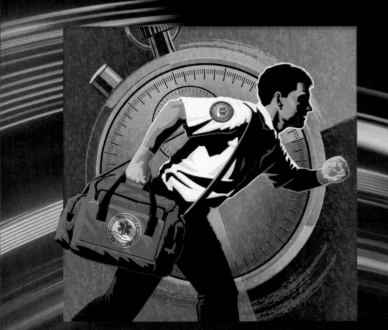

Prevention

CHAPTER 16 **Injury Prevention**

© Ralf Hiemisch/Getty Images

Injury Prevention

Lead Editors
Heidi Abraham, MD, EMT-B, EMT-T, FAEMS
Thomas Colvin, NREMT-P
Nancy Hoffmann, MSW

CHAPTER OBJECTIVES
At the completion of this chapter, you will be able to do the following:

- Describe the concept of energy as a cause of injury.
- Build a Haddon Matrix for a type of injury of interest.
- Relate the importance of accurate, attentive scene observations and documentation of data by prehospital care practitioners to the success of injury prevention initiatives.
- Assist in the development, implementation, and evaluation of injury prevention programs in your community or emergency medical services (EMS) organization.
- Describe the prevalence of intimate partner violence and what clues EMS should watch for.

- Describe and advocate for the role of EMS in injury prevention, including:
  - Individual
  - Family
  - Community
  - Professional
  - Organizational
  - Coalitions of organizations
- Identify strategies that prehospital care practitioners can implement that will reduce the risk of injury.

SCENARIO

You and your partner are on the scene of a motor vehicle collision and are working to rapidly extricate a patient who is overweight from the driver's seat of his vehicle. He was unrestrained in the vehicle during the collision. You and your partner are both wearing approved safety vests over your work gear because you are near the roadway. Law enforcement is on the scene to provide traffic control, and the ambulance is parked to maximize your protection from oncoming vehicles. The patient is properly secured onto your motorized stretcher, which is being used due to the patient's weight. The motorized stretcher allows you and your partner to lift the patient safely into the ambulance without putting excess strain on your bodies.

Once inside the ambulance, you secure yourself in the rear-facing chair and continue care of the patient while your partner maneuvers the vehicle safely into the lane and drives to the hospital. The ambulance arrives safely at the hospital, and you transfer the patient to the care of the emergency department (ED) staff.

(continues)

SCENARIO (CONTINUED)

While completing paperwork after the call, you consider the overall national injury and death statistics for prehospital care practitioners. You realize that thanks to the careful attention to all aspects of injury prevention that you and your partner demonstrated, the call was concluded safely for everyone involved.

- Is accident prevention a realistic approach in preventing injury and death in motor vehicle collisions and other causes of traumatic injury?
- Is there evidence that compliance with seat belt and safety seat laws has an impact in preventing injury and death?
- As prehospital care practitioners, what can we do to prevent deaths and injuries from motor vehicle collisions?

© National Association of Emergency Medical Technicians (NAEMT)

INTRODUCTION

A major impetus in the development of modern emergency medical services (EMS) systems was the publication of the 1966 white paper by the National Academy of Sciences/National Research Council (NAS/NRC), *Accidental Death and Disability: The Neglected Disease of Modern Society*. The paper spotlighted shortcomings in injury management in the United States and helped launch a formal system of on-scene care and rapid transport for patients injured as a result of "accidents." This educational initiative was instrumental in the creation of a more efficient system to deliver prehospital care to sick and injured patients.[1]

The incidence of death and disability from injury in the United States has fallen since the publication of the white paper.[2] Despite this progress, however, injury remains a major public health problem. In 2020, there were 278,345 recorded deaths from injury in the United States, and millions more are adversely affected to some degree.[3,4] Injuries remain a leading cause of death for all age groups.[5,6] For some age groups, particularly children, teenagers, and adults younger than 45, injury is the leading cause of death.[7]

Injury is a global problem as well. The World Health Organization (WHO) estimates that there are 4.4 million injury-related deaths annually and that approximately 3.1 million people worldwide died from preventable injuries in 2019 (not including homicide or suicide).[5,8]

The desire to care for patients stricken by injury draws many into the field of EMS. The Prehospital Trauma Life Support (PHTLS) course teaches prehospital care practitioners to be efficient and effective in patient assessment and injury management. The need for well-trained practitioners to care for injured patients will always exist. However, the most efficient and effective method to combat injury is to prevent it from happening in the first place. Healthcare practitioners at all levels play an active role in injury prevention to achieve the best results for not only the community at large but also for themselves.

In 1966, the authors of the NAS/NRC white paper recognized the importance of injury prevention when they wrote:

> The long-term solution to the injury problem is prevention. . . . Prevention of accidents involves training in the home, in the school, and at work, augmented by frequent pleas for safety in the news media; first aid courses and public meetings; and inspection and surveillance by regulatory agencies.[1]

Prevention of some diseases, such as rabies or measles, has been so effective that the occurrence of a single case makes front-page news. Public health officials recognize that prevention results in the greatest benefit toward the amelioration of disease. Curricula for prehospital care practitioners have long included formal instruction in scene safety and personal protective equipment as a means of self-injury prevention for the emergency medical services practitioner. To spur EMS systems to take a more active role in community prevention strategies, the *EMS Agenda for the Future*, developed by and for the EMS community, listed prevention as one of 14 attributes to develop further in order to "improve community health and result in more appropriate use of acute health resources."[9] The follow-up document, *EMS Agenda 2050: A People-Centered Vision for the Future of Emergency Medical Services*, outlines in its vision statement the role EMS plays in supporting ". . . the well-being of community residents and visitors through data-driven, evidence-based, and safe approaches to prevention, response, and clinical care."[10]

EMS systems are transforming themselves from a solely reactionary discipline to a broader, healthcare discipline that includes additional aspects, such as community paramedicine, and places more emphasis on prevention. Practitioners in the field support primary injury prevention (PiP) as part of the core mission of EMS, yet fewer than 50% of those surveyed implement PiP during clinical practice.[11] This chapter introduces key concepts of injury prevention to the prehospital care practitioner.

Concepts of Injury

Definition of Injury

A discussion of injury prevention should begin with a definition of the term **injury**. Injury is now commonly defined as a harmful event that arises from the release of specific forms of physical energy or barriers to the normal flow of energy.[12] The wide variability of the causes of injury initially represented a major hurdle in its study and prevention. For example, what does a fractured hip caused by an elderly person's fall have in common with a self-inflicted gunshot wound to the head of a young adult? Furthermore, how does one compare a femur fracture from a fall in an older woman to a femur fracture in a young man who crashed his motorcycle? All possible causes of injury—from vehicle crash, to stabbing, to suicide, to drowning—have one factor in common: the transfer of energy to the victim.

Injury as a Disease

The disease process has been studied for years. It is now understood that three factors must be present and interact simultaneously for an illness to occur: (1) an agent that causes the illness, (2) a host in which the agent can reside, and (3) a suitable environment in which the agent and host can come together. Once public health professionals recognized this "epidemiological triad," they discovered how to combat disease (**Figure 16-1**). Eradication of certain infectious diseases has been possible by vaccinating the host, destroying the agent with antibiotics, reducing environmental transmission through improved sanitation, or a combination of all three.

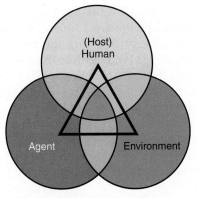

Figure 16-1 Epidemiological triad.
© National Association of Emergency Medical Technicians (NAEMT)

Only since the late 1940s has significant exploration of the **injury process** occurred. Pioneers in the study of injury demonstrated that despite the obviously different results, illness and injury are remarkably similar. Both require the presence of the three elements of the epidemiological triad, and therefore, both are treated as a disease:

1. For an injury to occur, a host (i.e., a human) must exist. As with illness, susceptibility of the host does not remain constant from individual to individual; it varies as a result of internal and external factors. *Internal* factors include intelligence, sex, or reaction time. *External* factors include intoxication or social beliefs. Susceptibility also varies over time within the same person.

2. As described previously, the agent of injury is *energy*. Velocity, shape, material, and time of exposure to the object that releases the energy all play a role in whether the host's tolerance level is overwhelmed.

3. The host and agent must come together in an environment that allows the two to interact. Typically, the environment is divided into physical and social components. *Physical* environmental factors can be seen and touched. *Social* environmental factors include attitudes, beliefs, and judgments. For example, teenagers are more likely to participate in risk-taking behavior (the physical component) because they have a greater sense of invincibility (the social component) than other age groups.

The characteristics of the host, agent, and environment change with time and circumstance. Public health professionals Tom Christoffel and Susan Scavo Gallagher describe this dynamic as follows:

> To illustrate, think of the components of the Epidemiological Triad as constantly turning wheels. Inside each wheel are pie-shaped sections, one for each possible circumstantial variable—good and bad. The three wheels turn at different rates, so different characteristics interact (meet) at different times and in different combinations. Some combinations predict that no injury will occur; some predict disaster.[13]

In the case of injury, the host might be a curious, mobile 2-year-old child; the agent of injury might be a swimming pool filled with water with a beach ball floating just beyond the edge; the environment might be a pool gate left open while the babysitter runs inside to check on a sibling. With the host, agent, and environment all coming together at the same time, an unintentional injury—in this case, drowning—can occur.

Haddon Matrix

Dr. William J. Haddon, Jr., is considered the father of the science of injury prevention. Working within the concept of the epidemiological triad, in the mid-1960s, he recognized that an injury can be broken down into the following three temporal phases:

1.   *Pre-event:* Before the injury
2.   *Event:* The point when harmful energy is released
3.   *Post-event:* The aftermath of the injury (see also Chapter 1, *PHTLS: Past, Present, and Future*).

By examining the three factors of the epidemiological triad during each temporal phase, Haddon created a nine-cell "phase-factor" matrix (**Table 16-1**). This grid has become known as the **Haddon Matrix**. It provides a means to depict graphically the events or actions that increase or decrease the odds that an injury will occur. It can also be used to identify prevention strategies. The Haddon Matrix demonstrates that *multiple* factors can lead to an injury, and therefore, multiple opportunities exist to prevent or reduce its severity. The matrix played a major role in dispelling the myth that injury is the result of a single cause, bad luck, or fate.

Table 16-1 depicts a Haddon Matrix for an ambulance crash. The components in each cell of the matrix are different, depending on the injury being examined. The *pre-event phase* includes factors that can contribute to the likelihood of a crash; however, energy is still under control. This phase may last from a few seconds to several years. The *event phase* depicts the factors that influence the severity of the injury. During this time, uncontrolled energy is released, and injury occurs if energy transfer exceeds the body's tolerance. The event phase is typically very brief; it may last only a fraction of a second and rarely lasts more than a few minutes. Factors in the *post-event phase* affect the outcome once an injury has occurred. Depending on the type of event, it may last from a few seconds to the remaining life span of the host. (See also Chapter 1, *PHTLS: Past, Present, and Future*.)

As mentioned previously, a key purpose of the Haddon Matrix is to recognize injury risks so that injury can be avoided. Public health programs have adopted the terminology of primary, secondary, and tertiary prevention.

*   *Primary prevention* is aimed at avoiding the injury before it occurs. This type of prevention activity involves education programs to help minimize risk-taking behaviors and the use of protective equipment such as helmets, child safety seats, and vehicle restraint systems.
*   *Secondary prevention* refers to those actions taken to prevent the progression of an acute injury once it has occurred—for example, avoiding the occurrence of hypoxia or hypotension after a traumatic brain injury or correcting it as rapidly as possible if it is already present.
*   *Tertiary prevention* is directed at minimizing death and the long-term disability following an injury (or disease). Active and aggressive rehabilitation programs fall into this category.

Swiss Cheese Model

British psychologist James Reason proposed another way of thinking about how accidents occur.[14] He likened the process to Swiss cheese. In every situation, a hazard exists that has the potential to cause injury or allow an error to occur. There are usually a series of safeguards or barriers to prevent this from happening. He suggested that each of these barriers or safeguards is like a piece of Swiss cheese. The holes in the cheese are flaws or failures that increase the potential for a hazard or error to cause injury. These flaws may be the result of deficiencies in the organization or administration or may occur following oversight of the system (latent conditions), or they may occur as a result of acts of omission or commission (active failures). Reason argued that every hazard has a trajectory, that a series of failures generally must occur in order for there to be subsequent harm, and that the trajectory must be such that it intersects with holes or failures that have aligned to allow all of the safeguards to fail and injury to occur (**Figure 16-2**).[14]

Classification of Injury

A common method to subclassify injuries is based on intent. Injury may result from either intentional or unintentional causes. Although this is a logical way to view injuries, it underscores the difficulty of injury prevention efforts.

Intentional injury is typically associated with an act of interpersonal or self-directed violence. Problems such as homicide, suicide, assault, sexual assault, domestic violence, child abuse, and war fall into this category.

In the past, **unintentional injuries** were called accidents. The authors of the NAS/NRC white paper appropriately referred to accidental death and disability; this was the vocabulary of the time.[1] Because we now believe that specific factors must come together for an injury to occur, healthcare practitioners now realize that the term *accidental* may not accurately portray the degree of preventability associated with unintentional injury resulting from events such as vehicle crashes, drownings, falls, and electrocutions. EMS systems have embraced this concept by using the term *motor vehicle collisions* or *crashes* (MVCs) rather than *motor vehicle accidents* (MVAs). However, public use of terminology has changed much more slowly. News reporters still describe persons injured in automobile accidents or accidental shootings. The term *accident* implies that a resulting injury was random and, therefore, unavoidable. The use of alternative language is intended to drive people to consider preventability in assessing incidents associated with injury.

It is also important to note that there may be overlap between these two common classifications of injury.[15]

Table 16-1 Haddon Matrix for an Ambulance Crash

Time Phases	Epidemiological Triad		
	Host Factors	Agent Factors	Environment Factors
Pre-event	Driver's visual acuity Experience and judgment Amount of time in the ambulance per shift Level of fatigue Proper nutrition Stress level Adherence to company and community driving laws Quality of driver education courses	Maintenance of brakes, tires, etc. Defective equipment Ambulance's high center of gravity Speed Ease of control	Visibility hazards Road curvature and gradient Surface coefficient of friction Narrow road shoulder Traffic signals Speed limits
Event	Safety belt use Physical conditioning Injury threshold Ejection	Speed capability Ambulance size Automatic restraints Hardness and sharpness of contact surfaces Hardness and sharpness of loose items (e.g., clipboards, flashlights) Steering column Practice of safe driving habits: speed, use of lights/siren, passing, intersections, backing Practice of good partner habits en route: watching road, clearing intersections Safe parking	Lack of guardrails Median barriers Distance between roadway and immovable objects Speed limits Other traffic Attitudes about safety belt use Maintaining an escape route Making no assumptions about an environment being safe (e.g., "nice part of town") Weather
Post-event	Age Physical condition Type or extent of injury	Fuel system integrity Entrapment	Emergency communication capability Distance to and quality of responding EMS Training of EMS personnel Availability of extrication equipment Trauma care system of the community Rehabilitation programs in the community

Data from Blau G, Chapman S, Boyer E, Flanagan R, Lam T, Monos C. Correlates of safety outcomes during patient ambulance transport: a partial test of the Haddon Matrix. *J Allied Health*. 2012;41(3):e69-72. PMID: 22968779.

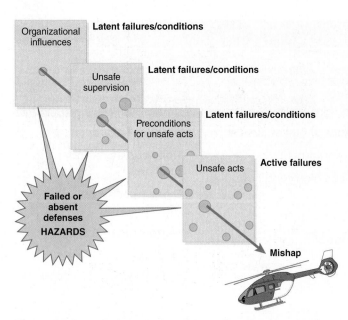

Figure 16-2 The Swiss cheese model of how defenses, barriers, and safeguards may be penetrated by an accident trajectory.

Reproduced from Reason J. *Human Error*. Cambridge University Press; 1990.

For example, a motor vehicle collision may have resulted from a driver attempting to commit suicide. Classifying the incident as an MVC alone implies no intent on the part of the driver to harm, whereas knowledge of the suicidal ideation of the driver clearly implies intent to cause the crash or collision.

Scope of the Problem

Injuries are a major health problem worldwide, resulting in 4.4 million deaths annually (**Box 16-1**), with road traffic accidents causing approximately 1.35 million, suicide nearly 700,000, and interpersonal violence around 520,000.[8,16-17] Causes of injury-related deaths vary among countries, both in terms of mechanism and age group impacted. Because of economic, social, and developmental issues, the causes of injury-related death vary from country to country and even from region to region within the same country.

For example, in low-income and middle-income countries of the Western Pacific, the leading injury-related

---

Box 16-1 Worldwide Injury-Related Statistics[17]

Injury Overall
- The top injury-related causes of mortality were:
  1. Road traffic injuries
  2. Acts of violence
  3. Falls
  4. Drowning
  5. Burns
  6. Poisonings
  7. Suicide
- Injuries accounted for 9% of the world's deaths and 16% of all disabilities.
- For persons ages 5 to 29 years, 3 of the top 10 leading causes of death were injury related.

Road Traffic Injury
- An estimated 1.35 million people die annually as a result of road traffic injuries, and between 20 and 50 million more were injured or disabled.
- Road traffic injury is the leading cause of death for children and youth ages 5 to 29 years.[18]
- Road traffic mortality for men younger than age 25 is almost three times higher than for women.

Burns[19]
- An estimated 180,000 deaths every year are caused by burns; the vast majority occur in low- and middle-income countries.
- Women in Southeast Asia have the highest fire-related burn mortality rates (due to open-fire cooking).

- Road traffic injuries are predicted to become the seventh leading cause of death by 2030.
- Twice as many men die from injury as women; fatal burn injuries are the notable exception.
- Men in Africa have the highest injury-related mortality rates.
- About 90% of all injury-related deaths occur in low-income and middle-income countries.
- Injury accounts for 12% of the total years of potential life lost either from premature death or from disability.

- Low-income countries account for more than three times the number of deaths from road traffic injuries than higher-income countries.[18]
- Africa and Southeast Asia account for the highest percentage of road traffic injury deaths.
- The likelihood of a crash and the severity of the consequences are directly linked to an increase in speed.

- Children younger than 5 years of age and elderly persons have the highest fire-related mortality rates.
- Nonfatal burn injuries are a leading cause of morbidity worldwide.

Drowning[20]

- In 2019, an estimated 236,000 people died from drowning.
- Over 90% of drowning deaths occurred in low- and middle-income countries.
- Among the various age groups, children younger than 5 years of age have the highest drowning mortality rates, accounting for more than 50% of drowning deaths.
- In the United States of America, drowning is the second leading cause of unintentional injury death in children ages 1 to 14 years.
- Official global data categorization does not factor in drowning deaths from flooding or water transport incidents, thus underestimating global drowning fatalities.

Falls[21]

- It is estimated that 684,000 people die as a result of falls annually.
- Over 80% of fall-related fatalities occur in low- and middle-income countries.
- In all regions of the world, adults older than 60 years of age, particularly women, have the highest fall mortality rate.
- Falls are now the second-leading cause of nonintentional injury fatalities.
- Globally, falls result in more years lived with injury than road traffic injuries, drowning, burns, and poisoning combined.

Poisoning

- According to WHO data, in 2016 an estimated 106,683 people died worldwide from unintentional poisoning.[22]
- More than 80% of fatal poisonings occurred in low- and middle-income countries.
- The European region accounts for more than one-third of all poisoning deaths worldwide.
- Snakebite is a largely unrecognized public health problem. While reliable data are hard to obtain, it has been estimated that over 5 million snakebites occur each year, resulting in up to 2.7 million envenomations and between 80,000 and 100,000 deaths.[23]

Interpersonal Violence[17]

- An estimated 415,000 people died worldwide in 2019 as a result of interpersonal violence.[24]
- The majority of deaths occurred in men and women ages 15 to 49.
- Of all homicides, 95% occurred in low- and middle-income countries.
- The highest interpersonal violence rates are found in the Americas among men ages 15 to 29 years.
- Among women, Africa has the highest mortality rate from interpersonal violence.

Suicide[25]

- Each year, approximately 700,000 people worldwide commit suicide.
- Of all suicides, 77% occurred in low- and middle-income countries.
- Suicide occurs throughout the life span.
- Around 20% of suicides globally are caused by pesticide self-poisoning.

causes of death are road traffic injuries, drowning, and suicide, whereas in Africa the leading causes are road traffic injuries, war, and interpersonal violence. In high-income countries of the Americas, the leading cause of death among people between 5 and 29 years of age is road traffic injuries. For this same age group in low-income and middle-income countries of the Americas, the leading cause is interpersonal violence.[6] **Figure 16-3** demonstrates that injury plays a leading role in the global burden of disease.

In 2019, over 36,000 people in the United States died in motor vehicle collisions.[26] Of those fatalities, 47% of passenger vehicle occupants were not wearing seatbelts.[27] Alcohol-related collision deaths accounted for 10,142 lives lost—a rate of 28 people per day, or one every 52 minutes.[28] In the United States, unintentional injuries are the overall fourth leading cause of death, accounting for approximately 200,000 deaths annually[29] (**Table 16-2**). Injury is an especially serious problem for the youth of America as well as of most industrialized nations of the world. In the United States, injury kills more children and young adults than all diseases combined and remains the leading cause of death for people ages 1 to 44 years.[30] Intentional injuries in this age group include suicide—the second leading cause of death—and homicide. Suicide numbers continue to climb.[30] Unintentional injury deaths in the same group include unintentional poisoning (e.g., opioid overdoses), MVCs, and unintentional falls. Opioid overdoses alone accounted for 49,860 deaths in 2019.[31]

Unfortunately, deaths from injury are only the tip of the iceberg. Injuries are also a leading cause of disability across all ages, ethnicities, and socioeconomic strata. Injuries require 29 million ED visits annually and have further impacts on family, friends, coworkers, and communities.[32]

The impact can be further realized by examining the number of **years of potential life lost (YPLL)** as a result of injury. YPLL is calculated by subtracting age at death from a fixed age of the group under examination, usually 65 or 70 years or the life expectancy of the group. The Organisation for Economic Co-operation and most U.S. federal and state agencies use 75 years as the benchmark. As an example, a person who dies at age 70 has 5 YPLL, whereas a child who dies at age 10 has 65 YPLL.[33] Thus, even though injury kills or disables people of all ages, it disproportionately affects children, youth, and young adults. That is, because injury is the leading killer of Americans between 1 and 44 years of age, it is responsible for more YPLL than any other cause of death. In 2020, injury stole an estimated 4.9 million *years* from its victims (**Figure 16-4**). Unintentional poisoning (predominantly opioid overdoses) accounted for 1.4 million of those years.

A third measure of injury severity can be demonstrated financially. The economics of injury are felt far beyond the patient and the immediate family. The cost of injury is spread across a wide spectrum. All members of society feel the effect because the costs of injury are borne by federal and other agencies, private insurance programs that pass the expense on to other subscribers, and employers as well as the patient. As a result, everyone pays when an individual is seriously injured. In 2019, the CDC estimated the cost of injuries to be $4.2 trillion, which includes direct medical care costs ($327 billion), as well as work loss, YPLL value, and quality of life loss costs.[34] Data from the WHO indicate that prevention activities are a good investment:

- Every U.S. dollar invested in motorcycle helmets results in a $32 savings of medical costs.

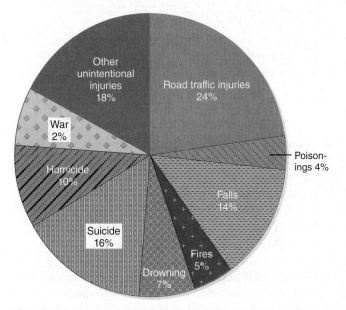

Figure 16-3 Distribution of global injury mortality by cause.

Data from World Health Organization. Injuries and violence: the facts 2014. n.d. https://apps.who.int/iris/bitstream/handle/10665/149798/9789241508018_eng.pdf

Table 16-2 Ranking of Causes of Injury-Related Deaths by Age Group, 2020											
	Age Group										
	+1	1–4	5–9	10–14	15–24	25–34	35–44	45–54	55–64	65 +	All Ages (number of deaths)
Unintentional Injury	4th	Leading	Leading	Leading	Leading	Leading	Leading	3rd	4th	8th	4th (200,955)
Intentional Injury											
Suicide	*	*	10th	2nd	3rd	2nd	4th	7th	9th	*	*
Homicide	*	3rd	4th	4th	3rd	2nd	7th	10th	*	*	*

*Data not applicable/available or not included in the top 10 causes of death.

Data from Centers for Disease Control and Prevention, National Center for Injury Prevention and Control. 10 leading causes of death, United States, 2020, all races, both sexes. Web-based Injury Statistics Query and Reporting System (WISQARS) website. Accessed March 2, 2022. https://www.cdc.gov/injury/wisqars/

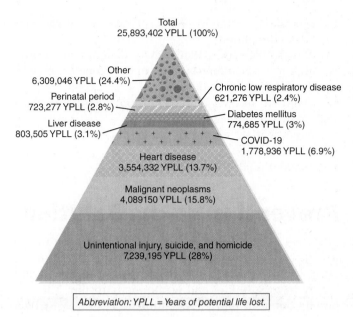

Figure 16-4 Years of potential life lost before age 75.

Data from Centers for Disease Control and Prevention, National Center for Injury Prevention and Control. Years of potential life lost (YPLL) before age 75, 2020 United States, all races, both sexes, all deaths. Web-based Injury Statistics Query and Reporting System (WISQARS) website. Accessed March 2, 2022. https://www.cdc.gov/injury/wisqars/

- Seat belts decrease the risk of ejection and of sustaining serious or fatal injury by 40% to 65% and saved an estimated 255,000 lives between 1975 and 2008.[35]

The toll of injury in terms of morbidity, mortality, and economic stress is excessive. As stated by Cristofell and Gallagher:

> Injuries have always been a threat to the public's well-being, but until the mid-twentieth century, infectious diseases overshadowed the terrible contribution injury made to human morbidity and mortality. Public health improvements . . . in other areas has left injury as a major threat to public health, one that has been termed "the neglected epidemic."[13]

Society is calling on all segments of the medical community to increase its prevention activities. With as many as 840,600 prehospital care practitioners in the United States alone, according to the American Ambulance Association, EMS systems can make a tremendous contribution to community-based injury prevention efforts.

Intimate Partner Violence

Intimate partner violence (IPV) is defined as physical violence, sexual violence, psychological aggressions, or stalking by a current or former intimate partner.[36] The CDC's National Intimate Partner and Sexual Violence Survey gathers data on sexual violence and IPV. In the United States, just over one-third (36.4%) of women experienced contact sexual violence (18.3%), physical violence (30.6%), and/or stalking (10.4%) by an intimate partner. Similarly, nearly one-third of men experienced contact sexual violence (8.2%), physical violence (31%), and/or stalking (2.2%) during their lifetime.[37] Finally, 36.4% of women said they had experienced at least one act of psychological aggression by an intimate partner as compared with men at 34.2%.[37]

Due to the nature of their profession, EMS practitioners are in a unique position to observe the dynamics between the patient and others at the scene. A few signs of intimate partner violence include the following:

- *Overly protective partners.* Abusers may be hesitant to leave their victim alone when they feel their victim might talk about the abuse.
- *Jealous or controlling behavior from the abuser.*
- *Overly timid patient.* You might encounter patients who avoid all eye contact or defer to their partner when asked a question.
- *Unexplained injuries or repeated injuries.* The patient may be unwilling to explain black eyes or bruising to the neck, may present with bruising to the body at various stages of healing, or may have a history of broken bones.

You should report any suspicions of intimate partner violence to the appropriate law enforcement agency. EMS practitioners are also in a unique position to become secondary victims on these calls. Pay particularly close attention to your own safety on these calls at all times and maintain a high level of situational awareness. Remember, it is not the EMS practitioner's duty to confront the assailant. That is a dangerous action.

Injury to EMS Personnel

EMS personnel are exposed to a wide variety of situations that can result in practitioner injury. Scenes are often unsecured, despite the best efforts of EMS personnel and law enforcement, because these scenes involve people in emotional and physical crisis. There are regular reports of EMS practitioners being assaulted on the job, shot at, or otherwise targeted. The very nature of the emergency work presents many opportunities for injury. Just driving to the scene can be hazardous. Lifting, exposure to environmental hazards and infectious diseases, sleep deprivation, and the stress of the job also present significant opportunities for injury. The tragic situations encountered often contribute to depression, anxiety, and posttraumatic stress disorder (PTSD), which can have significant physical effects on practitioners, as well as causing additional psychological stress.

Sleep deprivation is an important factor that clearly affects prehospital care practitioner well-being and performance.[38] The longer a person is awake, the greater the resulting fatigue and drowsiness; the greater the impairment in reaction time, medical decision making, and judgment; and the greater the likelihood of mistakes, injury to self or others, and even fatality.[39] Sleep deprivation has been compared to alcohol intoxication, with no sleep for 18 hours approximating a blood alcohol concentration (BAC) of 0.05 and no sleep for 24 hours approximating a BAC of 0.1.

In addition, sleep deprivation can have profound effects on the health of the prehospital care practitioner and can interfere with important personal and family relationships. Lack of sleep can lead to irritability, anxiety, and depression.

A study published in 2011 reviewed fatal and nonfatal injuries to EMTs and paramedics during the period from 2003 to 2007.[40] The authors reviewed data from the Bureau of Labor Statistics Census of Fatal Occupational Injuries as well as the occupational portion of the National Electronic Injury Surveillance System. For that time period, they found 99,400 nonfatal injuries and 65 fatalities. Most of the fatalities were transportation related, either motor vehicle collisions (45%) or aircraft crashes (31%). The fatality rate for full-time equivalents EMS workers was 7.0 per 100,000.[41] Among paid EMS personnel in general, the fatality rate was 6.3 per 100,000.[40] In comparison, the fatality rate for fire fighters was 6.1 per 100,000 and for all workers was 4.0 per 100,000 during this same period.[41] The only good news in this report is that the fatality figure is lower than that documented in the report from 10 years prior.

These numbers reveal a disturbing truth. According to Garrison:

> . . . the most dangerous times for EMS personnel are when they are inside their ambulance when it is moving or when they are working at a crash scene near other moving vehicles.[42]

It is critical that EMS personnel know and understand the concepts of injury and injury prevention so that the risks inherent in EMS can be identified and corrected. From the first day of training, students are taught that no one is more important at the scene than the prehospital care practitioner, so personnel safety must come first. Seat belt use in the ambulance is the first step toward safety.

The National EMS Culture of Safety project was prompted by a recommendation in 2009 from the National Emergency Medical Services Advisory Council (NEMSAC) for the Department of Transportation's National Highway Traffic Safety Administration (NHTSA) to create a strategy for improved safety in EMS. The American College of Emergency Physicians (ACEP) and the EMS for Children (EMSC) program, along with other key players from fire and EMS groups, were part of the project that agreed on a strategy involving six key elements:

- Just culture, which encourages reporting of mistakes and near-misses, so that errors can be avoided in the future

- Coordinated support and resources among agencies across the nation
- A responder and patient safety data system, allowing for better understanding of the scope of some of these issues
- Evolution of EMS education to include better training on these topics
- Promulgation of safety standards based on good evidence
- Incident reporting and investigation[43]

Prevention as the Solution

The ideal is to prevent an injury from occurring in the first place, thus obviating the need to treat it after it occurs. When injury is prevented, it spares the patient and family from suffering and economic hardship. The National Center for Injury Prevention and Control (NCIPC) of the Centers for Disease Control and Prevention (CDC) estimates that up to 40% of deaths from the top five leading causes are preventable.[44]

Because of the variability among the host, agent, and environment at any given time, healthcare practitioners cannot always predict or prevent every individual injury. However, it is possible to identify high-risk populations (which include prehospital care practitioners), high-risk products, and high-risk environments. Prevention efforts focused on high-risk groups or settings influence as wide a range of society as possible. Healthcare practitioners can pursue prevention in multiple ways. Some strategies have proven successful across the United States and around the world. However, other strategies work in one region but not in another. Before implementing an injury prevention strategy, efforts must focus on determining whether it will work. Although it is not necessary to "reinvent the wheel," healthcare practitioners may need to modify a prevention strategy to improve its chances of success. Methods for doing this are examined in the following section.

Concepts of Injury Prevention

Goal

The goal of injury prevention programs is to bring about a change in knowledge, attitude, and behavior on the part of a previously identified segment of society. Simply providing information to potential victims is not enough to prevent injury. A program must be implemented in a manner that will influence society's attitudes and—most important—change behavior. The hope is that any change in behavior will be long term. This task is monumental but not insurmountable.

Opportunities for Intervention

Prevention strategies can be arranged according to their effect on the injury event. They coincide with the temporal phases of the Haddon Matrix. Pre-event interventions, known as primary interventions, strive to prevent the injury from occurring. Actions intended to keep intoxicated drivers off the road, laws to prevent texting while driving, and measures to install traffic lights are designed to prevent crashes from occurring. Event phase interventions are intended to reduce injury severity by softening the blow of injuries that occur. Requiring safety belts, installing cushioned dashboards and airbags in vehicles, and enforcing child safety seat laws are means to reduce the severity of injury sustained in crashes. Post-event interventions provide a means to improve the likelihood of survival for those who are injured. Encouraging physical fitness, designing fuel systems for vehicles that do not explode on impact, and implementing high-quality EMS systems are intended to reduce the recovery time for persons who are injured.

Prehospital systems have traditionally limited their community involvement to the post-event phase. Although countless lives have been saved, the limitations inherent in waiting until injury has occurred mean that the best results have not been achieved. EMS systems must explore entering the injury cycle earlier. Using the Haddon Matrix, EMS systems can identify opportunities to collaborate with other public health and public safety organizations to prevent injuries from occurring or to soften their blow.

Potential Strategies

No single strategy provides the best approach to injury prevention. The most effective options depend on the type of injury under study. However, Haddon developed a list of 10 generic strategies designed to break the chain of injury-producing events at numerous points (**Table 16-3**). These strategies represent ways that the release of uncontrolled energy can be prevented, or at least reduced, to amounts the body can better tolerate. Table 16-3 also presents countermeasures that can be taken in the pre-event, event, and post-event phases and that are directed toward the host, agent, or environment. This list is not complete and merely serves as a starting point to help determine the most effective options for the particular problem under study.

Most injury prevention strategies are either active or passive. **Passive strategies** require little or no action on the part of the individual; sprinkler systems and vehicle airbags are examples. **Active strategies** require the cooperation of the person being protected; examples include manual seat belts and choosing to wear a motorcycle or bicycle helmet. Passive measures are generally more effective because people do not need to consciously do anything to take advantage of the protection. Nonetheless, passive strategies are usually more difficult to implement because they can be expensive or require legislative or regulatory action. Sometimes a combination of active and passive strategies is the best option.

Strategy Implementation

Four common approaches to implementing an injury prevention strategy have become known as the Four Es of injury prevention—education, enforcement, engineering, and equity. Each of these elements is described here.

Education

Educational strategies are meant to impart information. The target audience may be individuals who engage in high-risk activities, policy makers who have the authority to enact further prevention legislation or regulation, or prehospital care practitioners learning to become active participants in injury prevention.

Education once was the primary means of implementing prevention programs because society believed that most injuries were simply the result of human error. Although this assumption is true to a certain extent, many failed to recognize the role that energy and the environment play in causing injury. Education is still often used, however, and is probably the easiest of the four strategies to implement.

Experience has demonstrated that educational strategies have not met with overwhelming success for several reasons. For starters, the target audience may never hear the message. If the message is heard, some may reject it outright or not embrace it enough to alter behavior. Those who embrace it may do so sporadically or with declining enthusiasm over time.[45] However, education still can be particularly useful in reducing injury in the following four areas:

1. *Teaching young children basic safety behaviors and skills that stay with them later in life.* Examples include responding appropriately when a smoke detector sounds an alarm, calling 911 for help in an emergency, or fastening seat belts.
2. *Teaching about certain types and causes of injuries for certain age groups.* Education may be the only strategy available for these groups.
3. *Altering the public's perception of risk and acceptable risk to change social norms and attitudes.* This approach was used regarding drinking and driving and occurs now regarding wearing a helmet when riding a bicycle, scooter, or skateboard or using rollerblades.
4. *Promoting policy change and educating consumers to demand safer products.*[45]

Table 16-3 Basic Strategies for Injury Countermeasures

Strategy	Possible Countermeasures
Prevent initial creation of the hazard.	Do not produce firecrackers, three-wheeled all-terrain vehicles, or various poisons. Eliminate spearing in high school football.
Reduce amount of energy contained in the hazard.	Limit the horsepower of motor vehicle engines. Package toxic drugs in smaller, safer amounts. **Obey speed limits.** Mandate improved public transportation to reduce the number of privately owned vehicles on the road. **Encourage reduction of temperature on home hot water heaters.** Limit the muzzle velocity of guns. Limit the amount of gunpowder in firecrackers.
Prevent release of a hazard that already exists.	**Store firearms in locked containers or use gun locks.** Close pools and beaches when no lifeguard is on duty. **Encourage use of nonslip surfaces in bathtubs and showers.** **Require childproof containers for all hazardous household drugs and chemicals.** **Limit cell phone use in vehicles, or use hands-free models.** Require safety shields on rotating farm machinery. Improve vehicle handling.
Modify rate or spatial distribution of the hazard.	**Require use of seat belts and child safety seats.** Provide antilock brakes. Encourage use of short cleats on football shoes so feet rotate rather than transmit sudden force to the knees. Require vehicle airbags. Provide hydraulic bumpers on vehicles. Provide safety harnesses to protect workers from falls. **Encourage use of flame-retardant pajamas.**
Separate in time or space the hazard from that which is to be protected.	Provide pedestrian overpasses at high-volume crossings. Keep roadsides clear of poles and trees. Do not have play areas near unguarded bodies of water. Install bike paths. Spray pesticides at a time when people are not present. Install sidewalks. Route trucks carrying hazardous material along low-density roads. **Encourage use of smoke detectors in the home.**

Strategy	Possible Countermeasures
Separate the hazard from that which is to be protected by a material barrier.	Install fencing around all sides of swimming pools. **Encourage use of protective eyewear for sports and occupational hazards.** Build highway medians. Build protective shields around hazardous machinery. Install guardrails between sidewalks and roads. Install reinforced panels in vehicle doors. **Require healthcare workers to place used needles directly into a sharps container.** **Require use of helmets for motorcyclists, bicyclists, and high-risk sporting activities.**
Modify basic nature of the hazard.	Provide airbags in motor vehicles. Provide collapsible steering columns. Provide breakaway poles. Make crib slats too narrow to strangle a baby. Adopt breakaway baseball bases. **Remove throw rugs in homes of the elderly.**
Make what is to be protected more resistant to the hazard.	**Encourage calcium intake to reduce osteoporosis.** **Promote campaigns such as Stop the Bleed, hands-only CPR, and other educational events to teach the public how to mitigate emergencies.** Encourage musculoskeletal conditioning in athletes. Prohibit alcohol sales and consumption near recreational water areas. Treat medical conditions such as epilepsy to prevent episodes that can result in burns, drownings, and falls. Check earthquake-resistant building codes in susceptible areas.
Begin to counter the damage already done by the hazard.	**Provide emergency medical care.** **Stock AEDs in public locations such as airports, gyms, and schools.** Employ systems to route injured persons to appropriately trained prehospital care practitioners. **Develop school protocols for responding to injury emergencies.** **Provide first-aid training to residents.** Install automatic sprinkler systems.
Stabilize, repair, and rehabilitate the object of the damage.	Develop rehabilitation plans at an early stage of injury treatment. Make use of occupational rehabilitation for paraplegic patients.

*The examples listed are for illustrative purposes only and are not necessarily the official recommendations of PHTLS, the National Association of EMTs, or the American College of Surgeons Committee on Trauma.

Bold indicates opportunities for EMS personnel to provide education and leadership.

As a singular approach to injury prevention, educational programs have had disappointing results. Like many medications, education needs to be "re-dosed" after a period of time in order to have a continued effect. However, when coupled with other forms of implementation strategies, education can be a valuable tool. Education often serves as a starting point to pave the way for enforcement and engineering strategies.

Enforcement

Enforcement seeks to tap the persuasive power of law to compel adherence to simple but effective prevention strategies. Statutory commands can either require or prohibit, and they can be directed at individual behavior (people), products (things), or environmental conditions (places), as follows:

- Legal requirements that apply to people are mandatory seat belt, child restraint, and helmet laws.
- Prohibitions that apply to people are drunk driving laws, speed limits, and assault laws.
- Legal requirements that apply to products include design and performance standards, such as the federal Motor Vehicle Safety Standards.
- Prohibitions that apply to products include restrictions on dangerous animals and flammable fabrics.
- Legal requirements that apply to places include the installation of breakaway signposts along highways and fencing around swimming pools.
- Prohibitions that apply to places include the outlawing of firearms in schools and airport terminals.
- Legal requirements that apply to specific target groups and locations include the federal requirements that public safety and emergency responders wear high-visibility clothing at high-traffic crash sites.[13]

Enforcement is also an active countermeasure because people must obey the law to benefit from it. The target audiences may be less likely to comply if they believe the directive infringes on personal freedom, if they have little chance of getting caught, or if they will not face consequences of violating the law.

Because society as a whole tends to obey laws or at least stay within narrow limits around them, enforcement is often more effective than education. Enforcement in tandem with education appears to produce better results than either initiative alone. Motorcycle helmet laws provide an interesting case study in the role of enforcement in injury prevention. In states in which helmet laws have been repealed for motorcyclists, the rate of serious injuries and fatalities has increased.[46-48]

Engineering

Often the most effective means of injury prevention are those in which destructive energy release is permanently separated from the host. Passive countermeasures accomplish this goal with little or no effort on the part of the individual. Engineering strategies strive to build injury prevention into products or environments so that the host does not have to act differently to be protected. Engineering strategies help the people who actually need them, and they do so every time. Measures such as automatic sprinkler systems in buildings, flotation hulls in boats, and backup alarms on ambulances all are intended to save lives with little or no effort on the part of the host.

Engineering seems to be the perfect answer to injury prevention. It is passive, effective, and usually the least disruptive of the Four Es. Unfortunately, it is often the most expensive to implement. Designing safety into a product usually makes it more expensive and may require legislative or regulatory initiation. The price may be more than the manufacturer is willing to absorb or the customer is willing to pay. Society dictates how much safety it wants built into a product and how much it is willing to support the endeavor financially.

Education initiatives should precede enforcement and engineering strategies. Ultimately, the most effective countermeasures may be those that incorporate all four implementation strategies.

Equity

Equity is often described as the fourth E of injury prevention. It is distinct from the other three in that is it is applied across each of the others when working to decrease disparities in injury risk within the population.

From an education standpoint, efforts must be made to ensure that education is directed at the highest risk populations. If the message is going to effectively reach the target audience, it must be delivered in a format that audience is likely to access and in a culturally competent way.

Helping people understand the risk of space heaters in a home, for example, is not effective if efforts are not also in place to ensure alternative methods of heating a home are available. Attempts to alter the public perception about risk require conversations in the community about risk magnitude and mitigation. Telling someone not to use a skateboard without a helmet is less effective than it would be if combined with providing accurate information about the consequences of head injury and skateboard accidents as well as access to helmets.

Notably, the equity lens should be applied to every set of interventions to mitigate the risk of injury due to trauma as inequities often result from failure to consider the differential challenges faced by at-risk populations.

Public Health Approach

Much has been learned about injury and injury prevention. Unfortunately, a wide discrepancy exists between what is known about injury and what is being done about it.[49] Injury is a complex problem in all societies of the world. Unfortunately, a single person or single agency will usually have little impact. Taking a public health approach has achieved success in dealing with diseases, and this same approach is also making progress with injury prevention. EMS agencies that have joined forces with other public and private organizations have been able to accomplish as much, or more, than they could on their own. Partnerships bring together a community's expertise to tackle a complex and perplexing issue.

A public health approach creates a community-based coalition to combat a community-based disease through a four-step process, as follows:

1. Surveillance
2. Risk factor identification
3. Intervention evaluation
4. Implementation

The coalition comprises experts from such diverse fields as epidemiology, the medical community, schools of public health, public health agencies, community advocacy programs, economics, sociology, and criminal justice. EMS systems have an important place in a public health approach to injury prevention. Participating in a coalition to improve playground safety may not have the immediate effect of providing care at the scene of a horrific vehicle crash, but the results will be much more widespread.

Surveillance

Surveillance is the process of collecting data within a community. Collection of population-based data aids in the discovery of an injury's true magnitude and effect on the community. A community can be a neighborhood, city, county, state, or even the ambulance service itself. Support for the program, proper allocation of resources, and even knowing who to include on the interdisciplinary team depend on understanding the scope of the problem.

Sources of information available within a community include the following:

- Mortality data
- Hospital admission and discharge statistics
- Medical records
- Trauma registries
- Police reports
- EMS run sheets
- Insurance reports
- Unique surveillance data collected solely for the study at hand

Risk Factor Identification

After a problem is identified and researched, it is necessary to know who is at risk in order to direct a prevention strategy at the correct population. "Shotgun" approaches to injury prevention are less successful than targeted ones. Identification of causes and risk factors determines who is injured; what types of injuries are sustained; and where, when, and why those injuries occur.[50] Sometimes a risk factor is obvious, such as the presence of alcohol in fatal vehicle crashes. At other times, research is required to discover the true risk factors involved in injury events. EMS systems can serve as the "eyes and ears" of public health at the scene of injuries to identify risk factors that no one else may be able to uncover. Risk factors can then be charted on a Haddon Matrix as they are properly identified.

Intervention Evaluation

As risk factors become clear, intervention strategies begin to emerge. Haddon's list of 10 injury prevention strategies serves as a starting point (see Table 16-3). Even though communities have different characteristics, with modification, an injury prevention initiative from one community may work in another. Once a potential intervention has been selected, a pilot program using one or more of the Four Es may give indications of the success of full-scale implementation.

Implementation

The final steps in the public health approach are implementation and evaluation of the intervention. Detailed implementation procedures are prepared so that others interested in implementation of similar programs will have a guide to follow. Collection of evaluation data measures the effectiveness of a program. Answering the following three questions may help determine the success of a program:

1. Have attitudes, skills, or judgment changed?
2. Has behavior changed?
3. Does behavioral change lead to a favorable outcome?[12]

The public health approach provides a proven means to combat a disease such as injury. Through a multidisciplinary, community-based effort, it is possible to identify the "who, what, where, when, and why" of an injury problem and develop a plan of action. EMS systems need to play a much more substantial role in helping to close the gap between what is known about injury and what is being done about it. This approach can be thought of as a continuous loop. Continued surveillance occurs after implementation of an injury control strategy. These data are then used to modify or change the strategy. Successes in injury prevention can be broadened to wider populations that may be at risk.

Evolving Role of EMS in Injury Prevention

Traditionally, the role of the prehospital care practitioner in health care focused almost exclusively on post-event, one-on-one treatment of the individual. Little emphasis was placed on understanding the causes of the injuries or what a practitioner could do to prevent them. As a result, patients may return to the same environment only to be injured again. In addition, information that could aid in the development of a communitywide prevention program to keep others from becoming injured in the first place may not be documented and, therefore, may remain unavailable to other sectors of public health.

The public health approach to injury is more proactive. It works to determine how to alter the host, agent, and environment to prevent injuries. Through coalitions that conduct surveillance and implement interventions, public health works to develop communitywide prevention programs. The *EMS Agenda for the Future* envisions closer ties between EMS systems and public health that would make both sectors of health care more effective.[9] The practice of community paramedicine is one way that EMS has become more involved in this aspect of injury (and illness) prevention.

Prehospital care practitioners can take a more active role in the development of communitywide injury prevention programs. EMS systems enjoy a unique position in the community. With over 1 million practitioners in the United States alone,[51] basic and advanced practitioners are widely distributed at the community level. Practitioners enjoy a credible reputation in the community, making them high-profile role models. In addition, they are readily welcomed into homes and businesses. All phases of the public health approach to injury prevention benefit from an EMS presence.

One-on-One Interventions

EMS systems do not have to give up their one-on-one approach to patient care to conduct valuable injury prevention interventions. The one-on-one approach makes EMS systems uniquely able to conduct injury prevention initiatives. Prehospital care practitioners can bring injury prevention messages directly to high-risk individuals. One indicator of a successful educational program is that the information is received with enough enthusiasm to change behavior. Practitioners can use their role model status to deliver important prevention messages. Implicitly, people look up to role models, listen to what they have to say, and emulate what they do.

On-scene prevention counseling takes advantage of a "teachable moment." A teachable moment is the time when a patient who does not require critical medical interventions or the patient's family members are in a state that makes them more receptive to what a role model says. The prehospital care practitioner may think of the on-scene time as wasted when it becomes apparent that little or no medical interventions are necessary. However, this may be the best time to deliver primary prevention.[52]

Not every call allows for injury prevention counseling. Serious and life-threatening calls require concentration on acute care. However, as many as 95% of ambulance calls are not life threatening. A significant proportion of EMS calls require minor, if any, treatment. One-on-one prevention counseling may be appropriate during these noncritical calls.

Patient interactions are typically short encounters, especially those that require little or no treatment. However, they do provide enough time to discuss and demonstrate to patients and family members practices that may prevent an injury in the future. Prehospital care practitioners are in a unique position in that they are the only healthcare worker who enters the patient's environment, thereby viewing situations that may predispose to injury. A role model who discusses the importance of replacing a burned-out lightbulb and removing a slippery throw rug in a dimly lit hallway may prevent a fall by an elderly resident. Practitioners have an attentive audience during the ride to a hospital. Prevention is a more valuable topic to discuss than the weather or the local sports team. Teachable moments take 1 to 2 minutes to complete and do not interfere with treatment or transport.

Educational programs have been developed to train prehospital care practitioners to administer on-scene injury prevention counseling.[53] These types of programs must be further developed and evaluated to discover which are the most valuable and, therefore, worthy of inclusion in the primary education of a practitioner.

Communitywide Interventions

The public health approach to injury prevention is community based and involves a multidisciplinary team. Prehospital care practitioners have the expertise to be valuable members of that team. Communitywide prevention strategies depend on data to address properly the "who, what, when, where, and why" of an injury problem. Multiple sources of information, as described previously, provide the needed data. Practitioners, perhaps more than any other team member, have the opportunity to examine patient interaction with the environment at the time of the injury. This may allow identification of a high-risk individual, high-risk attitude, or high-risk behavior that is not present by the time the patient arrives at the ED.

The prehospital care practitioner can use documentation acquired en route to a medical facility in the following two ways:

1. Data can be used immediately by emergency personnel who receive the patient. Emergency physicians and nurses are also being called on to improve and increase their role in injury prevention. Their "teachable moment" can reinforce and supplement the practitioner's on-scene counseling if they know what has already been discussed or demonstrated.

2. Others in public health can use injury data from practitioners retrospectively to help develop a comprehensive, communitywide injury prevention program.

Prehospital care practitioners usually do not practice documentation to help support a communitywide prevention program. Knowing what to acquire and when to document information beneficial to the development of communitywide prevention programs requires opening a dialogue with other members of the public health team. Leaders in the EMS system need to build a coalition with others in public health to develop documentation policies that promote complete documentation of injuries.

EMS can be the spearhead for workable, effective injury prevention programs that make a profound impact in a community. Programs have been created out of the desire of a small group of EMS professionals to prevent childhood fatalities.[54,55] Services and individuals in North Carolina, Florida, South Carolina, Oregon, and Virginia have been recognized for their efforts in designing, coordinating, and conducting injury prevention programs through the Nicholas Rosecrans Award for best practices in injury prevention in EMS.[56,57]

Even though opportunities exist for prehospital care practitioners to educate patients, one study by Dr. David Jaslow and colleagues suggests that a minority of prehospital practitioners utilize the teachable moment. They found that only 33% routinely educate their patients on how to modify injury risk behaviors, and only 19% routinely provide instruction about proper use of protective devices.[57]

Injury Prevention for EMS Practitioners

"Who's the most important person at an incident scene?" EMS students are always asked this question early in their training to make them think about their own safety. Invariably, one or two students will say "the patient," which is what the instructor wanted to hear. This incorrect response provides a teachable moment for the instructor to begin the course-long directive to reinforce the point that self-injury prevention is the most valuable service a prehospital care practitioner can deliver.

Hostile environments resulting from terrorist activities or hazardous materials spills unfortunately make the news too often. Many terrorist attacks include secondary explosions designed to kill or injure first responders as they are arriving on the scene. However, even the everyday activities of prehospital practitioners provide sufficient opportunity for injuries that could end a career or life. The Bureau of Labor Statistics paints an accurate picture of the "normal" dangers in EMS:

> EMTs and paramedics work both indoors and outdoors, in all types of weather. They are required to do considerable kneeling, bending, and heavy lifting. These workers risk noise-induced hearing loss from sirens and back injuries from lifting patients. In addition, EMTs and paramedics may be exposed to diseases such as hepatitis B and AIDS, as well as violence from drug overdose victims or mentally unstable patients. The work is not only physically strenuous but also stressful, involving life-or-death situations and suffering patients.[58]

Prehospital care practitioners are at substantial risk for injury or death while responding to, managing the patient at, and transporting from an emergency medical call. The risks associated with injury both on scene and in a moving ambulance can be minimized by utilizing proper preventive measures such as seat belts or reflective clothing.

Prehospital care practitioners can become complacent toward the everyday dangers of the job. Complacency is a feeling of security or safety in the unacknowledged face of potential danger. Compounding the situation are the idealism and invincibility of youth typical of some EMS personnel.[59] Management is needed to create a culture of injury prevention or, better, a culture of safety by instituting prevention policy, maintaining adherence to procedure, and rewarding positive performance. The practitioners themselves must be equally committed to the principles of injury prevention. Failure in this initiative by either management or practitioners can have potentially devastating effects.

Other factors to consider are the experience level of personnel and their degree of fatigue. Drivers must be adequately prepared and trained to operate vehicles safely, and EMS personnel must be monitored to ensure they have adequate sleep to maintain safe operations. In a study that looked at common factors in EMS personnel involved in ambulance crashes, the odds were greater that the drivers involved in emergency vehicle crashes would be younger EMS personnel and those EMS personnel reporting sleep problems.[60]

Dr. Neil Stanley of the British Sleep Society noted, "Nobody should be doing anything really important for 15 to 30 minutes after they wake up." This has serious implications for EMS, considering that EMS personnel must respond immediately, no matter what time of night it is, whether awake or asleep, and be expected to function "normally." The National Highway Transportation Safety Administration supported a Fatigue in EMS project that created a panel to review evidence related to fatigue in EMS and develop recommendations for fatigue risk management. Five of the panel's recommendations are as follows:

- Use fatigue/sleepiness survey instruments to measure and monitor fatigue in EMS personnel.
- Have EMS personnel work shifts shorter than 24 hours in duration.
- Allow EMS personnel to have access to caffeine as a fatigue countermeasure.
- Provide EMS personnel with the opportunity to nap while on duty to mitigate fatigue.
- Provide EMS personnel with education and training to mitigate fatigue and fatigue-related risks.

The panel noted that implementation of a fatigue mitigation program in EMS systems would require multiple strategies to achieve true effectiveness.[61] However, the prevalence of fatigue and the importance of fatigue mitigation on both practitioner and patient safety should outweigh the obstacles to implementation.

In a prehospital service, employees are not only the most valuable asset but also the most expensive. The service, community, and, most important, the prehospital care practitioner benefit when the employee remains uninjured. An in-house injury prevention program is worthwhile on its own merits. Many EMS and law enforcement agencies are realizing the benefits of having athletic trainers on their staff, for immediate treatment and rehabilitation of injuries. Of these agencies, 96% reported that the athletic trainer made an impact on their

workers' compensation costs within 1 year, reducing overall medical costs by as much as 50%. The significantly faster return to duty also has a tremendous psychological benefit for the practitioner.[62,63]

Dr. Janet Kinnane and colleagues mention in-house prevention programs that utilize education, enforcement, and engineering implementation strategies.[52] The wide variability of the programs demonstrates the dangers involved in EMS systems and the need for prevention initiatives. It also demonstrates the variability among EMS communities. Even though all EMS systems are similar, individual services (communities) have different risk factors and different prevention priorities.

The Four Es equally apply to EMS practitioners. Education programs enhance wellness, prevent back injury, and increase awareness of the potential for violent patients. Enforcement programs introduce mandatory fitness programs and establish protocols to safely and effectively handle violent patients. Engineering initiatives address increasing seat belt use in the back of the ambulance by evaluating the position of equipment and location of the seat. Preemployment screening and physical strengthening help to reduce back injury.

A small-scale, in-house injury prevention program may reap rewards beyond the most important outcome of improved employee health. Small successes lay the groundwork for participation in larger, more complicated endeavors. They provide a valuable on-the-job learning tool about injury prevention for all employees. In addition, in-house prevention programs provide an introduction of the EMS system to other public health agencies in the community that assist with in-house program implementation and evaluation.

SUMMARY

- The most efficient and effective method to combat injury is to prevent it from happening in the first place.
- Illness and injury are similar. Both require the presence of the three elements of the epidemiological triad: host, agent, and environment.
- The Haddon Matrix helps predict injury risk by examining the three factors of the epidemiological triad during each event phase—pre-event, event, and post-event.
- According to the Swiss cheese model, every hazard has a trajectory, and a series of failures generally must occur for there to be subsequent harm.
- Injury is classified as intentional or unintentional.

- Because of economic, social, and developmental issues, the causes of injury-related death vary from country to country and even region to region within the same country.
- Injury is the leading killer of Americans between ages 1 and 44 years. It is responsible for more years of potential life lost than any other cause of death.
- Intimate partner violence is defined as physical violence, sexual violence, psychological aggressions, or stalking by a current or former intimate partner. Practitioners must report any suspicions of intimate partner violence to the appropriate law enforcement agency.
- Injury prevention programs seek to bring about a change in knowledge, attitude, and behavior on the part of a previously identified segment of society.

SUMMARY (CONTINUED)

- Most injury prevention strategies are either active (requiring the cooperation of the person being protected) or passive (not requiring conscious effort).
- The Four Es of injury prevention are education, enforcement, engineering, and equity.
- A public health approach creates a community-based coalition to combat a community-based disease through a four-step process: (1) surveillance, (2) risk factor identification, (3) intervention evaluation, and (4) implementation.

- Prehospital care practitioners can take a more active role in the development of communitywide injury prevention programs. They can use their role model status to deliver important prevention messages and should take advantage of "teachable moments."
- Self-injury prevention is the most valuable service a prehospital care practitioner can provide.

SCENARIO RECAP

You and your partner are on the scene of a motor vehicle collision and are working to rapidly extricate a patient who is overweight from the driver's seat of his vehicle. He was unrestrained in the vehicle during the collision. You and your partner are both wearing approved safety vests over your work gear because you are near the roadway. Law enforcement is on the scene to provide traffic control, and the ambulance is parked to maximize your protection from oncoming vehicles. The patient is packaged properly and secured onto your motorized stretcher, which is being used due to the patient's weight. The motorized stretcher allows you and your partner to lift the patient safely into the ambulance without putting excess strain on your bodies.

Once inside the ambulance, you secure yourself in the rear-facing chair and continue care of the patient while your partner maneuvers the vehicle safely into the lane and drives to the hospital. The ambulance arrives safely at the hospital, and you transfer the patient to the care of the ED staff.

While completing paperwork after the call, you consider the overall national injury and death statistics for prehospital care practitioners. You realize that thanks to the careful attention to all aspects of injury prevention that you and your partner demonstrated, the call was concluded safely for everyone involved.

- Is accident prevention a realistic approach in preventing injury and death in motor vehicle collisions and other causes of traumatic injury?
- Is there evidence that compliance with seat belt and safety seat laws has an impact in preventing injury and death?
- As prehospital care practitioners, what can we do to prevent deaths and injuries from motor vehicle collisions?

SCENARIO SOLUTION

You and your partner remained safe while at the motor vehicle collision scene because you recalled and followed your department's safety protocols. You were aware that flashing or strobe lights are not always sufficient in attracting drivers' attention, so you wore your approved reflective vests to be more visible to other drivers while operating at the scene. You also recalled and followed proper lifting techniques and safety procedures, and you ensured your safety by wearing a seat belt while in the treatment area of the ambulance.

In addition, your department recently updated the reflective chevron design on the rear of the ambulance to enhance the visibility of the ambulance from a distance. To enhance night-time visibility, red and white lights on the exterior of the ambulance were replaced by additional blue lights. These measures have all proven to be very helpful in reducing scene visibility concerns and ensuring crew member safety.

References

1. National Academy of Sciences/National Research Council. *Accidental Death and Disability: The Neglected Disease of Modern Society.* National Academy of Sciences/National Research Council; 1966.
2. National Center for Health Statistics. *Health, United States, 2000—With Adolescent Health Chartbook.* National Center for Health Statistics; 2000.
3. National Center for Health Statistics, Centers for Disease Control and Prevention. All injuries. Updated January 22, 2022. Accessed March 2, 2022. https://www.cdc.gov/nchs/fastats/injury.htm
4. National Center for Health Statistics, Centers for Disease Control and Prevention. Accidents or unintentional injuries. Reviewed January 24, 2022. Accessed March 2, 2022. https://www.cdc.gov/nchs/fastats/accidental-injury.htm
5. National Safety Council. International overview. Accessed March 2, 2022. https://injuryfacts.nsc.org/international/international-overview/
6. Peden M, McGee K, Sharma G. *The Injury Chart Book: A Graphical Overview of the Global Burden of Injuries.* World Health Organization; 2002.
7. Centers for Disease Control and Prevention, National Center for Injury Prevention and Control. Ten leading causes of death by age group, United States—2018. Accessed March 2, 2022. https://www.cdc.gov/injury/images/lc-charts/leading_causes_of_death_by_age_group_2018_1100w850h.jpg
8. National Safety Council. Injury Facts: International overview. Published 2020. Accessed April 7, 2022. https://injuryfacts.nsc.org/international/international-overview/#:~:text=According%20to%20the%20World%20Health,3%2C159%2C000%20died%20from%20preventable%20injuries%20
9. National Highway Traffic Safety Administration, U.S. Department of Health and Human Services, Health Resources and Services Administration, Maternal and Child Health Bureau. *Emergency Medical Services Agenda for the Future.* National Highway Traffic Safety Administration; 1999.
10. EMS Agenda 2050 Technical Expert Panel.. *EMS Agenda 2050: A People-Centered Vision for the Future of Emergency Medical Services* (Report No. DOT HS 812 664). National Highway Traffic Safety Administration; 2019.
11. Jaslow D, Ufberg J, Marsh R. Primary injury prevention in an urban EMS system. *J Emerg Med.* 2003;25(2):167-170. doi: 10.1016/s0736-4679(03)00165-3. PMID: 12902003
12. Martinez R. Injury control: a primer for physicians. *Ann Emerg Med.* 1990;19:72-77.
13. Christoffel T, Gallagher SS. *Injury Prevention and Public Health: Practical Knowledge, Skills, and Strategies.* Aspen; 1999.
14. Reason J. Human error: models and management. *BMJ.* 2000;320:768-770.
15. Cohen L, Miller T, Sheppard MA, Gordon E, Gantz T, Atnafou R. Bridging the gap: bringing together intentional and unintentional injury prevention efforts to improve health and well being. *J Safety Res.* 2003;34:473-483.
16. Centers for Disease Control and Prevention. Road traffic injuries and deaths: a global problem. Last reviewed December 14, 2020. Accessed March 2, 2022. https://www.cdc.gov/injury/features/global-road-safety/index.html
17. World Health Organization. Injuries and violence. Published March 19, 2021. Accessed March 2, 2022. https://www.who.int/news-room/fact-sheets/detail/injuries-and-violence
18. World Health Organization. Global status report on road safety 2018: summary. World Health Organization; 2018. https://www.who.int/publications/i/item/9789241565684
19. World Health Organization. Burns. https://www.who.int/news-room/fact-sheets/detail/burns#:~:text=Burns%20are%20a%20global%20public,and%20South%2DEast%20Asia%20regions. Published March 5, 2018. Accessed March 28, 2022.
20. World Health Organization. Drowning. Published April 27, 2021. Accessed March 2, 2022. https://www.who.int/news-room/fact-sheets/detail/drowning
21. World Health Organization. Falls. Published April 26, 2021. Accessed March 2, 2022. https://www.who.int/news-room/fact-sheets/detail/falls
22. World Health Organization. Guidelines for establishing a poison centre. Published January 14, 2021. Accessed March 2, 2022. https://www.who.int/publications/i/item/9789240009523
23. World Health Organization. Snakebite envenoming. Published May 17, 2021. Accessed March 2, 2022. https://www.who.int/news-room/fact-sheets/detail/snakebite-envenoming
24. Institute for Health Metrics and Evaluation. Interpersonal violence: level 3 cause. Accessed March 2, 2022. https://www.healthdata.org/results/gbd_summaries/2019/interpersonal-violence-level-3-cause
25. World Health Organization. Suicide. Published June 17, 2021. Accessed March 2, 2022. https://www.who.int/news-room/fact-sheets/detail/suicide
26. Federal Highway Administration. *Highway statistics, 2019.* U.S. Department of Transportation; 2020.
27. Department of Transportation, National Highway Traffic Safety Administration. Seat belts. Accessed March 2, 2022. https://www.nhtsa.gov/risky-driving/seat-belts
28. Department of Transportation, National Highway Traffic Safety Administration. Drunk driving. Accessed March 2, 2022. https://www.nhtsa.gov/risky-driving/drunk-driving
29. Centers for Disease Control and Prevention, National Center for Injury Prevention and Control. Fatal injury data. Web-based Injury Statistics Query and Reporting System (WISQARS). Reviewed February 10, 2022. Accessed March 2, 2022. https://www.cdc.gov/injury/wisqars/fatal.html

30. Centers for Disease Control and Prevention, National Center for Injury Prevention and Control. Injuries and violence are leading causes of death. Reviewed February 28, 2022. Accessed March 2, 2022. https://www.cdc.gov /injury/wisqars/animated-leading-causes.html

31. Centers for Disease Control and Prevention. Drug overdose deaths. Reviewed March 3, 2021. Accessed March 2, 2022. https://www.cdc.gov/drugoverdose/deaths /index.html

32. U.S. Department of Health and Human Services. Injury and violence. Accessed March 2, 2022. https://www.healthy people.gov/2020/leading-health-indicators/2020-lhi-topics /Injury-and-Violence

33. Organisation for Economic Co-operation and Development. Potential years of life lost. Accessed March 2, 2022. https://data.oecd.org/healthstat/potential-years-of-life -lost.htm

34. Peterson C, Miller GF, Barnett SB, Florence C. Economic Cost of Injury—United States, 2019. *Morb Mortal Wkly Rep.* 2021;70:1655-1659.

35. Houry D. Saving lives and protecting people from injuries and violence. *Ann Emerg Med.* 2016 Aug;68(2):230-232.

36. National Center for Injury Prevention and Control, Division of Violence Prevention. Intimate partner violence: definitions. Reviewed October 9, 2021. Accessed March 2, 2022. https://www.cdc.gov/violenceprevention/intimate partnerviolence/index.html

37. Smith SG, Zhang X, Basile KC, Merrick MT, Wang J, Kresnow M, Chen J. National Intimate Partner and Sexual Violence survey: 2015 data brief – updated release. Published November 2018. Accessed March 2, 2022. https://www.cdc.gov/violenceprevention/pdf/2015data -brief508.pdf

38. VanDale K. Sleep deprivation in EMS. Fire Engineering website. Published February 1, 2013. Accessed March 2, 2022. https://www.fireengineering.com/firefighting/sleep -deprivation-in-ems/

39. Patterson PD, Weaver MD, Frank RC, et al. Association between poor sleep, fatigue, and safety outcomes in emergency medical services providers. *Prehosp Emerg Care.* 2012;16:86-97.

40. Reichard A, Marsh S, Moore P. Fatal and nonfatal injuries among emergency medical technicians and paramedics. *Prehosp Emerg Care.* 2011;15(4):511-517.

41. Page D. Studies show dangers of working in EMS. *Journal of Emergency Medical Services.* Published October 31, 2011. Accessed March 2, 2022. https://www.jems.com /operations/studies-show-dangers-working-ems/

42. Garrison HG. Keeping rescuers safe. *Ann Emerg Med.* 2002;40:633-635.

43. Erich J. Creating a culture of safety. *EMS World.* 2014; 42(1):15-16.

44. Centers for Disease Control and Prevention. Up to 40 percent of annual deaths from each of five leading US causes are preventable. Published May 1, 2014. Accessed March 2, 2022. https://www.cdc.gov/media/releases/2014 /p0501-preventable-deaths.html

45. National EMS Advisory Council. Strategy for a national EMS culture of safety DRAFT 3.1. Published May 16, 2012. Accessed March 2, 2022. https://www .ems.gov/pdf/nemsac/may2012/ems_culture_of_safety -draft_3-1_05162012.pdf

46. Mertz KJ, Weiss HB. Changes in motorcycle-related head injury deaths, hospitalizations, and hospital charges following repeal of Pennsylvania's mandatory motorcycle helmet law. *Am J Public Health.* 2008;98(8):1464-1467.

47. Bledsoe GH, Li G. Trends in Arkansas motorcycle trauma after helmet law repeal. *South Med J.* 2005;98(4):436-440.

48. Chenier TC, Evans L. Motorcyclist fatalities and the repeal of mandatory helmet wearing laws. *Accid Anal Prev.* 1987;19(2):133-139.

49. Centers for Disease Control and Prevention. Ambulance crash-related injuries among emergency medical services workers—United States, 1991–2002. *Morb Mortal Wkly Rep.* 2003;52(8):154-156.

50. Todd KH. *Accidents Aren't: Proposal for Evaluation of an Injury Prevention Curriculum for EMS Providers—A Grant Proposal to the National Association of State EMS Directors.* Department of Emergency Medicine, Emory University School of Medicine; 1998.

51. National Association of State EMS Officials. 2020 National Emergency Medical Services Assessment. Published May 27, 2020. Accessed March 2, 2022. https://nasemso .org/wp-content/uploads/2020-National-EMS-Assessment _Reduced-File-Size.pdf

52. Kinnane JM, Garrison HG, Coben JH, et al. Injury prevention: is there a role for out-of-hospital emergency medical services? *Acad Emerg Med.* 1997;4(4):306-312.

53. California Paramedic Foundation. EPIC Medics. Accessed March 2, 2022. https://caparamedic.org/epic-medics/

54. Hawkins ER, Brice JH, Overby BA. Welcome to the world: findings from an emergency medical services pediatric injury prevention program. *Pediatr Emerg Care.* 2007;23(11):790-795.

55. Griffiths K. Best practices in injury prevention. *J Emerg Med Serv.* 2002;27(8):60-74.

56. Krimston J, Griffiths K. Best practices in injury prevention. *J Emerg Med Serv.* 2003;28(9):66-83.

57. Jaslow D, Ufberg J, Marsh R. Primary injury prevention in an urban EMS system. *J Emerg Med.* 2003;25(2):167-170.

58. U.S. Department of Labor. Emergency medical technicians and paramedics. In: U.S. Department of Labor, Bureau of Labor Statistics, eds. *Occupational Outlook Handbook, 2004–2005 Edition.* U.S. Department of Labor; 2004.

59. Federal Emergency Management Agency, U.S. Fire Administration. *EMS Safety: Techniques and Applications.* International Association of Fire Fighters, FEMA contract EMW-91-C-3592. Federal Emergency Management Agency; 1994.

60. Studnek JR, Fernandez AR. Characteristics of emergency medical technicians involved in ambulance crashes. *Prehosp Disaster Med.* 2008;23(5):432-437.

61. Patterson PD, Higgins JS, Van Dongen HPA, et al. Evidence-based guidelines for fatigue risk management in

emergency medical services. *Prehosp Emerg Care*. 2018;22 (Suppl 1):89-101.

62. Kilpatrick D. Athletic trainers: a new hope for firefighter recovery. Fire Engineering website. Published December 1, 2016. Accessed March 2, 2022. https://www.fireengineering.com/firefighting/athletic-trainers-a-new-hope-for-firefighter-recovery/

63. Kilpatrick D. The cost efficiency of athletic trainers. Firehouse website. Published December 1, 2016. Accessed March 2, 2022. https://www.firehouse.com/safety-health/health-fitness/article/12268580/the-cost-efficiency-of-athletic-trainers

Suggested Reading

American College of Surgeons Committee on Trauma. *Advanced Trauma Life Support, Student Course Manual*. 10th ed. American College of Surgeons; 2018.

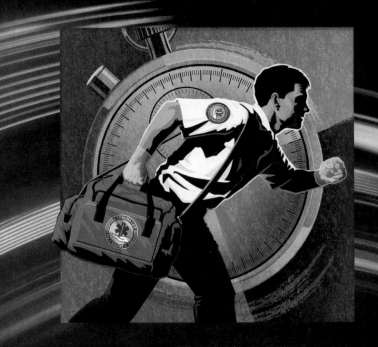

Mass Casualties and Terrorism

CHAPTER **17**

Disaster Management

Lead Editor
Faizan H. Arshad, MD

CHAPTER OBJECTIVES

At the completion of this chapter, you will be able to do the following:

- Identify the five phases of the disaster cycle.
- Explain the comprehensive emergency management process.
- Discuss common pitfalls encountered during disaster response.

- Understand and discuss the components that constitute the medical response to a disaster.
- Recognize how disaster response may affect the psychological well-being of prehospital care practitioners.

SCENARIO

You are dispatched to a local high school that has been placed into service as a shelter following community-wide flooding from a large weather event. Your community's mayor and other dignitaries are in attendance at the school to address the community's concerns about closed roads and power outages.

While en route to the scene, dispatch updates you there are multiple reports of numerous casualties after the collapse of elevated bleachers in the gym that were being used as seating during the mayor's community address. Police and fire resources are also en route to the scene but have limited available resources due to other ongoing weather-related public safety incidents.

- What safety and security concerns would you expect to encounter?
- What triage system should be utilized?
- How should the response to this incident be organized?

INTRODUCTION

Disasters, in comparison to traditional emergency response, can be time consuming, may encompass multiple agencies, and include medical and psychosocial challenges. Furthermore, there may be prolonged phases to disaster response, including rebuilding infrastructure, that may continue well after the initial response has concluded.

The United Nations Office for Disaster Risk Reduction defines a disaster as follows:

> A serious disruption of the functioning of a community or a society causing widespread human, material, economic, or environmental losses which exceed the ability of the affected community or society to cope using its own resources.[1]

This broad definition does not provide specific reference to medical issues or the emergency medical response but is inclusive of the overall community and sociopolitical response to any disaster of significant magnitude.

From a medical perspective, the definition can be further refined. A disaster is defined as a situation in which the number of patients presenting for medical assistance exceeds the capacity of the emergency medical system with the usual resources at hand and thus requires additional, and sometimes external, assistance.[2] This concept applies to all medical care settings, including both hospitals and the prehospital setting. This situation is commonly referred to as a **mass-casualty incident (MCI)**. The abbreviation MCI has also been used to refer to "multiple-casualty incidents," which are events that involve more than one casualty but may be handled with standard local resources. In this text, MCI will be used to refer to mass-casualty incidents that overwhelm the community's available resources.

It is important to understand that these definitions illustrate two key concepts: (1) A disaster is not dependent on a specific number of victims, and (2) the impact of the disaster exceeds the available resources of the medical response and there is typically disruption of infrastructure. Simply stated, all MCIs are a component of a disaster, but not all disasters are MCIs.

It is difficult to predict the time, location, or complexity of the next disaster. Nevertheless, all disasters, regardless of etiology, have similar medical and public health consequences. Disasters differ in the degree to which these consequences occur and the degree to which they disrupt the medical and public health infrastructure of the disaster locale. A guiding principle of disaster response is to do the greatest good for the greatest number of people with the resources available. This objective differs from "conventional" nondisaster-related medical care, which is to do the greatest good for the individual patient.

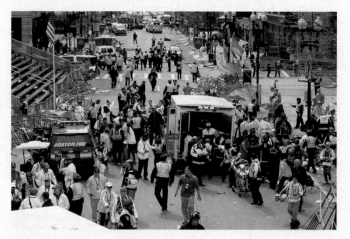

Figure 17-1 Mass-casualty management at the scene of the Boston Marathon bombings.
© Charles Krupa/File/AP Photo

Natural disasters and human-made disasters, including acts of terror, encompass the spectrum of possible disaster threats. **Weapons of mass destruction (WMDs)**, which create large numbers of casualties while possibly also contaminating the environment, represent particularly ominous threats. (See Chapter 18, *Explosions and Weapons of Mass Destruction*.)

An approach to disaster management that is consistent, principled, and ideally, rehearsed is becoming the accepted practice worldwide. This strategy forms the framework for **mass-casualty incident (MCI) response**. The primary objective of the MCI response is to reduce the morbidity (injury and disease) and mortality (death) caused by the disaster. All prehospital care providers need to incorporate the key principles of MCI response into their training, given the potential complexity posed by patient care, scene management, and continued operational threats (**Figure 17-1**).

The Disaster Cycle

A theoretical framework has been proposed for disasters. The sequence of events in a disaster can be analyzed using this framework. This conceptual description not only provides an overview of the natural history of a disaster, it also provides the basis for the development of the response process.[3] The five phases of disaster response are described as follows:

1. The **quiescent period**, or **interdisaster period**, represents the time in between disasters or MCIs during which risk assessment and mitigation activities should be undertaken and plans for the response to potential events are developed, tested, and implemented. Intelligence gathering is also a component of the interdisaster period.

2. The second phase is the **prodrome (predisaster) phase**, or **warning phase**. At this point, a specific event has been identified as impending or highly likely to occur. This could reflect a natural weather condition (e.g., hurricane) or the active unfolding of a hostile and potentially violent situation, such as an active shooter or hostile assailant event. During this period, specific steps may be taken to mitigate the effects of the ensuing events. These defensive maneuvers may include such actions as fortifying physical structures, initiating evacuation plans, and mobilizing public health resources to mount a post-event response. It must be noted, however, that not all incidents will have a warning phase. For example, an earthquake may occur without warning.

3. The third phase is the **impact phase**, or the occurrence of the actual event. During this period, there is often little that can be done to alter the impact or outcome of what is occurring.

4. The fourth phase is the **rescue, emergency, or relief phase**, which is the period immediately following the impact. The response occurs during this phase, and appropriate management and intervention can help reduce otherwise preventable deaths. The skills of emergency medical responders, prehospital care practitioners, rescue teams, and medical support services will be brought to bear to maximize the number of survivors of the event.

5. The fifth phase is the **recovery or reconstruction phase**, during which community resources are called upon to endure, emerge from, and rebuild after the effects of the disaster through the coordinated efforts of the medical, public health, and community infrastructure (physical and political). This period is by far the longest, sometimes lasting months, and perhaps years, before a community fully recovers.

Understanding the disaster cycle (**Figure 17-2**) allows prehospital care practitioners to evaluate the preparations that have been made in anticipation of the likely hazards and events encountered in their community. After an incident has occurred, there follows an opportunity for critical evaluation of the after-action report and assessment of the practitioner's individual response, as well as the response of others, to determine the efficiency of the process and identify areas for future improvement. These concepts apply to all disasters, regardless of size.

The duration of each phase of the disaster life cycle will vary depending on the frequency with which incidents occur in a given community, the nature of the incident, and the degree to which the community is prepared.

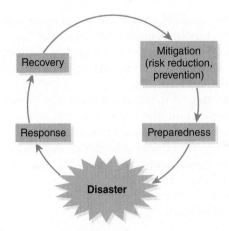

Figure 17-2 The life cycle of a disaster. The quiescent phase is represented by the mitigation and preparedness arrows. The warning phase comes just before the impact of the event. It is followed by the rescue and recovery phases.
© National Association of Emergency Medical Technicians (NAEMT)

For example, the quiescent period in some locations can be extremely long (measured in years), whereas in other communities it may be measured in months or days (e.g., hurricanes). The southeastern states in the United States prepare for hurricanes annually with a quiescent period between events of approximately 6 to 8 months. In contrast, although hurricanes have struck the New England states, they are a rare event with a longer quiescent period. Similarly, the rescue and recovery phases can vary significantly depending on the particular incident. The rescue and recovery from something like a plane crash will be measured in hours, or sometimes days, whereas the rescue and recovery from a major flood may take weeks to months, or longer.

Comprehensive Emergency Management

Knowledge of the life cycle of disasters can be used to implement the steps involved in **comprehensive emergency management**. Comprehensive emergency management defines the specific steps needed to manage an incident and consists of five components: mitigation, preparedness, response, recovery, and prevention.

- **Mitigation:** This component of emergency management generally occurs during the quiescent phase of the disaster cycle. Potential hazards or likely etiologies of MCIs in the community are identified and assessed. Steps are then taken to prevent these hazards from causing an incident or to minimize their effect should something unexpected occur.

- **Preparedness:** This step involves the advance identification of an incident and the specific supplies needed, including the needs of the population, durable medical equipment for persons with special needs; response equipment; personnel that would be needed to manage the incident; and the specific incident action plan that would be employed if a particular scenario unfolds.

- **Response:** This phase involves the activation and deployment of the various resources identified in the preparedness phase in order to manage an active incident. Traditional emergency prehospital practitioners typically operate during this period.
- **Recovery:** This component addresses the actions necessary to return the community to its preincident functional status.

Although this process is typically applied to the management of a disaster, these same steps may also be used for the individual emergency preparedness of each emergency responder.

Personal Preparedness

Just as it is vital that each community and agency undertake a comprehensive planning process to be prepared for the challenges of a potential disaster, each prehospital care practitioner must be ready to face, on a personal and professional level, the many issues the disaster may present.

Prehospital care practitioners must have a complete understanding of the many potential hazards that may accompany a disaster response in advance of the actual incident and be prepared to take the necessary steps to protect themselves from these dangers. Gaps in knowledge about such issues as building collapse, hazardous materials incidents, active shooter/hostile events, WMDs and their potential effects on patient treatment, appropriate personal protective equipment, and overall incident management should be identified in advance and addressed. Regular training and interagency drills are proactive ways to maintain skills and competencies and practice a concerted response with first responders of different disciplines.

Disasters may extend beyond a typical operating period, and prehospital care practitioners must discuss with their families their own roles, responsibilities, and potentially prolonged absence. This discussion includes preparing their families for what they should do and where they should go during such an event to ensure their safety. Just as the local emergency medical services (EMS) system procures supplies and equipment before a disaster, practitioners should ensure that adequate supplies are available at home to meet their families' needs (**Box 17-1, Box 17-2,** and **Box 17-3**). Practitioners should plan for who would care for children and pets during an extended tour

---

Box 17-1 Emergency Supply List

All homes should have some basic supplies on hand (at least 3 days' worth) for emergencies. The following is a list of some basic items that emergency supply kits should include. It is important that individuals review this list and consider where they live and the unique needs of their family in order to create an emergency supply kit that will meet their specific needs. Individuals should also consider having at least two emergency supply kits, one full kit at home and smaller portable kits in their workplace, vehicle, or other places where they spend time. Prescription medications are also an important aspect to consider when planning one's emergency kit.

- Water—1 gallon per person and pet, per day (3-day supply for evacuation, 2-week supply for home)
  - Consider storing more water than this for hot climates, for pregnant women, and for persons who are sick.
  - Consider adding an effective water filter.
- Food—nonperishable, easy-to-prepare items, including food for pets (3-day supply for evacuation, 2-week supply for home) (see Box 17-2)
  - Remember, it is better to have extra food that you can share than to run out of food during an emergency.

- Cell phone with chargers
- Battery-powered or hand-cranked National Oceanic and Atmospheric Administration (NOAA) weather radio with tone alert and extra batteries
- Flashlight and extra batteries
- First aid kit (see Box 17-3)
- Whistle to signal for help
- Dust mask, to help filter contaminated air, and plastic sheeting and duct tape to shelter in place
- Moist towelettes, garbage bags, and plastic ties for personal sanitation
- Wrench or pliers to turn off utilities (or multitool device that includes both)
- Can opener for food (if kit contains nonperishable food)
- Local maps

Additional items to consider adding to an emergency supply kit:

- *Items for infants*, including formula, diapers, bottles, pacifiers, powdered milk, and medications not requiring refrigeration
- *Items for seniors, persons with special needs, or anyone with serious allergies*, including special foods, denture items, extra eyeglasses, hearing

aid batteries, prescription and nonprescription medications that are regularly used, inhalers, and other essential equipment
- Prescription medications and glasses
- Important family documents such as copies of insurance policies, identification, important medical records, and bank account records in a waterproof, portable container
- Cash and change
- Emergency reference material such as a first aid book or information from www.ready.gov
- Sleeping bag or warm blanket for each person (Consider additional bedding if you live in a cold-weather climate.)
- Complete change of clothing, including a long-sleeved shirt, long pants, and sturdy shoes (Consider additional clothing if you live in a cold-weather climate.)
- Household chlorine bleach and medicine dropper (When diluted 9 parts water to 1 part bleach, bleach can be used as a disinfectant. In an emergency, you can use it to treat water by using 16 drops of regular household liquid bleach per gallon of water. Do not use bleaches that are scented or color safe or that have added cleaners.)
- Fire extinguisher (A-B-C type)
- Matches in a waterproof container
- Paper and pencil
- Entertainment—including games and books, favorite toys, and stuffed animals for small children
- Kitchen accessories—a manual can opener; mess kits or disposable cups, plates, and utensils; utility knife; salt and sugar; aluminum foil and plastic wrap; resealable plastic bags; paper towels
- Sanitation and hygiene items—shampoo, deodorant, toothpaste, toothbrushes, comb and brush, lip

balm, sunscreen, contact lenses and supplies, any medications regularly used, toilet paper, moist towelettes, soap, hand sanitizer, liquid detergent, feminine supplies, plastic garbage bags (heavy duty) and ties (for personal sanitation uses), medium-sized plastic bucket with tight lid, disinfectant, household chlorine bleach
- Needles and thread
- A map of the area marked with places you could go and their telephone numbers
- An extra set of keys and IDs—including keys for cars and any properties owned and copies of driver's licenses, passports, and work identification badges
- Copies of credit cards
- Copies of medical prescriptions
- A small tent, compass, and shovel

Pack the items in easy-to-carry containers, such as a 5-gallon bucket, label the containers clearly, and store them where they would be easily accessible. Duffle bags, backpacks, and covered trash receptacles are good candidates for containers. In a disaster situation, a family may need access to the disaster supply kit quickly—whether sheltering at home or evacuating. Ensuring that family vehicles are filled with gasoline and electric vehicles are charged will allow for immediate evacuation to a safe location. Following a disaster, having the right supplies can help a household endure home confinement or evacuation.

Make sure the needs of everyone who would use the kit are covered, including infants, seniors, and pets. It is a good idea to involve whoever may use the kit, including children, in assembling it. Kits should be updated yearly to account for children's growth and development as well as changes to prescriptions and review of expiration dates.

Data from Federal Emergency Management Agency. Ready America. n.d. www.ready.gov. https://www.ready.gov/kit; and Centers for Disease Control and Prevention. All-Hazards Preparedness Guide. n.d. https://www.cdc.gov/cpr/documents/AHPG_FINAL_March_2013.pdf

Box 17-2 Food Kit

- Store at least a 3-day supply of nonperishable food.
- Select foods that require no refrigeration, preparation, or cooking and little or no water.
- Pack a manual can opener and eating utensils.
- Avoid salty foods, as they will make you thirsty.
- Choose foods your family will eat.
- Suggested foods include the following:
  - Ready-to-eat canned meats, fruits, and vegetables
  - Protein or fruit bars
  - Dry cereal or granola
  - Peanut butter

- Dried fruit
- Nuts
- Crackers
- Canned juices
- Nonperishable pasteurized milk
- High-energy foods
- Vitamins
- Food for infants
- Comfort/stress foods
- Bring a propane stove or grill for cooking (with extra propane tank).

Data from Federal Emergency Management Agency. Ready America. n.d. www.ready.gov; and Centers for Disease Control and Prevention. Emergency preparedness and response. n.d. https://emergency.cdc.gov/

Box 17-3 First Aid Kit

In any emergency, a family member may be cut or burned or may suffer other injuries. An emergency kit should include the following:

- Two pairs of latex gloves or other sterile gloves (if anyone has latex allergies)
- Sterile dressings to stop bleeding
- Cleansing agent/soap and antibiotic towelettes to disinfect
- Antibiotic ointment to prevent infection
- Burn ointment to prevent infection
- Adhesive bandages in a variety of sizes
- Eye wash solution to flush the eyes or to use as a general decontaminant
- Thermometer
- Daily prescription medications such as insulin, cardiac medications, and asthma inhalers (Periodically rotate medicines to account for expiration dates.)
- Prescribed medical supplies such as glucose and blood pressure monitoring equipment and supplies
- Any durable medical equipment like canes or walkers. Special thought should be given to powering durable medical equipment during a power outage (e.g., ventilator, continuous positive airway pressure [CPAP] machine, scooter, chair lift).

Other useful things to include:

- Cell phone with charger
- Scissors
- Tweezers
- Tube of petroleum jelly or other lubricant
- Nonprescription medications:
  - Aspirin or nonaspirin pain reliever (acetaminophen)
  - Antidiarrheal medication
  - Antacid (for upset stomach)
  - Laxative

Data from Federal Emergency Management Agency. Ready America. n.d. www.ready.gov; and Centers for Disease Control and Prevention. Emergency preparedness and response. n.d. https://emergency.cdc.gov/

of duty. Taking these actions will help reassure both the practitioner and family members—allowing the practitioner to continue operating during a disaster if needed, especially during an extended response.

An additional resource with information about personal and family preparation in the event of a disaster, including how to create a family communication plan, is the Ready campaign sponsored by the Federal Emergency Management Agency (FEMA), available online at www.ready.gov.

Mass-Casualty Incident Management

An important premise of disaster response is to remember that all disasters are local. The variability of available resources will vary tremendously from urban, to suburban, to rural locales. In general, the severity and diversity of injuries, in addition to the total number of victims, will be major factors in determining whether an MCI requires resources and assistance from outside the impacted community.

Today's complex disasters, especially those involving terrorism and WMDs (chemical, biologic, radiologic, or nuclear), may result in an austere and/or hazardous environment. An **austere environment** is a setting in which resources, supplies, equipment, personnel, transportation, and other aspects of the physical, political, social, and economic environments are limited. As a result of these limitations, constraints on the availability and adequacy of immediate care for the population can be variable, again, depending on one's location and resource infrastructure. Prehospital care practitioners should anticipate not being able to offer the same level of care provided to an individual sick or injured patient when responding to a disaster. Meaningful interventions provided expediently to patients who meet specific criteria are most likely to optimize outcomes for salvageable patients.[4]

Emergency medical concerns related to MCIs include the following five elements:

- *Search and rescue.* This activity involves the process of systematically looking for those individuals who have been impacted by an event and rescuing them from hazardous situations. Depending on the situation, this often requires the use of specially trained teams, particularly when extrication issues are involved.
- *Triage and initial stabilization.* This is the process of systematically evaluating and categorizing each victim according to the seriousness of the injury or illness and providing initial medical care to address immediate life- or limb-threatening concerns.
- *Patient tracking.* This is a system by which patients are uniquely identified and followed through their initial contact with search and rescue, evacuation, triage and transport, and ultimately disposition to definitive care.
- *Definitive medical care.* This component involves the provision of the specific medical care needed to treat the patient's injuries. This care will usually be provided at hospitals; however, alternate care facilities may be used in major events when hospitals are overwhelmed with casualties or when hospitals have been directly impacted and/or damaged by the incident.

- *Evacuation.* This is the process of transporting disaster victims and injured patients away from the disaster site, either to a safe location or to a definitive care facility.

Public health concerns related to MCIs include the following:

- Water (ensuring a supply of safe, potable water)
- Food (ideally nonperishable and needing neither refrigeration nor cooking)
- Shelter (a place for cover, protection, and refuge)
- Sanitation (protection from contact with human and animal feces, solid waste, and wastewater)
- Security and safety
- Transportation
- Communication (dissemination of information to the affected population, including information about communicable diseases)
- Endemic and epidemic diseases (Endemic diseases are ones that are always present in a given area or population but that usually occur with low frequency, whereas an epidemic disease is one that develops and spreads rapidly to the population at risk.)

Both medical and public health disaster-response activities are coordinated through one organizational structure: the incident command system.

The National Incident Management System

The U.S. National Incident Management System (NIMS) was developed to provide a template for a comprehensive nationwide, systematic approach to managing an incident, regardless of cause, size, location, or complexity. NIMS offers a set of preparedness concepts and principles for all hazards and events. It outlines the essential principles for a common operating structure and interoperability of communications and information management systems. It also provides standardized resource management procedures. NIMS uses the incident command system to oversee the direct response to an incident.

Incident Command System

Many different organizations may participate in the response to a disaster. The **incident command system (ICS)** was created to allow different types of agencies (fire, police, EMS, etc.) and multiple jurisdictions of similar agencies (e.g., city, county, state) to work together effectively, using a common language and organizational structure to manage the response to a disaster or other major incident (**Figure 17-3**). (Further information can be found in Chapter 5, *Scene Management.*) Representatives from the various responding agencies will usually come together

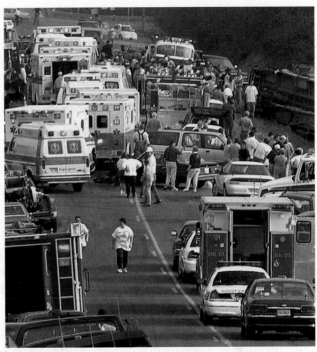

Figure 17-3 The incident command system (ICS) allows integration of fire, police, and EMS assets at a disaster scene.
© David Crigger/Bristol Herald Courier/AP Photo

in an incident command post to facilitate interagency communications and decision making and work together to unify the command process.

The ICS recognizes that, regardless of the specific nature of the incident or the primary responding agency (police, fire, or medical), there are a number of functions that must always happen. The ICS is organized around these necessary functions. Its components are:

- Command
- Safety officer
- Information officer
- Liaison officer
  - Planning
  - Logistics
  - Operations
  - Finance

These functions apply in varying degrees to all incidents and are now used in medical settings of all types, from prehospital to in-hospital, to organize the response to a disaster.

From a medical perspective, several important ICS principles will help during an MCI response:

1. ICS must be established early, preferably upon arrival of the first emergency responder to the scene. Establishing command is an important first step for any responder, and it is important to remember command can be transitioned to supervising officers as they arrive on scene.

2. Medical and public health responders, often tasked with working independently, should implement the principles of ICS management to better integrate their response with other agencies during an MCI.

3. Implementing ICS will allow for the effective integration of the medical response within the overall response to the incident.

Detailed information and training about the ICS is available on the FEMA website.[5]

Characteristics of the Incident Command System

An ICS provides a standard, professional, organized approach to managing emergency incidents. The use of an ICS enables an emergency response agency to operate more safely and effectively. A standardized approach facilitates and coordinates the use of resources from multiple agencies, working toward common objectives. It also eliminates the need to develop a unique approach for each situation, saving valuable time during an MCI or disaster. While often thought of in reference to larger events, the ICS can also be used during everyday MCIs that occur more frequently in our local communities and require the integration of multiple first responder agencies. For example, traffic events involving two to three vehicles are an example of an everyday MCI.

Effective management of incidents requires an organizational structure to provide both a hierarchy of authority and responsibility, as well as to establish formal channels of communications. Through the use of the command structure, the specific responsibilities and authority of everyone in the organization are clearly delineated and predefined, allowing heterogeneous groups to operate together with greater ease.

Jurisdictional Authority

Jurisdictional authority is usually not a problem at an incident with a single focus. Matters can become more complicated when several jurisdictions are involved or multiple agencies within a single jurisdiction have authority for various aspects of the incident. When there are overlapping responsibilities, the ICS may employ a **unified command**. This approach brings representatives of different agencies together to work on one plan and ensures that all actions are fully coordinated. *Command*, although the chosen term of the ICS, is perhaps misleading. It is important to remember that incidents are managed; personnel are commanded. *Incident command*, whether conducted by an individual or through unified command, is a management and leadership position. The command structure is responsible for setting strategic objectives and maintaining a comprehensive understanding of the impact of an incident as well as identifying the

strategies required to manage the scene effectively. The command function is structured in one of two ways: single or unified.

Single command is the most traditional command function and leads to the term **incident commander**. When an incident occurs within a single jurisdiction, and when there is no jurisdictional or functional agency overlap, a single incident commander should be identified and designated with overall incident management responsibility by the appropriate jurisdictional authority. This does not mean that other agencies do not respond or do not have a role in supporting the management of the incident.

Single command is best used when a single discipline in a single jurisdiction is responsible for the strategic objectives associated with managing the incident. Single command also is appropriate in the later stages of an incident that was initially managed through unified command. Over time, as many incidents stabilize, the strategic objectives become increasingly focused within a single jurisdiction or discipline. In this situation, it is appropriate to transition from unified command to single command.

It is also acceptable, if all agencies and jurisdictions agree, to designate a single incident commander in multiagency and multijurisdictional incidents. In this situation, however, command personnel should be carefully chosen. The incident commander is responsible for developing the strategic incident objectives on which the **incident action plans (IAPs)** will be based. An IAP is an oral or written plan containing general objectives that reflect the overall strategy for managing an incident. The incident commander is responsible for the IAP and all requests pertaining to the ordering and releasing of incident resources.

When multiple agencies with overlapping jurisdictions or legal responsibilities are involved in the same incident, unified command provides several advantages. In this approach, representatives from each agency cooperate to share command authority. They work together and are directly involved in the decision-making process. Unified command helps ensure cooperation, avoids confusion, and guarantees agreement on goals and objectives. An example of unified command could include a situation involving release of hazardous materials. The fire department has responsibility for fire control, containment of hazardous materials, and rescue; the police department has responsibility for evacuation and area security; and public works has responsibility for site clean-up.[6]

All-Risk and All-Hazard System

The ICS has evolved into an all-risk, all-hazard system that can be applied to manage resources at fires, floods, tornadoes, plane crashes, earthquakes, hazardous materials incidents, active shooter or hostile assailant events, public health emergencies, explosions, or any other type of emergency situation. This kind of system has also been used to manage many nonemergency events, such as large-scale public or mass-gathering events, that have similar requirements for command, control, and communications. The flexibility of the ICS enables the management structure to expand as needed, using whichever components are required. The operations of multiple agencies and organizations can be integrated smoothly in the management of the incident.

Everyday Applicability

An ICS can and should be used for everyday operations as well as major incidents. Command should be established at every incident. Regular use of the system ensures familiarity with standard procedures and terminology. It also increases the users' confidence in the system. Frequent use of ICS for routine situations makes it easier to apply to larger incidents.

Unity of Command

Unity of command is a management concept in which each person has only one direct supervisor. All orders and assignments come directly from that supervisor, and all reports are made to the same supervisor. This approach eliminates the confusion that can result when a person receives orders from more than one boss. Unity of command reduces delays in solving problems as well as the potential for life and property losses. By ensuring that each person has only one supervisor, unity of command can increase overall accountability, prevent freelancing, improve the flow of communication, assist with the coordination of operational issues, and enhance the safety of the practitioner. An ICS is not necessarily a rank-oriented system. The best-qualified person should be assigned to the appropriate level for each situation, even if that means a lower ranking individual is temporarily assigned to a higher level position. This concept is critical for the effective application of the system and must be embraced by all participants. Additionally, a critical component of NIMS is a series of national credentialing standards for ICS positions such as command and section chiefs in the operations, planning, logistics, and finance/administration sections.

Span of Control

Span of control refers to the number of subordinates who report to one supervisor at any level within the organization. Span of control relates to all levels of ICS—from the strategic level to the operational/tactical level as well as to the task level.

In most situations, one person can effectively supervise only three to seven people or resources. Because of the dynamic nature of emergency incidents, an individual who has command or supervisory responsibilities in an ICS normally should not directly supervise more than five people. The actual span of control should depend on the complexity of the incident and the nature of the work being performed. For example, in a complex incident involving hazardous materials, the span of control might be only three; during less intense operations, the span of control could be as high as seven.

Modular Organization

The ICS is designed to be flexible and modular. The ICS organizational structure—command, operations, planning, logistics, and finance/administration—is predefined, ready to be staffed and made operational as needed. Indeed, an ICS has often been characterized as an organizational toolbox, where only the tools needed for the specific incident are used. In an ICS, these tools consist of position titles, job descriptions, and an organizational structure that defines the relationships between positions. Some positions and functions are used frequently, whereas others are needed only for complex or unusual situations. Any position can be activated simply by assigning someone to the intended role.

Common Terminology

ICS promotes the use of common terminology both within an organization and among all agencies involved in emergency incidents. Common terminology means that each word has a single definition, and no two words used in managing an emergency incident have the same definition. Everyone uses the same terms to communicate the same thoughts, so everyone understands what is meant. Each job comes with one set of responsibilities, and everyone knows who is responsible for each duty.

Integrated Communications

Integrated communications ensure that everyone at an emergency can communicate with both supervisors and subordinates. The ICS must support communication up and down the chain of command at every level. A message must be able to move efficiently through the system from command down to the lowest level and from the lowest level up to the command level.

Consolidated Incident Action Plans

An ICS ensures that everyone involved in the incident is following one overall plan. Different components of the organization may perform different functions, but all of their efforts contribute to the same overarching goals and objectives. Everything that occurs is coordinated within the overall response. At smaller incidents, command develops an action plan and communicates the incident priorities, objectives, strategies, and tactics to all of the operating units. Representatives from all participating agencies meet regularly to develop and update the plan. In both large and small incidents, those involved in the incident understand what their specific roles are and how they fit into the overall plan.

Designated Incident Facilities

Designated incident facilities are assigned locations where specific functions are always performed. For example, command will always be based at the incident command post. The staging area, rehabilitation area, casualty collection point, treatment area, base of operations, and helispot (landing zone) are all designated areas where particular functions take place. The facilities required for the specific incident are established according to the specific IAP or a predefined ICS plan.

Resource Management

Resource management entails the use of a standard system of assigning and keeping track of the resources involved in the incident. The resource management system of the ICS keeps track of the various resource assignments. At large-scale incidents, units are often dispatched to a **staging area** rather than going directly to the incident location. A staging area is a location close to the incident scene where a number of units can be held in reserve, ready to be assigned if needed.

Organization of the Incident Command System

The ICS structure identifies a full range of duties, responsibilities, and functions that are performed at emergency incidents. Some components are used on almost every incident, whereas others apply to only the largest and most complex situations. The five major components of an ICS organization are command, operations, planning, logistics, and finance/administration.

An ICS organization chart may be basic or add complexity as greater components are needed. Each block on an ICS organization chart refers to a functional area or a job description. Positions are staffed as they are needed by incident command, who decides which additional components are needed for the given situation.

Command

On an ICS organization chart, the first component is **command** (**Figure 17-4**). Command is the only position in the ICS that must always be filled for every incident, as having a clearly defined leader has several advantages to incident management. Command is established when the first unit arrives on the scene and is maintained until the last unit leaves the scene.

In the ICS structure, command (either single or unified) is ultimately responsible for managing an incident

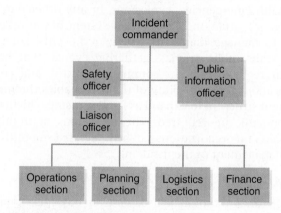

ICS Organizational Structure

Figure 17-4 The ICS organization chart.
© National Association of Emergency Medical Technicians (NAEMT)

and has the necessary authority to direct all activities at the incident scene. Command is directly responsible for the following tasks:

- Determining strategy
- Selecting incident tactics
- Setting the action plan
- Developing the ICS organization
- Managing resources and requesting additional resources
- Coordinating resource activities
- Providing for scene safety
- Releasing information about the incident
- Coordinating with outside agencies

Incident Command Post

The **incident command post** is the headquarters for the incident. Command functions are centered within the headquarters; thus, command and all direct support staff should always be located at the incident command post. The location should be broadcast to all units as soon as the post is established.

Relative to the incident scene, the command post should be in a protected nearby location. Often, for a major incident, the location is a special vehicle or building. This location enables the command staff to function without needless distractions or interruptions. For large incidents that are geographically spread out, the command post may be some distance from the emergency incident.

Command Staff

Individuals on the **command staff** perform functions that report directly to command and cannot be delegated to other major sections of the organization. The safety officer, liaison officer, and public information officer are always part of the command staff. In addition, aides, assistants, and advisors may be assigned to work directly for members of the command staff.

SAFETY OFFICER

The **safety officer** is responsible for ensuring that safety issues are managed effectively at the incident scene. This individual is the eyes and ears of command in terms of safety—identifying and evaluating hazardous conditions, watching out for unsafe practices, and ensuring that safety procedures are followed appropriately. The safety officer is appointed early during an incident. As the incident becomes more complex and the number of resources present at the scene increases, additional qualified personnel can be assigned as assistant safety officers.

LIAISON OFFICER

The **liaison officer** is a representative of command who serves as a point of contact for representatives from outside agencies. This member of the command staff is responsible for exchanging information with representatives from those agencies. During an active incident, command may not have time to meet directly with everyone who comes to the incident command post. The liaison officer functions as the representative of command under these circumstances, obtaining and providing information or directing people to the proper location or authority. The liaison area should be adjacent to, but not inside, the command post.

PUBLIC INFORMATION OFFICER

The **public information officer (PIO)** is responsible for gathering and releasing incident information to the news media and other appropriate agencies. At a major incident, communicating with the public and news media is very important for information dissemination. Because command must make managing the incident the top priority, the PIO serves as the contact person for media requests, which frees up command to concentrate on the incident. A media headquarters should be established near—but not within—the command post. The information presented to the media by the PIO needs to be approved by the incident commander. Employing a PIO also helps disseminate a consistent and coordinated message, especially during a complex event involving multiple agencies.

General Staff Functions

The incident commander has the overall responsibility for the entire incident command organization, although some elements of the incident commander's responsibilities can be handled by the command staff. When the incident is too large or too complex for one person to manage effectively, the incident commander may appoint someone to oversee parts of the operation. Everything that occurs at an emergency incident can be divided among the major functional components within ICS:

- Operations
- Planning
- Logistics
- Finance/administration

The chiefs of these four sections are known collectively as the **ICS general staff**. Command decides which (if any) of these four positions needs to be activated, when to activate it, and who should be placed in each position. Recall that the blocks on the ICS organization chart refer to functional areas or job descriptions, not to positions that must always be staffed.

The four section chiefs on the ICS general staff, when they are assigned, may run their operations from the main incident command post, although this structure is not required. At a large incident, the four functional sections may operate from different locations, but they will always be in direct contact with command.

Operations

The **operations section** is responsible for the management of all actions that are directly related to mitigating the incident. The operations section rescues any trapped individuals, treats any injured patients, and does whatever else is necessary to alleviate the emergency situation.

For smaller incidents, command may directly supervise the functions of the operations section. At complex incidents, a separate **operations section chief** takes on this responsibility so that command can focus on overall strategy while the operations section chief focuses on the tactics that are required to get the job done.

Operations are conducted in accordance with an IAP that outlines what the strategic objectives are and how emergency operations will be conducted. At most incidents, the IAP is relatively simple and can be expressed in a few words or phrases. The IAP for a large-scale incident can be a lengthy document that is regularly updated and used for daily briefings of the command staff.

Planning

The **planning section** is responsible for the collection, evaluation, dissemination, and use of information relevant to the incident. The planning section works with preincident plans, building construction drawings, maps, aerial photographs, diagrams, reference materials, and status boards. It is also responsible for developing and updating the IAP. The planning section develops what needs to be done by whom and identifies which resources are needed.

Command activates the planning section when information needs to be obtained, managed, and analyzed. The **planning section chief** reports directly to command. Individuals assigned to planning examine the current situation, review available information, predict the probable course of events, and prepare recommendations for strategies and tactics. The planning section also keeps track of resources at large-scale incidents and provides command with regular situation and resource status reports.

Logistics

The **logistics section** is responsible for providing supplies, services, facilities, and materials during the incident. The **logistics section chief** reports directly to command and serves as the supply officer for the incident. Among the responsibilities of this section are keeping vehicles fueled, providing food and refreshments for emergency responders, and arranging for specialized equipment.

Finance/Administration

The **finance/administration section** is the fourth major ICS component managed directly by command. This section is responsible for the accounting and financial aspects of an incident, as well as any legal issues that may arise in its aftermath. This function is not staffed at most incidents, because cost and accounting issues are typically addressed after the incident. Nevertheless, a finance/administration section may be needed at large-scale and long-term incidents that require immediate fiscal management, particularly when outside resources must be procured quickly. A finance/administration section may also be established during a natural disaster or during a hazardous materials incident where reimbursement may come from the shipper, carrier, chemical manufacturer, or insurance company. An excellent example of this is the response that most healthcare agencies launched to address the COVID-19 pandemic. Each individual hospital, nursing home, EMS agency, or other entity that used the NIMS structure likely established a finance/administration section to address the plethora of financial challenges associated with the response, including the need to track expenses for reimbursement from state or federal sources, some of which had not even been defined at the time the finance/administration section was first launched.

Medical Response to Disasters

While there may be multiple simultaneous goals of disaster response, the specific components of medical response, when combined, will help minimize the mortality and morbidity of victims of the event. Although these actions will be discussed sequentially in this chapter, it is important to remember that during an actual disaster many of the actions will occur concurrently (**Box 17-4**). Additionally, it is important to mention that the overall response may depend on the location of the incident and local protocols as well as available resources. The command structure or framework for response may vary considerably for international deployments.

Box 17-4 The Basic Steps in Medical Response to Disasters

Medical response to a disaster involves the following basic steps:

1. Notification and activation of EMS
2. Initial response
3. EMS response to the scene
4. Assessment of the situation
   a. Cause
   b. Number of casualties
   c. Additional resources
      i. Medical
      ii. Other
5. Communication of the situation and needs
6. Activation of the medical community
   a. Notification of receiving facilities
7. Search and rescue
8. Triage (treatment of airway and hemorrhage life threats)
9. Casualty collection
10. Treatment
11. Transport
12. Retriage

© National Association of Emergency Medical Technicians (NAEMT)

Initial Response

The first step is notification and activation of the EMS response system. This is usually performed by witnesses to the event who call the local emergency dispatch center seeking response by appropriate police, fire, and emergency medical agencies (**Figure 17-5**).

The first prehospital care practitioners to arrive at the incident have a number of important functions to fulfill that will set the stage for the entire emergency medical response. Counterintuitive to normal operations as a first responder, these actions do not include initiating patient care. The first practitioners on scene must perform an overall scene assessment. The goals of this assessment are to assess any potential hazards, estimate the total number of casualties, determine what additional medical resources will be needed at the scene, and evaluate whether any specialized equipment or personnel, such as search-and-rescue teams, will be required. Depending on the incident, practitioners should also be watchful for signs of a secondary device designed to intentionally harm emergency responders.

Once a basic assessment is complete, the information gathered should be efficiently communicated to the dispatch center, which will work to enlist the needed resources for a coordinated response. After this, the prehospital care practitioners shift their focus to identifying

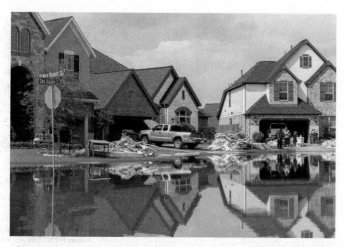

Figure 17-5 Natural disasters, such as hurricanes and floods, result in an influx of calls into local emergency dispatch centers. A view of the storm damage from Hurricane Harvey in Texas in 2017.

© Michelmond/Shutterstock

appropriate locations to perform triage, to collect casualties, and to stage incoming ambulances, personnel, and supplies so as not to impede rapid access and egress to and from the scene or to expose responding assets to potential hazards from the event.

It is also essential that the responding EMS agency notify the likely receiving hospitals in the community regarding the event, communicating the estimated number of casualties and their respective levels of criticality so that the receiving centers may prepare appropriately and consider activating their internal hospital-specific disaster plans. The field component of the disaster response is the first link in the overall chain of survival for the victims of a disaster, and EMS agencies are responsible for the timely notification to receiving centers.

Search and Rescue

At this point, the on-scene process of initiating patient care can begin. Generally, this will start with a search-and-rescue effort to identify and evacuate casualties from the impacted site to a safer location. The local population near a disaster site, as well as survivors themselves if they are able, are often the immediate search-and-rescue resource and may have already begun to search for victims before the arrival of any public safety personnel.[7] Experience has demonstrated that the local community may respond to a disaster site and begin the process of aiding victims.

Many countries and communities have developed formal, specialized search-and-rescue teams as an integral part of their national and local disaster-response plans. Members of these teams receive specialized

training in confined-space environments and are activated as needed for a particular event. These search-and-rescue units generally include the following:

- A cadre of medical specialists
- Technical specialists knowledgeable in hazardous materials, structural engineering, heavy equipment operation, and technical search-and-rescue methods (e.g., listening equipment, remote cameras)
- Trained canines and their handlers

Importantly, activation of specialized teams may take time, and in austere environments improvisation is often necessary. For example, at an MCI at a building site, local construction companies may provide valuable search-and-rescue assets including equipment, tools, and materials that can be used at the disaster site to assist in moving heavy debris.

Triage

As patients are identified and evacuated, they are brought to the triage site, where they can be assessed and a triage category assigned. The term *triage* is a French word that means "to sort." From a medical perspective, triage means sorting casualties based on the severity of their injuries. This process was first described in the early 1800s by Baron Dominique Larrey, who was surgeon-in-chief to Napoleon and left his legacy by developing the prototype ambulance during the Napoleonic Wars. Larrey stated:

> Those who are dangerously wounded should receive the first attention, without regard to rank or distinction. They who are injured in a less degree may wait until their brethren in arms, who are badly mutilated, have been operated on and dressed, otherwise the latter would not survive many hours; rarely, until the succeeding day.[8]

This concept, which has been further researched and expanded since Larrey, serves to prioritize patients who need immediate medical care and lifesaving interventions.

Triage is one of the most important missions of any disaster medical response. As noted previously, the objective of conventional triage in the nondisaster setting is to do the greatest good for the individual patient. This imperative usually means treating the sickest patient. The objective of mass-casualty triage is to do the greatest good for the greatest number of people. Mass-casualty triage in the field should be overseen by a trained triage officer. A **triage officer** should have a wide breadth of clinical experience in the assessment and management of field injuries, as potentially challenging decisions may be made about patients who will be deemed critical versus those who will be classified as mortally wounded or expectant. A paramedic with significant field experience usually meets this requirement. A trained physician with experience in the field may also function in this capacity.[9,10] Nevertheless, all prehospital practitioners should be able to perform the basic functions of triage and be well rehearsed in the application of an agency-specific triage algorithm. Specialized training to address vulnerable populations such as children and those with special needs can be invaluable.

A number of different methodologies exist for evaluating and assigning the triage category.[11] One method involves a rapid physiologic and mental status evaluation. This triage process is referred to as the **START triage algorithm** (**S**imple **T**riage **A**nd **R**apid **T**reatment). This system evaluates the respiratory status, perfusion status, and mental status of the patient in making a prioritization for initial transfer to definitive care facilities.[10,12] (See Box 5-6 in Chapter 5, *Scene Management*.) Other triage systems include the MASS (**M**ove, **A**ssess, **S**ort, **S**end), Smart, Jump-START (pediatric algorithm), and Sacco triage methods.

In an effort to provide national guidance and bring uniformity to the triage process, the Centers for Disease Control and Prevention (CDC) in the United States convened a multidisciplinary group of experts to develop a consensus-based triage system, now known as SALT.[10] (See Box 5-7 in Chapter 5, *Scene Management*.) This triage system involves **S**orting the patient based on the patient's ability to move, **A**ssessing the patient for the need for **L**ifesaving interventions, performing those interventions, and ultimately, **T**reatment and **T**ransport.

Regardless of the exact triage method used, all triage systems ultimately classify patients into one of (usually) four injury-severity categories. The highest priority patients are those who are identified as having critical, but likely survivable, injuries and are usually categorized as *immediate* and color-coded *red*. Patients with moderate injuries (who may be nonambulatory) and can potentially tolerate a short delay in care are categorized as *delayed* patients and color-coded *yellow*. Patients with relatively minor injuries, often referred to as the "walking wounded," are classified as *minimal* victims and color-coded *green*. Patients who have expired on the scene or whose injuries are so severe that death is inevitable are categorized as *dead* or *expectant* and color-coded *black*. Of note, some triage systems, particularly SALT, specifically separate those patients classified as mortally wounded from those who are dead, color coding the expectant as *gray*. Certain urban response agencies, due to the density of the population and response area, have also noted the importance of identifying medical patients involved during an incident (orange tag). For example, a patient suffering an exacerbation of chronic obstructive pulmonary disease following a structural collapse due to inhaled debris may not have a traumatic injury but still has need for urgent transport.[13] Because trauma patients may overwhelm trauma-capable facilities, identifying nontrauma conditions allows those patients to be directed to alternative facilities.

All these color codes refer to the use of "disaster tags" at disaster scenes and are attached to patients once they have been triaged. The color code provides an immediate visual reference to the patient's triage category. Some triage systems also use a classification system in which immediate, delayed, minimal, and dead or expectant patients are referred to as Class I, Class II, Class III, and Class IV, respectively.

It is important that triage personnel avoid the temptation to pause their triage function in favor of treating a critically injured patient whom they encounter. During this initial triage phase, medical interventions are limited to those actions that are performed easily and rapidly and are not labor intensive. Generally, this means performing only procedures such as manual airway opening, chest needle decompression, administration of a chemical antidote, and external hemorrhage control including wound packing and tourniquet application. Interventions such as bag-mask ventilation, closed chest compression, establishing intravenous (IV) access, and endotracheal intubation are often deferred during the triage process. One limited exception to this principle is that supraglottic airway devices are sometimes used during the response to tactical events.

Once patients have been triaged, they are brought together at **casualty collection points** according to their triage priority. Specifically, all of the immediate patients (red) are grouped, as are the delayed (yellow) and minimal (green) patients. Casualty collection points should be located close enough to the disaster site that the victim can be easily carried to them and treatment rapidly provided, but far enough away from the impact site to be safe from any ongoing hazard. Important considerations include the following:

- Proximity to the disaster site
- Safety from hazards and uphill and upwind from contaminated environments
- Protection from climatic conditions (when possible)
- Easy visibility for disaster victims and assigned personnel
- Convenient entry and exit routes for ground, air, and water evacuation
- Safe distance from staging ambulance exhaust fumes

As additional medical staff and resources arrive and become available on scene, medical care and interventions are provided at the casualty collection points according to the triage priority. These are appropriate locations to which physicians responding to the scene may be assigned to further evaluate and treat injured patients.

Finally, as transportation resources become available, patients are transported for definitive care according, once again, to their triage priority (**Figure 17-6**). Immediate patients are not held on scene for the provision of further medical care if transport is available (**Figure 17-7**).

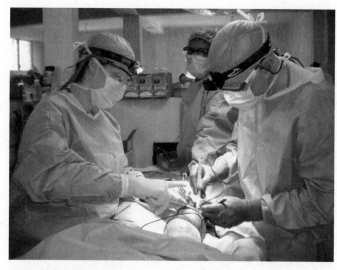

Figure 17-6 Definitive medical care at a Haitian hospital after the earthquake of 2010.

Courtesy of Andrew Pollak, MD.

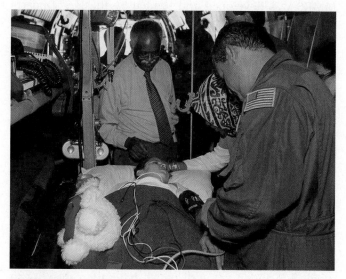

Figure 17-7 Interior of a military transport plane converted for medical evacuation with patient litters.

© Evan Vucci/AP Photo

Needed medical interventions should be conducted during transport to the definitive care facility.

Because of visible, critical injuries, emergency responders often tend to move individual patients forward for immediate treatment and transport and bypass the triage process. This tendency should be avoided so that all victims can be sorted, reserving treatment for salvageable victims first. Nevertheless, bypassing the triage process can be considered in certain scenarios:

1. Inclement weather, posing excessive risk to the responder and casualties
2. Darkness or impending nightfall without the capability of supplemental illumination

3. The continued risk of injury as a result of natural or unnatural events
4. No triage facility or triage officer immediately available
5. Any tactical situation in a law enforcement scenario in which the victims are rapidly moved from the impact site to the collection point for transport[12,14]

Finally, triage should be thought of as a dynamic and ongoing process. Once a patient is evaluated and categorized, the patient may not carry that triage category for the remainder of care. Instead, as the patient's condition changes, the triage category may change as well. For example, a patient with a major extremity wound and hemorrhage may initially be categorized as an immediate patient; however, after pressure is applied to the wound and the bleeding is controlled, the patient may be retriaged as delayed. Alternatively, a patient initially categorized as immediate could deteriorate rapidly and subsequently be retriaged as expectant.

Retriage should occur on the scene while patients are waiting for transport resources. In addition, patients will undergo retriage upon arrival at the receiving destination and again as they are prioritized for emergent surgery.

Treatment

Because the number of patients will initially exceed the available resources, treatment on the scene is generally limited to manually opening the airway, decompressing tension pneumothoraces, controlling external hemorrhage, and administering chemical agent antidotes. Only when adequate resources have arrived on scene or during transport to the hospital should additional interventions be provided, such as IV access and splinting of fractures.

Transport

The transport and tracking of patients from an MCI to the receiving hospitals involves a coordinated effort using a variety of transport vehicles. Immediate and delayed patients will be taken to the hospital in ambulances or helicopters (if available and conditions permit). Those incidents that result in large numbers of patients, particularly patients in the minimal category, may be more easily and expeditiously managed by using nontraditional transport vehicles such as buses and vans, and in some cases, patients may be transported to nonhospital sites for evaluation and treatment. It is important to remember, however, that when such alternate transport mechanisms are used, prehospital care practitioners with adequate supplies and equipment must be assigned to accompany the casualties in that vehicle. Each patient's movement and destination should be accurately recorded on a patient tracking log or via commercially available tracking systems.

Another important issue in effectively responding to an MCI relates to the decision-making process for patient destination once transport is initiated.[15] Recent events have demonstrated that patients who can easily move or be moved will often depart the disaster site using any available means of transportation and make their own way to surrounding hospitals.[6] Often this results in large numbers of "walking wounded" arriving at the hospital closest to the disaster site. The 2017 Las Vegas Harvest music festival shooting, for example, was notable for the use of application-based taxi services such as Uber and Lyft.

Prehospital care practitioners must understand that the hospital closest to a disaster scene may be overwhelmed with patients even before the arrival of the first transporting ambulance. Before taking a patient to the closest hospital, communication channels should be established to ascertain the status of the emergency department (ED) and its ability to accept and treat patients transported by ambulance. If the closest hospital is overwhelmed, the EMS system may transport patients to more distant facilities when needed. Dispersal of patients to multiple institutions will ultimately better preserve the ability of all the receiving hospitals to optimize the patient care they are able to provide. Consideration for specialty receiving facilities should also be given due consideration if the patient's condition warrants, including trauma, burn, and reimplantation centers.

However, in those communities that have limited numbers of hospitals, EMS may have no option but to transport patients to the nearest hospital. In some municipalities, Disaster Medical Control Centers directly communicate with hospitals to determine their capabilities for handling acutely injured patients.

Medical Assistance Teams

If the disaster is of significant proportion that additional on-scene resources are needed, some hospitals have developed disaster-response teams to help augment the EMS field response and provide on-site care, thus allowing prehospital care practitioners to be freed from the task of providing medical care at casualty collection points and, instead, performing patient transport. Agencies may have preexisting arrangements with surrounding communities and employ mutual aid to help provide additional prehospital capacity (**Figure 17-8**). Additionally, if outside resources are needed from the state or federal government, other emergency medical response teams are available in many municipalities. Statewide "Go-teams" or other specialty response teams, and even the National Guard, are assets that can be mobilized for a response by local authorities.

As a result of the Metropolitan Medical Response System (MMRS) in the United States, MMRS task forces

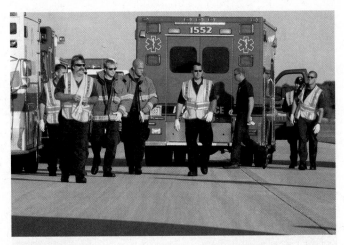

Figure 17-8 Agencies from surrounding communities may provide mutual aid during a large-scale emergency.
© Nancy G Fire Photography, Nancy Greifenhagen/Alamy Stock Photo

or strike teams have been created in many cities. The MMRS was developed and funded by the U.S. Department of Health and Human Services (DHHS) to help respond to terrorist or public health emergencies. The goal is to help integrate the various local response agencies and services to enhance the response to such an event. These response assets comprise medical personnel from emergency medicine, trauma surgery, surgical subspecialties, and nursing. MMRS task forces can respond with resources that have been purchased through state and federal funds. These strike teams can be used to augment and backfill medical facilities or to staff mobile medical facilities that are established to provide surge capacity and medical care to patients.

On a larger scale, the U.S. government has capabilities through the National Disaster Medical System to mobilize disaster medical assistance teams (DMATs). DMATs are able to provide field care as well as create mobile medical facilities, some of which have the capability to perform surgical interventions and meet the critical care needs of patients, when local resources have been overwhelmed. A request for DMATs must come through the appropriate channels, usually from the local emergency manager to the state emergency management authority and the governor's office through the federal government to the DHHS, which houses the National Disaster Medical System's response program. Some states have similarly organized and structured teams that can respond to statewide emergencies.

Threat of Terrorism and Weapons of Mass Destruction

Terrorism may present some of the most challenging MCIs for emergency responders. The spectrum of terrorist threats is limitless, ranging from suicide bombers, to conventional weapons or explosives, to military weapons, to WMDs (chemical, biologic, radiologic, and nuclear). Terrorist events have the greatest potential of all human-made disasters to generate large numbers of casualties and fatalities. (See Chapter 18, *Explosions and Weapons of Mass Destruction*, for detailed information about specific weapons.)

Terrorists have unfortunately demonstrated remarkable ingenuity in creating civilian casualties. During the terrorist attacks on September 11, 2001, the terrorists used passenger jets replete with fuel to generate massive destruction of life and property.

One of the unique features of a terrorist threat, especially involving WMDs, is that psychological casualties usually predominate. Terrorists do not need to kill a large number of people to achieve their goals; they only need to create a climate of fear and panic to overwhelm the medical infrastructure. In the March 1995 sarin attacks in Tokyo, 5,000 total patients presented to hospitals. Of these, fewer than 1,000 had physical effects from the sarin gas; the remaining presented with psychological stress and desire for physician evaluation and assessment. The 2001 anthrax incidents in the United States also dramatically increased the number of individuals presenting to EDs with nonspecific respiratory symptoms that ultimately did not result from actual anthrax exposure.

Explosions and bombings continue to be the most frequent cause of mass casualties in disasters caused by terrorists worldwide, both as a primary event and when secondary devices are staged to inflict damage upon emergency responders. The majority of these bombings consist of relatively small explosives that produce low mortality rates. However, when strategically placed in buildings, pipelines, or moving vehicles, their impact can be much greater (**Figure 17-9**). The high morbidity and mortality rates are related not only to the intensity of the blast but also to the subsequent structural damage that leads to the collapse of the targeted buildings. A greater threat could include conventional explosives combined with a chemical, biologic, or radiologic agent, such as a "dirty bomb," which combines a conventional incendiary with radioactive material.

The WMDs that create contaminated environments may prove to be the greatest logistical challenge. Emergency responders can be limited regarding patient transport due to contamination risks. Prehospital care practitioners must be prepared and equipped to perform triage, not only to determine the extent of the injuries but also to assess the potential for contamination and need for decontamination and initial stabilization. At the same time, practitioners need to take appropriate steps to protect themselves from potential contamination by using the appropriate personal protective equipment.

Decontamination

Decontamination is an important consideration for all disasters involving hazardous materials and WMDs (**Figure 17-10**). Terrorist events with large numbers of victims, unknown substances, and multitude of "worried well," significantly increase the specter of contaminated or potentially contaminated casualties. (See Chapter 18, *Explosions and Weapons of Mass Destruction*, for additional information.) As a general rule, if patients are deemed

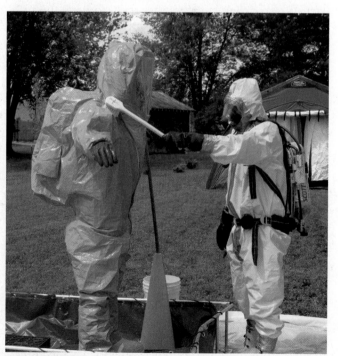

Figure 17-10 Decontamination of personnel in level A personal protective equipment in the "warm zone" by personnel in level B personal protective equipment.
© Jones & Bartlett Learning

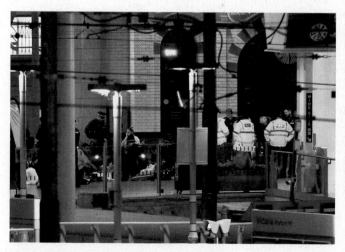

Figure 17-9 Manchester bombing, 2017.
© Dave Thompson/Getty Images News/Getty Images

to be contaminated, decontamination procedures should occur prior to transport to definitive care. Site security and manpower are important considerations during the decontamination process as is containing and safely disposing of the contaminated materials.

Treatment Area

When responding to a disaster involving hazardous materials and WMDs, it is critical that the triage and casualty collection points be appropriately positioned upwind and uphill of the contaminated area (300 yards [275 meters]).

Psychological Response to Disasters

Psychological trauma and other adverse psychological **sequelae** are frequent side effects of events such as natural disasters and unintentional disasters caused by humans.[16] In contrast, one of the objectives of terrorism is to inflict psychological pain, trauma, and disequilibrium. Maintaining good mental health is just as important as maintaining good physical health for all emergency responders.

Characteristics of Disasters That Affect Mental Health

Not all disasters have the same level of psychological impact. Disaster characteristics that seem to have the most significant mental health impact include the following:

- Little or no warning preincident
- Serious threat to personal safety
- Potential unknown health effects
- Uncertain duration of the event
- Human error or malicious intent
- Symbolism related to the terrorist target

Factors Impacting Psychological Response

Everyone who experiences a disaster, either as a victim or as an emergency responder, is affected to some degree. Fortunately, this does not mean that most individuals will develop a mental health disorder. It does mean, however, that all affected individuals, both victims and emergency responders, will have some type of psychological or emotional response to the event.

Similarly, there are both individual and collective reactions that can promote resilience and help communities recover from these extraordinary events. Factors affecting individual response to disasters include the following:

- Physical and psychological proximity to the event
- Exposure to gruesome or grotesque situations

- Diminished health status before or because of the disaster
- Magnitude of loss
- History of previous trauma

Factors impacting collective response to trauma include the following:

- Degree of community disruption
- Predisaster family and community stability
- Community leadership
- Cultural sensitivity of recovery efforts

Psychological Sequelae of Disasters

Postdisaster psychological responses are wide ranging, from mild stress responses to full-blown **posttraumatic stress disorder (PTSD)**, major depression, acute stress disorder, or suicide.[16] PTSD is a mental health condition that results from exposure to horrific or terrifying events and can manifest as flashbacks to the incident, nightmares, anxiety, heightened startle response, sensitivity to noise or touch, and uncontrollable thoughts about the incident.

Interventions

A number of relatively simple actions can help individuals to minimize the psychological effects of an event and assist them in returning to predisaster levels of function.

- Individuals should return to usual, daily activities as soon as possible.
- In persons with no diagnosed mental health disorder, it may be helpful to provide educational materials that explain psychological responses to disasters and how those responses can impact individuals and their families.
- Crisis counseling should be available, followed by referral when treatment is indicated.
- When a mental health condition is diagnosed, therapeutic interventions can be helpful, including cognitive-behavioral therapy, trauma-informed care, eye movement desensitization and reprocessing therapy, and prescription medications.

Emergency Responder Stress

Emergency responders can become secondary victims of stress and experience other psychological sequelae. These consequences can adversely affect their performance during and after an event. Personal well-being as well as family and professional relationships may be negatively impacted. Supervisory personnel and colleagues should be alert for the development or manifestations of stress and psychological distress in individuals who were involved in an incident response.

A number of intervention strategies are often used in an effort to help prevent and manage stress after an incident. These include debriefing, defusing, and grief management sessions. Collectively, these processes have been referred to as **critical incident stress management (CISM)**. The value of CISM has been questioned, primarily in those instances where CISM has been a mandated intervention for emergency responders.[17] CISM can be offered as an option to those emergency responders who feel inclined to participate but should never be mandated for all emergency responders as it may actually cause harm in some circumstances. Alternative programs such as Psychological First Aid, chaplaincy, peer support, employee-assistance programs, and wellness checks address some of the limitations of CISM and provide teams with effective tools for immediate intervention in situations where practitioners have psychologically related complaints or are showing signs of distress and are amenable to assistance.

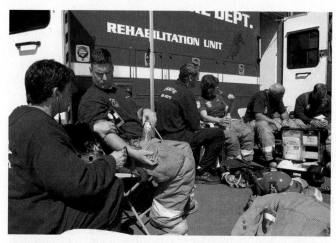

Figure 17-11 Adequate rest periods on scene can help relieve stress.
© Jones & Bartlett Learning. Courtesy of MIEMSS.

Signs of Stress in Workers

Some common signs of stress in emergency responders include physiologic, emotional, cognitive, and behavioral elements.

Physiologic Signs

- Fatigue, even after rest
- Nausea
- Fine motor tremors
- Tics
- **Paresthesias**
- Dizziness
- Gastrointestinal upset
- Heart palpitations
- Choking or smothering sensations

Emotional Signs

- Anxiety
- Irritability
- Feeling overwhelmed
- Unrealistic anticipation of harm to self or others
- Apathy
- Guilt

Cognitive Signs

- Memory loss
- Decision-making difficulties
- Anomia (inability to name common objects or familiar people)
- Concentration problems or distractibility
- Reduced attention span
- Calculation difficulties

Behavioral Signs

- Insomnia
- Hypervigilance
- Crying easily
- Inappropriate humor
- Ritualistic behavior
- Avoidance/social isolation

Managing Stress On-Site

The following on-site interventions can assist in reducing stress:

- Limited exposure to traumatic stimuli
- Reasonable operational hours
- Adequate rest periods (**Figure 17-11**)
- Reasonable diet
- Regular exercise program
- Private time
- Speaking with empathic colleagues
- Monitoring signs of stress

Disaster Education and Training

The development and implementation of a formal education and training program will improve the prehospital care practitioner's ability to respond effectively to an MCI. The practitioner may fulfill a variety of roles in disaster and mass-casualty management, including mitigation and preparedness, search and rescue, triage, acute medical care, transport, and post-event recovery. Preparedness with regard to education and training can be accomplished in various structured, as well as unstructured, learning environments. Each has its individual advantages and disadvantages, as measured by educational impact and comparative cost.

Independent learning is the foundation of disaster preparedness. A multitude of resources are available through printed literature as well as via the internet. The CDC, public health agencies, FEMA, the Center for Domestic Preparedness, and the military forces all offer internet-based learning opportunities and resources to individuals. Courses can be completed on an independent basis on a time-flexible schedule. This modality, however, does not allow for direct hands-on experience.

Group training is directed at specific teams with regard to disaster response. Training programs are broadly available and include understanding incident command structure and WMD preparedness. Numerous professional and paraprofessional organizations have developed training programs and modules specific to their scope of professional practice, including public health, emergency medicine, critical care, and surgical and medical specialties, as well as all levels of prehospital care practitioners. One example of this type of program for prehospital care practitioners is NAEMT's All Hazards Disaster Response course (**Box 17-5**).

Simulations provide a training opportunity that brings together many individuals from varied backgrounds who are essential to an effective disaster response. Two examples include tabletop exercises and a fully active field-training drill. Tabletop exercises are cost-effective and highly useful methods to test and evaluate a disaster response. As the name suggests, these exercises are conducted around a table, with the various participants verbally indicating what the expected response actions would be. Tabletop exercises allow for real-time communications and interaction among multidisciplinary agencies. These activities require direction in the form of an experienced facilitator guiding the participants through the objectives and providing constructive feedback to the group at the conclusion of the exercise.

Field exercises are the most realistic training events, involving the actual execution and performance of the community disaster-response plan. The field exercise allows for a real-time assessment of the physical capacity to meet the objectives as defined in writing. Ideally, the exercises will involve moving victims from the point of impact and injury through the EMS response system and into definitive care at medical facilities. These events, however, are labor intensive, long in duration, and potentially costly.

It is imperative that interdisciplinary training events are conducted at regular intervals and include all the appropriate agencies and participants that would be expected during an actual response. In this way, each agency will have the opportunity to learn about and understand their respective roles, responsibilities, and capabilities during a disaster.

Common Pitfalls of Disaster Response

After-action inquiries following MCIs have identified consistent challenges associated with the medical response to these events.[18,19] Identification of these challenges has resulted from subsequent evaluations of the response to these incidents as well as from communities that have performed risk, vulnerability, and needs assessments mandated by the U.S. government in order to receive funding to enhance the disaster-response infrastructure.[20]

Preparedness

As emergency responders in a community, prehospital care practitioners prepare for the devastation that can occur in a mass-casualty event and plan for such events in a variety of ways. Although a tabletop drill can be a valuable method of preparing, it does not truly test the ability of the practitioners to perform the necessary duties or the ability of the EMS agency to bring resources and assets to the site in a timely and efficient manner. Realistic functional disaster drills—during which victims are triaged, evaluated, "treated," transported, and tracked through the emergency medical response system to a hospital facility's doors in a realistic fashion—better test the emergency medical response that will be required. The ability to provide for *surge capacity* (the ability to expand services to meet a sudden influx of patients) and for supplying the large number of staff, ambulances, and other equipment needed for victims must be appropriately addressed by the entire medical community.

Unfortunately, few agencies regularly test surge capacity response in real time; instead, they rely on tabletop drills as a measure of their capability. Community-wide drills that involve multiple agencies more reliably predict an organization's level of preparedness for MCI response.

Box 17-5 All Hazards Disaster Response

The National Association of Emergency Medical Technicians (NAEMT) offers the 8-hour continuing education program All Hazards Disaster Response (AHDR). AHDR utilizes realistic scenarios to prepare first responders to best manage patients during a disaster. AHDR features an activity that assists participants in performing a hazard vulnerability analysis for their communities.

Moreover, MCIs can be highly varied—a response to a large alarm fire is vastly different from a response to an active shooter incident. A fundamental approach to responding to all hazards includes performing a hazard vulnerability analysis to identify and prioritize potential MCI or disaster scenarios most likely to affect a specific locale. Hazard vulnerability analysis is a systemic risk assessment tool that facilitates identifying hazards or risks that are most likely to have an impact on the surrounding community. This analysis also tailors response initiatives and resources to best address events that are most likely to occur or those that present the greatest disruption to the community.

Communications

The lack of a unified communication system significantly hinders the ability to mount a coordinated response to an MCI. Individual communication systems are effective, but relying on a single modality for communication is a setup for failure. The use of cellular phones, for example, was ineffective following disruption of the central communication center located in the World Trade Center on September 11, 2001. Also, the inability of police, fire, and EMS agencies to communicate with each other because of different radio technologies or frequencies is a limitation that may reduce the ability to effectively respond to MCIs.

Redundancy in the system is paramount, regardless of the chosen source for primary communications. Landlines, hardwired phone systems, cellular phone systems, satellite phone systems, VHF radios, and 800- to 900-MHz frequency systems all have some degree of vulnerability and could be compromised by a particular incident. Thus, having multiple communication options is crucial to ensuring ongoing and effective communications.

The following two principles are essential to maintain communications capability:

1. A unified communication system must exist to which all pertinent emergency responders in the community have access.
2. There must be system redundancy such that if one modality of communication fails or is disabled another source can be used efficiently and effectively as a backup.

Another common problem is the use of codes as a form of communication shorthand. Unfortunately, there is no single agreed-upon set of emergency codes for all agencies to use; thus, a responding agency may find itself at a scene with other agencies, all of whom are using codes that may have different meanings. It is for this reason that ICS and NIMS recommend the use of plain English during an incident to avoid any confusion in meaning.

Scene Security

Scene security has become an ever-increasing problem in MCIs. Scene safety and security are important for the following reasons:

1. To protect the emergency response teams from a second incident, resulting in further casualties (e.g., secondary device targeting first responders)
2. To provide for the safe ingress and egress of emergency responders and victims unencumbered by bystanders
3. To protect and facilitate securing the scene and potential physical evidence

Scene security may become a significant challenge during a disaster, because resources may potentially be spread thin due to response to the event. Coordination with local law enforcement leaders is essential for the prehospital and medical community to ensure that security and force protection will be available if necessary.

Self-Dispatched Assistance

In some MCIs, public safety and EMS agencies (as well as medical responders of all types) from adjacent and even distant communities have responded to the scene without any formal request for assistance from the impacted jurisdiction.[4] These "self-dispatched" emergency responders, although well intentioned, could add complexity to an ongoing event. With self-dispatched assistance, coordinated rescue efforts can be strained by inability to effectively integrate with the incident command structure. Communications issues can also be more challenging by incompatible radio systems brought by the self-dispatched emergency responders.

Ideally, public safety and EMS agencies should respond to a disaster site only if they have been specifically requested to do so by the responsible jurisdiction and the incident commander.[21] In addition, it is helpful if access to the scene is controlled and a staging area is established as soon as possible to which all responding units and volunteers can be directed to be credentialed and better incorporated into the incident response.

Supply and Equipment Resources

Most EMS agencies have plans for the routine use of supplies and have purchased supplies based on the expected daily demand. Events of large magnitude will rapidly exhaust these resources and may disrupt conventional supply chains. Having backup resources for the replenishment of supplies during a disaster is essential for the ongoing mission of high-quality patient care. Supplies

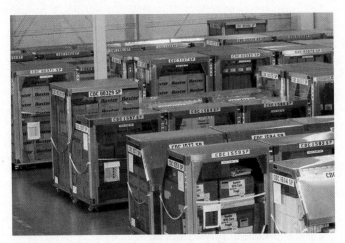

Figure 17-12 In communities that have been designated to receive MMRS funds, community stockpiles of pharmaceuticals have been or are being purchased in preparation for such events.

Courtesy of Strategic National Stockpile Communications Team/Centers for Disease Control and Prevention

must be available in a timely fashion, and appropriate mechanisms must be in place for distribution. Distribution plans should not depend on deployed prehospital care practitioners, as they may be tasked with other operational assignments.

The EMS agency must also have a plan in place for pharmaceutical replenishment. In those communities that have been designated to receive MMRS funds, community stockpiles of pharmaceuticals have been or are being purchased in preparation for such events (**Figure 17-12**).

Failure to Notify Hospitals

In the confusion of responding to an MCI, as well as performing the numerous tasks that must be accomplished in initiating the prehospital medical response to such an event, contacting receiving hospitals directly to prepare for the influx of patients is often overlooked. Hospital notification and activation should be integral parts of the EMS agency's MCI plan; otherwise, hospitals may not be informed or may be informed too late to optimize the influx of patients. It is essential that EMS agencies include hospital notification as part of their MCI plan so that a coordinated, seamless transition from field care to hospital care can occur. Just as first responders implement the ICS, hospitals also have a unique ICS referred to as H-ICS—the Hospital Incident Command System, which can be activated and tasked with leveraging additional resources for the healthcare facility. Furthermore, ongoing communication from the field to the hospital and from the hospital to the field is important for monitoring the status of the event and the patient load at hospitals.

Media

The media are often seen as a detriment to the physical and operational process of disaster response. However, EMS agencies are encouraged to partner with the media, including social media, because these outlets can be an asset during a disaster response when used responsibly. The media can help disseminate accurate information to the general population, giving them directions on appropriate actions before, during, or after an event. The media's purpose is to broadcast information to the public, and prehospital agencies have the responsibility to partner with the media to ensure the information provided is timely and accurate as well as helpful to the response process.

Having a designated PIO who is trained to deal with the media and authorized to speak about the incident is an important method of communicating with the various media representatives seeking information about the incident. Of particular importance is the recognition that each responding agency will likely have a PIO present. Under the unified command concept, ideally, one consistent message should be delivered by a single PIO; however, any messages given out by PIOs of the various agencies must be consistent with each other. As always, caution should be exercised by individual responders in sharing pictures of a potential scene on social media. Adherence to social media policies is always a consideration during operational response and a request for information from media should be deferred to the designated PIO within the agency.

SUMMARY

- Disasters result from natural climactic or geologic events; however, they may also result from intentional or unintentional acts of humans.
- Although disasters may be unpredictable, adequate preparation can turn an unthinkable event into a manageable situation.

- The incident command system (ICS) allows different types of agencies (e.g., fire, police, EMS) and multiple jurisdictions of similar agencies (e.g., city, county, state) to work together effectively, using a common language and organizational structure to manage the response to a disaster or other major incident.

SUMMARY (CONTINUED)

- Prehospital care practitioners must understand the concepts of triage to ensure they can do the greatest good for the greatest number of people with the resources available.
- Transport must take into consideration factors such as whether nearby hospitals have the capacity to meet demands and whether certain patients would benefit from extended transport to a trauma center more capable of meeting their needs.
- Despite the fact that disasters occur in varying sizes and result from many different causes, common pitfalls have been identified that hinder management of such events, including:
  - Inadequate preparedness
  - Communications failures
  - Inadequate scene safety measures
  - Self-dispatched assistance
  - Supply and equipment shortages
  - Poor media relations
- Disaster response may take a psychological toll on those involved, both victims and emergency responders. Agencies should consider voluntary debriefing with affected personnel to help practitioners maintain good mental health, which is just as important as maintaining good physical health. As the importance of mental health becomes even more relevant, agencies are offering a greater number of resources, including employee assistance programs, peer-to-peer counseling, crisis hotlines, greater mental health and resilience education and awareness, chaplaincy programs, and ongoing surveillance and wellness checks.
- Understanding the disaster cycle is important to preparation and prevention efforts. There are generally five phases in a disaster response: quiescent, or interdisaster, period; prodrome (warning) phase; impact phase; rescue, emergency, or relief phase; and recovery or reconstruction phase.
- The best outcomes in response to MCIs result from the creation of a well-devised disaster plan that has been rehearsed, tested, and critiqued to identify and improve problem areas.

SCENARIO RECAP

You are dispatched to a local high school that has been placed into service as a shelter following community-wide flooding from a large weather event. Your community's mayor and other dignitaries are in attendance at the school to address the community's concerns about closed roads and power outages.

While en route to the scene, dispatch updates you there are multiple reports of numerous casualties after the collapse of elevated bleachers in the gym that were being used as seating during the mayor's community address. Police and fire resources are also en route to the scene but have limited available resources due to other ongoing weather-related public safety incidents.

- What safety and security concerns would you expect to encounter?
- What triage system should be utilized?
- How should the response to this incident be organized?

SCENARIO SOLUTION

While responding to the high school, preplanned mutual aid resources are simultaneously dispatched to assist. The local hospitals are also updated about the evolving MCI. As the first-arriving EMS unit, you report to the incident command post where a unified command structure is being assembled. As practiced, you conduct an overall assessment of the scene and the medical needs and relay that information back to your dispatch.

(continues)

SCENARIO SOLUTION (CONTINUED)

Triage team leaders begin sorting through the casualties. Treatment areas are established a safe distance from the collapse. As casualties arrive at the treatment areas, they are organized by severity of injury. Prehospital care practitioners begin appropriate care and secondary triage of the injured. As mutual aid resources arrive at staging areas, they are assigned tasks and placed into service. Transport vehicles arrive, and the injured are transported to hospitals. All patients are tracked and accounted for through each step of this process. There is ongoing communication with the hospitals regarding capacity and patient count.

Once all casualties have left the scene, fire services, code inspection services, and police begin to investigate the origin of the collapse.

References

1. United Nations Office for Disaster Risk Reduction. Disaster. Accessed January 18, 2022. https://www.undrr.org/terminology/disaster

2. Starr GA, Allen TW, Stewart CE. Chapter 4. Disaster Medicine. In: Stone C, Humphries RL, eds. *CURRENT Diagnosis & Treatment Emergency Medicine*. 7th ed. McGraw Hill; 2011. Accessed January 31, 2022. https://accessemergencymedicine.mhmedical.com/content.aspx?bookid=385&sectionid=40357217

3. Cuny FC. Introduction to disaster management: lesson 5–technologies of disaster management. *Prehosp Disaster Med*. 1993;6:372-374.

4. Phillips SJ, Knebel A, eds. *Mass Medical Care with Scarce Resources: A Community Planning Guide*. Prepared by Health Systems Research, Inc., an Altarum company, under contract No. 290-04-0010. AHRQ Publication No. 07-0001. Agency for Healthcare Research and Quality; 2007.

5. Federal Emergency Management Agency. ICS resource center. Accessed January 18, 2022. http://training.fema.gov/EMIWeb/IS/ICSResource/index.htm

6. U.S. Department of Agriculture. ICS 300 – Lesson 4: Unified Command. Accessed January 18, 2022. https://www.usda.gov/sites/default/files/documents/ICS300Lesson04.pdf

7. Auf der Heide E. The importance of evidence-based disaster planning. *Ann Emerg Med*. 2006;47:34-49.

8. Larrey DJ. *Memoires de Chirurgie Militaire, et Campagnes*. Vols. 1-4. J. Smith, Publisher; 1812-1817.

9. Burkle FM, ed. *Disaster Medicine: Application for the Immediate Management and Triage of Civilian and Military Disaster Victims*. Medication Examination Publishing; 1984.

10. Burkle FM, Hogan DE, Burstein JL. *Disaster Medicine*. Lippincott, Williams & Wilkins; 2002.

11. Lerner EB, Schwartz RB, Coule PL, et al. Mass casualty triage: an evaluation of the data and development of a proposed national guideline. *Disaster Med Public Health Preparedness*. 2008;2(Suppl 1):S25-S34.

12. Super G. *START: A Triage Training Module*. Hoag Memorial Hospital Presbyterian; 1984.

13. Arshad FH, Williams A, Asaeda G, et al. A modified Simple Triage and Rapid Treatment algorithm from the New York City (USA) Fire Department. *Prehosp Disaster Med*. 2015;30(2):1-6.

14. Burkle FM, Newland C, Orebaugh S, et al. Emergency medicine in the Persian Gulf: part II–triage methodology lessons learned. *Ann Emerg Med*. 1994;23:748-754.

15. Bloch YH, Schwartz D, Pinkert M, et al. Distribution of casualties in a mass-casualty incident with three local hospitals in the periphery of a densely populated area: lessons learned from the medical management of a terrorist attack. *Prehosp Disast Med*. 2007;22:186-192.

16. Hick JL, Ho JD, Heegaard WG, et al. Emergency medical services response to a major freeway bridge collapse. *Disaster Med Public Health Preparedness*. 2008;2(Suppl 1):S17-S24.

17. Bledsoe BE. Critical incident stress management (CISM): benefit or risk for emergency services? *Prehosp Emerg Care*. 2003;7(2):272-279. doi: 10.1080/10903120390936941

18. Assistant Secretary for Preparedness and Response. Tracie Healthcare Emergency Preparedness Information Gateway. Lessons Learned From the Pulse Nightclub Shooting: An Interview with Staff from Orlando Regional Medical Center. Accessed April 8, 2022. https://files.asprtracie.hhs.gov/documents/aspr-tracie-lessons-learned-from-the-pulse-nightclub-shooting-508.pdf

19. Assistant Secretary for Preparedness and Response. Tracie Healthcare Emergency Preparedness Information Gateway. Healthcare Response to a No-Notice Incident: Las Vegas. Published March 28, 2018. Accessed April 8, 2022. https://files.asprtracie.hhs.gov/documents/aspr-tracie-no-notice-incident-las-vegas-webinar-ppt-508.pdf

20. Assistant Secretary for Preparedness and Response. Tracie Healthcare Emergency Preparedness Information Gateway. ASPR TRACIE Technical Assistance (TA) Request. August 9, 2019. Accessed April 8, 2022. https://files.asprtracie.hhs.gov/documents/aspr-tracie-ta---after-action-reports--real-life-events---8-9-19-final.pdf

21. American College of Emergency Physicians. Unsolicited medical personnel volunteering at disaster scenes. Published June 2002. Reaffirmed October 2008. Revised October 2017. Accessed January 18, 2022. https://www.acep.org/patient-care/policy-statements/unsolicited-medical-personnel-volunteering-at-disaster-scenes/

Suggested Reading

Briggs SM. *Advanced Disaster Medical Response: Manual for Providers*. 2nd ed. Cine-Med Inc; 2014.

De Boer J, Dubouloz M. *Handbook of Disaster Medicine: Emergency Medicine in Mass Casualty Situations*. Van der Wees; 2000.

Eachempati SR, Flomenbaum N, Barie PS. Biological warfare: current concerns for the health care provider. *J Trauma*. 2002;52:179-186.

Emergency Medicine Clinics of North America. 1996;14(2) (entire issue).

Feliciano DV, Anderson GV Jr., Rozycki GS, et al. Management of casualties from the bombing at the Centennial Olympics. *Am J Surg*. 1998;176(6):538-543.

Hirshberg A, Holcomb JB, Mattox KL. Hospital trauma care in multiple-casualty incidents: a critical view. *Ann Emerg Med*. 2001;37(6):647-652.

Hogan DE, Burstein JL, eds. *Disaster Medicine*. 2nd ed. Lippincott, Williams & Wilkins; 2016.

Slater MS, Trunkey DD. Terrorism in America: an evolving threat. *Arch Surg*. 1997;132(10):1059-1066.

Stein M, Hirshberg A. Medical consequences of terrorism: the conventional weapon threat. *Surg Clin North Am*. 1999;79(6):1537-1552.

U.S. Department of Homeland Security, Federal Emergency Management Agency. Accessed January 18, 2022. www.fema.gov

CHAPTER **18**

Explosions and Weapons of Mass Destruction

Lead Editors
Daniel P. Nogee, MD
Faizan H. Arshad, MD

CHAPTER OBJECTIVES

At the completion of this chapter, you will be able to do the following:

- Discuss the essential considerations regarding mitigation of a weapon of mass destruction (WMD) event:
  - Scene assessment
  - Incident command
  - Personal protective equipment
  - Patient triage
  - Principle of decontamination

- Describe the mechanisms of injury, evaluation and management, and transport considerations associated with specific categories of WMD agent:
  - Explosive and incendiary agents
  - Chemical agents
  - Biologic agents
  - Radiologic agents
- Know how to access and utilize resources for further study.

SCENARIO

It is a warm summer evening, and you are dispatched to the scene of a reported explosion outside a popular café. You know this café is usually busy and typically seats patrons inside and outside on the patio. Dispatch informs you the number of victims is not yet known, although they have received multiple emergency calls regarding this incident. Other public safety agencies have also been dispatched to the location.

Upon arrival at the location, you observe you are the first prehospital care practitioner on scene. No incident command has yet been established. Dozens of people are running away from the cafe. Many are imploring you to assist victims who have obvious bleeding. Other victims are lying on the ground with variable states of consciousness.

- What will you do first?
- What are your priorities as you determine your course of action?
- How will you care for so many people?

INTRODUCTION

Preparing to manage an incident that potentially involves a weapon of mass destruction (WMD) is a challenge for emergency medical services (EMS) systems. Although a number of different mnemonics are used to recall the various types of WMDs, perhaps the easiest to remember is CBRNE, which stands for **C**hemical, **B**iologic, **R**adiologic, **N**uclear, and **E**xplosive.

History has demonstrated these incidents can occur without warning anywhere.

- The 1995 bombing of the Murrah Federal Building in Oklahoma City resulted in 168 deaths and 700 casualties. Eighty percent of the deaths resulted from the collapse of the building rather than the direct effects of the explosive. One-third of the patients brought to one Oklahoma City hospital were transported by EMS. Of these transported patients, 64% required admission to the hospital, whereas only 6% of self-referred patients to the emergency department (ED) required admission.
- The September 11, 2001, World Trade Center attacks in which terrorists used passenger aircraft as flying bombs resulted in over 1,100 injured survivors, with almost one-third of those casualties transported to the hospital by prehospital care practitioners. Emergency responders accounted for 29% of the casualties.
- The multiple train bombings in Madrid, Spain, in 2004 caused 190 deaths and 2,051 injuries.
- The mass transit attack in London in 2005, in which bombs exploded in three subway trains and one double-decker bus, caused 52 deaths and more than 779 injuries.
- The Boston Marathon bombings in 2013 resulted in 3 deaths and approximately 264 injuries.
- The 2015 attacks in Paris, France, perpetrated by both gunmen and suicide bombers, killed 130 people and injured hundreds more.
- In June 2016, a gunman opened fire on the crowd at the Pulse Nightclub in Orlando, Florida, killing 49 adults and wounding 53 others.
- In 2016 in Nice, France, a terrorist deliberately drove a large cargo truck through crowds of people who had gathered to celebrate Bastille Day, resulting in 86 deaths and 458 injuries.
- The Manchester Arena bombing in 2017 resulted in 22 deaths and approximately 250 injuries. Many of the victims in this incident were children.
- A 2017 attack in New York City, in which a terrorist deliberately drove a rented work truck through a bicycle path, resulted in the deaths of 8 people and 12 injuries.
- The October 2017 Route 91 Harvest country festival shootings killed 58 people and injured more than 500 others in what has been deemed the worst mass shooting in U.S. history.

Although conventional explosives are the most commonly used and most likely form of WMD event, EMS systems worldwide have also been challenged by chemical and biohazard events. The 1995 sarin gas attack in the Tokyo subway system killed 12, and more than 5,000 people sought medical attention, many of whom were asymptomatic but concerned about possible exposure. The Tokyo Fire Department sent 1,364 firefighters to the 16 affected subway sites, and 135 emergency responders (10%) were affected by direct or indirect exposure to the nerve agent. Multiple alleged chemical attacks during the Syrian civil war have been investigated by the United Nations, including the use of the potent chemical weapons sarin (2015), chlorine (2014), and sulfur mustard (2015), resulting in many civilian and first responder casualties.

No life-threatening bioterrorism assault in the United States has yielded a large number of casualties, but this does not mean that EMS systems have not been challenged to prepare for bioterrorism threats. During 1998 and 1999, almost 6,000 people across the United States were affected by a series of anthrax-related hoaxes in more than 200 incidents. The letters containing anthrax delivered in the fall of 2001 resulted in only 22 cases of clinical anthrax but generated countless calls for public safety agencies to respond to suspicious packages and powders.

Although not a bioterrorist event, the COVID-19 pandemic placed significant strain on EMS and disaster response resources at local, regional, and national levels. Early in the pandemic, many nursing homes and assisted living facilities were hit with large waves of cases,[1] resulting in EMS agencies and disaster response organizations, including state National Guard units and federal Disaster Medical Assistance Teams (DMAT), providing mass casualty triage, logistical support, and patient care.[1,2] Limited availability of effective personal protective equipment (PPE) resulted in many responders, including EMS and emergency department staff, contracting COVID-19 early in the pandemic, causing further strain on limited medical resources.[3] Although other infectious disease outbreaks have placed similar localized strain on medical resources, such as severe acute respiratory syndrome (SARS) in Toronto in 2003, and Ebola virus disease (EVD) in West Africa in 2013–2016, the massive scale of the COVID-19 pandemic highlighted the strain that infectious disease outbreaks can place on EMS and other medical resources. The global disruption caused by the COVID-19 pandemic has shed light on the potential impact of an intentional release of such an infectious virus from a lab focused on viral gain-of-function research.

The threat that EMS may one day have to respond to a radiologic WMD event grows, with increasing speculation that terrorists may detonate a radiologic dispersion device ("dirty bomb") that would generate injuries and panic about radioactive contamination.

Weapons of mass destruction, while traditionally thought of as the previously mentioned CBRNE classes, can take on many different forms and shapes. For example, the "intentional vehicular assault," in which terrorists intentionally drive a wheeled vehicle into a crowd of pedestrians, unfortunately has become more common in the past several years, likely owing to the ease of obtaining a weapon (vehicle) and a target (crowd) relative to traditional CBRNE attacks.

Additionally, "active shooter" or "public mass shooting" events, involving one or more people attacking civilian targets with small arms (i.e., handguns, rifles, and other available nonmilitary or military firearms) have become increasingly common and severe within the United States and abroad.[4] Although not considered a WMD per se, active shooter events are considered in the context of WMD events as they present very similar challenges for EMS responders.

Compared to smaller-scale shootings, active shooter events may result in more casualties due to massive hemorrhage, possibly due to a longer length of time between injury of victims and treatment by medical personnel and overwhelming of local medical resources due to large numbers of victims. Prehospital practitioners responding to active shooter events may be directly targeted by the perpetrators, raising concerns of scene safety.

The 2013 Hartford Consensus Conference resulted in the creation of the THREAT framework to prepare for and mitigate mass shooting events: **T**hreat suppression, **H**emorrhage control, **R**apid **E**xtrication, **A**ssessment by medical practitioners, and **T**ransport to definitive care.[5] Multifaceted approaches including "Stop the Bleed" campaigns to provide trauma-focused medical education to civilians, prepositioning of mass-trauma care resources (tourniquets, bandages, etc.) in areas likely to be targeted, active shooter–specific medical training for prehospital practitioners such as Tactical Combat Casualty Care (TCCC)/Tactical Emergency Casualty Care (TECC), and response drills in conjunction with law enforcement/public safety agencies may help to reduce casualties in mass shooting incidents.

General Considerations

Scene Assessment

The ability of prehospital care practitioners to assess the scene properly is crucial to ensuring personal safety and the safety of other emergency responders. WMD events pose significant threats to responding emergency services. In the case of a high-explosives detonation, there may be fire, spilled hazardous materials, power line hazards, and risk of falling debris or *subsidence* (the creation of craters). One emergency responder was killed by falling debris in response to the Oklahoma City bombing.[6] Many emergency responders were killed in the 2001 World Trade Center attack, including 343 firefighters, 15 emergency medical technicians, and 3 law enforcement officers, when the buildings collapsed.

Chemical attacks potentially expose the prehospital care practitioner to the offending agent, not only from the primary source—the weapon—but also from secondary exposure to contamination of victims' skin, clothing, and personal belongings. Biologic agents, depending on the form of their delivery, pose a risk of illness from the offending agent (e.g., aerosolized anthrax spores) or from transmission of a communicable disease (e.g., plague or smallpox). A further risk to practitioners and patients alike is the possibility of additional devices. For example, a second bomb could be placed at the scene of the incident, set to explode after the arrival of emergency responders, with the intention of increasing not only injury but also confusion and panic.

All of these factors must be taken into consideration when prehospital care practitioners are dispatched to the scene of a possible explosive or WMD event and are evaluating the scene. Before entering any such scene, all responding units from all involved agencies should approach from an upwind and uphill direction and stage at a safe distance from the incident site. Approaching from an upwind direction is important because many of the WMDs, particularly the chemical and biologic agents, pose an inhalation risk, and inadvertent exposure is more likely at a downwind location. An uphill location is chosen to avoid exposure to runoff at an incident involving the release of liquid chemicals.

Prehospital care practitioners should then conduct a critical evaluation, ideally from a safe distance, of the scene, looking for clues that would warn them of potential hazards. The presence of visible vapors, spilled liquid, or possible ongoing dispersion should be noted; such observations are indicative of an active danger. Looking to see how patients are presenting must be included as part of the scene assessment, with particular attention to the signs and symptoms of patient presentation, such as seizures in multiple casualties, suggesting a possible chemical or biologic agent release. Practitioners need to communicate their observations through the chain of command so that proper steps can be taken to mount an appropriate and safe response, to increase the protective measures for the emergency responders, and to ensure the effective delivery of care to patients.

Access to and egress from the potentially contaminated site must be controlled. Concerned bystanders and well-meaning volunteers must not be allowed to enter the scene, as they may contribute to the casualty count if they expose themselves to the agent. Victims of the

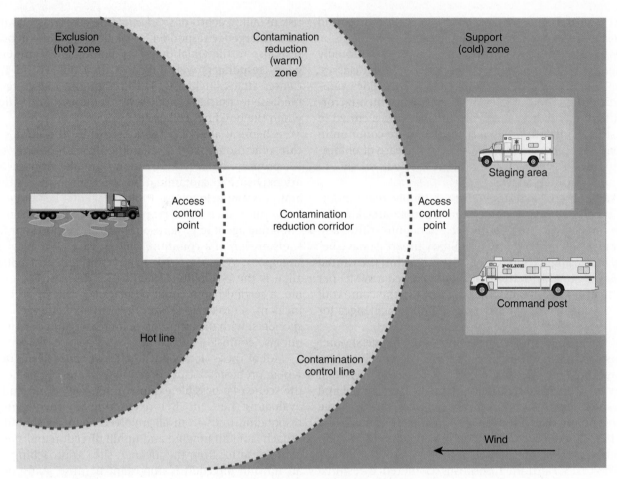

Figure 18-1 The scene of a WMD or hazardous materials incident is generally divided into hot, warm, and cold zones. The command post and staging area should both be located within the cold zone.
© National Association of Emergency Medical Technicians (NAEMT)

incident must also be contained as they seek to evacuate the scene, because self-transport may further disseminate a dangerous chemical or substance to unsuspecting contacts or hospital EDs. Similar to a hazardous materials incident, scene control zones (hot, warm, cold) should be established with controlled access points and transit corridors to prevent spread of the contaminants and inadvertent exposure and to provide safe areas for patient assessment and management (**Figure 18-1**; see the "Personal Protective Equipment" section).

Incident Command System

The incident command system (ICS) offers a management structure that coordinates all available resources to ensure an effective response. The ICS is discussed in detail in Chapter 5, *Scene Management,* and Chapter 17, *Disaster Management.* All incidents, regardless of size or complexity, will have a designated incident commander, who may be the first responding prehospital care practitioner until relieved by some other competent authority. It is essential that practitioners be familiar with and have

the opportunity to practice implementation of the ICS, ideally in interagency settings.

Personal Protective Equipment

When responding to WMD events, the proper personal protective equipment (PPE) needs to be worn. Requirements for PPE may range from the standard daily uniform to a fully encapsulated suit with **self-contained breathing apparatus (SCBA)**, depending on the specific agent involved and the specific role and training level of the prehospital care practitioner. This equipment is designed to protect the emergency responder from exposure to offending agents by providing defined levels of protection of the respiratory tract, skin, and mucous membranes. When dealing with hazardous substances of any type, PPE has generally been described in terms of the following levels (**Figure 18-2**):

- *Level A*. This level offers the highest amount of respiratory and skin protection. The respiratory tract is protected by an SCBA or **supplied air respirator (SAR)**

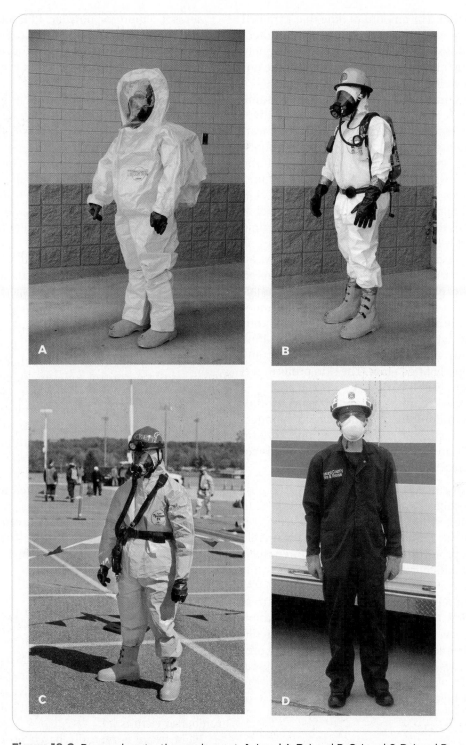

Figure 18-2 Personal protective equipment. **A.** Level A. **B.** Level B. **C.** Level C. **D.** Level D.

A-C. Courtesy of Rick Brady; **D.** © Jones & Bartlett Learning. Courtesy of MIEMSS.

delivering air to the emergency responder with posi-tive pressure. A chemical-resistant barrier that com-pletely encapsulates the wearer protects the skin and mucous membranes. It takes considerable time to don this protection, thus delaying the practitioner's

ability to access and help patients. Patience on the part of the prehospital care practitioners responding to the chaos of this type of event is essential. Addi-tional resources also need to be committed to assist emergency responders with donning and doffing this level of protection. The amount of time that a trained emergency responder can spend in Level A protection is also limited by both the available air supply and the buildup of heat and humidity within the enclosed suit, as well as specific agency protocols.

- *Level B.* The respiratory tract is protected in the same manner as in Level A protection, with positive-pressure-supplied air. Nonencapsulated chemical-resistant garments, including suit, gloves, and boots, which provide splash protection only, protect the skin and mucous membranes. The highest respiratory protection is afforded, with a lower level of skin protection. Similar to Level A protection, Level B protection takes time to don and doff, and work time within the suit is limited.

- *Level C.* The respiratory tract is protected by an **air-purifying respirator (APR)**. This may be a **powered air-purifying respirator (PAPR)**, which draws ambient air through a filter canister and delivers it under positive pressure to a face mask or hood, or a nonpowered APR, which relies on the wearer to draw ambient air through a filter canister by breathing through a properly fitted mask. The skin protection is the same as for Level B.

- *Level D.* This level represents standard work clothes (i.e., standard uniform for the emergency responder) and may also include a gown, gloves, and surgical mask. Level D provides minimal respiratory protection and minimal skin protection.

It might be concluded that the best protective posture for a prehospital care practitioner is always to respond in the highest level of protection, Level A, regardless of the threat. This is, however, not a reasonable response. Level A protection is cumbersome, often making manual tasks difficult to perform. Significant training and experience are required when using an SCBA. Level A protection puts the wearer at risk for heat stress and physical exhaustion. It can make communication between emergency responders and victims difficult. Appropriate PPE must be selected based on the presumed threat, the level of training, and the operational responsibilities of the practitioner. Most important, the practitioner must be trained and practiced in the use of the PPE selected.

Control Zones

PPE is selected based on the known (or suspected) hazards of the environment and proximity to the threat. Proximity to the threat has often been described in terms of the following control zones:

- The *hot zone* is the area where there is immediate threat to health and life. This includes an environment contaminated with a hazardous gas, vapor,

aerosol, liquid, or powder. PPE adequate to protect the emergency responder is determined based on potential routes of exposure to the substance and the likely agent. Level A protection is most often used in the hot zone.

- The *warm zone* is characterized as an area where the concentration of the offending agent is limited. In the case of a WMD scene, this is the area to which victims are brought from the hot zone and where decontamination takes place. The prehospital care practitioner is still at risk for exposure if working in this area as the agent is carried from the hot zone on victims, emergency responders, and equipment. PPE is recommended based on potential routes of exposure to the substance.

- The *cold zone* is the area outside the hot and warm zones that is not contaminated, where there is no risk of exposure, and thus no specific level of PPE is required beyond standard universal precautions.

It is important to note that it is often difficult to define these control zones and that they may be dynamic rather than static. Factors that contribute to the dynamics of the control zones include the activity of the victims and emergency responders and ambient conditions. For example, unless completely incapacitated, contaminated victims might walk toward prehospital care practitioners in the cold zone or leave the scene completely, either in panic or with the intention of seeking medical aid at a nearby hospital. By design, warm zones and cold zones are designated upwind of the hot zone, but if wind direction changes, practitioners would be at risk of exposure if they were unable to don the proper PPE or to rapidly retreat. These contingencies must be anticipated when planning for or responding to a WMD event.

Patient Triage

Prehospital care practitioners will potentially face a large and overwhelming number of victims who will require evaluation and treatment after a WMD event. Every EMS system should identify and rehearse a mechanism for rapidly triaging victims. The objective of patient triage in a WMD incident is to do the greatest good for the greatest number of victims.

Field triage is typically based on easily measurable physiologic criteria that assign patients to severity categories in order to identify those victims who require treatment and transport to a medical treatment facility most urgently.[7] Several triage schemes and criteria are available.[8] Triage systems include the START (**S**imple **T**riage **A**nd **R**apid **T**reatment) system, the MASS (**M**ove, **A**ssess, **S**ort, **S**end) system, and the SALT (**S**ort by ability to move, **A**ssess need for **L**ifesaving interventions, **T**riage and **T**ransport) system advocated by the

Centers for Disease Control and Prevention (CDC).[9] (For more information about triage, see Chapter 17, *Disaster Management*.)

Whatever patient triage system is used, it must be employed in routine EMS operations to promote familiarity and to ensure recognition among prehospital care practitioners at all levels of care, including the hospital or trauma center.

Principles of Decontamination

Patients and prehospital care practitioners alike may require decontamination after exposure to agents that may pose a risk to health. These individuals should have decontamination procedures performed in the field in a designated decontamination area. Decontamination areas are typically upwind and uphill of the affected area when conditions allow. Known exposure to only vapor or gases does not require decontamination to prevent secondary contamination, although the victim's clothing should be removed.

Decontamination is a two-step process that first involves removal of all clothing, jewelry, and shoes, which are bagged, tagged, and secured for later identification. These items may serve as evidence in incident investigation and may be returned to the owner if successfully decontaminated. The simple act of removing clothing achieves removal of the majority of contamination. Any remaining solid contaminant should be carefully brushed away, and any liquid contamination should be blotted off. The second step involves washing the skin surfaces with water or water and a mild detergent to ensure removal of all substances from the skin. Avoid using harsh detergents or bleach solutions on skin, and scrub gently. Chemically or physically aggravating the skin may contribute to increased absorption of the offending agent. When washing, skin folds, axillae, groin, buttocks, and feet must receive special attention because contaminants can collect in these areas and may be overlooked. Decontamination during a radiologic event is almost always dry, as washing may lead to contaminated runoff, and dry decontamination is largely effective in removing secondary contamination.

Specialized decontamination agents, including Reactive Skin Decontamination Lotion, fuller's earth, and various other products, contain active ingredients that may neutralize hazardous chemical agents before they can be fully absorbed through the skin. The exact mechanism of action and application procedures vary by product, but in general they are incorporated as part of the skin decontamination process and are used in place of or in addition to traditionally used soap-and-water or diluted sodium hypochlorite (bleach) solutions. Lab and animal models have suggested usage of these specialized decontamination agents can reduce systemic toxicity and improve survival.[10,11] Individual EMS agencies should consider adding one or more of these products to their decontamination setup; the U.S. Department of Health and Human Services maintains the "Chemical Hazards Emergency Medical Management" website, which contains a helpful database of medical countermeasures and links to supporting research.[12]

Decontamination should be performed in a systematic manner to avoid missing areas of contaminated skin. Contact lenses should be removed from the eyes, and the mucous membranes should be irrigated with copious amounts of water or saline, especially if the patient is symptomatic. Ambulatory patients should be able to perform their own decontamination under instruction from prehospital care practitioners. Nonambulatory patients will require the assistance of emergency responders properly outfitted with appropriate PPE to decontaminate patients on litters. Timely and effective decontamination is critical to improving patient outcomes, but requires large amounts of resources and trained personnel, including site security (to ensure contaminated patients do not wander into "clean" areas), "hot-zone" medical staff (to stabilize patients prior to decontamination when feasible), and enough decontamination teams to maintain a sustainable work-rest cycle (performing decontamination in full PPE can be physically exhausting, particularly in warm ambient temperatures).[13]

Expeditious decontamination may be warranted in the effort to decrease exposure time to various life-threatening substances. All prehospital care practitioners need to be familiar with a hasty decontamination procedure that may be executed even before arrival of the formal hazardous materials/decontamination team, to minimize exposure time for both patients and emergency responders.

When planning for and setting up a decontamination area, the issues to consider include the following:

- Offering privacy for all patients or responders required to disrobe
- Having warm water available when possible for irrigation and showering
- Providing a suitable substitute for clothing at the completion of decontamination
- Assuring victims that their personal belongings will be secure until a final disposition is made regarding their return or necessary disposal
- Appropriately disposing of waste water, if practical

After the victim has been decontaminated, there must be a method in place for documenting that the patient has undergone decontamination. At this point, the victim is not released but is instead observed for a period to note whether signs of toxicity occur or reoccur, indicating incomplete removal of the offending agent and the need for repeat washing and treatment.

Explosions, Explosives, and Incendiary Agents

Understanding injury from explosives is essential for all prehospital care practitioners in both civilian and military settings. Practitioners need to understand the pathophysiology of injury resulting from unintentional and industrial explosive devices and from the wide range of antipersonnel explosive devices such as letter bombs, shaped-charge warheads, rocket-propelled grenades, antipersonnel land mines, aerial-delivered cluster bombs, enhanced blast weapons, and improvised explosive devices (IEDs). A study of the 36,110 bombing incidents in the United States reported by the Bureau of Alcohol, Tobacco, and Firearms (ATF) between 1983 and 2002 concluded that "the U.S. experience reveals that materials used for bombings are readily available [and] healthcare providers . . . need to be prepared."[14]

Explosions occur in homes (primarily due to gas leaks or fires) and are an occupational hazard of many industries, including mining, demolition, chemical manufacturing, or the handling of fuel or dust-producing substances such as grain. Industrial explosions result from chemical spills, fires, faulty equipment maintenance, or electrical/machinery malfunctions, and they may produce fires, toxic fumes, building collapse, secondary explosions, falling debris, and large numbers of casualties. Another common cause of explosion is the rupture of a pressurized containment vessel, such as a boiler, when the internal pressure exceeds the capability of the container to withstand the elevated pressure. Illicit manufacture of methamphetamine, resulting in fires and explosions, has increased in the last two decades and can result in both blast and chemical hazards to first responders.[15] Analyses of workplace-associated fatalities from 1995 to 2010 identified 2,373 incidents of unintentional fires and explosions causing at least one fatality, with fewer than 12% of incidents causing multiple fatalities.[16]

Terrorists worldwide are increasingly using bombs, especially IEDs, against civilian targets. These devices are inexpensive, are made from easily obtained materials, and result in the devastating havoc that focuses international exposure on their efforts. An emergency responder is much more likely to encounter injury from conventional explosives than from a chemical, biologic, or nuclear attack. Globally, over 58,000 terrorist attacks involving the use of explosive devices were identified between 1970 and 2014, with a significant increase in the number of terrorist explosions occurring annually starting in the early 2000s. Of these attacks, approximately 5% were suicide bombings and were associated with significantly increased numbers of fatalities and injuries per attack.[17]

Because both civilian and military emergency responders may be called upon during a bomb attack on civilian populations, all prehospital care practitioners need to be familiar with their roles during these increasingly frequent occurrences.

At present, although the United States is not typically exposed to as many bomb attacks as other countries, explosion incidents (including intentional bombings, accidental explosions, and incidents of undetermined intent or still under investigation) totaled 715 in 2019; these incidents resulted in 86 injuries and 16 fatalities.[18]

Categories of Explosives

Prehospital care practitioners need to consider the type of explosive device and its location when evaluating casualties of terrorist blast incidents.[19] Explosives fall into one of two categories based on the velocity of detonation: high explosives and low explosives.

High Explosives

High explosives react almost instantaneously. Because they are designed to detonate and release their energy very quickly, high explosives are capable of producing a *shock wave*, or **overpressure phenomenon**, which can result in primary blast injury. The initial explosion creates an instantaneous rise in pressure, creating a shock wave that travels outward at supersonic speed, but decays very rapidly.[20] Overpressures from high explosions can exceed 4 million pounds per square inch (psi), compared with 14.7 psi ambient pressure. The shock wave is the leading front and an integral component of the *blast wave*, which is created on the rapid release of enormous amounts of energy, with subsequent propulsion of fragments, generation of environmental debris, and often intense thermal radiation (**Box 18-1**). The shock wave, or pressure wave, propagates from the point of origin, rapidly dissipating as the distance from the point of detonation increases. This wave is not to be confused with wind generated by a blast.

Common examples of high explosives are 2,4,6-trinitrotoluene (TNT), nitroglycerin, dynamite, ammonium nitrate–fuel oil, and the more recent polymer-bonded explosives that have 1.5 times the power of TNT, such as gelignite and the plastic explosive Semtex. High explosives have a sharp, shattering effect (*brisance*) that can pulverize bone and soft tissue, create blast overpressure injuries (*barotrauma*), and propel debris at ballistic speeds (*fragmentation*). It is also important to note that a high explosive may result in a low-order explosion, particularly if the explosive has deteriorated as a result of age (Semtex) or, in some cases, has become wet (dynamite). The reverse, however, is not true; a low explosive cannot produce a high-order explosion.

Low Explosives

Low explosives (e.g., gunpowder), when activated, change relatively slowly from a solid to a gaseous state (in an action more characteristic of burning than of detonation), generally creating a blast wave that moves less than 6,500 ft/sec (2,000 m/sec). Examples of low explosives include pipe bombs, gunpowder, and pure petroleum-based bombs such as Molotov cocktails.[21] Explosions resulting from container rupture and ignition of volatile compounds fall into this category as well. Because they release their energy much more slowly, low explosives are not capable of producing overpressure.

The type and amount of explosive will determine the size of the blast associated with detonation of the device. This fact makes the approach to the scene and the location for staging emergency responders and equipment a critical decision. When responding to a scene that involves either a suspicious device or a potential secondary device, all emergency responders must stage at a safe distance from the site in the event of a second detonation. (See Table 5-1 in Chapter 5, *Scene Management*, for guidelines regarding safe distances depending on the possible size of the explosion.)

Mechanisms of Injury

Traumatic injury after explosions has generally been divided into three categories: primary, secondary, and tertiary blast injury.[22] In addition to the injuries that result directly from the blast, additional categories of injuries classified as quaternary and quinary have been described and result from complications or toxic effects that are related to the explosive or contaminants. Although these injuries are described separately, they may occur in combination in victims of explosions. (Table 4-1 in Chapter 4, *The Physics of Trauma*, summarizes the effects of explosions on the human body.)

Primary Blast Injury

Primary blast injury results from high-order explosive detonation and the interaction of the blast overpressure wave with the body or tissue to produce stress and shear waves. **Stress waves** are supersonic, longitudinal pressure waves that (1) create high local forces with small, rapid distortions; (2) produce microvascular injury; and (3) are reinforced and reflected at tissue interfaces, thereby enhancing injury potential, especially in gas-filled organs such as the lungs, ears, and intestines. Injuries from the stress waves are caused by (1) pressure differentials across delicate structures such as the alveoli of the lung, (2) rapid compression of and subsequent reexpansion of gas-filled structures, and (3) reflection of the wave at the tissue–gas interface.

Shear waves are transverse waves with a lower velocity and longer duration that cause asynchronous movement of tissues. The degree of damage depends on the extent to which the asynchronous motions overcome inherent tissue elasticity, resulting in tearing of tissue and possible disruption of attachments. However, muscle, bone, and solid-organ injury are much more likely to result from the secondary, tertiary, and quaternary effects of the explosion than from the shock wave alone.[23,24]

Depending on the proximity of the victim to the explosion, as well as shielding from or augmentation to the shock wave if the explosion occurs in a closed space, a victim may suffer primary blast injury.

Primary blast injury occurs in gas-filled organs such as the lung, bowel, and middle ear. The injury to the tissue occurs at the gas–fluid interface, presumably from a rapid compression of the gas in the organ, causing violent collapse of that organ, followed by an equally rapid and violent expansion, resulting in tissue injury. Damage to the lung manifests as pulmonary contusions, or possibly *hemopneumothoraces*, resulting in hypoxemia if the patient does not immediately succumb to the injuries (**Box 18-2**). The alveolar–capillary interface can also become disrupted, resulting in arterial gas emboli, which may cause cerebral or cardiac embolic complications. Damage to the bowel may include hematomas of the bowel wall or even perforation of the bowel. Tympanic membrane rupture or disruption of the middle ear ossicles also may occur and is the most common form of primary blast injury. (See Chapter 4, *The Physics of Trauma*.) Loss of hearing is common after an explosion and may be temporary or permanent.

Evidence of primary blast injury to the lung (or BLI) is found more often in patients who die minutes after the explosion from associated injuries than those who survive; however, pulmonary primary blast injury has been noted with greater frequency among surviving victims of confined-space explosions.[25-27] Primary blast injury has also been associated with other severe injuries and is indicative of increased mortality risk in survivors of the initial event. After an open-air explosion in Beirut, only 0.6% of survivors had evidence of primary blast injury, and 11% of those died.[28] In a confined-space explosion in Jerusalem, 38% of survivors had evidence of primary blast injury, with a similar mortality rate of approximately 9%.[29] Similarly, two of the three bombs that were detonated in the London subway system exploded in wide tunnels, resulting in 6 and 7 fatalities, respectively. The third device detonated in the subway system was exploded in a narrow tunnel, causing 26 fatalities. This difference in mortality between open- and closed-space bombings results from the reflection of the blast wave back onto the victims rather than the dispersal of the blast wave into the surrounding area.

Secondary Blast Injury

Secondary blast injury is caused by flying debris and bomb fragments. Secondary blast injury is the most common category of injury in terrorist bombings and low explosions. These projectiles may be components of the bomb itself, as in military weapons designed to fragment, or they may be parts of improvised bombs augmented with nails, screws, and bolts. Secondary blast injury is also caused by debris that is carried by the *blast wind* (Box 18-1). The force required to create enough overpressure to rupture 50% of exposed tympanic membranes (approximately 5 psi) can briefly generate blast winds of 145 miles per hour (233 km per hour). Blast winds associated with an overpressure resulting in significant primary blast injury may exceed 831 miles per hour (1,337 km per hour).[23] Although brief in duration, these blast winds can propel debris with great force and for great distances, causing both penetrating and blunt trauma.

Tertiary Blast Injury

Tertiary blast injury is caused by the blast wind throwing the victim's body, resulting in tumbling and collision with stationary objects. This can result in the whole spectrum of injuries associated with blunt trauma and even penetrating trauma, such as an impalement.

Quaternary and Quinary Effects

Following the blast itself, *quaternary effects* may be seen.[22] These injuries include burns and toxicities from fuel, metals, trauma from structural collapse, and septic syndromes from soil and environmental contamination of wounds.

The increasing threat of radiation-, chemical-, or biologic-enhanced explosives (i.e., dirty bombs) has given rise to a fifth (*quinary*) category of effects, which includes injuries caused by radiation, chemicals, or biologic agents and projectiles such as bone fragments of a suicide bomber.[30,31]

Injury Patterns

The prehospital care practitioner will be confronted with a combination of familiar penetrating, blunt, and thermal injuries and possibly survivors with primary blast injury.[32] The numbers and types of injuries will depend on multiple factors, including explosion magnitude, composition, environment, and location and number of potential victims at risk.

Various mortality rates have been associated with different types of bombings. One study that examined terrorist bombings showed that 1 of 4 victims died immediately after structural-collapse bombings, 1 of 12 died immediately in closed-space bombings, and 1 of 25 died immediately after open-space bombings.[20,33] Additional studies have found that mortality is higher when an explosion occurs in an enclosed space.[34,35] Soft-tissue injuries, orthopedic trauma, and traumatic brain injury are predominant among survivors (**Box 18-3**).

Box 18-2 Blast Lung Injury: What Prehospital Care Practitioners Need to Know

Few civilian prehospital care practitioners in the United States have experience treating patients with explosion-related injuries. **Blast lung injury (BLI)** presents unique triage, diagnostic, and management challenges and is a direct consequence of the blast wave from high-explosive detonations upon the body. Persons in enclosed space explosions or those in close proximity to the explosion are at a higher risk. BLI is a clinical diagnosis characterized by respiratory difficulty and hypoxia. BLI can occur, although rarely, without obvious external injury to the chest. It is often not an immediate manifestation but develops over several hours during the overall course of resuscitation.

Clinical Presentation

- Symptoms may include dyspnea, hemoptysis, cough, and chest pain.
- Signs may include tachypnea, hypoxia, cyanosis, apnea, wheezing, decreased breath sounds, and hemodynamic instability.
- Victims with greater than 10% body surface area burns, skull fractures, and penetrating torso or head injuries may be more likely to have BLI.
- Hemothoraces or pneumothoraces may occur.
- Due to tearing of the pulmonary and vascular tree, air may enter the arterial circulation (*air emboli*) and result in embolic events involving the central nervous system, retinal arteries, or coronary arteries, resulting in stroke-like symptoms.
- Clinical evidence of BLI is often present at the time of initial evaluation; however, it more typically presents several hours after initial injury during the course of resuscitation and has been reported to occur as late as 24 to 48 hours after an explosion.
- Other injuries may often be present.

Prehospital Management Considerations

Although scene safety is always a major consideration for prehospital care practitioners, incidents such as these often require emergency responders of all types to enter the scene before it can be declared completely secure. Practitioners must remain aware of their surroundings, be observant for possible additional devices, and consider other hazards that may have resulted as a consequence of the primary explosion. Patient assessment and management steps are as follows, assuming direct and indirect threat potential has been mitigated and practitioners have a safe operating environment consistent with the instruction in TCCC and TECC:

- Initial triage, trauma resuscitation, and transport of patients should follow standard protocols for multiple injured patients or mass casualties, including assessment and treatment following the XABCDE primary survey or MARCH algorithm (control Massive hemorrhage, Airway, Respiration, Circulation, and Head and Hypothermia).
- Note the patient's location and the surrounding environment. Explosions in a confined space result in a higher incidence of primary blast injury, including lung injury.
- All patients with suspected or confirmed BLI should receive supplemental high-flow oxygen sufficient to prevent hypoxemia.
- Impending airway compromise requires immediate intervention.
- If ventilatory failure is imminent or occurs, patients should be intubated; however, prehospital care practitioners must realize that mechanical ventilation and positive pressure may increase the risk of alveolar rupture, pneumothorax, and air embolism in BLI patients.
- High-flow oxygen should be administered if air embolism is suspected, and the patient should be placed in a semi–left lateral or left lateral position.
- Clinical evidence of or suspicion for a hemothorax or pneumothorax warrants close observation. Chest decompression should be performed for patients clinically presenting with a tension pneumothorax. Close observation is warranted for any patient with suspicion of BLI who is transported by air.
- Fluids should be administered judiciously, as overzealous fluid administration in the patient with BLI may result in volume overload and the worsening of pulmonary status.
- Patients with BLI should be transported rapidly to the nearest appropriate facility, in accordance with community response plans for mass-casualty events.

Data from Centers for Disease Control and Prevention, National Center for Injury Prevention and Control, Division of Injury Response. Blast injuries: fact sheets for professionals. Published March 1, 2012. Accessed January 26, 2022. https://stacks.cdc.gov/view/cdc/21571

For example, of 592 survivors of the Oklahoma City bombing, 85% had soft-tissue injuries (lacerations, puncture wounds, abrasions, contusions), 25% had sprains, 14% had head injuries, 10% had fractures/dislocations, 10% had ocular injuries (9 with ruptured globes), and 2% had burns.[36] The most common location for soft-tissue injury was the extremities (74%), followed by head and neck (48%), face (45%), and chest (35%).

- Musculoskeletal injury accounts for the great majority of surgical procedures in survivors.
- Blast lung predominates among casualties who die (17% to 47%).
- Blast-induced brain and eye trauma is common despite the small surface area of those organs.
- External injuries to four or more body areas or extensive burns (> 10% body surface area) are indicators of serious internal injuries.
- Ear injury (tympanic membrane perforation) is commonly encountered and is bilateral much of the time.
- Mortality rate is significantly higher in closed- versus open-space explosions (15.8% vs. 2.8%).

Data from Frykberg ER, Tepas JJ III. Terrorist bombings: lessons learned from Belfast to Beirut. *Ann Surg.* 1988;208:569-576; Turégano-Fuentes F, Caba-Doussoux P, Jover-Navalón JM, et al. Injury patterns from major urban terrorist bombings in trains: the Madrid experience. *World J Surg.* 2008;32(6):1168-1175.

Eighteen survivors had severe soft-tissue injuries, including carotid artery and jugular vein lacerations; facial and popliteal artery lacerations; and severed nerves, tendons, and ligaments. Seventeen survivors had serious internal organ injury, including partial bowel transection; lacerated kidney, spleen, and liver; pneumothorax; and pulmonary contusion. Of patients with fractures, 37% had multiple fractures. Of those diagnosed with a head injury, 44% required admission to the hospital.[35]

Evaluation and Management

The general evaluation and management of trauma victims are applicable to the casualty from a WMD and are addressed in other chapters. Unique to this patient population, however, is the possibility of primary blast injury. Primary blast injuries might increase the likelihood that prehospital care practitioners will encounter patients with hemoptysis and pulmonary contusions, pneumothorax or tension pneumothorax, or even arterial gas embolism. Among survivors of primary blast injury, clinical manifestations may be present immediately[37,38] or may have a delayed onset of 24 to 48 hours.[39] Intrapulmonary hemorrhage and focal alveolar edema result in frothy bloody secretions and lead to ventilation–perfusion mismatch, increased intrapulmonary shunting, and decreased compliance. Hypoxia results, with increased work of breathing. This is similar in pathophysiology to pulmonary contusions induced by other mechanisms of nonpenetrating thoracic trauma.[40] The presence of rib fractures should

increase suspicion of tertiary or quaternary injury to the thorax.

Primary blast injuries are often not immediately apparent, and, therefore, care at the scene should include (1) monitoring for frothy secretions and respiratory distress, (2) sequential oxygen saturation (SpO_2) measurements, and (3) provision of oxygen. Decreased SpO_2 is a "red flag" for early BLI even before symptoms begin. Fluid administration must be carefully managed, with care taken to avoid fluid overload.[6]

The likelihood of multisystem trauma is increased in bomb victims.[41] The management principles for these patients are similar to those for trauma from other mechanisms. As nuances of the environment of injury can greatly affect the relative predominance of primary versus secondary and higher-order injuries, patients may present with internal injuries out of proportion to their external appearance. For example, a patient close to the blast but shielded by a concrete wall may have significant internal injuries from primary blast effects but appear less severely injured on initial exam than a patient located farther away from the explosion with secondary blast injuries from flying debris resulting in many superficial lacerations. Prehospital practitioners should closely monitor all casualties, reassess vital signs frequently, and retriage to higher categories as indicated.

Transport Considerations

Patients requiring transport must be brought to an appropriate medical treatment facility for further evaluation and management. These patients often require the services of a designated trauma center. Prehospital care practitioners should be aware of the epidemiology of patient transport after an explosives event. Patient arrival at hospitals is usually *bimodal*, with ambulatory patients arriving first and more critically ill patients arriving later by ambulance.

This bimodal patient transport was demonstrated in the Oklahoma City bombing. Patients began to arrive in the EDs 5 to 30 minutes after the bombing, with patients who were more seriously injured taking longer to arrive. Also, the geographically closest hospitals in Oklahoma City received the majority of victims, as seen with other disasters. Nearby hospitals that are overwhelmed by the first wave of patients may experience some difficulty managing the critically ill patients who arrive in the second wave. In Oklahoma City, the aggregate peak arrival rate of patients to EDs was 220 per hour at 60 to 90 minutes; 64% of patients visited EDs within a 1.5-mile radius of the event. Prehospital care practitioners should consider this latter fact when determining the destination of patients transported by ambulance from the bomb scene.[6] In bombings that have occurred where many of the hospitals closest to the bombing have sustained substantial damage themselves, the distribution patterns have been much more complex and harder to predict. For instance, during the 2020 Beirut Port ammonium nitrate explosion, three hospitals closest to the port sustained enough structural damage that they could not receive victims of the blast and in fact had to transfer patients and injured staff to other facilities. Other hospitals (those within a 5-km radius) were so overwhelmed with patients in the 54 hours following the blast that some only recorded those patients admitted to the operating room or intensive care unit. Patients who received primary care (e.g., wound suture or stapling) were unregistered casualties, creating a significant undercount of those affected by the explosion.[42]

Incendiary Agents

Incendiary agents are typically encountered in the military and are used to burn equipment, vehicles, and structures. Terrorists may use them to increase the lethality of improvised explosive devices. The three incendiary agents most often recognized are thermite, magnesium, and white phosphorus. All three are highly flammable compounds that burn at extremely high temperatures.

Thermite

Thermite is powdered aluminum and iron oxide that burns furiously at 3,600°F (1,982°C) and scatters molten iron.[43] Its primary mechanism of injury is partial-thickness or full-thickness burns. The primary and secondary surveys are performed with intervention directed at treating burns. Thermite wounds can be irrigated with copious amounts of water and any residual particles or material subsequently removed.

Magnesium

Magnesium is also a metal in powdered or solid form that burns furiously hot. In addition to its ability to cause partial-thickness or full-thickness burns, magnesium can react with tissue fluid and cause alkali burns. The same chemical reaction produces hydrogen gas, which can cause the wound to bubble or can result in subcutaneous emphysema. Inhalation of magnesium dust can produce respiratory symptoms, including cough, tachypnea, hypoxia, wheeze, pneumonitis, and airway burns. Residual magnesium particles in a wound will react with water, so irrigation is discouraged until the wounds can be debrided and the particulates removed. If irrigation is required for other reasons, such as decontamination of another suspected material, care should be taken to ensure flushing or removal of magnesium particles from the wound.[43]

White Phosphorus

White phosphorus (WP) is a solid that spontaneously ignites when exposed to air, causing a yellow flame and white smoke. WP that comes in contact with skin can quickly result in partial-thickness or full-thickness burns. WP can become embedded in the skin, propelled by the blast of WP munitions. The substance will continue to burn in the skin if exposed to air. Prehospital care practitioners can decrease the likelihood of combustion in the skin by immersing the affected areas in water or applying saline-soaked dressings to the area. Oily or greasy dressings are avoided in these patients because WP is lipid soluble, and application of these dressings may increase the likelihood of systemic absorption and toxicity. Systemic absorption can lead to lethal heart, liver, and kidney injury. Contaminated clothing should be removed, as it may catch fire if the WP reignites. WP fluoresces under ultraviolet light, which can be used to ensure thorough decontamination. Copper sulfate has historically been used to neutralize WP and facilitate its removal because the reaction results in a black compound, which is easier to identify in the skin. Copper sulfate has fallen out of favor, however, because of complications from its use—specifically, intravascular hemolysis (breakdown or rupture of red blood cells within blood vessels); topical application of silver nitrate may be safer and more effective in decontaminating WP embedded in skin and wounds.[44]

Chemical Agents

Many scenarios could expose the prehospital care practitioner to chemical agents (**Box 18-4**), including an industrial complex accident, a spilled tanker truck or railway car, unearthed military ordnance, or a terrorist attack. The 1984 Union Carbide industrial accident in Bhopal, India, and the sarin gas attack in Tokyo in 1995 are examples of such incidents.

Physical Properties of Chemical Agents

The physical properties of a substance are affected by its chemical structure, the environmental temperature, and ambient pressure. These factors will determine whether a substance exists as a solid, liquid, or gas. Understanding the physical state of a chemical agent is important for the prehospital care practitioner because it gives clues about

Box 18-4 Classification of Chemical Agents

- Cyanides (blood agents or asphyxiants)
  - Hydrogen cyanide, cyanogen chloride
- Nerve agents
  - Tabun (GA), sarin (GB), soman (GD), cyclosarin (GF), VX, some agricultural pesticides
- Lung toxicants (choking or pulmonary agents)
  - Chlorine, phosgene, diphosgene, ammonia
- Vesicants (blistering agents)
  - Sulfur mustard, lewisite
- Incapacitating agents
  - BZ (3-quinuclidinyl benzilate)
- Lacrimating agents (riot control agents)
  - CN and CS (tear gas agents), oleoresin capsicum (OC or pepper spray)
- Vomiting agents
  - Adamsite

© National Association of Emergency Medical Technicians (NAEMT)

the likely route of exposure and the potential for transmission and contamination.

A solid is in a state of matter that has a fixed volume and shape; a powder is an example of a solid. When heated to its melting point, solids become liquids. Liquids that are heated to their boiling point become a gas. Solid particles and liquid particles can become suspended in the air, similar to a dust particle or a liquid mist. This is considered an **aerosol**. A **vapor** is simply a solid or liquid that is in a gaseous state but technically would be expected to be found as a solid or liquid at standard temperature and pressure, defined as 32°F (0°C) and normal atmospheric pressure (1 atmosphere, 14.7 psi). Some solids and liquids can, therefore, emit vapors at room temperature. The process of solids emitting vapors, bypassing the liquid state, is called **sublimation**. The likelihood that solids or liquids vaporize into a gaseous form at room temperature is defined as the **volatility** of the substance. Highly volatile substances easily convert into a gas at room temperature.

These physical properties have implications for primary and secondary contamination and possible routes of exposure. **Primary contamination** is defined as exposure to the chemical agent at its point of release. For example, primary contamination occurs, by definition, in the hot zone. Gases, vapors, liquids, solids, and aerosols can all play a role in primary contamination.

Secondary contamination is defined as exposure to a chemical agent after it has been carried away from the point of origin, whether by a victim, an emergency responder, or a piece of contaminated equipment or debris. Secondary contamination generally occurs in the warm zone, although it may happen at more remote locations if the exposed victim is able to self-evacuate. Solids and liquids (and sometimes aerosols) generally contribute to secondary

contamination. Gases and vapors do not typically play a role in secondary contamination because they cause injury by inhalation of the substance and do not deposit on skin. However, vapors can become trapped in clothing and then off-gas to potentially expose others to the hazard.

Volatility plays a significant role in the risk of secondary contamination. More volatile substances are considered "less persistent," meaning that because they vaporize, the likelihood of long-lasting physical contamination is unlikely. These chemical agents will readily disperse and be carried away by the wind. Less volatile substances are considered "more persistent." These substances do not vaporize, or do so at a very slow rate, thereby remaining on exposed surfaces for a long time, increasing the risk of secondary contamination. For example, the nerve agent sarin is a nonpersistent agent, whereas the nerve agent VX is a persistent agent.[45]

Personal Protective Equipment

PPE is selected based on the threat of exposure to the chemical agent. Level A is appropriate for emergency responders entering the hot zone, until specific agents in use and their concentrations are known. Once the agent has been identified, incident command may make the decision to move to lower levels of PPE (B or C), particularly for responders tasked with carrying out decontamination or working in the "warm zone." Of note, agency-specific protocols should always determine the zone in which responders are able to operate safely.

Evaluation and Management

After ensuring the safety of the scene, the prehospital care practitioner must first confirm that victims are undergoing decontamination. Patients with likely skin exposure to the liquid form of a chemical will require decontamination with water. If available, soap may be used as well, but showering with copious amounts of water will generally suffice. Exposure to a gas does not mandate decontamination by shower, but it does mandate removal from any ongoing exposure and removal of any clothing that may have trapped residual vapors, which can subsequently off-gas and pose a hazard to care practitioners in the field or in the hospital.

Once the victim has been properly decontaminated, the prehospital care practitioner will likely encounter patients with signs and symptoms of exposure to a hazardous substance that has not yet been specifically identified. Victims of chemical agents can manifest signs and symptoms of exposure that affect the following areas:

- The respiratory system, affecting oxygenation and ventilation
- The mucous membranes, causing eye and upper airway injury

- The nervous system, resulting in seizures or coma and altered levels of consciousness
- The gastrointestinal (GI) tract, causing vomiting or diarrhea
- The skin, causing burning and blistering

It is important to evaluate the presenting signs and symptoms and whether they are improving or progressing. Patients with worsening clinical findings likely had incomplete cleansing of the contaminant and should undergo repeat decontamination to assure complete removal.

Patients require a primary survey to determine what lifesaving intervention may be immediately required. A secondary survey may then assist in the identification of symptom constellations that might indicate the nature of the chemical agent and suggest a specific antidote. This constellation of clinical signs and symptoms suggesting exposure to a certain class of chemical or toxin is called a **toxidrome**.[46]

The *irritant gas toxidrome* includes mucous membrane burning and inflammation, coughing, and difficulty breathing. Agents responsible might include chlorine, phosgene, or ammonia.

The *asphyxiant toxidrome* is caused by cellular oxygen deprivation. This can result from inadequate oxygen availability, as in an oxygen-poor atmosphere; inadequate oxygen delivery to the cells, as in carbon monoxide poisoning; or inability to utilize oxygen at the cellular level, as in cyanide poisoning. Signs and symptoms include shortness of breath, chest pain, dysrhythmias, syncope, seizures, coma, and death.

The *cholinergic toxidrome* is characterized by rhinorrhea, respiratory secretions, difficulty breathing, nausea, vomiting, diarrhea, profuse sweating, pinpoint pupils, possible altered mental status, seizures, and coma. Pesticides and nerve agents can cause these cholinergic signs and symptoms.[47,48]

Most often, prehospital care practitioners will initiate supportive therapy without knowing the specific chemical cause of the injury. If the offending agent is properly identified, or if its identity is suggested by the toxidrome or clinical presentation, therapy specific to the agent may be delivered. Cyanide and nerve agent victims are examples of patients who can benefit from agent-specific antidote therapy.

Transport Considerations

Contaminated patients should not be transported until they have been decontaminated. Transporting contaminated patients results in cross-contamination of the transporting vehicle and personnel, thus taking them out of service until they have been decontaminated. This leads to compromise of the response capability of the ambulance service and may prolong the scene time and management of ill or injured patients. This same concern about not transporting contaminated patients applies to air medical services.

Patients must be brought to an appropriate medical treatment facility for further evaluation and management. Transporting to the optimal facility is particularly important because some chemical toxic effects may not become apparent for 8 to 24 hours. Communities may identify preferred hospitals for the management of chemical casualties. These facilities may be more capable of managing these patients by virtue of specialized training or availability of critical care services and specific antidotes. Considerations similar to those previously noted for explosive incidents regarding transport epidemiology also apply to these patients.

Nearby EDs may become overwhelmed by ambulatory, self-evacuated, self-transported patients. Of the 640 patients presenting to one hospital in Tokyo after the sarin incident, 541 arrived without EMS assistance.[49] Hospitals closest to the event will likely receive the largest number of ambulatory patients. These factors should be considered in determining the destination of patients transported via ambulance.

Selected Specific Chemical Agents

Cyanides

Prehospital care practitioners encounter cyanides most commonly when responding to a fire in which certain plastics or textiles are burning or to certain industrial complexes, where they may be found in large quantities. Cyanides are used in chemical syntheses, electroplating, mineral extraction, dyeing, printing, photography, agriculture, and the manufacture of paper, textiles, and plastics. However, cyanide also has been inventoried in military stockpiles, and some terrorist websites have provided instructions for making a cyanide dispersal device.

Hydrogen cyanide is a highly volatile liquid and, thus, will most often be encountered as a vapor or gas. Therefore, it has greater potential for mass casualties in a confined space with poor ventilation than if released outdoors. Although a smell of bitter almonds has been associated with this agent, this is not a reliable indicator of hydrogen cyanide exposure, and not everyone can detect this odor.[50]

Cyanide's mechanism of action is arrest of metabolism or respiration at the cellular level, quickly resulting in cell death. Cyanide binds in the mitochondria of cells, preventing oxygen usage in cellular metabolism. Victims of cyanide poisoning actually are able to inhale and absorb oxygen into the blood but are unable to use it at the cellular level. Thus, patients who are ventilating will present with evidence of acyanotic hypoxia.

The organs most affected are the central nervous system (CNS) and the heart. Symptoms of mild cyanide poisoning include headache, dizziness, drowsiness, nausea, vomiting, and mucosal irritation. Severe cyanide poisoning includes alteration of consciousness, dysrhythmias, hypotension, seizures, and death. Death can occur within a few minutes after inhalation of high levels of cyanide gas.

Management

Supportive therapy is important, including high-concentration oxygen delivery, correction of hypotension with fluids or vasopressors, and management of seizures. Cyanide antidote kits are available for patients with known or suspected cyanide poisoning.

Hydroxocobalamin (pro-vitamin B_{12}) is the preferred field antidote for cyanide poisoning because it is easy to use, it involves a single medication administration instead of two, and it does not create an intermediate chemical that is itself a poison. Modern cyanide antidote kits contain IV hydroxocobalamin, which binds with cyanide to form cyanocobalamin (vitamin B_{12}), which is nontoxic.

The traditional, now antiquated, cyanide antidote treatment kit involved treatment with two medications, a nitrite followed by thiosulfate. The administration of inhaled amyl nitrite, or preferably intravenous (IV) sodium nitrite, creates methemoglobin (itself a poison that in high enough concentrations can kill), which binds cyanide in the bloodstream, making it less available to poison the patient's cellular respiration. The nitrite is followed by IV administration of sodium thiosulfate to assist the body in the conversion of cyanide to harmless thiocyanate, which is excreted by the kidneys.

Nerve Agents

Nerve agents were originally developed as insecticides, but once their effects on humans were recognized, numerous different types were developed in the early to mid-1900s. These deadly chemicals can be found in the military stockpiles of many nations. Nerve agents have also been produced and used by terrorist organizations, the most notorious releases occurring in Matsumoto, Japan, in 1994 and in the Tokyo, Japan, subway system in 1995. More recently, United Nations inspectors confirmed the use of the nerve agent sarin against civilians in the Syrian civil war in 2013, resulting in multiple casualties, including first responders.[51] Commonly available pesticides (e.g., malathion, carbaryl [Sevin]) and common therapeutic medications (e.g., physostigmine, pyridostigmine) share properties with nerve agents, causing similar clinical effects.

Nerve agents are usually liquids at room temperature. Sarin is the most volatile of the group. VX is the least volatile and is found as an oily liquid. The main routes of intoxication are through inhalation of the vapor (usually the volatile or nonpersistent agents) and

absorption through the skin (usually VX). Nerve agents can injure or kill at very low doses. A single small drop the size of a pinhead of VX, the most potent nerve agent developed, placed on the skin could kill a victim. Because nerve agents are liquids, they pose a risk for secondary contamination from contact with contaminated clothes, skin, and other objects.

The mechanism of action of nerve agents is inhibition of the enzyme acetylcholinesterase, an enzyme required to break down acetylcholine. **Acetylcholine** is a neurotransmitter that stimulates cholinergic receptors. Acetylcholine receptors are found in smooth muscles, skeletal muscles, the CNS, and most exocrine (secretory) glands. Some of these cholinergic receptors are termed **muscarinic sites** (because experimentally they are stimulated by muscarine) and are mostly found in smooth muscles and glands. Others are termed **nicotinic sites** (because experimentally they are stimulated by nicotine) and are mostly found in skeletal muscle. The mnemonic **DUMBELS** (**D**iarrhea, **U**rination, **M**iosis, **B**radycardia, **B**ronchorrhea, **B**ronchospasm, **E**mesis, **L**acrimation, **S**alivation, **S**weating) represents the constellation of symptoms associated with the muscarinic effects of nerve agent toxicity. The mnemonic **MTWHF** (**M**ydriasis [rarely seen], **T**achycardia, **W**eakness, **H**ypertension, **H**yperglycemia, **F**asciculations) represents the constellation of symptoms associated with stimulation of nicotinic receptors (**Box 18-5**). The CNS effects, a result of both muscarinic and nicotinic receptors, include confusion, convulsions, and coma.

The clinical effects depend on the dose and route of nerve agent exposure (inhalation or dermal) and whether the muscarinic or nicotinic effects predominate. Small amounts of vapor exposure primarily cause irritation to eyes, nose, and airways. Large amounts of vapor exposure can quickly lead to loss of consciousness, seizures, apnea, and muscular flaccidity. *Miosis* (constricted pupils) is the most sensitive marker of exposure to vapor. Symptoms of dermal exposure also vary according to dose and time of onset. Small doses may not result

---

Box 18-5 Nerve Agent Mnemonics

The mnemonic DUMBELS (**D**iarrhea, **U**rination, **M**iosis, **B**radycardia, **B**ronchorrhea, **B**ronchospasm, **E**mesis, **L**acrimation, **S**alivation, **S**weating) represents the constellation of symptoms associated with the muscarinic effects of nerve agent toxicity.

The mnemonic MTWHF (**M**ydriasis [rarely seen], **T**achycardia, **W**eakness, **H**ypertension, **H**yperglycemia, **F**asciculations) represents the constellation of symptoms associated with stimulation of nicotinic receptors.

in symptoms for up to 18 hours. Fasciculations of the underlying muscles and localized sweating at the site of the skin exposure may occur, followed by GI symptoms, nausea, vomiting, and diarrhea. Large dermal doses will result in onset of symptoms in minutes, with effects similar to a large vapor exposure.

Clinical symptoms of nerve agents include *rhinorrhea* (runny nose), chest tightness, miosis (pupil is pinpoint, and patient complains of blurry or dim vision), shortness of breath, excessive salivation and sweating, nausea, vomiting, abdominal cramps, involuntary urination and defecation, muscle fasciculations, confusion, seizures, flaccid paralysis, coma, respiratory failure, and death.

Management

Management of nerve agent poisoning includes decontamination (**Figure 18-3**), a primary survey, administration of antidotes, and supportive therapy. Ventilation and oxygenation of the patient may be difficult because of bronchoconstriction and copious secretions. The patient will likely require frequent suctioning. These symptoms improve after sufficient quantities of antidotes are administered. The three therapeutic medications for the management of nerve agent poisoning are atropine, pralidoxime chloride, and benzodiazepines.

Atropine is an anticholinergic medication that reverses most of the muscarinic effects of the nerve agent via competitive antagonism at the receptor site, although it has little effect on the nicotinic sites. Atropine is indicated for exposed victims with pulmonary complaints. Miosis alone is not an indication for atropine, and furthermore, atropine will not correct the ocular abnormalities. Atropine is given according to local system protocols. It is titrated until the patient's ability to breathe or ventilate is improved or there is drying of pulmonary secretions. In moderate to severe exposures, it is not unusual to start with an initial dose of 4 to 6 milligrams (mg) and give as much as 10 to 20 mg of atropine over a few hours.

Pralidoxime chloride (2-PAM chloride) is an oxime. Pralidoxime works by uncoupling the bond between the nerve agent and acetylcholinesterase, thereby reactivating the enzyme and helping to reduce the effects of the nerve agent, primarily on nicotinic receptors. The oxime therapy needs to be initiated within minutes to a few hours of the exposure to be effective, depending on the nerve agent released; otherwise, the bond between acetylcholinesterase and the nerve agent will become permanent ("aging"), delaying recovery of the patient.

Benzodiazepine therapy is initiated to manage the seizures and help to reduce the brain injury and other life-threatening effects associated with status epilepticus. It is recommended for all patients with signs of significant nerve agent poisoning whether or not they have begun to seize. Midazolam (Versed) is the preferred benzodiazepine medication due to its rapid high bioavailability after intramuscular or intravenous injection. Evidence from animal models suggests the seizure-terminating and neuroprotective effects are lessened if administration is delayed after the initial poisoning.[52] If midazolam is unavailable, diazepam (Valium) or lorazepam (Ativan) are alternative agents, but they may be less effective than midazolam.[53,54]

Atropine and pralidoxime come packaged together in a single autoinjector called DuoDote. The dose of atropine is 2.1 mg, and the dose of pralidoxime is 600 mg. This autoinjector is intended for rapid intramuscular injection in the event of a nerve agent exposure. Total dosage is determined by protocol and titration of these medications to effect. In the past, the atropine and pralidoxime were supplied in individual autoinjectors marketed as the "Mark-1" kit. These kits have largely been supplanted by the single autoinjector containing both antidotes. Diazepam is also available as a 10-mg autoinjector, marketed as the Convulsant Antidote for Nerve Agents (CANA; **Figure 18-4**).

Treatment with up to 6 mg of atropine via 1 to 3 autoinjectors given at 5- to 10-minute intervals should be sufficient to treat most minor to moderate severity nerve agent casualties to the clinical endpoint of drying respiratory secretions. However, more severely poisoned cases are likely to require significantly larger quantities of atropine, pralidoxime, and benzodiazepines than carried by most prehospital practitioners. If patients have not reached clinical stability within several minutes of use of multiple autoinjectors, consider administering additional atropine and benzodiazepines intravenously until definitive care can be undertaken at a hospital.[48] The CHEMPACK system, administered by the Strategic National Stockpile, has distributed large quantities of nerve agent medical countermeasures, including autoinjectors and multidose vials of atropine, pralidoxime, and benzodiazepines, in order to allow for rapid and effective treatment of nerve agent

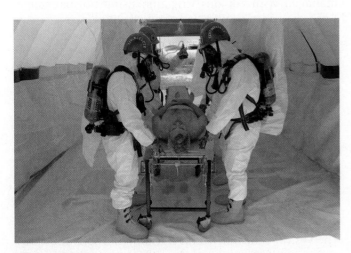

Figure 18-3 Decontamination from nerve agents.
© Jones & Bartlett Learning. Photographed by Glen E. Ellman.

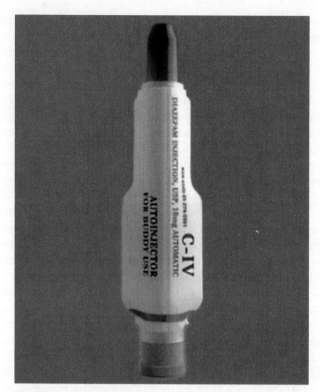

Figure 18-4 Convulsant Antidote for Nerve Agents (CANA).
Courtesy of the USDHHS Radiation Emergency Medical Management.

mass-casualty incidents.[55] Prehospital practitioners should familiarize themselves with the locations of the nearest CHEMPACK resources for consideration of where to transport severe or large numbers of nerve agent casualties.

Lung Toxicants

Lung toxicants, including chlorine, phosgene, ammonia, sulfur dioxide, and nitrogen dioxide, are present in numerous industrial manufacturing applications. Phosgene has been stockpiled for military applications and was the most lethal chemical warfare agent used in World War I. United Nations investigators researching chemical attacks during the Syrian civil war suspected, but could not absolutely confirm, that chlorine was used as a weapon in multiple incidents.[56]

Lung toxicants that are chemical pulmonary agents may be gases, vapors, aerosolized liquids, or solids. The properties of the agent influence its ability to cause injury. For example, aerosolized particles of 2 micrometers (μm) or smaller readily access the alveoli of the lung, causing injury there, whereas larger particles are filtered out before reaching the alveoli. Water solubility of an agent also affects the injury pattern. Ammonia and sulfur dioxide, which are highly water soluble, cause irritation and injury to the eyes, mucous membranes, and upper airways. Phosgene and nitrogen oxides, which have low water solubility, tend to cause less immediate irritation

and injury to the eyes, mucous membranes, and upper airways, thus providing little warning to the victim and allowing for prolonged exposure to these agents. Prolonged exposure makes it more likely that the alveoli will be injured, resulting not only in upper-airway injury, but also in alveolar collapse and noncardiogenic pulmonary edema. Moderately water-soluble agents, such as chlorine, can cause both upper airway and alveolar irritation.

The mechanisms of injury vary among the lung toxicants. Ammonia, for example, combines with the water in the mucous membranes to form a strong base, ammonium hydroxide. Chlorine and phosgene, when combined with water, produce hydrochloric acid, causing injury to the tissues. Lung toxicants are not systemically absorbed but compromise the victim by damaging components of the pulmonary system, from the upper airway to the alveoli.

The agents with high water solubility cause burning of the eyes, nose, and mouth. Tearing, rhinorrhea, coughing, dyspnea, and respiratory distress secondary to glottic irritation or laryngospasm are possible. Bronchospasm can result in coughing, wheezing, and dyspnea. Agents with low water solubility, causing injury to the alveoli, can immediately injure the alveolar epithelium in the case of a large exposure, leading to death from acute respiratory failure, or, with less massive exposure, can result in a delayed onset (24 to 48 hours) of respiratory distress, secondary to development of mild noncardiogenic pulmonary edema to fulminant acute respiratory distress syndrome, depending on the dose.

Management

Management of lung toxicants includes removal of the patient from the offending agent, decontamination with copious irrigation (if solid, liquid, or aerosol exposure, especially for ammonia), primary survey, and supportive therapy, which will likely require interventions to maximize ventilation and oxygenation. Eye irritation can be managed with copious irrigation using normal saline. Contact lenses should be removed. Expect to manage profuse airway secretions, which will require suctioning. Bronchospasm may respond to inhaled beta-adrenergic agonists. Hypoxia will require correction with high-flow oxygen and possibly intubation with positive-pressure ventilation. Prehospital care practitioners need to be prepared to encounter difficult airway management secondary to copious secretions, inflammation of glottic structures, and laryngeal spasm. All victims exposed to phosgene should be transported for evaluation because of the likelihood of delayed symptoms.

Vesicant Agents

The vesicants include sulfur mustard, nitrogen mustards, and lewisite. These agents have been stockpiled for military operations by many countries. Sulfur mustard was first introduced to the battlefield in World War I. It was reportedly used by Iraq against its Kurdish population and also in its conflict with Iran in 1980. More recently it is suspected to have been used in warfare in Syria. It is relatively easy and inexpensive to manufacture.

Sulfur mustard is an oily, clear to yellow-brown liquid that can be aerosolized by a bomb blast or a sprayer. Its volatility is low, allowing it to persist on surfaces for a week or more. This persistence allows for easy secondary contamination. The agent is absorbed through the skin and mucous membranes, resulting in direct cellular damage within 3 to 5 minutes of the exposure, although clinical symptoms and signs may take 1 to 12 hours (usually 4 to 6 hours) after exposure to develop. The delayed onset of symptoms often makes it difficult for the victim to recognize that the exposure occurred and, therefore, increases the potential for secondary contamination. Warm, moist skin increases the likelihood of skin absorption, making the groin and axillary regions particularly susceptible. The eyes, skin, and upper airways can develop a range of findings, from erythema and edema to vesicle development to full-thickness necrosis. Upper airway involvement can result in cough and bronchospasm. High-dose exposures can result in nausea and vomiting, as well as bone marrow suppression.

Management for sulfur mustard involves decontamination using soap and water, primary survey, and supportive therapy; no antidote exists for the effects of mustard agents. In fact, it is important to note that because the cellular damage from sulfur mustard occurs within several minutes of the exposure, decontamination will not change the clinical course of the exposed patient. It is primarily intended to prevent inadvertent cross-contamination. Eyes and skin should be decontaminated with copious amounts of water as soon as exposure is recognized to minimize further absorption of the agent and prevent secondary contamination. The fluid in resulting vesicles and blisters is not a source of secondary contamination. Pulmonary bronchoconstriction may benefit from nebulized beta-agonists. Skin wounds should be treated as burns, with regard to local wound care.

Lewisite has a similar constellation of symptoms, but the onset of action is much quicker than with sulfur mustard, resulting in immediate pain and irritation to the eyes, skin, and respiratory tract. Unlike sulfur mustard, lewisite does not cause bone marrow suppression. Also unique to this agent is "lewisite shock," the result of intravascular volume depletion secondary to capillary leakage.

As with sulfur mustard, prehospital management of these exposed patients involves decontamination, primary survey, and supportive care. British anti-lewisite is an antidote available for the in-hospital treatment of lewisite-exposed patients. It is administered intravenously for patients with hypovolemic shock or pulmonary symptoms. Applied topically, British anti-lewisite ointment has

been reported to prevent mucous membrane and skin injury. Care practitioners should be careful to avoid coming in contact with the fluid inside skin blisters caused by lewisite, as it may contain toxic arsenic compounds and active lewisite or dangerous breakdown products.[57]

Biologic Agents

Biologic agents in the form of contagious disease exposure represent a threat to prehospital care practitioners on a daily basis (**Box 18-6**). Proper infection control procedures must be in place to prevent the contraction or transmission of tuberculosis, influenza, human immunodeficiency virus (HIV), methicillin-resistant *Staphylococcus aureus* (MRSA), SARS variants, meningococcus, and myriad other organisms.

Referenced here are diseases as we currently understand their contagion capabilities. However, viral function can potentially be manipulated in the lab. It is possible that such manipulation could result in production of viral variants with substantially increased infectivity and virulence. Intentional or accidental release of such pathogens into the environment could trigger a pandemic as large or larger than the recent COVID-19 pandemic. While there is no proof that allows for a definitive conclusion as to whether the SARS CoV-2 virus responsible for the COVID-19 pandemic was released from a laboratory versus transmitted to humans from an animal reservoir, the resulting impact certainly reminds us of the potential for

---

Box 18-6 Classification of Biologic WMD Agents

- Bacterial agents
  - Anthrax
  - Brucellosis
  - Glanders
  - Plague
  - Q fever
  - Tularemia
- Viral agents
  - Smallpox
  - Venezuelan equine encephalitis
  - Nipah virus
  - Viral hemorrhagic fevers (Ebola virus, yellow fever, hantavirus)
  - New threats related to viral gain-of-function research[58]
- Biologic toxins
  - Botulinum
  - Ricin
  - Staphylococcal enterotoxin B
  - T-2 mycotoxins

such an event in the future, resulting from either an intentional deployment of virus to cause a pandemic or a lab accident occurring in the context of an attempt to manipulate or even just to study a virus.

Preparing for bioterrorist events increases the complexity of EMS system preparation. An intentional terrorist act might include delivery of a biologic agent with the potential to cause disease or illness, such as aerosolized spores, aerosolized live organisms, or an aerosolized biologic toxin. Patients with pathogens not typically seen by prehospital care practitioners, such as plague, anthrax, and smallpox, might be encountered, requiring appropriate PPE and precautions. Familiar infection control procedures will be effective in the safe management of these potentially contagious patients. If the practitioner is responding to an overt release event, appropriate precautions regarding decontamination of victims and PPE are required, similar to other hazardous materials events. However, this entire process becomes much more complicated in the context of delayed presentation. Variability in incubation periods makes determination of sources of contamination and control of spread more difficult to achieve.

Concentrated Biohazard Agent Versus Infected Patient

Prehospital care practitioners can experience bioterrorism in two ways. The first scenario involves the overt release of a material that is either identified as, or thought to be, a biologic agent. The anthrax hoaxes of 1998 and 1999 and the anthrax letters of 2001 are good examples. Practitioners responded on countless occasions to individuals covered in "white powder" or suspected anthrax. In this situation, the practitioner will encounter an environment or a patient contaminated with a suspicious substance. EMS systems may be summoned to suspicious activity, such as a device delivering an unknown aerosol agent. The nature of the threat at these events is usually unknown, and precautions for personal safety should always be paramount. These incidents must be respected and treated as a WMD incident until proven otherwise. If the suspicious substance is in fact a concentrated aerosol of an infectious organism or toxin, PPE appropriate for the biologic agent and decontamination are required.

In this situation, prehospital care practitioners will be caring for victims contaminated with a suspected biologic agent on their skin or clothing. Any person, patient, or practitioner coming in direct physical contact with a suspected biologic agent should remove all exposed articles of clothing and perform a thorough washing of exposed skin with soap and water.[59] Clinically significant re-aerosolization of material from victims' skin or clothing is unlikely, and the risk to the practitioner is negligible.[60] However, as a matter of routine practice, potentially

contaminated clothing normally removed by pulling the item over the face and head should instead be cut off to minimize any risk of inadvertent inhalation of contaminant. Decontamination may then proceed using water or soap and water. Consultation with appropriate public health and law enforcement officials will then determine the need for antibiotic prophylaxis.

The second scenario involves a response to a patient who is a victim of a remote, covert bioterrorist event. Perhaps the patient inhaled anthrax spores after a covert attack at work and now, several days later, is manifesting signs of pulmonary anthrax. Perhaps a terrorist has self-inoculated with smallpox, and you are summoned to assist a person with a suspicious rash. In these cases, personal and public safety can be ensured by knowledge of proper infection control procedures and the proper donning and removal of PPE appropriate for the biohazard (**Box 18-7** and **Box 18-8**). Decontamination of the patient in this scenario is not necessary because the exposure occurred several days in the past.

All prehospital care practitioners should be familiar with PPE for infection-control purposes. Different types of PPE are recommended, depending on the potential for transmission and the likely route of transmission.

Box 18-7 Sequence for Putting on PPE

The type of PPE used will vary based on the level of precautions required (e.g., standard precautions and contact, droplet, or airborne infection isolation).

1. Gown
   - Fully cover torso from neck to knees, arms to end of wrists, and wrap around the back.
   - Fasten in back of neck and waist.
2. Mask or respirator
   - Secure ties or elastic bands at middle of head and neck.
   - Fit flexible band to nose bridge.
   - Fit snug to face and below chin.
   - Fit-check respirator.
3. Goggles or face shield
   - Place over face and eyes and adjust to fit.
4. Gloves
   - Extend to cover wrist of isolation gown.

Use safe work practices to protect yourself and limit the spread of contamination:

- Keep hands away from face.
- Limit surfaces touched.
- Change gloves when torn or heavily contaminated.
- Perform hand hygiene.

Reproduced from Centers for Disease Control and Prevention. PPE sequence. October 16, 2014. https://www.cdc.gov/hai/pdfs/ppe/ppe-sequence.pdf

Box 18-8 Sequence for Removing PPE

Except for the respirator, remove PPE at the doorway or in an anteroom of the involved room. Remove the respirator after leaving the contaminated room and closing the door.

1. Gloves
   - The outside of the glove is contaminated!
     - Grasp outside of glove with opposite gloved hand; peel off.
     - Hold removed glove in gloved hand.
     - Slide fingers of ungloved hand under remaining glove at wrist.
     - Peel glove off over first glove.
     - Discard gloves in waste container.
2. Goggles
   - The outside of the goggles or face shield is contaminated!
     - To remove, handle by headband or ear pieces.
     - Place in designated receptacle for reprocessing or in waste container.
3. Gown
   - The gown front and sleeves are contaminated!
     - Unfasten gown ties.
     - Pull away from neck and shoulders, touching inside of gown only.
     - Turn gown inside out.
     - Fold or roll into a bundle and discard in waste container.
4. Mask or respirator
   - The front of the mask/respirator is contaminated—do not touch!
     - Grasp bottom, then top ties or elastics, and remove.
     - Discard in waste container.

Once PPE is removed, wash hands. If hands become contaminated during any step of removing PPE, immediately wash hands or use an alcohol-based sanitizer.

Data from Centers for Disease Control and Prevention, Atlanta. Sequence for putting on personal protective equipment (PPE). https://www.cdc.gov/hai/pdfs/ppe/ppe-sequence.pdf

Transmission-based PPE is used in addition to the standard precautions, which are used in the care of all patients. These include contact, droplet, and aerosol precautions.

Contact Precautions

This level of protection is recommended to reduce the likelihood of transmission of microorganisms by direct or indirect contact. Contact precautions include the use of gloves and a gown.

Commonly encountered organisms that require contact precautions include viral conjunctivitis, MRSA, scabies, and herpes simplex or zoster virus. Organisms that require strict contact precautions that might be encountered as a result of bioterrorism include bubonic plague or the viral hemorrhagic fevers, such as Marburg or Ebola, as long as the patient does not have pulmonary symptoms or profuse vomiting and diarrhea, in which case airborne precautions should also be taken.

Droplet Precautions

This level of protection is recommended to reduce the likelihood of transmission of microorganisms that are known to be transmitted by large droplet nuclei (greater than 5 µm) expelled by an infected person in the course of talking, sneezing, or coughing or during routine procedures, such as suctioning. These droplets infect by landing on the exposed mucous membranes of the eyes, nose, and mouth. Because the droplets are large, they do not remain suspended in air, and therefore, contact must be in close proximity, usually defined as 3 feet (0.9 meters) or less. Droplet precautions include the contact precautions of gloves and gown and additional eye protection and a surgical mask. Because the droplets do not remain suspended in air, no additional respiratory protection or air filtration is required.

Typically encountered organisms in this category include influenza, *Mycoplasma pneumoniae*, and invasive *Haemophilus influenzae* or *Neisseria meningitidis*, causing sepsis or meningitis. Pneumonic plague is an example of a possible agent encountered as a result of a bioterrorist event.

Aerosol Precautions

This level of protection is recommended to reduce the likelihood of transmission of microorganisms by the airborne route. Some organisms can become suspended in the air attached to small droplet nuclei (less than 5 µm) or attached to dust particles. In this case, microorganisms can become widely dispersed by air currents immediately around the source or more distant from the source, depending on environmental conditions. To avoid such dispersion, these patients are kept in negative-pressure isolation rooms in a hospital in which the exhaust ventilation can be filtered.

Aerosol precautions include gloves, gown, eye protection, and a fit-tested high-efficiency particulate air (HEPA) filter mask, such as the N95 (**Box 18-9**). Examples of illnesses typically encountered that would require aerosol precautions include tuberculosis, measles, chickenpox, and SARS and its variants, including SARS-CoV-2. Smallpox and viral hemorrhagic fever with pulmonary symptoms are examples that could possibly be related to a bioterrorist event.

Box 18-9 Biologic Agent Precautions

Note that many illnesses associated with biologic events require no additional protection beyond standard precautions, provided there is no risk of exposure to a concentrated agent. Examples include patients with inhalational anthrax or a biologic toxin such as botulinum. However, in most cases, the specific biologic agent will likely not be identified for several days. Although some agents, such as anthrax, are not spread from person to person, prehospital care practitioners must assume the worst—that the biologic agent is contagious—and use all available precautions, including aerosol precautions.

© National Association of Emergency Medical Technicians (NAEMT)

Selected Agents

The CDC categorizes bioterrorism agents by priority level, based on their impact to the public (**Table 18-1**).

Anthrax

Anthrax is a disease caused by the bacterium *Bacillus anthracis*. *B. anthracis* is a spore-forming bacterium and, thus, can exist as either a vegetative cell or as a spore. The vegetative cell lives well in a host organism but cannot survive long outside the body, unlike the spore, which can remain viable in the environment for decades.

The disease is naturally occurring, contracted most often by persons in contact with infected animals or anthrax-contaminated animal products resulting in the cutaneous form of the disease. The spores have been weaponized and are known to be inventoried in several nations' military stockpiles. The accidental release of aerosolized anthrax spores from a Soviet military facility at Sverdlovsk in 1979 resulted in approximately 79 cases of pulmonary anthrax with 68 reported deaths. Letters contaminated with anthrax spores were sent through the U.S. Postal Service in 2001 to prominent legislators and media outlets. Although only 22 cases (11 pulmonary, 11 cutaneous) and 5 deaths resulted, thousands of people required prophylaxis with antibiotics. A hypothetical release of 220 pounds (100 kilograms [kg]) of anthrax spores over Washington, D.C., is estimated to be capable of causing 130,000 to 3 million deaths.[61]

Routes of exposure to anthrax include the respiratory tract, the GI tract, and breaks in the skin. Exposure to anthrax through the respiratory tract leads to inhalational or pulmonary anthrax. Exposure through the GI tract causes gastrointestinal anthrax, and skin infection causes cutaneous anthrax.

Gastrointestinal anthrax is rare and would result from ingesting food substances contaminated with spores. Patients have nonspecific symptoms of nausea, vomiting, malaise, bloody diarrhea, and acute abdomen; mortality is approximately 50%. Cutaneous anthrax follows deposition of spores or organisms into a break in the skin. This results in a papule, which subsequently ulcerates and causes a dry, black eschar with local edema. If not treated with antibiotics, mortality approaches 20%; with antibiotics, mortality is rare.[62]

For maximal effectiveness in a terrorist attack, anthrax would likely be disseminated in its spore form. Anthrax spores are approximately 1 to 5 µm in size, which allows the spores to be suspended in air as an aerosol. Aerosolized spores can be inhaled into the lungs and deposited in the alveoli. They are then consumed by macrophages and carried to the mediastinal lymph nodes, where they germinate, manufacture toxins, and cause *acute hemorrhagic mediastinitis* (bleeding into the lymph nodes in the middle of the chest cavity) and often death. The onset of symptoms after inhalation of spores varies, with most victims developing symptoms within 1 to 7 days, although there may be a latency period of as long as 60 days. Symptoms initially are nonspecific, including fever, chills, dyspnea, cough, chest pain, headache, and vomiting. After a few days, symptoms improve, followed by a rapidly deteriorating course of fever, dyspnea, diaphoresis, shock, and death.[59,62,63] Before the 2001 anthrax attacks, mortality from inhalational anthrax was thought to be 90%, but outcomes from those incidents suggest that with early antibiotic therapy and critical care services, mortality may be significantly lower.[62]

Inhalational anthrax is not contagious and does not pose a risk to the prehospital care practitioner. Only exposure to aerosolized spores poses a risk of infectivity. Caring for patients known to be infected with inhalational anthrax requires only standard precautions; however, if the specific agent is unknown, aerosol precautions are warranted. The practitioner should provide supportive therapy and transport ill patients to facilities in which critical care services are available.

Management

Anthrax spores are extremely difficult to destroy and can be easily transported on victims' skin or clothes, presenting an infectious hazard to practitioners. Victims of known or suspected anthrax releases (e.g., letters containing suspicious white powders) should be decontaminated on scene by responders wearing level A PPE, to avoid contamination of transport equipment or infection of practitioners by anthrax spores carried on victims' skin or clothes.

Table 18-1 CDC Risk Categories for Bioterrorism Agents

Category	Risks	Agents
A	Category A agents are those that pose a risk to national security due to: ■ Ease of dissemination or transfer from person to person ■ Risk of high mortality rates ■ Potential for major public health impact ■ Risk for widespread public panic and social disruption ■ Requirement of special action(s) for public health preparedness	Anthrax Botulism Plague Smallpox Tularemia Viral hemorrhagic fevers ■ Filoviruses ■ Arenaviruses
B	Category B agents are those that pose a risk due to: ■ Ease of dissemination ■ Resultant moderate morbidity rates and low mortality rates ■ Requirement of specific enhancements of the CDC's diagnostic capacity and disease surveillance	Brucellosis *Clostridium perfringens* Food safety threats (e.g., *Salmonella* species, *Escherichia coli*) Glanders Melioidosis Psittacosis Q fever Ricin toxin Staphylococcal enterotoxin B Typhus fever Viral encephalitis Water safety threats (e.g., *Vibrio cholerae, Cryptosporidium parvum*)
C	Category C agents are those identified as emerging pathogens and pose a risk due to: ■ Potential to be engineered for mass dissemination ■ Availability ■ Ease of production ■ Potential for high morbidity and mortality rates ■ Potential for major health impact	Emerging infectious disease ■ Hantavirus ■ Nipah virus

Data from Centers for Disease Control and Prevention. Bioterrorism agents/diseases. Accessed December 3, 2021. https://emergency.cdc.gov/agent/agentlist-category.asp

Prophylaxis with antibiotics is required only for individuals who have been exposed to spores. Local public health officials will determine the appropriate antibiotic and length of prophylactic treatment. The latest recommendations suggest 60 days of therapy with oral ciprofloxacin or doxycycline and postexposure vaccination.[64]

An anthrax vaccine does exist, and an immunization program for U.S. military forces was instituted in 1998. The current regimen requires a series of six initial shots and annual boosters. It is currently recommended only for military personnel and for laboratory and industrial workers at high risk for exposure to spores. The CDC has purchased tens of thousands of doses of the anthrax vaccine for the Strategic National Stockpile that would be made available to emergency responders in the event of an anthrax incident with risk of exposure.

Plague

Plague is a disease caused by the bacterium *Yersinia pestis*. It is naturally occurring, found in fleas and rodents. If an infected flea bites a human, the person can develop *bubonic plague*. If this local infection goes untreated, the patient can become systemically ill, resulting in septicemia and death. A number of patients may proceed to develop pulmonary symptoms (*pneumonic plague*). Plague was responsible for the Black Death of 1346, which killed 20 to 30 million people in Europe, approximately one-third of its population at that time. *Y. pestis* has been weaponized for military stockpiles with techniques developed to aerosolize the organism directly, bypassing the animal vector. The World Health Organization reports that in a worst-case scenario, 110 pounds (50 kg) of *Y. pestis*, released as an aerosol over a city of 5 million, would result in 150,000 cases of pneumonic plague and 36,000 deaths.[65]

Naturally occurring plague, resulting from the bite of an infected flea, causes symptoms in 2 to 8 days, with onset of fever, chills, weakness, and acutely swollen lymph nodes (buboes) in the neck, groin, or axilla. Untreated patients can deteriorate to systemic illness and death. Twelve percent have been described as developing pneumonic plague, with complaints of chest pain, dyspnea, cough, and hemoptysis, and these patients can also succumb from systemic illness.

Plague occurring from terrorist deployment of a weapon would likely result from aerosolized organisms, and thus, it would clinically present as the pneumonic form of the disease. Inhalation of *Y. pestis* aerosol would result in symptoms in 1 to 6 days. Patients will present with fever, cough, and dyspnea, with bloody or watery sputum. They may also develop nausea, vomiting, diarrhea, and abdominal pain. Buboes are not typically present. Without antibiotics, death occurs in 2 to 6 days after the development of respiratory symptoms.[66]

Currently, no vaccine is available to protect from pneumonic plague. Treatment of the disease includes antimicrobial and supportive therapy, often requiring critical care services. Antibiotic regimens are also recommended for individuals with unprotected close exposure to patients with known pneumonic plague.

Patients with plague represent a communicable disease risk. If patients present with only cutaneous signs and symptoms (bubonic plague), contact precautions are adequate to protect the prehospital care practitioner. If patients present with pulmonary signs of plague (pneumonic plague), a more likely scenario after a terrorist attack, practitioners must wear PPE

suitable for respiratory droplet protection. Droplet precautions include a surgical mask, eye protection, gloves, and a gown. Responders to the scene of an overt *Y. pestis* aerosol delivery, which would not likely be a recognized event, would require level A PPE suitable for a hazardous environment if entering the hot zone or warm zone.

Management

Plague victims are treated in the field with supportive therapy. Communication with the receiving facility is vital before arrival to ensure that the pneumonic plague patient can be properly isolated in the ED and that staff are prepared with the appropriate PPE. Asking the patient to wear a surgical mask, if tolerated, may decrease the likelihood of secondary transmission.

Decontamination of the vehicle and equipment is similar to that required after transport of any patient with communicable disease. Contact surfaces should be wiped down with disinfectant approved by the Environmental Protection Agency (EPA) or 1:1,000 diluted bleach solution. There is no evidence to suggest that *Y. pestis* poses a long-term environmental threat after dissolution of the primary aerosol.[66] The organism is sensitive to heat and sunlight and does not last long outside the living host. *Y. pestis* does not form spores.

Smallpox

Smallpox is also known as *variola major* and *variola minor*, depending on the severity of the illness. This naturally occurring viral disease was eradicated in 1977 but still exists in at least two laboratories—Russia's Institute of Virus Preparations and the CDC. It was alleged that the Soviet government began a program in 1980 to produce large quantities of smallpox virus for use in bombs and missiles, as well as to develop more virulent strains of the virus for military purposes. There is concern that smallpox virus may have changed hands after the dissolution of the Soviet Union.[67]

The smallpox virus infects its victim by entering the mucous membranes of the oropharynx or respiratory mucosa. After a 12- to 14-day incubation period, the patient develops fever, malaise, headache, and backache. The patient then develops a **maculopapular rash** that starts on the oral mucosa and quickly progresses to a generalized skin rash with characteristic round, tense vesicles and pustules. The rash tends to affect the head and extremities more densely than the trunk (centrifugal), with the stage of the lesions appearing uniform (**Figure 18-5**). This presentation distinguishes smallpox from *varicella*, or chickenpox (**Box 18-10**), which begins on and is denser on the trunk (centripetal) and has lesions at various stages of development (new lesions appear

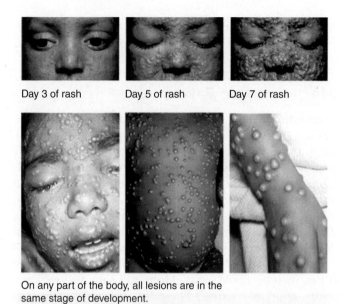

Day 3 of rash   Day 5 of rash   Day 7 of rash

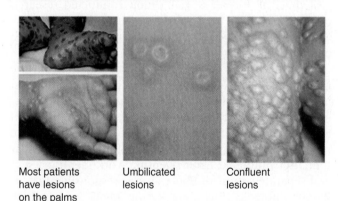

On any part of the body, all lesions are in the same stage of development.

Most patients have lesions on the palms or soles   Umbilicated lesions   Confluent lesions

Figure 18-5 Smallpox.
Courtesy of the Centers for Disease Control and Prevention.

with older, crusted lesions) (**Figure 18-6**). Mortality from naturally occurring smallpox was approximately 30%.[67] Little is known about the natural course of the disease in immunocompromised patients, such as those with HIV.

Smallpox is a contagious disease that is primarily spread by droplet nuclei projected from the oropharynx of infected patients and by direct contact. Contaminated clothing and bed linens can also spread the virus. Patients are contagious beginning slightly before the onset of the rash, although this might not always be obvious if the rash is subtle in the oropharynx. When managing a patient with smallpox, prehospital care practitioners must wear PPE appropriate for contact and aerosol precautions. This includes an N95 mask, eye protection, goggles, and gown. Ideally, persons managing patients with smallpox will have been immunized.[68]

The smallpox vaccination program in the United States was stopped in 1972. The residual immunity provided by this vaccination program is unknown, and it is suggested that individuals whose last immunization was 40 years ago will likely now be susceptible to contracting smallpox.[67] Vaccination for the smallpox virus is available to certain U.S. Department of Defense and State Department members. It was also made available under a Department of Health and Human Services program to develop public health Smallpox Response Teams. It is currently available to the general public only for participants in clinical trials. In case of a public health emergency, the United States has stockpiles of vaccine that can be released for mass immunization of the public. Vaccination within 4 days of the exposure has been shown to offer some protection against contracting the illness and substantial protection against a fatal outcome.[67]

Management

To manage a patient with smallpox, prehospital care practitioners provide supportive care. The recommended PPE must be worn at all times, and it is imperative that there is no breach in infection-control procedures. Hospitals with the appropriate isolation facilities and properly trained staff should be identified in the community. The receiving facility must be contacted to inform the

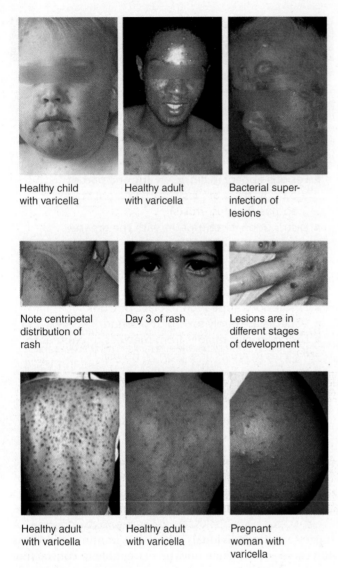

Healthy child with varicella

Healthy adult with varicella

Bacterial super-infection of lesions

Note centripetal distribution of rash

Day 3 of rash

Lesions are in different stages of development

Healthy adult with varicella

Healthy adult with varicella

Pregnant woman with varicella

Figure 18-6 Chickenpox
Courtesy of the Centers for Disease Control and Prevention.

staff of the intention to transport the confirmed or suspected case of smallpox to their facility so that proper precautions can be taken to prevent transmission of the virus. The identification of a patient with smallpox would be considered a public health emergency of enormous significance.

Proper removal of PPE without breach in infection control procedures is important for the safety of the prehospital care practitioner. All contaminated disposable medical waste must be properly bagged, labeled, and disposed of as other regulated medical waste. Reusable medical equipment must be cleaned after use according to standard protocol, either by autoclaving or by subjecting the equipment to high-level disinfection. Environmental surfaces need to be cleaned by an approved EPA-registered

detergent-disinfectant. Air decontamination or fumigation of the emergency vehicle is not required.[69]

Ebola Virus and Other Viral Hemorrhagic Fevers

Viral hemorrhagic fevers (VHFs) are a clinical syndrome caused by several different viruses and typified by the clinical presentation of fever, malaise, and hemorrhagic symptoms, including coagulopathy, bleeding from venipuncture sites and mucous membranes, petechiae, and ecchymoses in the most severe cases. Case fatality rates, defined as the percentage of infected people who die from the infection, vary significantly among different VHF viruses and even among outbreaks of the same virus but can exceed 90%. Examples of viruses that cause VHFs include Ebola virus, Marburg virus, yellow fever virus, and Lassa virus.[70] There is some evidence to suggest that the former Soviet Union conducted research on weaponized VHF viruses, and currently terrorist organizations may be developing their own programs to exploit VHFs.[71]

Ebola virus is a type of filovirus (named for the filament-like shape of viral particles in this family), first isolated and identified in 1976 from patients in two outbreaks of VHFs near the borders of current-day South Sudan and the Democratic Republic of the Congo. The name *Ebola* comes from the name of a small river near the latter outbreak. Later scientific work identified several separate strains of Ebola viruses responsible for different outbreaks, including Reston Ebola virus, which caused an outbreak among research monkeys housed in a quarantine facility in Reston, Virginia, in 1989. Unlike smallpox, Ebola virus is thought to have a natural reservoir in animals, most likely bats, meaning new outbreaks could occur at any time.[70,72] Ebola virus gained worldwide attention in 2014 when an outbreak spread throughout West Africa causing over 11,000 deaths among over 28,000 reported cases between 2013 and 2016, including several in the United States and other Western countries.[73]

Clinically, infection with Ebola virus causes Ebola virus disease (EVD), a VHF, which initially manifests after a 2- to 21-day incubation period with fevers, chills, generalized malaise, and muscle aches, and progresses to GI symptoms with abdominal pain, vomiting, and diarrhea, as well as neurologic symptoms, including headache and confusion, and respiratory symptoms including cough, chest pain, and shortness of breath. At the peak of illness, severe cases may develop hemorrhagic symptoms and generalized coagulopathy. Death occurs from multiorgan failure, sepsis, electrolyte abnormalities, and hypovolemic shock, primarily from gastrointestinal volume loss.[72]

Although the case fatality rate varies significantly among strains and different outbreaks, the 2013–2016 West African outbreak had a final case fatality rate of below 40%, versus around 75% at the start of the outbreak, and over 90% in some prior outbreaks. It is suspected that the improvement in this rate was due to improvements in caring for patients with EVD, primarily aggressive replacement of gastrointestinal volume and electrolyte losses.[74]

Management

Transport of suspected EVD victims poses a significant risk to EMS personnel, due to the highly infectious nature of the virus. Body fluids from symptomatic patients contain extremely large amounts of active virus, and only a small exposure is needed to infect an individual. Review of the West African outbreak showed that 3.9% of cases were among healthcare workers who became infected while caring for EVD patients.[74] The CDC has published specific guidelines on PPE use for transporting EVD patients, based on the best currently available evidence; in short, the CDC recommends skin protection with multiple layers (disposable scrubs, impermeable gown, over-apron, multiple layers of gloves, and boot covers) and respiratory/mucous membrane protection with a preference for a PAPR and hood over N95 mask and eye protection, analogous to OSHA level C. These recommendations may be updated if another outbreak occurs.[75] Extensive training on EVD PPE and direct supervision of donning/doffing procedures by experienced observers are strongly recommended.

EMS agencies affiliated with Grady Hospital in Atlanta, Georgia, and Nebraska Medical Center in Omaha, Nebraska, developed equipment and plans for transporting critically ill patients with highly contagious disease prior to the 2013–2016 EVD outbreak and afterward published reports on their experiences treating and transporting actual and suspected EVD patients. These reports made many specific and helpful recommendations for transporting EVD patients, including the following:

- Use of appropriate PPE (with strict attention paid to donning/doffing procedure and recommendation for a PAPR over negative-pressure mask for better practitioner protection and comfort during long transports)
- Isolation of the driver compartment of the ambulance from the patient compartment with an improvised positive-pressure system
- Covering of all equipment and surfaces within the patient compartment of the ambulance with thick plastic sheets to limit contamination
- Further isolation of patients within a contamination-limiting suit or capsule

- Careful decontamination of ambulance and equipment afterward with use of disinfectant wipes (as opposed to spraying down surfaces with pressurized water, which could aerosolize virus particles)[76,77]

Based on experience gained in the 2013–2016 outbreak, medical management of EVD patients now focuses primarily on symptom control and oral repletion of GI fluids and electrolyte losses. There are multiple new therapies that may improve survival rates, including antiviral and immunomodulatory medications and vaccines, but their efficacy is still under investigation. Advance supportive care interventions, such as IV fluids; lab monitoring of electrolytes, cell counts, and viral levels; antibiotics; and intubation/ventilation may also be helpful, but these measures significantly increase the risk of infection to healthcare practitioners.[74]

Botulinum Toxin

Botulinum toxin is produced by the bacterium *Clostridium botulinum* and is the most poisonous substance known. It is 15,000 times more toxic than the nerve agent VX and 100,000 times more toxic than sarin.[78] Botulinum toxin has been weaponized for military use by the United States; the former Soviet Union; Iraq; and probably Iran, Syria, and North Korea.[79] The Aum Shinrikyo cult, responsible for the Tokyo subway sarin attack, attempted, without success, to deliver an aerosol of botulinum toxin in 1995. Despite the reported difficulty of concentrating and stabilizing the toxin for dissemination, it is estimated that a terrorist point-source delivery of botulinum aerosol could incapacitate or kill 10% of persons downwind 0.3 mile (0.5 km).[79] The toxin could also be introduced into the food supply in an attempt to poison large numbers of people.

Three forms of botulism exist naturally. *Wound botulism* occurs when toxins are absorbed from a dirty wound, often with devitalized tissue, in which *C. botulinum* is present. *Foodborne botulism* occurs when improperly prepared or home-canned foods allow the bacteria to grow and produce toxin, which is ingested by the victim. *Intestinal botulism* occurs when toxin is produced and absorbed within the GI tract. In addition to these three naturally occurring forms, a man-made form of botulism, called *inhalational botulism*, can occur as a result of aerosolized botulinum toxin.

Regardless of the route, botulinum toxin is carried to the neuromuscular junction where it binds irreversibly, preventing normal release of the neurotransmitter acetylcholine and causing a descending flaccid paralysis. Onset of symptoms is several hours to a few days. All patients will present with diplopia (double vision) and multiple cranial nerve deficits, causing difficulty with sight, speech, and swallowing. The extent and rapidity of the descending paralysis depend on the dose of the toxin. Patients become fatigued, lose the ability to control the muscles of the head and neck, may lose their gag reflex, or may progress to paralysis of the muscles of respiration and develop respiratory failure, requiring intubation and months of mechanical ventilation. Untreated patients usually die of mechanical upper airway obstruction or inadequate ventilation. The classic triad of botulinum toxicity is (1) descending symmetric flaccid paralysis with cranial nerve deficits, (2) lack of fever, and (3) a clear sensorium. After weeks to months, patients may recover as new axon buds develop to innervate the denervated muscles.

Management

Care for the patient with botulism is supportive, with administration of antitoxin in the hospital. Early use of antitoxin will minimize further deterioration but cannot reverse existing paralysis. This antitoxin is available from the CDC.

Prehospital care practitioners caring for victims of botulism would need to be vigilant about airway compromise and insufficient ventilation. Patients may not be able to manage their secretions or maintain a patent airway. Because of diaphragm paralysis, patients may not be able to generate an adequate tidal volume. This may be exacerbated by having the patient in a supine or semi-recumbent position. Patients experiencing respiratory difficulty should be intubated and adequately ventilated.

Standard precautions are adequate for the management of patients experiencing the effects of botulinum toxicity, because it is not a contagious disease. Botulism aerosols degrade readily in the environment, and it is anticipated that after delivery in a terrorist incident, substantial inactivation will occur after 2 days. Responders to an overt aerosol dissemination event would require level A PPE suitable for a hazardous environment if working in the hot zone or warm zone.

Because the aerosol can persist for approximately 2 days under average weather conditions, victims who have been exposed to botulinum aerosol require decontamination by clothing removal and washing with soap and water. Equipment can be decontaminated using a 0.1% hypochlorite bleach solution.[79] Patients will not require isolation after arrival at the hospital, but critical care services may be needed for patients requiring mechanical ventilation.

Radiologic Disasters

Since the terrorist attacks of September 11, 2001, new consideration has been given to the likelihood of EMS systems needing to manage a radiologic emergency. Historically, planning has focused on civil-defense preparation for a strategic exchange of military nuclear weapons or the rare occurrence of a nuclear power plant accident. Currently, however, there is increasing awareness of the possibility that terrorists could deploy an improvised nuclear detonation device, or perhaps more likely, a radiologic dispersion device, that uses conventional explosives to disseminate radioactive material into the environment. Although the large-scale nuclear exchanges feared during the Cold War seem less likely today, the proliferation of nuclear weapons in the past few decades among smaller nations has led to concerns of rogue states or terrorist groups obtaining nuclear weapons and using them to attack civilian populations.

Although radiologic accidents are rare, there have been 243 radiation accidents since 1944 in the United States, with 1,342 casualties that met criteria for significant exposure. Worldwide, 403 accidents have occurred, with 133,617 victims, 2,965 with significant exposure, and 120 fatalities. The Chernobyl disaster of 1986 was responsible for 116,500 to 125,000 exposed casualties and close to 50 deaths as of 2005, although it is estimated that the total number of deaths could reach as many as 4,000 as additional cancer victims succumb.[80,81] In the 1987 Goiania, Brazil, incident, a canister of cesium-137, a highly radioactive isotope used for medical radiation therapy, was broken open and the radioactive material inside disseminated. Of the 129 people who were contaminated, 20 were hospitalized and 4 died; approximately 125,000 people were screened for radiation contamination. The release of the radioactive isotope was not realized until 16 days after the canister was opened, when victims presented to local hospitals with symptoms of radiation poisoning; this delay in recognition likely increased the number of victims contaminated.[82] The Fukushima nuclear power plant in Japan was seriously damaged after a nearby earthquake and tsunami in 2011, resulting in the destruction of several reactors and the release of radiation into the environment. It will take years and even decades before the health impact of this incident on the surrounding population and environment can be fully evaluated.

Radiation disasters can generate fear and confusion in both victims and emergency responders. Familiarization with the hazard and management principles will help to ensure an appropriate response and help to reduce panic and disorder (**Box 18-11**).

Exposure to ionizing radiation and radioactive contamination may result from several different scenarios: (1) detonation of a nuclear weapon, whether high grade or an improvised low-yield device; (2) detonation of a dirty bomb or radiologic dispersion device, in which there is no nuclear detonation, but rather conventional explosives are detonated to disperse a *radionuclide* (radioactive material); (3) sabotage or accident at a nuclear reactor site; and (4) mishandled nuclear waste.

1. Assess the scene for safety.
2. All patients should be medically stabilized from their traumatic injuries before radiation injuries are considered. Patients are then evaluated for their external radiation exposure and contamination.
3. An external source of radiation, if great enough, can cause tissue injury, but it does not make the patient radioactive. Patients with even lethal exposures to external radiation are not a threat to prehospital care practitioners.
4. Patients can become contaminated with radioactive material deposited on their skin or clothing. More than 90% of surface contamination can be removed by removal of clothing.[74] The remainder can be washed off with soap and water.
5. Prehospital care practitioners should protect themselves from radioactive contamination by observing, at a minimum, standard precautions, including protective clothing, gloves, and a mask.
6. Patients who develop nausea, vomiting, or skin erythema within 4 hours of exposure have likely received a high external radiation exposure.
7. Radioactive contamination in wounds should be treated as dirt and irrigated as soon as possible. Avoid handling any metallic foreign body.
8. Potassium iodide (KI) is of value only if there has been a release of radioactive iodine. KI is not a general radiation antidote.
9. The concept of time/distance/shielding is key in the prevention of untoward effects from radiation exposure. Radiation exposure is minimized by decreasing time in the affected area, increasing distance from a radiation source, and using metal or concrete shielding.

Modified from Department of Homeland Security Working Group on Radiological Dispersion Device (RRD) Preparedness. Medical preparedness and response subgroup. May 1, 2003. https://www.hsdl.org/?abstract&did=437718

Medical Effects of Radiation Catastrophes

The injuries and risks associated with a radiologic catastrophe would be multifactorial. In the case of a nuclear detonation, casualties would be produced by the explosion, resulting in primary, secondary, and tertiary blast injuries; thermal injury; and structural collapse. Victims

may be further subjected to radiation injury from *irradiation*, in which radiation passes through the body causing damage but does not result in contamination (similar to getting an x-ray); from external radioactive contamination, which can be deposited on skin and clothing from fallout; or from internal radiation through radioactive particulate contamination, which victims may inhale, ingest, or have deposited in wounds.

Accidents at nuclear reactors could generate large doses of ionizing radiation, without a nuclear detonation, especially under circumstances in which the reactor reaches a point of "criticality." Explosions, fire, and gas release could also result in radioactive gas or particulate matter, which could expose emergency responders to the risk of exposure to contamination with radioactive particles.

Detonation of a **radiological dispersal device (RDD)** typically would not deliver enough radiation to cause immediate injury. However, RDDs would complicate management for prehospital care practitioners by distributing radioactive particulates that could contaminate victims and emergency responders and make it difficult to manage the injuries caused by the conventional explosive. RDDs could cause confusion and panic in the public and among emergency responders concerned about radioactivity, hindering efforts to assist victims.

Ionizing radiation causes injury to cells by interacting with atoms and depositing energy. This interaction results in **ionization**, which can damage the cell nucleus either directly, causing cell death or malfunction, or indirectly, damaging cell components by interacting with water in the body and producing toxic molecules. Acute exposure to large doses of penetrating ionizing radiation (irradiation with gamma rays and neutrons) in a short time can result in acute radiation illness. Types of ionizing radiation include alpha particles, beta particles, gamma rays, and neutrons.

Alpha particles are relatively large and cannot penetrate even a few layers of the skin. Intact skin or a uniform offers adequate protection from external contamination emitting alpha particles. Ionizing radiation from alpha particles is a concern only if it is internalized by inhaling or ingesting alpha-particle emitters. When internalized, alpha-particle radiation can cause significant local cellular injury to adjacent cells.

Beta particles are small charged particles that can penetrate more deeply than alpha particles and can affect deeper layers of the skin with the ability to injure the base of the skin, causing a *beta burn*. Beta-particle radiation is found most frequently in nuclear fallout. Beta particles also result in local radiation injury.

Gamma rays are similar to x-rays and can easily penetrate tissue. Gamma rays are emitted with a nuclear detonation and with fallout. They also could be emitted from

Diagnosis
Be alert to the following:

1. The acute radiation syndrome follows a predictable pattern after substantial exposure or catastrophic events (Table 18-2).
2. Individuals may become ill from contaminated sources in the community and may be identified over much longer periods based on specific syndromes (Table 18-3).
3. Specific syndromes of concern, especially with a 2- to 3-week prior history of nausea and vomiting, are:
   · Thermal burn-like skin effects without documented thermal exposure
   · Immunologic dysfunction with secondary infections
   · Tendency to bleed (epistaxis, gingival bleeding, petechiae)
   · Marrow suppression (neutropenia, lymphopenia, and thrombocytopenia)
   · Epilation (hair loss)

Understanding Exposure
Exposure may be known and recognized or clandestine and may occur by the following means:

1. Large recognized exposures, such as a nuclear bomb or damage to a nuclear power station
2. Small radiation source emitting continuous gamma radiation, producing group or individual chronic intermittent exposures (e.g., radiologic sources from medical treatment devices, environmental water or food pollution)
3. Internal radiation from absorbed, inhaled, or ingested radioactive material (internal contamination)

This information is not meant to be complete and is intended as a quick guide only; please consult other references and expert opinion.

Modified from Department of Veterans Affairs Employee Education System for Office of Public Health and Environmental Hazards. *Terrorism with ionizing radiation: general guidance pocket guide.* May 16, 2002. Accessed April 22, 2022. https://www.greenbeltmd.gov/home/showpublisheddocument/824/636639777504570000

some radionuclides that might be present in an RDD. Gamma radiation can result in what is termed *whole-body exposure*. Whole-body exposure can result in acute and chronic radiation illnesses (**Box 18-12**, **Table 18-2**, and **Table 18-3**).

Neutrons can penetrate tissue easily, with 20 times the destructive energy of gamma rays, disrupting the atomic structure of cells. Neutrons are released during a nuclear detonation but are not a fallout risk. Neutrons also contribute to whole-body radiation exposure and can result in acute radiation illness. Neutrons can convert stable metals into radioactive isotopes. This ability has significance in patients with metal hardware or those in possession of metal objects at the time of exposure.

Whole-body exposure is measured in terms of the *gray* (Gy). The *rad* (radiation absorbed dose) was a familiar dose unit that was replaced by the gray; 1 Gy equals 100 rad. The rem (radiation equivalent–man) describes the dose in rad multiplied by a "quality factor," which takes into account the intrinsic special deposition pattern of different types of radiation. The rem has been replaced with the *sievert* (Sv); 1 Sv equals 100 rem.

Radiation affects rapidly dividing cells most readily, resulting in injury to the bone marrow and GI tract where high cell turnover rates occur. Higher doses can affect the CNS directly. The dose of whole-body exposure determines the medical consequences of the exposure. Patients receiving up to 1 Gy of whole-body irradiation would typically not exhibit signs of injury. At 1 to 2 Gy, less than half of patients will develop nausea and vomiting, many will subsequently develop *leukopenia* (decreased white blood cell count), and deaths will be minimal. Most victims receiving greater than 2 Gy will become ill and require hospitalization; at greater than 6 Gy, mortality becomes high. At doses greater than 30 Gy, neurologic signs are manifest, and death is most likely.[24]

Acute radiation syndrome generally follows a defined progression that first manifests in a prodromal phase characterized by malaise, nausea, and vomiting. This is followed by a latent phase, in which the patient is essentially asymptomatic. The length of the latent phase depends on the total absorbed dose of radiation. The greater the dose of radiation, the shorter the latent phase. The latent phase is followed by the subsequent illness phase, manifested by the organ system that has been injured. Damage to the bone marrow occurs with total doses of 0.7 to 4.0 Gy and results in decreasing levels of white blood cells and decreased immunity to infection over several days to weeks. Decreased platelets can result in easy bruising and bleeding. Decreased red blood cells will result in anemia. At 6 to 8 Gy, the GI tract will be affected, resulting in diarrhea, volume loss, and hematochezia (bloody stools). Above 30 Gy, the patient will manifest symptoms of the neurovascular syndrome, experiencing the prodromal phase of nausea and vomiting, a short latent phase lasting only a few hours, followed by a rapid deterioration of mental status, coma,

Table 18-2 Acute Radiation Syndrome						
	Effects of Whole-Body Irradiation or Internal Absorption, by Dose Range in rad (1 rad = 1 centigray; 100 rad = 1 gray)					
Feature	**0–100 (0–1 Gy)**	**100–200 (1–2 Gy)**	**200–600 (2–6 Gy)**	**600–800 (6–8 Gy)**	**800–3,000 (8–30 Gy)**	**> 3,000 (> 30 Gy)**
Prodromal Phase of Syndrome						
Nausea, vomiting	None	5–50%	50–100%	75–100%	90–100%	100%
Time of onset	—	3–6 hr	2–4 hr	1–2 hr	< 1 hr	N/A
Duration	—	< 24 hr	< 24 hr	< 48 hr	48 hr	N/A
Lymphocyte count	Unaffected	Minimally decreased	< 1,000 at 24 hr	< 500 at 24 hr	Decreases within hours	Decreases within hours
CNS function	No impairment	No impairment	Routine task performance. Cognitive impairment for 6–20 hr	Simple, routine task performance. Cognitive impairment for > 24 hr	Rapid incapacitation; may have a lucid interval of several hours	
Latent Phase of Syndrome						
No symptoms	> 2 wk	7–15 d	0–7 d	0–2 d	None	None
Manifest Illness						
Signs/symptoms	None	Moderate leukopenia	Severe leukopenia, purpura, hemorrhage, pneumonia, hair loss after 300 rad		Diarrhea, fever, electrolyte disturbance	Convulsions, ataxia, tremor, lethargy
Time of onset	—	> 2 wk	2 d to 4 wk	2 d to 4 wk	1–3 d	1–3 d
Critical period	—	None	4–6 wk; greatest potential for effective medical intervention		2–14 d	1–46 hr
Organ system	None	—	Hematopoietic; respiratory (mucosal) systems		GI tract. Mucosal systems	CNS
Hospitalization duration	0%	< 5%. 45–60 d	90%. 60–90 d	100%. 100+ d	100%. Weeks to months	100%. Days to weeks
Mortality	None	Minimal	Low with aggressive therapy	High	Very high; significant neurologic symptoms indicate lethal dose	

Abbreviations: CNS, central nervous system; d, day(s); GI, gastrointestinal; hr, hour(s); N/A, not available; wk, week(s)

Modified from Armed Forces Radiobiology Research Institute. *Medical Management of Radiological Casualties.* Author; 2003.

Table 18-3 Symptom Clusters as Delayed Effects After Radiation

General	Gastrointestinal	Dermatological	Hematological
Headache	Anorexia	Partial-thickness and full-thickness skin damage	Lymphopenia
Fatigue	Nausea	Epilation (hair loss)	Neutropenia
Weakness	Vomiting	Ulceration	Thrombocytopenia
	Diarrhea		Purpura
			Opportunistic infections

Modified from Armed Forces Radiobiology Research Institute. *Medical Management of Radiological Casualties.* Author; 2003.

and death, sometimes accompanied by hemodynamic instability. Doses this high can occur after a nuclear detonation, but the victim will most likely have been killed by injuries associated with the blast. Victims could also be exposed to these high doses at a nuclear power facility where no blast has occurred, but a reactor core has reached criticality.[24]

Not all radiation accidents or terrorist events will result in high-dose radiation exposure. Low-dose radiation exposure, as would most likely occur after an RDD detonation, probably would not produce acute injury secondary to radiation. Dependent on dose, the patient may have an increased future risk of developing cancer. The acute effects of RDD detonation, besides the effects of the detonation of the conventional explosive, will likely be psychological, including stress reactions, fear, acute depression, and psychosomatic complaints, which would significantly strain the EMS agencies and medical infrastructure.

Patients can become contaminated with material that emits alpha, beta, and even gamma radiation, but the most common contaminants will emit alpha and beta radiation. Only gamma radiation contributes to whole-body irradiation, as previously described. Alpha and beta radiation have limited ability to penetrate, but still can cause local tissue injury. Patients can easily be decontaminated by clothing removal and washing with water or soap and water. It is impossible for a patient to be so contaminated as to be a radiologic hazard to prehospital care practitioners caring for the individual, so management of traumatic life-threatening injury is an immediate priority and should not be delayed pending decontamination.[24]

As described, radioactive particles can be inhaled, ingested, or absorbed through the skin or contaminated wounds. This type of exposure to radiation will not result in acute effects of radiation exposure but can result in delayed effects. Any victims or emergency responders who operate in an area at risk for airborne radioactive particles without the benefit of respiratory protection would require subsequent evaluation to identify internal contamination, which could require medical intervention to dilute or block the effects of the inhaled radionuclide.

Personal Protective Equipment

Prehospital care practitioners would be operating in an environment with risk of exposure to ionizing radiation after a radiologic disaster. The radiation risk would depend greatly on the type of radiologic event.

The PPE available to prehospital care practitioners for use in chemical and biologic hazards will offer some protection from radioactive particulate contamination. However, it will not provide protection from high-energy radiation sources, such as a damaged reactor or nuclear blast at ground zero.

Radioactivity can be present in gases, aerosols, solids, or liquids. If radioactive gases are present, SCBA will offer the highest protection. If aerosols are present, an APR may be adequate to prevent internal contamination caused by inhalation of contaminated particles. An N95 mask will offer some protection from inhaled particulates. A standard splash-resistant suit will protect against particulates that emit alpha radiation and will offer some protection from beta radiation but will provide no protection from gamma radiation or neutrons. This type of barrier protection will assist in the decontamination of particulate matter from an individual, but it does not protect against the risks of acute radiation illness when the person is exposed to high-energy sources of external radiation.

None of the typical PPE carried by prehospital care practitioners protects from a high-energy point source of radiation. This type of radiation is encountered during the first minute of a nuclear detonation, in a critical reactor core, or with a high-energy radiation source such as cesium-137, which may be dispersed in an RDD. The best protection from these sources is decreased time of exposure, increased distance from the source, and shielding. New materials that may offer some protection from low-level gamma radiation for emergency responder PPE are under investigation.

Unlike insufficient PPE worn to protect against chemical agents, the inhalation, ingestion, or skin absorption of radiation-emitting gas or particulate will not immediately incapacitate a prehospital care practitioner or victim. All practitioners who operated in an environment potentially contaminated with radioactive material would have to undergo a radiation survey to determine if internal contamination had occurred and undergo active management if warranted.

Dose rate meters or alarms should be worn if available. Standards exist for acceptable doses of ionizing radiation in the occupational environment under normal and emergency conditions.[18] Dose rates of ionizing radiation can be measured to prevent emergency responders from putting themselves at risk for acute radiation illness or an unacceptably higher incidence of cancer. The incident commander should be approached for guidance on radiation-exposure readings and limits.

Assessment and Management

Patients who have been injured in a radiologic catastrophe should receive primary and secondary surveys as dictated by the mechanism of injury. Prehospital care practitioners can expect to evaluate patients who have sustained blast injury and thermal injury in the case of a nuclear detonation or from the conventional high-explosive detonation of an RDD (**Box 18-13**). Priority should be given to management of traumatic injuries with the radiologic aspects of the case receiving secondary consideration. Decontamination of the victim is recommended to eliminate radioactive particulate contamination but should not delay the care of patients requiring immediate intervention for their traumatic injuries. If the patient does not show signs of serious injury requiring immediate intervention, the patient can be decontaminated first.

If radioiodine is present in the environment, as might be encountered in a nuclear reactor, following a spent fuel rod accident, or following detonation of a nuclear device, then giving potassium iodide to emergency responders and victims may help prevent accumulation of radioiodine in the thyroid, where it can increase the likelihood of cancer. Other *blocking* and *decorporation therapy* may be recommended by the hospital or federal assistance agencies when more information about the catastrophe is available. Blocking therapy is designed to interfere with the effects of the

---

Box 18-13 Treatment and Decontamination Considerations for Radiation Exposure

Treatment Considerations
- If trauma is present, treat.
- If external radioactive contaminants are present, decontaminate (after treatment of life-threatening problems).
- If radioiodine (e.g., reactor accident) is present, consider giving prophylactic potassium iodide (Lugol's solution) within first 24 hours only (ineffective later).
- See www.orau.gov/reacts/guidance.htm.

Decontamination Considerations
- Exposure without contamination requires no decontamination.
- Exposure with contamination requires standard (universal) precautions, removal of patient clothing, and decontamination with water.
- Internal contamination will be determined at the hospital.
- Treating contaminated patients before decontamination may contaminate the facility; plan for decontamination before arrival.
- For a patient with a life-threatening condition, *treat*, then decontaminate.
- For a patient with a non–life-threatening condition, *decontaminate*, then treat.

Modified from Armed Forces Radiobiology Research Institute. *Medical Management of Radiological Casualties.* Author; 2003.

---

radiologic agent, whereas decorporation treatment is targeted at removing the agent from the body using medications that combine with the agent and allow for its elimination.

Transport Considerations

Patients should be transported to the nearest appropriate medical center that is capable of managing trauma and radiation injuries. All hospitals are required to have a plan for management of a radiologic emergency, but communities may have identified institutions that have decontamination facilities, are capable of managing trauma, and have staff trained to deal effectively with possible external or internal radioactive contamination, as well as the complications of whole-body exposure to ionizing radiation.

SUMMARY

- Weapons of mass destruction manufactured by terrorist regimes pose a significant threat to civilized society.
- Prehospital care practitioners may come in contact with explosions and with chemical and radiologic material as the result of industrial mishaps.
- The safety of prehospital care practitioners is paramount. They should possess a working knowledge of levels of personal protective equipment and the fundamentals of decontamination.
- Explosive agents and firearms have predominated in recent terrorist attacks. High explosives produce primary blast injuries in survivors who are in close proximity to the blast, and secondary injuries result from flying debris.
- Not only may chemical agents injure the skin and pulmonary system, but they may also result in systemic illness, manifesting as a specific toxidrome that yields clues to the agent. Antidotes are used for some of these agents.
- Biologic agents can be highly virulent bacteria or viruses or toxins produced by living organisms. The types of protective precautions used by practitioners vary with the specific agents.
- Several types of radiation exist. Exposure to these agents may result in acute radiation illness, which is typically a function of the type of radiation and the length of exposure.

SCENARIO RECAP

It is a warm summer evening, and you are dispatched to the scene of a reported explosion outside a popular café. You know this café is usually busy and typically seats patrons inside and outside on the patio. Dispatch informs you the number of victims is not yet known, although they have received multiple emergency calls regarding this incident. Other public safety agencies have also been dispatched to the location.

Upon arrival at the location, you observe you are the first prehospital care practitioner on scene. No incident command has yet been established. Dozens of people are running away from the cafe. Many are imploring you to assist victims who have obvious bleeding. Other victims are lying on the ground with variable states of consciousness.

- What will you do first?
- What are your priorities as you determine your course of action?
- How will you care for so many people?

SCENARIO SOLUTION

As always, the first priority is safety. Assess the scene. Look for evidence of a secondary device that may pose a threat to emergency responders. Are there other hazards? Look for hanging debris, downed or exposed power lines, or hazardous materials spills.

Communicate with your chain of command, and use the incident command system (ICS). Because you are the first emergency responder to the scene, the communications center will be relying on you for information. Describe pertinent details of the scene, observed hazards, numbers of victims, and likely number of resources required to manage the scene and victims. Carefully observe the crowd for evidence of a toxidrome. Is there an unusually high proportion of respiratory difficulty? Are victims vomiting and seizing? Is there evidence of agent dispersal in addition to the explosive blast? Based on your observations, the communications center and the on-duty supervisor can apprise other units and agencies of your situation and dispatch the necessary resources. A predefined disaster response plan may be activated.

SCENARIO SOLUTION (CONTINUED)

Once the personal safety of all emergency responders has been ensured and information has been communicated, prepare to serve as the incident commander until relieved by another competent authority.

As soon as is feasible, don PPE appropriate for the incident, and then approach the victims with the intention of triaging them for treatment and transport using the START algorithm. Without engaging in the medical management of victims initially, sort the victims into immediate, urgent, delayed, and expectant categories. Remember, blast victims may not be able to hear directions or questions from emergency responders. As other assistance arrives, direct personnel to assume roles of the ICS until supervisory personnel arrive to assume command and control functions.

References

1. Chason R, Wiggins O, Tan R. Dozens of cases, and 10 deaths. Inside Maryland's worst coronavirus outbreak. W*ashington Post*. April 5, 2020. Accessed October 31, 2021. https://www.washingtonpost.com/local/maryland-news/pleasant-view-coronavirus-outbreak-carroll-county/2020/04/04/4a4bb2c2-7520-11ea-87da-77a8136c1a6d_story.html

2. Torrey J, Orr J, Florance J. Rapid deployment of national guard alternative healthcare facility with isolation unit capabilities in response to covid-19. *Mil Med*. 2021;186(1-2):258-264.

3. Weiden MD, Zeig-Owens R, Singh A, et al. Pre-COVID-19 lung function and other risk factors for severe COVID-19 in first responders. *ERJ Open Res*. 2021;7(1):00610-2020. doi: 10.1183/23120541.00610-2020

4. Turner CD, Lockey DJ, Rehn M. Pre-hospital management of mass casualty civilian shootings: a systematic literature review [published correction appears in *Crit Care*. 2017 Apr 13;21(1):94]. *Crit Care*. 2016;20(1):362. doi:10.1186/s13054-016-1543-7

5. Jacobs LM, Wade DS, McSwain NE, et al. The Hartford Consensus: THREAT, a medical disaster preparedness concept. *J Am Coll Surg*. 2013;217(5):947-953. doi: 10.1016/j.jamcollsurg.2013.07.002

6. Hogan DE, Waeckerle JF, Dire DJ, et al. Emergency department impact of the Oklahoma City terrorist bombing. *Ann Emerg Med*. 1999;34:160-167.

7. Kennedy K, Aghababian R, Gans L, et al. Triage: techniques and applications in decision making. *Ann Emerg Med*. 1996;28(2):136-144.

8. Garner A, Lee A, Harrison K. Comparative analysis of multiple-casualty incident triage algorithms. *Ann Emerg Med*. 2001;38:541-548.

9. Lerner EB, Schwartz RB, Coule PL, et al. Mass casualty triage: an evaluation of the data and development of a proposed national guideline. *Disaster Med Public Health Preparedness*. 2008;2(suppl 1):S25-S34.

10. Thors L, Koch M, Wigenstam E, Koch B, Hägglund L, Bucht A. Comparison of skin decontamination efficacy of commercial decontamination products following exposure to VX on human skin. *Chem Biol Interact*. 2017;273:82-89.

11. Taysse L, Daulon S, Delamanche S, Bellier B, Breton P. Skin decontamination of mustards and organophosphates: comparative efficiency of RSDL and fuller's earth in domestic swine. *Hum Exp Toxicol*. 2007;26(2):135-141.

12. U.S. Department of Health and Human Services. Medical Countermeasures Database. Chemical Hazards Emergency Medical Management website. Updated August 16, 2021. Accessed January 31, 2022. https://chemm.hhs.gov/medical_countermeasures.htm

13. Hurst G, ed. *Field Management of Chemical and Biological Casualties Handbook*. 5th ed. Borden Institute, Walter Reed Army Medical Center; 2016.

14. Kapur GB, Hutson HR, Davis MA, Rice PL. The United States twenty-year experience with bombing incidents: implications for terrorism preparedness and medical response. *J Trauma*. 2005;59:1436-1444.

15. Melnikova N, Orr MF, Wu J, Christensen B. Injuries from methamphetamine-related chemical incidents—five states, 2001–2012. *Morb Mortal Wkly Rep*. 2015;64(33):909-912.

16. Pierce B. How rare are large, multiple-fatality work-related incidents? *Accid Anal Prev*. 2016;96:88-100.

17. Edwards DS, Mcmenemy L, Stapley SA, Patel HD, Clasper JC. 40 years of terrorist bombings: a meta-analysis of the casualty and injury profile. *Injury*. 2016;47(3):646-652.

18. U.S. Bomb Data Center. *Explosives Incident Report (EIR)—2019*. Redstone Arsenal, AL: U.S. Bomb Data Center; 2019. https://www.atf.gov/file/143481/download

19. Arnold J, Halpern P, Tsai M. Mass casualty terrorist bombings: a comparison of outcomes by bombing type. *Ann Emerg Med*. 2004;43:263-273.

20. DePalma RG, Burris DG, Champion HR, et al. Blast injuries. *N Engl J Med*. 2005;352(13):1335-1342.

21. Centers for Disease Control and Prevention. Explosions and blast injuries: a primer for clinicians. Updated May 9, 2003. Accessed January 31, 2022. https://www.cdc.gov/masstrauma/preparedness/primer.pdf

22. Wightman JM, Gladish JL. Explosions and blast injuries. *Ann Emerg Med*. 2001;37:664-678.

23. Armed Forces Radiobiology Research Institute (AFRRI). *Medical Management of Radiological Casualties*. AFRRI; 2003.

24. Plurad DS. Blast injury. *Mil Med*. 2011 Mar;176(3):276-282. doi: 10.7205/milmed-d-10-00147

25. Almogy G, Mintz Y, Zamir G, et al. Suicide bombing attacks: can external signs predict internal injuries? *Ann Surg.* 2006;243(4):541-546.

26. Garner MJ, Brett SJ. Mechanisms of injury by explosive devices. *Anesthesiol Clin.* 2007;25(1):147-160.

27. Avidan V, Hersch M, Armon Y, et al. Blast lung injury: clinical manifestations, treatment, and outcome. *Am J Surg.* 2005;190(6):927-931.

28. Frykberg ER, Tepas JJ, Alexander RH. The 1983 Beirut Airport terrorist bombing: injury patterns and implications for disaster management. *Am Surg.* 1989;55:134-141.

29. Katz E, Ofek B, Adler J, et al. Primary blast injury after a bomb explosion in a civilian bus. *Ann Surg.* 1989;209:484-488.

30. Kluger Y, Nimrod A, Biderman P, et al. Case report: the quinary pattern of blast injury. *J Emerg Mgmt.* 2006;4(1):51-55.

31. Sorkine P, Nimrod A, Biderman P, et al. The quinary (Vth) injury pattern of blast (Abstract). *J Trauma.* 2007;56(1):232.

32. Nelson TJ, Wall DB, Stedje-Larsen ET, et al. Predictors of mortality in close proximity blast injuries during Operation Iraqi Freedom. *J Am Coll Surg.* 2006;202(3):418-422.

33. Mallonee S, Shariat S, Stennies G, et al. Physical injuries and fatalities resulting from the Oklahoma City bombing. *JAMA.* 1996;276:382-387.

34. Arnold JL, Tsai MC, Halpern P, et al. Mass-casualty, terrorist bombings: epidemiological outcomes, resource utilization, and time course of emergency needs (Part I). *Prehosp Disaster Med.* 2003;18(3):220-234.

35. Halpern P, Tsai MC, Arnold JL, et al. Mass-casualty, terrorist bombings: implications for emergency department and hospital emergency response (Part II). *Prehosp Disaster Med.* 2003;18(3):235-241.

36. U.S. Bomb Data Center. *Explosive incidents 2007: 2007 USBDC explosives statistics.* U.S. Bomb Data Center; 2007.

37. Caseby NG, Porter MF. Blast injury to the lungs: clinical presentation, management and course. *Injury.* 1976;8:1-12. doi: 10.1016/0020-1383(76)90002-4

38. Leibovici D, Gofrit ON, Shapira SC. Eardrum perforation in explosion survivors: is it a marker of pulmonary blast injury? *Ann Emerg Med.* 1999;34:168-172.

39. Coppel DL. Blast injuries of the lungs. *Br J Surg.* 1976;63:735-737.

40. Cohn SM. Pulmonary contusion: review of the clinical entity. *J Trauma.* 1997;42:973-979.

41. Peleg K, Limor A, Stein M, et al. Gunshot and explosion injuries: characteristics, outcomes, and implications for care of terror-related injuries in Israel. *Ann Surg.* 2004;239(3):311-318. doi: 10.1097/01.sla.0000114012.84732.be

42. Mansour HA, Bitar E, Fares Y, Makdessi AA, et al. The Beirut Port explosion: injury trends from a mass survey of emergency admissions. *Lancet.* 2021;398:21-22.

43. Tappan J. Magnesium and thermite poisoning. Medscape. Updated August 22, 2019. Accessed January 31, 2022. http://emedicine.medscape.com/article/833495-overview

44. Irizarry L. White phosphorus exposure. Medscape. Updated January 6, 2022. Accessed January 31, 2022. http://emedicine.medscape.com/article/833585-overview

45. Sidell FR, Takafuji ET, Franz DR, eds. *Medical Aspects of Chemical and Biological Warfare, TMM Series. Part 1: Warfare, Weaponry and the Casualty.* Office of the Surgeon General, TMM Publications; 1997.

46. Walter FG, ed. *Advanced HAZMAT Life Support.* 2nd ed. Arizona Board of Regents; 2000.

47. U.S. Army, Medical Research Institute of Chemical Defense. *Medical Management of Chemical Casualties Handbook.* U.S. Army Research Institute; 2000.

48. Greenfield RA, Brown BR, Hutchins JB, et al. Microbiological, biological and chemical weapons of warfare and terrorism. *Am J Med Sci.* 2002;323(6):326-340.

49. Okumura T, Takasu N, Ishimatsu S, et al. Report on 640 victims of the Tokyo subway sarin attack. *Ann Emerg Med.* 1996;28(2):129-135.

50. Centers for Disease Control and Prevention. Emergency Preparedness and Response—Specific Hazards: Facts about Cyanide. Last reviewed April 4, 2018. Accessed March 23, 2022. https://emergency.cdc.gov/agent/cyanide/basics/facts.asp#:~:text=Cyanide%20sometimes%20is%20described%20as,CK%20(for%20cyanogen%20chloride)

51. Sellstrom A, Cairns S, Barbeschi M. Report of United Nations Mission to Investigate Allegations of the Use of Chemical Weapons in the Syrian Arab Republic on the Alleged Use of Chemical Weapons in the Ghouta Area of Damascus on 21 August 2013. United Nations. Published September 16, 2013. Accessed January 31, 2022. https://digitallibrary.un.org/record/756814?ln=en

52. Reddy SD, Reddy DS. Midazolam as an anticonvulsant antidote for organophosphate intoxication—a pharmacotherapeutic appraisal. *Epilepsia.* 2015;56(6):813-821.

53. Rotenberg JS, Newmark J. Nerve-agent attacks on children: diagnosis and management. *Pediatrics.* 2003;112:648-658.

54. McDonough JH, Capacio BR, Shih TM. Treatment of nerve-agent-induced status epilepticus in the nonhuman primate. In: *U.S. Army Medical Defense—Bioscience Review, June 2–7.* U.S. Army Medical Research Institute; 2002.

55. U.S. Department of Health and Human Services. CHEMPACK: Chemical Hazards Emergency Medical Management. Updated August 16, 2021. Accessed October 31, 2021. https://chemm.hhs.gov/chempack.htm

56. United Nations, Security Council. Organization for the Prohibition of Chemical Weapons-United Nations Joint Investigative Mechanism. Fourth report of the Organization for the Prohibition of Chemical Weapons-United Nations Joint Investigative Mechanism. Published October 21, 2016. Accessed January 31, 2022. http://undocs.org/S/2016/888

57. Tuorinsky SD. *Textbooks of Military Medicine: Medical Aspects of Chemical Warfare.* Borden Institute, Walter Reed Army Medical Center; 2008.

58. Lipsitch M. Why Do Exceptionally Dangerous Gain-of-Function Experiments in Influenza? *Methods Mol Biol.* 2018;1836:589-608. doi: 10.1007/978-1-4939-8678-1_29

59. Ingelsby TV, Henderson DA, Bartlett JG, et al. Anthrax as a biological weapon: medical and public health management. *JAMA.* 1999;281(18):1735-1745.

60. Keim M, Kaufmann AF. Principles for emergency response to bioterrorism. *Ann Emerg Med.* 1999;34(2):177-182.

61. U.S. Congress, Office of Technology Assessment. Proliferation of weapons of mass destruction, Pub. No. OTA-ISC-559. U.S. Government Printing Office; 1993.

62. Inglesby TV, O'Toole T, Henderson DA, et al. Anthrax as a biological weapon, 2002: updated recommendations for management. *JAMA.* 2002;287:2236-2252.

63. Kman NE, Nelson RN. Infectious agents of bioterrorism: a review for emergency physicians. *Emerg Med Clin North Am.* 2008;26:517-547.

64. Stern EJ, Uhde KB, Shadomy SV, Messonnier N. Conference report on public health and clinical guidelines for anthrax. *Emerging Infect Dis.* 2008;14(4). https://wwwnc-origin.cdc.gov/eid/article/14/4/07-0969-f1

65. World Health Organization. Health Aspects of Chemical and Biological Weapons. World Health Organization; 1970.

66. Inglesby TV, Dennis DT, Henderson DA. Plague as a biological weapon: medical and public health management. *JAMA.* 2000;283(17):2281-2290.

67. Henderson DA, Inglesby TV, Bartlett JG. Smallpox as a biological weapon: medical and public health management. *JAMA.* 1999;281(22):2127-2137.

68. Centers for Disease Control and Prevention. *Smallpox Response Plan and Guidelines.* Version 3.0, Guide C, Part 1. Centers for Disease Control and Prevention; 2008:1-13.

69. Centers for Disease Control and Prevention. *Smallpox Response Plan and Guidelines.* Version 3.0, Guide F. Centers for Disease Control and Prevention; 2003:1-10.

70. Basler CF. Molecular pathogenesis of viral hemorrhagic fever. *Semin Immunopathol.* 2017;39(5):551-561.

71. Cenciarelli O, Gabbarini V, Pietropaoli S, et al. Viral bioterrorism: learning the lesson of Ebola virus in West Africa 2013–2015. *Virus Res.* 2015;210:318-326.

72. Feldmann H, Geisbert TW. Ebola haemorrhagic fever. *Lancet.* 2011;377:849-862.

73. Coltart CE, Lindsey B, Ghinai I, Johnson AM, Heymann DL. The Ebola outbreak, 2013–2016: old lessons for new epidemics. *Philos Trans R Soc Lond B Biol Sci.* 2017;372(1721):20160297. doi: 10.1098/rstb.2016.0297

74. Duraffour S, Malvy D, Sissoko D. How to treat Ebola virus infections? A lesson from the field. *Curr Opin Virol.* 2017;24:9-15.

75. Centers for Disease Control and Prevention, National Center for Emerging and Zoonotic Infectious Diseases, Division of Healthcare Quality Promotion. Guidance on personal protective equipment (PPE) to be used by healthcare workers during management of patients with confirmed Ebola or persons under investigation (PUIs) for Ebola who are clinically unstable or have bleeding, vomiting, or diarrhea in U.S. hospitals, including procedures for donning and doffing PPE. Reviewed August 30, 2018. Accessed January 31, 2022. https://www.cdc.gov/vhf/ebola/healthcare-us/ppe/guidance.html

76. Lowe JJ, Jelden KC, Schenarts PJ, et al. Considerations for safe EMS transport of patients infected with Ebola virus. *Prehosp Emerg Care.* 2015;19(2):179-183.

77. Isakov A, Miles W, Gibbs S, Lowe J, Jamison A, Swansiger R. Transport and management of patients with confirmed or suspected Ebola virus disease. *Ann Emerg Med.* 2015;66(3):297-305.

78. Franz DR, Jahrling PB, Friedlander AM, et al. Clinical recognition and management of patients exposed to biological warfare agents. *JAMA.* 1997;278(5):399-411.

79. Arnon SS, Schechter R, Inglesby TV, et al. Botulinum toxin as a biological weapon: medical and public health management. *JAMA.* 2001;285:1059-1070.

80. Hogan DE, Kellison T. Nuclear terrorism. *Am J Med Sci.* 2002;323(6):341-349.

81. World Health Organization, International Atomic Energy Agency, United Nations Development Programme. Chernobyl: the true scale of the accident. Published September 5, 2005. Accessed January 31, 2022. https://www.who.int/news/item/05-09-2005-chernobyl-the-true-scale-of-the-accident

82. Flynn DF, Goans RE. Nuclear terrorism: triage and medical management of radiation and combined-injury casualties. *Surg Clin North Am.* 2006;86(3):601-636.

Suggested Reading

Centers for Disease Control. Blast injuries: fact sheet for professionals. http://www.emergency.cdc.gov/blastinjuries

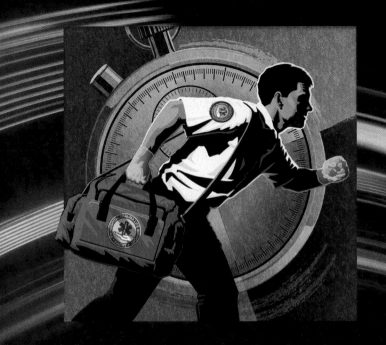

Special Considerations

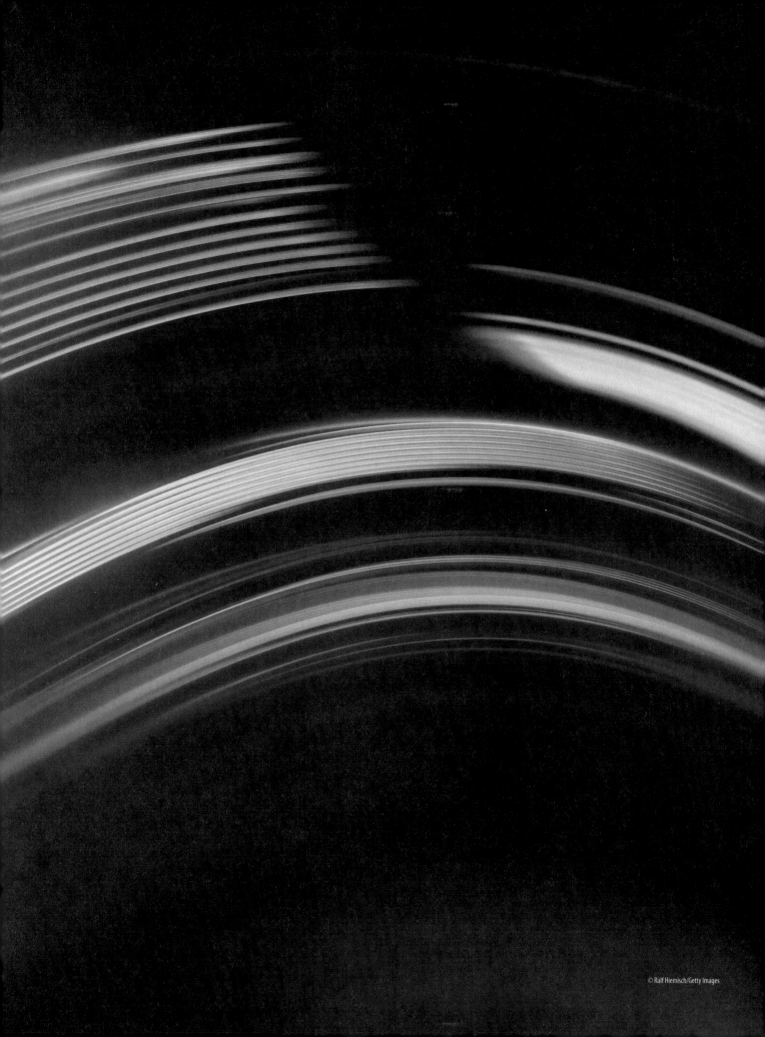

CHAPTER **19**

Environmental Trauma I: Heat and Cold

Lead Editors
Seth Hawkins, MD
R. Bryan Simon, RN

CHAPTER OBJECTIVES

At the completion of this chapter, you will be able to do the following:

- Explain why heatstroke is considered an emergent life-threatening condition.
- Identify the similarities and differences between heatstroke and exercise-associated hyponatremia.
- Describe the two most effective and rapid cooling procedures for heatstroke.
- List the five factors that place prehospital care practitioners at risk for heat illness.

- Discuss the fluid hydration guidelines and how they can be applied to prevent dehydration in warm or cold environments.
- Identify the differences in the management of mild hypothermia from that of severe hypothermia.
- List the signs of mild, moderate, and severe frostbite and discuss how to prevent its progression.
- Explain reasons for actively warming hypothermic patients in cardiopulmonary arrest.

SCENARIO

It is a hot summer afternoon with temperatures reaching 102°F (38.9°C). Over the past 30 days, it has been very humid, with temperatures reaching over 100°F (37.8°C) daily. The ambient temperature has resulted in many heat-related conditions that have required emergency medical services (EMS) personnel to transport numerous patients to the emergency departments (EDs) of the inner city.

At 1700 hours, your ambulance unit responds to a dispatch for an unresponsive male patient in a vehicle. As your ambulance unit arrives on scene, you observe a 76-year-old man who appears to be unconscious and uninjured in a vehicle parked outside of a department store. Your rapid assessment of the patient's airway, breathing, and circulation (ABCs) and level of consciousness reveals that the patient is verbal, but he is saying things that are illogical and irrational.

- What are the potential causes for this patient's decreased level of consciousness?
- What hallmark signs support a heat-related diagnosis?
- How would you emergently manage this patient at the scene and en route to the emergency department?

INTRODUCTION

This chapter focuses on recognizing and treating exposure to both hot and cold temperatures. The most significant morbidity and mortality in the United States from all environmental traumas are caused by thermal trauma.[1-5]

Environmental extremes of heat and cold have a common outcome of injuries and potential death that can affect many individuals during the peak summer and winter months. It is critical to know that mortality increases significantly when a traumatized patient presents in the hospital with either hypothermia (core body temperature less than 95°F [35°C]) or with a heat-related illness (hyperthermia) with core body temperature usually greater than 101°F [38.5°C]).[6,7] Individuals who are especially susceptible to both highs and lows of temperature are very young persons, the older adult population, people living in urban areas and in poverty, people who take specific medications, people in occupational groups that work outdoors (e.g., agricultural workers), people with chronic illnesses, and those with alcoholism or other addictions.[3-5,8-11] Although the relative risk of experiencing a heat-related or cold-related emergency may be higher in wilderness settings, most EMS responses in the United States for heat and cold injuries occur in urban settings. For this reason, all EMS practitioners need to be familiar with these topics (**Box 19-1**).[12] Additionally, expanding interest in recreational and high-risk adventure activities in the wilderness backcountry during periods of environmental extremes places more individuals in wilderness areas at risk for heat-related and cold-related injuries and fatalities.[6,13-15]

Epidemiology

Heat-Related Illness

Approximately 618 people die each year in the United States from conditions relating to extreme heat.[3] The year 2020 tied the year 2016 as the warmest documented year in recorded history (since 1880); it and the preceding 7 years were the hottest 7 years ever recorded, continuing a trend of climate change that has resulted in measurable and consequential global warming.[16] More deaths are caused by heat stress than by hurricanes, lightning, tornadoes, floods, and earthquakes combined.[2,17] Furthermore, morbidity and mortality can be extremely high when periodic seasonal heat waves occur (more than three consecutive days of air temperatures 90°F [32.2°C] or higher). The Centers for Disease Control and Prevention (CDC) reported a total of 10,527 deaths (2004 to 2018) resulting from exposure to extreme heat (annual mean = 702).[17]

Cold-Related Illness

Mild to severe cold weather conditions cause an average of 774 deaths per year in the United States.[4,18] Almost one-half of these deaths occurred in persons age 65 years and older.[4,16] When adjusted for age, death from hypothermia occurred approximately 2.5 times more often in men than in women. The incidence of hypothermia-related deaths progressively increases with age, and it is three times higher in males than in females after age 15 years. Major contributing factors for accidental hypothermia are urban poverty, socioeconomic conditions, alcohol intake, malnutrition, and age (very young and older adults).[4,9]

Even though hypothermia is typically associated with cool or colder weather, it may occur in conditions that one would ordinarily not consider cold but that allow the body's temperature to fall below 96°F (35.6°C). For example, the elderly and infants may develop hypothermia in summertime if the air conditioning in their home is too cold for their limited adaptive mechanisms. Swimmers and surfers can become hypothermic in the summer when exposed to water that is cooler than body temperature, and the combination of low, but not freezing, temperatures, along with high winds and rain, can result in conditions conducive to hypothermia.[19] It is therefore important to appreciate that hypothermia is not just a cold weather disease.

Anatomy

The Skin

The skin, the largest organ of the body, interfaces with the external environment and serves as a layer of protection. It prevents the invasion of microorganisms, maintains fluid balance, and regulates temperature. Skin is composed of three tissue layers: the epidermis, dermis, and subcutaneous tissue (**Figure 19-1**). The outermost layer, the epidermis, is made up entirely of epithelial cells, with no blood vessels. Underlying the epidermis is the thicker dermis. The dermis is 20 to 30 times thicker than the

---

Box 19-1 Prehospital Versus Out-of-Hospital

Although this text focuses on prehospital care, the term *prehospital* is not accurate in all scenarios. Studies have demonstrated that most of the people cared for in wilderness and other remote outdoor environments are not transferred to a hospital, given that typically a hospital is not immediately accessible. Thus, some organizations refer to medical care provided in such environments as *out-of-hospital* care.

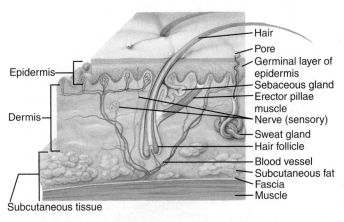

Figure 19-1 The skin is composed of three tissue layers—epidermis, dermis, and subcutaneous tissue—and associated muscle. Some layers contain structures such as glands, hair follicles, blood vessels, and nerves. All of these structures are interrelated with the maintenance, loss, and gain of body temperature.

© Jones & Bartlett Learning

epidermis. It is made up of a framework of connective tissues that contain blood vessels, blood products, nerves, sebaceous glands, and sweat glands. The innermost layer, the subcutaneous layer, is a combination of elastic and fibrous tissue as well as fatty deposits. Below this layer is skeletal muscle. The skin, nerves, blood vessels, and other underlying anatomic structures have major roles in regulating body temperature.

Physiology

Thermoregulation and Temperature Balance

Humans are considered **homeotherms**, or warm-blooded animals. A key feature of homeotherms is that they can regulate their own internal body temperature at a constant level, often above the level of their environment, and independent of varying environmental temperatures.

The human body is essentially divided into a warmer inner core and an outer shell. The brain and the thoracic and abdominal organs are included in the inner core, and the skin and subcutaneous layer make up the outer shell. The outer shell plays a critical role in the regulation of the body's **core temperature**. The core temperature is regulated through a balance of heat-production and heat-dissipation mechanisms. The temperature of the skin's surface and the "thickness" of the outer shell depend on the **environmental temperature**. The outer shell becomes "thicker" in colder temperatures and "thinner" in warmer temperatures based on the shunting of blood away from or to the skin, respectively. This outer shell, or tissue insulation, as induced by vasoconstriction, has

been estimated to offer about the same level of protection as wearing a light business suit.

Metabolic heat production will vary based on activity levels. Independent of the variation of external temperature, the body normally functions within a narrow temperature range, known as **environmental temperature**, of about 1°F (0.6°C) on either side of 98.6°F (37°C ± 0.6°C). Normal body temperature is maintained in a narrow range by homeostatic mechanisms regulated in the brain's hypothalamus. The **hypothalamus** is known as the **thermoregulatory center** and functions as the body's thermostat to control neurologic and hormonal regulation of body temperature. Trauma to the brain can disrupt the hypothalamus, which in turn causes an imbalance in the regulation of body temperature.

Humans have two systems to regulate body temperature: **behavioral regulation** and **physiologic thermoregulation**. Behavioral regulation is governed by the individual's thermal sensation and comfort, and the distinguishing feature is the conscious effort to reduce thermal discomfort (e.g., adding or shedding clothing, seeking shelter in cold environments). The processing of sensory feedback to the brain of thermal information in behavioral regulation is not well understood, but the feedback of thermal sensation and comfort responds more quickly than physiologic responses to changes in environmental temperature.[20]

Heat Production and Thermal Balance

Basal metabolic rate is the heat produced primarily as a by-product of metabolism, mostly from the large organs of the core and from skeletal muscle contraction. The heat generated is transferred throughout the body by blood in the circulatory system. Heat transfer and its dissipation from the body by the cardiopulmonary system are important in the assessment and management of heat illness, as discussed later in the chapter.

Shivering increases the metabolic rate by increasing muscle tension, which leads to repeated bouts of muscular contraction and relaxation, and it is the most powerful of the body's heat production mechanisms. Although shivering can occur due to skin cooling at core temperatures measuring 98.6°F (37°C), typically shivering begins when the core temperature drops to between 94°F and 97°F (34.4°C to 36.1°C) and continues until the core temperature is 86°F (30°C).[7] With maximal shivering, heat production is increased by five to six times the resting level.[21,22]

The physiologic thermoregulation systems that control heat production and heat loss responses are well documented.[20,22,23] Two principles in thermoregulation are key to understanding how the body regulates core temperature: **thermal gradient** and **thermal equilibrium**.

A thermal gradient is the difference in temperature (high vs. low temperature) between two objects. Thermal equilibrium is the state at which two objects in contact with one another are at the same temperature; it is achieved by the transfer of heat from a warmer object to a colder object until the objects are the same temperature.

When body temperature rises, the normal physiologic response is to increase skin blood flow and to begin sweating. Most body heat is transferred to the environment at the skin surface by conduction, convection, radiation, and evaporation. Because heat is transferred from greater temperature to lower temperature, the human body can gain heat by radiation and conduction during hot weather conditions.

Methods to maintain and dissipate body heat are important concepts for prehospital care practitioners. They must understand how both heat and cold are transferred to and from the body so that they can effectively manage a patient who has hyperthermia or hypothermia (**Figure 19-2**). The methods of heat and cold transfer are described as follows:

- **Radiation** is the loss or gain of heat in the form of electromagnetic energy; it is the transfer of energy from a warm object to a cooler one. A patient with heat illness can acquire additional body heat directly from the sun. Sources of radiant heat must be understood and managed by the prehospital care practitioner when assessing and treating the patient, as they will impact interventions to cool or warm a patient.
- **Conduction** is the transfer of heat between two objects in direct contact with each other, such as a patient lying on a frozen lawn after a fall. A patient will generally lose heat faster when lying on the cold ground than when exposed to cold air. Therefore, prehospital care practitioners need to protect and insulate the patient from colder ground temperatures rather than merely covering the patient with a blanket.
- **Convection** is the transfer of heat from a solid object to a medium that moves across that solid object, such as air or water over the body. The movement of cool air or water across the warmer skin provides for the continuous transfer of heat from the body. The body will lose heat 25 times faster in water than in air of the same temperature. A patient with wet clothing will lose body heat rapidly in mild to cold temperatures, so prehospital care practitioners should remove wet clothing and keep a patient dry to maintain body heat. When prehospital care practitioners effectively manage a patient with heat illness, they use the principle of convective heat loss by moistening and fanning the patient to dissipate body heat quickly.
- **Evaporation** of sweat from a liquid to a vapor is an extremely effective method of producing heat loss

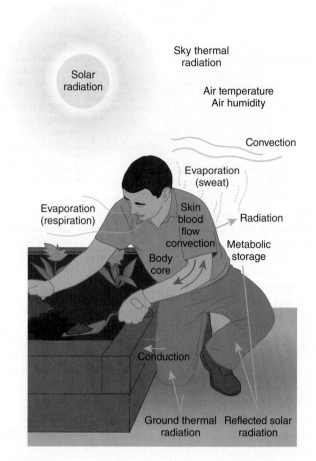

Figure 19-2 How humans exchange thermal energy with the environment.
© National Association of Emergency Medical Technicians (NAEMT)

from the body, depending on the relative humidity or moisture in the air. A **basal level** of both water and accompanying heat loss from exhaled air, skin, and mucous membranes is called **insensible loss** and is caused by evaporation. This insensible loss is normally about 10% of basal heat production, but when the body temperature rises, this process becomes more active (sensible), and sweat is produced. Evaporative heat loss increases in cool, dry, and windy conditions such as deserts. Collectively, convection and evaporation are more important than other methods of heat transfer because they are regulated by the body to control core temperature.[5]

Increases (hyperthermia) and decreases (hypothermia) in body temperature beyond the steady-state range (98.6°F ± 1°F [37°C ± 0.6°C]) can result from different internal and external causes, and return to steady-state temperature can occur without complications.[24] Hyperthermia occurs primarily in one of three ways:

- As a normal response to sustained exercise, in which the heat produced elevates core temperature and

is the stimulus for heat-dissipating responses (e.g., sweating, increased blood flow to the skin)
- When the sum of heat production and heat gained from the environment is greater than the body's heat dissipation capability
- From a fever

Unlike the first two ways, fever usually occurs in response to inflammation because of a change in the *thermoregulatory set point* (body temperature setting) of the brain, and the body responds by elevating body temperature to a higher value (100°F to 106°F [37.8°C to 41.1°C]). Heat production increases temporarily to achieve a new thermoregulatory set point temperature in an attempt to make the environment less hospitable for the invading infection.[23]

Homeostasis

These anatomic structures and physiologic systems are designed to interact in such a way that the body functions appropriately when exposed to temperature changes. The body is in a constant state of neurologic feedback from peripheral and internal regions to the thermoregulatory center and other regions in the brain and consequent responses. All of these systems interact to maintain constant, stable internal conditions, called homeostasis, in the body. However, at times, homeostasis is not achieved. For example, an imbalance may occur in the cardiovascular and thermoregulatory adjustments to eliminate excessive body heat, one outcome of which is the loss of excessive body fluid through sweating that causes acute dehydration and may lead to signs and symptoms of heat illness.

Risk Factors in Heat Illness

Numerous studies on humans have demonstrated large individual differences in tolerance to hot environments.[24] These differences can be partially explained by both physical characteristics and medical conditions that are associated with an increased risk for heat illness (**Box 19-2**). It is important to realize that any situation in which heat production exceeds the body's ability to dissipate heat may result in heat injury.

Key risk factors that contribute to the onset of heat illness are alcohol consumption, medications, dehydration, higher body mass index, obesity, inadequate diet, improper clothing, low fitness, sleep loss, extremes of age, cardiovascular disease, skin injuries, previous heat-related illness, sickle cell trait, cystic fibrosis, sunburn, viral illness, and exercise during the hottest hours of day.[18,19,25,26,28,29] Transient conditions include those affecting individuals who travel from cooler climates and are not heat-acclimatized to warmer climates on arrival. Other transient factors that place individuals at risk for

---

Box 19-2 Heat Illness Risk Factors

Factors That Increase Internal Heat Production
- Physical exertion
- Response to infection (fever)
- Hyperthyroidism
- Agitated and tremulous states (Parkinson, psychosis, mania, drug withdrawal—opiate and alcohol)
- Drug overdoses (such as cocaine, caffeine, LSD, phencyclidine hydrochloride, methamphetamine, ecstasy)

Factors That Interfere With Heat Dissipation
- High ambient temperature
- High humidity
- Obesity (insulation effect, less efficient dissipation)
- Impaired vasodilation
- Diabetes
- Alcoholism
- Medications (diuretics, tranquilizers, beta blockers, antihistamines, phenothiazines, antidepressants)
- Impaired ability to sweat (cystic fibrosis, skin diseases, healed burns)
- Heavy or tight clothing

Factors That Impair the Body's Response to Heat Stress Dehydration
- Prior episode of heatstroke
- Recent GI or respiratory infections
- Hypokalemia
- Cardiovascular disease

Abbreviations: GI, gastrointestinal; LSD, lysergic acid diethylamide.

Data from Hawkins SC, Simon RB, Beissinger JP, Simon D. *Vertical Aid: Essential Wilderness Medicine for Climbers, Trekkers, and Mountaineers.* The Countryman Press; 2017; Hall B, Hall J. *Sauer's Manual of Skin Diseases.* 10th ed. Lippincott Williams & Wilkins; 2010; Krakowski A, Goldenberg A. Exposure to radiation from the sun. In: Auerbach PS, ed. *Auerbach's Wilderness Medicine.* 7th ed. Mosby Elsevier; 2017; and Lipman GS, Gaudio FFG, Eifling KP, Ellis MA, Otten EM, Grissom CK. Wilderness Medical Society practice guidelines for the prevention and treatment of heat-related illness: 2019 update. *Wilderness Environ Med.* 2019;30(4):S33-S46.

---

heat illness are common illnesses, including colds and other conditions that cause fever, vomiting, and diarrhea, along with poor dietary and fluid intake.[30,31] Cumulative exposure is also a known risk factor for members of the military or firefighters, with risk increasing with additional days of exposure unless relieved.[32]

Factors considered to be chronic conditions that place individuals at greater risk for heat illness are fitness level, body size, age, medical condition, and medication use.

Obesity, Fitness, and Body Mass Index

Obesity and low levels of physical fitness caused by genetic factors or a sedentary lifestyle with inadequate daily physical activity will reduce tolerance to heat exposure. Physical fitness provides a cardiovascular reserve to maintain cardiac output as needed to sustain thermoregulation, and it allows individuals to acclimatize more quickly through sustained tolerance for physical activity and increased sweat production while hyperthermic.[27,33,34] Individuals who are overweight have a normal response to heat exposure—vasodilation of skin blood vessels and increased sweating. However, the combination of low fitness, lack of heat acclimatization, increased thermal insulation, and altered sweat gland distribution increases the energy cost of movement and places them at greater risk for heat illness.

Age

Thermoregulatory capacity and tolerance to heat diminish with age, particularly in those individuals age 65 years or older. These individuals can improve their heat tolerance by maintaining a low body weight and attaining an improved level of physical fitness.

Special consideration must be given for infants and young children because their body surface area makes up a much greater proportion of their overall weight compared to that of an adult, causing them to face a much greater risk of heat-related illness. Furthermore, infants have an immature thermoregulatory capacity that does not allow them to adequately maintain body temperature when exposed to high heat.

Medical Conditions

Underlying medical conditions such as diabetes mellitus, thyroid disorders, and renal disease can increase the risk for heat intolerance and heat illness. Cardiovascular disease and circulatory problems that increase cutaneous blood flow and circulatory demand are aggravated by heat exposure. In these extreme environmental conditions, heart disease and pulmonary diseases may be the presenting signs and symptoms aggravated by high ambient temperatures. A mild form of heat illness seen in individuals is miliaria rubra (prickly heat, heat rash, sweat rash), which has been shown to cause reduced heat tolerance through blocked or inflamed sweat pores.[19,33]

Medications

The use of specific prescription or over-the-counter medications can place individuals at a greater risk for heat illness (see Box 19-2). Certain medications can increase metabolic heat production, suppress body cooling and thirst, reduce cardiac reserve, and alter renal electrolyte and fluid balance.[6,33] Sedative and narcotic drugs affect mental status and can affect logical reasoning and judgment, potentially suppressing decision-making ability when the individual is exposed to heat.

Dehydration

Total body water (TBW) is the largest component of the human body, representing 50% to 70% of body weight.[35] For example, a 165-pound (lb; 75-kilogram [kg]) man contains approximately 45 liters of water, representing 60% of body weight. Excessive changes in the normal body water balance (*euhydration*) resulting from either overconsumption of water (*hyperhydration*) or fluid deficit (*hypohydration*) alter homeostasis, producing specific signs and symptoms. Dehydration, defined as the hypotonic hypovolemia caused by a net loss of hypotonic body fluids, can be a serious outcome of both heat and cold exposure, and it is also seen as a dangerous side effect of diarrhea, vomiting, and fever.[35]

Dehydration is a common finding in cases of heat illness occurring over many days, as seen in geriatric patients, or during physical activity, as seen with profuse sweating in athletes, members of the military, and firefighters. In the elderly, dehydration is often due to low fluid consumption, whereas athletes, military personnel, and firefighters consume inadequate volumes of fluid during daily activities and thus do not replace depleted TBW. Children (younger than 15 years) and persons older than 65 years are particularly susceptible to dehydration.

Body water is lost daily through sweat, tears, urine, and stool. Normally, drinking fluids and eating foods that contain water replace these losses. When a person becomes sick with fever, diarrhea, or vomiting, or an individual is exposed to heat, dehydration occurs. Occasionally, drugs that deplete body fluids and electrolytes, such as diuretics, can cause dehydration.

During heat exposure, body water is primarily lost as sweat, as this is the primary means of heat removal from the body. Individuals can sweat 0.8 to 1.4 liters per hour (liters/hr), and it has been reported that some elite athletes who are heat-acclimatized can sweat up to 3.7 liters/hr during competition in hot environments.[36] The keys to avoiding the onset of heat illness are to maintain a body fluid balance and to minimize dehydration during daily activities, particularly during any physical activity in moderate to high heat exposure. Signs and symptoms of dehydration are nonspecific and at times difficult to identify.

With mild to moderate levels of acute dehydration (2% to 6% body weight), individuals experience thirst, weakness, fatigue, headache, lightheadedness, irritability, decreased heat tolerance, dark odorous urine, diminished urine output, and cognitive deterioration, along with reductions in strength and aerobic physical capacity.[33,35,37,38] Severely dehydrated patients will present with signs and symptoms similar to those of hypovolemic shock: rapid pulse, pale, sweaty skin, weakness, and nausea.[33]

When individuals are encouraged to drink fluids frequently during heat exposure, the rate at which fluids can be replaced by mouth is limited by the rate of gastric emptying and the rate of fluid absorption in the small intestine.[39] Fluids empty from the stomach to the small intestine, where absorption occurs into the bloodstream, at a maximal rate of approximately 1 to 1.2 liters/hr.[38] Furthermore, gastric emptying rates are decreased approximately 20% to 25% when sweat-induced weight loss causes dehydration of 5% of total body weight (e.g., 5% of a 200-lb male = 10-lb weight loss [5% of a 100-kg male = a 5-kg weight loss).[40] Various hydration strategies and considerations are discussed in more detail later in this chapter.

Signs and Symptoms of Dehydration

The following are the most common signs and symptoms of dehydration in infants, children, and adults, although people may experience different symptoms[33,35]:

- Less frequent urination and dark color urine
- Thirst
- Dry skin
- Fatigue
- Lightheadedness
- Headache
- Dizziness
- Confusion
- Dry mouth and mucous membranes
- Increased heart rate and breathing

In infants and children, additional symptoms may include the following:

- Dry mouth and tongue
- No tears when crying
- No wet diapers for more than 3 hours
- Sunken abdomen, eyes, or cheeks
- Sunken fontanelles (in infants)
- High fever
- Listlessness
- Irritability
- Skin that does not flatten when pinched and released (*skin tenting*)

Injuries Caused by Heat

Heat-related disorders can range from minor to severe in patients with heat illness.[29,41] It is important to note that prehospital care practitioners may or may not see a progression of signs and symptoms, starting with minor syndromes (e.g., miliaria rubra, exercise-associated muscle cramps) and advancing to major heat-related illness (e.g., heatstroke). In most heat exposures, the patient can dissipate core body heat adequately and maintain core temperature within the normal range. However, when heat-related conditions result in a call for EMS assistance, the minor heat-related conditions may be apparent to the prehospital care practitioner during patient assessment, along with signs and symptoms of a major heat illness (**Table 19-1**).

Minor Heat-Related Disorders

The minor heat-related disorders include miliaria rubra, heat edema, exercise-induced muscle (heat) cramps, and heat syncope. These are not life-threatening problems, but they do require assessment and treatment.

Miliaria Rubra

Miliaria rubra, also known as "prickly heat" and "heat rash," is a red, *pruritic* (itchy), *papular* (raised bumps) rash normally seen on the skin in areas of restrictive clothing and heavy sweating (**Figure 19-3**). This condition is caused by inflammation of the sweat glands that blocks the sweat ducts. As a result, affected areas cannot sweat, putting individuals at increased risk of heat illness, depending on the amount of skin surface involved.[13,19,25,27]

Management

Treatment begins by cooling and drying the affected area(s) and by preventing further conditions that cause sweat in these areas. For example, get the patient out of the heat and humidity and into a cooler, dryer environment. A cool shower and "dab" drying the area will help resolve these rashes. Antihistamines may be administered to relieve itching.[13,19,25,27]

Heat Edema

Heat edema is a mild, dependent edema in the hands, feet, and ankles seen during early stages of heat acclimatization when plasma volume is expanding to compensate for the increased need for thermoregulatory blood flow. This form of edema does not indicate excessive fluid intake or cardiac, renal, or hepatic disease. In the absence of other diseases, this condition is of no clinical significance and is self-limited. Heat edema is observed more often in females.

Management

Treatment consists of loosening any constricting clothing, removing any tight or constricting jewelry, and elevating the legs. Diuretics are not indicated and may increase the risk of heat illness.

Exercise-Associated Muscle (Heat) Cramps

Exercise-associated muscle cramps can occur at any temperature and are not related specifically to elevated body

Table 19-1 Common Heat-Related Disorders

Disorder	Cause/Problem	Signs/Symptoms	Treatment
Exercise-associated muscle (heat) cramps	Failure to replace fluids and electrolytes lost through sweating; electrolyte and muscle problems	Painful, spasmodic muscle cramps, usually in heavily exercised muscles such as calves, thighs, and abdominals	Move to cool place; rest; encourage drinking sport drinks or drinks with NaCl (e.g., tomato juice). Transport those with signs or symptoms listed for dehydration, heat exhaustion, heatstroke, or exercise associated hyponatremia.
Dehydration	Failure to replace sweat loss with fluids	Thirst, nausea, excessive fatigue, headache, hypovolemia, decreased thermoregulation; reduced physical and mental capacity	Replace sweat loss with lightly salted fluids; rest in cool place until body weight and water losses are restored. In some patients, intravenous (IV) rehydration is necessary.
Heat exhaustion	Excessive heat strain with inadequate water intake; cardiovascular problems with venous pooling, decreased cardiac filling time, reduced cardiac output; untreated, may progress to heatstroke	Low urine output, tachycardia, tachypnea, weakness, malaise, unstable gait, extreme fatigue, pale/cool/clammy skin, headache, dizziness (fainting possible), nausea/vomiting, temperature normal or mildly elevated, sweating	Stop exertion, remove from heat stress, and place patient in prone position in cooler location; remove restrictive clothing; cool body with water and fanning; encourage drinking lightly salty fluids (e.g., sport drinks); administer IV 0.9% NaCl or lactated Ringer's solution.
Heatstroke	High core temperatures > 105°F (40.5°C); cellular disruption; dysfunction of multiple organ systems common; neurologic disorder with thermoregulatory center failure	Mental status changes, including confusion, irrational behavior, or delirium; possible shivering; tachycardia initially, then bradycardia late; hypotension; rapid and shallow breathing; dry or wet, hot skin; loss of consciousness; seizures and coma	Emergency: Apply rapid, immediate cooling by water immersion or wetting patient, or wrap patient in cool, wet sheets and fan vigorously. Apply ice packs to the entire body, or chemical cold packs to the cheeks, palms, and soles.[27] Continue until core temperature is 102.2°F (39°C).[27] Treat for shock if necessary once core temperature is lowered. Protect the airway and immediately transport to emergency department.
Exercise-associated hyponatremia	Low plasma sodium concentration (< 135 mmol/L); typically seen in individuals during prolonged activity in	Headache, nausea, vomiting, malaise, dizziness, ataxia, altered mental status, polyuria, pulmonary edema, signs of intracranial pressure,	Restrict hypotonic and isotonic fluid intake; give salty foods/saline. Unresponsive patients receive standard resuscitative care, 15 liters/min oxygen by nonrebreathing

Disorder	Cause/Problem	Signs/Symptoms	Treatment
	hot environments; drinking water (> 1.5 liters/hr) or that exceeds sweat rate; inappropriate arginine vasopressin secretion; failure to replace sodium loss in sweat	seizures, coma; core temperature < 102.2°F (39°C); mimics signs of heat exhaustion and dehydration	mask. If serum sodium levels can be measured and are below 130 mmol/L, provide IV hypertonic saline, 100-mL bolus of 3% hypertonic saline, every 10-minutes for three doses or until neurologic symptoms end. Transport immediately with alert patient in sitting position or left-lateral position if unresponsive.

Modified from Schimelpfenig T, Richards G, Tartar S. Management of heat illnesses. In: Hawkins SC, ed. *Wilderness EMS.* Wolters Kluwer; 2018; Bennett BL, Hew-Butler T, Rosner MH, Myers T, Lipman GS. Wilderness Medical Society Practice guidelines for treatment of exercise-associated hyponatremia: 2019 update. *Wilderness Environ Med.* 2020;31(1):50-62.

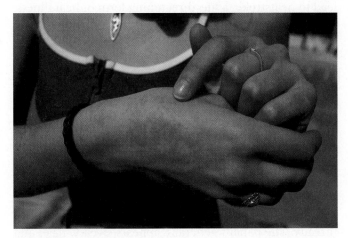

Figure 19-3 Heat rash.
© Ian west/Alamy Stock Photo

temperature. They manifest as short-term, painful muscle contractions frequently seen in the calf (gastrocnemius) muscles, but also in the voluntary muscles of the abdomen and extremities, and are commonly observed following prolonged physical activity, often in warm to hot temperatures. These cramps occur in individuals during exercise that produces profuse sweating or during the exercise-recovery period. Smooth muscle, cardiac, diaphragm, and *bulbar* muscles (muscles involved with speech, chewing, and swallowing) are not involved. Muscle cramps can occur alone or in association with heat exhaustion.

The cause of muscle cramping is unknown, but it is believed to be related to a combination of neuromuscular fatigue along with body water loss and sodium and other electrolyte losses. It is more commonly seen when individuals exercise in hot, humid environments without proper heat acclimatization, exercise beyond their physical fitness level, or experience profuse sweating.[13,27,33]

Management

Treatment consists of rest in a cool environment, prolonged stretching of the affected muscle, massage, and consuming oral fluids and food containing sodium chloride (e.g., 1/8 to 1/4 teaspoon of table salt added to 10 to 16 ounces [oz; 300 to 500 milliliters (mL)] of fluids or sport drinks, 1 to 2 salt tablets with 10 to 16 oz [300 to 500 mL] of fluid, or salty snacks). Intravenous (IV) fluids are rarely needed, but prolonged and severe diffuse muscle cramps can be resolved more rapidly with IV normal saline (NS). Avoid the use of salt tablets by themselves because they can cause gastrointestinal (GI) distress.[13,27,33]

Heat Syncope

Heat syncope is seen with prolonged standing in warm environments and is caused by low blood pressure that results in dizziness, weakness, or brief and transient loss of consciousness. Heat exposure causes peripheral vasodilation and orthostatic venous blood pooling in the legs, causing low blood pressure. Heat syncope often occurs to soldiers in formation or during a parade and can be seen in athletes after completion of a long duration exercise. Another common name for heat syncope is heat-associated postural hypotension.[27,33]

Management

Remove from the heat stress to a cool environment, and rest the patient in a recumbent position. Loosen or remove constrictive clothing, and if dehydration is suspected, provide oral or IV rehydration. If a fall occurred, patients should be thoroughly evaluated for injury. Patients with a significant history of cardiac or neurologic disorders need further evaluation for the cause of their syncopal episode. Monitoring of vital signs and the electrocardiogram (ECG) during transport is essential.[27,33]

Major Heat-Related Disorders

The major heat-related disorders include exercise-associated collapse, heat exhaustion, and heatstroke (classic and exertional forms) and may pose a life threat if allowed to progress.

Exercise-Associated Collapse

This disorder occurs when an individual collapses after strenuous exercise.[42-48] During exercise, contraction of the muscles of the lower extremities assists in augmenting venous blood return to the heart. When exercise stops, such as at the end of a jog, the muscle contraction that assisted blood return to the heart slows significantly. This in turn causes venous blood return to the heart to decrease, resulting in a decreased cardiac output to the brain. This disorder is often seen at the completion of marathons, ultramarathons, and triathlons.[49]

Assessment

Signs and symptoms include difficulty standing and walking, nausea, lightheadedness, dizziness, or syncope. Patients may feel better when lying down but become lightheaded when they attempt to stand or sit (*orthostatic hypotension*). Profuse sweating is not unusual. Ventilation and pulse rates may be rapid. The patient's core body temperature may be normal or slightly elevated. It is difficult to rule out dehydration, but this type of postexercise collapse is not from hypovolemia. In contrast, collapse that occurs during exercise requires immediate evaluation for other causes (e.g., cardiovascular).

Management

The patient is removed to a cool environment to rest in a recumbent position with legs elevated. IV rehydration is provided if truly needed for moderate to severe dehydration; otherwise provide cool fluids by mouth. Because many of these patients experienced collapse because of the decreased venous return at the end of exercise and not from dehydration, it is highly recommended to withhold IV therapy until further assessment and passive "cooldown" are completed. As with any form of collapse, further evaluation is necessary to rule out other disorders (e.g., heatstroke, exercise-associated hyponatremia, cardiac or neurologic causes). Monitoring of vital signs and ECG during transport is essential to detect cardiac dysrhythmias.

Heat Exhaustion

Heat exhaustion is the most common heat-related disorder seen by prehospital care practitioners. This condition can develop over days of exposure (often seen in elderly persons) or acutely (often seen in athletes). Heat exhaustion results from cardiac output that is insufficient to support the increased circulatory load caused by competing demands of thermoregulatory heat dissipation, increased skin blood flow, reduced plasma volume, reduced venous return to the heart from vasodilation, and sweat-induced depletion of salt and water.[31] Heat exhaustion often occurs to older adults due to a combination of high temperatures, medication use (e.g., diuretics), inadequate water intake, and preexisting cardiac insufficiency.[13,33]

Distinguishing severe heat exhaustion from heatstroke often may be difficult, but a quick mental status assessment will determine the level of neurologic involvement. If heat exhaustion is not effectively treated, it may lead to heatstroke, a life-threatening form of heat illness. Heat exhaustion is a *diagnosis of exclusion* when there is no evidence of heatstroke. These patients will need further physical and laboratory evaluation in the ED.

Assessment

Signs and symptoms of heat exhaustion are neither specific nor sensitive. They include fatigue, dizziness, headache, vomiting, malaise, hypotension, and tachycardia. Core body temperatures may measure from 101.3°F to 104°F (38.5°C to 40°C), although they can be normal or only slightly elevated.[13] During the acute stage of heat exhaustion, the blood pressure is low, and the pulse and ventilatory rates are rapid. The radial pulse may feel thready. The patient generally appears sweaty, pale, and ashen.

It is important to obtain a good history of prior heat illness and the current heat exposure incident because these patients may display signs and symptoms of other conditions of fluid and sodium loss (e.g., hyponatremia; see later discussion). Reassessment is critical because heat exhaustion may progress to heatstroke. Continuously look for any changes in mentation and personality (e.g., confusion, disorientation, irrational or unusual behavior). Any such change should be taken as a progressive sign of hyperthermia indicating heatstroke—*an immediately life-threatening condition!*

Management

Immediately remove the patient from the hot environment (e.g., sun, hot pavement, hot vehicle) to a cooler location either in the shade or air-conditioned space (e.g., ambulance). Place the patient in a recumbent position. Remove clothing and anything restricting heat dissipation, such as blankets. Assess the patient's heart rate, blood pressure, ventilatory rate, and rectal temperature (if a thermometer is available and conditions permit) and be alert particularly for central nervous system (CNS) status changes as an early indicator of life-threatening heatstroke.

Oral rehydration with electrolytes should be considered for any patient who can take fluids by mouth and who is not at risk of aspirating. Sport drinks are the ideal choice, but the drinks should be diluted to half-strength due to their high sugar content when undiluted. Large amounts of oral fluids may increase bloating, nausea, and vomiting. Normally IV fluids are not needed if blood pressure, pulse, and rectal temperature are normal. However, in patients who are not able to consume fluids by mouth, IV fluids provide rapid recovery from heat exhaustion.[29] If IV fluids are needed, lactated Ringer's (LR) solution or NS should be used. IV solutions produce more rapid fluid recovery than do fluids by mouth due to delays in gastric emptying and absorption in the small intestine caused by dehydration.

In exertional heat exhaustion, most exercising patients recover with recumbent rest and oral fluids. Before making any decision regarding IV therapy for these patients, the prehospital care practitioner needs to conduct a thorough assessment for signs and symptoms of dehydration, *orthostatic* (postural) pulse, blood pressure changes, and the ability to ingest oral fluids. Ongoing mental status changes should prompt further evaluation for heatstroke, hyponatremia, hypoglycemia, and other medical problems. In the exertional heat exhaustion patient, the recommended IV fluids are NS or 5% dextrose in NS for patients who are mildly hypoglycemic. However, practitioners must exercise caution to ensure that large amounts of IV fluids are not administered to a patient who has been participating in prolonged exercise (greater than 4 hours), especially individuals who do not have obvious clinical signs of dehydration, or in a collapsed athlete with suspected heat exhaustion who has been drinking a large amount of water. This type of patient may have exercise-associated hyponatremia (low serum sodium level), and providing oral and/or IV fluids will cause further *dilutional hyponatremia*, potentially precipitating a life-threatening condition.[50,51] See the discussion on exercise-associated hyponatremia for information on how best to correctly assess the patient for heat-related illness or exercise-associated hyponatremia.

Because heat exhaustion may be difficult to distinguish from heatstroke and because patients with heatstroke should be cooled rapidly to reduce core temperature, the best course of action is to provide some active cooling procedures to all patients with heat exhaustion. Active cooling can be done simply and quickly by wetting the head and upper torso with water or a wet cloth and then fanning or positioning the patient into the wind to increase convective body heat dissipation. Body-cooling procedures will also improve mental status.

Rapidly transport all patients who are unconscious, or who do not recover rapidly, as this is a sign of an immediately life-threatening heatstroke condition. Proper environmental temperature control and monitoring of vital signs and mental status are essential during transport.

Heatstroke

Heatstroke is considered the most emergent and life-threatening form of heat illness and is one of the most time-sensitive life-threatening conditions that prehospital care practitioners encounter. Heatstroke is a form of hyperthermia resulting in failure of the thermoregulatory system—a failure of the body's physiologic systems to dissipate heat and cool down. Heatstroke is characterized by an elevated core temperature of 104°F (40°C) or greater and CNS dysfunction, resulting in delirium, convulsions, or coma.[40,44,52]

The most significant difference in heatstroke compared with heat exhaustion is neurologic disability, which presents to the prehospital care practitioner as mental status changes. Pathophysiologic changes often result in multiple organ failure.[41,53] These pathophysiologic changes occur when organ tissue temperatures rise above a critical level. Cell membranes are damaged, leading to disruption in cell volume, metabolism, acid–base balance, and membrane permeability that causes cellular and a whole-organ dysfunction with ultimate cell death and organ failure.[29] The degree of complications in patients with heatstroke is not entirely related to the magnitude of core temperature elevation.

This whole-body pathophysiologic dysfunction is the underlying reason for the need for early heatstroke recognition by prehospital care practitioners. With early recognition, aggressive whole-body cooling to rapidly reduce core temperature and decrease the associated heatstroke morbidity and mortality is possible.

Morbidity and mortality are directly associated with the duration of elevated core temperature, and a positive patient outcome is directly related to how fast the core temperature can be decreased below 102°F (38.9°C). Even with aggressive prehospital intervention and in-hospital management, heatstroke is often fatal, and many patients who survive have permanent neurologic disability.

Heatstroke has two different clinical presentations: classic heatstroke and exertional heatstroke (**Table 19-2**).

Classic heatstroke is a disorder most commonly seen in infants, febrile children, people who are homeless or cannot afford adequate air conditioning, older adults, people with alcoholism, and patients with chronic illnesses. It may be compounded by the risk factors listed in Box 19-2 (e.g., medications). A classic presentation is a patient who is exposed to elevated humidity and high room temperatures over several days without air

Table 19-2 Classic Versus Exertional Heatstroke

	Classic	Exertional
Patient characteristics	Elderly	Men (15 to 45 years)
Health status	Chronically ill	Healthy
Concurrent activity	Sedentary	Strenuous exercise
Drug use	Diuretics, antidepressants, antihypertensives, anticholinergics, antipsychotics	Usually none
Sweating	May be absent	Usually present
Lactic acidosis	Usually absent; poor prognosis if present	Common
Hyperkalemia	Usually absent	Often present
Hypocalcemia	Uncommon	Frequent
Hypoglycemia	Uncommon	Common
Creatine	Mildly elevated	Greatly elevated
Rhabdomyolysis	Mild	Frequently severe

Modified from Knochel JP, Reed G. Disorders of heat regulation. In: Kleeman CR, Maxwell MH, Narin RG, eds. *Clinical Disorders of Fluid and Electrolyte Metabolism.* McGraw-Hill; 1987.

Box 19-3 Common Causes of Death From Exertional Heatstroke (EHS)

1. *Inaccurate temperature assessment or misdiagnosis.* This is often due to the inability to rule out other similar medical conditions. Oral, axillary, and tympanic temperature measurements may underestimate the degree of temperature elevation; therefore, prehospital care practitioners should rely only on the rectal temperature to determine the degree of hyperthermia and maintain a high index of suspicion in high-risk patients.[55]
2. *No care or a treatment delay.* Failing to recognize the potential for EHS and delaying the response to provide effective care can have disastrous results.
3. *Inefficient whole-body cooling techniques.* Rapid reduction of core temperature to below 104°F (40°C) within 30 minutes is critical. This goal is recognized as the "golden half-hour" of heatstroke management and is the standard to meet with rapid whole-body cooling.[56]
4. *Immediate transport.* With EHS, it is critical to begin whole-body cooling to reduce the core temperature at the scene and not to transport until this treatment has begun. Cooling should continue during transport with rectal temperature assessment to ensure core temperature drops below 104°F (40°C).

conditioning, leading to dehydration and high core temperature. Often this patient's sweating mechanism has stopped, known as **anhidrosis**. This is especially common in large cities during summer heat waves, when effective home ventilation is either not possible or not used.[54] Scene assessment will provide information helpful in the identification of classic heatstroke.

Exertional heatstroke (EHS) is a preventable disorder often seen when people who lack the requisite physical fitness or heat acclimatization engage in short-term, strenuous physical activity (e.g., industrial workers, athletes, military recruits, firefighters, and other public safety personnel) in a hot, humid environment. These conditions can rapidly elevate internal heat production and limit the body's ability to dissipate heat. Almost all

EHS patients exhibit sweat-soaked and pale skin at the time of collapse as compared to dry, hot, and flushed skin in the classic heatstroke patient.[29] Even though drinking fluids can slow the rate of dehydration during strenuous activity and reduce the rate at which core temperature rises, hyperthermia and EHS may still occur in the absence of significant dehydration.

With aggressive treatment, no one should die from EHS if prompt care begins within 10 minutes of collapse. Some of the common reasons that death from EHS may occur are listed in **Box 19-3**.[42-44] The motto to "cool first, transport second" is meant to avoid any delays in initiating the lowering of core temperature.

Assessment

The appearance of signs and symptoms depends on the degree and duration of hyperthermia.[36] Patients with heatstroke typically present with hot, flushed skin. They may or may not be sweating, depending on where they are found and whether they have classic or exertional heatstroke. Blood pressure may be elevated or diminished, and the radial pulse is usually tachycardic and thready; 25% of these patients are hypotensive. The patient's level of consciousness can range from confused to unconscious, and seizure activity may also be present, particularly during cooling.[57] As confirmed in hospitals, rectal temperature may range from 104°F to 116°F (40°C to 46.7°C), but patients can have heatstroke with body temperatures lower than 104°F (40°C).[41,57,58]

The key to distinguishing heatstroke from one of the other heat-related conditions is altered mental status. Temperature is usually elevated and often is quite high. Any patient who is warm to the touch with an altered mental status (confused, disoriented, combative, or unconscious) should be presumed to have heatstroke and managed immediately and aggressively to reduce core temperature.

Management

Heatstroke is a true time-sensitive emergency. Immediately remove the patient from the source of heat. Cooling the patient should begin immediately in the field by one prehospital care practitioner while another practitioner assesses and stabilizes the patient's ABCs. Cooling of the patient begins immediately with whatever means are available (e.g., garden hose, bottled water, IV saline liter bags), even before removing clothing. Application of ice and cold-water immersion are the fastest two methods of cooling, but these approaches may be limited in the prehospital setting.[43,59-61]

Since the late 1950s, it has been thought that cold- or ice-water immersion will cause vasoconstriction sufficient to decrease heat loss from the body and cause the onset of shivering so that internal heat is produced, thus limiting the exchange of heat. Current empirical evidence refutes the concern that cooling rates in these patients would be blunted. Therefore, this form of cooling, if available, should not be withheld from a patient with heatstroke.[47] Many protocols and curricula recommend that temperature not be actively dropped below 102.2°F (39°C) to avoid rebound shivering (increasing body temperature) or "overshoot" or "afterdrop," causing the patient to become hypothermic.[46,61] The evidence-based Wilderness Medical Society Practice Guidelines for Hyperthermia Management note that there is no evidence to support a risk of either of these theoretical concerns; however, they cite 102.2°F (39°C) as the threshold to stop active cooling in heatstroke.[27]

If cold water and ice are not immediately available, remove the patient's excess clothing, wet down the patient from head to toe, and provide continuous fanning of the skin. It is essential that this procedure begin immediately and not be delayed before preparing to transport the patient from the scene to the ambulance. Patient wetting and fanning are the next most effective cooling techniques, causing evaporation and convective heat loss.[59] Individuals who rapidly become lucid during whole-body cooling usually have the best prognosis. The most important intervention prehospital care practitioners can deliver to a patient with heatstroke (along with management of ABCs) is immediate and rapid whole-body cooling to reduce core temperature.

During transport, the patient should be placed in a prepared, air-conditioned ambulance. It is an error to place a patient with heatstroke into a hot internal cabin of an ambulance, even if transfer time to the hospital is short. Remove any additional clothing, cover the patient with a sheet, and wet down the sheet with irrigation fluids along with providing continuous fanning, ideally by powered fans from the cabin overhead. Ice packs, if available and time allows, can be placed in the groin area, in the axillae, and around the anterior-lateral neck because blood vessels are closest to the skin surface in these areas. The widespread recommendation of using only ice packs is a much less effective core cooling technique. Ice packs alone are insufficient to rapidly lower core body temperature unless they cover the entire body and should be considered only as an extra cooling method and not a priority in patient care.[4,27,57,59]

If possible, the patient's rectal temperature should be measured every 5 to 10 minutes during transport to ensure effective cooling. Other means to assess the patient's temperature (e.g., oral, skin, axillary) should not be used for treatment decisions because they do not adequately reflect the patient's core temperature.[29,62]

Provide high-flow oxygen, support ventilations with a bag-mask device as needed, and monitor the patient's cardiac rhythm.

Patients with heatstroke generally do not require extensive fluid resuscitation and typically are initially given IV fluids consisting of 1.0 to 1.5 liters of NS. Provide a 500-mL fluid challenge and assess vital signs. Fluid volume should not exceed 1 to 2 liters in the first hour, or follow local medical protocol. Monitor blood glucose because these patients are frequently hypoglycemic and may require a bolus of 50% dextrose IV. Seizures can be managed with 5 to 10 milligrams (mg) of diazepam or other benzodiazepines as per local protocol. Transport the patient in a right or left lateral recumbent position to maintain an open airway and to avoid aspiration.

Exercise-Associated Hyponatremia

Exercise-associated hyponatremia (EAH), also known as water intoxication, is a life-threatening condition that has been increasingly described after prolonged physical exertion in recreational hikers, climbers, marathoners, ultra-marathoners, triathletes, adventure racers, and military infantry personnel.[49,63-67] With the increasing popularity of these outdoor activities, the incidence of mild to severe EAH has steadily increased since it was first reported in the mid-1980s.[66] It is now known to be one of the most severe medical complications of endurance activities and is an important cause of event-related fatalities.[50,51]

EAH is commonly associated with excessive consumption of water (1.5 quarts [qt; 1.4 liters] or greater per hour) during prolonged activities.[67] Two major pathogenic mechanisms largely account for the development of EAH: (1) excessive fluid intake and (2) impaired urinary water excretion due largely to persistent secretion of *arginine vasopressin (AVP)*, also referred to as antidiuretic hormone (ADH).[50,51] EAH can take two forms, mild or severe, depending on presenting symptoms.

In the severe form, low plasma sodium concentration disturbs the osmotic balance across the blood–brain barrier, resulting in the rapid influx of water into the brain, which causes cerebral edema.[49-51,66,68] In similar fashion to the signs and symptoms of increased intracranial pressure in head trauma (see Chapter 8, *Head and Neck Trauma*), a progression of neurologic symptoms from hyponatremia will occur, including headache, vomiting, malaise, confusion, and seizures, progressing to coma, permanent brain damage, brain stem herniation, and death.[50,51,66] These individuals are said to have **exercise-associated hyponatremic encephalopathy (EAHE)**.[50,51,66]

Symptomatic EAHE patients generally have a serum sodium concentration below 126 milliequivalents (mEq)/liter (normal range, 135 to 145 mEq/liter) with rapidly developing (less than 48 hours) hyponatremia, as seen frequently in prolonged endurance activities.[50,51,63,67] Alternatively, the milder form of EAH generally presents with isolated serum sodium levels of 135 to 128 mEq/liter, without easily discernable symptoms (i.e., weakness, nausea/vomiting, headache, or no symptoms), and is self-limiting with rest, food, and electrolyte fluids. Even with the initial presenting mild signs and symptoms of EAH, a patient can progress into EAHE. It has been suggested that there is an acute drop in serum sodium concentration at the end of an endurance event caused by the absorption of water retained in the GI tract.[50,51] This may account for a transient lucid period after finishing an endurance activity followed by the acute development of clinic signs of EAHE within about 30 minutes following the cessation of the activity.

Studies have reported that 18% to 23% of ultramarathoners and 29% of the Hawaiian Ironman Triathlete finishers had EAH.[46,53-55,57-71] In 2003, 32 cases of EAH were reported in hikers in the Grand Canyon National Park (GCNP), and 19% of all nonfatal heat-related incidents in GCNP from 2004 to 2009 were attributed to hyponatremia.[72-74]

EAH can occur in the following situations:

1. Excessive sodium and water loss in sweat throughout an endurance event, resulting in dehydration and sodium depletion

2. Overhydration solely with water while maintaining plasma sodium, creating a dilution of sodium concentration

3. Combination of excessive sodium and fluid loss in sweat and an excessive overhydration with water only

The evidence indicates that EAH is a result of fluid retention in the extracellular space (*dilutional*) rather than fluid remaining unabsorbed in the intestine.[63] Typically, these patients have not consumed sport electrolyte drinks, have consumed energy food supplements containing no salt, or have consumed salt in insufficient quantity to balance the loss of sodium in sweat or the dilution from excessive water intake.

The following are a few key risk factors that have been linked to the development of EAH[42,43,49,75]:

1. Activity or exercise duration (greater than 4 hours) or slow running/exercise pace
2. Female gender (may be explained by lower body weight)
3. Low or high body mass index
4. Excessive drinking (greater than 1.5 liters/hr) during an event or activity
5. Use of nonsteroidal anti-inflammatory drugs, which decrease renal filtration

EAH has been described as the "other heat-related illness" because the symptoms are nonspecific and are similar to those exhibited in minor and major heat-related disorders.[72] Many endurance events and multiday adventure activities are conducted in warm to hot environments; therefore, it is assumed that the signs and symptoms of EAH are some form of heat illness, and patients are managed with standard protocols that address the presumed hypovolemia and excessive body heat. Standard protocols that provide body cooling and IV fluid challenge to correct hyperthermia, sweat-induced dehydration, and mental status changes can complicate the dilutional hyponatremia and place the patient at further risk for seizure and coma. Treating a patient with EAH with fluids and rest will worsen the patient's condition, unlike the heat exhaustion patient.

This "other heat-related disorder" is becoming more widely recognized and correctly treated today by EMS and ED personnel, largely because of an increased effort to educate medical personnel and the public in its prevention, early recognition, and management (**Box 19-4**). Prehospital care practitioners directly supporting or responding to calls at physical endurance events in urban or wilderness settings need to be aware that EAH is more frequently reported today. It is important to remember that, in general, dehydration is more common in prolonged exertional activities and that it can lead to impaired performance during exercise or work-related tasks and to serious heat illness; however, symptomatic hyponatremia brought on by overdrinking is more dangerous and potentially a life-threatening illness.[75] This distinction illustrates a tension in hydration strategies: Waiting for thirst as an indicator to hydrate may predispose individuals to mild dehydration, whereas set regimens for hydration regardless of thirst risk may predispose individuals to overhydration and EAH. See the "Hydration" section later in this chapter for further discussion of this issue.

Assessment

A wide range of signs and symptoms may be found in the endurance-athlete population with hyponatremia (see Table 19-1). Core temperature is usually normal but can be low or slightly elevated, depending on the ambient temperature, body heat dissipation, and recent exercise intensity at assessment. Heart rate and blood pressure can be low, normal, or elevated, depending on core temperature, exercise intensity, hypovolemia, or shock. Ventilatory rate ranges from within normal limits to slightly elevated. Hyperventilation observed with EAH can account for vision disturbances, dizziness, tingling in hands, and paresthesias in the extremities. The hallmark assessment and findings are mental status changes, fatigue, malaise, headache, and nausea. Other forms of neurologic changes include slowed speech, ataxia, and cognitive changes, including irrational behavior, combativeness, and fear. These patients often report that they have a sense of "impending doom."

Management

The first step in treatment is recognizing the disorder and determining the severity. Management is based on the severity of EAH and what portable diagnostic tools are available to measure serum sodium.[49] **Figure 19-4** provides an algorithm for assessing patients to determine whether EAH or a heat-related illness is present. Mild symptoms should be managed conservatively by observing the patient to ensure no further progression to EAHE and waiting for normal diuresis of excessive fluid.

Place symptomatic patients in an upright position to maintain their airway and to minimize any positional effect on intracranial pressure. These patients are known to have projectile vomiting when transported. Place unconscious patients in the left lateral recumbent position, anticipate vomiting, and consider active airway management. Provide high-flow oxygen, establish IV access at the keep vein open (KVO) rate, and monitor for seizures.

As needed, administer anticonvulsant therapy (e.g., titrate benzodiazepines IV, per medical protocol). Check with medical control for volume of NS fluid, if any, to be administered, depending on patient severity and transport time to the hospital. Because these patients are already fluid overloaded, infusion of IV hypotonic fluids is contraindicated, as this can worsen the degree of hyponatremia and fluid overload.[76]

Patients with extensive signs and symptoms of EAHE (i.e., cerebral edema and pulmonary edema) need to have their plasma sodium concentration increased. The current consensus for management in the prehospital setting is to provide a 100-mL bolus infusion of 3% hypertonic saline over 10 minutes to acutely reduce brain edema. Each dose will raise sodium by 2 to 3 mEq/liter, if this solution is available.[58,76] If no clinical improvement is noted, up to two additional 100-mL, 3% bolus infusions can be given per medical protocol.[49,76] These severe cases of EAHE have a poor outcome if patients do not receive hypertonic saline.[77] Keep the patient calm while en route to the ED, and continue to monitor for mental status changes or seizures.

Prevention of Heat-Related Illness

Because heat stress is a significant public health factor in the United States, methods for preventing heat illness are vital to any community, particularly for those individuals who must work in high-heat occupational settings. For example, from 2006 to 2015, a total of 1,000 firefighters (including volunteer, career, and wildland firefighters) were killed in the line of duty in the United States,[78] for a yearly average of 100 firefighter deaths. In 2015, 90 firefighters were killed in the line of duty, with 60 (66.7%) deaths occurring at the scene due to stress or overexertion; heat illness is included as a cause of death in this category.[78]

Prehospital care practitioners and their EMS agencies are a good resource as partners for community education on heat stress prevention strategies in many different formats, including workshops, educational handouts, agency website or newsletter, community presentations, and local newspaper.

As with the general public, heat-related illness in prehospital care practitioners represents an occupational risk; therefore, EMS and other public safety personnel need to use prevention strategies and prepare for exposure to high ambient temperature when appropriate

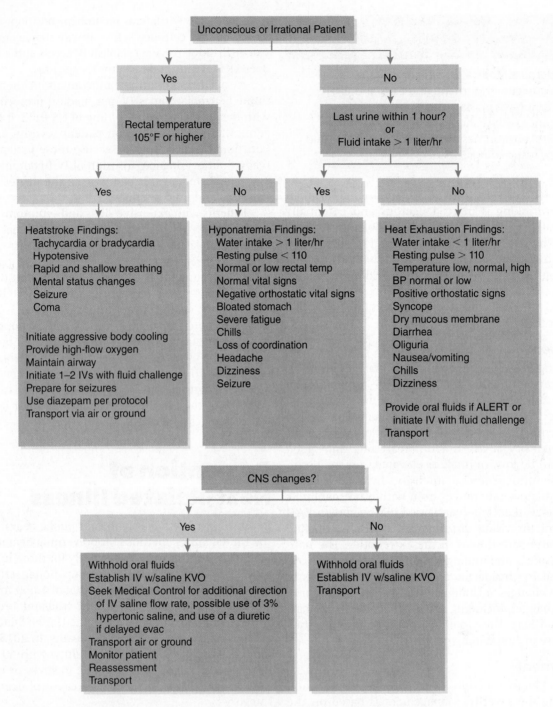

Figure 19-4 Treatment algorithm for heat exhaustion, heatstroke, and hyponatremia.
© National Association of Emergency Medical Technicians (NAEMT)

and relevant. These strategies, which include administrative policies, procedures, engineering controls, use of equipment, and medical surveillance programs, are designed to help minimize the overall impact from acute or chronic heat exposure. The implementation of simple preventive procedures can have a dramatic impact on lowering the incidence of heat illness. Box 19-5 provides

an overview of heat stress prevention strategies for prehospital care practitioners, firefighters, and other public safety personnel.[79]

A complex interaction of factors that combine to exceed the tolerance limits for individual heat exposure can eventually lead to the onset of signs and symptoms of heat-related illness. The capacity of humans to work

Box 19-5 Prevention of Heat-Related Disorders in Prehospital Care Practitioners

You can prevent the serious consequences of heat disorders by improving your level of fitness and becoming acclimated to the heat.

Maintaining a high level of aerobic fitness is one of the best ways to protect yourself against heat stress. The fit prehospital care practitioner has a well-developed circulatory system and increased blood volume. Both are important to regulate body temperature. Fit practitioners start to sweat sooner, so they work with a lower heart rate and body temperature. They adjust to the heat twice as fast as unfit practitioners. They lose acclimatization more slowly and regain it quickly.

The time required for heat acclimatization varies depending on timing and frequency of exposure, and it has been shown to occur within 10 to 14 days of heat exposure as the body changes in the following ways[13,80-82]:

- Increases sweat production
- Improves blood distribution
- Decreases heart rate
- Lowers skin and body temperatures

As a prehospital care practitioner, you can acclimatize by gradually increasing work time in the heat, taking care to replace fluids, and resting as needed. Acclimatization is maintained with periodic work or exercise in a hot environment.

On the Job

The heat stress index (see **Figure 19-5**) illustrates how temperature and humidity combine to create moderate-heat or high-heat stress conditions. Be alert for heat stress when radiant heat from the sun

or nearby flames is high, when the air is still, or when working hard and therefore creating large amounts of metabolic heat. The heat stress index does not consider the effects of long hours of hard work, dehydration, or the impact of personal protective clothing and equipment.

When heat stress conditions exist, you must modify the way you work or exercise. Pace yourself. There are individual differences in fitness, acclimatization, and heat tolerance. Push too hard and you will become a candidate for a heat-related illness.

When possible, you should do the following:

- Avoid working close to heat sources.
- Do harder work during cooler morning and evening hours.
- Change tools or tasks to minimize fatigue.
- Take frequent rest breaks.
- Most important, maintain hydration by replacing lost fluids.

Hydration

Maintaining body fluids is essential for sweating and the removal of internal heat generated during physical activities. To minimize dehydration and the risk of heat illness, you must hydrate before, during, and after exercise or physical work. The Wilderness Medical Society now recommends *ad libitum* (drink to thirst) fluid intake to ensure proper hydration while preventing excessive fluid intake and onset of EAH. Prehospital care practitioners must monitor their own level of thirst throughout the day and drink fluids in an amount necessary to prevent a loss of body weight greater than 2%.[49,58] Individual characteristics

Temperature (°F) Versus Relative Humidity (%)

°F	90%	80%	70%	60%	50%	40%
80	85	84	82	81	80	79
85	101	96	92	90	86	84
90	121	113	105	99	94	90
95		133	122	113	105	98
100			142	129	118	109
105				148	133	121
110						135

High	Possible Heat Disorder
80–90°F	Fatigue possible with prolonged exposure and physical activity.
90–105°F	Sunstroke, heat cramps, and heat exhaustion possible.
105–130°F	Sunstroke, heat cramps, and heat exhaustion likely, and heatstroke possible.
130°F or greater	Heatstroke highly likely with continued exposure.

Due to the nature of the heat index calculation, the values in the tables have an error ± 1.3°F.

Figure 19-5 Heat stress index.

Courtesy of the National Weather Service, Pueblo, Colorado. https://www.weather.gov/pub/

(*continues*)

(e.g., body weight, genetic predisposition, heat acclimatization state, and metabolic state) will influence sweat rate for a given activity. These factors will result in large individual sweat rates and total sweat loss. For example, long-distance running is known to cause an average sweat rate of 1.5 to 2 qt (1.4 to 1.9 liters) per hour in summer months, whereas football players (large body mass and wearing protective gear) are known to sweat on average over 2 qt (1.9 liters) per hour and up to 9 qt (8.5 liters) per day.[63] A commitment to frequent hydration breaks is required to ensure dehydration does not exceed greater than 2% of body weight (based on preactivity nude body weight) throughout the duration of physical activity.

Before work, you should take extra fluids to prepare for the heat. Drink 8 to 16 oz (200 to 500 mL) of water, juice, or a sport drink before work. Avoid excess caffeine; it hastens fluid loss in the urine. There is no physiologic advantage to excessively consuming large amounts of fluid prior to physical activity. The American College of Sports Medicine now recommends prehydrating slowly for several hours before a physical activity and consuming 0.16 to 0.24 oz (approximately 5 to 7 mL) per kg of body weight.[35] The goal is to produce urine output that is clear to straw color in appearance and prevent starting an activity in a dehydrated state.

While working, take several fluid breaks every hour based on recognition of thirst. Individual sweat rates will vary, as will the amount of water needed to be consumed per hour. Caution should be used to prevent consumption of excessive fluids greater than 1.5 qt/hr (1.4 liters/hr) for prolonged periods unless you have determined your individualized sweat loss rate per hour. The American College of Sports Medicine now recommends a starting point of 14 to 28 oz (0.4 to 0.8 liters) on average per hour for exercise activities (e.g., marathon running) and adjusting the amount consumed based on individual lower or higher sweat rates for activities in cool or warm temperature conditions and for lighter or heavier individuals.[63]

Water is the body's greatest need during work in the heat. Studies show that workers drink more when lightly flavored beverages are available. Providing a portion of fluid replacement with a carbohydrate/electrolyte sport beverage will help to retain fluids and maintain energy and electrolyte levels. Unfortunately, many sport drinks contain large amounts of sugar, which can actually slow absorption of ingested fluid.

After work, you need to continue drinking to replace fluid losses. To achieve rapid and complete recovery for activities resulting is large sweat loss (i.e., firefighting), drink approximately 24 oz for each pound of body weight loss (1.5 liters for each kilogram of body weight loss).[63] Rehydration is enhanced when fluids contain sodium and potassium or when foods with these electrolytes are consumed along with the fluid.

Make potassium-rich foods such as potatoes, prune juice, carrot juice, bananas, and citrus fruits a regular part of your diet, and vary your intake of fluids to include lemonade, orange juice, or tomato juice. Limit the amount of caffeine drinks such as coffee and colas because caffeine increases fluid loss in the urine, although moderate amounts have no negative effect.[49] Avoid alcoholic drinks because they also cause dehydration. To avoid common viruses, avoid sharing water bottles except in emergencies.

Hydration can be reassessed by observing your urine's volume, color, and concentration. Low volumes of dark, concentrated urine and painful urination indicate a serious need for rehydration. Other signs of dehydration include a rapid heart rate, weakness, excessive fatigue, and dizziness. Rapid loss of several pounds of body weight is a certain sign of dehydration. Rehydrate before returning to work. Continuing to work in a dehydrated state can lead to serious consequences, including heatstroke, muscle breakdown, and kidney failure.

Clothing
Personal protective clothing strikes a balance between protection and comfort. Australian researchers have concluded that the task for personnel wearing personal protective equipment (PPE) is not to keep heat out, but to let it out. About 70% of the heat load comes from within, from metabolic heat generated during hard work. Only 30% comes from the environment. Wear loose-fitting garments to enhance air movement. Wear cotton T-shirts and underwear to help sweat evaporate in hot environments. Avoid extra layers of clothing that insulate, restrict air movement, and contribute to heat stress.

Individual Differences
Individuals differ in their response to heat. Some emergency responders, such as firefighters, are at greater risk for heat disorders due to their environment and gear requirements. Other reasons include inherited differences in heat tolerance

and sweat rate; excess body weight, which raises metabolic heat production; and illness, illicit drugs, and medications, which can also influence the body's response to work in a hot environment. Check with your physician or pharmacist if you are using prescription or over-the-counter medications, or if you have a medical condition.

You should always train and work with a partner who can help in the event of a problem. Remind each other to drink fluids, and watch each other. If your partner develops a heat disorder, begin treatment immediately.

Summary
Prevention
- Improve or maintain aerobic fitness.
- Acclimate to the heat.

On the job
- Be aware of conditions (temperature, humidity, air movement).
- Take frequent rest breaks and drink fluids regularly to relieve thirst.

- Avoid extra layers of clothing.
- Maintain a steady pace.

Hydrate
- The hydration goal is to prevent dehydration (sweat loss) of greater than 2% of nude body weight.
- Before work, drink several cups of water, juice, or a sport drink.
- During work, take frequent fluid breaks.
- After work, keep drinking to ensure rehydration.
- Remember, "Only you can prevent dehydration."

Partners
- Always work or train with a partner.

Drinks
- Sport drinks with carbohydrates (5% to 10%) and electrolytes (e.g., sodium 20 to 30 mEq/liter and potassium 2 to 5 mEq/liter) encourage fluid intake, provide energy, and diminish urinary water loss. The carbohydrates also help maintain immune function and mental performance during prolonged, arduous work. Drinks with caffeine and alcohol interfere with rehydration by increasing urine production.

Modified from U.S. Department of Agriculture, U.S. Forest Service: Heat Stress Brochure, American College of Sports Medicine. Position stand: exercise and fluid replacement. *Med Sci Sports Exerc.* 2007;39(2):377.

in moderate to hot environments can be maximized through advanced preparation of physical fitness, heat acclimatization, living and working conditions, personal hygiene, and use of food and beverages to maintain and replace electrolytes and water in the body. Environment, fluid hydration, physical fitness, and heat acclimatization are essential factors to understand.

Environment

Prehospital care practitioners and other public safety personnel are subjected to high heat environments as part of their occupational requirements. During training or an emergency response, many personnel will encounter high levels of heat stress while working in PPE (impermeable clothing), such as turnout gear, hazardous material suit, or chemical/biologic protective garment. This heat stress is further compounded by the need to enter poorly ventilated or confined spaces or to work on a multivehicle crash in the sun on a hot, humid day.

PPE compromises the body's ability to dissipate body heat and prevents the evaporation of sweat during a heavy workload. With high sweat rates from internal heat production during physically demanding tasks and the external heat exposure, personnel are at a high risk of dehydration and heat illness. Thus, the use of PPE diminishes the physiologic advantage gained through heat acclimatization and physical fitness.

These risks can be minimized by measuring the environmental heat conditions and, when applicable, following the recommended work/rest and hydration guidelines for work in highly thermal environments.[24,83]

One traditional tool for measuring the thermal load is the **heat stress index** (Figure 19-5). This index uses the combination of ambient temperature (read on a thermometer) and relative humidity. This is a better method of predicting potential systemic heat injury than the ambient temperature alone. If working in direct sunlight, near surfaces that radiate large amounts of heat, or in heavy protective clothing, 10°F (~5.5°C) should be added to the value in the table.

A more widely used method for measurement of environmental heat strain used in many industrial and military settings is the *wet-bulb globe temperature (WBGT) index*[24,84] (**Table 19-3**). This index uses the combination of a dry bulb for ambient temperature, wet bulb for humidity measurement, black globe for radiant heat, and air movement to provide a more accurate impact of the environmental conditions. Integrated in the five-level WBGT index range of temperatures are hourly work/rest (minutes) and hydration (quarts) guidelines. A color flag (no flag, green, yellow, red, or black) represents each of the five WBGT ranges of temperatures. The WBGT can be monitored hourly and the corresponding color flag placed on a flagpole outdoors for all personnel to see throughout the day. When applicable, the appropriate adjustments of clothing, physical activity, work/rest

Table 19-3 Fluid Replacement Guidelines for Warm-Weather Training

Heat Category	WBGT Index (°F)	Easy Work		Moderate Work		Hard Work	
		Work/Rest (minutes)	Water Intake (qt/hr)	Work/Rest (minutes)	Water Intake (qt/hr)	Work/Rest (minutes)	Water Intake (qt/hr)
1	78 to 81.9	NL	1/2	NL	3/4	40/20	3/4
2	82 to 84.9	NL	1/2	50/10	3/4	30/30	1
3	85 to 87.9	NL	3/4	40/20	3/4	30/30	1
4	88 to 89.9	NL	3/4	30/30	3/4	20/40	1
5	> 90	50/10	1	20/40	1	10/50	1
		Easy Work		**Moderate Work**		**Hard Work**	
		Walking on hard surface at 2.5 mph; 4 kph), less than 31-lb (14 kg) load		Walking on hard surface at 3.5 mph (5 kph), less than 40-lb (19 kg) load		Walking on hard surface at 3.5 mph (6 kph), greater than 40-lb (18 kg) load	
				Walking in loose sand at 2.5 mph (4 kph), no load; calisthenics		Walking in loose sand at 2.5 mph (4 kph) with load	

Abbreviations: kph, kilometers per hour; lb, pound; mph, miles per hour; NL, no limit to work time; WBGT, wet-bulb globe temperature.

Note: The work/rest times and fluid replacement volumes will sustain performance and hydration for at least 4 hours of work in the specified heat category. Individual water needs will vary. Rest means minimal physical activity (sitting or standing), accomplished in shade if possible.

Caution: Hourly fluid intake should not exceed 1.5 qt (1.4 liters). Daily fluid intake should not exceed 12 qt (11.4 liters). When wearing body armor: Add 5°F (~2.75°C) to WBGT index in humid climates. When wearing PPE over garment: Add 10°F (~5.5°C) to WBGT index for easy work and 20°F (~11°C) for moderate and hard work.

Current version of WBGT, hydration, and work/rest guidelines as updated by U.S. Army Research Institute for Environmental Medicine (USARIEM) and published by Montain SJ, Latzka WA, Sawka MN. *Mil Med.* 1999;64:502.

cycles, and fluid intake can then be made based on these WBGT conditions. This integrated WBGT system and related policies can easily be developed at various public safety locations and training sites to ensure that effective heat illness prevention programs are in use to reduce fatigue, injuries, and heat illness.

Hydration

If the WBGT flag system is not used to provide guidelines for hydration, another excellent resource is published by the American College of Sports Medicine, based on years of research.[75] These guidelines are easily applied to any individual engaged in physical activity. Hydration guidelines should be established within an agency to prevent excessive dehydration (greater than 2% body weight loss) by creating easy access to water and sport electrolyte

drinks, particularly during activity in warm environments and when the individual feels thirsty (**Box 19-6**). Ideally, fluid-replacement programs should be customized based on individualized sweat rate loss, body mass, and exercise intensity as determined from a pre- or post-physical activity nude body weight loss measurement.

Fitness

To increase heat tolerance effectively in high-heat conditions, prehospital care practitioners should increase their aerobic fitness through individualized programs (e.g., walking, jogging, biking, swimming, stair stepping, using elliptical exercise machines).[84] These programs will provide the cardiac reserve to sustain the cardiac output required to meet the competing demands of physical (muscular) work and heat dissipation mechanisms

Box 19-6 Hydration Guidelines to Minimize Dehydration

General Principles

It is important to maintain hydration, especially when exercising or performing activities that involve heavy physical exertion. A person's hydration needs will differ depending on how heavily the person sweats. General principles to remember include the following:

1. Drink before and during exertion and when thirsty.
2. Use water and electrolyte drinks to replace lost fluids.
3. Note your weight before and after exertion to help track whether your fluid intake is sufficient, deficient, or excessive.

Make sure you drink sufficiently even when not exercising. If you postpone drinking during your regular day, your body may dehydrate more quickly once you exert yourself.

Weight

Weight is a factor used to determine hydration (or dehydration). It is important to replace fluid lost during physical exertion. If people do not replace this fluid, they will weigh less after exertion. Conversely, if they drink excessive amounts during physical exertion, they may gain weight due to the fluid intake. Ideally, a person will weigh approximately the same before and after exercise; this indicates that the person maintained the appropriate fluid level.

When you do not drink enough during exertion, be sure to replenish fluids afterward. Do not use dehydration as a weight-loss technique.

Type of Drink

In addition to remembering to drink sufficient amounts, it is important to know what type of fluid to drink. Drinking only water during heavy exertion can lead to electrolyte imbalance. Sport electrolyte drinks are designed to replace electrolytes lost through sweat. However, most commercial sport drinks have excessive carbohydrates; oral hydration solutions should not have more than 6% carbohydrate content.[58] Many commercial sports drinks can be diluted with water to reach this carbohydrate concentration. During exercise, stay alert for swelling of the hands and feet, headache, and bloating, which could indicate hyponatremia.

In addition, if you are an athlete or work in a profession that requires heavy exertion, include a moderate amount of salt in your diet to help fulfill your body's increased need for sodium chloride.

Fluid Intake Recommendations

Recommendations for replacing fluid (with water and sport electrolyte drinks) are as follows (**Table 19-4**):

Table 19-4 Fluid Intake Recommendations

Time Frame	Quantity
4 hours before exercise	16–20 oz (0.5–0.6 liters)
10–15 minutes before exercise	8–12 oz (0.2–0.4 liters)
During exercise for less than 60 minutes	3–8 oz (0.1–0.2 liters) every 15–20 minutes
During exercise for greater than 60 minutes	3–8 oz (0.1–0.2 liters) of a sport beverage every 15–20 minutes
Postexercise (within 2 hours)	20–24 oz (0.6–0.7 liters) every 1 lb (0.5 kg) lost

Data from American College of Sports Medicine. Selecting and effectively using hydration for fitness. Accessed October 25, 2021. https://www.yumpu.com/en/document/read/46203304/selecting-and-effectively-using-hydration-for-fitness-american

(thermoregulation) in a high-temperature environment.[85,86] The American College of Sports Medicine, American Heart Association, and Department of Health and Human Services have collaborated to establish updated nationwide physical activity recommendations to maintain health and well-being.[86]

Heat Acclimatization

A policy and protocol for heat acclimatization should be provided within a public safety organization.[87] Heat acclimatization can be achieved with 60 to 120 minutes of heat-exposed exertion per day for approximately

8 to 14 days.[35,49,88] The benefits of heat acclimatization are increased work performance, improved heat tolerance, and reduced physiologic strain. These adjustments include increased blood volume, increased stroke volume, decreased heart rate at a given activity level, reduced sodium concentration in sweat, sodium conserved in the body, earlier onset of sweating, and increased sweat volume rate (Box 19-7). These changes improve the transfer of body heat from the core to the skin in an effort to increase the heat transfer from the skin to the environment. Although heat tolerance is improved in these individuals (e.g., endurance athletes, military infantry personnel) and is considered desirable, the greater sweat-volume production of 1.1 to 2.1 qt/hr (1 to 2 liters/hr) results in large fluid losses, leading to dehydration. Consequently, the greater volume of sweat loss in heat-acclimatized individuals increases the hydration requirements during heat exposure, particularly when the person does not adhere to a rigorous oral hydration schedule. Box 19-8 provides an overview of heat acclimatization guidelines.

Box 19-7 Benefits of Heat Acclimatization

1. Thermal comfort: improved
2. Core temperature: reduced
3. Skin blood flow: earlier
4. Heart rate: lowered
5. Salt losses (sweat and urine): reduced
6. Exercise performance: improved
7. Sweating: earlier and greater
8. Body heat production: lower
9. Thirst: improved
10. Organ protection: improved

Reproduced from the Heat Acclimatization Guide, Ranger and Airborne School Students. Accessed October 25, 2021. https://www.usariem.army.mil/assets/docs/partnering/HeatAcclimatizationGuide.pdf

---

Box 19-8 Heat Acclimatization Guidelines

The following is a modified version of the heat acclimatization guidelines designed for healthy and physically fit infantry personnel in preparation for physical activity in hot environments.

Should You Be Concerned About Hot Weather?
If you are used to working in cool or temperate climates, exposure to hot weather will make it much more difficult to complete your work. Hot weather will make you feel fatigued, make it more difficult to recover, and increase your risk of heat illness. Individuals with the same abilities but who are used to working in hot weather will have a greater heat tolerance and physical ability during heat exposure.

What Is Heat Acclimatization?
Heat acclimatization refers to biologic adaptations that reduce physiologic strain (e.g., heart rate, body temperature), improve physical work capabilities, improve comfort, and protect vital organs (brain, liver, kidneys, muscles) from heat injury. The most important biologic adaptation from heat acclimatization is an earlier and greater sweating response, and for this response to improve, it needs to be invoked.

Heat acclimatization is specific to the climate and physical activity level. Individuals who perform only light or brief physical work will achieve the level of heat acclimatization needed to perform that task. If they attempt a more strenuous or prolonged task, additional acclimatization and improved physical fitness will be needed to perform that task successfully in the heat.

How Do You Become Heat Acclimatized?
Heat acclimatization occurs when repeated heat exposures are sufficiently stressful to elevate body temperature and provoke profuse sweating. Resting in the heat, with physical activity limited to that required for existence, results in only partial acclimatization. Physical exercise in the heat is required to achieve optimal heat acclimatization for that exercise intensity in a given hot environment.

Generally, about 8 to 14 days of daily heat exposure is needed to induce heat acclimatization. Heat acclimatization requires a minimum daily heat exposure of 1 to 2 hours (can be broken into two 1-hour exposures) combined with physical exercise that requires cardiovascular endurance (e.g., jogging) rather than strength training. Gradually increase the exercise intensity or duration each day. Work up to an appropriate physical training schedule adapted to the required physical activity.

The benefits of heat acclimatization will be retained for about 1 week and then decay, with about 75% lost by about 3 weeks, once heat exposure ends. One or 2 days of intervening cool weather will not interfere with acclimatization to hot weather.

How Quickly Can You Become Heat Acclimatized?
For the average individual, heat acclimatization requires about 8 to 14 days of heat exposure and progressive increases in physical work. By the second day of acclimatization, significant reductions in physiologic strain are observed. By the end of the first week and second week, greater than 60% and greater than 80% of the physiologic adaptations are complete, respectively. Less fit individuals or those unusually susceptible to heat exposure may require several additional days or weeks to fully acclimatize.

Physically fit individuals should be able to achieve heat acclimatization in about 1 week. However, several weeks of living and working in the heat (seasoning) may be required to maximize tolerance to high body temperatures.

What Are the Best Heat Acclimatization Strategies?

1. Maximize physical fitness and heat acclimatization before hot weather exposure. Maintain physical fitness with maintenance programs tailored to the environment, such as physical training in the cooler morning or evening hours.
2. Integrate training and heat acclimatization. Train in the coolest part of the day, and acclimatize in the heat of the day. Start slowly by reducing your usual training intensity and duration (compared to what you could achieve in temperate climates). Increase training and heat exposure volume as your heat tolerance permits. Use interval training to modify your activity level.
3. If the new climate is much hotter than what you are accustomed to, recreational activities may be appropriate for the first 2 days with periods of run/walk. By the third day, you should be able to integrate training runs (20 to 40 minutes) at a reduced pace.
4. Consume sufficient water to replace sweat losses. Sweat rates of more than 1 qt (0.9 liter) per hour are common. Heat acclimatization increases the sweating rate and, therefore, increases water requirements. As a result, heat-acclimatized individuals will dehydrate faster if they do not consume fluids. Dehydration negates many of the thermoregulatory advantages conferred by heat acclimatization and high physical fitness.

Data from Sawka MN, Kolka MA, Montain SJ. *Ranger and Airborne School Students' Heat Acclimatization Guide.* U.S. Army Research Institute of Environmental Medicine; 2003.

Emergency Incident Rehabilitation

Even when taking appropriate precautions (e.g., hydration, heat acclimatization) while working in extremely hot settings, EMS practitioners will sometimes be pushed to their physical limits. Firefighters, in particular, may wear a wide range of PPE, depending on the capacity in which they are working. This PPE is often heavy and restrictive and can add greatly to the heat stress experienced on scene.[89] Rehabilitation must occur before the point of overexertion, not after.

Rehabilitation involves the following principles[89]:

- Relief from extreme climatic conditions
- Rest and recovery
- Cooling or rewarming (as needed)
- Rehydration (fluid replacement)
- Calorie and electrolyte replacement
- Medical monitoring
- Tracking team members (accountability)

Injuries Produced by Cold

Dehydration

Dehydration occurs very easily in the cold, particularly with increased physical activity. This occurs for three primary reasons:

- Evaporation of sweat
- Increased respiratory heat and fluid losses caused by the dryness of cold air
- Cold-induced diuresis

Cold-induced diuresis is a normal physiologic response resulting from skin vasoconstriction from prolonged cold exposure. This is the body's response to reduce body heat loss by shunting blood away from the colder periphery to deeper veins within the body. This response causes a central blood volume expansion, which results in a rise in the mean arterial pressure, stroke volume, and cardiac output.[90] The expanded blood volume can produce a diuresis, manifested by frequent urination. Cold-induced diuresis can reduce plasma volume by 7% to 15%, resulting in hemoconcentration and acute dehydration from an almost twofold fluid loss over normal.

As with exposure to heat, adherence to fluid hydration guidelines and access to liquids when thirsty while working in cold environments are necessary to minimize dehydration along with the associated fatigue and physical and cognitive changes. Because thirst is suppressed in cold environments, dehydration is a significant risk.

Minor Cold-Related Disorders

Contact Freeze Injury

When cold material contacts unprotected skin, it can produce local **frostbite** immediately. Do not touch any metal surface, alcohol, gasoline, antifreeze, ice, or snow with the hands; see the "Frostbite" section for assessment and management (**Box 19-9**).

Frostnip

Frostnip is often a precursor to frostbite and produces reversible signs of skin blanching and numbness in localized tissue. It is typically seen on the cheeks, nose, and earlobes. Frostnip is a self-limited and nonfreezing tissue injury as long as cold exposure does not continue; it does not require prehospital care practitioner intervention and transport.

Cold Urticaria

Cold urticaria ("hives") is a disorder characterized by the rapid onset (within minutes) of itchiness, redness, and swelling of the skin after exposure to cold. The sensation of burning may be a prominent feature. This condition, caused by a local release of histamine, is sometimes observed when ice is applied directly to the skin during cold therapy for sprains and strains. Individuals with a history of cold urticaria are advised to avoid cold-water immersion, which could potentially cause death from systemic anaphylaxis. Treatment includes avoiding the cold and possibly taking antihistamines.

Chilblains (Pernio)

Chilblains are a nonfreezing cold injury that presents as small skin lesions that are itchy and tender, appearing as bluish-red bumps that occur on the extensor skin surface of the finger or any skin surface (most commonly the feet, hands, legs, and thighs) from chronic cold exposure (**Figure 19-6**). Chilblains occur several hours after exposure to the cold in temperate humid climates. They are sometimes aggravated by sun exposure. Cold causes constriction of the small arteries and veins in the skin, and rewarming results in leakage of blood into the tissues and swelling of the skin.

Chilblains are more likely to develop in those with poor peripheral circulation. Some contributing factors are a familial tendency and peripheral vascular disease caused by diabetes, smoking, hyperlipidemia (increased serum lipid levels), poor nutrition (e.g., anorexia nervosa), connective tissue disease, and bone marrow disorders. Each chilblain comes up over a few hours as an itchy, bluish-red swelling and subsides over the next 7 to 14 days. In severe cases, blistering, pustules, scabs, and ulceration can occur. Occasionally the lesions may be ring shaped. They may become thickened and persist for months.

Symptoms will subside with removal of the individual from the cold. Management involves protection from cold with appropriate gloves and clothing.

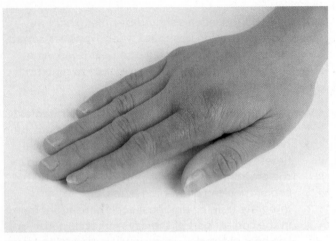

Figure 19-6 Chilblains most commonly affects the feet, hands, legs, and thighs.
© kungfu01/Shutterstock

Ultraviolet (Solar) Keratitis (Snow Blindness)

Without protection from exposure to bright reflections on snow, the risk of ultraviolet burns to skin and eyes increases. This risk is greatly enhanced at higher altitudes. **Solar keratitis** is insidious during the exposure phase, with corneal and conjunctival epithelium burns occurring in as little as 2 hours but not becoming apparent until 6 to 12 hours after exposure.[19]

Management of snow blindness is based on symptoms, which include excessive tearing, severe pain, redness, swollen eyelids, pain when looking at light, headache, a gritty sensation in the eyes, and decreased (hazy) vision. Prehospital care practitioners need to consider patching affected eyes if there is no other method to prevent further ultraviolet exposure (e.g., sunglasses) and then transport the patient. Topical ophthalmic anesthetic drops, if available, may be used to provide symptomatic relief. Medical attention is required to determine the level of severity and the need for antibiotics and analgesics.[91]

Major Cold-Related Disorders

Localized Cutaneous Cold Injury

Cold injuries occur at peripheral sites on the body and are classified as either freezing (e.g., frostbite) or nonfreezing (e.g., frostnip, chilblains, immersion foot) injuries. Localized cold injuries are preventable with proper preparation for cold exposure, early recognition of cold injury, and effective medical care. However, frostbite, the most serious form of freezing injury because of the risk of limb loss, is the primary injury of concern in this section.

Prevention of cold injury through an understanding of the contributing factors is key. Nicotine, alcohol intoxication, homelessness, and major psychiatric disorders remain important predisposing factors.[92] Tight or constricting clothes, too many socks, and tight-fitting footwear are predictable factors in the onset of frostbite. With an increase in adventure sports and other recreational activities conducted in the winter season, localized cold injuries are seen more often.

Prehospital care practitioners need to prevent body heat loss and protect exposed skin from frostbite in patients during prolonged exposure to cold conditions. For example, in patients needing vehicular extrication, in scenarios resulting in the inability to move the patient, and in patients in cold environments with soft-tissue swelling, impaired circulation can lead to an increased incidence of localized cold injury. The priority of care for all patients presenting with frostbite or other cold injuries is to protect them from further exposure to the elements and focus on hypothermia prevention and treatment.

Nonfreezing Cold Injury

Nonfreezing cold injury (NFCI) is a syndrome that causes damage to tissues in cold, but not freezing, temperatures. Most often associated with immersion foot and trench foot, this syndrome can affect any extremity. NFCI results from damage to peripheral tissues caused by prolonged (hours to days) wet/cold exposure, does not involve freezing of tissue, but may coexist with a freezing injury such as frostbite.[93-96] This syndrome primarily involves the feet and is reflected in two types of NFCI. Even though the following injuries are clinically identical, they are caused by different environmental conditions. **Trench foot** occurs primarily in military personnel during infantry operations and is related to the combined effects of prolonged cold exposure and restricted circulation in the feet; it does not involve immersion in water.[92] **Immersion foot** is caused by prolonged immersion of extremities in moisture that is cool to cold. Prehospital care practitioners may see immersion foot in persons who are homeless, persons with alcoholism, or elderly persons; in hikers and hunters; in multiday adventure sport athletes; and in ocean survivors.[93,97,98] Frequently, this syndrome goes unrecognized during assessment of individuals who have been exposed to cold or wet conditions because of failure to remove boots or shoes and examine the feet and because of the lack of formal medical training in NFCI.[93] Immersion foot may extend to the knees and above, depending on the depth of immersion.[97]

This syndrome occurs as a result of many hours of cooling of the lower extremities in temperatures ranging from 32°F to 59°F (0°C to 15°C).[99] Soft-tissue injury occurs to the skin of the feet, known as **maceration**. The breakdown of the skin predisposes individuals to infection. The greatest injury is seen to the peripheral nerves

and blood vessels, caused by secondary ischemic injury. Mild NFCI is self-limited initially, but with continued prolonged cold exposure, it becomes irreversible. When the feet are wet and cold, they are at increased risk, and the injury's course is accelerated because wet socks insulate poorly and water cools more effectively than air at the same temperature. Any factors that reduce circulation to the extremities will contribute to the injury, such as constrictive clothing, boots, prolonged immobility, hypothermia, and crouched posture.

NFCI is classified in four degrees of severity, as follows:

- *Minimal.* Hyperemia or engorgement caused by an increase in blood flow to the feet and slight sensory change will remain 2 to 3 days after injury. The condition is self-limited, and no signs of injury remain after 7 days. Occasionally, cold sensitivity will remain.
- *Mild.* Edema, hyperemia, and slight sensory change remain 2 to 3 days after injury. Seven days after injury, anesthesia is found on the plantar surface of the foot and tips of the toes and lasts 4 to 9 weeks. Blisters and skin loss are not observed. Ambulation is possible when walking does not cause pain.
- *Moderate.* Edema, hyperemia, blisters, and mottling are present 2 to 3 days after injury. At 7 days, anesthesia to touch is present to both dorsal and plantar surfaces and toes. Edema persists 2 to 3 weeks, and pain and hyperemia last up to 14 weeks. Some blister sloughing occurs but no loss of deep tissue. Some patients will have permanent injury.
- *Severe.* Severe edema, blood forced into surrounding tissues (*extravasation*), and gangrene are present 2 to 3 days after injury. Complete anesthesia of the entire foot remains at 7 days, with paralysis and muscle wasting in the affected extremities. The injury goes beyond the foot into the lower leg. This severe injury produces significant tissue loss, resulting in *autoamputation* (nonsurgical amputation of dead tissue). Gangrene is a constant risk until tissue loss is complete. The patient is expected to have prolonged convalescence and a permanent disability.[93]

ASSESSMENT

Because the patient has experienced mild or moderate cold exposure, it is essential to rule out hypothermia and assess for dehydration. Even though this is not a freezing injury, NCFI still is an insidious and potentially disabling injury; the common finding with these two localized cold injuries is that the extremity is cooled to the point of anesthesia or numbness while the injury is occurring.

The key to management of NFCI is detection and recognition during assessment. During the primary assessment, injured tissue appears macerated, edematous, pale/yellowish white, anesthetized, pulseless, and immobile but not frozen. Patients complain of clumsiness and stumbling when attempting to walk. After removal from cold, and during or after rewarming, peripheral blood flow increases as reperfusion of ischemic tissue begins. Extremities change color from white to mottled pale blue while remaining cold and numb. The diagnosis of trench foot or immersion foot is generally made when these signs have not changed after passive rewarming of the feet. From 24 to 36 hours after rewarming, a marked hyperemia develops, along with severe burning pain and reappearance of sensation proximally but not distally. This is caused by venous vasodilation. Edema and blisters develop in the injured areas as perfusion increases. Skin will remain poorly perfused after hyperemia appears, and the skin is likely to slough as the injury evolves. Any pulselessness after 48 hours in the injured extremity suggests severe, deep injury and a greater chance of substantial tissue loss and the development of gangrene.

MANAGEMENT

Once a possible NFCI is detected, the priorities are to eliminate any further cooling of the patient or the extremity, prevent further trauma at the site of injury, and transport the patient. Do not allow the patient to walk on an injured extremity. Carefully remove the footwear and socks. Cover the injured part or extremity with a loose, dry, sterile dressing; protect it from the cold; and begin passive rewarming of injured tissue during transport. The affected area may be aggravated by the weight of a blanket. No active rewarming is necessary. Do not massage the affected area because doing so may cause further tissue damage. As needed, treat the patient for dehydration with a bolus of IV fluids, and reassess. Depending on length of transport, severe pain may develop during passive rewarming as tissues begin to reperfuse.

Freezing Cold Injury

On the continuum of further peripheral cold tissue exposure beginning with frostnip (no tissue loss), frostbite ranges from mild to severe tissue destruction and possibly the loss of tissue due to intense vasoconstriction.[9,10,14] The most susceptible body parts for frostbite are those tissues with large surface-to-mass ratios, such as the ears and nose, or areas farthest from the body's core, such as the hands, fingers, feet, toes, and male genitalia. The feet and toes are the most commonly affected areas.[99] These structures are most susceptible to cold injury because they contain many arteriovenous capillary **anastomoses** (connections) that easily shunt blood away during vasoconstriction. The body's normal response to lower-than-desirable temperatures is to reduce blood flow to the skin surface to reduce heat exchange with the environment. The body accomplishes this by vasoconstriction of peripheral blood vessels to shunt warm blood to the body's core to maintain a normal body temperature.

Reduction of this blood flow greatly reduces the amount of heat delivered to the distal extremities.

The longer the period of exposure to the cold, the more the blood flow is reduced to the periphery. The body conserves core temperature at the expense of extremity and skin temperature. The heat loss from the tissue becomes greater than the heat supplied to that area.

When an extremity is cooled to 59°F (15°C), maximal vasoconstriction and minimal blood flow occur. If cooling continues to 50°F (10°C), vasoconstriction is interrupted by periods of **cold-induced vasodilation (CIVD)** and an associated increase in tissue temperature caused by an increase in blood flow. CIVD recurs in 5- to 10-minute cycles to provide some protection from the cold. Individuals show differences in susceptibility to frostbite when exposed to the same cold conditions, which may be explained by the amount of CIVD.

Tissue does not freeze at 32°F (0°C) because cells contain electrolytes and other solutes that prevent tissue from freezing until skin temperature reaches approximately 28°F (–2.2°C). In cases of below-freezing temperatures, when the extremities are left unprotected, the intracellular and extracellular fluids can freeze. This results in the formation of ice crystals. As the ice crystals form, they expand and cause damage to local tissues. Blood clots may form, further impairing circulation to the injured area.

The type and duration of cold exposure are the two most important factors in determining the extent of freezing injury. Frostbite is classified by depth of injury and clinical presentation.[14] The degree of injury in many cases will not be known for at least 24 to 72 hours after thawing, except in very minor or severe exposures. Skin exposure to cold that is short but intense will create a superficial injury, whereas severe frostbite to a whole extremity can occur during prolonged exposures. Direct cold injury is usually reversible, but permanent tissue damage occurs during rewarming. In more severe cases, even with appropriate rewarming of tissue, microvascular thrombosis can develop, leading to early signs of gangrene and necrosis. If the injured site freezes, thaws, and then refreezes, the second freezing causes a greater amount of severe thrombosis and vascular damage and tissue loss. For this reason, prehospital care practitioners need to prevent any frozen tissue that thaws during initial field treatment from refreezing.

Traditional methods of frostbite classification present four degrees of injury (similar to burns) based on initial physical findings after freezing and advanced imaging in the hospital after rewarming (**Figure 19-7** and **Figure 19-8**), as follows:

- **First-degree frostbite.** This epidermal injury is limited to skin that has brief contact with cold air or metal. The skin appears white or as yellowish plaque at the site of injury. There is no blister or tissue loss.

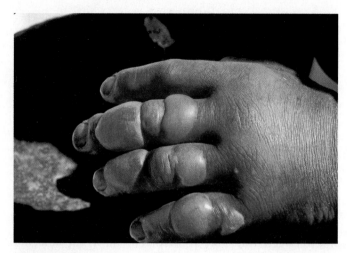

Figure 19-7 Edema and blister formation 24 hours after frostbite injury.
© ANT Photo Library/Science Source

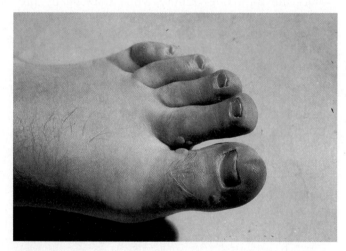

Figure 19-8 Deep second-degree and third-degree frostbite with hemorrhagic blebs, one day after thawing.
© ANT Photo Library/Science Source

Skin thaws quickly, feels numb, and appears red with surrounding edema; healing occurs in 7 to 10 days.

- **Second-degree frostbite.** This degree of injury involves all of the epidermis and superficial dermis. It initially appears similar to first-degree injury; however, frozen tissues are deeper. Tissue feels stiff to the touch, but tissue beneath gives way to pressure. Thawing is rapid; after thawing, superficial skin blister or vesiculation occurs, with clear or milky fluid after several hours, surrounded by erythema and edema. There is no permanent loss of tissue. Healing occurs in 3 to 4 weeks.
- **Third-degree frostbite.** This degree of injury involves the epidermis and dermis layers. Frozen skin is stiff, with restricted mobility. After tissue thaws, skin

swells along with a blood-filled blister (*hemorrhagic bulla*), indicating vascular trauma to deep tissues; swelling restricts mobility. Skin loss occurs slowly, leading to mummification and sloughing. Healing is slow.

- **Fourth-degree frostbite.** At this level, frozen tissue involves full thickness completely through the dermis, with muscle and bone involvement. There is no mobility when frozen and passive movement when thawed, with no intrinsic muscle function. Skin perfusion is poor, and blisters and edema do not develop. Early signs of necrotic tissue are evident. A slow mummification process will occur along with sloughing of tissue and autoamputation of nonviable tissue.

Although traditional classification of frostbite is by the four degrees of injury, it is easiest for practitioners in the prehospital setting to classify as either superficial or deep.[100-102] **Superficial frostbite** (first and second degree) affects the skin and subcutaneous tissues, resulting in clear blisters when rewarmed. **Deep frostbite** (third and fourth degree) affects skin, muscle, and bone, and the skin has hemorrhagic blisters when rewarmed. The level of severity and anticipated tissue loss may vary within a single extremity.[103] An additional classification method has been introduced that examines the frozen tissue after rewarming in an effort to identify amputation risk.[104]

In certain situations, frostbite may occur rapidly, and prehospital care practitioners may respond to the following:

- Hydrocarbon fluid spills on skin (e.g., gasoline, butane, propane) will cause rapid evaporation and conduction in below-freezing temperatures
- Touching extremely cold metal with warm skin
- Intense windchill on exposed skin caused by rotary wind from a medical helicopter

ASSESSMENT

On arrival, assess scene safety and then the patient for ABCs. Move the patient from the cold to an area protected from moisture, cold, and wind to prevent further cooling. Many frostbite victims may have additional associated medical conditions, such as dehydration, hypovolemia, hypothermia, hypoglycemia, and traumatic injury. Remove any wet clothing to minimize further body heat loss. *When in doubt, treat hypothermia first.* Superficial frostbite is usually assessed through a combination of recognizing the environmental conditions, locating the patient's chief complaint of pain or numbness, and observing discolored skin in the same area. The environmental conditions during exposure must be below freezing.

Frostbite injuries are insidious because the patient may have no pain at the injury site when skin is frozen and covered by a glove or footwear. Detection of the affected area requires direct visual inspection of highly suspect body regions, as previously listed. Gentle palpation of the area can determine if the underlying tissue is compliant or hard. Ensure that the patient or prehospital care practitioner does not rub or massage the affected skin, because this will cause further cellular damage to frozen tissues. The patient with superficial freezing will usually complain of discomfort during the manipulation of the frostbitten area. In patients with deep frostbite, the frozen tissue will be hard and usually is not painful when touched. After inspection of the affected area, a decision is necessary regarding the method of rewarming, which is usually based on transport time to the ED.

The state of Alaska EMS protocol for frostbite rewarming in the prehospital phase states the following[105]:

1. If transport time is short (1 to 2 hours at most), then the risks posed by improper rewarming or refreezing in the prehospital phase outweigh the risks for delaying treatment for deep frostbite.

2. If transport time will be prolonged (more than 1 to 2 hours), frostbite will often thaw spontaneously. It is more important to prevent hypothermia than to rewarm frostbite rapidly in warm water. This does not mean that a frostbitten extremity should be kept in the cold to prevent spontaneous rewarming. Anticipate that frostbitten areas will rewarm as a consequence of keeping the patient warm; protect them from refreezing at all costs.

MANAGEMENT

Patients with superficial frostnip or frostbite should be placed with the affected area against a warm body surface, such as covering the patient's ears with warm hands or placing affected fingers into armpits, axillae, or groin regions. Superficial frostbite only needs to be warmed at normal body temperatures.

Management of deep frostbite in the prehospital setting includes first assessing and treating the patient for hypothermia, if present.[103,106] Provide supportive care and appropriate shelter for the patient and the affected part to minimize heat loss. Do not allow the patient to walk on affected feet. Protect fragile tissues from further trauma during patient movement. Assess the frostbite area. Remove any clothing and jewelry from the affected area, and check for loss of sensation.

If there is frostbite distal to a fracture, attempt to align the limb unless there is resistance. Splint the fracture in a manner that does not compromise distal circulation.

Air dry the affected area, and do not rub the tissues. Cover the affected area with a loose, dry, bulky sterile dressing that is noncompressive and nonadherent. Fingers and toes should be individually separated by and protected with sterile cotton gauze. Do not drain any blisters. Hands and feet should be splinted and elevated to reduce edema.

Analgesics may be required for pain relief and should be initiated before the tissues have thawed. Initiate IV NS with a 250-mL bolus to treat dehydration and reduce blood viscosity and capillary sludging. Ensure early transport to an appropriate facility.

Attempts to begin rewarming of deep frostbite patients in the field can be hazardous to the patient's eventual recovery and are not recommended unless prolonged transport times (over 2 hours) are involved. If prolonged transport is involved, thaw the affected part in a warm water bath at a temperature no greater than 98.6°F to 102.2°F (37°C to 39°C) on the affected area until the area becomes soft and pliable to the touch (~30 min).[99,106] If refreezing is a concern, do not thaw. Protect the injured extremity while thawing by preventing any area from touching the sides or bottom of the water bath as sensation is diminished or absent in frostbitten tissue and additional damage can occur.[19]

Administer ibuprofen (12 mg/kg up to 800 mg) or aspirin (75–81 mg) if available and permissible given local protocols.[104] Nonsteroidal medications such as ibuprofen help decrease inflammation and pain and inhibit the production of substances that cause vasoconstriction.

During transport, hydrate the patient by providing something warm (and nonalcoholic) if it is available, depending on the patient's level of consciousness and other injuries. Tobacco use (smoking, chewing, using nicotine patches) should be discouraged because nicotine causes further vasoconstriction.

Accidental Hypothermia

Hypothermia is defined as the condition in which the core body temperature is 95°F (35°C) or below, as measured by a rectal thermometer probe placed at least 6 inches (15 cm) into the rectum.[15,49] Hypothermia can be viewed as a decrease in core temperature that renders a patient unable to generate sufficient heat production to return to homeostasis or normal body functions.

Hypothermia can occur in many different situations, resulting from cold ambient air, cold-water immersion, or cold-water submersion, and can be intentionally induced during surgery, or as a therapeutic measure in some conditions such as traumatic brain injury.[15,107,108] Hypothermia can also occur in more moderate environments, especially in the context of trauma patients. Immersion ("head out") hypothermia typically occurs when an individual is accidentally placed into a cold environment without preparation or planning. For example, a person who has fallen into ice water is immediately in danger of submersion injury, resulting from cold shock gasp reflex, loss of motor skills, hypothermia, and drowning. These unique aspects of submersion incidents can lead to hypoxemia and hypothermia. (See later discussion and Chapter 20, *Environmental Trauma II: Lightning, Drowning, Diving, and Altitude.*)

The progression of hypothermia in cold air or cold water can be delayed if the metabolic heat production can match the loss of heat. Surviving an overwhelming cold exposure is possible, with many reported cases of survival at sea and in other extreme situations.[109,110] Many factors are known to affect survival after cold exposure, including age, gender, body composition (e.g., body surface area to body mass ratio), onset and intensity of shivering, level of physical fitness, nutritional state, and alcohol consumption.

Hypoglycemia can occur during progressive phases of hypothermia and may be more common in immersion hypothermia. This occurs due to the rapid depletion of the fuel sources—blood glucose and muscle glycogen—by the contracting muscles during the shivering process. As the blood glucose stores are depleted through shivering, the brain's hypothalamus, which acts as the body's thermoregulatory center, is deprived its primary fuel. Consequently, a person who has consumed alcohol is at greater risk for hypothermia because alcohol blocks the production of glucose in the body and inhibits maximal shivering for heat production.[15] Thus, rapid assessment and effective management of low blood glucose in the patient with hypothermia are essential to achieve effective increase in metabolism and shivering during rewarming.

Unlike frostbite, hypothermia leading to death can occur in environments with temperatures well above freezing. **Primary hypothermia** generally occurs when healthy individuals are in adverse weather conditions, they are unprepared for overwhelming acute or chronic cold exposure, and there is an involuntary drop of core temperature (below 95°F [35°C]). Deaths by primary hypothermia are a direct result of cold exposure and are documented by the medical examiner as accident, homicide, or suicide.[14]

Secondary hypothermia is considered a normal consequence of a patient's systemic disorders, including hypothyroidism, hypoadrenalism, trauma, carcinoma, and sepsis. See **Box 19-10** for a wide variety of medical conditions associated with secondary hypothermia. If unrecognized or improperly treated, this type of hypothermia can be fatal, in some cases within 2 hours. Death in patients with secondary hypothermia is often caused by the underlying disease and is potentiated by hypothermia. Mortality is greater than 50% in cases of secondary hypothermia caused by complications of other injuries and in severe cases in which the core body temperature is below 89.6°F (32°C).[15]

Box 19-10 Conditions Associated With Secondary Hypothermia

Impaired Thermoregulation
- Central failure
- Anorexia nervosa
- Cerebrovascular accident
- Central nervous system trauma
- Hypothalamic dysfunction
- Metabolic failure
- Neoplasm
- Parkinson disease
- Pharmacologic effects
- Subarachnoid hemorrhage
- Toxins
- Peripheral failure
- Acute spinal cord transection
- Decreased heat production
- Neuropathy
- Endocrinologic failure
- Alcoholic or diabetic ketoacidosis
- Hypoadrenalism
- Hypopituitarism
- Lactic acidosis
- Insufficient energy
- Extreme physical exertion
- Hypoglycemia
- Malnutrition
- Neuromuscular compromise
- Recent birth and advanced age with inactivity
- Impaired shivering

Increased Heat Loss
- Dermatologic disorder
- Burns
- Medications and toxins
- Iatrogenic cause
- Emergency childbirth
- Cold infusions
- Heatstroke treatment
- Other associated clinical states
- Carcinomatosis
- Cardiopulmonary disease
- Major infection (bacterial, viral, parasitic)
- Multisystem trauma
- Shock

Data from ECC Committee, Subcommittees and Task Forces of the American Heart Association. 2005 American Heart Association Guidelines for cardiopulmonary resuscitation and emergency cardiovascular care. *Circulation.* 2005;112(24): ivi-203; and American Heart Association. 2010 guidelines for cardiopulmonary resuscitation and emergency cardiovascular care. *Circulation.* 2010;122:S640-S656.

The prehospital care practitioner must rapidly act to prevent further body heat loss in the traumatic patient, as mild hypothermia is very common following injury in all weather conditions.

Hypothermia and the Trauma Patient

It is all too common to receive patients with hypothermia at a trauma center and to have these patients experience further body heat loss occur during the primary assessment.[111,112] The development of hypothermia that begins in the prehospital setting is related to the effect of trauma on thermoregulation and the inhibition of shivering as a primary mechanism for heat production.[113] In many patients, heat loss continues after arrival at the hospital due to a multitude of reasons: an exposed patient in a cold ED or trauma center, administration of cool resuscitation fluids, open abdominal or thoracic cavities, the use of anesthetic and neuromuscular blocking agents that prevent heat-producing shivering, and cold exposure in an operating room environment.[114,115]

In the prehospital setting, the trauma patient should be moved off of cold ground as soon as possible and placed in a warm ambulance. The temperature in the ambulance should be adjusted to minimize heat loss from the patient and maximize performance of prehospital care practitioners, whose work may be impaired by too hot an ambient work environment. The Wilderness Medical Society recommends an in-compartment ambulance temperature of 75°F (24°C) as an ideal balance of these two considerations.[7] Warmed (100°F to 108°F [37.8°C to 42.2°C]) IV fluids will also help to maintain the patient's body temperature.

One cause of higher mortality in hypothermic trauma patients is related to the combination of *hypothermia*, *acidosis*, and *coagulopathy* (inability of blood to clot normally). This is known as the *lethal triad* in trauma patients.[116] It is essential to assess and treat patients for both trauma and hypothermia because the coagulopathy is reversible with patient rewarming.[112] In one study, 57% of the trauma patients admitted to a level I trauma center were hypothermic at some point in the continuum of care. The mortality rate has been reported to range from 40% to 100% when core temperature falls below 90°F (32.2°C) in a trauma patient. This rate contrasts with a mortality of 20% in a primary hypothermic (nontraumatic) patient at moderate core temperature levels (82°F to 90°F [27.8°C to 32.2°C]).[115] Consequently, the mortality rate associated with hypothermia in the trauma victim is very significant, such that some researchers have created a special trauma hypothermia classification beyond the standard definition of mild, moderate, and severe hypothermia (**Table 19-5**).[116,117]

This relationship of trauma, hypothermia, and increased mortality has been reported for decades, including recently in combat casualty patients.[118] However, recent clinical studies have reported that hypothermia is not an independent risk factor for mortality in trauma patients but is more closely related to injury severity or multiple organ dysfunction syndrome.[119-122] One study

Table 19-5 Classifications of Hypothermia

Classification	Core Body Temperature
Mild hypothermia	95–89.6°F (35–32°C)
Moderate hypothermia	89.5–82.4°F (32–28°C)
Severe hypothermia	82.3–75.2°F (28–24°C)
Profound hypothermia	< 75.2°F (< 24°C)

Data from Zafren K, Giesbrecht GG, Danzl DF, et al. Wilderness Medical Society practice guidelines for the out-of-hospital evaluation and treatment of accidental hypothermia. *Wilderness Environ Med.* 2014;25:426.

reported that certain prehospital care practices can influence the severity of hypothermia in trauma patients. These practices include anticipating hypothermia, avoiding undressing patients, taking frequent temperature measurements, maintaining warm mobile cabin temperatures, and maintaining and providing only warm IV fluids.[121] The potential therapeutic benefits of intentionally induced hypothermia are currently under study (**Box 19-11**).

Immersion Hypothermia

During immersion, if there is no heat gain or heat loss by the body, water temperature is considered *thermoneutral*. Thermoneutral water temperature is 91.4°F to 95°F (33°C to 35°C), at which temperatures a naked individual passively standing in neck-level water can maintain a nearly constant core temperature for at least 1 hour.[115,130,131] Individuals in thermoneutral water are at almost no risk for the initial immersion cold shock and hypothermia experienced in sudden cold-water exposure.[132]

When immersion occurs in water temperature colder than the lower thermoneutral limit, the immediate physiologic changes are a rapid decline in skin temperature, peripheral vasoconstriction resulting in shivering, and increased metabolism, ventilation, heart rate, cardiac output, and mean arterial pressure. To offset any heat loss in water, heat production must occur by increasing physical activity, shivering, or both. If not, core temperature continues to fall and shivering ceases, and these physiologic responses decrease proportionally with the fall in core temperature.[108]

The greatest risk of immersion hypothermia usually begins in water temperature less than 77°F (25°C).[131] Because the heat dissipation capacity of water is 25 times greater than that of air, individuals are at risk for more rapid hypothermia in water. However, continued physical activity (i.e., swimming to keep warm) in cold water

Box 19-11 Therapeutic Hypothermia

It is well established that the detrimental *lethal triad* in trauma victims increases mortality. However, there is some developing early evidence to suggest that intentionally induced hypothermia may have a beneficial role in select circumstances of shock, organ transplantation, nontraumatic cardiac arrest, and control of intracranial pressure from traumatic brain injury.[117,123]

Although the value of initiating therapeutic hypothermia (TH) in the prehospital setting has not been demonstrated, the fastest growing application of this therapy is for victims of sudden nontraumatic cardiac arrest.[117,124,125] It is well known that the outcome following cardiac arrest is very poor, with only 3% to 27% of all cardiac arrest patients surviving to discharge. However, there is a growing amount of evidence for increased survival rate with TH following nontraumatic cardiac arrest. These statements recommended intentional cooling of the patient to 89.6°F to 93.2°F (32°C to 34°C) for 12 to 24 hours in unconscious adults with spontaneous circulation after nontraumatic (often fibrillatory) cardiac arrest with evidence of subsequent neurologic compromise.[123,125,126]

Currently, evidence regarding TH in the multiple trauma patient is conflicting. Preclinical studies suggest that TH may be useful in hypotensive penetrating trauma patients. There is potential for TH to be used in cases of blunt trauma, but it has not been well studied. Clinical trials have conflicting results, or results with uncertain clinical significance, in the case of traumatic brain injury (TBI)[127,128] and spinal cord injuries. TH cannot be definitively recommended for general trauma patients until better clinical research is available.[129] There is presently no role for TH in the prehospital setting for survivors of traumatic cardiac arrest or for trauma patients.

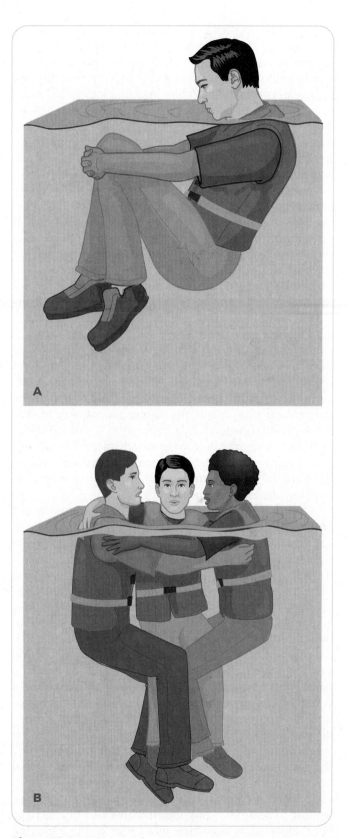

will eventually become a detriment by increasing convective heat loss to the colder water surrounding the body, resulting in a faster onset of hypothermia. This understanding has led to the recommendation for individuals to minimize heat loss during cold-water immersion by using the *heat escape lessening posture* (HELP) or the *huddle position* when multiple immersion victims are together (**Figure 19-9**).[131]

The lowest recorded core temperature for an infant with an intact neurologic recovery from accidental hypothermia is 59°F (15°C).[125] In an adult, 56.6°F (13.7°C)

Figure 19-9 Techniques for decreasing cooling rates of survivors in cold water. **A.** Heat escape lessening posture (HELP). **B.** Huddle technique.

is the lowest recorded core temperature for a survivor of accidental hypothermia. This occurred in a 29-year-old female who struggled to self-rescue for more than 40 minutes before symptoms of severe hypothermia affected muscular contraction.[110] She was immersed for more than 80 minutes before a rescue team arrived and cardiopulmonary resuscitation (CPR) was initiated during transport to a local hospital. After 3 hours of continuous rewarming, her core temperature returned to normal, and she survived with normal physiologic function.

Because vital signs may have decreased to a nearly imperceptible level, the initial impression of hypothermic patients may be that they are dead. Prehospital care practitioners managing patients with hypothermia should not stop treatment interventions and declare the patient dead until the patient has been rewarmed to over 95°F (35°C) and still has no evidence of cardiorespiratory and neurologic function, or signs of nonsurvivability are present (ice in airway, frozen chest wall, decapitation, etc.). The 29-year-old hypothermia survivor is just one example of a patient being discharged from the hospital with full neurologic function after prolonged CPR in the field. The lesson from this case, and others with a similar outcome, is that although the initial impression of a hypothermic patient may be that the individual is dead, this impression is not sufficient justification to withhold basic or advanced life support unless signs of irrevocable nonsurvivability are present. Keep the following phrase in mind: *Patients are not dead until they are warm and dead.*

Whether intentional or unintentional, cold-water immersion (head out) occurs throughout the year in the United States because of recreational and commercial activities, as well as from accidents. If individuals survive the initial submersion incident without fatally drowning, they are at risk for hypothermia, depending on the water temperature. It is important to note that the public generally underestimates the amount of time required to become hypothermic in very cold water, believing that it occurs rapidly, with a short time until death. However, rapid death from immersion often is the result of panic or cold shock response leading to aspiration of water or transient muscular paralysis/dysfunction and fatal drowning, not hypothermia. The key points to understand are that (1) cold shock is initially the greatest threat and (2) patients should focus more on controlling the gasp reflex and their breathing to survive this initial physiologic response (**Box 19-12**). The body's responses to cold-water immersion can be divided into four phases, leading to death. It is important to note that deaths have been reported as occurring in all four of the following phases[131]:

- *First phase—cold shock response.* This phase begins with a cardiovascular reflex known as *cold shock response* that

---

Box 19-12 The 1-10-1 Principle

When a person becomes immersed in ice-cold water, the onset of cold shock or hypothermia depends on several factors, including body size, water temperature, and the amount of the person's body that is immersed. Generally speaking, however, the physiologic response to cold water immersion can be described by the 1-10-1 principle.[111,131]

- *1 minute.* The threat of cold shock will pass in about 1 minute. The person should avoid panicking and focus on gaining control of breathing and keeping the airway clear.
- *10 minutes.* After about 10 minutes, a person will not be able to move arms, legs, and other body parts. The person should use this time to self-rescue, if possible, or establish a survivable position until rescuers arrive.
- *1 hour.* A person has up to 1 hour before becoming unconscious from hypothermia. Panicking or struggling unnecessarily will reduce this time. Wearing a personal flotation device could allow another hour before the heart stops beating.

---

occurs quickly (within 1 to 2 minutes) after immersion (may occur in water colder than 68°F [20°C]). It begins with rapid skin cooling, peripheral vasoconstriction, a gasp reflex and the inability to breath-hold, hyperventilation, and tachycardia.[92,107,131] The gasp response may lead to aspiration and drowning, depending on the individual's head location above or below water. These responses can lead to immediate sudden death or death within minutes following immersion because of several conditions, including syncope or convulsions resulting in drowning, vagal arrest, and ventricular fibrillation.[108,131,133-135]

- *Second phase—cold incapacitation.* If a victim survives the cold shock phase, significant cooling of peripheral tissues, especially in the extremities, occurs over the next 5 to 15 minutes of immersion. This cooling has a deleterious effect on gross and fine motor skills of the extremities, causing finger stiffness, poor coordination, and loss of muscle power, making it nearly impossible to swim, grasp a rescue line, or perform other survival motor skills.[108,131]

- *Third phase—onset of hypothermia.* Surviving the first two phases without drowning places an individual at risk of hypothermia from continued heat loss and core temperature reduction from immersion longer than 30 minutes.[131] If the victim is not able to remain above the water surface because of fatigue and

<table>
<tr><td>

Box 19-13 Cold Water Survival Guidelines

</td><td>

Box 19-14 Self-Rescue

</td></tr>
</table>

Box 19-13 Cold Water Survival Guidelines

The U.S. Coast Guard and other search-and-rescue (SAR) organizations use guidelines to assist in estimating how long individuals can survive in cold water. These guidelines are mathematical models that estimate core temperature cooling rate based on the influence of the following variables:

- Water temperature and sea state
- Clothing insulation
- Body composition (amount of fat, muscle, and bone)
- Amount of the body immersed in water
- Behavior (e.g., excessive movement) and posture (e.g., HELP, huddle) of the body in the water
- Shivering thermogenesis[137-139]

Box 19-14 Self-Rescue

Early studies in the 1960s to 1970s suggested that during accidental immersion in cold water, it was a better option not to self-rescue by attempting to distance-swim to safety but to stay in place, float still in lifejackets, or hang on to wreckage and not swim around to keep warm. More recent research has suggested that self-rescue swimming during accidental immersion in cold water (50°F to 57°F [10°C to 13.9°C]) is a viable option based on the following conditions:

- The victim has initially survived the cold-shock phase within the first few minutes of cold-water exposure.
- The victim has decided early to attempt self-rescue or wait for rescue since decision-making ability will become impaired as hypothermia progresses. After 30 minutes of submersion, the likelihood of success is significantly lower.
- There is a low probability for rescue by emergency responders in the area.
- The victim can reach shore within 45 minutes of swimming based on fitness level and swimming ability.[131]
- On average, a cold-water immersion victim wearing a personal flotation device should be able to swim approximately a half mile (800 m) in 50°F (10°C) water before incapacitation due to muscle cooling and fatigue of the arms, rather than general hypothermia, occurs.
- Cold-water swim distance is about one-third of the distance covered in warmer water.[140]

hypothermia, aspiration and drowning results.[92,111] How long an individual can survive in cold water depends on many factors. It has been estimated that a submersion victim cannot survive for more than 1 hour at a water temperature of 32°F (0°C); and at a water temperature of 59°F (15°C), survival is uncommon after 6 hours.[136]

- *Fourth phase—circumrescue collapse.* In this phase, fatalities have been observed during all periods of survivor rescue (before, during, and after) despite the apparent stable and conscious condition. Symptoms range from fainting to cardiac arrest and have been referred to as rewarming shock or postrescue collapse, with deaths occurring at any stage after rescue, up to 24 hours. The three proposed reasons for circumrescue collapse are (1) afterdrop of core temperature, (2) collapse of arterial blood pressure, and (3) changes in hypoxia, acidosis, or rapid changes in pH that induce ventricular fibrillation. It is noted that up to 20% of those who are recovered alive during the fourth phase will die due to circumrescue collapse.[131]

For more information about surviving cold-water immersion, see **Box 19-13** and **Box 19-14**.

Pathophysiologic Effects of Hypothermia on the Body

Whether from exposure to a cold environment or immersion, the influence of hypothermia on the body affects all major organ systems, particularly the cardiac, renal, and central nervous systems. As the body's core temperature decreases to 95°F (35°C), maximal rate of vasoconstriction, shivering, and metabolic rate occurs, with increases in heart rate, respiration, and blood pressure. Cerebral metabolism oxygen demand decreases by 6% to 10% per 1.8°F (~1°C) drop in core temperature, and cerebral metabolism is preserved.

When core temperature falls to between 86°F (30°C) and 95°F (35°C), cognitive function, cardiac function, metabolic rate, ventilatory rate, and shivering rate are all significantly decreased or completely inhibited. At this point, the limited physiologic defensive mechanisms to prevent heat loss from the body are overwhelmed, and core temperature falls rapidly.

At a core temperature of 85°F (29.4°C), cardiac output and metabolic rate are reduced approximately 50%. Ventilation and perfusion are inadequate and do not keep up with the metabolic demand, causing cellular hypoxia, increased lactic acid, and, eventually, metabolic and respiratory acidosis. Oxygenation and blood flow are maintained in the core and brain.

Bradycardia occurs in a large percentage of patients as a direct effect of cold on the depolarization of cardiac pacemaker cells and their slower propagation through the conduction system. It is important to note that the use of atropine, as well as other cardiac medications, is often ineffective to increase the heart rate when the myocardium is cold.[9] When core temperature falls below 86°F (30°C), the myocardium becomes irritable. The PR, QRS, and QTC intervals are prolonged. ST-segment and T-wave changes and J (or Osborn) waves may be present and may mimic other ECG abnormalities, such as an acute myocardial infarction. The J waves are a striking ECG feature in hypothermic patients and are seen in approximately one-third of moderate to severe hypothermia patients (less than 90°F [32.2°C]). The J wave is described as a "humplike" deflection between the QRS complex and the early part of the ST segment.[131,141] The J wave is best viewed in the aVL, aVF, and left precordial leads (**Figure 19-10**).

Atrial fibrillation and extreme bradycardia develop and may continue between 83°F and 90°F (28.3°C to 32.2°C). When the core temperature reaches 80°F to 82°F (26.7°C to 27.8°C), any physical stimulation of the heart can cause ventricular fibrillation (VF). CPR or rough handling (patient assessment and movement) of the patient could be sufficient to cause VF. At these extremely low core temperatures, pulse and blood pressure are not detectable, the joints are stiff, and the pupils become fixed and dilated. Remember, a patient should not be assumed to be dead until rewarming has been completed and signs of life are still absent.

With acute cold exposure, renal blood flow increases because of the shunting of blood during vasoconstriction. This may result in a phenomenon known as *cold diuresis* in which patients produce more urine and may, as a result, become dehydrated. At 80.6°F to 86°F (27°C to 30°C), renal blood flow is depressed by 50%. At this moderate to severe hypothermic level, the decrease in cardiac output causes a fall in renal blood flow and glomerular filtration rate, which in turn results in acute kidney failure.[131]

Assessment

It is imperative to assess scene safety on arrival. All emergency responders need to maximize their safety and protection from cold exposure while working in this environment. There should be a high suspicion for hypothermia even when the environmental conditions are not highly suggestive (e.g., wind, moisture, temperature).

Protect patients from further cooling, either by carefully moving them to shelter or by insulating them in place from the elements. Doing so prevents further heat loss. Assess the patient's ABCs. Take up to 60 seconds to carefully evaluate the patient's pulse, which may present as very weak or absent in a patient with moderate to severe hypothermia. Some patients who are alert may present with vague complaints of fatigue, lethargy, nausea, and dizziness. Neurologic function is assessed and monitored frequently. Patients with severe hypothermia generally present with bradypnea, stupor, and coma.

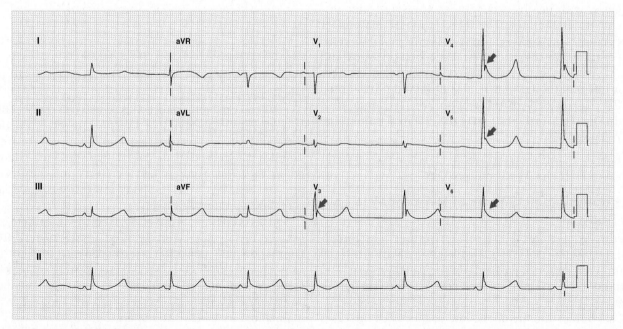

Figure 19-10 Osborn or J wave in hypothermic patient.
Data from *12-Lead ECG: The Art of Interpretation*, courtesy of Tomas B. Garcia, MD.

To accurately measure hypothermic temperatures, a low-range rectal thermometer is often necessary. However, rectal temperatures are not usually assessed in the field or widely used as a vital sign in most prehospital systems. Ambulances that do have access to a thermometer usually carry a standard-range oral or rectal (for infants) thermometer with a lower limit of 96°F (35.6°C). Electronic thermometers are not useful in hypothermic situations for accurate readings. Tympanic membrane infrared temperature measurement is generally accurate if careful technique is used to assure aiming the probe at the tympanic membrane and not the ear canal, which can affect the reading. In addition, the ear must be clear of cerumen (ear wax) and blood. Therefore, prehospital care practitioners need to rely on scene size-up, patient mental status, skin vitals, and ABCS. **Table 19-6** provides the anticipated physiologic responses with decreasing core temperature.

Signs of shivering and mental status change are important in the assessment of suspected hypothermia. Patients with mild hypothermia (core temperature greater than 90°F [32.2°C]) will be shivering and usually show signs of altered level of consciousness (e.g., apathy, confusion, slurred speech, altered gait, clumsiness). They

Table 19-6 Characteristics of Hypothermia

Classification	Core Body Temperature	Physiologic Response
Mild hypothermia	95–89.6°F (35–32°C)	Shivering, foot stamping
		Constricted blood vessels
		Increased respiratory rate
		Flat affect
		Dysarthria
		Ataxia
		Cold diuresis
Moderate hypothermia	89.5–82.4°F (32–28°C)	Shivering ceases; progressively weaker and stiffer muscles with loss of coordination
		Slowed respiratory rate
		Slow pulse
		Profound hypoventilation
		Decline in protective airway reflexes
		Oxygen consumption decreases by half
		Confusion
		Lethargy
Severe hypothermia	82.3–75.2°F (28–24°C)	Decrease in minute volume
		Increase in tracheobronchial secretions
		Bronchospasm may occur
		Weak pulse
		Dysrhythmia
		Slow respirations
		Coma
Profound hypothermia	< 75.2°F (< 24°C)	Apparent death
		Cardiac arrest

© National Association of Emergency Medical Technicians (NAEMT)

will be slow in their actions and are usually found in a nonambulatory state, sitting or lying. Law enforcement personnel and prehospital care practitioners may misinterpret this condition as drug or alcohol intoxication or, in geriatric patients, as cerebrovascular accident (stroke). However, a patient's level of consciousness is not a reliable indicator of the degree of hypothermia; some patients have remained conscious at core temperature below 80°F (26.7°C).

When the patient's core temperature falls below 90°F (32.2°C), moderate hypothermia is present, and the patient will probably not complain of feeling cold. Shivering may be absent, and the patient's level of consciousness will be greatly decreased, possibly to the point of unconsciousness. The patient's pupils will react slowly or may be dilated and fixed. The patient's palpable pulses may be diminished or absent, and the patient will have mild to moderate hypotension. The patient's ventilations may have slowed to as few as 2 breaths/minute. An ECG may show atrial fibrillation, the most common dysrhythmia. Other arrhythmias may be present with prolonged PR, QR, and QTC intervals. J (Osborn) waves may be present. As the myocardium becomes progressively colder and more irritable at about 82°F (27.8°C), VF is observed more often.

Because of the changes in cerebral metabolism, evidence of *paradoxical undressing* may be observed before the patient loses consciousness. This is an attempt by the patient to remove the clothing while in the cold environment, and it is thought to represent a response to an impending thermoregulatory failure.

Management

Prehospital care of the patient with hypothermia consists of preventing further heat loss, gentle handling, initiating rapid transport, and rewarming. This includes moving the patient away from any cold source to a warm ambulance or to a warm shelter if transportation is not immediately available (see the "Prolonged Transport" section). After assessing pulse and finding no signs of life, CPR should immediately be started.[142] Any wet clothing should be removed by cutting with trauma shears to avoid unnecessary movement and agitation of the patient. Concern for initiating ventricular dysrhythmia based on the handling of the patient should not delay any critical interventions. This concern becomes more realistic in severe hypothermia patients (core temperature below 86°F [30°C]). The patient's head and body should be insulated from the cold ground and covered completely with warm blankets or sleeping bags, followed by an outer windproof layer to prevent conductive, convective, and evaporative heat loss.

Patients who are conscious and alert should avoid drinks containing alcohol or caffeine. Anticipate hypoglycemia, and assess the patient's blood glucose level. For the patient with mild hypothermia with normal glucose levels, provide warm, high-caloric or glucose-containing fluids. For patients with moderate hypothermia with low blood glucose concentration, establish IV fluids and administer dextrose IV per local medical protocol, and repeat glucose determination every 5 minutes to determine the need for an additional dextrose bolus.

Hypothermic patients may benefit from supplemental oxygen because they have decreased oxygen delivery to the tissues. The oxyhemoglobin dissociation curve shifts to the left with a decrease in core temperature. This means that a pulse oximetry reading suggesting adequate levels of hemoglobin saturation may not reflect adequate oxygenation at the cellular level. Ideally, the patient may benefit more if the oxygen can be warmed and humidified (108°F to 115°F [42.2°C to 46.1°C]).

In unresponsive hypothermic patients, passive rewarming will be insufficient to increase core temperature. These patients will need an airway adjunct to protect the airway, and this should be initiated depending on jaw rigidity. The prehospital care practitioner should not hesitate to definitively support the airway since there is a low risk of triggering a fatal dysrhythmia during an advanced airway procedure.[111] If endotracheal intubation cannot be successfully achieved without rough handling, continue ventilation with a bag-mask device, and consider another advanced airway device (e.g., King supraglottic airway, laryngeal mask airway, nasal intubation). At a minimum, use an oral or nasal pharyngeal airway with bag-mask ventilation.

Intravenous NS, ideally with 5% dextrose, should be warmed to 109°F (42.8°C) and administered without agitating the patient. The patient with hypothermia should not be given "cold" (room-temperature) fluids because this could make the patient colder or could delay rewarming. When NS and dextrose solutions are unavailable, any warm crystalloid solution is satisfactory. Provide a fluid challenge of 500 to 1,000 mL, and prevent the solution from freezing or becoming colder by placing the IV bag under the patient to infuse warm fluids under pressure. The rewarming effect of warmed IV fluids is minimal at best, and the prehospital care practitioner should use good judgment to decide whether fluids (orally or IV) are worth the risks of aspiration, coughing, and painful stimuli to the patient. Hot packs or massaging of the patient's extremities is not recommended.[7]

Typically, active external rewarming occurs only to the thoracic region, with no active rewarming of the extremities. This approach will prevent increased peripheral circulation, which can cause an increased amount of colder blood to return from the extremities to the thorax before central core rewarming. Increased return of peripheral blood can increase acidosis and hyperkalemia and can decrease the core temperature (afterdrop). This complicates resuscitation and may precipitate VF.

2020 American Heart Association Guidelines for Cardiopulmonary Resuscitation and Emergency Cardiovascular Care Science

Cardiac Arrest in Special Situations—Accidental Hypothermia

Guidelines for resuscitation of a patient with hypothermia have evolved over many decades. The most recent revision of the emergency cardiovascular care guidelines by the American Heart Association (AHA) were published by the AHA in the journal *Circulation* in 2020. These guidelines did not change those published in 2015 with regard to cardiac arrest secondary to accidental hypothermia.[142,143]

The victim with hypothermia can present many challenges to the prehospital care practitioner, particularly the unconscious patient with moderate to severe hypothermia. Because severe hypothermia is defined by a core temperature of less than 86°F (30°C), the patient can present as clinically dead with no detectable pulse or respiration because of the reduced cardiac output and decreased arterial pressure. Historically, the challenge has been to determine whether to initiate basic life support (BLS) or advanced life support (ALS) interventions on these patients based on the viability of the patient. Furthermore, it may be difficult to determine from bystanders whether these patients had a primary hypothermic exposure or whether a medical event or traumatic injury preceded the hypothermia. Other concerns for a prehospital care practitioner are protecting the hypothermic patient with a potential irritable myocardium from any rough handling and initiating chest compression for the patient with nondetectable pulse, in whom both these interventions may initiate VF.[142]

Independent of any scenario that created the primary or secondary hypothermia, lifesaving procedures should generally not be withheld on the basis of clinical presentation, whether in an urban setting with short transport distances or in the backcountry environment with potentially significant delays in transport, in which scenario, extended patient care may be necessary (see later discussion).

Basic Life Support Guidelines for Treatment of Mild to Severe Hypothermia

Patients with hypothermia should be kept in a horizontal position when possible, and certainly during initial care, to avoid aggravating hypotension and afterdrop.[7] These patients are often volume depleted from cold diuresis. It may be difficult to feel or detect respiration and a pulse in the patient with hypothermia. Therefore, it is recommended initially to assess for breathing and then check for a pulse for up to 60 seconds to confirm one of the following:

- Respiratory arrest
- Pulseless cardiac arrest (asystole, ventricular tachycardia, VF)
- Bradycardia (requiring CPR)

If the patient is not breathing, start rescue breathing immediately unless the victim is obviously dead (e.g., decapitation, rigor mortis). Start chest compressions immediately in any patient with hypothermia who is pulseless and has no detectable signs of circulation.[142] If there is a doubt about detecting a pulse, begin compressions. Never withhold BLS interventions until the patient is rewarmed. If the patient is determined to be in cardiac arrest, use the current BLS guidelines.

An automated external defibrillator (AED) should be used if pulseless ventricular tachycardia or VF is present. The current emergency cardiovascular care guidelines (see **Figure 19-11**) recommend that these patients be treated by providing up to five cycles (2 minutes) of CPR (one cycle is 30 compressions to 2 breaths) before checking the ECG rhythm and attempting to shock when an AED arrives.[144] If a shockable rhythm is determined, give one shock, and then continue five cycles of CPR. If the patient with hypothermia does not respond to one shock with a detectable pulse, further attempts to defibrillate the patient should be deferred and efforts directed toward effective CPR with an emphasis on rewarming the patient to above 86°F (30°C) before attempting further defibrillation.[144]

When performing chest compressions in a patient with hypothermia, a greater force is required because chest wall elasticity is decreased when cold.[145] If core temperature is below 86°F (30°C), the conversion to normal sinus rhythm does not normally occur until rewarming above this core temperature is accomplished.[146]

The importance of not declaring a patient dead until the patient has been rewarmed and remains unresponsive cannot be overemphasized. Studies of victims of hypothermia indicate that cold exerts a protective effect on the vital organs.[146,147]

Advanced Cardiac Life Support Guidelines for Treatment of Hypothermia

The treatment of severe hypothermia in the field remains controversial.[142] However, the guidelines for administering advanced cardiovascular life support (ACLS) procedures are different from those with a normothermic patient. Unconscious patients with hypothermia need a

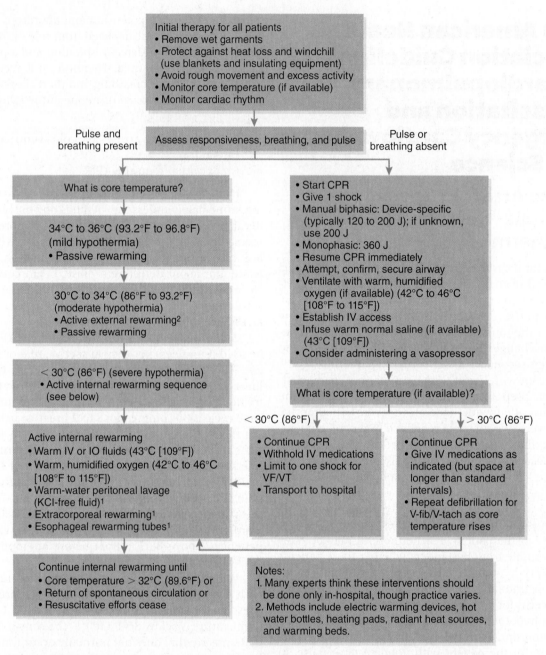

Figure 19-11 Modified from American Heart Association (AHA) hypothermia algorithm from the 2010 Cardiopulmonary Resuscitation and Emergency Cardiovascular Care guidelines. Note: Peritoneal lavage, extracorporeal rewarming, and esophageal rewarming tubes are usually hospital-only procedures.

Data from American Heart Association. Environmental trauma I: heat and cold. In *Handbook of Emergency Cardiovascular Care for Healthcare Providers.* AHA; 2006.

protected airway and should be intubated. Do not delay airway management based on the concern of initiating VF. As noted earlier, if a shockable rhythm is detected, defibrillate once at 120 to 200 biphasic joules or 360 monophasic joules, resume CPR, and then defer cardiac drugs and subsequent defibrillation attempts until core temperature is above 86°F (30°C). If possible, initiate active rewarming procedures with warm, humidified

oxygen and warm IV solutions, and package the patient for transport in a way that will prevent further heat loss. It is important to note that passive rewarming is adequate for patients with mild hypothermia. However, patients with moderate to severe hypothermia need active rewarming that is generally limited to procedures performed in an ED, operating room, or critical care unit. Passive rewarming procedures alone for these patients are totally inadequate to increase core temperature in the prehospital setting, and EMS personnel should focus on effective techniques in preventing further heat loss.[15]

The challenge with ACLS procedures in a patient with hypothermia is that the heart may be unresponsive to ACLS drugs, pacing, and defibrillation.[148] Furthermore, ACLS drugs (e.g., epinephrine, amiodarone, lidocaine, procainamide) can accumulate to toxic levels in the circulation with repeated administration in the patient with severe hypothermia, particularly when the patient rewarms.[142] Consequently, it is recommended to withhold IV medications in patients with a core temperature below 86°F (30°C). If a patient with hypothermia initially presents with a core temperature above 86°F (30°C), or if a patient with severe hypothermia has been rewarmed above this temperature, IV medications may be administered. However, longer intervals between drug administration are recommended than with standard drug intervals in ACLS.[142] The use of repeated defibrillation is indicated if the core temperature continues to rise above 86°F (30°C), consistent with the current ACLS guidelines.[144]

Finally, BLS/ACLS procedures performed in the field should be withheld only if the patient's injuries are incompatible with life, if the body is frozen such that chest compressions are impossible, or if the mouth and nose are blocked with ice.[15,142] Figure 19-11 provides an algorithm of mild, moderate, and severe hypothermia guidelines for both patients with a pulse and pulseless patients.[121]

Prevention of Cold-Related Injuries

The prevention of cold injuries in patients, yourself, and other prehospital care practitioners is vital when on the scene. Recommendations to prevent cold-related injuries include the following:

1. Note the risk factors generally associated with cold injury:
   * Fatigue
   * Dehydration
   * Undernutrition
   * Lack of cold weather experience
   * African ancestry
   * Tobacco use
   * Windchill
2. When you cannot stay dry in cold, wet, and windy conditions, seek shelter as soon as possible.
3. Remember that individuals with a history of cold injury are at a greater risk of a subsequent cold injury.
4. Avoid dehydration.
5. Avoid alcohol in cold environments.
6. Use the huddle technique with others if accidental water immersion in cold water occurs. You are more likely to survive if you remain still in cold water less than 68°F (20°C) and do not attempt to swim to shore unless it is nearby (< 45 minutes away).
7. Increase your likelihood of survival in cold environments by:
   * Maintaining a will to survive
   * Being adaptable and improvising
   * Staying optimistic and believing that the event is only a temporary situation
   * Maintaining a calm outlook and even a sense of humor
8. Use body heat to warm extremities that are cold or nearly frozen by placing fingers in the armpits or groin area. Toes and feet can be placed on another person's stomach.
9. Keep protective cold weather clothing (e.g., boots, socks, gloves, winter hat, insulated pants and jacket, windproof outer shell) in your car for unexpected car emergencies during cold weather months. Avoid clothing that absorbs moisture, as wet clothing will exacerbate heat loss (e.g., use wool or fleece).
10. Always wear gloves. Frostbite can occur rapidly when touching metal objects in the cold with your bare hands. Mittens are more effective than gloves at trapping warm air around all fingers.
11. Understand that the windchill index (**Figure 19-12**) is composed of wind speed and air temperature, and dress for extreme cold with insulated clothing and a windproof garment.
12. Keep feet dry with socks that transfer moisture from your feet to footwear.
13. Do not walk through snow with low-cut shoes. If you lack appropriate shoes and protective clothes, attempt to stay in a protected area.
14. Do not lie or rest directly on snow. Insulate with tree boughs, a sleeping pad, a poncho, or any material available. Use a sleeping bag outdoors.
15. Do not wear clothing that will absorb and retain sweat; any sweat retained in your clothes will increase heat loss and cause shivering.
16. When using lotion, use oil-based products (e.g., ChapStick, Vaseline). Water-based lotions on the face, hands, and ears will increase the risk for frostnip and frostbite.
17. When protecting the lower extremities from cold weather, be sure to protect the genital region. Use sweatpants, long underwear, Lycra tights, Gore-Tex pants, or any combination of these garments.

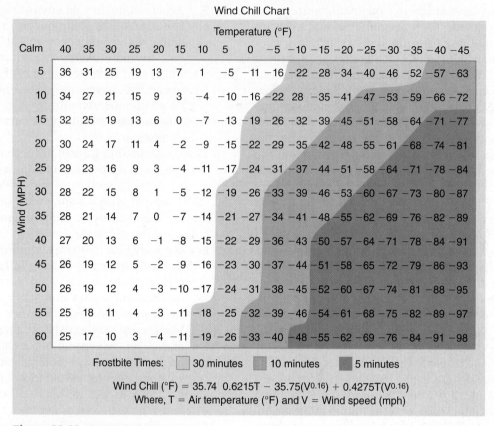

Figure 19-12 Windchill index.
Courtesy of the National Weather Service.

18. To prevent frostbite:
- Do not wear tight clothing, gloves, or boots that restrict circulation.
- Exercise fingers, toes, and face periodically to keep them warm and to detect numb areas.
- Work or exercise with a partner, who watches for warning signs of cold injury and hypothermia.
- Wear properly insulated clothing, and keep it dry; always carry extra undergarments, socks, and shoes.
- Watch for numbness and tingling.[149]

Prolonged Transport

At times, the location of a patient will result in a delay in transport or a prolonged transport to an appropriate facility, necessitating extended prehospital care. Consequently, practitioners may need to consider management options beyond what would be used with a rapid transport. How the patient is managed will depend on the time to definitive care, approved medical protocols, equipment and supplies on hand, additional personnel and resources, and location of the patient and severity of the injuries.

Some extended care considerations for moderately to severely injured patients from each of the environments discussed in this chapter are provided here. As with all patient care, it is understood that the first priorities are scene safety, XABCDEs (eXsanguinating hemorrhage, Airway, Breathing, Circulation, Disability, Expose/Environment)—sometimes also expressed as MARCH (Massive hemorrhage, Airway, Respirations, Circulation, Hypothermia),[19] and the use of standard assessment and management procedures appropriate to these environments. Specific attention must be paid to removal of the environmental stress (heat or cold). If medical control is available, always obtain a consult early, and communicate routinely throughout the extended care period. Any of the procedures listed that fall outside an individual's scope of practice are to be used only by other, credentialed medical practitioners.

It is important to know that all agencies have established guidelines for discontinuation of CPR. The AHA published a discussion on the ethical issues arising from withholding or withdrawing BLS or ALS resuscitation efforts.[144] The Wilderness Medical Society recommends that once CPR is initiated, it should be continued until resuscitation is successful with an awake patient, until rescuers are exhausted, until rescuers are placed in danger, until the patient is turned over to more definitive care, or until the patient does not respond to prolonged (30 minutes) resuscitative efforts.[150] The National Association of EMS Physicians also provides guidelines for the termination of CPR in the out-of-hospital environment (see Chapter 6, *Patient Assessment and Management*).[151] If medical control is available, begin patient consult early, if possible, for consideration of CPR termination after a total time of 20 minutes, depending on special patient circumstances.[151] (See Chapter 20, *Environmental Trauma II: Lightning, Drowning, Diving, and Altitude*, for additional situations [e.g., cold water submersion, lightning strike] in which CPR may be extended longer than 20 to 30 minutes.)

Heat-Related Illness

Heatstroke

Provide whole-body cooling as quickly as possible. Consider using any available access to water. Immerse the body to neck level in cool water (maintain body control and protect the airway), or spray the whole body with water (e.g., IV fluids, saline, water bottles, water from hydration backpacks), and provide a source of continuous wind current (e.g., natural wind current, fanning with towel, fire ventilation fans). When possible, stay in contact with medical control to keep them informed of the patient's status and to receive further medical directions. Stop body cooling when rectal temperature reaches 102°F (38.9°C). Then protect the patient from shivering and hypothermia. If an athletic trainer has already instituted treatment with an ice bath prior to EMS arrival, consider continuation of the ice bath until the patient's rectal temperature reaches 102.2°F (39°C), and advise medical control of the situation.

As you are cooling the patient, manage the airway in unresponsive patients, and initiate good ventilation with a bag-mask device with high-flow oxygen. Insert an IV line, provide a 500-mL NS fluid challenge, and assess vital signs. Patients should have vital signs assessed after every 500 mL. Total fluid volume should not exceed 1 to 2 liters in the first hour. An additional liter can be considered during the second hour if prehospital care is extended.

The next priorities are to manage any seizure activity and hypoglycemia per medical protocol with diazepam and dextrose, respectively. Place the patient in the recovery position, and continue the assessment to include level of consciousness, vital signs, rectal temperature, and blood glucose. Provide supportive care and basic bodily needs throughout the remaining extended care period.

Exercise-Associated Hyponatremia

Correct the presumed low blood sodium concentration. If the patient can take food by mouth and if such food is available, provide potato chips, pretzels, or other salty food or a sport electrolyte or other sodium-containing beverage. An oral sodium solution has been demonstrated to be an appropriate hypertonic saline treatment.[152] In the field, this solution could be prepared by dissolving three to four bouillon cubes in a half cup of water (125 mL) (~9% saline). Salt tablets given alone are not recommended; additional fluid must accompany the tablets, and there is the risk of increasing sodium levels too much.

Next, establish an IV line and start NS with a flow rate set to KVO. Check with medical control to consider a flow rate of 250 mL/hr or greater based on the estimated delay in transporting the patient to the hospital or the presence of severe dehydration or **rhabdomyolysis**. Do not use hypotonic IV fluids because they will exacerbate cerebral edema and could potentiate the condition, leading to seizure, coma, and death. In a patient with severe signs or symptoms (seizure or coma), consider administration of furosemide (a diuretic, if available) to reduce extracellular body water content while providing some sodium by infusing NS, 250 to 500 mL/hr IV.

Assess cerebral edema and increased intracranial pressure. Establish a baseline Glasgow Coma Scale score, and reassess every 10 minutes as an indicator of progressive cerebral edema and increased intracranial pressure (manage per recommendations for cerebral edema). (For further details, see Chapter 8, *Head and Neck Trauma*.)

Be prepared to manage nausea and projectile vomiting. Take one side of a large trash bag and make a hole for the patient's head about 12 inches (30 centimeters) below the rim of the bag. Place the patient's head through the hole so that the patient can look down into the center of the bag. Also be prepared to manage urine when diuresis begins. Use a large trash bag as a diaper or use a bucket or other container.

Give supplemental oxygen (2 to 4 liters/minute by nasal cannula) if the patient shows signs of pulmonary distress or if patients are lethargic or obtunded. Manage the airway of unresponsive patients, and initiate good ventilation with a bag-mask device (no hyperventilation) with oxygen at 10 breaths/minute. (For further details, see Chapter 8, *Head and Neck Trauma*.)

Assess the patient's blood glucose level, and provide IV dextrose per protocol to hypoglycemic patients. Monitor for seizures, and administer an anticonvulsant (e.g., diazepam, initially 2 to 5 mg IV/intramuscular, and titrate per medical protocol). Place unconscious patients in a left lateral recumbent position. Continue ongoing assessment of the patient.

Cold-Related Illness

Frostbite

Protect and treat the patient for hypothermia, if present. Start IV fluid hydration, or at least establish an IV, before initiation of rewarming procedures. If a vein cannot be accessed, the intraosseous route is an alternative. In a situation of significant transport delay, active rewarming should be considered. Rapid, active rewarming can reverse the direct injury of ice crystals in tissues, but it may not change the injury severity. It is critical to keep the thawed tissue from refreezing because this significantly worsens the outcome compared with passive thawing. When and where to begin active rewarming are key considerations, if active rewarming is to be done at all.

A standard rewarming procedure is to immerse the affected extremity in circulating water warmed to a temperature between 98.6°F and 102.2°F (37°C and 39°C) in a large enough container to accommodate the frostbitten tissues without their touching the sides or bottom of the container.[104,105] Water should feel warm, but not hot, to the normal hand. (Note that the temperature range given here is lower than that previously recommended; this temperature range decreases pain for the patient while only slightly slowing the rewarming phase.) If available, an oral or rectal thermometer should be used to measure water temperature. A temperature below that recommended will thaw tissue but is less beneficial for rapid thawing and for tissue survival. Any greater temperature will cause greater pain and may cause a burn injury. Do not rewarm with intense sources of dry heat (e.g., placing near campfire). Continue immersion until tissue is soft and pliable, which may take up to 30 to 60 minutes. Active motion of the extremity during immersion is beneficial, without direct rubbing or massaging of the affected part. If immersion warming is not available, the affected parts may be wrapped in loose, bulky sterile dressings with sterile cotton gauze placed between fingers or toes to avoid further tissue damage. Blisters should not be ruptured.[106]

Extreme pain is experienced during rapid thawing. Treat with IV analgesics and titrate as needed and based on local protocols. (Aspirin is contraindicated in pediatric patients because of the risk of Reye's syndrome.)

The return of normal skin color, warmth, and sensation in the affected part are all favorable signs. Dry all affected parts with warm air (do not towel dry affected parts), and ideally, apply topical aloe vera on skin, place sterile gauze between toes or fingers, bandage, splint, and elevate the extremity. Cover any extremity with insulating material, and wrap a windproof and waterproof material (e.g., trash bag) as the outer layer, particularly if continuing patient extraction outdoors to a transport location.

Hypothermia

Start active rewarming procedures. The key point is to prevent further heat loss by insulating the patient from the environment and removing wet clothing and replacing it with dry clothing. Administer heated IV fluids (104°F to 107.6°F [40°C to 42°C]).

Shivering is the single best way for rewarming non-trauma patients with mild hypothermia in the traditional prehospital setting with short transport times compared with external methods of rewarming. Patients with hypothermia who are able to shiver maximally can increase their core temperature by up to 6°F to 8°F (~3°C to 4°C) per hour. External heat sources are often used but may provide only minimal benefit.[93] For the patient with moderate to severe hypothermia, these heat sources remain important considerations in the extended-care situation when used in combination with the hypothermia insulation wrap (described later). Some considerations regarding external heat sources include the following:

- Warmed (maximum 108°F [42.2°C]), humidified oxygen by mask can prevent heat loss during ventilation and provide some heat transfer to the chest from the respiratory tract.
- Body-to-body contact has merit for heat transfer, but many studies fail to show any advantage except in patients with mild hypothermia.
- Electric and portable heating pads provide no additional advantage.
- Forced-air warming has some benefit in minimizing post-cooling core temperature (afterdrop); it provides an effective warming rate comparable to shivering for patients with mild hypothermia.

Insulate all patients with hypothermia in the remote setting to minimize heat loss. Prepare a multilayer hypothermia wrap. Place a large, waterproof plastic sheet on the floor or ground. Add an insulation layer of a sleeping pad, blankets, or a sleeping bag on top of the waterproof layer. Lay the patient on top of the insulation layer along with any external heat sources. Add a second insulating layer on top of the patient. The left side of the hypothermia wrap is folded over the patient first, then the right side. The patient's head is covered to prevent heat loss, keeping an opening at the face to allow patient assessment.[19,153]

Assess the patient for hypoglycemia. Providing dextrose will ensure that adequate fuel (sugar) is available for muscular metabolism during shivering and will prevent further hypoglycemia. Alert patients can consume warm, sugary fluids by mouth.

SUMMARY

- Prehospital care practitioners will inevitably be faced with environmental encounters such as those described in this chapter.
- To provide rapid assessment and treatment in the prehospital setting, practitioners must possess basic knowledge of common environmental emergencies. They must also understand how the body regulates temperature, including the role of the skin and the thermoregulatory mechanisms in the brain.
- Methods to maintain and dissipate body heat are important concepts for prehospital care practitioners. Practitioners must understand how both heat and cold are transferred to and from the body (i.e., radiation, conduction, convection, evaporation) so that they can effectively manage a patient who has hyperthermia or hypothermia.
- For heat-related illness, practitioners should treat patients with heatstroke with effective, rapid, whole-body cooling to reduce core temperature quickly.
- For cold-related illness, practitioners should manage all patients with moderate to severe

hypothermia gently, taking the time to remove them from the cold environment, and begin passive rewarming while monitoring core temperature. The key is to prevent further body heat loss.
- Practitioners must remember that drugs and defibrillation are generally ineffective when core temperature is less than 86°F (30°C).
- Patients are not dead until they are warm and dead, unless signs are present of obvious futility of resuscitation (e.g., frozen chest, decapitation, ice in airway).
- Practitioners must know how to protect themselves from heat- and cold-related injuries and how to advocate for the safety of others. Important prevention concepts include hydration, physical fitness, heat acclimatization, adequate clothing for cold weather, and avoidance of risk factors.
- Remember that you must maintain your own safety to be an effective rescuer. In too many cases, practitioners have lost their lives while attempting a rescue.

SCENARIO RECAP

It is a hot summer afternoon with temperatures reaching 102°F (38.9°C). Over the past 30 days, it has been very humid, with temperatures reaching over 100°F (37.8°C) daily. The ambient temperature has resulted in many heat-related conditions that have required EMS personnel to transport numerous patients to the EDs of the inner city.

At 1700 hours, your ambulance unit responds to a dispatch for an unresponsive male patient in a vehicle. As your ambulance unit arrives on scene, you observe a 76-year-old man who appears to be unconscious in a vehicle parked outside of a department store. Your rapid assessment of the patient's ABCs and level of consciousness reveals that the patient is verbal, but he is saying things that are illogical and irrational.

- What are the potential causes for this patient's decreased level of consciousness?
- What hallmark signs support a heat-related diagnosis?
- How would you emergently manage this patient at the scene and en route to the ED?

SCENARIO SOLUTION

This 76-year-old man has been waiting in his car for his spouse to return from the shopping center. He has been exposed to high heat without effective hydration to offset fluid loss (sweat) and is dehydrated. The patient has a body mass index over 30, placing him at greater risk of heat-related illness because of obesity.

On the wife's return, she provided additional history indicating that he is taking a diuretic for hypertension, a beta blocker for coronary heart disease, and an anticholinergic for Parkinson disease. All three medications

(continues)

SCENARIO SOLUTION (CONTINUED)

are known risk factors for heat-related illness. This patient needs quick assessment of his ABCs and level of consciousness using the AVPU (**A**lert, responds to **V**erbal stimulus, responds to **P**ainful stimulus, **U**nresponsive) scale, as he was found in a non–air-conditioned car. Due to his irrational and illogical verbal statements, his age, and the location, you have a high suspicion for heatstroke.

You rapidly assess for blunt or penetrating trauma and find none. Next, geriatric patients must be assessed for exacerbation of any underlying medical disease, such as cardiac disease or a neurologic disorder (e.g., stroke). All three of his medical conditions are known to be made worse with hyperthermia, thereby increasing his mortality risk. It is essential that this patient receive whole-body cooling immediately.

You move the patient out of the direct sunlight on the front seat and remove any excess clothing. You use the saline water bottles from the trauma bag to begin wetting him down from his head to toes. You have your partner start the fan and place the air conditioning on high to increase airflow across the patient's body to increase convective heat transfer. The stretcher is readied to transfer the patient to the ambulance. Ice water and cool moist towels are readied in the back of the ambulance for this patient with hyperthermia.

You quickly transfer the patient from his vehicle to the ambulance. As transport is initiated, the patient's whole body is wetted down with cold wet towels, and the overhead fans are directed at the patient. The patient is placed on high-flow oxygen, ECG is monitored, and an IV is established at a KVO rate initially. You are prepared to evaluate rectal temperature to confirm hyperthermia (greater than or equal to 104°F [40°C]). If confirmed, you will provide a 500-mL saline IV bolus. You take a set of vital signs and inform medical control to prepare for a 76-year-old male patient with heatstroke.

References

1. Centers for Disease Control and Prevention/National Center for Health Statistics. Compressed mortality file. Updated November 19, 2018. Accessed October 25, 2021. https://www.cdc.gov/nchs/data_access/cmf.htm

2. Centers for Disease Control and Prevention. Heat-related deaths—Chicago, Illinois, 1996–2001, and United States, 1979–1999. *Morb Mortal Wkly Rep.* 2003;52(26):610.

3. National Center for Environmental Health (NCEH)/Agency for Toxic Substances and Disease Registry (ATSDR), Coordinating Center for Environmental Health and Injury Prevention (CCEHIP). Natural disasters and severe weather: extreme heat. Updated June 30, 2021. Accessed October 25, 2021. https://www.cdc.gov/disasters/extremeheat/index.html

4. Meiman J, Anderson H, Tomasallo C. Hypothermia-related deaths—Wisconsin, 2014, and United States, 2003–2013. *Morb Mortal Wkly Rep.* 2015;64(6):141-143.

5. Centers for Disease Control and Prevention. Hypothermia-related deaths—United States, 2003. *Morb Mortal Wkly Rep.* 2004;53(8):172.

6. O'Brien KK, Leon LR, Kenefick RW. Clinical management of heat-related illnesses. In: Auerbach PS, ed. *Auerbach's Wilderness Medicine.* 7th ed. Mosby Elsevier; 2017.

7. Dow J, Giesbrecht GG, Danzl DF, et al. Wilderness Medical Society practice guidelines for the out-of-hospital evaluation and treatment of accidental hypothermia: 2019 Update. *Wilderness Environ Med.* 2019;30(Suppl 4):S47-S69.

8. Lugo-Amador NM, Rothenhaus T, Moyer P. Heat-related illness. *Emerg Med Clin North Am.* 2004;22:315-327.

9. Ulrich AS, Rathlev NK. Hypothermia and localized injuries. *Emerg Med Clin North Am.* 2004;22:281-298.

10. Centers for Disease Control and Prevention. Hypothermia-related deaths—United States, 2003. *Morb Mortal Wkly Rep.* 2004;53(8):172.

11. Brown DJA, Brugger H, Boyd J, et al. Accidental hypothermia. *N Engl J Med.* 2012;367(20);1930-1938.

12. Hawkins SC. Wilderness EMS systems. In: Hawkins SC, ed. *Wilderness EMS.* Wolters Kluwer; 2018.

13. Leon LR, Kenefick RW. Pathophysiology of heat-related illnesses. In: Auerbach PS, ed. *Auerbach's Wilderness Medicine.* 7th ed. Mosby Elsevier; 2017.

14. Freer L, Handford C, Imray CHE. Frostbite. In: Auerbach PS, ed. *Auerbach's Wilderness Medicine.* 7th ed. Mosby Elsevier; 2017.

15. Danzl DF, Huecker MR. Accidental hypothermia. In: Auerbach PS, ed. *Auerbach's Wilderness Medicine.* 7th ed. Mosby Elsevier; 2017.

16. National Aeronautics and Space Administration. 2020 Tied for Warmest Year on Record, NASA Analysis Shows. Published January 14, 2021. Accessed October 25, 2021. https://www.nasa.gov/press-release/2020-tied-for-warmest-year-on-record-nasa-analysis-shows

17. Vaidyanathan A, Malilay J, Schramm P, Saha S. Heat-related deaths—United States, 2004–2018. *Morb Mortal Wkly Rep.* 2020;69:729-734. doi: 10.15585/mmwr.mm6924a1

18. Centers for Disease Control and Prevention. Hypothermia-related deaths—United States, 1999–2002 and 2005. *Morb Mortal Wkly Rep.* 2006;55(10):282-284.

19. Hawkins SC, Simon RB, Beissinger JP, Simon D. *Vertical Aid: Essential Wilderness Medicine for Climbers, Trekkers, and Mountaineers*. The Countryman Press; 2017.

20. Hardy JD. Thermal comfort: skin temperature and physiological thermoregulation. In: Hardy JD, Gagge AP, Stolwijk JAJ, eds. *Physiological and Behavioral Temperature Regulation*. Charles C. Thomas; 1970.

21. Pozos RS, Danzl DF. Human physiological responses to cold stress and hypothermia. In: Pandolf KB, Burr RE, eds. *Medical Aspects of Harsh Environments*. Vol 1. Office of the Surgeon General, Borden Institute/TMM Publications; 2001:351-382.

22. Stocks JM, Taylor NAS, Tipton MJ, Greenleaf JE. Human physiological responses to cold exposure. *Aviat Space Environ Med*. 2004;75:444-457.

23. Wenger CB. The regulation of body temperature. In: Rhoades RA, Tanner GA, eds. *Medical Physiology*. Little, Brown; 1995.

24. Nunnelely SA, Reardon MJ. Prevention of heat illness. In: Pandolf KB, Burr RE, eds. *Medical Aspects of Harsh Environments*. Vol 1. Office of the Surgeon General, Borden Institute/TMM Publications; 2001:209-230.

25. Hall B, Hall J. *Sauer's Manual of Skin Diseases*. 10th ed. Lippincott Williams & Wilkins; 2010.

26. Krakowski A, Goldenberg A. Exposure to radiation from the sun. In: Auerbach PS, ed. *Auerbach's Wilderness Medicine*. 7th ed. Mosby Elsevier; 2017.

27. Lipman GS, Gaudio FFG, Eifling KP, Ellis MA, Otten EM, Grissom CK. Wilderness Medical Society practice guidelines for the prevention and treatment of heat-related illness: 2019 update. *Wilderness Environ Med*. 2019;30(4):S33-S46.

28. Yeo T. Heat stroke: a comprehensive review. *AACN Clin Issues*. 2004;15:280-293.

29. Wenger CB. Section I: human adaption to hot environments. In: Pandolf KB, Burr RE, eds. *Medical Aspects of Harsh Environments*. Vol 1. Office of the Surgeon General, Borden Institute/TMM Publications; 2001:51-86.

30. Sonna LA. Practical medical aspects of military operations in the heat. In: Pandolf KB, Burr RE, eds. *Medical Aspects of Harsh Environments*. Vol 1. Office of the Surgeon General, Borden Institute/TMM Publications; 2001:293-309.

31. Tek D, Olshaker JS. Heat illness. *Emerg Med Clin North Am*. 1992;10(2):299-310.

32. Wallace RF, Kriebel D, Punnett L, et al. The effects of continuous hot weather training on risk of exertional heat illness. *Med Sci Sports Exerc*. 2005;37(1):84-90.

33. Schimelpfenig T, Richards G, Tartar S. Management of heat illnesses. In: Hawkins SC, ed. *Wilderness EMS*. Wolters Kluwer; 2018.

34. Bedno SA, Li Y, Han W, et al. Exertional heat illness among overweight U.S. Army recruits in basic training. *Aviat Space Environ Med*. 2010;81(2):107-111.

35. Kenefick RW, Cheuvront SN, Leon LR, O'Brien KK. Dehydration and rehydration. In: Auerbach PS, ed. *Auerbach's Wilderness Medicine*. 7th ed. Mosby Elsevier; 2017.

36. Armstrong LE, Hubbard RW, Jones BH, Daniels JT. Preparing Alberto Salazar for the heat of the 1984 Olympic marathon. *Phys Sportsmed*. 1986;14:73-81.

37. Johnson RF, Kobrick JL. Psychological aspects of military performance in hot environments. In: Pandolf KB, Burr RE, eds. *Medical Aspects of Harsh Environments*. Vol 1. Office of the Surgeon General, Borden Institute/TMM Publications; 2001.

38. Sawka MN, Pandolf KB. Physical exercise in hot climates: physiology, performance, and biomedical issues. In: Pandolf KB, Burr RE, eds. *Medical Aspects of Harsh Environments*. Vol 1. Office of the Surgeon General, Borden Institute/TMM Publications; 2001.

39. Dutchman SM, Ryan AJ, Schedl HP, et al. Upper limits of intestinal absorption of dilute glucose solution in men at rest. *Med Sci Sport Exerc*. 1997;29:482-488.

40. Neufer PD, Young AJ, Sawka MN. Gastric emptying during exercise: effects of heat stress and hypohydration. *Eur J Appl Physiol*. 1989;58:433-439.

41. Bouchama A, Knochel JP. Medical progress: heatstroke. *N Engl J Med*. 2002;346(25):1978-1988.

42. Adams T, Stacey E, Stacey S, Martin D. Exertional heat stroke. *Br J Hosp Med (London)*. 2012;73(2):72-78.

43. Case DJ, Armstrong LE, Kenny GP, O'Connor FG, Huggins RA. Exertional heat stroke: new concepts regarding cause and care. *Curr Sports Med Rep*. 2012;11(3):115-123.

44. Casa DJ, McDermott BP, Lee E, Yeargin SW, Armstrong LE, Maresh CM. Cold-water immersion: the gold standard for exertional heat stroke treatment. *Exerc Sport Rev*. 2007;35(3):141-149.

45. Holtzhausen LM, Noakes TD. Collapsed ultra-endurance athlete: proposed mechanisms and an approach to management. *Clin J Sport Med*. 1997;7(4):292-301.

46. Gardner JW, Kark JA. Clinical diagnosis, management and surveillance of exertional heat illness. In: Pandolf KB, Burr RE, eds. *Medical Aspects of Harsh Environments*. Vol 1. Office of the Surgeon General, Borden Institute/TMM Publications; 2001:231-279.

47. Asplune CA, O'Connor FG, Noakes TD. Exercise-associated collapse: an evidence-based review and primer for clinicians. *Br J Sports Med*. 2011;45:1157-1162.

48. Nichols AW. Heat-related illness in sports and exercise. *Curr Rev Musculoskelet Med*. 2014;7:355-365.

49. Bennett BL, Hew-Butler T, Rosner MH, Myers T, Lipman GS. Wilderness Medical Society practice guidelines for treatment of exercise-associated hyponatremia: 2019 update. *Wilderness Environ Med*. 2020;31(1):50-62.

50. Rosner MH. Exercise-associated hyponatremia. *Semin Nephrol*. 2009;29(3):271-281.

51. Rosner M, Bennett B, Hoffman M, Hew-Butler T. Exercise induced hyponatremia. In: Simon E, ed. *Hyponatremia: Evaluation and Treatment*. Springer; 2013.

52. Leon LR, Helwig BG. Heat stroke: role of the systemic inflammatory response. *J Appl Physiol*. 2010;109(6):1980-1988.

53. Gaffin SL, Hubbard RW. Pathophysiology of heatstroke. In: Pandolf KB, Burr RE, eds. *Medical Aspects of Harsh Environments*. Vol 1. Office of the Surgeon General, Borden Institute/TMM Publications; 2001:161-208.

54. Semenza JC, Rubin CH, Flater KH, et al. Heat-related deaths during the July 1995 heat wave in Chicago. *N Engl J Med*. 1996;335(2):84-90.

55. Miller KC, Casa DJ, Adams WM, et al. Roundtable on preseason heat safety in secondary school athletics: prehospital care of patients with exertional heat stroke. *J Athl Train*. 2021;56(4):372-382.

56. Belval LN, Casa DJ, Adams WM, et al. Consensus statement: prehospital care of exertional heat stroke. *Prehosp Emerg Care*. 2018;22(3):392-397. doi: 10.1080/10903127.2017.1392666

57. Knochel JP, Reed G. Disorders of heat regulation. In: Narins RE, ed. *Maxwell and Kleenman's Clinical Disorders of Fluid and Electrolyte Metabolism*. 5th ed. McGraw-Hill; 1994.

58. Hawkins SC. Environmental emergencies. In: Pollak AN, ed. *Caroline's Emergency Care in the Streets*. 8th ed. Jones & Bartlett Learning; 2018.

59. Armstrong LE, Crago AE, Adams R, et al. Whole-body cooling of hyperthermic runners: comparison of two field therapies. *Am J Emerg Med*. 1996;14:335-358.

60. Costrini A. Emergency treatment of exertional heatstroke and comparison of whole-body cooling techniques. *Med Sci Sports Exerc*. 1984;22:15-18.

61. Gaffin SL, Gardner J, Flinn S. Current cooling method for exertional heatstroke. *Ann Intern Med*. 2000;132:678. doi: 10.7326/0003-4819-132-8-200004180-00023

62. Miller KC, Casa DJ, Adams WM, et al. Roundtable on preseason heat safety in secondary school athletics: prehospital care of patients with exertional heat stroke. *J Athl Train*. 2021;56(4):372-382.

63. Speedy DB, Noakes TD. Exercise-associated hyponatremia: a review. *Emerg Med*. 2001;13(1):17-27.

64. Backer HD, Shopes E, Collins SL, Barkan H. Exertional heat illness and hyponatremia in hikers. *Am J Emerg Med*. 1999;17(6):532-539.

65. Gardner JW. Death by water intoxication. *Mil Med*. 2002; 164(3):432-434.

66. Noakes TD, Goodwin N, Rayner BL, et al. Water intoxication: a possible complication during endurance exercise. *Med Sci Sports Exerc*. 1985;17:370-375.

67. Rosner MH, Kirven J. Exercise-associated hyponatremia. *Clin J Am Soc Nephrol*. 2007;2:151-161.

68. Adrogue HJ, Madias NE. Hyponatremia. *N Engl J Med*. 2000;342(21):1581-1589.

69. Hiller WDB. Dehydration and hyponatremia during triathlons. *Med Sci Sports Exerc*. 1989;21(Suppl 5):S219-S221.

70. Speedy DB, Noakes TD, Rodgers IR. Hyponatremia in ultra-distance triathletes. *Med Sci Sports Exerc*. 1999;31: 809-815.

71. Laird RH. Medical care at ultra-endurance triathlons. *Med Sci Sports Exerc*. 1989;21(Suppl 5):S222-S225.

72. Collins S, Reynolds B. The other heat-related emergency. *JEMS*. 2004;29(7):74-88.

73. Backer HD, Shopes E, Collins SL, Barkan H. Exertional heat illness and hyponatremia in hikers. *Am J Emerg Med*. 1999;17:532-539.

74. Noe RS, Choudhary E, Cheng-Dobson J, Wolkin AF, Newman SB. Exertional heat-related illnesses at the Grand Canyon National Park, 2004–2009. *Wilderness Environ Med*. 2013;24:422-428.

75. American College of Sports Medicine. Position stand: exercise and fluid replacement. *Med Sci Sports Exerc*. 2007;39(2):377-390.

76. Hew-Bulter T, Ayus JC, Kipps C, et al. Statement of Second International Exercise-Associated Hyponatremia Consensus Development Conference, New Zealand, 2007. *Clin J Sport Med*. 2008;18(2):111-121.

77. Ayus JC, Arieff A, Moritz ML. Hyponatremia in marathon runners. *N Engl J Med*. 2005;353:427.

78. U.S. Fire Administration. Firefighter fatalities in the United States in 2015. Federal Emergency Management Agency. Published October 2016. Accessed October 25, 2021. https://www.usfa.fema.gov/downloads/pdf/publications/ff_fat15.pdf

79. U.S. Department of Agriculture, U.S. Forest Service. Heat stress brochure. Accessed October 25, 2021. http://www.fs.fed.us/fire/safety/fitness/heat_stress/hs_pg1.html

80. Brazaitis M, Skurvydas A. Heat acclimation does not reduce the impact of hyperthermia on central fatigue. *Eur J Appl Physiol*. 2010;109:771-778.

81. Cheung SS, McLellan TM. Heat acclimation, aerobic fitness, and hydration effects on tolerance during uncompensable heat stress. *J Appl Physiol*. 1998;84:1731-1739.

82. Garrett AT, Goosens NG, Rehrer NJ, Patterson MJ, Cotter JD. Induction and decay of short-term heat acclimation. *Eur J Appl Physiol*. 2009;107:659-670.

83. Montain SJ, Latzka WA, Sawka MN. Fluid replacement recommendations for training in hot weather. *Mil Med*. 1999;164(7):502-508.

84. Parson KC. International standards for the assessment of the risk of thermal strain on clothed workers in hot environments. *Ann Occup Hyg*. 1999;43(5):297-308.

85. American College of Sports Medicine. Position stand on the recommended quantity and quality of exercise for developing and maintaining cardiorespiratory and muscular fitness, and flexibility in adults. *Med Sci Sports Exerc*. 1998;30(6):975-981.

86. Haskell WL, Lee IM, Pate RR, et al. Physical activity and public health: updated recommendation for adults from the American College of Sports Medicine and the American Heart Association. *Med Sci Sports Exerc*. 2007;39(8): 1423-1424.

87. Sawka MN, Kolka MA, Montain SJ. *Ranger and Airborne School Students' Heat Acclimatization Guide*. U.S. Army Research Institute of Environmental Medicine; 2003.

88. Eichna LW, Park CR, Nelson N, et al. Thermal regulation during acclimatization in a hot, dry (desert type) environment. *J Appl Physiol*. 1950;163:585-597.

89. Federal Emergency Management System, U.S. Fire Administration. Emergency Incident Rehabilitation. Published February 2008. Accessed October 25, 2021. http://www.usfa.fema.gov/downloads/pdf/publications/fa_314.pdf

90. Hostler D. First responder rehab: good, better, best. *JEMS*. 2007;32(12):98-112; quiz 114.

91. Paterson R, Drake B, Tabin G, Butler FK Jr, Cushing T. Wilderness Medical Society practice guidelines for treatment of eye injuries and illnesses in the wilderness: 2014 update. *Wilderness Environ Med*. 2014;25:S19-S29.

92. Ulrich AS, Rathlev NK. Hypothermia and localized injuries. *Emerg Med Clin North Am*. 2004;22(2):281-298.

93. Thomas JR, Oakley EHN. Nonfreezing cold injury. In: Pandolf KB, Burr RE, eds. *Medical Aspects of Harsh Environments*. Vol 1. Office of the Surgeon General, Borden Institute/TMM Publications; 2001:467-490.

94. Montgomery H. Experimental immersion foot: review of the physiopathology. *Physiol Rev*. 1954;34(1):127-137.

95. Francis TJR. Nonfreezing cold injury: a historical review. *J R Nav Med Serv*. 1984;70:134-139.

96. Imray CHE, Handford C, Thomas OD, Castellani JW. Nonfreezing cold-induced injuries. In: Auerbach PS, ed. *Auerbach's Wilderness Medicine*. 7th ed. Mosby Elsevier; 2017.

97. Wrenn K. Immersion foot: a problem of the homeless in the 1990s. *Arch Intern Med*. 1991;151:785-788.

98. Ramstead KD, Hughes RB, Webb AJ. Recent cases of trench foot. *Postgrad Med J*. 1980;56:879-883.

99. Laskowski-Jones L, Jones L. Management of cold injuries. In: Hawkins SC, ed. *Wilderness EMS*. Wolters Kluwer, 2018.

100. Biem J, Koehncke N, Classen D, Dosman J. Out of cold: management of hypothermia and frostbite. *Can Med Assoc J*. 2003;168(3):305-311.

101. Vogel JE, Dellon AL. Frostbite injuries of the hand. *Clin Plast Surg*. 1989;16:565-576.

102. Mills WJ. Clinical aspects of freezing injury. In: Pandolf KB, Burr RE, eds. *Medical Aspects of Harsh Environments*. Vol 1. Office of the Surgeon General, Borden Institute/TMM Publications; 2001.

103. McIntosh SE, Hamonko M, Freer L, et al. Wilderness Medical Society Practice guidelines for the prevention and treatment of frostbite. *Wilderness Environ Med*. 2011;22;156-166.

104. Cauchy E, Davis CB, Pasquier M, Meyer EF, Hackett PH. A new proposal for management of severe frostbite in the austere environment. *Wilderness Environ Med*. 2016;27:92-99.

105. Zafren K, Giesbrecht G. State of Alaska Cold Injuries Guidelines. Department of Health and Social Services, Juneau, Alaska. Revised July 2014. Accessed October 25, 2021. http://mra.org/wp-content/uploads/2016/05/Alaska-DHSS-EMS-Cold-Injuries-Guidelines-June-2014.pdf

106. McIntosh SE, Freer L, Grissom CK, Pandey P, Dow DD, Hackett PH. Wilderness Medical Society practice guidelines for the prevention and treatment of frostbite: 2019 update. *Wilderness Environ Med*. 2019;30(4):S19-S32.

107. Sessler DI. Mild preoperative hypothermia. *N Engl J Med*. 1997;336:1730-1737.

108. Giesbrecht GG. Cold stress, near drowning and accidental hypothermia: a review. *Aviat Space Environ Med*. 2000;71:733-752.

109. Stocks JM, Taylor NAS, Tipton MJ, Greenleaf JE. Human physiological responses to cold exposure. *Aviat Space Environ Med*. 2004;75:444-457.

110. Gilbert M, Busund R, Skagseth A, et al. Resuscitation from accidental hypothermia of 13.7°C with circulatory arrest. *Lancet*. 2000;355:375-376.

111. Danzl DF, Pozos RS, Auerbach PS. Multicenter hypothermia survey. *Ann Emerg Med*. 1987;16(9):1042-1055.

112. Tsuei BJ, Kearney PA. Hypothermia in the trauma patient. *Injury Int J Care Injured*. 2004;35:7-15.

113. Stoner HB. Effects of injury on the responses to thermal stimulation of the hypothalamus. *J Appl Physiol*. 1972;33(5):665-671.

114. Ferrara A, MacArthur J, Wright H. Hypothermia and acidosis worsen coagulopathy in the patient requiring massive transfusion. *Am J Surg*. 1990;160:515-518.

115. Epstein M. Renal effects of head-out immersion in man: implications for understanding volume homeostasis. *Physiol Rev*. 1978;58:529-581.

116. Jurkovich G. Hypothermia in the trauma patient. *Adv Trauma*. 1989;4:111-140.

117. Jurkovich GJ. Environmental cold-induced injury. *Surg Clin N Am*. 2007;87(1):247-267.

118. Bennett BL, Giesbrect G, Zafren K, et al. Management of hypothermia in tactical combat casualty care: TCCC guideline proposed change 20-01 (June 2020). *J Spec Oper Med*. 2020;20(3):21-35.

119. Beilman GJ, Blondett JJ, Nelson AB. Early hypothermia in severely injured trauma patients is a significant risk factor of multiple organ dysfunction syndrome but not mortality. *Ann Surg*. 2009;249:845-850.

120. Mommsen P, Andruszkow H, Fromke C, et al. Effects of accidental hypothermia on posttraumatic complications and outcome in multiple trauma patients. *Injury*. 2013;44(1):86-90.

121. Lapostolle F, Sebbah JL, Couvreur J. Risk factors for the onset of hypothermia in trauma victims: the Hypotrauma study. *Crit Care*. 2012;16(4):R142. doi: 10.1186/cc1144

122. Trentzsch H, Huber-Wagner S, Hildebrand F, et al. Hypothermia for prediction of death in severely injured blunt trauma patients. *Shock*. 2012;37(2):131-139.

123. Nolan JP, Morley PT, Vanden Hoek TL, et al. Therapeutic hypothermia after cardiac arrest: an advisory statement by the Advance Life Support Task Force of the International Liaison Committee on Resuscitation. *Circulation*. 2003;108:118-121.

124. Alzaga AG, Cerdan M, Varon J. Therapeutic hypothermia. *Resuscitation*. 2006;70:369-380.

125. Nolan JP, Neumar RW, Adrie C, et al. Post-cardiac arrest syndrome: epidemiology, pathophysiology, treatment, and prognostication: a scientific statement from the International Liaison Committee on Resuscitation; the American Heart Association Emergency Cardiovascular Care Committee; the Council on Cardiovascular Surgery and Anesthesia; the Council on Cardiopulmonary, Perioperative, and Critical Care; the Council on Clinical Cardiology; the Council on Stroke. *Resuscitation*. 2008;79:350-379.

126. Nolan JP, Hazinski MF, Billi JE, et al. Part 1: executive summary: 2010 International Consensus on Cardiopulmonary Resuscitation and emergency cardiovascular care science with treatment recommendations. *Resuscitation*. 2010;81S:e1-e25.

127. Crompton EM, Lubomirova I, Cotlarciuc I, Han T, Sharma SD, Sharma P. Meta-analysis of therapeutic hypothermia for traumatic brain injury in adult and pediatric patients. *Crit Care Med*. 2017;45(4):575-583.

128. Andres PJD, Sinclair HL, Rodriguez A, et al. Hypothermia for intracranial hypertension after traumatic brain injury. *N Engl J Med*. 2015;373:2403-2412.

129. Finkelstein RA, Alam HB. Induced hypothermia for trauma: current research and practice. *J Intensive Care Med*. 2010;25(4):205-206.

130. Carlson LD. Immersion in cold water and body tissue insulation. *Aerospace Med*. 1958;29:145-152.

131. Giesbrecht GG, Steinman AM. Immersion into cold water. In: Auerbach PS, ed. *Auerbach's Wilderness Medicine.* 7th ed. Mosby Elsevier; 2017.

132. Wittmers LE, Savage M. Cold water immersion. In: Pandolf KB, Burr RE, eds. *Medical Aspects of Harsh Environments.* Vol 1. Office of the Surgeon General, Borden Institute/TMM Publications; 2001:531-552.

133. Tipton MJ. The initial responses to cold-water immersion in man. *Clin Sci.* 1989;77:581-588.

134. Keatinge WR, McIlroy MB, Goldfien A. Cardiovascular responses to ice-cold showers. *J Appl Physiol.* 1964;19: 1145-1150.

135. Mekjavic IB, La Prairie A, Burke W, Lindborg B. Respiratory drive during sudden cold water immersion. *Respir Physiol.* 1987;70(1):121-130.

136. Sempsrott J, Schmidt AC, Hawkins SC, Cushing TA. Drowning and submersion injuries. In: Auerbach PS. *Auerbach's Wilderness Medicine.* 7th ed. Mosby Elsevier; 2017.

137. Wissler EH. Probability of surviving during accidental immersion in cold water. *Aviat Space Environ Med.* 2003;74:47-55.

138. Tikuisis P. Predicting survival time at sea based on observed body cooling rates. *Aviat Space Environ Med.* 1997;68:441-448.

139. Hayward JS, Errickson JD, Collis ML. Thermal balance and survival time prediction of man in cold water. *Can J Physiol Pharmacol.* 1975;53(1):21-32.

140. Ducharme MB, Lounsbury DS. Self-rescue swimming in cold water: the latest advice. *Appl Physiol Nutr Metab.* 2007;32:799-807.

141. Van Mieghem C, Sabbe M, Knockaert D. The clinical value of the ECG in noncardiac conditions. *Chest.* 2004;125(4): 1561-1576.

142. Vanden Hoek TL, Morrison LJ, Shuster M, et al. Part 12.9: cardiac arrest in special situations: accidental hypothermia: 2010 American Heart Association guidelines for cardiopulmonary resuscitation and emergency cardiovascular care. *Circulation.* 2010;122:S829-S861.

143. Panchal AR, Bartos JA, Cabañas JG, et al. Part 3: adult basic and advanced life support: special circumstances of resuscitation: accidental hypothermia. 2020 American Heart Association guidelines for cardiopulmonary resuscitation and emergency cardiovascular care. *Circulation.* 2020;142(16):S366-S468.

144. Morrison LJ, Kierzek G, Diekema DS, et al. Part 3: Ethics. 2010 American Heart Association Guidelines for cardiopulmonary resuscitation and emergency cardiovascular care. *Circulation.* 2010;122:S665-S675.

145. Danzl DF, Lloyd EL. Treatment of accidental hypothermia. In: Pandolf KB, Burr RE, eds. *Medical Aspects of Harsh Environments.* Vol 1. Office of the Surgeon General, Borden Institute/TMM Publications; 2001:491-529.

146. Southwick FS, Dalglish PH. Recovery after prolonged asystolic cardiac arrest in profound hypothermia: a case report and literature review. *JAMA.* 1980;243:1250-1253.

147. Bernard MB, Gray TW, Buist MD, et al. Treatment of comatose survivors of out-of-hospital cardiac arrest with induced hypothermia. *N Engl J Med.* 2002;346(8): 557-563.

148. Reuler JB. Hypothermia: pathophysiology, clinical setting, and management. *Ann Intern Med.* 1978;89:519-527.

149. Armstrong LE. Cold, windchill, and water immersion. In: Armstrong LE. *Performing in Extreme Environments.* Human Kinetics; 2000.

150. Wilderness Medical Society. Myocardial infarction, acute coronary syndromes, and CPR. In: Forgey WW, ed. *Practice Guidelines for Wilderness Emergency Care.* 5th ed. Globe Pequot Press; 2006.

151. National Association of EMS Physicians. Position paper of the National Association of EMS Physicians: termination of resuscitation in nontraumatic cardiac arrest. *Prehosp Emerg Care.* 2011;15(4):542. doi: 10.3109/10903127 .2011.598621

152. Siegel AJ, d'Hemecourt P, Adner MM, Shirey T, Brown JL, Lewandrowski KB. Exertional dysnatremia in collapsed marathon runners: a critical role for point-of-care testing to guide appropriate therapy. *Am J Clin Pathol.* 2009;132(3):336-340.

153. Auerbach PS, Constance BB, Freer L. *Field Guide to Wilderness Medicine.* 4th ed. Mosby Elsevier; 2013.

Suggested Reading

Auerbach PS, ed. *Auerbach's Wilderness Medicine.* 7th ed. Mosby Elsevier; 2017.

Hawkins SC, Simon RB, Beissinger JP, Simon D. *Vertical Aid: Essential Wilderness Medicine for Climbers, Trekkers, and Mountaineers.* The Countryman Press; 2017.

Hawkins SC. *Wilderness EMS.* Wolters Kluwer; 2017.

CHAPTER **20**

Environmental Trauma II: Lightning, Drowning, Diving, and Altitude

Lead Editors
Seth C. Hawkins, MD
Justin Sempsrott, MD

CHAPTER OBJECTIVES
At the completion of this chapter, you will be able to do the following:

- Explain safety hazards associated with outdoor lightning strikes.
- Describe the use of "reverse" triage for multiple lightning casualties.
- Identify the key risk factors for high-altitude illness.
- Explain appropriate initial ABC (airway, breathing, and circulation) management of a drowning incident.
- Describe the management of a nonfatal drowning incident.

- Identify five methods for preventing a drowning incident.
- Contrast the signs and symptoms of type I and type II decompression sickness.
- Describe two primary treatment interventions for type II decompression sickness and arterial gas embolism.
- Discuss the similarities and differences between acute mountain sickness and high-altitude cerebral edema.

SCENARIO

In a coastal town, a family of four was strolling on the beach with their dog during a chilly winter day. The son tossed a rubber ball toward the water's edge, and the dog gave chase. In an instant, a large shore-breaking wave swallowed up the dog in the rough surf. The 17-year-old son was first into the water to attempt to save the dog, only to be overtaken by the water. He was seen struggling in the rough, surging surf by his parents and sister.

The boy's father and mother grabbed a nearby flotation device stationed on the beachfront and followed him into the surf to help. Their 19-year-old daughter remained on shore and called for help on her cell phone. The dog eventually made it back to the shore. The parents pulled their son out of the cold water after finding him submerged and unresponsive. Your paramedic unit arrives to the scene within 7 minutes of the daughter's call.

As you exit the ambulance, you observe an unconscious teenage boy lying partially prone with his face rotated to the side in sand with surging water close by. He is still in the surf zone and could be submersed by a wave. You join with arriving fire department emergency responders to approach the victim.

- How should you approach the patient in this setting?
- If the patient has no pulse or respirations, what is the next immediate intervention?
- What other concerns do you have for the patient that need to be addressed on scene?

INTRODUCTION

Each year worldwide, significant morbidity and mortality are caused by a variety of environmental conditions, including lightning strikes, drowning, recreational scuba diving, and high-altitude climbing. (See Chapter 19, *Environmental Trauma I: Heat and Cold*, for heat and cold conditions.) Prehospital care practitioners must know the disorders associated with each type of environment; understand the anatomy, physiology, and pathophysiology involved; and know how to rapidly perform patient assessment and management. At the same time, they must know how to prevent injury to themselves and other public safety personnel.

Lightning-Related Injuries

Lightning is the most widespread threat to people and property during the thunderstorm season and is second only to floods in causing storm-related deaths in the United States since 1959.[1] Over 50,000 thunderstorms occur daily in the world, with lightning striking the earth more than 100 times each second.[2] Lightning is reported to start approximately 75,000 forest fires annually and starts 40% of all fires.[3] The most destructive form of lightning is the cloud-to-ground strike (**Figure 20-1**). Based on real-time lightning-detection systems in the United States, it is estimated that cloud-to-ground lightning strikes occur approximately 20 million times per year, with as many as 50,000 flashes per hour during a summer afternoon.[4,5] In the United States, lightning occurs most frequently from June through August but occurs in Florida and along the southeastern coast of the Gulf of Mexico throughout the year, with Florida and Texas accounting for 25% of

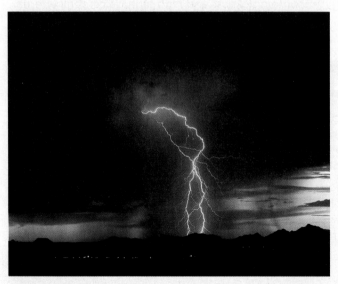

Figure 20-1 A cloud-to-ground lightning strike, with streak lightning pattern.
© Jhaz Photography/Shutterstock

lightning deaths.[6,7] Worldwide, rural populations are at the greatest risk due to the lack of lightning-safe structures and prevention education. Consequently, it is estimated that 24,000 fatalities occur annually, and lightning causes about 10 times more injuries than deaths worldwide.[7,8]

Since the 1950s, the number of deaths from lightning in the United States has decreased, possibly because of fewer people working outdoors in rural areas, improved warning systems for approaching storms, increased public education on lightning safety, and improved medical care.[9] While the early part of the 20th century saw as many as 400 annual deaths from lightning, the average number of annual deaths from 1968 to 2010 was 79, and the latest reports indicate that lightning now kills only about 30 individuals each year and injures about 400.[3,7,10-12] Based on a study of 2006–2019 data, the common belief that golfers are responsible for the majority of lightning deaths was shown to be a myth; during this time individuals fishing accounted for four times as many fatalities as golfers, and beach activities/camping accounted for twice as many fatalities as golfers. June through August were by far the peak months for lightning activity and lightning deaths, with weekend days (Friday–Sunday) being the most common.[12]

The greatest threats from lightning strikes are neurologic and cardiopulmonary injuries. Practice guidelines from the Wilderness Medical Society (WMS) are available for the prevention and treatment of lightning injuries for prehospital and in-hospital care.[13] These recommendations for medical management are graded based on the quality of the supporting evidence. (See Chapter 2, *Golden Principles, Preferences, and Critical Thinking*.)

Epidemiology

Based on National Oceanic and Atmospheric Administration (NOAA) data, in the years from 2006 to 2019, there were 418 deaths due to lightning. Of these fatalities, 79% were male.[12]

Cranial or leg burn involvement indicates a greater risk for death, and some analyses show that about 74% of lightning strike survivors have permanent disabilities.[14] However, this finding is controversial, with other studies reporting much less permanent injury.[11,15] Of the individuals who died from a lightning strike, 52% were outside (25% of whom were at work). Death occurred within 1 hour in 63% of the lightning victims in one review of Florida lightning incidents.[9]

Mechanism of Injury

Injury from lightning can result from the following six mechanisms:[11,13,14]

- *Direct strike* occurs when a person is in an open environment unable to find shelter. It accounts for only 3% to 5% of lightning strikes involving people.[7]

- *Side flash* or *splash contact* occurs when lightning hits an object (e.g., ground, building, tree) and splashes onto a victim or multiple victims. The current will jump from the primary strike object and can splash over to a person. Splashes occur from person to person, tree to person, and even indoors from telephone wire to a person talking on the phone (this can sometimes be direct rather than splash contact, depending on phone and wire proximity to face).

- *Contact* occurs when a person is in direct contact with an object that is struck directly or by a splash. It accounts for one-third of all lightning injuries. For rescue personnel who may have metal gear on their body (such as carabiners) or who are tied into a rescue system such as a belay during a climbing rescue that could involve a thunderstorm, the WMS and climbing medicine experts recommend tying off individually. Also, metal objects such as carabiners, ice tools, or hiking/ski poles should be isolated and direct contact avoided.[7,13]

- *Step voltage* occurs when lightning hits the ground or a nearby object and the current spreads outward radially, passing through a person's body in the process. Human tissue provides less resistance than the ground, and the current will travel, for example, up one leg and down the other, following the path of least resistance. Ground current accounts for the majority of lightning injuries. Step voltage is also known as *stride voltage* or *ground current*.

- *Upward streamer* occurs when current passes up from the ground and through the victim but does not connect with the downward lightning streamer. The energy in this streamer is less, compared to a full lightning strike, and accounts for approximately 1% to 15% of lightning injuries. Upward streamer is a more recently identified form of lightning contact.

- *Blast injury* or other blunt trauma can occur from a shock wave produced by lightning, which can propel a person up to 30 feet (9.1 meters [m]). In addition, injuries can result from lightning that causes forest fires, building fires, and explosions.[3,16,17]

The following are six known factors that determine the injury severity from electrical and lightning current:

- Type of circuit
- Duration of exposure
- Voltage
- Amperage
- Resistance of tissue
- Current pathway

Once lightning or another high-voltage electrical source contacts the human body, the heat generated within the body is directly proportional to the amount of current, tissue resistance, and duration of contact. As resistance of various tissues increases (e.g., nerve < blood < muscle < skin < fat < bone), so does the heat generated by the passage of current.

It is easy to assume that lightning injuries are like high-voltage electrical injuries. However, significant differences exist between the two mechanisms of injury. A lightning strike is direct current (DC) as opposed to alternating current (AC), which is responsible for industrial and household electrical injuries. Lightning produces millions of volts of electrical charge, with currents ranging from 30,000 to 50,000 amperes, and the duration of exposure to the body is instantaneous (10 to 100 milliseconds). The temperature of lightning varies with the diameter, but the average temperature is approximately 14,430°F (8,000°C).[10] In comparison, high-voltage electrical exposure tends to be a much lower voltage than lightning. However, the key factor that distinguishes lightning injury from high-voltage electrical injury is the duration of current exposure within the body.[16] The result is a more prolonged electrical injury exposure with deeper resultant burn injury, and more extensive risk of deep muscle and kidney injury. The resultant cardiac dysrhythmia is more commonly ventricular fibrillation,

At times, lightning can show injury patterns like those seen with high-voltage electricity because of a rare lightning pattern that produces a prolonged strike lasting up to 0.5 second. This type of lightning, called *hot lightning*, can cause deep burns to human tissue, explode trees, and set fires. Lightning can show entry and exit wounds on the body, but a more common pathway of lightning once it strikes a victim is to pass over the body. This is referred to as a *flashover* current. A flashover current can also enter the eyes, ears, nose, and mouth. It is theorized that the flashover current flow is the reason why many victims survive lightning strikes. It is also known that a flashover current may vaporize moisture on skin or blast a part of clothing or shoes off a victim. The immense flashover current generates large magnetic fields, which can, in turn, induce secondary electric currents within the body and are thought to cause cardiac arrest and other internal injuries.[18,19]

Injuries From Lightning

Lightning injuries range from minor, superficial wounds to major multisystem trauma and death. **Table 20-1** lists common signs and symptoms of lightning injury. As a tool to determine the likely recovery or prognosis from lightning strikes, victims can be placed in one of three injury categories: minor, moderate, and severe.[13,20]

Minor Injury

Patients with minor injury are awake and report an unpleasant and abnormal sensation (*dysesthesia*) in the affected extremity or extremities. In a more serious lightning strike, victims report they have been hit in the head or state that an

Table 20-1 Lightning Injury: Common Signs, Symptoms, and Treatment

Injuries	Signs/Symptoms	Treatment
Minor	Feeling of strange sensation in extremity; confusion; amnesia; temporary unconsciousness, deafness, or blindness; tympanic membrane rupture	Scene safety; XABCDEs; medical history and secondary survey; monitor ECG; give oxygen and transport all patients with mild injuries.
Moderate	Disorientation, combativeness, paralysis, fractures, blunt trauma, absent pulses in lower extremities, spinal shock, seizures, temporary cardiorespiratory arrest, comatose	Scene safety; XABCDEs; medical history and secondary survey; monitor ECG; CPR (CAB) early when needed; give oxygen and transport all patients.
Severe	Any of the above, otorrhea (fluid leak) in ear canal, cardiac fibrillation or cardiac asystole	CPR (CAB) and advanced lifesaving procedures; use "reverse" triage with multiple patients.

Abbreviations: CAB, circulation, airway, breathing; CPR, cardiopulmonary resuscitation; ECG, electrocardiogram; XABCDE, exsanguinating hemorrhage, airway, breathing, circulation, disability, expose/environment.

Data from O'Keefe Gatewood M, Zane RD. Lightning injuries. *Emerg Med Clin North Am.* 2004;22:369-403; and Cooper MA, Andrews CJ, Holle RL, Blumenthal R, Aldana NN. Lightning-related injuries and safety. In: Auerbach PS, ed. *Auerbach's Wilderness Medicine.* 7th ed. Mosby Elsevier; 2017:71-118.

explosion hit them, because they are unsure of the source. A patient may present at the scene with the following:

- Confusion (short term or hours to days)
- Amnesia (short term or hours to days)
- Temporary deafness
- Blindness
- Temporary unconsciousness
- Temporary paresthesia
- Muscular pain
- Cutaneous burns (rare)
- Transient paralysis

Victims present with normal vital signs or with mild, transient hypertension, and recovery is usually gradual and complete.

Moderate Injury

Victims with moderate injury have progressive single or multisystem injuries, some of which are life threatening. Some patients in this category can have a permanent disability. Patients may present at the scene with the following:

- Immediate effects
  - Seizures
  - Deafness
  - Cardiac arrest and cardiac injuries
  - Pulmonary injuries
  - Confusion, amnesia
  - Blindness
  - Dizziness
  - Contusion from shockwave
  - Blunt trauma (e.g., fractures)
  - Chest pain, muscle aches
  - Tympanic membrane rupture
  - Headache, nausea, postconcussion syndrome
- Delayed effects
  - Neurologic symptoms and signs
  - Memory deficits
  - Attention deficits
  - Neuropsychological changes
  - Coding and retrieval problems
  - Distractibility
  - Personality changes
  - Irritability
  - Chronic pain
  - Seizures

Depending on the location of the lightning strike, a strike affecting the respiratory center of the brain can result in prolonged respiratory arrest that may lead to secondary cardiac arrest as a result of hypoxemia.[14] Victims in this category may experience immediate cardiopulmonary arrest, although the inherent automaticity of the heart may produce a spontaneous return to normal sinus rhythm.[14] Because immediate cardiopulmonary arrest is the greatest threat, prehospital care practitioners need to address immediate life threats in a CAB (circulation, airway, breathing) sequence immediately for all lightning strike victims and continuously monitor the electrocardiogram (ECG) for secondary cardiac events, which may occur as far out as 3 days after the incident.[13]

Severe Injury

The mechanism for sudden death from lightning strike is simultaneous cardiac and respiratory arrest. Victims with severe injury from a direct lightning strike (cardiovascular or neurologic injuries) or delays in cardiopulmonary resuscitation (CPR) have a poor prognosis. On arrival at the scene, the prehospital care practitioner may find the patient in cardiac arrest with asystole or ventricular fibrillation. Lightning causes a massive DC countershock, which simultaneously depolarizes the entire myocardium.[18] The American Heart Association (AHA) recommends vigorous resuscitation measures for those who appear dead on initial evaluation. This is based on many reports of excellent recovery after lightning-induced cardiac arrest and on the fact that victims in this category are typically young and without heart disease.[17] Data published in 1980 suggested that only 23% of lightning strike patients receiving CPR survived[14]; this statistic is still shared in contemporary medical literature but may not account for more recent innovations in CPR-based resuscitation. Of all causes of cardiopulmonary arrest, lightning may have one of the most promising prognoses for recovery, because the initial insult is temporary and may be reversible.

It is not uncommon to observe the initial cardiac arrest with spontaneous recovery of electrical activity following the lightning strike, but any ongoing respiratory arrest due to a paralyzed medullary respiratory center may cause secondary hypoxemic cardiac arrest.[17,21] If prolonged cardiac and neurologic ischemia has occurred, it may be very difficult to resuscitate these patients.[10] Other common findings are tympanic membrane rupture with cerebrospinal fluid and blood in the ear canal; ocular injuries; and various forms of blunt trauma from falls, including soft-tissue contusions and fractures of the skull, ribs, extremities, and spine. Many patients in this category have no evidence of burns. In those patients presenting with cutaneous burns caused by lightning, it is generally reported to be less than 20% total body surface area.

Injury to the central nervous system (CNS) is common in a lightning victim and has been classified into four groups of CNS injuries[14]:

- *Group 1 CNS effects* (immediate and transient): Loss of consciousness (75%); paresthesias (80%); weakness (80%); confusion, amnesia, and headaches
- *Group 2 CNS effects* (immediate and prolonged): Hypoxic ischemic neuropathy; intracranial hemorrhage; postarrest cerebral infarction
- *Group 3 CNS effects* (possible delayed neurologic syndromes): Motor neuron diseases and movement disorders
- *Group 4 CNS effects* (trauma from fall or blast): Subdural and epidural hematomas and subarachnoid hemorrhage

Assessment

On arrival at the scene, as with any other call, the priority is the safety of the prehospital care practitioners and other public safety personnel. Emergency responders must determine whether there is still a chance of lightning in the area. Even when a storm approaches or has passed, there still is a source of danger that is not always apparent, because lightning remains a real threat as far as 10 to 15 miles away from the main storm cell—hence its nickname, the "bolt from the blue." Indeed, this reality is a source of the popular saying "out of the blue" or "out of the clear blue sky" for an unexpected event.[7,14]

The mechanism of injury may be unclear without a witness because lightning can strike during a sunny day. When in doubt about the mechanism of injury, immediately assess for XABCDEs (eXsanguinating hemorrhage, Airway management, Breathing, Circulation, Disability, Expose/environment) and any life-threatening conditions, as for any emergency. Patients who were struck by lightning (as opposed to those electrocuted as a result of other mechanisms) do not carry an electrical charge, and touching them poses no risk in providing patient care. Assess the victim's heart rhythm with the ECG. It is common to see nonspecific ST-segment and T-wave changes such as QT interval prolongation and transient T-wave inversions, but more specific evidence of myocardial infarction with Q-wave or ST-segment elevation is rarely seen.[22]

Once the patient is stable, a detailed head-to-toe assessment is necessary to identify the wide range of injuries that can occur with this type of trauma. Assess the patient's situational awareness and the neurologic function of all extremities, because the upper and lower extremities may experience transient paralysis (known as *keraunoparalysis*). Lightning victims have been known to have an autonomic dysfunction that causes dilated pupils, which mimics head trauma.[21] Assess the eyes because more than half of victims have some form of ocular injury. Look for blood and cerebrospinal fluid in the ear canals; half of these victims will have one or two ruptured tympanic membranes. All victims of lightning injury have a high probability of blunt trauma from being thrown against a solid object or being struck by falling objects or other musculoskeletal injury such as dislocation from muscle spasm. Possibility of spinal injury should be considered during the assessment and corresponding management steps implemented as determined by local protocol.

Assess the skin for signs of burns, ranging from superficial to full thickness. Lightning burns may or may not be apparent in the field because they develop within the first few hours. Burns occur in less the one-half of lightning survivors and in most cases are superficial.[13,14] It is common to see a feathering appearance in the skin,

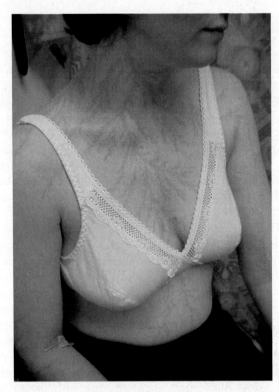

Figure 20-2 Lichtenberg figures.

known as **Lichtenberg figures**, but these patterns are not burns and resolve in 24 hours (**Figure 20-2**). It is more common to see burns caused by igniting of clothes and heating of jewelry or other objects.

If the incident involves multiple victims, the principles of triage should be implemented immediately. The normal rules of triage are to focus limited personnel and resources on patients with moderate and severe injuries and quickly bypass those patients without respiration and circulation. However, with multiple lightning strike patients, the rule changes to use "reverse" triage and "resuscitate the dead," because these patients are either in respiratory arrest or cardiac arrest and have a high probability of recovery if managed expeditiously.[7,10,11,14,23] In contrast, other patients who have survived a lightning strike have little likelihood of deteriorating, unless there is associated trauma and occult hemorrhage.[10]

Management

The priorities for managing a lightning victim are to ensure scene safety for yourself and your crew and to assess any victim for XABCDE. If spontaneous respiration or circulation is absent, initiate effective CPR up to five cycles (2 minutes), and evaluate the heart rhythm with an automated external defibrillator (AED) or cardiac monitor based on current guidelines.[17] AEDs have proven helpful in some documented cases.[10] Use advanced life support (ALS)

measures to manage lightning-induced cardiopulmonary arrest based on current AHA guidelines for advanced cardiovascular life support (ACLS) and pediatric advanced life support (PALS), as discussed elsewhere.[17] Evaluate and treat for shock and hypothermia. Apply high-flow oxygen for all moderately and severely injured patients. Intravenous fluids should be started at a keep vein open (KVO) rate, because patients who have been injured by lightning, unlike conventional high-voltage electrical-injured patients, do not have massive tissue destruction and burns requiring a larger amount of fluids. Patients who show unstable vital signs or who have sustained associated trauma may have their fluids titrated as appropriate.

Stabilize any fractures and package the blunt trauma patient, keeping spinal motion restriction principles in mind and avoiding cervical extrication collar and backboard unless indicated.[24] Lightning strike victims with minor to severe injuries need to be transported to an emergency department (ED) for further evaluation and observation. Transport the patient by either ground or air, as determined by availability, distance, and time to the hospital and overall risk to the flight crew and benefit to the patient.

As mentioned previously, lightning strike victims have a higher probability of a positive outcome from early and effective resuscitation. However, there is little evidence to suggest that these patients can regain a pulse from prolonged basic life support (BLS) or ALS procedures lasting longer than 20 to 30 minutes.[3] Before terminating resuscitation, all efforts should be made to stabilize the patient by establishing an airway, supporting ventilation, and correcting any hypovolemia, hypothermia, and acidemia.

Prevention

With numerous thunderstorms throughout the year, lightning ground strikes are common. Both prehospital care practitioners and the general public must be educated about prevention and the many lightning myths and misconceptions (**Box 20-1**). Numerous lightning-prevention resources are provided by agencies such as the National Weather Service/NOAA, National Lightning Safety Institute, American Red Cross, and Federal Emergency Management Agency.[25-27]

Official guidelines are published for lightning-injury prevention and treatment by both national and international medical commissions and organizations, including the WMS, the AHA, the International Commission for Mountain Emergency Medicine, and the medical commission of the International Climbing and Mountaineering Federation (**Box 20-2**).[13,17,28]

Prehospital care practitioners and other public safety personnel should establish procedures for a severe weather watch that provides storm warnings and is updated throughout the day as one method of prevention. There is no place that is 100% safe outdoors. The

Box 20-1 Myths and Misconceptions About Lightning

General Myths

All of the following common beliefs about lightning are *false*:

- Lightning strikes are invariably fatal.
- A major cause of death is burns.
- A victim struck by lightning bursts into flames or is reduced to ashes.
- Victims remain charged or electrified after they are struck.
- Individuals are only at risk for being struck when there are storm clouds overhead.
- Occupying a building during the storm affords 100% protection from lightning.
- Lightning never strikes the same place twice.
- Wearing rubber-soled shoes and a raincoat will protect a person.
- Rubber tires in a vehicle are what protect a person from injury.
- Wearing metal jewelry increases the risk of attracting lightning.
- Lightning always hits the highest object.
- There is no danger from lightning unless it is raining.
- Lightning can occur without thunder.

Misconceptions Regarding Patient Care

Some myths and misconceptions held by prehospital care practitioners can adversely affect the care and outcomes of their patients.

- Victims who are not immediately killed by lightning will be okay.
- If the victim has no outward signs of injury, the damage cannot be that serious.
- Lightning injuries should be treated similar to other high-voltage electrical injuries.
- Lightning victims who undergo resuscitation efforts for several hours might still recover successfully.

Data from O'Keefe Gatewood M, Zane RD. Lightning injuries. *Emerg Med Clin North Am.* 2004;22(2):369-403.

Box 20-2 Prevention Guidelines for Prehospital Care Practitioners in Mountainous Regions

Prehospital care practitioners servicing mountainous regions are at greater risk for lightning strike, especially those who serve as park rangers, SAR members, and other public safety personnel in high-altitude and remote areas. Some general prevention guidelines for these practitioners include the following:

- Take note of the weather forecast, because thunder and lightning in the mountains occur mainly during summer months in the late afternoons and night. Thus, the saying, "Up by noon and down by 2:00 p.m." is used to remind individuals to return to lower elevations by the middle to late afternoon to decrease the risk for lightning strike.
- The best place to get out of a lightning storm in the mountains is a hut or mountain refuge. Stay away from open doors and windows.
- Tents do not provide any protection from lightning strike, and tent poles may act as lightning rods.
- Larger caves and valleys are protective, but small caves provide little protection if the person is near the opening and sidewalls.
- Wet stream beds are more dangerous than open areas.
- Stay off mountain ridges and summits, power lines, and ski lifts.
- Stay clear of the base of taller trees since lightning will travel down the trunk to the base. In a forest, it is best to get into a cluster of smaller trees.
- If caught in the open, do not sit or lie flat. It is best to crouch down with feet or knees together and keep contact with as small an area of the ground as possible to minimize injury from ground current. Prehospital care practitioners should try to use some insulation between themselves and the ground, such as a dry pack on which to kneel or sit.
- If in a group, stay apart from each other, but within sight, to reduce the number of people injured by ground current or side flashes between persons.
- Consider the use of small, portable lightning detectors so that advance warning is received and prevention steps can be implemented before the storm arrives.

© National Association of Emergency Medical Technicians (NAEMT)

ambulance is the safest shelter if the practitioners are near it when no large building is available.

One public education motto used is, "If you see it, flee it; if you hear it, clear it." Another useful rule is the "30–30 rule." When the time between seeing lightning and hearing thunder is 30 seconds or less, individuals are in danger and need to seek appropriate shelter. Following this rule, it is considered safe to resume outdoor activity only after 30 minutes following the last lightning or thunder, because a thunderstorm still is a threat and lightning can strike up to 10 to 15 miles from the main storm cell even after the storm has passed.[7,27,29] Another measure of lightning proximity is the "flash-to-bang" rule, which states that 5 seconds = 1 mile (1.6 kilometers [km]); that is, following lightning, for every 5 seconds until the sound of thunder, the lightning is 1 mile (1.6 km) away. Note that some erroneous teaching of

---

Box 20-3 Lightning Safety Guidelines

The following are guidelines for lightning safety as a storm develops:

- Find a lightning-safe vehicle or a lightning-safe structure.[25,29]
  - An automobile that is a fully enclosed metal vehicle is a lightning-safe shelter. Other all-metal mobile transportation-related vehicles such as airplanes, buses, vans, and construction equipment with enclosed, mostly metal cabs are also safe. A cautionary note, however, will emphasize that the "outer metal shield" of a vehicle should not be compromised. This means:
    - Windows need to be rolled up.
    - Contact must not be made with any interior objects such as radio dials, metal door handles, two-way radio microphones, etc., that connect with external objects.
  - All other objects that penetrate from inside to outside should be avoided.
  - Unsafe vehicles include those made of fiberglass and other plastics, plus small riding machinery or vehicles without enclosed canopies, such as motorcycles, farm tractors, golf carts, and all-terrain vehicles.
  - Metal buildings are lightning-safe places. So, too, are large, permanent structures made of masonry and wood. Once again, the caveat is to not become part of the pathway conducting lightning. This means avoiding all electrical circuits, switches, powered equipment, metal doors and windows, hand rails, and so on. Small post-supported structures, such as bus stops, picnic shelters, or baseball field dugouts, are not safe.

The following are guidelines for lightning safety when indoors:

- Stay away from windows, open doors, fireplaces, bath and shower, and metal objects such as sinks and appliances.

- Turn off the radio and computer and avoid hardwired telephones; use a telephone only in an emergency.
- Turn off all faucets, electrical appliances, and devices before a storm arrives.

The following are guidelines for lightning safety when outdoors:

- Avoid using handheld radios, cell phones, or other electronic signal/communication devices, if possible.
- Avoid metal objects such as bikes, tractors, and fences.
- Avoid tall objects such as trees, and make yourself small.
- Avoid areas near pipelines, power lines, and ski lifts.
- Avoid open fields.
- Avoid open shelters (e.g., carport, bus shelter), depending on overall size, because side flashes or ground strikes can occur.
- Drop ski poles and golf clubs, which may attract lightning.
- In large public outdoor events, seek out nearby buses or minivans.
- Seek to make the smallest contact with ground, if possible, to minimize ground contact. In the "lightning position," the individual squats with the feet together, hands covering the ears; a ground pad, backpack, or some insulation material is placed under the feet. An alternative position of comfort is to kneel or sit cross-legged.
- Do not stand, hug, squat, or huddle near tall trees; seek out a low area of lower trees or saplings.
- Seek out ditches unless there is contact with water.
- If on water, seek shore immediately and move inland, away from the water. Avoid swimming, boating, or being near the tallest object on water.[1,10]

---

the 30–30 rule suggests that 30 minutes following the last thunderclap, the storm cell is 30 miles or more away. As the "flash-to-bang" rule explains, when the time between the flash and the boom is 30 seconds or less, the storm is only 6 miles (9.7 km) away, well within the 10- to 15-mile (16.1–24.1 km) distance for lightning strike outside the main storm cell.[7]

For more information about preventing lightning strike, see **Box 20-3**. See **Box 20-4** for information about support for lightning strike survivors.

Box 20-4 Survivors of Lightning Injury

Support for survivors of lightning injury is available from Lightning Strike and Electric Shock Survivors International, Inc. (LS&ESSI, Inc.). This nonprofit support group comprises survivors, their families, and other interested parties. There are members throughout the United States and in more than 13 other countries (www.lightning-strike.org).

Drowning

Drowning is common in the United States, accounting for over 4,000 deaths annually.[30] Drowning remains a leading cause of preventable death across all age groups but is an epidemic among children.[31-34] The World Health Organization estimates that approximately 236,000 deaths occurred in 2019 from drowning, accounting for 7% of all injury-related deaths globally, making it the third leading cause of unintentional injury death.[30,31,35] This statistic likely underestimates the actual global burden of drowning, as it does not include nonfatal drownings, or deaths from drowning due to floods, suicide, or homicide; furthermore, in many middle- and low-income countries, patients may die from drowning and never reach a hospital.[30,35]

Previously, *drowning* was defined as the *outcome* by which air-breathing mammals *died* due to submersion in a liquid. We now understand drowning as a process, not an outcome. Multiple modifier terms were historically used, including *dry drowning*, *wet drowning*, *secondary drowning*, *delayed drowning*, and *near-drowning*.[30] None of these terms has a universal or accepted medical definition, particularly across cultural and international contexts. The updated definition adopted at the 2002 World Congress of Drowning states that drowning is the process of respiratory impairment as a result of submersion or immersion in a liquid medium, usually water.[36-39]

There has always been a desire to define and classify those patients who were submerged or immersed but initially survived, only to later die. Classification schemes based on salinity or the presence of water in the lungs at autopsy distract from the primary pathophysiology and final common pathway of drowning, namely cerebral anoxia. Just as someone who survives a stroke, regardless of morbidity, would not be said to have had a "near stroke," there is no role for terms like dry drowning, secondary drowning, and near-drowning, a position which has also been adopted by the World Health Organization, the International Liaison Committee on Resuscitation, the WMS, the U.S. Centers for Disease Control and Prevention (CDC), the AHA, the American Red Cross, and the American College of Emergency Physicians.[36,40]

The drowning process begins with respiratory impairment as the person's airway goes below the surface of the water (submersion) or water splashes over the face (immersion, with injury through aspiration).[41] The drowning process has only three outcomes or modifiers: fatal drownings (the patient dies), nonfatal drownings with morbidity (the patient lives but sustains injury or illness), and nonfatal drownings without morbidity (there is no death or apparent significant injury or illness).[30,37,42] Further considerations involving the classification of drowning include the following:

- Incidents involving patients who experience submersion or immersion *without* respiratory impairment, but who require retrieval from the water, should be considered a water rescue and not a drowning.
- As with lightning, the WMS has developed consensus-driven practice guidelines for drowning that are helpful in evaluating the most current recommendations and their evidence within the wilderness medicine community.[43]

Epidemiology

Drowning is the fifth leading cause of unintentional injury death for all ages in the United States, but it overwhelmingly affects younger age groups.[30,44] Drowning is the leading cause of death by unintentional injury for ages 1 to 4 years, the second leading cause of injury death for ages 5 to 14 years, and the third leading cause of injury death for ages 15 to 24 years.[45] It is the third leading cause of injury death in infants (younger than age 1 year), who are often at risk for drowning in bathtubs, buckets, and toilets.[32,46] The CDC reported that from 2010 to 2019 there were an average of 3,957 cases of unintentional fatal drownings in the United States each year, and an estimated 8,080 cases were treated in U.S. hospital EDs each year for nonfatal drowning.[32,33] An additional 347 people died each year from drowning in boating-related incidents.[32]

Fatal incidents occur most often in natural water settings (lakes, rivers, and oceans), followed by pools and bathtubs.[32] In comparison, unintentional nonfatal drownings treated in EDs in the United States were highest for pools, followed by natural settings and bathtubs. The nonfatal and fatal injury rates were the highest for children 4 years or younger and for males of all ages. The nonfatal rate for males was almost twice that of females, and 80% of fatal drowning patients are males.[44]

For every child who fatally drowns, four others seek emergency care for nonfatal drowning, with outcomes ranging from no to varying degrees of irreversible brain injury.[30,34,44,46]

Devastating neurologic injury is the most feared outcome for drowning survivors of all ages and demonstrates the axiom that drowning is truly a neurologic disease with a pulmonary pathway. The major determinant of survival and long-term functionality following drowning is the extent of CNS injury.[30]

Risk Factors for Drowning

Specific factors place individuals at an increased risk for drowning.[30,36,46-48] Recognizing these factors will increase awareness and assist in the creation of preventive strategies and policies to minimize these occurrences. For infants and young children, the major risk factor is inadequate supervision; for adolescents and adults, it is risky behavior and use of drugs or alcohol.[46]

Drowning risk factors include the following:

- *Breathing behaviors leading to hypoxic blackout.* To increase their underwater swim distance, some swimmers will intentionally hyperventilate immediately before going underwater, lowering their partial pressure of arterial carbon dioxide ($PaCO_2$). Because the body's carbon dioxide level provides the stimulus to breathe in patients without chronic obstructive pulmonary disease,[49] a decrease in $PaCO_2$ decreases the feedback to the respiratory center in the hypothalamus to take a breath during breath holding. However, these swimmers are at risk of drowning because the partial pressure of arterial oxygen (PaO_2) does not change significantly with hyperventilation. As the individual continues to swim underwater, PaO_2 will decrease significantly and cause a possible loss of consciousness and cerebral hypoxia. This condition has been called shallow water blackout,[50,51] hypoxia of ascent (in a diving context), surface blackout, and static apnea blackout,[52] although the terms "hypoxic blackout" and "hypoxic loss of consciousness" are commonly used terms for this condition.[53-55]

- *Accidental cold-water immersion leading to cold shock.* Another situation that places individuals at greater risk of drowning is cold-water immersion (*head out*). The physiologic changes that occur with cold-water immersion can have either a disastrous outcome or a protective effect on the body, depending on many circumstances.[30] Adverse outcomes are more common, resulting from both cardiovascular collapse and sudden death within minutes of cold-water immersion, a condition known as "cold shock." (See Chapter 19, *Environmental Trauma I: Heat and Cold*, for more information.)

- *Age.* Drowning is recognized as a young person's epidemic, with toddlers as the largest group, based on their inquisitive nature and momentary lapses in adult supervision. Children younger than 4 years have the highest drowning rate.[32,56]

- *Gender.* Males account for 80% of drownings, with two age-related peak incidences.[44] The first peak incidence occurs in males at age 2 years, which decreases until age 10 years and then rises rapidly to peak again at age 18 years. Older males may be more at risk for drowning because of higher exposure rates to aquatic activities, higher alcohol consumption while at the waterfront, and more risk-taking behavior.[30,57]

- *Race.* Due to the history of segregation in the United States, many older African Americans were denied access to pools and swimming lessons. If a grandparent or parent does not swim, swimming lessons for children may become a lower priority for the family. Today, African American children drown more often than white children. African American children tend to drown in ponds, lakes, and other natural sources of water.[31] However, when drowning occurs in a swimming pool, African American children from age 5 to 19 years fatally drown 5.5 times more often than white children, with the greatest disparity in the 11- to 12-year-old subset, where African American children drown 10 times more often than white children.[44] Overall, the drowning rate of African American male children has been estimated to be as high as three times that of white males, and in the military, African American soldiers drown 62% more often than white soldiers.[58,59] Drowning rates are also higher for immigrants, Hispanics, and other minority groups for multiple reasons that are poorly understood.

- *Location.* Drowning typically occurs in backyard swimming pools and in natural areas such as lakes, ponds, and the ocean, but it also occurs in buckets and bathtubs.[30,60] Houses in rural areas with open wells increase the risk of a young child drowning sevenfold.[30] Other hazardous locations are water barrels, fountains, and underground cisterns.

- *Alcohol and drugs.* Alcohol is often associated with drowning,[30,61,62] likely because it impairs judgment.[47] As many as 20% to 30% of adult boating fatalities and drownings involve alcohol use in which the occupants used poor judgment, were speeding, failed to wear life jackets, or handled the watercraft recklessly.[30,63]

- *Underlying disease or trauma.* The onset of illness from underlying disease can lead to drowning. Hypoglycemia, myocardial infarction, cardiac dysrhythmia, depression and suicidal thoughts, and syncope predispose individuals to drowning incidents.[46] A study reported that the risk of drowning in people with epilepsy is raised 15- to 19-fold compared to people in the general population.[64] Polypharmacy in the elderly has led to increased rates of drowning in persons age 65 years and older. Cervical spine injuries and head trauma should be suspected in all unwitnessed incidents and injuries involving body surfers, board surfers, and victims diving in shallow water or water with submerged objects such as rocks or trees. Note that long backboard immobilization in or out of water is no longer recommended by leading lifeguard organizations or wilderness EMS authorities, although backboards may be useful as a transportation tool in moving patients.[65-69] (See Chapter 9, *Spinal Trauma*, for a detailed discussion of spinal protection.)

- *Child abuse.* A high incidence of nonaccidental trauma from drowning is reported, particularly in bathtubs. A study of children sustaining bathtub drowning deaths between 1982 and 1992 found that 67% had historical or physical findings compatible with a diagnosis of abuse or neglect.[48] Consequently, it is highly recommended that any suspicious child-drowning bathtub incident be reported to local social services for appropriate investigation.

- *Hypothermia.* Drowning may result directly from prolonged immersion leading to hypothermia. (See the "Cold-Related Disorders" section in Chapter 19, *Environmental Trauma I: Heat and Cold*, for further discussion of accidental hypothermia.) Hypothermia is defined as a core (central) body temperature less than 95°F (35°C). Immersion into water allows for rapid loss of body heat into the usually cooler water, thus precipitating hypothermia, although most deaths in cold water are due directly to drowning, not secondary to hypothermia. Any time boating or other nonswimming activities are done in cold water, a personal flotation device (PFD) must be available and, ideally, should be worn during any operation that could lead to immersion or submersion.

- Interestingly, *ability to swim* is not a consistent risk factor for drowning.[30] This may be because nonswimmers may avoid water, while highly talented swimmers (like surfers or military personnel routinely deployed in aquatic environments) might take higher risks. White men have a higher incidence of drowning than white women, even though they are reported to have better swimming ability.[30] On the other hand, one study reported that nonswimmers or beginners accounted for 73% of drownings in home swimming pools and 82% of incidents in canals, lakes, and ponds.[70] Although, statistically speaking, the ability to swim might not correlate with a reduced risk of drowning, swimming instruction is nonetheless recommended and encouraged as a preventive measure against drowning. One study suggests that children ages 1 to 4 years with some formal swim instruction are more than eight times less likely to die by drowning than matched controls.[71] However, for young children, far more protective than swimming lessons is vigilant adult supervision.[30] In addition, in many nontechnical water exposures (e.g., not surf or whitewater), survival ability may be linked to one's ability to stay afloat, not swim, emphasizing the importance of PFDs or other flotation devices, as well as directing educational opportunities for those seeking survival skills (flotation) rather than true swimming skills.

Mechanism of Injury

A common scenario of *head-out immersion* in water or a whole-body submersion incident begins with a situation that creates a panic response, leading to breath holding, air hunger, and increased physical activity in an effort to stay or get above the water surface. According to most bystander reports, submersion victims are rarely seen screaming and waving for assistance while struggling to stay above the surface of the water. Rather, they are seen either floating on the surface or in a motionless position, or they dive underwater and fail to come up. As the drowning process progresses, a reflex inspiratory effort draws water into the pharynx and larynx, causing a choking response. Drowning experts report that laryngospasm is very rare, probably occurring in 3% of cases or less.[41,66] In the vast majority of cases, it is water aspiration and subsequent hypoxemia that causes unconsciousness.[41]

As noted earlier, archaic and historical dialogues about the pathophysiology of drowning persist in modern medicine, mostly concerning differences between drowning in freshwater versus saltwater and whether water did or did not enter the lungs.[37,46,60] Regardless, the final common pathway is cerebral anoxia, and these distinctions are not medically helpful.

For prehospital care practitioners, the common denominator in any drowning is brain hypoxia. Whether hypoxemia results from submersion, laryngospasm, or aspiration is not meaningful to patient management or outcome. The whole drowning process from immersion or submersion to hypoxemia, apnea, loss of consciousness, cardiac arrest, pulseless electrical activity, and asystole usually occurs in seconds to a few minutes.[41] For those who survive, patient management should be aimed at quickly reversing hypoxemia and subsequent tissue hypoxia (especially in the brain) in drowning patients, thereby preventing cardiac arrest or brain damage. The most important factor that determines outcome is the duration of submersion. Age, salinity, water temperature, or witnessed status do not predict outcome.[72]

Surviving Cold-Water Immersion or Submersion

There are four phases that describe the body's responses and mechanisms of death during cold-water immersion. These phases correlate to the 1-10-1 principle[73]:

1. *Initial immersion and the cold shock response.* The victim has 1 minute to get the breathing rate under control.
2. *Short-term immersion and the loss of performance.* The victim has 10 minutes of meaningful movement to get out of the water.
3. *Long-term immersion and the onset of hypothermia.* Victims have up to 1 hour until they become unconscious from hypothermia.
4. *Circumrescue collapse just before, during, or after rescue.* If the victim survives the first three phases, up to 20% may experience this type of collapse during rescue.

In each of these phases, there is wide individual variation due to body size, water temperature, and the amount of the body that is immersed. Each phase is accompanied by specific survival hazards for the immersion victim that originate from or are influenced by a variety of pathophysiologic mechanisms. Deaths have occurred during all four phases.

In rare cases of prolonged submersion—one case for as long as 66 minutes—patients have presented to the hospital with severe hypothermia and recovered with either partial or full neurologic function.[74,75] In these submersion incidents, the lowest recorded core temperature of a survivor is 56.6°F (13.7°C) in an adult woman.[76] In another case, a child survived fully intact after submersion in ice water for 40 minutes, with a core temperature of 75°F (23.9°C). After 1 hour of resuscitation, spontaneous circulation returned.[77] While this case is noteworthy as an exceptional outlier, the survivor demonstrated that from a population-based perspective, the only variable that can predict outcome is submersion time (longer submersion time equates to a lower chance of survival).[72]

No definitive explanation exists for such cases. Hypothermia due to slow cooling over the course of several minutes to hours leads to worse outcomes and is not protective. One factor that may explain why some young children survive is the mammalian diving reflex (**Box 20-5**). The **mammalian diving reflex** slows heart rate and shunts blood to the brain. Recent evidence suggests that the diving reflex present in various mammals is active in only 15% to 30% of human subjects, so while it cannot be considered the lone explanation of why some children survive, it still may explain part of this phenomenon.[30]

There is often much discussion about whether to dedicate resources to search and rescue (SAR) or recovery, or if resuscitation should be started after rescue. As previously stated, the only validated factor that determines outcome is duration of submersion. Some sources cite 60 minutes of known submersion time to transition to recovery or not perform resuscitation once rescued.[78] This is a difficult discussion that must ultimately fall to the individual jurisdiction based on local human, political, and financial resources. With unlimited access to all three, we would continue each SAR operation indefinitely without having

to transition to recovery. Previously, much attention has been given to the "cold" water drowning, with case reports of survival with prolonged submersion in cold water. However, duration of submersion alone is predictive of outcome without regard to water temperature.[72] The cited review acknowledges that they excluded those outlier case reports of survival after prolonged submersion. Tipton and Golden performed a review to determine a protocol that would have captured all of the outliers that were excluded.[78] This work informed the development of the protocol for the United Kingdom Fire and Rescue Services (UKFRS).[79] The UKFRS guideline calls for a dynamic risk assessment (DRA) at time zero; at 30 minutes, the search only continues if water temperature is less than 43°F (6°C), then another 30 minutes if it is a small child (i.e., younger than 12 years).

Ultimately, a protocol has to be developed that includes some time frame to transition from SAR with resuscitation to recovery without attempted resuscitation. These are difficult decisions, and there has to be a balanced interpretation of the literature and humanism. The key is for local medical directors and rescue teams to have these discussions before an incident and develop protocols that fit within the locally available resources.

Water Rescue

Many water safety organizations recommend the use of highly skilled professionals who regularly train for water rescue, retrieval, and resuscitation. If no professional water rescue teams are available, however, prehospital care practitioners must consider their own safety and the safety of all emergency responders before attempting an in-water rescue. The following guidelines are recommended to safely rescue a victim out of the water. All of these steps follow an initial, top-priority attempt to provide flotation to the victim; in most aquatic rescue scenarios, this intervention potentially interrupts the drowning process and buys time to plan further rescue interventions.

- *Reach*. Attempt to perform the water rescue by reaching out with a pole, stick, paddle, or anything so that the rescuer stays on land or on a boat. Use caution to avoid being inadvertently pulled into the water.
- *Throw*. When reaching is not possible, throw something to a victim, such as a life preserver or rope so that it floats to the victim.
- *Tow*. Once the victim has a rescue line, tow the victim to safety.
- *Row*. If water entry is necessary, it is preferable to use a boat or paddleboard to reach the victim and to wear a PFD.[30]
- *Go (Don't Go)*. The riskiest technique is to deploy a rescue swimmer. Some wilderness EMS texts describe this risk by naming this step "Go (Don't Go)," indicating that the "Go" step should be initiated only following proper training and a complete risk–benefit

---

Box 20-5 Mammalian Diving Reflex

The mammalian diving reflex is a condition likely present in all vertebrates, although it is most studied in large aquatic mammals. Its purpose is to conserve intrinsic oxygen stores (oxygen bound to hemoglobin and myoglobin) during underwater submersion. Bradycardia is the primary component and dramatically reduces cardiac output. Massive peripheral vasoconstriction counteracts the blood pressure drop this would normally cause, which redistributes available blood (and thus oxygen) to the CNS and heart. This allows the organism to exist on far less oxygen than would normally be required. This reflex appears to be present in infant humans but wanes with age.

analysis suggesting the benefit exceeds the risk.[43,67,80] Rescuers should wear a PFD if entering the water and ideally be leashed to a belay system capable of self-release for swift-water environments.[30,66,67,80]

- *Helo.* In some parts of the country, a helicopter may be equipped to assist with flood or swift-water water rescue and is thus labeled in this algorithm.[67] Helicopter rescue is listed as the final step because helicopters tend to introduce a level of complexity and risk to an operation and require additional risk–benefit analysis. Helicopter rescue is rarely available for rapid deployment and is usually part of a longer rescue operation where immediate fatal drowning risk has been contained.

Swimming rescues are not recommended unless the prehospital care practitioner has been trained appropriately to manage a victim who can rapidly turn violent from panic, creating a potential double drowning. Too many well-intentioned emergency responders have become victims because their own safety was not the priority; some studies suggest as many as 5% of drowning fatalities are would-be rescuers.[81,82] See **Figure 20-3** for a few options for in-water rescue systems, equipment for a submersion and/or trauma victim, and movement when in deep water.

Predictors of Survival

The following are important factors that help predict outcome in resuscitation of a person who has drowned.[41]

1. Early BLS is crucial. For cardiac arrest patients or unresponsive drowning patients, early application of oxygen and rescue breathing or CPR as indicated is critically important to outcome.
2. The greater the duration of submersion, the greater the risk of death or severe neurologic impairment after hospital discharge:
   - 0 to 5 minutes = 10%
   - 6 to 10 minutes = 56%
   - 11 to 25 minutes = 88%
   - Greater than 25 minutes = 100%
3. Signs of brain stem injury predict death or severe neurologic impairment and deficits.

Assessment

The initial priorities for any drowning patient include the following[30,41]:

1. Prevent injuries to the patient and emergency responders; ensure access to flotation devices for all individuals in the water.
2. Initiate plans early for water extraction, availability of at least BLS-level EMS management, and rapid transport to the ED.
3. Conduct a safe water rescue (consider a possible diving-related cause and the need for spinal

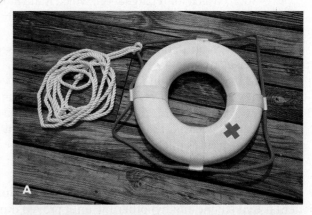

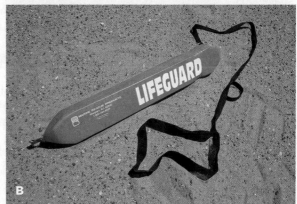

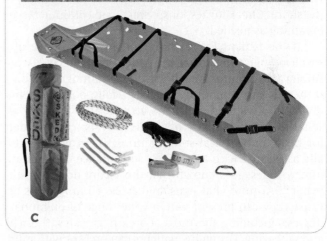

Figure 20-3 Options for in-water rescue equipment and patient packaging. **A.** Rescue throw lines. **B.** Tow device. **C.** In-water patient packaging equipment.

A and B. Courtesy of Rick Brady; **C.** © National Association of Emergency Medical Technicians (NAEMT)

motion restriction). Consider in-water resuscitation if trained in this modality.[43]

4. Due to hypoxemia, assess the ABCs (airway, breathing, circulation) using the traditional approach, not CAB (circulation, airway, breathing).
5. Reverse hypoxemia and acidemia with five rescue breaths initially, followed by 30 chest compressions, and continue with two breaths thereafter

(30:2). Watch for regurgitation, which is the most common complication during rescue breathing and during CPR.

6. CPR with only chest compression is not advised in persons who have drowned.

7. Restore or maintain cardiovascular stability.

8. Prevent further loss of body heat and initiate rewarming efforts in hypothermic patients, bearing in mind that therapeutic hypothermia temperatures might be considered in postarrest patients.

Initially, it is safest to presume that the submersion patient is hypoxemic and hypothermic until proved otherwise. Consequently, efforts should be made to establish effective respirations during water rescue, because cardiac arrest from drowning is primarily the result of lack of oxygen. Submersion patients in respiratory arrest usually respond after a few rescue breaths. Attempts to provide chest compressions when in the water are ineffective, so taking time to assess for the presence of a pulse is meaningless and will only delay getting the patient to land.

Remove the patient from the water safely. Once on land, the patient should be placed in a supine position with the trunk and head in line and at the same level, which is usually parallel (on sloping beaches or banks) to the shore. Check for responsiveness, and continue rescue breathing as needed.

If the patient is breathing and in the absence of a suspicion of trauma, place the patient in the recovery position, and monitor for effective respirations and pulse. If there is suspicion of trauma (e.g., falls, boat accidents, diving into water with underwater hazards), quickly assess the patient for any other life threats, and evaluate for head and cervical spine injuries. Drowning is actually associated with a relatively low chance of traumatic injury, unless it is known that the victim dove into the water.[83] Acquire vital signs, and assess all lung fields because they can present with a wide range of pulmonary distress, including shortness of breath, crackles, rhonchi, and wheezing. Drowning patients can present with minimal symptoms initially and then deteriorate rapidly with signs of pulmonary edema. However, there has never been a case published in the medical literature of a patient who was initially completely asymptomatic on clinical examination who then died hours later of abrupt, late-onset symptoms.[36]

Assess the patient's oxygen saturation with pulse oximetry and monitor the end-tidal carbon dioxide ($ETCO_2$) levels. Assess for cardiac rhythm disturbances because submersion patients often have dysrhythmias secondary to hypoxia and hypothermia. Assess for altered mental status and neurologic function of all extremities because many submersion patients develop

sustained neurologic damage. Determine the patient's blood glucose level, as hypoglycemia may have been the cause for the submersion incident. Acquire a baseline Glasgow Coma Scale (GCS) score and continue to assess for trends. Always suspect hypothermia and minimize further heat loss. Remove all wet clothing and assess temperature (if the appropriate thermometers are available and the situation permits) to determine the level of hypothermia, and initiate steps to minimize further heat loss. (See Chapter 19, *Environmental Trauma I: Heat and Cold*, for management of hypothermia.)

Management

Figure 20-4 presents a management tool for persons who have drowned based on a six-grade classification system and a guide for medical intervention for each grade.[41] A patient who has experienced some form of submersion incident, but who is not presenting with any signs or symptoms at the time of the primary survey, still needs follow-up care in a hospital after assessment at the scene due to the potential for delayed onset of symptoms. Many asymptomatic patients (Grade 2) are released in 6 to 8 hours, depending on clinical findings in the hospital. In one study of 52 swimmers who experienced a submersion incident and were all initially asymptomatic immediately after the incident, 21 (40%) went on to develop shortness of breath and respiratory distress due to hypoxemia within 4 hours.[84] In general, all symptomatic patients are admitted to the hospital for at least 24 hours for supportive care and observation because the initial clinical assessment can be misleading. It is critical to obtain a good history of the incident, detailing the estimate of submersion time and any past medical history.

All suspected drowning patients should receive high-flow oxygen (15 liters/minute) independent of their initial breathing status or oxygen saturation, based on the concern for worsening pulmonary distress, particularly if the patient develops shortness of breath. Monitor the patient's oxygen saturation for evidence of progressive hypoxia. Apply and monitor the ECG, particularly for pulseless electrical activity or asystole. Obtain intravenous (IV) access, and provide normal saline (NS) or lactated Ringer (LR) solution at a KVO rate unless the patient is hypotensive. Then provide a 500-milliliter (mL) fluid bolus and reassess vital signs.

Transport all drowning patients to the ED for evaluation. Because many drowning patients are asymptomatic, some may refuse transport because they have no immediate chief complaint. If so, take the time necessary to provide good patient education, explaining that even minimal difficulty breathing can be a sign of aspiration and may worsen over the next few hours. Firm and persistent persuasion is needed for the patient to agree to be

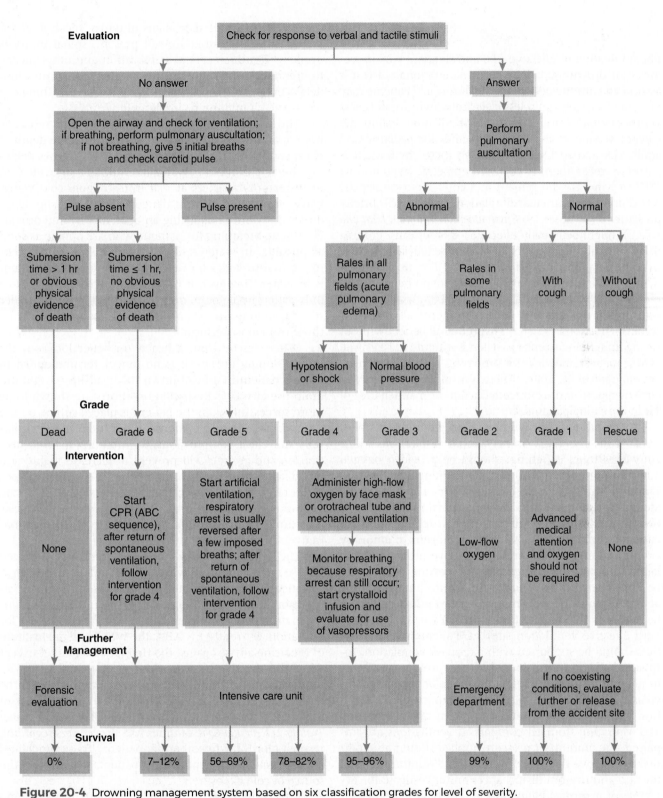

Figure 20-4 Drowning management system based on six classification grades for level of severity.

Reproduced from Szpilman D, Bierens JJ, Handley AJ, Orlowski JP. Drowning. *N Eng J Med.* 2012;366(22):2102–2110. https://doi.org/10.1056/NEJMra1013317. © 2012 Massachusetts Medical Society. Reprinted with permission from Massachusetts Medical Society.

transported or to report to the closest ED for further evaluation and observation. If the patient is adamant about refusing care, the patient must be informed of the potential ramifications of refusing care, and a signed refusal of care against medical advice must be obtained. The largest study of drowning patients to date showed a mortality rate of 0.6% to 5% for patients with only minimal or moderate initial symptoms.[85]

Patient Resuscitation

Rapid initiation of effective BLS and standard ALS procedures for drowning patients in cardiopulmonary arrest is associated with the best chance of survival.[60] Patients may present in asystole, pulseless electrical activity, or pulseless ventricular tachycardia/ventricular fibrillation. Follow the current version of the AHA guidelines for pediatric and adult ALS and ACLS for managing these rhythms. It is currently recommended to use therapeutic hypothermia (TH) in patients who remain in a coma from cardiac arrest caused by ventricular fibrillation. (This topic is briefly presented in Chapter 19, *Environmental Trauma I: Heat and Cold*.) It might be equally effective for other causes of cardiac arrest, but it has not been proven beneficial to induce hypothermia for submersion patients.[86] For drowning patients who are already hypothermic, hypothetical arguments could be made that they should be warmed only to standard TH temperature, per local protocol, although this recommendation is based on hypothetical benefit without strong underlying science to defend or refute it.[30,43,66] The WMS Practice Guidelines for Drowning, with a recommendation grade of 2C, state, "There is insufficient evidence to either support or discourage induction or maintenance of TH in drowning patients."[43]

A symptomatic drowning patient who presents with signs of distress (e.g., anxiety, rapid respirations, difficulty breathing, coughing) should be provided oxygen and transported to the hospital for additional evaluation. Emphasis should be placed on correcting hypoxemia, acidemia, and hypothermia. Provide spinal motion restriction in all suspected trauma patients. In unresponsive patients, copious volumes of noncardiogenic pulmonary edema (foam) may be present. Positive-pressure ventilation and positive end-expiratory pressure (PEEP) can be effective ways to manage this foam, but suctioning at the expense of oxygenation and ventilation should be avoided. Hypoxemia and acidemia can be corrected with effective ventilation support. Patients who are apneic should be supported with bag-mask ventilation. Intubation should be considered early to protect the airway in patients who are apneic or cyanotic or who have decreased mental status, because drowning patients swallow large amounts of water and are at risk of vomiting and aspirating stomach contents. If ventilations are impaired, the amount of pressure applied should be modified to improve the ease of ventilation. Monitor the ECG for rate and rhythm disturbances and investigate for evidence of a cardiac event that might have preceded or followed the submersion incident. Provide 100% oxygen (15 liters/minute) with a nonrebreathing mask. Obtain IV access and provide NS or LR solution at a KVO rate. Provide transport to the local ED.

Routine attention to spinal cord restriction during in-water rescue is not necessary unless the reasons leading to the submersion indicate that trauma is likely (e.g.,

diving, use of water slide, signs of injury, alcohol use).[86] When these indicators are not present, spinal injury is unlikely. Routine cervical stabilization and other means to immobilize the spine during a water rescue can cause delays in opening the airway so that rescue breathing can begin and should not be implemented.[66,67,80]

The use of compressions during in-water rescue is not recommended for many reasons.[43] First, the depth of chest compressions is ineffective in water. Besides delaying effective CPR out of water, attempting to provide CPR in water puts rescuers at risk from fatigue, cold water, wave, surge, and current dangers. Emphasis should be directed toward establishing an open airway and providing rescue breathing for patients who are apneic as soon as possible. In-water resuscitation is a recognized technique that provides for rescue breathing while a patient is in water. However, it has been shown to be effective only when implemented by trained practitioners under specific circumstances, and should be attempted only by those trained to perform it.[43]

When rescue from a beach (or other location) involves sloping terrain, it is no longer recommended to place a patient in a head-down (or head-up) position to drain the airway.[80] Resuscitation efforts are shown to be more successful when the patient is placed supine on the ground, parallel to the shoreline, with effective ventilation and chest compressions. Maintaining a level position on the ground will prevent a decrease in forward blood flow during chest compressions in the head-up position or an increase in intracranial pressure (ICP) in the head-down position. Furthermore, no evidence suggests that lung drainage is effective with any particular maneuver and may be harmful.

The Heimlich maneuver has been previously suggested for use in drowning. However, the Heimlich maneuver is designed for airway obstruction and does not remove water from the airway or lungs. Rather, it may induce vomiting in drowning patients and place them at greater risk for aspiration. Currently, the AHA, the WMS, and the Institute of Medicine advise against the Heimlich maneuver except when the airway is blocked with foreign material.[43,87] Victims who recover with spontaneous breathing should be placed in a lateral recumbent position to reduce the risk of aspiration if the patient vomits. (Chapter 19, *Environmental Trauma I: Heat and Cold*, outlines ALS procedures regarding resuscitation of a hypothermic patient. These guidelines are the same for all hypothermic patients regardless of the source of cold exposure.)

Most drowning patients have copious froth coming out of the mouth, which is a result of water mixing with surfactant in the lungs as well as possibly other debris. There is no benefit to suctioning this froth, and, in fact, time spent trying to clear the airway of this material is time lost in establishing oxygenation for the patient. The froth can be breathed back into the lungs after any large, solid foreign bodies are removed from the airway.[30,66]

Because of the critical nature of oxygenation and ventilation in drowning patients in cardiac arrest, the preference would be to intubate cardiac arrest drownings as soon as possible. Supraglottic airway devices are of unproven benefit in drowning due to high airway resistance.[88-90]

Prevention of Drowning

Prevention strategies are vital in the effort to lower the rates of drowning incidents in the United States. It is estimated that 85% of all cases of drowning can be prevented by supervision, swimming instruction, technology regulations, and public education.[41] Many education programs emphasize the reduction of unintentional water entry of infants and children by encouraging the installation of various types of barriers around pools (e.g., isolation fences, pool covers, alarms) and the use of PFDs such as life vests.[47] Furthermore, CPR initiated by a bystander before the arrival of prehospital care personnel is associated with improved patient prognosis, so community CPR training can certainly be considered a preventive intervention for drowning.[91]

Prehospital care practitioners have great opportunities to be advocates of water safety and education in their respective communities, with an emphasis on communication of the risk factor areas previously identified. Furthermore, prevention should be emphasized to practitioners and other public safety personnel who arrive on the scene so that they do not become additional submersion victims. A panicked and struggling victim can be a danger to an unprepared in-water rescuer, potentially resulting in a double drowning. Practitioners need to assess the problem quickly, control the scene to prevent bystanders from entering the water, and ensure their own safety.

Community education regarding submersion incidents should include the following recommendations:

- Beaches
  - Always swim near a lifeguard.
  - Ask a lifeguard about a safe place to swim.
  - Always swim with others.
  - Do not overestimate your swimming capability.
  - Always watch your children.
  - Swim away from piers, rocks, and stakes.
  - Don't drink alcohol.
  - Take lost children to the nearest lifeguard tower.
  - Be aware that the majority of ocean drownings occur in rip currents.
  - Know the weather conditions before going into water.
  - Never try to rescue someone without knowing what you are doing; many people have died in such attempts.
  - If you are fishing on rocks, wear a lifejacket.
  - Always enter shallow water feetfirst.
  - Do not dive in shallow water; injury to the cervical spine could result.
  - Keep away from marine animals.
  - Read and heed signs and flags posted on the beach.
- Residential pools and other water sources
  - Ensure constant, continuous, uninterrupted adult supervision of children.
  - Set rules for water safety.
  - Never leave a child alone near a pool or a source of water, such as a bathtub or bucket.
  - Install a four-sided fence that is at least 4 ft (1.2 m) tall around the pool with a self-closing and self-latching gate.
  - Do not allow children to use arm buoys or other air-filled swim aids.
  - Use an approved life jacket.
  - Avoid toys that will attract children around pools.
  - Use two drains 3 ft (9 m) apart and anti-hair covers, or turn off pump filters when using pools.
  - Use cordless or mobile phones near pools to prevent leaving the poolside to answer the telephone elsewhere.
  - Keep rescue equipment (e.g., shepherd's hook, life preserver) and a telephone by the pool.
  - Do not try or allow hyperventilation to increase underwater swim time.
  - Do not dive in shallow water.
  - Provide swimming lessons for all children by age 4 years but preferably by age 1 year.[30,92]
  - After children have finished swimming, secure the pool so they cannot return (locks or audible alarms on gates are recommended).
  - All family members and others watching children should learn water safety, first aid, and age-appropriate CPR.[14]

Communities can also prevent drowning by educating the public about the dangers of driving through floodwaters. As intense flood-causing storms become more common, this message is becoming increasingly important. If drivers do find themselves in a submerged vehicle, they will need to know how to promptly, safely free themselves (**Box 20-6**).

Recreational Scuba-Related Injuries

Recreational diving using **self-contained underwater breathing apparatus (scuba)** is a common activity enjoyed by people in many age groups. The popularity of this activity continues to grow, with more than 400,000 new certified divers each year, now totaling nearly 4 million recreational scuba divers in the United States.[97,98] Relative to the increasing number of new divers each year, the injury rate is low, but the concern for medical fitness to dive has increased because of the diversity of divers, increasing age, low physical fitness, and underlying medical conditions. Water is an unforgiving environment when

Studies suggest that as many as 10% of drownings occur in submerging or submerged vehicles and that 10% of motor vehicle–related deaths during disasters are due to submerged vehicles.[30,93,94] Many erroneous strategies have been shared in the media about how to escape a vehicle filling with water, including waiting for it to fill with water before trying to escape so that the doors will open, breathing trapped air, or kicking out the windshield.[66,94] However, recent thorough investigations of these strategies have proven them to be dangerous and ineffective and have resulted in a more evidence-based set of instructions for escaping a submerging vehicle.[93]

Vehicles float for about 30 to 120 seconds before sinking. During this time, the windows should be rolled down and the vehicle exited as rapidly as possible. Studies have shown that three adults can escape a vehicle in this way, while also releasing a child manikin in a back seat, within 51 seconds.[95] Emergency medical dispatchers in particular should be aware of advising callers to escape a submerging vehicle before further action is taken, especially in light of numerous drowning deaths from submerging vehicles while callers were on the phone with a dispatcher.[96] The series of actions that should be taken by an individual in a submerging vehicle, or by someone attempting a rescue of individuals in a submerging vehicle, are as follows[30]:

1. *Seat belts:* Unfasten.
2. *Windows:* Open.
3. *Children:* If present, release from restraints and bring close to an adult who can assist in their escape.
4. *Out:* Children should be pushed out the window first and then followed immediately.

problems occur. Currently, there are medical guidelines that indicate relative and temporary health risks and absolute contraindications for scuba diving.[98-103]

Injuries to divers occur from many underwater hazards (e.g., shipwrecks, coral reefs) or from handling hazardous marine life. However, more often, prehospital care practitioners respond to scuba-related injuries and fatalities caused by **dysbarism**, or altered environmental pressure, which accounts for most serious diving medical disorders. The mechanism of injury is based on the principles of gas laws when breathing compressed gases (e.g., oxygen, helium, nitrogen) at varying underwater depths and pressures, as will be described in detail in subsequent sections.

The associated causes for diving fatalities have not changed significantly in recent history. The most frequently cited problem is insufficient gas (air) or running out of gas. Other common factors included entrapment or entanglement, buoyancy control, equipment misuse or problems, rough water, and emergency ascent. The principal injuries or causes of death included drowning or asphyxia due to inhalation of water, air embolism, and cardiac events. Older divers were at greater risk of cardiac events, with men at higher risk than women, although the risks were equal at age 65 years.[104]

Most scuba-related injuries caused by dysbarism present with signs (e.g., ear squeeze on descent) and symptoms either immediately or within 60 minutes after surfacing, but some symptoms are delayed up to 48 hours after individuals depart the dive site and return home. Consequently, with the increasing number of scuba divers today flying to and from popular dive sites in the United States, the Caribbean, and other remote locations, there is a greater possibility of responding to diving-related injuries at locations distant from the actual dive site. Prehospital care practitioners need to recognize these scuba-related disorders, provide initial treatment, and initiate plans early for transport to the local ED or for treatment at the closest recompression chamber.[101]

Epidemiology

Divers Alert Network (DAN) compiles an extensive morbidity and mortality database derived from casualty data provided by participating recompression chambers in North America. Diving-associated death rates peaked in the 1970s, with annual rates as high as 150, but since then have remained stable at much lower annual death rates ranging from 77 to 91.[98,104] DAN publishes these data in annual reports, which can be found on their website.[105] The number of U.S. fatalities reported to DAN usually increases as summer approaches, peaks around July, and then diminishes as winter approaches. North America has the most reported diving deaths, with Europe coming in a distant second. Three to four times more men are injured when diving than women.

Males account for 81% of deaths, with most of the deaths occurring in divers between 40 and 59 years of age. Drowning was the most common cause of death. Cardiovascular disease was the second most common cause of death and the most common cause of disabling injury. Both these causes were significantly more common as causes of death and disabling injury than arterial gas embolism (AGE), the third most common condition.[105] Even though drowning was the leading cause of fatalities, it is unclear what led to the drowning, such as cardiac events, equipment issues, lack of air, entanglement, narcosis, panic, disorientation, hypothermia, or AGE. Some drowning deaths during scuba diving are the result of AGE.[104]

Mechanical Effects of Pressure

Scuba-related diving injuries incurred by the changing atmospheric pressure, or dysbarism, can be separated into two types: (1) the conditions when a change in pressure from the underwater environment results in tissue trauma or barotrauma in closed air spaces in the body (e.g., ears, sinuses, intestines, lungs) and (2) the problems that occur from breathing compressed gases at elevated partial pressure, such as decompression sickness.

Barotrauma associated with scuba diving relates directly to the pressure effects of air and water on the diver. When standing at sea level, the atmospheric pressure is 760 torr, which is essentially the same as 760 millimeters of mercury [mm Hg]) or 14.7 pounds per square inch (psi) on the body. This amount of pressure is also known as 1 atmosphere (1 atm). As a diver descends deeper in water, the absolute pressure increases 1 atm for every 33 ft (10 m) of seawater. Consequently, a depth of 33 ft of seawater is equivalent to 2 atm (air [1 atm] and 33 ft of water [1 atm]) of pressure on the body. **Table 20-2** lists common units of pressure in the underwater environment.

When a diver descends under the increasing pressure of seawater, the effect of the forces exerted on the body differs depending on the tissue compartments. The force applied to solid tissue acts in similar fashion to a fluid medium, and the diver is generally unaware of compressive force. In the air-containing spaces of the body, however, gases are compressed as the diver descends. Conversely, these gases expand as the diver ascends toward the surface. Boyle's law and Henry's law explain the effects of pressure on the body when underwater.

Boyle's Law

Boyle's law states that the volume of a given mass of gas is inversely proportional to the absolute pressure found in that environment. Stated another way, as a diver

descends in the water to a greater depth, the pressure increases and the volume of the gas (e.g., the volume in the lung or ear) decreases. The reverse is also true, the volume of the gas (e.g., in the lung or ear) increases in size when the diver ascends toward the surface. This is the principle behind the effects of barotrauma and AGE in the body. **Figure 20-5** shows the effects of pressure on the volume and diameter of a gas bubble.

Henry's Law

Henry's law states that at a constant temperature, the amount of gas that will dissolve in a liquid is directly proportional to the partial pressure of that gas outside the liquid. Henry's law is fundamental to understanding how gas from a compressed air cylinder (scuba tank) behaves in the body as the diver descends in the water. For example, the increasing partial pressure of nitrogen will cause it to dissolve in the fluids of the body's tissues as the pressure increases during descent. On return toward the surface, nitrogen will "bubble out" of the fluid solution in the tissues. A slower ascent allows the nitrogen to dissipate rather than form bubbles. Thus, Henry's law describes the principle that explains why decompression sickness occurs.

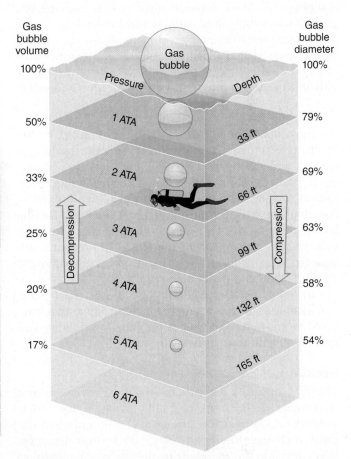

Table 20-2 Common Units of Pressure in Underwater Environment			
Depth (FSW)	PSIA	ATA	Torr or mm Hg (absolute)
Sea level	14.7	1	760
33	29.4	2	1,520
66	44.1	3	2,280
99	58.8	4	3,040
132	73.5	5	3,800
165	88.2	6	4,560
198	102.9	7	5,320

Abbreviations: ATA, atmosphere absolute; FSW, feet seawater; mm Hg, millimeters of mercury; PSIA, pounds per square inch absolute.

Figure 20-5 Boyle's law. The volume of a given quantity of gas at constant temperature varies inversely with pressure.

Barotrauma

Barotrauma, also known as *squeeze*, is the most common form of scuba-related diving injury.[106] Although many forms of barotraumas cause pain, most resolve spontaneously and do not require EMS involvement or recompression chamber therapy. However, some pulmonary overpressurization injuries are very serious. During scuba diving, barotrauma occurs within noncompressible, gas-filled body cavities (e.g., sinuses). If the pressure in these spaces cannot equalize during a dive as ambient pressure increases, vascular engorgement, hemorrhage, and mucosal edema result from decreasing air volume when the diver descends, and tissue disruption results from increasing air volume when the diver ascends. The various forms of barotraumas are described next.

Barotrauma of Descent

Mask Squeeze

This form of barotrauma generally occurs in inexperienced divers who fail to equalize the pressure in their face mask to the external water pressure during their descents. Examine the soft tissue around the patient's eyes and conjunctival tissues for capillary rupture. Signs and symptoms of mask squeeze include skin ecchymoses, periorbital swelling, and conjunctival hemorrhage. Mask barotrauma is self-limited, and treatment is no diving until the tissue damage clears. Management includes providing a cold compress over the eyes, encouraging the patient to rest, and providing pain medication as needed.

Tooth Squeeze

An infrequent finding, this form of barotrauma occurs in divers when gas is trapped in the interior portion of a tooth after receiving a dental filling, recent tooth extractions, or a root canal or with defective dental restorations. During descent, the tooth can fill with blood or can implode with increasing external pressure. During ascent, any air forced into the tooth will expand, causing either pain or explosion of the tooth. To prevent tooth squeeze, it is recommended that divers do not dive for 24 hours after any dental treatment.

Examine the affected tooth to see if it is intact. Signs and symptoms of tooth squeeze include pain and a fractured tooth. Refer the patient for dental evaluation and give pain medication as needed.

Middle-Ear Squeeze

This type of squeeze occurs in 40% of scuba divers and is considered the most common diving injury.[107] Ear squeeze occurs near the surface of the water, when the greatest changes in pressure occur as the diver descends. Divers need to begin equalizing their middle ear early as they start to descend so a pressure differential across the tympanic membrane (TM) leading to severe pain and then rupture of the eardrum does not occur. The diver will experience vertigo if the TM ruptures, allowing water to enter the middle ear. Divers with upper respiratory infection or allergies may have difficulty equalizing their middle ear during a dive.

Examine the ear canal for blood caused by ruptured TM. Signs and symptoms of middle-ear squeeze include pain, vertigo, conductive hearing losses with TM rupture, and vomiting. If examination of the external auditory canal is possible, redness of the TM will often be present.

No pressure changes are permitted (e.g., diving or flying) in patients with middle-ear squeeze. Patients may need decongestants if the TM has not ruptured to open up the eustachian tube and allow the pressure to equalize. Antiemetics such as prochlorperazine or ondansetron may be necessary for vertigo and vomiting. Transport the patient in an upright position or position of comfort. Antibiotics may be prescribed with ruptured TM to prevent infection. The patient should be referred for audiometric evaluation to assess possible hearing loss.

Sinus Squeeze (Sinus Barotrauma)

Normally, pressure in the sinuses equalizes easily as the diver is descending and ascending. Pressure develops by the same mechanism as the middle ear squeeze, but sinus squeeze is not as common. As a diver descends, there is an inability to maintain pressure in the sinuses, and a relative vacuum develops in the sinus cavity, causing intense pain, mucosal wall trauma, and bleeding in the sinus cavity. This squeeze may be caused by congestion, sinusitis, *mucosal hypertrophy* (enlargement or thickening), rhinitis, or nasal poyps.[106] A reverse sinus squeeze during ascent can occur as well (see later discussion in the section "Reverse Squeeze").

Examine the patient's nose for discharge. Signs and symptoms of sinus squeeze include severe pain over the affected sinus or bloody discharge from the affected sinus.

No specific management is needed at the scene. Since the bleeding is from the mucosa of the sinus, treating the patient for epistaxis (nosebleed) by pinching firmly on the fleshy part of the patient's nostrils just below the nasal bones may not be effective, but it represents the only prehospital option. Transport in a position of comfort.

Reverse Squeeze

This form of sinus squeeze can occur on ascent when any form of blockage in the sinus openings prevents expanding gas from escaping. The expanding gas puts pressure on the mucosal lining of the sinus, causing pain with hemorrhage. Sinus barotrauma occurs in divers with upper respiratory infections or allergies.

Examine the nose for discharge. Signs and symptoms of sinus barotrauma include severe pain over the affected sinus and bloody discharge.

Decongestants may help with reducing mucosal edema and promote drainage of the sinus. No other specific management is needed at the scene unless extensive bleeding is observed, in which case treat for epistaxis by pinching firmly on the fleshy part of the patient's nostrils, just below the nasal bones. This may be of minimal benefit as the bleeding is from the sinus not the anterior nasal plexus. Transport the patient in a position of comfort.

Inner-Ear Barotrauma

Although much less common than middle-ear squeeze, this is the most serious form of ear barotrauma because it may lead to permanent deafness.[107] Inner-ear barotrauma occurs when a diver descends and has failed attempts to equalize the middle ear. Further forceful attempts can result in a large rise in middle-ear pressure and can rupture the round window structure.

Examine the ear canal for any discharge. Signs and symptoms include roaring tinnitus, vertigo, hearing loss, a feeling of fullness or "blockage" in the affected ear, nausea, vomiting, pallor, diaphoresis (sweating), disorientation, and ataxia (loss of muscular coordination).

The patient should avoid activities that raise ICP, strenuous activities, Valsalva-like maneuvers, and loud noises, with no pressure changes (e.g., diving or flying). Transport the patient in an upright position. Early medical consultation with DAN or an ED is recommended because it may be difficult to determine if the patient is experiencing inner-ear decompression sickness and if there is an immediate need for recompression chamber therapy. The patient should also be urgently referred for evaluation by an ear, nose, and throat specialist.

Barotrauma of Ascent

Alternobaric Vertigo

This is a type of barotrauma that occurs as expanding gas moves through the eustachian tube and unequal pressure develops in the middle ear, which can cause vertigo. Although the symptoms are brief, vertigo can trigger panic in divers, leading to other forms of injury caused by a rapid ascent to the surface (e.g., air embolism, drowning).

Examine the ear canal for any discharge; assess any hearing loss. Signs and symptoms of alternobaric vertigo are short in duration, resulting in transient vertigo, pressure in the affected ear, tinnitus, and hearing loss.

No specific intervention is required if the patient is asymptomatic after the dive and no equalization problems are found. Provide decongestants as needed and according to the EMS system's policies and procedures. No transport to the ED is needed if symptoms resolve quickly and completely, and the patient may follow up with a primary care provider. If symptoms persist, transport for evaluation is appropriate.

Gastrointestinal Squeeze

This type of barotrauma occurs when expanding gas in the gut becomes trapped as the diver surfaces. Gastrointestinal (GI) barotrauma occurs in divers who frequently perform Valsalva maneuvers in the head-down position, swallow air during breathing, or consume gas-producing foods prior to diving, which increases the amount of air in the stomach at depth that expands on ascent.

Examine the abdominal quadrants. Signs and symptoms of GI squeeze include abdominal fullness, belching, and flatulence.

GI squeeze normally resolves on its own and rarely needs medical attention. If the pain and fullness do not resolve, transport for evaluation is appropriate.

There are other causes of abdominal pain after surfacing, including spinal cord decompression sickness. Abdominal pain that does not resolve on the surface needs prompt attention in the ED.

Pulmonary Overinflation Barotrauma

Pulmonary overinflation is a serious form of barotrauma resulting from the expansion of gas in the lungs during ascent. Normally the diver eliminates expanding gas with normal exhalations when returning to the surface. If the expanding gas does not escape, alveoli will rupture. This causes any one of several forms of injuries, depending on the amount of air that escapes outside the lung and its final location. A common scenario is a diver who has a rapid and uncontrollable ascent to the surface caused by running out of air, panic, or a dropped weight belt. These types of injuries are collectively called "pulmonary overinflation syndrome" (POIS) or *burst lung*. Recompression therapy is contraindicated for all forms of POIS except AGE.

The five forms of POIS are as follows:

1. Overdistension with local injury
2. Mediastinal emphysema
3. Subcutaneous emphysema
4. Pneumothorax
5. AGE

OVERDISTENSION WITH LOCAL INJURY

This is lung barotrauma that is found without extrapulmonary air or overt lung injury. Auscultate the lung fields for diminished breath sounds. Chest pain may or may not be present. If blood is seen in the sputum (hemoptysis), then prompt attention in the ED is warranted.

Ensure that the patient rests in a position of comfort, and treat the patient's symptoms as needed. Monitor the patient's vital signs and oxygen saturation with pulse oximetry; provide high-flow, 100% oxygen. Transport the patient in a position of comfort. The patient needs further medical evaluation to rule out a more severe form of POIS and should avoid further pressure exposure (e.g., diving or commercial flying).

MEDIASTINAL EMPHYSEMA

Mediastinal emphysema is another form of POIS that is caused by escaping gas from ruptured alveoli entering the interstitial space to the mediastinum. This condition can be benign. Examine the lung fields for diminished breath sounds. Signs and symptoms include hoarseness, neck fullness, and minor substernal chest pain; often a dull ache or tightness is present that worsens with breathing and coughing. Examine the patient's chest and neck for subcutaneous emphysema. In severe cases, the diver presents with chest pain, dyspnea, and difficulty swallowing.

Ensure that the patient rests in a position of comfort. Monitor the patient's vital signs and oxygen saturation with pulse oximetry; provide high-flow oxygen. Usually, mediastinal emphysema requires no specific treatment. However, patients may need to be medically evaluated to rule out other causes of chest pain and severe forms of POIS. Transport the patient in a supine position. The patient should avoid further pressure exposure (e.g., diving or commercial flying).

SUBCUTANEOUS EMPHYSEMA

With subcutaneous emphysema, air escaping from ruptured alveoli continues to move superiorly into the neck and clavicle regions of the chest. Examine the lung fields for diminished breath sounds. Signs and symptoms of subcutaneous emphysema include swelling, crepitus, hoarseness, sore throat, and difficulty swallowing.

No specific treatment is required besides rest. Monitor the patient's vital signs and oxygen saturation with pulse oximetry, and provide high-flow oxygen. The patient will need further medical evaluation to rule out more severe forms of POIS. Transport the patient in the supine position. The patient should avoid further pressure exposure (e.g., diving or commercial flying).

PNEUMOTHORAX

Pneumothorax is not seen as often as other forms of POIS because air must escape through the visceral pleura around the lung, which presents greater resistance than air escaping through the interstitial space between the lung and visceral pleura. If the diver is at depth when a pulmonary rupture occurs, a tension pneumothorax can result as the volume of escaping gas expands as the diver continues toward the surface. Examine the lung fields for diminished breath sounds. Signs and symptoms will vary based on the size of the pneumothorax and include sharp chest pain, diminished breath sounds, breathlessness, subcutaneous emphysema, and dyspnea.

Provide ongoing assessment to monitor for conversion from simple to tension pneumothorax such as evidence of respiratory or hemodynamic collapse. Ensure rest in a position of comfort. Monitor the patient's vital signs and oxygen saturation with pulse oximetry, and provide 100% oxygen by nonrebreathing mask. Provide standard ALS management of tension pneumothorax with 14-gauge, 3.25-inch (8.5-centimeter) needle thoracostomy or finger thoracostomy as necessary. Transport the patient in a position of comfort. The patient needs further medical evaluation to rule out more severe forms of POIS and should avoid further pressure exposure (e.g., diving or commercial flying).

ARTERIAL GAS EMBOLISM

This is the most feared complication of POIS and, after drowning, is the next leading cause of death in divers, accounting for about 30% of fatalities.[108] AGE can occur in association with the four POIS conditions previously presented or in isolation as a result of air escaping and forming an air embolism. AGE typically occurs in divers who have an uncontrolled ascent to the surface without appropriate exhalation, causing an overinflation pulmonary injury. However, AGE can occur in divers who surface slowly without underlying lung pathology. During ascent, once the pulmonary overinflation bursts alveoli, air enters the pulmonary venous capillary circulation; the gas bubbles enter the left atrium and left ventricle, then exit the heart through the aorta, and are distributed to the cerebral, coronary, and other systemic vasculature. Gas bubbles can enter the coronary circulation, causing an occlusion resulting in cardiac dysrhythmia, cardiac arrest, or myocardial infarction.[109] If gas bubbles enter the cerebral circulation, the diver presents with signs and symptoms similar to an acute stroke.

Unlike decompression sickness, which can present with delayed symptoms hours after diving, symptoms of AGE appear either immediately at the water surface or, typically, within 10 to 15 minutes. Any loss of consciousness once a diver surfaces must be presumed to be AGE until proved otherwise.[109] The primary treatment for AGE is recompression chamber (hyperbaric) therapy.

Historically, it was recommended that patients with AGE be placed in the Trendelenburg position for transport, based on the belief that this would help keep bubbles from circulating in the systemic vasculature. However, evidence has shown that the head-down position does not prevent systemic circulation of nitrogen bubbles, makes it more difficult to oxygenate the patient, and may worsen cerebral edema.[110] Currently, it is recommended that all AGE patients be placed in a supine position in the field and during transport. High-flow, 100% oxygen by nonrebreathing mask and transport in the supine position provides nitrogen bubble washout in addition to other beneficial effects.[111,112]

Decompression Sickness

Decompression sickness (DCS) is directly related to Henry's law. When scuba divers breathe compressed air containing oxygen (21%) and nitrogen (79%), the amount of gas that will be dissolved in liquid is directly proportional to the partial pressure of gas in contact with liquid. Oxygen is used in the body for tissue metabolism when in solution and does not form gas bubbles during ascent from depth.

Nitrogen, an inert gas not used for metabolism, is the primary source of concern in DCS although helium can also be problematic if the diver is using a heliox tank. Nitrogen is five times more soluble in fat than in water and becomes dissolved in tissue proportionately to the increasing ambient pressure. Consequently, the deeper underwater the diver goes and the longer the diver stays at depth, the greater the amount of nitrogen that dissolves into tissue. As the diver ascends toward the surface, the absorbed nitrogen must be eliminated. If there is inadequate time to eliminate nitrogen during ascent, nitrogen comes out of solution in the tissues in the form of intravascular gas bubbles, causing obstruction of the vascular and lymphatic systems and tissue distension, and activating inflammatory responses.[113]

Most divers experience DCS within the first hour after surfacing, although some will present with symptoms up to 6 to 24 hours after surfacing. Traditionally, symptoms of DCS are categorized as type I, a mild form involving cutaneous, lymphatic, and musculoskeletal systems, or type II, a severe form involving the neurologic and cardiopulmonary systems (**Box 20-7**). Mild symptoms of DCS include fatigue and malaise. However, mild symptoms can be precursors to more severe signs and symptoms, such as numbness, weakness, and paralysis.

Studies now suggest that it is more important clinically to describe DCS by the region of the body affected and its evolution, and not as type I or type II.[98] This suggestion is applicable for prehospital care practitioners to ensure that even patients with mild DCS symptoms are treated aggressively with 100% oxygen and an early consult for recompression therapy. Some divers with the mild form of DCS will not seek medical assistance. Others may substantially delay seeking medical care because denial of DCS is a common finding in the scuba diving population.[116]

Several factors predispose a diver to DCS.[117,118] Some risk factors are known to enhance the uptake of nitrogen in tissues during descent and slow the release of nitrogen during ascent. Certain host and environmental factors, as well as improper decompression and aggressive diving practices, increase the risk for DCS.

Box 20-7 Decompression Illnesses

The term *decompression illness* (DCI) has been proposed to encompass type I and type II DCS and AGE.[114,115]

Limb Pain (Type I DCS)

This form of DCS results from bubble formation in the musculoskeletal system, typically occurring in one or more joints (often referred to as "the bends"). The most common joints involved are the shoulder and elbow, followed by the knee, hip, wrist, hand, and ankle.[97] This pain is described as a severe tendonitis—joint pain with a grating sensation on movement. The pain starts gradually, presenting as a deep, dull ache of mild to severe intensity. The pain-only form of DCS is not life threatening, but it requires neurologic evaluation to exclude more severe forms of DCS and timely treatment.

Cutaneous and Lymphatic (Type I DCS)

Cutaneous DCS is common, and it affects the skin or lymphatic systems. Cutaneous *skin bends* are usually not a serious symptom and are is classified as mild DCS, but are sometimes associated with neurologic symptoms. In some instances, signs of mottling and marbling minutes following a dive can be considered precursors of a serious DCS hit.[119,120] Symptoms include an intense rash that progresses to a red patchy or bluish discoloration of the skin of the torso and proximal extremities.[111] Lymphatic obstruction can result in swelling and an orange-peel appearance (*peau d'orange*). It can be associated with capillary leakage and hypovolemic syndrome. Check vitals, perform a neurologic examination, and take a photo of skin changes.

Cardiopulmonary (Type II DCS)

This severe form of DCS is referred to as the *chokes* and results when venous bubbles overwhelm the pulmonary capillary system. Hypotension can occur from a massive venous air embolism in the lung. Symptoms include nonproductive cough, substernal chest pain, cyanosis, dyspnea, shock, and cardiopulmonary arrest. This disorder resembles acute respiratory distress syndrome.[121] (See Chapter 7, *Airway and Ventilation*, for further information.)

Spinal Cord (Type II DCS)

The white matter of the spinal cord is vulnerable to bubble formation, and nitrogen is highly soluble in spinal cord tissue (*myelin*). The most common site for this form of DCS is the lower thoracic spine, followed by the lumbar/sacral and cervical regions.[116] Common signs and symptoms include low back pain and "heaviness" in the legs. With this form of DCS, the patient often gives a vague statement in an effort to describe "strange sensations," or paresthesia, which can progress to weakness, numbness, and paralysis. Bowel and bladder dysfunction leading to urinary retention has also been reported.[122]

Assessment of AGE and DCS

A standardized approach for patients with AGE and DCS is provided to ensure that consistent care is given. It is recommended that all patients with scuba-related diving injuries be examined for signs and symptoms of AGE and DCS because the primary and essential lifesaving treatment is recompression chamber therapy, which requires specific planning and logistics to access.[52]

Arterial Gas Embolism

About 5% of all AGE patients present with immediate apnea, unconsciousness, and cardiac arrest. Others present with signs and symptoms similar to acute stroke, with loss of consciousness, stupor, confusion, hemiparesis, seizure, vertigo, visual changes, sensory changes, and headache.

Decompression Sickness

Type I DCS is characterized by deep pain in a joint, including minor forms of cutaneous pruritus (severe itching) and obstruction of lymph vessels (lymphedema). Type II DCS is characterized by symptoms involving the CNS, ranging from weakness and numbness to paralysis.

Obtain a dive profile and medical history of the events that led to the diving-related injury from a fellow diver, including the following:

- Time of onset of signs and symptoms
- Source of breathing medium (e.g., air or mixed gases; heliox)
- Dive profile (dive activity, depth, duration, dive frequency, surface interval, interval between dives)
- Dive location and water conditions
- Dive risk factors
- Underwater medical and equipment problems on ascent and descent
- Whether the diver was attempting a no-decompression dive or a decompression dive
- Rate of ascent
- Decompression stop(s)
- Post-dive activity level
- Post-dive aircraft travel or altitude exposure, with type and duration
- Past and present medical history (especially a history of previous DCS)
- Medication use
- Current use of alcohol or illicit drugs[123]

Management

Ensure the ABCs, protect the patient's airway, and initiate BLS or ALS procedures as required. Initiate 100% oxygen at 12 to 15 liters/minute and give NS or LR (no dextrose) IV fluid therapy (1 to 2 mL/kg/hour). Monitor the patient's vital signs, pulse oximetry, and ECG. Check and treat the patient's blood glucose level as required. Control any seizures. Protect the patient from hypothermia, and consult early with local medical control or DAN for the closest hospital with a recompression chamber

(primary treatment). Note that recompression chambers willing to treat divers can be rare—for example, in the entire state of Florida there are only four—meaning that specific planning, and ideally preplanning before an incident, is needed to ensure rapid transport to the closest appropriate facility.[52] See **Box 20-8** for DAN contact information. Standard recompression therapy with 100% hyperbaric oxygen is given according to the U.S. Navy treatment tables.[124] Transport the patient in a supine position. For any scuba-related diving injury, if air evacuation is provided by helicopter or other nonpressurized aircraft, it is recommended to fly as low as safely possible (e.g., 500 ft [150 m]), and certainly not to exceed 1,000 ft (300 m), to minimize further expansion of air bubbles (Boyle's law) and potential exacerbation of the decompression insult.[52,99,103,112]

Definitive treatment for AGE or DCS is to administer 100% oxygen at two to three times the atmospheric pressure in a recompression chamber following standard protocols.[124] For further discussion of recompression chamber treatment methods for scuba-related diving injuries, see the *U.S. Navy Diving Manual* or other sources.[98,124] The patient immediately benefits, based on the principles of Boyle's law, by increasing the ambient pressure and decreasing the size of bubbles formed and increasing the oxygen concentration in tissues. **Box 20-9** describes the benefits of recompression and hyperbaric oxygen therapy.

For the transporting prehospital team, it is critical to ensure that the receiving ED or other facility knows that diving-related conditions such as DCS and AGE are true emergencies and that a detailed examination, including a neurologic examination, will need to be completed as soon as possible by a facility-based emergency clinician. There are additional reading resources that describe

---

Box 20-8 Divers Alert Network (DAN) Contact Information for Diving Emergencies

After EMS is notified, call the Divers Alert Network (DAN)

Emergency Number: 919-684-9111

Nonemergency Medical Questions
919-684-2948 Ext. 6222

Monday–Friday, 8:30 a.m. to 5:00 p.m. (EST)

Address
Divers Alert Network

6 West Colony Place

Durham, NC 27705 USA

Data courtesy of Divers Alert Network® (DAN®).

Box 20-9 Recompression Therapy for Scuba-Related Diving Injuries

The goals of recompression therapy for scuba-related diving injuries caused by pulmonary overinflation barotrauma and DCS are to compress the bubbles and increase oxygen delivery to tissues. Recompression therapy includes the following mechanisms:

- Reduces volume of the bubbles where they are circulated to the pulmonary capillaries and filtered out
- Promotes reabsorption of bubbles in solution
- Increases oxygen delivery to the tissues
- Corrects hypoxia
- Provides an increased diffusion gradient for nitrogen
- Reduces edema
- Reduces blood vessel permeability

All divers with AGE and DCS must be considered early for recompression in a hyperbaric treatment facility because the treatment is more successful if started within 6 hours after the onset of symptoms. Divers are not always near a recompression chamber when symptoms occur, and there can be considerable delays getting to a chamber by ground or by arranging for air transport. Contact the Divers Alert Network to consult for diving medical assistance and to determine the closest recompression chamber.

In the meantime, place the patient in a supine position. Nitrogen washout can be increased by providing 100% oxygen by mask and by starting an IV fluid line with normal saline or lactated Ringer solution at 1 to 2 mL/kg/hr to ensure adequate intravascular volume and capillary perfusion. During recompression treatment, patients with AGE or DCS normally will receive recompression treatment at 2.8 atm for 2 to 4 hours while breathing 100% oxygen. Longer and repeated treatment will be necessary if the patient has no clinical improvement of symptoms.

Recompression treatment principles include the following:

- Any painful or neurologic signs or symptoms occurring within 24 hours of a dive are caused by DCS until proved otherwise.
- Any painful or neurologic signs or symptoms occurring within 48 hours of flying after diving are caused by DCS until proved otherwise.
- Contact the DAN 24-hour emergency hotline for consultation at 919-684-9111.
- Every diver with signs or symptoms of DCS should receive recompression treatment.
- Never fail to treat cases when in doubt about the diagnosis.
- Early treatment generally improves outcomes, whereas delayed treatment may worsen outcomes.
- Long delays should be discussed with a diving medicine physician before recompression treatment, because divers may respond to recompression therapy days after injury.
- Monitor the patient closely for signs of relief from or progression of symptoms.
- Inadequate treatment can lead to a recurrence.
- Continue to treat until clinical plateau.

Data from Tibbles PM, Edelsberg JS. Hyperbaric oxygen therapy. *N Engl J Med*. 1996;334(25):1642; Barratt DM, Harch PG, Van Meter K. Decompression illness in divers: A review of the literature. *Neurologist*. 2002;8:186; and Van Hoesen KB, Bird NH. Diving medicine. In: Auerbach PS, ed. *Wilderness Medicine*. 6th ed. Mosby Elsevier; 2012.

techniques for optimizing team-to-team communication and hand-offs of this sort. See Chapter 6, *Patient Assessment and Management*, for more details on the patient hand-off process.

Table 20-3 summarizes signs and symptoms of barotrauma and its treatment. **Table 20-4** summarizes signs and symptoms of DCS and its treatment.

Prevention of Scuba-Related Diving Injuries

Certified scuba divers need frequent skill refresher training to prevent and recognize scuba-related dive injuries. Many scuba professionals in the United States, such as lifeguards, fire and law enforcement personnel, SAR members, Coast Guard members, and Department of Defense employees, depend on local prehospital care practitioners to provide initial and follow-up medical care and transport to local hospitals or recompression chambers. Collaboration among dive teams and local EMS agencies to develop medical scenarios during dive training is strongly encouraged.[52] This should include frequent scuba training in varying underwater conditions and locations, along with in-water rescue scenarios and initial medical care, which are paramount to responding safely and effectively for in-water swimmer/diver rescues and recoveries. Scuba training coordination among medical dive team members and local practitioners will ensure effective communication and appropriate continuity of field care. This training should include scenario-based consults with local medical control and DAN.

Medical Fitness to Dive

Although prehospital care practitioners do not certify fitness to dive, they should be aware of the factors used by physicians in determining fitness to dive.

Table 20-3 Barotrauma: Common Signs, Symptoms, and Treatment

Type	Signs/Symptoms	Urgency	Treatment*
Mask squeeze	Corneal injection, conjunctival hemorrhage	Nonurgent	Self-limited; rest, cold compresses, pain medication
Sinus squeeze	Pain, bloody nasal discharge Rare retro-orbital emphysema or pneumocephalus	First aid, evaluation as convenient	Pain medication, decongestants, antihistamines
Middle-ear squeeze	Pain, vertigo, tympanic membrane rupture, hearing loss, vomiting	First aid, evaluation as convenient	Decongestants, antihistamines, pain medication; may need antibiotics; avoid diving and flying
Inner-ear barotraumas	Tinnitus, vertigo, ataxia, hearing loss	Urgent	Bed rest; elevate head; avoid loud noises; stool softeners; avoid strenuous activity; no diving or flying for months
External-ear barotraumas	Difficulty with Valsalva maneuver, earache, bloody discharge, possible tympanic membrane rupture	First aid, evaluation as convenient	Maintain dry ear canal; antibiotics may be needed for infection
Tooth squeeze	Tooth pain while diving	First aid, evaluation as convenient	Self-limited; pain medication
Alternobaric vertigo	Pressure, pain in affected ear, vertigo, tinnitus	First aid, evaluation as convenient	Usually short lived; decongestants; prohibit diving until resolution with normal hearing
Pulmonary barotraumas	Substernal pain, voice change, dyspnea, subcutaneous emphysema	Urgent	Assess ABCs, neurologic functions; 100% oxygen 12 to 15 liters/minute nonrebreathing mask; transport patient lying supine; need to rule out AGE
Subcutaneous emphysema	Substernal pain and crepitus, brassy voice, neck swelling, dyspnea, bloody sputum	Urgent	Rest; avoid diving and flying; oxygen and recompression therapy only in severe cases
Pneumothorax	Sharp chest pain, dyspnea, diminished breath sounds	Emergency	100% oxygen 12 to 15 liters/minute nonrebreathing mask; monitor pulse oximetry; transport in position of comfort; assess for tension pneumothorax
Tension pneumothorax	Cyanosis, distended neck veins, tracheal deviation	Emergency	14-gauge needle thoracentesis; 100% oxygen 12 to 15 liters/minute nonrebreathing mask; monitor pulse oximetry

Type	Signs/Symptoms	Urgency	Treatment*
AGE	Unresponsiveness, confusion, headache, visual disturbances, seizure	Emergency	Assess ABCs, neurologic functions; initiate BLS/ALS; control seizures; 100% oxygen 12 to 15 liters/minute nonrebreathing mask; transport patient lying supine; glucose-free IV fluid therapy (1 to 2 mL/kg/hr); monitor ECG; consult DAN (919-684-9111) for closest recompression chamber (primary treatment)

*Good patient education on scene for minor barotrauma injuries is important because some of these injuries are self-limiting and others need physician evaluation; others need patient referral to the family physician or ED and will not necessitate EMS transport.

Abbreviations: ABCs, airway, breathing, circulation; AGE, arterial gas embolism; ALS, advanced life support; BLS, basic life support; DAN, Divers Alert Network; ECG, electrocardiogram.

Data from Clenney TL, Lassen LF: Recreational scuba diving injuries. *Am Fam Physician*. 1996;53(5):1761-1764; Salahuddin M, James LA, Bass ES. SCUBA medicine: A first-responder's guide to diving injuries. *Curr Sports Med Rep*. 2011;10(3):134-139; and Van Hoesen KB, Bird NH. Diving medicine. In: Auerbach PS, ed. *Wilderness Medicine*, 6th ed. Mosby Elsevier; 2012.

Table 20-4 Decompression Sickness: Common Signs, Symptoms, and Treatment

Condition	Signs/Symptoms	Treatment
DCS Type I		
Skin bends	Intense itching (pruritus); red rash patches over shoulders and upper chest; skin marbling may precede burning sensation and itching over shoulders and torso; localized cyanosis and pitting edema.	Self-limiting; resolves on its own; observe for delayed signs of limb-pain DCS. Neurologic evaluation mandatory.
Limb-pain DCS	Large joint tenderness; mild to severe joint or extremity pain; pain is usually steady but may throb and present in 75% of cases; grating sensation on joint motion; worse with movement. DCS type I may progress to DCS type II.	Mild pain only: often resolves on its own, observe 24 hours; Moderate to severe pain: start with 100% oxygen, 12 to 15 liters/minute nonrebreathing mask; transport all patients in supine position; glucose-free IV fluid therapy (1 to 2 mL/kg/hr); consult DAN (919-684-9111) early for closest recompression chamber for a timely definitive treatment.
DCS Type II		
Cardiopulmonary "chokes"	Substernal pain, mild cough, dyspnea, nonproductive cough, cyanosis, tachypnea, tachycardia, shock and cardiac arrest	ABCs; 100% oxygen, 12 to 15 liters/minute nonrebreathing mask; BLS or ALS as needed; glucose-free IV fluid therapy (1 to 2 mL/kg/hr); transport all patients in supine position; consult DAN (919-684-9111) early for closest recompression chamber for definitive treatment; emergency.
Neurologic		
Brain	Many visual changes, headache, confusion, disorientation, nausea and vomiting	
Spinal cord	Back pain, heaviness or weakness, numbness, paralysis, urine retention, fecal incontinence	
Inner ear	Vertigo, ataxia	

Abbreviations: ABCs, airway, breathing, circulation; ALS, advanced life support; BLS, basic life support; DAN, Divers Alert Network; DCS, decompression sickness; IV, intravenous.

Modified from Barratt DM, Harch PG, Van Meter K. Decompression illness in divers: A review of the literature. *Neurologist*. 2002;8:186-202; and Van Hoesen KB, Bird NH: Diving medicine. In: Auerbach PS, ed. *Wilderness Medicine*. 6th ed. Mosby/Elsevier; 2012.

Furthermore, prehospital care practitioners responding to diving-related incidents must assess divers, in all age groups, not only for primary diving disorders related to a submersion incident (e.g., DCS, AGE) but also for underlying medical conditions (e.g., cardiac, pulmonary, neurologic, endocrine, psychiatric, or a combination of both medical and dysbaric disorders). Ideally, all new divers should be seen by a diving medical physician before the start of scuba training, but this often does not occur. Five general medical screening recommendations for identifying individuals who are at an increased risk for a diving-related problem are listed here. These recommendations are based on the consensus of medical diving specialists.[98,103,125] Recommendations include the following:

- Inability to equalize pressure in one or more of the body's air spaces increases the risk for barotrauma.
- Medical or behavioral conditions may manifest underwater or at a remote diving site and can endanger the diver's life because of the condition itself, because it occurs in the water, or because adequate medical help is not available.
- Impaired tissue perfusion or diffusion of inert gases increases the risk of DCS.

- Poor physical condition increases the risk of DCS or exertion-related medical problems. The factors compromising physical condition may be physiologic or pharmacologic.
- In women who are pregnant, the fetus may be at increased risk of dysbaric injury.

For many years, people with diabetes have questioned the diving medical experts about scuba diving waivers for individuals who have control of their blood glucose levels. In June 2005, an international workshop was held in the United States that was jointly sponsored by the Undersea and Hyperbaric Medical Society (UHMS) and DAN. They brought together over 50 medical and research experts from around the world to develop guidelines for recreational divers with diabetes.[126] The panel indicated that dive candidates who use medication (oral hypoglycemic agents or insulin) to treat diabetes but who are otherwise qualified to dive may undertake recreational scuba diving. However, they stated that strict criteria need to be met before diving. The panel agreed that people with diabetes who are using dietary control will easily meet the new guidelines. The consensus guidelines (**Box 20-10**) consist of 19 points, under the categories of

---

Box 20-10 Guidelines for Recreational Diving With Diabetes

Selection and Surveillance
- Individual must be at least 18 years of age (16 years if in special training program).
- Diving will be delayed after starting/changing medication, as follows:
  - Three months with oral hypoglycemic agents
  - One year after initiation of insulin therapy
- There must be no episodes of hypoglycemia or hyperglycemia requiring intervention from a third party within at least 1 year.
- There must be no history of hypoglycemia unawareness.
- A glycated hemoglobin (HbA1c) test result of ≤ 9% must be recorded no more than 1 month prior to initial assessment and at each annual review.
  - Values > 9% indicate the need for further evaluation and possible modification of therapy.
- There must be no significant secondary complications from diabetes.
- A physician/diabetologist should carry out an annual review and determine that the diver has a good understanding of the disease and the effect of exercise in consultation with an expert in diving medicine, as required.
- An evaluation for silent cardiac ischemia for candidates older than 40 years must be performed.

- After initial evaluation, periodic surveillance for silent cardiac ischemia can be in accordance with accepted local/national guidelines for the evaluation of diabetics.
- Candidate must document intent to follow protocol for divers with diabetes and to cease diving and seek medical review for any adverse events during diving possibly related to diabetes.

Scope of Diving
- Diving should be planned to avoid:
  - Depths > 100 ft (30 m) seawater
  - Durations > 60 minutes
  - Compulsory decompression stops
  - Overhead environments (e.g., cave, wreck penetration)
  - Situations that may exacerbate hypoglycemia (e.g., prolonged cold and arduous dives)
- Individuals must have a dive buddy/leader informed of diver's condition and steps to follow in case of problem.
  - Dive buddy should not have diabetes.

Glucose Management on the Day of Diving
- Individuals should perform a general self-assessment of fitness to dive.
- Blood glucose must be ≥ 150 milligrams per deciliter (mg/dL; 8.3 millimoles per liter [mmol/L]), stable or rising, before entering the water.

- · Complete a minimum of three predive blood glucose tests to evaluate trends at 60 minutes, 30 minutes, and immediately prior to diving.
- · Alterations in dosage of oral hypoglycemic agent or insulin on evening prior or day of diving may help.
- ■ Delay dive if blood glucose is:
  - · < 150 mg/dL (8.3 mmol/L)
  - · > 300 mg/dL (16.7 mmol/L)
- ■ Rescue medication considerations include:
  - · Carry readily accessible oral glucose during all dives.
  - · Have parenteral glucagon available at the surface.

- ■ If hypoglycemia is noticed underwater, the diver should surface (with buddy), establish positive buoyancy, ingest glucose, and leave the water.
- ■ Check blood glucose frequently for 12 to 15 hours after diving.
- ■ Ensure adequate hydration on days of diving.
- ■ Log all dives, including blood glucose test results and all information pertinent to diabetes management.

Data courtesy of Divers Alert Network® (DAN®).

Box 20-11 Current Guidelines Recommended by Diver's Alert Network for Flying Safely After Diving

The following guidelines are the consensus of attendees at the 2002 Flying After Diving Workshop. They apply to dives followed by flights at cabin altitudes of 2,000 to 8,000 ft (610 to 2,440 m) for divers who do not have symptoms of DCS. The recommended preflight surface intervals do not guarantee avoidance of DCS. Longer surface intervals will reduce DCS risk further.

- ■ For a single no-decompression dive, a minimum preflight surface interval of 12 hours is suggested.
- ■ For multiple dives per day or multiple days of diving, a minimum preflight surface interval of 18 hours is suggested.

For dives requiring decompression stops, there is little evidence on which to base a recommendation, and a preflight surface interval substantially longer than 18 hours appears prudent.

Data courtesy of Divers Alert Network® (DAN®).

selection and surveillance, scope of diving, and glucose management on the day of diving.

Flying After Diving

Because diving is conducted at many popular dive locations in the United States and at remote locations outside the United States, persons may dive the day before flying. Because of Boyle's law, flying too soon after a dive can increase the risk of DCS during flight or after arriving at the destination because of the reduced atmospheric pressure in either a pressurized or a nonpressurized commercial aircraft. **Box 20-11** lists the current guidelines recommended by DAN for flying safely after diving.[98]

High-Altitude Illness

In the United States, more than 40 million people each year travel above 8,200 ft (2,500 m) without acclimatization to participate in activities that include snowboarding, alpine skiing, hiking, camping, festivals, climbing, work, and many others. Thus, many people are at risk for altitude-related illness, which can develop within hours to days after they arrive at altitude.[127] Prehospital care practitioners and ED staff need to become familiar with the predisposing factors, signs and symptoms, medical management, and education and prevention techniques to reduce the morbidity and mortality of high-altitude illness.

This section presents three medical conditions directly caused by high-altitude environments and highlights specific underlying medical conditions that worsen as a result of high-altitude–induced hypoxia (altitude-exacerbated preexisting medical conditions).

Epidemiology

High-altitude illness is a term that encompasses cerebral and pulmonary syndromes: (1) acute mountain sickness (AMS), (2) high-altitude cerebral edema (HACE), and (3) high-altitude pulmonary edema (HAPE). AMS and HACE are mild and severe ends of a spectrum, whereas HAPE involves separate processes. Even though the risks of acquiring high-altitude illness are low, once it develops, progression can be fatal.[128,129]

Acute mountain sickness (AMS) is a mild form of high-altitude illness, rarely experienced at altitudes below 6,540 ft (2,000 m), but the incidence increases to 1.4% to 25% with increasing altitudes of 6,750 to 8,000 ft (2,060 to 2,440 m).[130,131] AMS develops in 20% to 25% of cases above 8,200 ft (2,500 m) and in 40% to 50% of cases at 14,000 ft (4,270 m). The incidence of AMS is greater than 90% when the rate of ascent to approximately 14,000 ft (4,270 m) occurs over hours versus days.[132] Furthermore, a small number of AMS cases (5% to 10%) progress from mild symptoms to become high-altitude cerebral edema, a severe form of AMS.[129]

High-altitude cerebral edema (HACE) is a severe neurologic form of high-altitude illness. It has a low incidence rate (0.01%) in the general population at an altitude above 8,200 ft (2,500 m); this rate increases to 1% to 2% in more physically active individuals and is even higher above 13,120 ft (4,000 m) with rapid ascent.[127]

High-altitude pulmonary edema (HAPE) is generally rare outside of certain high-altitude operations but accounts for the most deaths from high-altitude illness; it is easily reversed if recognized early and managed correctly. HAPE typically presents within 2 to 5 days after arrival at altitude.[129] The incidence rate for HAPE is 0.01% to 0.1% at 8,200 ft (2,500 m) in the general population and increases to 2% or more in climbers at an altitude of 13,120 ft (4,000 m).

Hypobaric Hypoxia

There are three defined levels of altitude. **High altitude** is defined as an elevation of 5,000 to 11,480 ft (1,500 to 3,500 m). This is a common altitude in the western mountain ranges of the United States, where high-altitude illness is reported with greater frequency than in other regions, and whose ski areas are generally higher than in areas such as the European Alps.[133] **Very high altitude** is defined as an elevation of 11,480 to 18,045 ft (3,500 to 5,500 m) and is the more common altitude for serious forms of high-altitude illness.[134] **Extreme altitude** is defined as elevations higher than 18,045 ft (5,500 m).[129] With a progressive increase in altitude, the environment

becomes very hostile to any person who is not acclimatized to the decreased availability of oxygen, causing a condition known as **hypobaric hypoxia**. However, hypobaric hypoxia occurs at all altitudes to differing degrees.

High altitude is a unique environment because there is a decreased availability of oxygen for respiration, which results in cellular hypoxia. Even though the concentration of oxygen remains at 21% at all altitudes, decreased atmospheric pressure at higher altitude results in a decreased partial pressure of oxygen (PO_2). For example, PO_2 is 160 mm Hg at sea level (1 atm) and 80 mm Hg at 18,045 ft (0.5 atm at 5,500 m), resulting in less oxygen available during respiration. **Table 20-5** shows that as altitude increases from sea level to extreme altitude, there is a proportional decrease in barometric pressure, arterial blood gases, and arterial oxygen saturation (SaO_2). It is worth noting that SaO_2 remains, on average, above 91% in healthy, acclimatizing adults until reaching an altitude above 9,200 ft (2,800 m).

This relationship between increasing altitude and progressive hypoxia forms the basis for the acute physiologic adjustments in ventilatory rate and cardiac output and biochemical changes.[135] Consequently, it is the hypobaric hypoxia and hypoxemia that set up nonacclimatized individuals for high-altitude illness.[128]

Factors Related to High-Altitude Illness

The development of high-altitude illness depends on many factors specific to each high-altitude exposure, but key factors include rapid ascent, individual acclimatization

Table 20-5 Relationship of Altitude, Barometric Pressure (Pb), Arterial Blood Gases, and Oxygen Saturation*

Altitude (meters)	Altitude (feet)	Pb (mm Hg)	PaO₂ (mm Hg)	SaO₂ (%)	PaCO₂ (mm Hg)
Sea level	Sea level	760	100	98.0	40.0
1,646	5,400	630	73.0	95.1	35.6
2,810	9,200	543	60.0	91.0	33.9
3,660	12,020	489	47.6	84.5	29.5
4,700	15,440	429	44.6	78.0	27.1
5,340	17,500	401	43.1	76.2	25.7
6,140	20,140	356	35.0	65.6	22.0

*Data are mean values for subjects ages 20 to 40 years.

Note: PaCO₂, arterial carbon dioxide partial pressure; PaO₂, arterial oxygen partial pressure; SaO₂, arterial oxygen saturation.

Modified from Hackett PH, Roach RC. High-altitude medicine. In: Auerbach PS, ed. *Wilderness Medicine*. 6th ed. Mosby/Elsevier; 2012.

rate, physical exertion at altitude, young age, and history of prior altitude illness.[136] Additional factors include the following:

- *Increased altitude and ascent rate.* The incidence and severity of high-altitude illness are primarily related to the speed of ascent, altitude reached, and length of stay (in shorter durations; longer duration at altitude after a certain period of time equates to less risk), because these three factors increase the hypoxic stress in the body.[127,134]
- *Previous history of high-altitude illness.* A documented history of high-altitude illness is a valuable predictor of who is susceptible for subsequent high-altitude illness when returning to the same altitude at the same ascent rate.[137] Incidence rates for HAPE increase from 10% to 60% for those with a previous history of HAPE who abruptly ascend to an altitude of 14,960 ft (4,560 m).[138]
- *Preacclimatization.* Having a permanent residence above 2,950 ft (900 m) provides some preacclimatization and is associated with a lower rate of and severity of high-altitude illness when ascending to higher altitudes. However, this protection is limited if the ascent rate is rapid or reaches an extreme altitude.[133,134]
- *Age.* Age is a factor in developing AMS; the incidence is lower in those older than 50 years. HAPE occurs more frequently and with greater severity in children and young adults and is reported in equal proportions of men and women in these age groups.[128,139]
- *Physical fitness and exertion.* The onset and severity of high-altitude illness are independent of physical fitness; fitness does not accelerate altitude acclimatization. A high level of fitness does allow individuals to exert themselves more, but vigorous exertion on arrival at high altitude further exacerbates hypoxemia and hastens the onset of high-altitude illness.[133,140]
- *Medications and intoxicants.* Any substance that depresses ventilation and disrupts sleep patterns at altitude should be avoided because this will further exacerbate altitude-induced hypoxemia. These substances include alcohol, barbiturates, and opioids.[129,141]
- *Cold.* Exposure to cold ambient temperatures increases the risk for HAPE because cold increases the pulmonary arterial pressure.[142,143]

Preexisting medical conditions are another factor related to high-altitude illness. It is important to note that when clinical studies are used to determine the effective dose of medication for AMS and HACE, they generally include only healthy individuals without underlying medical problems. However, today many more high-altitude travelers and those who move their residence to higher altitudes have underlying diseases such as diabetes, hypertension, heart disease, or depression. The current medication recommendations for managing altitude illness may not be appropriate for these patients due to the potential for drug interactions and for those patients with renal and/or hepatic insufficiencies. A discussion of these issues can be found in a review article of the medications for the prevention and treatment of altitude illness (i.e., AMS, HAPE, and HACE) for healthy individuals and the drug selection and dosing for patients with underlying medical conditions.[143]

Table 20-6 lists conditions that increase the likelihood of developing high-altitude illness. Additionally,

Table 20-6 Risk Categories of High-Altitude Illness	
Risk Category	**Description**
Low	▪ Individuals with no prior history of altitude illness and ascending to < 9,200 ft (2,800 m) ▪ Individuals taking ≥ 2 days to arrive at 8,200 to 10,000 ft (2,500 to 3,000 m) with subsequent increases in sleeping elevation of less than 1,600 ft (500 m) per day
Moderate	▪ Individuals with prior history of AMS and ascending to 8,200 to 9,100 ft (2,500 to 2,800 m) in 1 day ▪ No history of AMS but ascending to > 9,100 ft (2,800 m) in 1 day ▪ All individuals ascending > 1,600 ft (500 m) per day at altitudes above 10,000 ft (3,000 m)
High	▪ History of AMS and ascending to ≥ 9,100 ft (2,800 m) in 1 day ▪ All individuals with prior history of HAPE or HACE ▪ All individuals ascending to > 11,500 ft (3,500 m) in 1 day ▪ All individuals ascending > 1,600 ft (500 m) per day at altitudes above 11,500 ft (3,500 m) ▪ Very rapid ascents

Abbreviations: AMS, acute mountain sickness; HACE, high-altitude cerebral edema; HAPE, high-altitude pulmonary edema.

Modified from Luk AM, McIntosh SE, Grissom, et al. Wilderness Medical Society consensus guidelines for the prevention and treatment of acute altitude illness. *Wilderness Environ Med.* 2010;21:146-155.

specific medical conditions known to increase susceptibility to high-altitude illness include the following:

- Cardiopulmonary congenital abnormalities: absent pulmonary artery, primary pulmonary hypertension, congenital heart defects
- Carotid artery surgery: irradiation or abolishing carotid bodies

Acute Mountain Sickness

AMS is a self-limited, nonspecific symptom complex that can be easily mistaken for a number of other conditions because of common symptoms, including influenza, hangover, exhaustion, and dehydration. A consensus panel defined AMS as the presence of headache in an unacclimatized person who has recently arrived at an altitude above 8,200 ft (2,500 m) and has one or more symptoms of AMS.[144] However, AMS can occur at levels as low as 6,600 ft (2,000 m). HACE is viewed as a severe form of AMS.[145,146] The majority of AMS cases do not progress to more severe forms of high-altitude illness.

The hallmark symptom of AMS is a mild to severe protracted headache believed to be caused by hypoxia-induced cerebral vasodilation.[147] Patients describe their headache as throbbing, as located in the occipital or temporal regions, and as worsening at night or on awakening. Other symptoms include nausea, vomiting, insomnia, dizziness, *lassitude* (weariness), fatigue, and difficulty sleeping. Malaise and lack of appetite may be present along with a decrease in urine output. It is important to recognize early symptoms of AMS so that continued ascent does not cause a preventable condition to progress into a severe form of HACE.

The onset of symptoms in AMS can occur as early as 1 hour after arriving at high altitude but typically occurs after 6 to 10 hours of exposure. Symptoms usually peak in 24 to 72 hours and subside in 3 to 7 days. If the onset of symptoms occurs beyond 3 days after arriving at altitude and does not include headache, and if oxygen therapy provides no benefit, the condition is probably not AMS.[128]

As with lightning and drowning management, the WMS has a consensus-derived set of practice guidelines regarding AMS. These guidelines are available online and should help practitioners determine evidence-based current best practices.[136]

Assessment

If patients are alert, the key is to obtain a good medical history, including the onset and severity of symptoms, rate of ascent, duration of exposure, use of medications that may cause dehydration, use of alcohol, and level of physical exertion. Obtain vital signs, including pulse oximetry. Also, assess the status of any underlying medical condition, as determined by the medical history.

Because a headache is the most common finding with AMS, assess for location and quality. Periodic breathing is a common finding in individuals who have ascended above about 10,000 ft (about 3,000 m). Assess neurologic function, and assess specifically for ataxia and excessive lethargy, as these symptoms are indicative of HACE.

Management

Descending 1,600 to 3,300 ft (500 to 1,000 m) will provide the quickest resolution of symptoms. Mild AMS will usually resolve on its own, but patients should avoid further ascent and any exertion until symptoms resolve. Provide analgesics for headache and antiemetics for nausea per local protocols. For moderate symptoms, descend to lower altitude. Assess pulse oximetry for SpO_2 greater than 90%. If lower than 90%, titrate oxygen by 1 to 2 liters/minute and reassess. However, this is altitude related; at 14,100 ft (4,300 m), a normal SpO_2 is in the mid-80s. Unexpectedly low SpO_2 might represent HACE, but SpO_2 readings are generally not very helpful in diagnosing AMS. For patients with neurologic symptoms, see management of HACE. Patients with underlying medical problems exacerbated by altitude should be transported on oxygen for medical evaluation of their primary illness and the secondary development of high-altitude illness.

See **Table 20-7** for a summary of the signs and symptoms, management, and prevention of AMS. See **Table 20-8** for dosing recommendations for children with AMS.

High-Altitude Cerebral Edema

HACE is a serious neurologic syndrome that can develop in individuals with AMS or HAPE, or that can develop on its own without relation to other altitude illnesses. At altitudes above 8,000 ft (2,440 m), cerebral blood flow increases as a result of hypoxia-induced vasodilation. The mechanism of injury appears to be related to a combination of sustained cerebral vasodilation, increased capillary permeability across the blood–brain barrier, and the inability to compensate sufficiently for the excess cerebral edema.[148]

HACE can occur at any time within 3 to 5 days after arrival at 9,000 ft (2,750 m), but most commonly it occurs at altitudes above 12,000 ft (3,600 m), with an onset of symptoms within hours. Some symptoms of AMS may be present, but the hallmark features of HACE are altered level of consciousness and ataxia, along with drowsiness, stupor, and confusion progressing to coma. Death results from brain herniation.[149]

Table 20-7 High-Altitude Illness (AMS, HACE, HAPE): Signs, Symptoms, Treatment, and Prevention

Signs/Symptoms	Treatment	Prevention
Acute Mountain Sickness (AMS)		
Mild: Headache, nausea, dizziness, and fatigue in first 12 hours	Oxygen 1 to 2 liters/minute by nasal cannula, and/or descend 1,600 to 3,300 ft (500 to 1,000 m); avoid further ascent until symptoms resolve; consider acetazolamide (250 mg PO bid) to speed acclimatization; give analgesics and antiemetics as needed	Ascend at slow rate; spend night at intermediate altitude; avoid overexertion; avoid direct transport above 9,840 ft (3,000 m) Consider acetazolamide 125 mg PO bid, starting day before ascent and continue for 2 days at maximum altitude Early AMS treatment may prevent subsequent complications
Moderate: Moderate to severe headache, marked nausea, vomiting, decreased appetite, dizziness, insomnia, fluid retention for $\geq$ 12 hours	Descend, consider dexamethasone* (4 mg PO/IM every 6 hours) and/or acetazolamide (250 mg PO bid); if unable to descend, vigilant observation for deterioration; oxygen (1 to 2 liters/minute) and/or portable hyperbaric therapy (2 to 4 psi) for a few hours, if available	Same as listed for mild illness, dexamethasone 2 mg every 6 hours, or 4 mg every 12 hours PO, starting day of ascent and discontinued cautiously after 2 days at maximum altitude, may be considered but should be used only if there is a high-risk ascent and acetazolamide is contraindicated
High-Altitude Cerebral Edema (HACE)		
AMS for $\geq$ 24 hours, ataxia, confusion, bizarre behavior, severe lassitude; usually symptoms of AMS also present with HACE	Immediately descend or evacuate $\geq$ 3,300 ft (1,000 m); give oxygen 2 to 4 liters/minute; titrate to maintain $SpO_2 \geq$ 90%; dexamethasone (8 mg IV/IM/PO initially, then 4 mg every 6 hours); hyperbaric therapy if cannot descend	As listed for AMS
High-Altitude Pulmonary Edema (HAPE)		
Dyspnea at rest, cough, crackles, severe exercise limitation, cyanosis, drowsiness, tachycardia, tachypnea, desaturation	Start oxygen 4 to 6 liters/minute, then titrate to maintain $SpO_2 \geq$ 90%; minimize exertion; keep warm; descend or evacuate 1,700 to 3,300 ft (500 to 1,000 m); consider nifedipine (30 mg sustained-release PO every 12 hours or 20 mg of sustained-release every 8 hours) if no HACE; consider inhaled beta-agonists (salmeterol, 125 mcg inhaled every 12 hours, or albuterol) in high-risk patients only; dexamethasone only if HACE develops	Ascend at a slow rate; avoid overexertion; consider nifedipine (30-mg sustained-release dose every 12 hours bid PO or 20 mg sustained-release every 8 hours) in person with repeated episodes of HAPE; start 1 day prior to ascent and continue for 2 days at maximum altitude

Abbreviations: bid, twice daily; EPAP, expiratory positive airway pressure; IM, intramuscular; IV, intravascular; m, meter; mcg, microgram; mg, milligram; PO, by mouth; psi, pounds per square inch; SaO_2, arterial oxygen saturation.

*Dexamethasone should be used only if no further ascent is contemplated; if for some operational reason the individual must ascend farther, dexamethasone is relatively contraindicated.

Data from Luks AM, Auerbach PS, Freer L, et al. Wilderness Medical Society consensus guidelines for the prevention and treatment of acute altitude illness: 2019 update. *Wilderness Environ Med.* 2019;30(4):S3-S18.

Table 20-8 Drug Dosing for Children With Altitude Illness

In 2001, the International Society for Mountain Medicine published a consensus statement recommending that adult treatment algorithms (for AMS, HACE, and HAPE) be followed with adjustments for pediatric drug dosages.

AMS	Acetazolamide 2.5 mg/kg/dose PO q 12 hours (maximum 250 mg per dose)
	Dexamethasone 0.15 mg/kg/dose PO q 6 hours up to 4 mg
HACE	Acetazolamide 2.5 mg/kg/dose PO q 12 hours (maximum 250 mg per dose)
	Dexamethasone 0.3 mg/kg per dose
HAPE	Dexamethasone 0.15 mg/kg/dose PO q 6 hours up to 4 mg

Abbreviations: kg, kilogram; mg, milligram; PO, by mouth; q, every.

Data from Pollard AJ, Niermeyer S, Barry PB, et al. Children at high altitude: an international consensus statement by an ad hoc committee of the International Society for Mountain Medicine. *High Alt Med Biol.* 2001;2:389-401; and Luks AM, Auerbach PS, Freer L, et al. Wilderness Medical Society consensus guidelines for the prevention and treatment of acute altitude illness: 2019 update. *Wilderness Environ Med.* 2019;30(4):S3-S18.

Assessment

The key is to obtain a good medical history, including the onset and severity of symptoms, rate of ascent, duration of exposure, and level of physical exertion. This can be gathered by questioning the patient's companions, or less commonly, the patient, if sufficiently alert. Obtain the patient's vital signs, including pulse oximetry. Also, assess the status of any underlying medical condition, as determined by the patient's medical history. It may be helpful to assess the patient's lung sounds and level of neurologic function because a strong association exists between HACE and HAPE. Although they are often found together, HAPE will manifest with dyspnea at rest, cough, and a low SpO_2, whereas HACE typically occurs without crackles.

Management

Do not delay planning for treatment and evacuation at the first signs or symptoms of HACE. The highest priority for any patient with HACE is immediate descent, along with initiation of high-flow oxygen (15 liters/minute) by nonrebreathing mask and monitoring of SpO_2 until 90% or greater. Unconscious patients should be managed as a patient with brain injury (see Chapter 7, *Airway and Ventilation,* and Chapter 8, *Head and Neck Trauma*), including intubation and other ALS procedures.[141] Dexamethasone should be administered, and a portable hyperbaric chamber may be used if supplemental oxygen is limited or absent.

See Table 20-7 for a summary of the signs and symptoms, management, and prevention of HACE. See Table 20-8 for dosing recommendations for children with HACE.

High-Altitude Pulmonary Edema

The onset of HAPE follows a pattern like that seen with AMS and HACE, occurring in unacclimatized individuals after a rapid ascent to high altitude. This high-altitude illness has a different mechanism of injury than AMS and HACE, however, because HAPE is induced by hypobaric hypoxia. HAPE is a form of noncardiogenic pulmonary edema associated with pulmonary hypertension and elevated capillary pressure.[137] More than 50% of patients with HAPE have AMS, and 14% have HACE.[150] The signs and symptoms most often appear in the morning after the second night (onset of 1 to 3 days) and rarely occur 4 days after arriving at a given altitude.[151] The development of HAPE and the rate of progression are hastened by cold exposure, vigorous exertion, and continued ascent. Compared with the other two high-altitude illnesses, HAPE accounts for the greatest number of fatalities.

Assessment

Patient assessment, including vital signs, lung sounds, and medical history, are vital in the determination of HAPE, which is defined by at least two or more symptoms (e.g., dyspnea at rest; cough, weakness, or decreased performance during exertion; chest tightness or congestion) and at least two signs (e.g., crackles or wheezing, central cyanosis or low SpO_2, tachypnea, or tachycardia).[152] Crackles are generally present in the lung fields, starting in the right axilla and eventually becoming bilateral. Assess the patient for fever; low fever may be seen with HAPE, whereas high fever might be suggestive of other conditions such as pneumonia. Late findings as HAPE progresses are resting tachycardia, tachypnea, and blood-tinged sputum. If treatment interventions are not provided, symptoms will progress over hours to days to include audible gurgling, respiratory distress, and eventually death.

Management

Descending or evacuating to a lower altitude by at least 1,700 to 3,300 ft (500 to 1,000 m) provides the fastest recovery, but initially patients show good improvement with rest and oxygen or hyperbaric treatment. Keep patients warm and prevent any exertion. These patients need to improve their arterial oxygenation, so start oxygen at 4 to 6 liters/minute or titrate oxygen flow until SaO_2 is 90% or greater. Reassess the patient's vital signs after starting oxygen because improved arterial oxygenation decreases the tachycardia and tachypnea. Because HAPE is a noncardiogenic form of pulmonary edema, diuretics have not been shown to be helpful. Anecdotal case reports have suggested favorable results with the use of continuous positive airway pressure (CPAP) for serious cases of HAPE, and the WMS suggests it can be considered as an adjunct to supplemental oxygen.[137,153,154]

See Table 20-7 for a summary of the signs and symptoms, management, and prevention of HAPE. See Table 20-8 for dosing recommendations for children with HAPE.

Prevention

Acute high-altitude illness in unacclimatized individuals is preventable. The common factor for the onset of AMS, HACE, and HAPE is the rate of ascent to higher altitude. Altitude illness may be experienced by skiers who travel by commercial airlines and take an early morning flight from continental American cities at sea level, arrive at high altitude around noon, and begin skiing by early afternoon at about 7,000 to 14,000 ft (2,100 to 4,500 m). Another scenario with risk of high-altitude illness is a call for mutual aid to various public safety personnel living below 3,300 ft (1,000 m). They assemble quickly and then arrive at 9,000 ft (2,750 m) or higher to assist local volunteer SAR teams trekking to higher altitudes in search of a missing backcountry hiker. Prehospital care personnel, whether ground crew or flight crew, who have responsibilities at high altitude for patient transfer to another hospital or for medical evacuation from the backcountry, need to possess the knowledge to minimize the risk of high-altitude illness for their own safety and the safety of coworkers (**Box 20-12** and **Box 20-13**).

Medications as Prophylaxis for High-Altitude Illness

In all cases, gradual ascent with specific logistical strategies for mitigation (such as "climb high and sleep low") are recommended for prevention of high-altitude illnesses of all types.[130,137,155-158]

AMS/HACE Pharmacologic Prevention

For the prevention of AMS and HACE, individuals traveling from sea level to over 9,850 ft (3,000 m) as their sleeping altitude in 1 day or individuals who have a history of AMS should consider prophylactic treatment. The WMS practice guidelines stratify risk, and

Box 20-12 Altitude Acclimatization Procedures

The following are key points for acclimatizing to high altitude:

- Ascend high enough to induce adaptions but not so high as to develop altitude illness.
- Unacclimatized individuals should ascend slowly and cautiously above 9,000 ft (2,800 m).
- Avoid heavy exertion for the first 3 days.
- Keep well hydrated with water.
- Avoid alcohol, sleeping pills, and other sedatives.
- Eat a high-carbohydrate diet.
- Avoid overexertion.
- Avoid smoking.
- Physical training is not preventive for high-altitude illness.

© National Association of Emergency Medical Technicians (NAEMT)

Box 20-13 Golden Rules of High-Altitude Illness

The "golden rules" of high-altitude illness are as follows:

1. If you are ill at altitude, your symptoms are caused by the altitude until proved otherwise.
2. If you have altitude symptoms, do not go any higher.
3. If you are feeling ill or are getting worse, or if you cannot walk heel to toe in a straight line, descend immediately.
4. A person ill with altitude illness must always be accompanied by a responsible companion who can accomplish or arrange for descent should it become necessary.[135]

© National Association of Emergency Medical Technicians (NAEMT)

the corresponding importance of prophylactic treatment, based on ascent plans and past medical history.[137] If pharmacologic prophylaxis is determined to be desirable, the drug of choice is oral acetazolamide, 125 mg twice daily, beginning 1 day before ascent and continuing for 2 days at maximum altitude or when starting descent.[137,155] An alternative drug is dexamethasone, 4 mg orally or intramuscularly (IM) every 6 hours and continuing for 2 days at maximum altitude (this dosing assumes active ascent with physical exertion).[155] The combination of both drugs may be more effective than either drug alone,[142,144] but the WMS and wilderness EMS experts recommend that this combination be restricted to emergency situations that mandate very rapid ascent.[137,156] Aspirin (325 mg) taken every 4 hours for three doses reduced the incidence of headache from 50% to 7% in one study.[146]

Two studies suggest a benefit from prophylactic use of ibuprofen 600 mg three times per day beginning 6 hours before ascending from 4,100 ft (1,250 m) up to 12,570 ft (3,800 m) as compared to a placebo treatment.[159,160] Lipman et al. reported that 43% of the participants in the ibuprofen group reported the development of AMS compared with 69% in the placebo group. Also, the placebo group reported that the severity of AMS was worse than reported in the ibuprofen group.[159] The benefit for using ibuprofen is that it provides a second-choice medication and can be taken the same day of ascent with no or low side effects when compared to the traditional use of acetazolamide for the prevention of AMS.[159] However, the drawback is that ibuprofen does not seem to speed acclimatization.[155] At least one wilderness EMS reference textbook argues that ibuprofen should not be recommended over acetazolamide until more data become available.[155] In addition, a single trial specifically comparing acetazolamide and ibuprofen found equal incidence of high-altitude headache and AMS in both groups.[161]

HAPE Pharmacologic Prevention

For the prevention of HAPE in individuals with a history of repeated episodes, prophylaxis with oral nifedipine, 60 mg daily divided into 2 or 3 doses (extended-release formulation), is recommended as a first-line intervention.[137,155] Salmeterol may also be considered as a supplement to nifedipine, at a dose of 125 mcg inhaled twice daily, but only in high-risk individuals with a clear history of recurrent HAPE.[137,155] Other medications being studied for HAPE prevention that show potential promise include sildenafil, tadalafil, and dexamethasone,[130] but further research is needed before they can be recommended for wilderness EMS purposes.[155]

Currently, prophylactic treatment should be avoided as a method to prevent altitude illness in children because of insufficient clinical studies.[162]

Prolonged Transport

Because environmental trauma often occurs in remote locations or in settings that do not easily accommodate ambulances, delivery of the patient to the nearest appropriate trauma center may be delayed. Prehospital care practitioners may need to continue managing the patient for an extended period while driving to the nearest hospital or waiting for helicopter arrival.

Drowning

Minimally symptomatic patients can become more symptomatic in an extended-care situation with a delay of 4 hours before worsening of symptoms. However, there is no case in the medical literature of a drowning patient presenting as initially completely asymptomatic and then deteriorating or dying hours or days later.[36] Initiate CPR for a drowning victim with five continuous breaths using the traditional ABC approach, not CAB, to begin correcting hypoxemia. Obtain a pulse oximetry reading before and after administration of oxygen. Provide high-flow oxygen via a nonrebreathing mask at 15 liters/minute.

Any patient with pulse oximetry values less than 92% (especially those with this level after initiation of oxygen), altered mental status, apnea, or coma may require early invasive airway management to protect from aspiration. Any patient who continues to be hypoxemic with pulse oximetry readings less than 92% after administration of high-flow oxygen is a candidate for CPAP or rapid-sequence intubation protocol. Use care with suction through the endotracheal tube as this may compromise oxygenation, although it may be needed if secretions are compromising ventilation. Consult with medical control, if available, to sedate and paralyze the patient (if permitted by protocols) to ensure successful intubation, oxygenation, and effective ventilation.

Another effective method to ensure effective oxygenation and ventilation is the use of PEEP for respiratory assistance.[30,46] PEEP recruits collapsed alveoli, improving the ventilatory–perfusion ratio and arterial oxygenation.

Determine the patient's GCS score, and assess routinely for trends because it is predictive of patient outcome. Monitor for hypothermia and hypoglycemia. Any comatose patient should have blood glucose measured or, if unable, receive IV dextrose. The placement of a nasogastric tube may be needed to reduce gastric content and water swallowed during submersion after a secure airway is achieved.

Lightning Injury

Victims of lightning may be in respiratory arrest, cardiac arrest, or both. Following CAB assessment, initiate CPR rapidly. When in an extended-care situation with multiple victims, use *reverse triage*, and first resuscitate those who appear dead. However, prolonged (multiple hours) CPR on these victims has a poor patient outcome, and there is little benefit from CPR or ACLS procedures lasting longer than 20 to 30 minutes. All measures to stabilize the patient to correct for hypoxemia, hypovolemia, hypothermia, and acidosis should be attempted before terminating resuscitative efforts.[3]

Assess the patient for cerebral edema and increased ICP. Establish a baseline GCS score, and reassess the patient every 10 minutes as an indicator of progressive cerebral edema and increased ICP (manage per recommendation for cerebral edema; see Chapter 8, *Head and Neck Trauma*).

Recreational Scuba-Related Diving Injuries

The standard treatment protocol for scuba-related injuries causing pulmonary overinflation syndrome (e.g., AGE, DCS) is to provide high-flow oxygen (15 liters/minute via nonrebreathing mask) at the scene and continue oxygen therapy during transport of the patient to the closest recompression chamber for hyperbaric oxygen therapy. Conduct an extensive neurologic evaluation and reassess the patient frequently for progression of signs and symptoms. Use analgesics for pain control per local protocols. Also consider giving aspirin (325 or 650 mg) for its antiplatelet activity.[99]

Contact DAN and local medical direction for the closest location of a functional recompression chamber. Before transporting a patient for hyperbaric oxygen therapy, contact the chamber directly because the status of chamber readiness can change without notification. When transporting by air, use aircraft that can preferably maintain sea-level atmosphere during flight. Any nonpressurized aircraft should maintain an altitude below 1,000 ft (300 m) en route to the chamber site.

High-Altitude Illness

Mild to moderate AMS can be managed with low-volume oxygen at 2 to 4 liters/minute by nasal cannula, titrated by 1 to 2 liters/minute (greater than 90% SpO_2), with a combination of analgesics (e.g., aspirin, 650 mg; acetaminophen, 650 to 1,000 mg; ibuprofen, 600 mg) for headache and prochlorperazine (5 to 10 mg IM) or ondansetron (4 mg orally dissolving tablet or IM) for nausea. Other medications used for treating mild to moderate AMS include oral acetazolamide (250 mg twice daily) and

dexamethasone (4 mg orally [PO] or IM every 6 hours) until symptoms resolve (although note that dexamethasone would be dangerous if contemplating further ascent).

Treat HACE with immediate descent, oxygen by nasal cannula to maintain greater than 90% SpO_2 (usually 2 to 4 liters/minute), and dexamethasone (8 mg PO, IV, or IM initially, then 4 mg every 6 hours). Consider using oral acetazolamide (250 mg twice daily) with prolonged delays to descent. Consider use of a hyperbaric chamber if descent is delayed. If a severe form of HACE develops and the patient is comatose, manage according to recommendations for cerebral edema (see Chapter 3, *Shock: Pathophysiology of Life and Death*).

Prolonged management of HAPE primarily consists of administering oxygen at 4 to 6 liters/minute by nasal cannula (greater than 90% SpO_2) until improvement of symptoms, then 2 to 4 liters/minute for conserving oxygen, or use a hyperbaric chamber. If oxygen is not available, give oral nifedipine (10 mg initially, then 30 mg extended-release dose every 12 to 24 hours). Consider CPAP. If the patient acquires HACE, add dexamethasone (8 mg PO or IM every 6 hours).

Use of portable hyperbaric chambers has been successful for treating high-altitude illness.[130] These lightweight, fabric pressure bags simulate descending to a lower altitude with or without the use of supplemental oxygen or medication (e.g., acetazolamide, dexamethasone, nifedipine). They inflate with manual pumps up to 2 psi, which is equivalent to descending a variable distance depending on the initial altitude and severity of HAPE. The use of these chambers for 2 to 3 hours can effectively improve symptoms. This is an ideal use of technology while waiting for transportation to definitive care, and sometimes a chamber represents the definitive care itself if the patient's symptoms resolve.

SUMMARY

- Basic knowledge of common environmental emergencies is necessary so that rapid assessment and treatment in the prehospital setting can be provided.
- Lightning
  - Lightning injuries range from minor superficial wounds to major multisystem trauma and death.
  - The mechanism for sudden death from lightning strike is simultaneous cardiac and respiratory arrest.
  - The priorities for managing a lightning victim are to ensure scene safety and to assess the

  XABCDEs, ensuring cardiac function, which will typically involve CPR and possibly defibrillation.
  - In circumstances with multiple casualties, the "reverse" triage approach is used, as patients in respiratory arrest or cardiac arrest have a high probability of recovery if managed expeditiously.
- Drowning
  - Prehospital care practitioners must understand the pathophysiologic process of drowning. The major determinant of survival and long-term functionality following drowning is the extent of CNS injury.
  - When managing drowned persons, all patients receive high-flow oxygen. Generally,

(continues)

SUMMARY (CONTINUED)

management involves IV access and fluid administration (normal saline or lactated Ringer solution), and transport to the ED for evaluation.

- Rapid initiation of effective BLS and standard ALS procedures for drowning patients in cardiopulmonary arrest is associated with the best chance of survival.
- Drowning prevention efforts that prehospital care practitioners can encourage in their communities include installing barriers around pools, monitoring children when near water, using personal flotation devices such as life vests, initiating CPR by bystanders before the arrival of prehospital care, and avoiding high-risk behaviors such as alcohol consumption when participating in water-related activities.

■ Recreational diving
- The type of recreational diving injury to which practitioners will most commonly respond is scuba-related injury or fatality caused by dysbarism (altered environmental pressure).
- Barotrauma can result in various types of pressure injuries. Examples of descent-related injuries include mask squeeze, tooth squeeze, middle-ear squeeze (most common), sinus squeeze, and inner-ear barotrauma. Ascent-related injuries include alternobaric

vertigo, sinus barotrauma, and pulmonary overinflation syndrome (POIS). Practitioners must be prepared to recognize these injuries to effectively evaluate and manage them.
- Management of diving injuries involves assessing the ABCs, protecting the patient's airway, and initiating BLS or ALS procedures.

■ High-altitude illness
- High-altitude illness is a term that encompasses cerebral and pulmonary syndromes: acute mountain sickness (AMS), high-altitude cerebral edema (HACE), and high-altitude pulmonary edema (HAPE).
- Prehospital care practitioners and ED staff need to become familiar with the predisposing factors, signs and symptoms, medical management, and education and prevention techniques to reduce the morbidity and mortality of high-altitude illness.
- Prehospital management for these conditions generally involves descent from high elevation, oxygen administration, and possible pharmacologic intervention (as indicated).

■ Due to the possibility of prolonged transport often relating to environmental trauma, prehospital care practitioners must be prepared to deliver ongoing patient management in the ambulance.

SCENARIO RECAP

In a coastal town, a family of four was strolling on the beach with their dog during a chilly winter day. The son tossed a rubber ball toward the water's edge, and the dog gave chase. In an instant, a large shore-breaking wave swallowed up the dog in the rough surf. The 17-year-old son was first into the water to attempt to save the dog, only to be overtaken by the water. He was seen struggling in the rough, surging surf by his parents and sister.

The boy's father and mother grabbed a nearby flotation device stationed on the beachfront and followed him into the surf to help. Their 19-year-old daughter remained on shore and called for help on her cell phone. The dog eventually made it back to the shore. The parents pulled their son out of the cold water after finding him submerged and unresponsive. Your paramedic unit arrives to the scene within 7 minutes of the daughter's call.

As you exit the ambulance, you observe an unconscious teenage boy lying partially prone with his face rotated to the side in sand with surging water close by. He is still in the surf zone and could be submersed by a wave. You join up with arriving fire department emergency responders to approach the victim.

- How should you approach the patient in this setting?
- If the patient has no pulse or respirations, what is the next immediate intervention?
- What other concerns do you have for the patient that need to be addressed on scene?

SCENARIO SOLUTION

Your plan is to have one fire fighter, equipped with a PFD, serve as a lookout for a threat of oncoming surf and for you, your partner, and two other fire fighters to approach the victim to pick him up by all four extremities and quickly carry him away from the surging waves. All individuals near or entering the water will have PFDs.

As the lead prehospital care practitioner, you direct the team to place the victim supine, parallel to the shore, so that the head and trunk are at the same level and then immediately check for responsiveness. The other emergency responders begin staging the emergency medical gear near the victim as you check the ABCs, remembering that in this case, an XABCDE sequence would be inappropriate. The patient may be apneic and need only rescue breathing or may need full CPR. In either situation, you know that the recommendation for drowning is now to provide five rescue breaths initially followed by 30 chest compressions and then to continue two breaths and 30 compressions until signs of life appear or resuscitation is terminated as futile.

The initial approach to the ABCs in drowning victims is essential to address the hypoxemia. High-flow oxygen is provided using a bag-mask device. You start an IV with crystalloids. In this case, spinal motion restriction is not needed because there was no mechanism of injury to suspect spinal trauma. Early intubation or assisted-mechanical ventilation, such as CPAP, may be indicated if the victim shows signs of deterioration with SpO_2 less than 92%. You transport the patient and his parents to the hospital for continued treatment and evaluation.

References

1. Curran EB, Holle RL, Lopez RE. Lightning fatalities, injuries and damage reports in the United States, 1959–1994. NOAA Tech Memo NWS SR-193; 1997.

2. Centers for Disease Control and Prevention. QuickStats: number of deaths from lightning among males and females— National Vital Statistics System, United States, 1968–2010. *Morb Mortal Wkly Rep*. Accessed January 18, 2022. https://www.cdc.gov/mmwr/preview/mmwrhtml/mm6228a6.htm

3. Gatewood MO, Zane RD. Lightning injuries. *Emerg Med Clin North Am*. 2004;22:369-403.

4. Huffines GR, Orville RE. Lightning ground flash density and thunderstorm duration in the continental United States: 1989–96. *J Appl Meteorol Climatol*. 1999;38(7):1013-1019.

5. Cummins KL, Krider EP, Malone MD. A combined TOA/MDF technology upgrade of the U.S. National Lightning Detection Network. *J Geophys Res*. 1998;103:9035-9044.

6. MacGorman, DR, Rust WD. Lightning strike density for the contiguous United States from thunderstorm duration records, Pub No NUREG/CR03759. Office of Nuclear Regulatory Research; 1984.

7. Hawkins SC, Simon RB, Beissinger JP, Simon D. *Vertical Aid: Essential Wilderness Medicine for Climbers, Trekkers, and Mountaineers*. The Countryman Press; 2017.

8. Cherington M, Walker J, Boyson M, Glancy R, Hedegaard H, Clark S. Closing the gap on the actual numbers of lightning casualties and deaths. 11th Conference on Applied Climatology. Dallas, TX: American Meteorological Society; 1999:379-380.

9. Dulcos PJ, Sanderson LM, Klontz KC. Lightning-related mortality and morbidity in Florida. *Pub Health Rep*. 1990;105:276-282.

10. Cooper MA, Andrews CJ, Holle RL, Blumenthal R, Aldana NN. Lightning-related injuries and safety. In: Auerbach PS, ed. *Auerbach's Wilderness Medicine*. 7th ed. Elsevier; 2017.

11. Nelson RD, McGinnis H. Lightning injuries and severe storms. In: Hawkins SC, ed. *Wilderness EMS*. Wolters Kluwer; 2018.

12. Jensenius JS. A detailed analysis of lightning deaths in the United States from 2006 through 2019. National Lightning Safety Council. Published February 2020. Accessed January 18, 2022. https://www.weather.gov/media/safety/Analysis06-19.pdf

13. Davis C, Engeln A, Johnson E, et al. Wilderness Medical Society practice guidelines for the prevention and treatment of lightning injuries: 2014 update. *Wilderness Environ Med*. 2014;25(4):S86-S95.

14. Cooper MA. Lightning injuries: prognostic signs of death. *Ann Emerg Med*. 1980;9:134-138.

15. Cooper MA, Edlich RF. Lightning injuries. Medscape. Updated September 17, 2021. Accessed October 25, 2021. http://emedicine.medscape.com/article/770642-overview

16. Andrews CJ, Darveniza M, Mackerras D. Lightning injury: a review of the clinical aspects, pathophysiology and treatment. *Adv Trauma*. 1989;4:241-287.

17. Ashish RP, Bartos JA, Cabañas JG, et al. 2020 American Heart Association guidelines for cardiopulmonary resuscitation and emergency cardiovascular care: cardiac arrest associated with electric shock and lightning strikes. *Circulation*. 2020;142(18):S366-S468.

18. Ritenour AE, Morton MJ, McManus JG, Barillo DJ, Cancio LC. Lightning injury: a review. *Burns*. 2008;34:585-594.

19. Beir M, Chen W, Bodnar E, Lee RC. Biophysical injury mechanisms associated with lightning injury. *Neurorehabilitation*. 2005;20(1):53-62.

20. Cooper MA. Electrical and lightning injuries. *Emerg Med Clin North Am*. 1984;2:489-501.

21. Casten JA, Kytilla J. Eye symptoms caused by lightning. *Acta Ophthalmol*. 1963;41:139-143.

22. Kleiner JP, Wilkin JH. Cardiac effects of lightning stroke. *JAMA*. 1978;240:2757-2759.

23. Taussig HB. Death from lightning and the possibility of living again. *Ann Intern Med*. 1968;68:1345-1353.

24. Hawkins SC, Williams J, Bennett BL, Islas A, Kayser DW, Quinn R. Wilderness Medical Society clinical practice guidelines for spinal cord protection. *Wilderness Environ Med*. 2019;30(4):S87-S99.

25. Zimmerman C, Cooper MA, Holle RL. Lightning safety guidelines. *Ann Emerg Med*. 2002;39:660-664.

26. National Lightning Safety Institute. Personal lightning safety. Accessed January 18, 2022. http://www.lightningsafety.com/nlsi_pls.html

27. National Weather Service. Lightning tips. Accessed January 18, 2022. https://www.weather.gov/safety/lightning-tips

28. Zafren K, Durrer B, Henry JP, Brugger H. Lightning injuries: prevention and on-site treatment in mountains and remote areas—official guidelines of the International Commission for Mountain Emergency Medicine and Medical Commission of the International Mountaineering and Climbing Federation (ICAR and UIAA MEDCOM). *Resuscitation*. 2005;65:369-372.

29. National Oceanic and Atmospheric Administration. Lightning myths. Accessed January 18, 2022. https://www.weather.gov/safety/lightning-myths

30. Sempsrott J, Schmidt AC, Hawkins SC, Cushing TA. Drowning and submersion injuries. In: Auerbach PS, ed. *Auerbach's Wilderness Medicine*. 7th ed. Elsevier; 2017.

31. Peden M, Oyegbite K, Ozanne-Smith J, et al., eds. World report on child injury prevention. World Health Organization; 2008.

32. Centers for Disease Control and Prevention. Nonfatal and fatal drowning in recreational water settings—United States, 2005–2009. *Morb Mortal Wkly Rep*. 2012;61(19):345.

33. Centers for Disease Control and Prevention. Drowning—United States, 2005–2009. *Morb Mortal Wkly Rep*. 2012;61(19);344-347.

34. Zuckerman GB, Conway EE Jr. Drowning and near-drowning. *Pediatr Ann*. 2000;29(6):360-366.

35. World Health Organization. Facts sheet: drowning. Updated April 27, 2021. Accessed October 25, 2021. https://www.who.int/news-room/fact-sheets/detail/drowning

36. Hawkins SC, Sempsrott J, Schmidt A. Drowning in a sea of misinformation: dry drowning and secondary drowning. *Emerg Med News*. 2017;39(8):1,39-40.

37. van Beeck EF, Branche CM, Szpilman D, et al. A new definition of drowning: towards documentation and prevention of a global public health program. *Bull World Health Organ*. 2005;83:853-856.

38. van Beeck EF, Branche CM, Szpilman D, et al. Definition of drowning. In: Bierens JJLM, ed. *Handbook on Drowning: Prevention, Rescue, Treatment*. Springer; 2006.

39. van Beek E, Branche C. Definition of drowning: a progress report. In: Bierens JJLM, ed. *Drowning: Prevention, Rescue, Treatment*. 2nd ed. Springer; 2014.

40. American College of Emergency Physicians. Death after swimming is extremely rare—and is NOT "dry drowning." Published July 11, 2017. Accessed January 18, 2022. https://www.prnewswire.com/news-releases/death-after-swimming-is-extremely-rare--and-is-not-dry-drowning-300486302.html

41. Szpilman D, Bierens JJLM, Handley A, Orlowshi JP. Drowning. *N Engl J Med*. 2012;366:2102-2110.

42. World Health Organization. Global report on drowning: preventing a leading killer. Published November 17, 2014. Accessed October 25, 2021. https://www.who.int/publications/i/item/global-report-on-drowning-preventing-a-leading-killer

43. Schmidt AC, Sempsrott JR, Hawkins SC, Arastu AS, Cushing TA, Auerbach PS. Wilderness Medical Society practice guidelines for the prevention and treatment of drowning: 2019 update. *Wilderness Environ Med*. 2019;30(4):S70-S86.

44. Centers for Disease Control and Prevention. Injury Center: Drowning Prevention: Drowning Facts. Accessed January 18, 2022. https://www.cdc.gov/drowning/facts/index.html. Last reviewed June 17, 2021.

45. Centers for Disease Control and Prevention. Leading causes of injury and death. Accessed January 18, 2022. https://www.cdc.gov/injury/wisqars/index.html

46. Olshaker JS. Submersion. *Emerg Med Clin North Am*. 2004;22:357-367.

47. Moran K, Quan L, Franklin R, Bennett E. Where the evidence and expert opinion meet: a review of the open-water recreational safety messages. *Int J Aquatic Res Educ*. 2011;5:251-270.

48. Lavelle JM. Ten-year review of pediatric bathtub near-drownings: evaluation for child abuse and neglect. *Ann Emerg Med*. 1995;25:344-348.

49. Craig AB Jr. Underwater swimming and loss of consciousness. *JAMA*. 1961;176:255-258.

50. Dickinson P. Shallow water blackout. In: Bierens JJLM, ed. *Drowning: Prevention, Rescue, Treatment*. 2nd ed. Springer; 2014.

51. International Life Saving Federation. Medical Position Statement—MPS 16: shallow water blackout. International Life Saving Federation position statements. https://medical.ilsf.org/shallow-water-blackout/

52. Chimiak JM, Buzzacott P. Management of diving injuries. In: Hawkins SC, ed. *Wilderness EMS*. Wolters Kluwer; 2018.

53. United States Lifesaving Association. *Open Water Lifesaving: The United States Lifesaving Association Manual*. 3rd ed. Pearson; 2017.

54. Pearn JH, Franklin RC, Peden AE. Hypoxic blackout: diagnosis, risks, and prevention. *Int J Aquatic Res Educ*. 2015;9:342-347.

55. Royal Life Saving Australia. Hypoxic blackout. Accessed October 25, 2021. https://www.royallifesaving.com.au/stay-safe-active/risk-factors/hypoxic-blackout

56. Jensen LR, Williams SD, Thurman DJ, Keller PA. Submersion injuries in children younger than 5 years in urban Utah. *West J Med*. 1992;157(6):641-644.

57. Howland J, Hingson R, Mangione TW, Bell N, Bak S. Why are most drowning victims men? Sex differences, aquatic skills and behaviors. *Am J Public Health.* 1996;86:93-96.

58. Schuman SH, Rowe JR, Glazer HM, et al. The iceberg phenomenon of near-drowning. *Crit Care Med.* 1976;4: 127-128.

59. Bell NS, Amoros PJ, Yore MM, et al. Alcohol and other risk factors for drowning among male active duty U.S. army soldiers. *Aviat Space Environ Med.* 2001;72(12):1086-1095.

60. DeNicola LK, Falk JL, Swanson ME, Kissoon N. Submersion injuries in children and adults. *Crit Care Clin.* 1997;13(3):477-502.

61. Howland J, Mangione T, Hingson R, et al. Alcohol as a risk factor for drowning and other aquatic injuries. In: Watson RR, ed. *Alcohol and Accidents: Drug and Alcohol Abuse Reviews.* Vol 7. Humana Press; 1995.

62. Howland J, Hingson R. Alcohol as a risk factor for drownings: a review of the literature (1950–1985). *Accid Anal Prev.* 1988;20(1):19-25.

63. Howland J, Smith GS, Mangione T, et al. Missing the boat on drinking and boating. *JAMA.* 1993;270:91-92.

64. Bell GS, Gaitatzis A, Bell CL, Johnson AL, Sander JW. Drowning in people with epilepsy. *Neurology.* 2008;71:578-582.

65. White J. *StarGuard: Best Practices for Lifeguards.* 5th ed. Human Kinetics; 2017.

66. Sempsrott J. Management of drowning. In: Hawkins SC, ed. *Wilderness EMS.* Wolters Kluwer; 2018.

67. Padgett J. Technical rescue interface: swiftwater rescue. In: Hawkins SC, ed. *Wilderness EMS.* Wolters Kluwer; 2018.

68. Smith B, Bledsoe B, Nicolazzo P. General management of trauma in the wilderness environment. In: Hawkins SC, ed. *Wilderness EMS.* Wolters Kluwer; 2018.

69. Smith W. Technical rescue interface introduction: principles of basic technical rescue, patient care integration, and packaging. In: Hawkins SC, ed. *Wilderness EMS.* Wolters Kluwer; 2018.

70. Rowe MI, Arango A, Allington G. Profile of pediatric drowning victims in a water-oriented society. *J Trauma.* 1977;17:587-591.

71. Brenner RA, Taneja GS, Haynie DL, et al. Association between swimming lessons and drowning in childhood: a case-control study. *Arch Pediatr Adolesc Med.* 2009; 163:203-210.

72. Quan L, Mack CD, Schiff MA. Association of water temperature and submersion duration and drowning outcome. *Resuscitation.* 2014;85(6):790-794. doi: 10.1016/j .resuscitation.2014.02.024

73. Giesbrecht GG, Steinman AM. Immersion into cold water. In: Auerbach PS, ed. *Wilderness Medicine.* 6th ed. Mosby Elsevier; 2012.

74. Bolte RG, Black PG, Bowers RS. The use of extracorporeal rewarming in a child submerged for 66 minutes. *JAMA.* 1988;260:377-379.

75. Lloyd EL. Accidental hypothermia. *Resuscitation.* 1996;32: 111-124. doi: 10.1016/0300-9572(96)00983-5

76. Gilbert M, Busund R, Skagseth A. Resuscitation from accidental hypothermia of 13.7°C with circulatory arrest. *Lancet.* 2000;355:375-376.

77. Siebke H, Breivik H, Rod T, et al. Survival after 40 minutes submersion without cerebral sequelae. *Lancet.* 1975;1: 1275-1277.

78. Tipton MJ, Golden FSC. A proposed decision-making guide for the search, rescue and resuscitation of submersion (head under) victims based on expert opinion. *Resuscitation.* 2011;82(7)819-824. doi: 10.1016/j.resuscitation .2011.02.021

79. National Fire Chiefs Council. National Operational Guidance: Rescue from water. Accessed March 11, 2022. https://www.ukfrs.com/scenarios/rescue-water

80. Schmidt A, Sempsrott J, Abo B. Technical rescue interface: open water rescue. In: Hawkins SC, ed. *Wilderness EMS.* Wolters Kluwer; 2018.

81. James Cook University. Drowning researchers look for help. Media Release, July 12, 2017. Published July 12, 2017. Accessed October 25, 2021. https://www.jcu.edu.au/news /releases/2017/july/drowning-researchers-look-for-help

82. Zhu Y, Jiang X, Li H, et al. Mortality among drowning rescuers in China, 2013: a review of 225 rescue incidents from the press. *BMC Pub Health.* 2015;15:631. doi: 10.1186/s12889-015-2010-0

83. Hwang V, Frances S, Durbin D, et al. Prevalence of traumatic injuries in drowning and near-drowning in children and adolescents. *Arch Pediatr Adolesc Med.* 2003;157(1):50-53.

84. Pratt FD, Haynes BE. Incidence of "secondary drowning" after saltwater submersion. *Ann Emerg Med.* 1986; 15(9):1084-1087.

85. Szpilman D. Near-drowning and drowning classification: a proposal to stratify mortality based on the analysis of 1,831 cases. *Chest.* 1997;112:660-665.

86. Kleinman ME, Brennan EE, Goldberger ZDD. Part 5: Adult Basic Life Support and Cardiopulmonary Resuscitation Quality. 2015 American Heart Association Guidelines Update for Cardiopulmonary Resuscitation and Emergency Cardiovascular Care. Accessed October 25, 2021. https://www.ahajournals.org/doi/full/10.1161/CIR .0000000000000259

87. Rosen P, Stoto M, Harley J. The use of the Heimlich maneuver in near-drowning: Institute of Medicine report. *J Emerg Med.* 1995;13:397-405.

88. Moran K, Quan L, Franklin R, Bennett E. Where the evidence and expert opinion meet: a review of open-water recreational safety messages. *Int J Aquatic Res Educ.* 2011;5(3):251-270.

89. Baker PA, Webber JB. Failure to ventilate with supraglottic airways after drowning. *Anaesth Intensive Care.* 2011;39:675-677.

90. Smith T, ed. *Clinical Procedures and Guidelines: Comprehensive Edition, 2019-2022.* Guideline 11.1: Drowning. Accessed October 25, 2021. https://www.stjohn.org.nz /globalassets/documents/health-practitioners/clinical -procedures-and-guidelines---comprehensive-edition.pdf

91. Kyriacou DN, Arcinue EL, Peek C, Kraus JF. Effect of immediate resuscitation on children with submersion injury. *Pediatrics.* 1994;94:137-142.

92. Denny SA, Quan L, Gilchrist J, et al. American Academy of Pediatrics Policy Statement. Prevention of drowning prevention. *Pediatrics.* 2019;143(4):e20. Published

May, 2019. Accessed October 25, 2021. https://pediatrics .aappublications.org/content/143/5/e20190850

93. Wintemute GJ, Kraus JF, Teret SP, Wright MA. Death resulting from motor vehicle immersions: the nature of the injuries, personal and environmental contributing factors, and potential interventions. *Am J Public Health*. 1990;80:1068-1070.

94. Hawkins SC. Submerged vehicles. *Wilderness Medicine Magazine*. Published February 26, 2015. Accessed October 25, 2021. www.wildernessmedicinemagazine.com/1137 /drowning-submerged-vehicles

95. McDonald GK, Giesbrecht GG. Vehicle submersion: a review of the problem, associated risks, and survival information. *Aviat Space Environ Med*. 2013;84:498-510.

96. Hawkins SC. Setting the record straight to reduce fatalities in sinking vehicles. *Emerg Med News*. 2015;37:5B.

97. Melamed Y, Shupak A, Bitterman H. Medical problems associated with underwater diving. *N Engl J Med*. 1992;326:30-35.

98. Van Hoesen KB, Lang MA. Diving medicine. In: Auerbach PS, ed. *Auerbach's Wilderness Medicine*. 7th ed. Mosby Elsevier; 2017.

99. Salahuddin M, James LA, Bass ES. SCUBA medicine: a first-responder's guide to diving injuries. *Curr Sports Med Rep*. 2011;10(3):134-139.

100. Lynch JA, Bove AA. Diving medicine: a review of the current evidence. *J Am Board Fam Med*. 2009;22:399-407.

101. Strauss MB, Borer RC Jr. Diving medicine: contemporary topics and their controversies. *Am J Emerg Med*. 2001; 19:232-238.

102. Morgan WP. Anxiety and panic in recreational scuba divers. *Sports Med*. 1995;20(6):398-421.

103. Della-Giustina D, Ingebretsen R. *Advanced Wilderness Life Support*. AdventureMed; 2013.

104. Divers Alert Network (DAN). Eleven-year trends (1987–1997) in diving activity: the DAN annual review of recreational SCUBA diving injuries and fatalities based on 2000 data. In: *Report on Decompression Illness, Diving Fatalities and Project Dive Exploration*. Divers Alert Network; 2000:17-29.

105. Divers Alert Network (DAN). *Report on Diving Fatalities: 2017 Edition*. Divers Alert Network; 2017.

106. Hardy KR. Diving-related emergencies. *Emerg Med Clin North Am*. 1997;15(1):223-240. doi: 10.1016/s0733-8627(05) 70292-3

107. Green SM. Incidence and severity of middle-ear barotraumas in recreational scuba diving. *J Wilderness Med*. 1993;4: 270-280.

108. Kizer KW. Dysbaric cerebral air embolism in Hawaii. *Ann Emerg Med*. 1987;16:535-541.

109. Cales RH, Humphreys N, Pilmanis AA, Heilig RW. Cardiac arrest from gas embolism in scuba diving. *Ann Emerg Med*. 1981;10(11):589-592.

110. Butler BD, Laine GA, Leiman BC, et al. Effect of Trendelenburg position on the distribution of arterial air emboli in dogs. *Ann Thorac Surg*. 1988;45(2):198-202.

111. Moon RE. Treatment of diving emergencies. *Crit Care Clin*. 1999;15:429-456.

112. Van Meter K. Medical field management of the injured diver. *Respir Care Clin North Am*. 1997;5(1):137-177.

113. Francis TJ, Dutka AJ, Hallenbeck JM. Pathophysiology of decompression sickness. In: Bove AA, Davis JC, eds. *Diving Medicine*. 2nd ed. Saunders; 1990.

114. Neuman TS. DCI/DCS: does it matter whether the emperor wears clothes? *Undersea Hyperb Med*. 1997;24(1):4-5.

115. Bove AA. Nomenclature of pressure disorders. *Undersea Hyperb Med*. 1997;24:1-2.

116. Spira A. Diving and marine medicine review: part II. diving diseases. *J Travel Med*. 1999;6:180-198.

117. Clenney TL, Lassen LF. Recreational scuba diving injuries. *Am Fam Physician*. 1996;53(5):1761-1774.

118. Kizer KW. Women and diving. *Physician Sportsmed*. 1981;9(2):84-92.

119. Lau AM, Johnston MJ, Rivard SC. Mottled, Blanching Skin Changes After Aggressive Diving. *J Spec Oper Med*. 2019;19(2):14-17. PMID: 31201746.

120. Estrada J, Meurer D, De Boer K, Huesgen K. Severe Decompression Illness: Case Report, Prehospital Recognition, and Regional Transport Considerations. *Case Rep Emerg Med*. 2017;2017:7203085. doi: 10.1155/2017/7203085. Epub 2017 Oct 4. PMID: 29109872; PMCID: PMC5646287.

121. Francis TJ, Dutka AJ, Hallenbeck JM. Pathophysiology of decompression sickness. In: Bove AA, Davis JC, eds. *Diving Medicine*. 2nd ed. Saunders; 1990.

122. Greer HD, Massey EW. Neurologic injury from undersea diving. *Neurol Clin*. 1992;10(4):1031-1045.

123. Kizer KW. Management of dysbaric diving casualties. *Emerg Med Clin North Am*. 1983;1:659-670.

124. Department of the Navy. *U.S. Navy Diving Manual*. Vol 1, Rev 4. U.S. Government Printing Office; 1999.

125. Davis JC. Hyperbaric medicine: critical care aspects. In: Shoemaker WC, ed. *Critical Care: State of the Art*. Society of Critical Care Medicine; 1984.

126. Pollock NW, Uguccioni DM, Dear GdeL, eds. Diabetes and recreational diving: guidelines for the future. Proceedings of the Undersea and Hyperbaric Medical Society/Divers Alert Network. June 19, 2005, Workshop. Divers Alert Network; 2005.

127. Gallagher SA, Hackett PH. High-altitude illness. *Emerg Med Clin North Am*. 2004;22:329-355.

128. Hackett PH, Roach RC. High-altitude illness. *N Engl J Med*. 2001;345(2):107-114. doi: 10.1056/NEJM200107123450206

129. Hackett PH, Luks AM, Lawley JS, Roach RC. High-altitude medicine and pathophysiology. In: Auerbach PS, ed. *Auerbach's Wilderness Medicine*. 7th ed. Mosby Elsevier; 2017.

130. Houston CS. High-altitude illness disease with protean manifestations. *JAMA*. 1976;236(19):2193-2195. doi:10.1001 /jama.1976.03270200031025

131. Montgomery AB, Mills J, Luce JM. Incidence of acute mountain sickness at intermediate altitude. *JAMA*. 1989; 261:732-734.

132. Gertsch JH, Seto TB, Mor J, Onopa J. Ginkgo biloba for the prevention of severe acute mountain sickness (AMS) starting day one before rapid ascent. *High Alt Med Biol*. 2002; 3(1):29-37.

133. Honigman B, Theis MK, Koziol-McLain J, et al. Acute mountain sickness in a general tourist population at moderate altitudes. *Ann Intern Med*. 1993;118(8):587-592.

134. Zafren K, Honigman B. High-altitude medicine. *Emerg Clin North Am*. 1997;15(1):191-222.

135. Hultgren HN. *High-Altitude Medicine*. Hultgren Publications; 1997.

136. Luks AM, Auerbach PS, Freer LF, et al. Wilderness Medical Society consensus guidelines for the prevention and treatment of acute altitude illness: 2019 update. *Wilderness Environ Med.* 2019;30(4):S3-S18.

137. Schneider M, Bernasch D, Weymann J, et al. Acute mountain sickness: influence of susceptibility, pre-exposure, and ascent rate. *Med Sci Sports Exerc.* 2002;34(12):1886-1891.

138. Bartsch P. High-altitude pulmonary edema. *Med Sci Sports Exerc.* 1999;31(suppl 1):S23-S27.

139. Roach RC, Houston CS, Honigman B. How well do older persons tolerate moderate altitude? *West J Med.* 1995;162(1):32-36.

140. Roach RC, Maes D, Sandoval D, et al. Exercise exacerbates acute mountain sickness at simulated high altitude. *J Appl Physiol.* 2000;88(2):581-585.

141. Roeggla G, Roeggla H, Roeggla M, et al. Effect of alcohol on acute ventilation adaptation to mild hypoxia at moderate altitude. *Ann Intern Med.* 1995;122:925-927.

142. Reeves JWJ, Zafren K, Honigman B, Schoene R. Seasonal variation in barometric pressure and temperature in Summit County: effect on altitude illness. In: Sutton JHC, Coates G, eds. *Hypoxia and Molecular Medicine.* Charles S. Houston; 1993:272-274.

143. Luks AM, Swenson ER. Medication and dosage considerations in the prophylaxis and treatment of high-altitude illness. *Chest.* 2008;133:744-755.

144. Roach RC, Bartcsh P, Oelz O, Hackett PH, Lake Louise Scoring Committee. The Lake Louise Acute Mountain Sickness Scoring System. In: Sutton JR, Houston CS, Coates G, eds. *Hypoxia and Molecular Medicine.* Charles S. Houston; 1993.

145. Muza SR, Lyons TP, Rock PB. Effect of altitude on exposure on brain volume and development of acute mountain sickness (AMS). In: Roach RC, Wagner PD, Hackett PH, eds. *Hypoxia: Into the Next Millennium: Advances in Experimental Medicine and Biology.* Vol 474. Kluwer-Academic/Plenum; 1999.

146. Hacket PH. High-altitude cerebral edema and acute mountain sickness: a pathological update. In: Roach RC, Wagner PD, Hackett PH, eds. *Hypoxia: Into the Next Millennium: Advances in Experimental Medicine and Biology.* Vol 474. Kluwer Academic/Plenum; 1999.

147. Sanchez del Rio M, Moskkowitz MA. High-altitude headache: lessons from aches at sea level. In: Roach RC, Wagner PD, Hackett PH, eds. *Hypoxia: Into the Next Millennium: Advances in Experimental Medicine and Biology.* Vol 474. Kluwer Academic/Plenum; 1999.

148. Hackett PH. The cerebral etiology of high-altitude cerebral edema and acute mountain sickness. *Wilderness Environ Med.* 1999;10(2):97-109.

149. Yarnell PR, Heit J, Hackett PH. High-altitude cerebral edema (HACE): the Denver/Front Range experience. *Semin Neurol.* 2000;20(2):209-217.

150. Hultgren HN, Honigman B, Theis K, Nicholas D. High-altitude pulmonary edema at ski resort. *West J Med.* 1996;164(3):222.

151. Stenmark KR, Frid M, Nemenoff R, et al. Hypoxia induces cell-specific changes in gene expression in vascular wall cells: implications for pulmonary hypertension. In: Roach RC, Wagner PD, Hackett PH, eds. *Hypoxia: Into the Next Millennium: Advances in Experimental Medicine and Biology.* Vol 474. Kluwer Academic/Plenum; 1999.

152. The Lake Louise consensus on the definition and quantification of altitude illness. In: Sutton JR, Coates G, Houston C, eds. *Hypoxia and Mountain Medicine.* Queen City Press; 1992.

153. Luks AM. Do we have a "best practice" for treating high-altitude pulmonary edema? *High Alt Med Biol.* 2008;9:111-114.

154. Koch RO, Burtscher M. Do we have a "best practice" for treating high-altitude pulmonary edema? [Letter to the Editor]. *High Alt Med Biol.* 2008;9:343-344.

155. Zafren K. Management of altitude illnesses. In: Hawkins SC, ed. *Wilderness EMS.* Wolters Kluwer; 2018.

156. Hackett PH, Rennie D, Levine HD. The incidence, importance, and prophylaxis of acute mountain sickness. *Lancet.* 1976;2:1149-1155.

157. Bartsch P, Maggiorini M, Mairbaurl H, et al. Pulmonary extravascular fluid accumulation in climbers. *Lancet.* 2002;360:571-572.

158. Singh I, Kapila CC, Khanna PK, et al. High-altitude pulmonary oedema. *Lancet.* 1965;191:229-234.

159. Lipman GS, Kanaan NC, Holck PS, et al. Ibuprofen prevents altitude illness: randomized controlled trial for prevention of altitude illness with nonsteroidal anti-inflammatories. *Ann Emerg Med.* 2012;59(6):484-490.

160. Gertsch JH, Corbett B, Holck PS, et al. Altitude sickness in climbers and efficacy of NSAIDs trial (ASCENT): randomized, controlled trial of ibuprofen versus placebo for prevention of altitude illness. *Wilderness Environ Med.* 2012;23:307-315.

161. Gertsch JH, Lipman GS, Holck PS, et al. Prospective, double-blind, randomized, placebo-controlled comparison of acetazolamide versus ibuprofen for prophylaxis against high altitude headache: the headache evaluation at altitude trial (HEAT). *Wilderness Environ Med.* 2010;21:236-243.

162. Pollard AJ, Niermeyer S, Barry PB, et al. Children at high altitude: an international consensus statement by an ad hoc committee of the International Society for Mountain Medicine. *High Alt Med Biol.* 2001;2(3):389-403.

Suggested Reading

Auerbach PS, ed. *Auerbach's Wilderness Medicine.* 7th ed. Mosby Elsevier; 2017.

Bechdel L, Ray S. *River Rescue: A Manual for Whitewater Safety.* 4th ed. CFS Press; 2009.

Bennett P, Elliott D. *Bennett and Elliots' Physiology and Medicine of Diving.* 5th ed. Saunders; 2003.

Bierens JJLM. *Drowning: Prevention, Rescue, Treatment.* 2nd ed. Springer; 2014.

Bove AA. *Bove and Davis' Diving Medicine.* 4th ed. Saunders; 2003.

Hawkins SC, ed. *Wilderness EMS.* Wolters Kluwer; 2018.

Hawkins SC, Simon RB, Beissinger JP, Simon D. *Vertical Aid: Essential Wilderness Medicine for Climbers, Trekkers, and Mountaineers.* The Countryman Press; 2017.

Rodway GW, Weber DC, McIntosh SE. *Mountain Medicine and Technical Rescue.* Carreg; 2016.

United States Lifesaving Association. *Open Water Lifesaving—The United States Lifesaving Association Manual.* 3rd ed. Pearson; 2017.

CHAPTER **21**

Wilderness Trauma Care

Lead Editors
Will Smith, MD, Paramedic, FAEMS
John Trentini, MD, PhD, FAWM

CHAPTER OBJECTIVES   At the completion of this chapter, you will be able to do the following:

- Explain the four principles of the LATE acronym, representing a simplified approach to wilderness emergency medical services (EMS) operations and trauma care.
- Identify levels of wilderness EMS care practitioners and how they should interface with the standard patient care continuum from the point of injury/illness to the hospital.
- Discuss the reasons for the dictum, "Every wilderness patient is hypothermic, hypoglycemic, and hypovolemic until proven otherwise."

- Describe escalating ways to manage bleeding wounds in the wilderness, in what situations to start with a tourniquet, and when to consider a tourniquet conversion (removal).
- Discuss the signs and symptoms of common bites and stings and medical management in the wilderness.
- Describe several operationally specific (expanded scope of practice) protocols that should be considered in wilderness trauma care.

SCENARIO

You are the medical and team leader for the local search and rescue team and have been dispatched to a popular canyoneering site in your jurisdiction. The only information you have is a global positioning system (GPS) location from a distress signal broadcast via an emergency satellite beacon. The time is about 1800 hours, and current temperature is 74°F (23°C). The weather forecast shows some building thunderstorms throughout the evening and an overnight low of 36°F (2°C). The team begins to plan the response using the LATE acronym: Locate, Access, Treat, Extricate.

Your team assembles the necessary gear, including the still-/swift-water and high-angle rescue kits, their own personal protective equipment, and the standard medical kit, and begins responding to the location. As the team leader, you interface with the incident commander and develop a communication plan with a staged team member to enable a communication relay from the top of the canyon back to the incident command post.

- What are the essential items for a team and individual medical kit to handle the most severe and most likely injuries for this type of rescue scenario?

(continues)

SCENARIO (CONTINUED)

- What operationally specific (expanded scope of practice) protocols would you want in place to care for patients in remote and/or prolonged care settings? Do you have standing orders, as you are expecting limited communication options?
- What safety concerns should you be considering for your rescue team? How do situational factors such as time of day, location of patient, and experience and training of your team affect safety?

You *locate* the GPS position and find a slot canyon with three known separate 100-foot (ft; 30-meter [m]) rappels. You attempt to yell and try to make contact but are unable to get any response. When you blow your whistle, you are able to hear a faint whistle blast in return. You and your team safely make your way toward the location. At the top of the second rappel, you find the two members of the party that set off the emergency beacon. They tell you one of their team members sustained an approximately 50-ft (15-m) fall deeper in the canyon at 1300 hours. They had to climb back up from the location to get a signal out on their emergency beacon. Another friend rappelled down to assess the victim and stated the injuries appear to be an angulated open femur fracture, with a lot of pooled blood, and that the patient appeared confused. The patient did not lose consciousness or show any other signs of head trauma. He was wearing a helmet. The friend has been holding pressure on a "pumper" with some continued bleeding.

You continue down the next rappel and establish verbal communication with the friend who is attending to the patient. You direct him to place an improvised tourniquet with 1-inch tubular webbing proximal to the wound that is continuing to bleed. You direct him to tighten the webbing by twisting a spare carabiner until the bleeding is stopped and to then secure it in place with another carabiner. The friend reports that the bleeding has been controlled.

Once your additional equipment reaches your location, you begin your final rappel to *access* the patient. Upon reaching the patient, you find a 25-year-old otherwise healthy male awake and now more alert with an obvious open deformed right femur fracture. The friend has tried to get extra clothing around the patient, but he is in a shallow pool of cold water and has wet clothing and is shivering. You begin planning and implementing the *treat* portion of your mission, but because it is getting dark, your team will have to wait until morning to *extricate* the patient.

- How can you direct others to provide care in a wilderness setting? Are you familiar with how dispatchers use emergency medical dispatch to assist with prearrival instructions during a 9-1-1 call, and can you remotely direct someone to provide initial care? What else would you direct the friend to perform if you have an additional delay in reaching the patient?
- What are your priorities of care in assessment and intervention? What are the prolonged patient care considerations?
- What is your plan to get this patient packaged and extricated?

© National Association of Emergency Medical Technicians (NAEMT)

INTRODUCTION

Delivery of medical care outside of the hospital in remote and austere environments describes the challenge of wilderness EMS. While multiple medical conditions can occur similarly in both wilderness and traditional EMS environments, many conditions can be exacerbated by the trauma associated with wilderness environments such as exposures to extremes of heat, cold, moisture, and altitude. Furthermore, challenging terrain increases the risk of falls and other injury mechanisms. Certain challenges associated with the wilderness environment are sufficiently unique and complex that entire areas of sub specialization certification have been devoted to wilderness EMS. Prehospital care practitioners with

responsibility for care delivery in such remote environments must be adequately prepared for the challenges they are likely to face.

Wilderness EMS Defined

Many terms are used to describe areas far from civilization (**Figure 21-1**), including wilderness, remote, backcountry, isolated, and austere. Emergency medical services (EMS) personnel tend to lump these terms together under the heading "wilderness." According to the dictionary, the following are definitions of *wilderness*[1]:

- A tract or region uncultivated and uninhabited by human beings

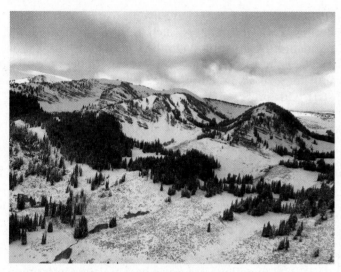

Figure 21-1 Wilderness is traditionally thought of as areas far from civilization, but similar surroundings may also occur in the street EMS settings when disasters or other resource-constrained events occur (e.g., mass-casualty incident).
Courtesy of Will Smith.

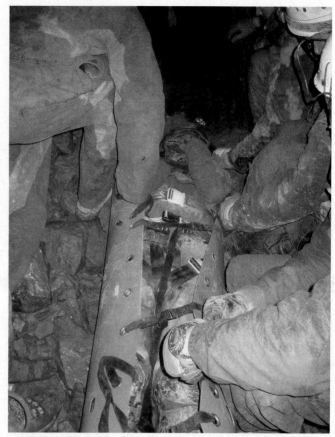

Figure 21-2 Patient care in a cave unquestionably represents wilderness EMS.
Courtesy of Will Smith.

- An area essentially undisturbed by human activity, together with its naturally developed life community
- An empty or pathless area or region

Because EMS is focused on patient care, the definition of *wilderness EMS* diverges slightly from the preceding definitions of wilderness. The *wilderness EMS* definition is really the application of medical care to patients in the wilderness. This chapter on wilderness trauma care provides guidance on questions such as, "When and where do we encounter wilderness EMS?" That is, "When should we think and work differently from the way we do in the traditional front country or street EMS settings?" The answer to this question goes beyond simple geography and involves many of the following considerations:

- Access to the scene
- Weather
- Daylight
- Terrain and elevation
- Special transport and handling needs
- Access and transport times
- Available personnel
- Communications
- Hazards present
- Medical and rescue equipment available
- Injury patterns for the specific environment

Numerous examples exist that expand the traditional view of wilderness EMS. For example, consider the following:

- In a city after an earthquake, it may be difficult to access those who are injured or trapped, there may be no roads for transport, and local EMS systems may be incapacitated and/or overwhelmed. In this situation, patients are likely to remain in their location for a considerable amount of time. They will have the same care requirements as a hiker who has fallen in the mountains and is hours or days away from a hospital.
- A person who has fallen in a large suburban park late in the evening during an ice storm is at risk from the same factors as a patient suffering the same type of fall in the wilderness. The patient may need a rescue team with ropes, crampons, and prehospital care practitioners who can anticipate and manage issues such as hypothermia, packaging, wound management, and difficult patient extrication.

Wilderness EMS Versus Traditional Street EMS

We often talk of how *wilderness* EMS differs from the traditional *street* EMS, but in reality, all aspects of EMS exist on a spectrum. At one end of the spectrum is an incident half a block from a level I trauma center, and at the other end of the spectrum is an incident in the deepest part of the Wind-Ice Cave system in western Wyoming (**Figure 21-2**). Wilderness EMS even goes beyond the rural and frontier EMS settings.[2] In the final analysis, where does the *street* end and the *wilderness* begin? The answer is, "It depends." It depends on the distance from the ambulance to the emergency department (ED). It depends on the weather. It depends on the terrain. It depends on the resources available and whether they remain intact and functional. Even more important, it depends on the nature of the injury and the capabilities of the EMS and rescue personnel on scene.

In recognizing these situational EMS variations, it is clear that wilderness EMS should be considered as part of the overall medical system, from the point of injury, to the definitive care provided at the trauma center, to the rehabilitation facility or home, until the patient has returned to baseline function. Documentation, quality assurance, medical oversight, protocols, skills validation, and other factors, all of which are mainstays of any traditional street EMS system, should also be components of a wilderness EMS system.

Wilderness EMS System

Several issues are critical for optimal wilderness patient care and are common problems for which management is different from on the street. This chapter provides an overview of the many issues involved in wilderness medical emergencies. Prehospital care practitioners who function in a formal capacity in the wilderness setting as wilderness medical practitioners should obtain specific training (**Box 21-1**).[3,4] In addition, oversight direction by a knowledgeable physician should be an integral component of wilderness medical activities.[5-7] In many regions of the United States, there is no medical oversight for wilderness medical practitioners on many search and rescue (SAR) teams.[8] While this is a suboptimal arrangement, there is a growing recognition that the best practice of providing medical oversight is essential for all prehospital EMS practitioners, including those who operate in wilderness and other austere settings.[6-8]

Training for Wilderness EMS Practitioners

Wilderness EMS practitioners traditionally have been set apart from traditional EMS. Some have viewed them as first aid providers and thus not under the scope of EMS

Box 21-1 Wilderness EMS Training

Prehospital care practitioners who may provide wilderness EMS care or who regularly travel in the backcountry are advised to take a specialized course or courses.

© National Association of Emergency Medical Technicians (NAEMT)

---

regulations. Some states have even excluded certain wilderness EMS practitioners, such as ski patrol, from EMS regulation. A growing realization is that any care provided at the point of injury/illness should be integrated into the overall system of care. This integration should start with prevention, and it should encompass immediate responders at the point of injury, who are probably providing traditional first aid care, to the traditional EMS and definitive hospital care. Wilderness-specific responders are generally trained at designated levels, although some of the traditional wilderness EMS training programs and certifications do not directly align with traditional street EMS models.[9] The National Association of EMS Physicians (NAEMSP) and other organizations have begun to help standardize the scope of practice of these practitioners, which in turn helps to standardize wilderness EMS operations to ensure best practices in training and patient care.[10]

Common wilderness EMS certifications include the following[3,4,11,12]:

- *Wilderness First Aid (WFA).* The basic level of wilderness EMS training. It is generally a 16- to 20-hour course.[4,13]
- *Wilderness Advanced First Aid (WAFA).* Training that builds on the WFA curriculum. It is generally a 36- to 40-hour course.
- *Wilderness Emergency Medical Responder (WEMR)/Wilderness First Responder (WFR).* The most common level of wilderness EMS practitioner. Many SAR teams as well as mountain and other guide services have individuals trained at this level. Some education models pair this with the National Registry of EMTs (NREMT) scope of practice to meet the emergency medical responder (EMR) certification to make a nationally recognized EMS standard. This is generally a 70- to 80-hour course. Some online and blended learning programs are being developed as well. This course focuses on the medical decision making needed in remote care environments, critical skills and patient care interventions, when to evacuate, and how to work safely.[4,14-16]
- *Wilderness EMT (WEMT).* A course that often consists of modules added to a traditional emergency medical technician (EMT) course, including WEMR/WFR decision making, skills, and wilderness protocols.
- *Outdoor Emergency Care (OEC).* A basic life support (BLS) course that is commonly taught by the National Ski Patrol and is generally 80 to 100 hours.[17] It has many similarities to a traditional EMT and WEMT training, but there remain some differences.[18,19] In many settings, ski patrollers interface with SAR teams, with both groups providing wilderness EMS care (**Figure 21-3**).
- *ParkMedic.* Generally an advanced emergency medical technician (AEMT)-level course with additional

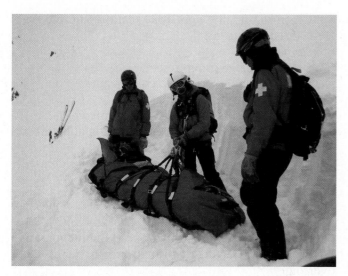

Figure 21-3 Ski patrollers and search and rescue teams often interface in wilderness EMS settings to provide optimal patient care.

Courtesy of Will Smith.

focused wilderness EMS skill sets required for optimal patient care in many of the remote National Park Service (NPS) locations.[20,21] The NPS has been training wilderness EMS practitioners for many years to this certification. It has been taught every other year in January at the University of California, San Francisco–Fresno Emergency Medicine program since the 1970s.

- *Wilderness AEMT, Wilderness Paramedic.* Generally training that is similar to the traditional EMS programs, followed by augmented training, through local and national conferences and courses, for advanced life support (ALS) providers.
- *Wilderness Physician Assistant (PA), Wilderness Advanced Practice Registered Nurse (APRN).* Training provided for those who may be involved with wilderness care and/or serve in formal roles in wilderness EMS systems. Many locations in the United States are staffed with PAs or APRNs, especially in remote or rural areas.
- *Wilderness Physician.* Training for physicians who are ordinarily identified by their primary and/or subspecialty board certification (e.g., emergency medicine, surgery, family medicine, etc.) but who, by chance, are exposed to caring for patients in the wilderness (i.e., on a good Samaritan basis), or who, in some cases, are members and medical directors for dedicated wilderness EMS teams. They not only give medical oversight to a team or agency but often provide direct patient care. Other allied health professionals (e.g., veterinarians, dentists) can also be involved in wilderness medical care, with the appropriate training and experience. There are multiple programs and organizations that provide this kind of education for physicians, from formal academic fellowships to other training programs.[4,22]

Wilderness EMS Medical Oversight

In this chapter, *front country* refers to any area in which conventional EMS can be delivered; it stands in contrast to *backcountry*, which refers to remote, often austere, locations. Just as front country EMS systems have medical oversight, so should wilderness EMS systems. In some regards, it is even more important, as the complex medical decision making and prolonged patient care virtually all require standing orders. Medical directors providing this oversight must be knowledgeable in the variables that affect care in these settings. They also must understand the scope of practice and limitations of their practitioners. In some settings, the medical director may even be providing direct medical oversight in the field and sometimes even direct patient care. If they enter the field, they must be fully trained and competent to manage themselves safely in these settings.[7,8,11,23,24]

Wilderness EMS Agencies

There are many agencies that practice wilderness EMS care. Examples of wilderness EMS agencies include the following[12,25,26]:

- SAR teams
- National, state, and local parks
- Ski patrols
- Expedition medical teams
- Specialized military teams

The Wilderness EMS Context

Key Wilderness EMS/SAR Principles: Locate, Access, Treat, Extricate (LATE)

In wilderness EMS, which is a common component of many SAR operations, a few key principles can help simplify the overall mission or callout. As discussed in the opening scenario, the acronym LATE can help organize the response—Locate, Access, Treat, Extricate.[25] Generally, every wilderness EMS operation will have some component of each (**Box 21-2**).

Locate is the first step in any event or callout. You have to find the patient before you can begin care. In some situations, this may be easy if a 9-1-1 call was made and you know the exact patient location. In other situations, this may be more difficult, and you will need to perform an extensive search operation.

Access can be a technical challenge. For example, a patient may be found but is on the opposite shore of a

---

Box 21-2 LATE

The acronym LATE (Locate, Access, Treat, Extricate) represents simplified principles in SAR and other wilderness EMS operations[25]:

- *Locate.* This is generally the first step in any wilderness EMS event. The patient must be located before the next steps of a rescue can be undertaken.
- *Access.* After a patient is located, the wilderness EMS practitioners must be able to access the location in order to begin patient care.
- *Treat.* This is the main function of wilderness EMS practitioners, but in some settings, extrication may become a higher priority, delaying care until the patient arrives at a safe location.
- *Extricate.* This is the final step of an SAR or other wilderness EMS operation. It involves removing the patient from the technical environment and transporting toward definitive care.

Modified from Smith WR. Principles of basic technical rescue, packaging, and patient care integration. In: Hawkins SC, ed. *Wilderness EMS.* Wolters Kluwer; 2018.

---

raging river. This type of situation is what distinguishes traditional street EMS from wilderness EMS.

Treat is often the phase in which the real definition of wilderness EMS care becomes clear. While some care may be identical to that performed in the street EMS setting, medical decision making, such as when to apply different treatment interventions, may be different in crucial ways. These decisions can dramatically change the duration of the next stage of the rescue, as well as the risk to the patient and rescuers.

Extricate is the last step in these simplified rescue principles. Although some of these principles can overlap, some may take priority over others. Just like in a hazardous materials or tactical situation, extrication may be a higher priority than standard treatment options, such as starting an intravenous (IV) line.

Technical Rescue Interface

Wilderness EMS practitioners must not only deliver appropriate care, but they must also be able to access patients in technical terrain safely. This means they must be able to navigate through the *technical rescue interface.*[25] This problem or interface is what often helps to define the wilderness EMS setting. Although rescue group structures can be quite varied, some examples of how wilderness EMS care is provided include the following:

- Self-rescue
- Companion rescue
- Bystander rescue

- Organized small group/strike team rescue (i.e., specialized SAR team)
- Ski patrol
- Organized large-group rescue
- Fire department technical rescue teams
- Industrial site rescue teams
- Military systems (e.g., Air Force pararescue)
- Multigroup/interagency rescue coordinating a complex response

Wilderness EMS Realms

There are many realms to wilderness EMS. A few potential scenarios are listed here, each with specific patient care considerations, patient access limitations, and other individual factors that often must be mitigated or overcome[25-27]:

- Space
- High angle (cliff/near vertical)
- Steep angle (side of a road on a mountain pass)
- Low angle
- Avalanche
- Cave, confined space, canyoneering
- Helicopter operations (long line, short haul)
- Still water, swift water, open water
- All-terrain vehicle, off-road vehicle, snowmobile, mountain bike
- Helicopter, fixed-wing rescue
- Snow, glaciated, crevasse rescue
- Mountaineering, climbing
- High altitude
- Diving

Wilderness Injury Patterns

Death from trauma has a trimodal (three-phase) distribution. See Chapter 1, *PHTLS: Past, Present, and Future,* for further details. The **first phase of death** is within seconds to minutes of injury. Deaths occurring during this first phase are usually caused by injuries to the brain, brain stem, high spinal cord, heart, aorta, or other large vessels and can best be managed by preventive measures such as helmets. Only a few of these patients can be saved, and then generally only in large urban areas where rapid emergency transport is available.

The **second phase of death** occurs within minutes to a few hours after injury. Rapid assessment and resuscitation are carried out to reduce this second phase of trauma deaths. Deaths occurring during this phase are usually caused by subdural and epidural hematomas, hemopneumothoraces, ruptured spleen, lacerations of the liver, pelvic fractures, or multiple injuries associated with significant blood loss. The fundamental principles of trauma care (hemorrhage control, airway management, balanced fluid resuscitation, and transport to an appropriate facility) can best be applied to these patients. The **third phase of death** occurs several days or weeks after the initial injury and is almost always caused by sepsis and organ failure.

Prehospital care practitioners focus mostly on saving patients from the second phase. In the wilderness, most of those who survive to be rescued have already passed the first phase of death and usually most of the second. However, the presence of medically trained individuals on an SAR team may be able to prevent deaths related to the second phase.[28,29] Often, this wilderness care focuses on, "What can we do *now* that will keep the patient from dying or having major complications later?" Wilderness EMS practitioners need to make sure the patient does not develop problems such as kidney failure from dehydration, overwhelming infection from poor resistance due to starvation, severe hypothermia, and skin necrosis from decubitus ulcers from unnecessary immobilization.

Preventive SAR programs have become an important focus to limit and decrease wilderness EMS encounters. Helmets and other safety features at ski areas have decreased the morbidity and mortality of users. The NPS and other programs, such as Back Country Zero, in partnership with Teton County SAR in Jackson, Wyoming, have extensive programs that promote education and prevention.

Safety

In the wilderness, even more so than on the street, scene safety is a critical consideration.[30] An injured or dead wilderness EMS practitioner distracts from the care of the patient and limits the possibility of a successful rescue mission. Street scene safety considerations apply even in the wilderness. In the wilderness, scene dangers can be less obvious than on the street, especially if the practitioner is not properly trained to function in the given environment.

The wilderness EMS practitioner and patient will be exposed to the environment and changes in weather. An incoming cold front with freezing rain, for example, may complicate the operation or even injure or kill the wilderness medicine practitioner and patient. If a rescue lasts for hours or days, the lack of food and water may cause debilitation. The wilderness terrain is often rugged, and dangerous technical terrain may complicate patient care and extrication (**Figure 21-4**). Wilderness EMS practitioners need to be aware of dangers specific to the environment, such as rockfall, avalanche risk, rising waters, high altitudes or altitude exposure, and recirculating eddies at the base of waterfalls.

Each member of the SAR team must take appropriate preparations and precautions to ensure the safety, health, and well-being of the SAR team collectively. All members must be educated regarding the hazards and dangers

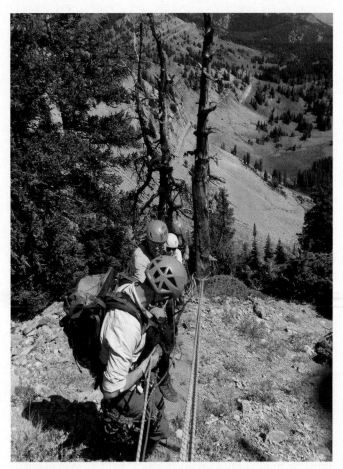

Figure 21-4 Steep slopes, cliffs, rockfall, and uneven footing are dangerous in wilderness rescue.
Courtesy of Will Smith.

of the specific environment in which they will be working. They must know their limitations and not exceed their capabilities trying to rescue an injured patient. Each member of the SAR team must be appropriately prepared with the necessary clothing and personal protective equipment (PPE) for the environmental conditions and rescue at hand. Finally, ensuring that the medical needs of the SAR team are met must be an integral component of the response effort. Appropriate supplies to address potential illness or injury of an SAR team member as well as enforcement of work–rest cycles will help maintain a well-functioning SAR team.

Proper Care Depends on Context

Our medical knowledge, understanding, and technology change as we make advances in medicine; however, some basic principles of medical care change little over the years and are independent of the patient's location. Prehospital Trauma Life Support (PHTLS) has long advocated that the critically injured patient be transported as quickly as possible to an appropriate destination,

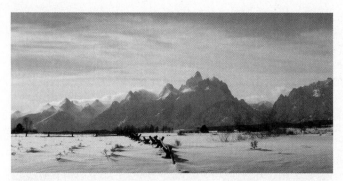

Figure 21-5 Wilderness terrain.
Courtesy of Will Smith.

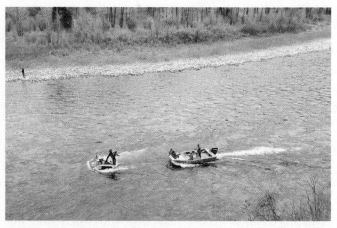

Figure 21-6 A patient trapped in a vehicle in the middle of a flowing river after a motor vehicle crash may need to be treated by modified protocols. Trauma care in the wilderness is often hampered by adverse environmental conditions, water, mud, underbrush, and confined spaces.
Courtesy of Brian Coe.

sometimes without detailed physical examination and treatment of noncritical conditions. However, *proper* care is somewhat context dependent. The definition of *detailed physical examination* and *noncritical conditions* may be different on an urban street than when deep in the wilderness (**Figure 21-5**). The situation, knowledge level, skill, scene conditions, and equipment available may alter medical decision making and management of the trauma patient.[20] (This concept is introduced in Chapter 2, *Golden Principles, Preferences, and Critical Thinking*.)

Ideal to Real Care

In wilderness EMS, complex medical decisions sometimes must be made based on an "ideal to real" care concept.[31] This decision-making process is what sets apart a wilderness EMS practitioner from a traditional street EMS practitioner. The ability to improvise is almost the standard in most wilderness EMS situations, and EMS practitioners must take the traditional ideal care protocol or treatment and adapt/improvise to meet the reality of the setting in which they find themselves.

Consider a patient with a complex fracture–dislocation of the shoulder. What is the proper care in the operating room (OR)? In many cases, it involves an open reduction and internal fixation (ORIF). However, proper care in the OR may not be proper care in the ED, where it would not be proper to attempt an open reduction. In the ED, x-ray films are taken to evaluate the fracture–dislocation, a short-acting pain medication is given, and a closed reduction of the dislocation is performed to reduce pain and swelling, to realign the bones grossly, and to decrease pressure on nerves and blood vessels. The definitive ORIF will occur later, in the OR.

Likewise, proper care in the ED may not be proper care in the street EMS setting. The prehospital care practitioners may not have the advantage of a large, warm, dry area to perform an assessment and provide treatment. They may be working in the rain, where the patient is hanging upside down inside a crushed vehicle while a rescue crew uses power tools to cut and remove metal to reach the patient. Once the patient is free, the prehospital care practitioner will assess the patient for other injuries, check the distal neurovascular status in the arm, immobilize the patient's shoulder, provide pain medication, and transport the patient rapidly to the ED. Similarly, on the street, it might not be proper care to attempt a closed or open reduction to reduce the fracture–dislocation (based on local protocols).

Finally, proper care on the street may not be proper care in the wilderness. What protocols may need to be modified for a patient who, following a motor vehicle crash, is trapped in a car that is in the middle of a flowing river or that is submerged (**Figure 21-6**)? In this case, swift-water rescue skills, techniques, and modified priorities must be performed in addition to patient care.[32] Examples such as this are why wilderness EMS protocols may require an operationally specific scope of practice for best patient care.[6,12]

For most conditions, however, proper care is proper care—whether it is performed in the OR, in the ED, on the street, or in the wilderness. Given a good fund of knowledge, critical-thinking skills, training, and understanding of key principles, prehospital care practitioners can perform medical decision making in the field to reflect the various situations in which they will encounter patients.

For a small but significant number of situations, noteworthy differences exist between proper street EMS care and proper wilderness EMS care. Such situations bring up the following important questions:

- Is street EMS care always optimal in the wilderness?
- If street EMS care is not optimal, how does the prehospital care practitioner know what the optimal care is? Is this established in local protocols?

- How do prehospital care practitioners deal with situations in the field when unsure precisely what the patient's injury might be? For example, how do wilderness medical practitioners determine that a fracture–dislocation is present when examining a patient who is hanging upside down from a rope deep within a cave?
- How does a prehospital care practitioner decide, for a particular patient in a particular situation, which is *more* proper, street or wilderness care?
- What makes a situation wilderness or street? What about all the in-between cases?

Definitive answers to all of these questions are not easy to provide. As stated previously, often the answer is, "It depends." However, at least good background information can be provided so that prehospital care practitioners may, as needed in a particular patient care situation, answer the questions in their respective setting. The PHTLS philosophy has always been that, given a good fund of knowledge and key principles, prehospital care practitioners are capable of making reasoned decisions regarding patient care. In the end, it is providing *real care* to the patient—based on the situation and resources at hand and based on the *ideal care*—that represents the standard in that setting.

Wilderness EMS Decision Making: Balancing Risks and Benefits

Experienced physicians, nurses, and prehospital care practitioners know that procedures such as airway management and wound management are the easy part of medicine. The difficult part is in knowing *when* to do *what*: critical thinking. Even more often than on the street, in the wilderness one risk needs to be weighed carefully against another and against the potential benefits. For *this* particular patient, in *this* particular setting, with *these* particular resources, and with *this* particular likelihood of *this* particular help arriving at *this* particular time in the future, what are the potential risks? What are the potential benefits? Wilderness EMS is largely the art of compromise: balancing the particular risks and benefits for each patient.

TCCC and TECC Principles Applied in Wilderness Trauma Care

The importance of considering the incident's context is evident in the combat and tactical settings of the Iraq and Afghanistan conflicts. Development and implementation of Tactical Combat Casualty Care (TCCC) guidelines have been clearly linked to improved casualty survivor rates.[33-37] Many of the concepts learned in the combat setting can be applied to the wilderness context. An entire preconference session was held on this topic at the Seventh World Congress of Wilderness Medicine in 2016 (Telluride, Colorado) and resulted in a publication: *Special Edition: Tactical Combat Casualty Care; Transitioning Battlefield Lessons Learned to Other Austere Environments*.[38] Although the sources of danger may not be the same (e.g., caring for a gunshot wound sustained in combat versus one sustained while hunting, or injuries from improvised explosive devices versus an avalanche), many of the same injury patterns and care priorities are shared by both rescuers and patients.[39]

Patient care priorities extrapolated from TCCC to wilderness settings have been widely adopted by many organizations. The NPS has a unique challenge in providing care in extremely diverse remote care settings (**Figure 21-7**). NPS rangers care for patients in remote, austere wilderness settings using both tactical and wilderness protocols.[20,21,40]

The TCCC tactical guidelines have been modified and adapted by the Committee on Tactical Emergency Casualty Care (TECC) for civilian and federal use.[41] TECC applies similar TCCC concepts across multiple all-hazard risk areas (tactical, hazardous materials, etc.) and to expanded populations (children, older adults, etc.). Many agencies have begun providing care based on TECC guidelines and have formalized programs such as rescue task force programs to blend this care into tactical and other hazardous situations (including wilderness and remote trauma care).[21,42]

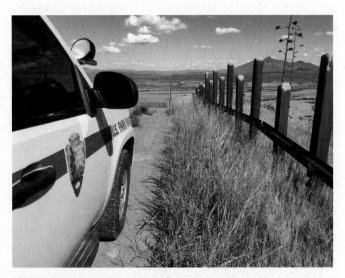

Figure 21-7 National Park Service ranger on patrol at the United States–Mexico border, a remote environment with the possibility of trauma-related injuries.
Courtesy of Will Smith.

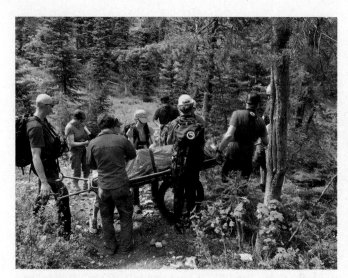

Figure 21-8 A wheeled litter is being used to transport an injured patient after a mountain bike crash. Although easier than directly carrying a nonambulatory patient, it still requires considerable resources.
Courtesy of Will Smith.

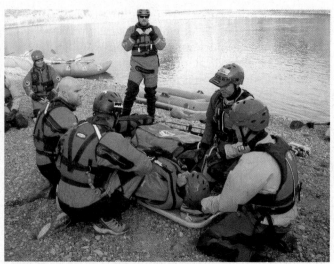

Figure 21-9 A personal flotation device is a mandatory packaging adjunct whenever you transport a patient over water.
Courtesy of Will Smith.

See further discussion on TCCC/TECC and patient care priorities in tactical settings in Chapter 22, *Civilian Tactical Emergency Medical Support (TEMS)*.

Principles of Basic Patient Packaging

Patient packaging becomes a paramount issue in wilderness EMS care, as ultimately, the patient needs to be extricated from the remote environment to definitive care. Sometimes this can be an easy task when managing an isolated injury. For example, an upper extremity injury can be splinted, and the patient can walk or be assisted out. However, other minor injuries, such as a lower extremity sprain or fracture, may require the patient to be carried out. More critical or life-threatening injuries always require some degree of patient packaging and more intensive extrication. Different rescue systems can be used to evacuate a nonambulatory patient in technical situations. **Figure 21-8** shows a patient packaged in a wheeled litter, a common rescue tool used to move patients when they are unable to walk. In overwater operations, care must be taken to ensure proper flotation for the patient (e.g., personal flotation device), in addition to the extrication capability (**Figure 21-9**). All of these factors must be considered when packaging patients in a wilderness EMS situation. Often patient packaging must employ more padding than usual and ongoing efforts to ensure a position of comfort for the patient, as the rescues are frequently prolonged.

Physiologic Splinting

Physiologic splinting is a concept that can be applied to virtually any injury in any EMS setting, not just the wilderness. It uses the premise of establishing normal physiologic alignment to the injured area and then immobilizing or supporting in that position. The same concepts of immobilizing the joint above and below a long-bone injury and the bone above and below a joint injury are incorporated.[12,25] Distal circulation, sensory, and motor assessments should be performed before and after any splinting and then continuously reassessed.

Wilderness application of *physiologic splinting* usually requires a great deal more padding than traditional EMS application. This is due mostly to the prolonged transport times to extract a patient from the remote setting. It is also important to make sure the patient packaging and physiologic splinting are done correctly at the outset. More padding not only reduces overall discomfort but also promotes normal neurovascular function and allows for expedited rescue operations. A hurried patient packaging without appropriate physiologic splinting and ample padding may lead to delays in the rescue if a patient must be repackaged.

The vacuum mattress (**Figure 21-10**) has become the standard of care for wilderness EMS patients requiring whole-body immobilization (including *spinal motion restriction/immobilization*). As with any specialized tool, it must be brought to the rescue scene; however, it is often more portable than the urban alternatives.[25] Smaller vacuum splints can be used for isolated extremity injuries. However, as with much of wilderness EMS, the ideal tools may not be available, and improvisation may

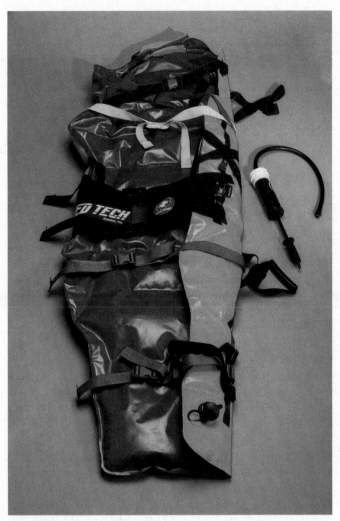

Figure 21-10 A full-body vacuum mattress used in physiologic splinting of the entire body.
Courtesy of David Bowers.

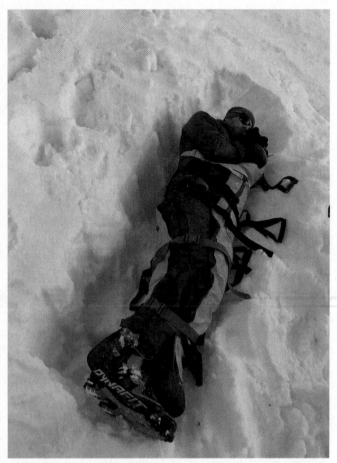

Figure 21-11 A patient packaged in a vacuum mattress in a lateral position to achieve physiologic splinting and to help maintain an open airway.
Courtesy of Will Smith.

be required to achieve the same patient care objective. This situation is another example of the *ideal* to *real* care concept, as previously discussed.

Airway Considerations

Airway management has been the utmost priority in EMS care, leading to the long-standing ABC (Airway, Breathing, Circulation) mantra. Wilderness EMS care must also consider airway management, but sometimes to an even higher degree. During extrication of an immobilized patient, especially when supine, a wilderness EMS practitioner may have a limited ability to monitor the airway and access the patient. Airway considerations with the potential for vomiting and airway compromise are of paramount concern. Elements of technical rescue and evacuation must be balanced with patient packaging and physiologic splinting. Lateral packaging is an option with

the vacuum mattress. This option would allow fluids and vomit to be more likely to drain from the airway based on gravity (**Figure 21-11**). Other considerations in prolonged patient care include anticipating potential problems, such as pretreating a patient with an antiemetic when there is a concern for vomiting. One easily administered option is ondansetron as an orally dissolving tablet. Typical antiemetic options such as promethazine and atypical agents such as diphenhydramine can be considered and have an additive effect. As always, medications should be managed by EMS practitioners at the appropriate skill level; a complete discussion is beyond the scope of this text.

Spinal Injuries and Spinal Motion Restriction

Much debate has occurred since the birth of EMS over the best care of both actual spine injuries and suspected injuries. Patients with a true spinal cord injury and obvious neurologic deficit have a relatively clear treatment pathway. They need to be packaged in the prehospital setting to limit further spinal motion until they reach definitive medical care. Ideally, in the context of prolonged transport times, that is with a vacuum mattress or other device that conforms to the shape of the spine rather than a rigid flat backboard.

The bigger dilemma occurs in wilderness trauma care when no clear neurologic deficit is present but there is a concern for a possible spine injury. For many years, patients were immobilized based on mechanism of injury alone, in anticipation that an unstable injury might lead to an actual spinal cord injury and long-term deficits. Treating for this concern of a possible spine injury became a mainstay of EMS training. The application of spinal motion restriction (also called spinal immobilization or spinal stabilization) was a hallmark feature of traditional EMS care. Many patients were immobilized over the years with the traditional hard backboard along with rigid cervical collars.

Numerous studies over the past few decades have led to revised treatment, limiting the number of patients immobilized for "possible spine injury." Research revealed that the rigid backboard and cervical collar were occasionally harming patients without providing the intended benefits. Studies have shown moderate pain even in healthy volunteers at 30 minutes and severe pain after about 45 minutes.[43] Other more concerning problems develop with prolonged immobilization, such as airway compromise, aspiration risk, and pressure sores. Rigid cervical collars can be associated with complications of increased intracranial pressure, decreased cerebral outflow, and cervical distraction in the context of incorrect application.[44-46] These complications become compounded by the additional factors encountered in prolonged care settings. For this reason, wilderness EMS systems and practitioners became early adopters of the limited use of spinal motion restriction.

Spinal motion restriction in the wilderness and remote care settings has dramatic implications on transport decisions, technical rescue risks, and other dynamics. This increase in risk to the patient and rescuers must be balanced with the small risk of a possible spinal cord injury (in many cases well under 1% with a normal neurologic exam).[47] To illustrate the wilderness EMS decision-making process, consider the following example:

A healthy 22-year-old woman was rock climbing along a river gorge when she fell 65 ft (20 m). Her anchors were placed in the cracks of the cliff and came out, one by one, slowing her fall slightly. But ultimately, she impacted the ground. She was wearing a helmet and did strike her head, experiencing a brief loss of consciousness. After an hour-long hike up the river gorge from where the ambulance could be parked, a wilderness EMS practitioner reaches the patient. She is now conscious and alert, complaining of only a mild

headache, with a normal neurologic examination and a normal physical examination. Friends had encouraged her to remain still and not move. It is late fall, it is getting dark, the nearest helicopter landing zone is back at the road an hour away, and the forecast is for a blizzard to start tonight. Does the patient need to undergo spinal motion restriction? Can she walk out assisted if she is able? Does the wilderness EMS practitioner need to call for an SAR team with a Stokes litter and proceed with a prolonged rescue lasting hours into the night? Do you have protocols to assess and treat patients in situations similar to this?

A number of trauma experts now maintain that rigid boards have no requisite role in wilderness EMS operations, even in cases of suspected spinal injury.[25,39] Vacuum mattresses, which have been used outside the United States for some time, are becoming the standard of care when spinal motion restriction is indicated. These devices are malleable and contour to the spine; they also can be used to limit motion of the head without a rigid cervical collar.

A patient with no detectable deficit but severe back pain after high-energy trauma may have an occult unstable spinal injury that is at risk. In general in the wilderness setting, if the patient is able to walk, it is safe to do so. Patients who are unable to walk should not be forced to do so.

An example of a death caused by spinal motion restriction occurred in Cornish, New Hampshire, in 2006. A patient who had tripped and injured her ankle was immobilized on a rigid backboard based on the concern of a possible head/spine injury and then transported on a rescue boat. When the boat sank, the patient died from the rescue and not her minor injuries.[48] Cases like this must remind wilderness EMS practitioners that the real risk of the rescue decisions and the potential risk from possible spine injury and blindly following rigid protocols must be balanced.[25] In general, if a patient is able to self-ambulate out of a technical wilderness situation with minimal pain and no neurologic symptoms, that is very likely the safest option to be considered.

Wilderness Extrication Options

Carrying patients in the wilderness is an extremely difficult, time-consuming, and potentially dangerous activity for both the patient and those doing the carrying. Those with no SAR experience generally underestimate the time and difficulty of a wilderness evacuation by at least half, or sometimes up to a factor of five, for more difficult evacuations, especially cave rescues. In some cases, helicopter evacuation may provide the most appropriate evacuation from remote or technical locations (**Figure 21-12**).[49]

If someone with no SAR experience says, "It'll take us about 2 hours to get the patient out of here," the time

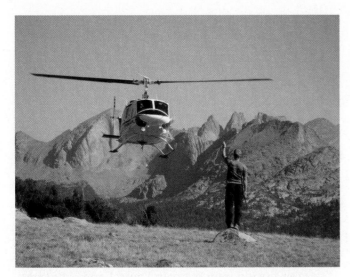

Figure 21-12 Helicopters can be used to balance the risk of exposing many rescuers to technical terrain for longer periods by using a potentially higher risk tool for a very short time. This balance of risk must constantly be evaluated for all wilderness extrications.

Courtesy of Will Smith.

frame is likely much, much longer. Wilderness EMS practitioners should expect it to take even longer if the patient is in a cave or other confined space, if the SAR team is short on people, if the terrain is particularly difficult, or if the weather is bad. This is especially important to remember if darkness is approaching or the weather is deteriorating.

Walking a patient out, even with several people helping, is almost always much faster. If the patient is able to and starts moving now, rather than waiting for a litter or SAR team, the evacuation will be much, much faster and completed much earlier. If the patient cannot walk (e.g., because of an ankle fracture), it may be possible to use a piggyback carry or to make an improvised stretcher out of sticks and rope.

Other Wilderness EMS Patient Care Considerations

Principles of Patient Assessment

While patient assessment is not unique in wilderness EMS settings, practitioners are generally with a patient for a much longer time. Vital sign trends, and especially mental status changes, give prolonged care practitioners much better insight into how treatments are affecting the patient's condition. Mental status is considered the most important vital sign; it ensures that the three main critical systems (circulatory, respiratory,

nervous) are functioning. Other traditional vital signs, such as blood pressure, may be completely impractical in some wilderness settings. Training to interpret a normal mental status and rate and presence of a radial pulse may offer all the details needed for a wilderness patient assessment.

MARCH PAWS

Initial patient assessment is the same regardless of the environment. The priority of attention is based on the major life threats that can be mitigated immediately at the point of injury. A systematic approach that is in accordance with PHTLS could follow the MARCH PAWS mnemonic, developed by the military. This approach has been gaining recognition in many military medicine settings.[50] Adaptations to MARCH PAWS for climbers and climbing rescue practitioners have also been published.[51]

  M—Massive hemorrhage. At the point of injury, the initial priority of care should be to identify and stop any massive hemorrhage. This is identified by doing an initial blood sweep of the extremities and proximal junctional hemorrhage sites (axilla and groin). A pelvic assessment is then performed with consideration of placement of a pelvic binder early if the pelvis is unstable.

  A—Airway. A simple assessment of the airway in conscious patients is accomplished by asking their name and to describe the situation. For unconscious patients, a simple jaw thrust can alleviate an obstructed airway. A nasopharyngeal airway is lightweight and can be placed for airway protection. In the case of severe maxillofacial trauma, a nasopharyngeal airway should be avoided. Sometimes lateral recumbent positioning may be all that is needed for a temporizing airway maneuver. Rapid sequence induction followed by intubation should be performed only by highly experienced and trained practitioners who have practiced intubation in austere environments. A surgical cricothyrotomy can be considered as an airway protection skill, by an appropriately trained and credentialed practitioner; however, it should be performed early if deemed clinically indicated and essential.

  R—Respirations. The assessment of respirations can be accomplished with traditional street EMS tools such as a stethoscope and pulse oximetry device, but in some wilderness settings, other patient assessment skills, such as physical palpation of the chest, may be needed. Secondary findings such as subcutaneous emphysema or crepitus associated with a rib fracture may lead to a clinical diagnosis of pneumothorax.

C—Circulation. A major goal of circulation assessment is to evaluate whether a patient is showing signs of shock. An overall assessment of the patient's circulatory status should be determined based on mentation and general appearance. An altered or confused patient should be considered to have signs of shock and treated accordingly. Careful attention should be made to assess and trend the presence of central (carotid, femoral) and distal (radial, posterior tibial, dorsalis pedis) pulses.

H—Head/Hypothermia. An initial gross neurologic examination should be conducted to assess the patient's level of consciousness. A patient can be described as Alert, responds to Verbal, responds to Pain, or is Unresponsive (AVPU). In the case of a suspected moderately or severely head-injured patient, the priority of care is to prevent hypoxia, hypotension, and hypoglycemia. During this phase of the assessment, the patient should be exposed for a full assessment. Wet clothes should be removed, and attention should be directed to prevent hypothermia by placing the patient in warm, dry clothes and off the ground using a sleeping pad or other barrier.

P—Pain. After the initial lifesaving interventions are completed in the MARCH assessment, you should next attend to managing the patient's pain. In an awake and alert patient, this can be accomplished by offering a dose of acetaminophen initially. Nonsteroidal anti-inflammatory drugs (NSAIDs) such as ibuprofen or naproxen should be avoided if there is a concern for hemorrhage, due to their antiplatelet effects. Meloxicam is an alternative long-acting NSAID that does not affect bleeding time and may be more safely used in trauma. Advanced practitioners who carry controlled substances such as fentanyl or ketamine should adhere to their local protocols for dosing and administrative guidance.

A—Antibiotics. Early antibiotics, ideally within 6 hours of a traumatic injury, may be indicated. A broad-spectrum antibiotic that covers the most likely pathogens for traumatic injuries should be used. Doxycycline is an excellent choice for travelers to carry, as it can be used to treat many conditions, including skin, respiratory, and gastrointestinal (GI) infections. Advanced practitioners who are providing point-of-injury care may administer ertapenem either intramuscularly or intravenously. If only one antibiotic is to be carried by an EMS team, some wilderness EMS infectious disease authorities recommend the use of ceftriaxone.[52] Practitioners must always check for known drug allergies prior to administering any medications to reduce the risk of inducing anaphylaxis

and thus further complicating the patient's condition and creating new care challenges.

W—Wounds. Irrigation and wound care should be accomplished prior to packaging and transporting a patient. A general rule is that as long as the water is potable, it is clean enough for wound irrigation. Gross decontamination and debris removal followed by copious volume irrigation should occur, and a sterile or clean dressing should be applied to the wound.

S—Splinting. Application of a modified splint provides immense pain relief for a patient with a fracture or severe soft-tissue injury. Simple immobilization, such as buttoning a wrist button to the chest for a shoulder dislocation or padding and immobilizing an ankle fracture using trekking poles for splints, can greatly improve pain control and ease transport of a casualty.

Prolonged Patient Care Considerations

As mentioned previously, wilderness EMS occurs in a wide variety of remote rescue settings that may be similar to military and other austere settings. With military theaters changing from Iraq and Afghanistan to other more remote areas of the world (e.g., Africa, the Pacific), the Prolonged Field Care (PFC) working group has been established to help focus on medical and trauma care in extended patient care settings ranging from hours to days. The group has identified 10 essential PFC capabilities to help focus training for these prolonged care settings (**Table 21-1**).[53] Virtually all patient care lessons learned can be bridged between the wilderness EMS practitioner and the military PFC settings.

Elimination (Urination/ Defecation) Needs

The truth described in a popular children's book, *Everyone Poops,*[54] applies to wilderness patients as well. Given the relatively short transport times in an urban setting, most patients do not have an elimination need. Trauma patients almost never defecate during their prehospital and ED care. However, if you are caring for a patient who has been in the wilderness for a day or more and it takes you several hours to get to the patient, it is much more likely that the patient will need to urinate or defecate, especially if there is a prolonged evacuation.

Having patient care supplies that include underpads for placing beneath the patient, having some sanitary wipes, carrying adult-type diapers that can be replaced after the patient has voided or defecated, or even stopping to let the patient urinate or defecate are all reasonable

Table 21-1 The 10 Core Capabilities as Identified by Prolonged Field Care (PFC) in Austere Locations

PFC Tasks	Minimum	Better	Best
1. Monitor the patient to create a useful vital sign trend.	Blood pressure cuff, stethoscope, pulse oximetry, Foley catheter (measure urine output), mental status, and understanding of vital sign interpretation	Add capnometry	Vital sign monitor to provide hands-free vital sign data at regular intervals
2. Resuscitate the patient beyond crystalloid or colloid infusion.	Field fresh whole blood (FWB) transfusion kits	Maintenance crystalloids also prepared for a major burn and/or closed head injury resuscitation (two to three cases of lactated Ringer's solution or PlasmaLyte A; hypertonic saline); consider adding lyophilized plasma as available; fluid warmer	Maintain a stock of packed red blood cells and fresh frozen plasma and have type-specific donors identified for immediate FWB draw
3. Ventilate/oxygenate the patient.	Provide positive end-expiratory pressure (PEEP) via bag-valve mask (you cannot ventilate a patient in the PFC setting [prolonged ventilation] without PEEP or the patient will be at risk of developing acute respiratory distress syndrome)	Provide supplemental oxygen via an oxygen concentrator	Portable ventilator with supplemental oxygen
4. Gain definitive control of the patient's airway with an inflated cuff in the trachea (and keep the patient comfortable).	Medic is prepared for a ketamine cricothyrotomy	Add ability to provide long-duration sedation	Add a responsible rapid-sequence intubation capability with subsequent airway maintenance skills, in addition to providing long-term sedation (to include suction and paralysis with adequate sedation)
5. Use sedation/pain control to accomplish the previous tasks.	Provide opiate analgesics titrated intravenously	Have training to sedate with ketamine (and adjunctive midazolam as needed)	Experienced with and maintains currency in long-term sedation practice using intravenous morphine, ketamine, midazolam, fentanyl, and so forth

(continues)

Table 21-1 The 10 Core Capabilities as Identified by Prolonged Field Care (PFC) in Austere Locations (*continued*)

PFC Tasks	Minimum	Better	Best
6. Use physical examination/diagnostic measures to gain awareness of potential problems.	Use physical examination without advanced diagnostics, maintain awareness of potential unseen injuries (e.g., abdominal bleed, head injury)	Have training to use advanced diagnostics such as ultrasound, point-of-care laboratory testing, and so forth	Experienced in both
7. Provide nursing, hygiene, and comfort measures.	Ensure the patient is clean, warm, dry, padded, and catheterized, and provide basic wound care	Elevate head of bed, debride wounds, perform washouts, wet-to-dry dressings, decompress stomach	Experienced in both
8. Perform advanced surgical interventions.	Chest tube, cricothyrotomy	Perform fasciotomy, wound debridement, amputation, and so forth	Experienced in both
9. Perform telemedicine consult.	Make reliable communications, present patient, pass trends of key vital signs	Add laboratory findings and ultrasound images	Video teleconference
10. Prepare the patient for flight.	Be familiar with physiologic stressors of flight	Have training in critical care transport	Experienced in critical care transport

Reproduced from Keenan S, Riesberg JC. Prolonged field care: beyond the "Golden Hour." *Wilderness Environ Med.* 2017;28(2S):S138.

measures (**Figure 21-13**). It is possible for people to urinate even while immobilized in a Stokes litter (**Figure 21-14**) with a full-body vacuum splint, if packaging is planned carefully and the litter is tipped up on the foot end. For women, a small funnel device, often carried by women when backpacking, will be needed to assist in elimination. In some rescue teams, a Foley catheter may even be used with the proper training.

Patients who are lying on their backs for a long time tend to develop decubitus ulcers. These sores may end up requiring surgery or debridement, resulting in longer hospital stays. Some patients will die from infection and other complications of the sores. Lying in one's own urine and feces for a long time (just hours, not even days) may make decubitus ulcers more likely. If patient care occurs for only a few minutes during a short transport, urine and feces are not a major issue. However, if a wilderness medicine practitioner has been taking care of a patient for several hours and delivers the patient to the ED lying

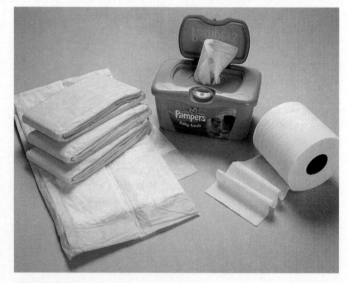

Figure 21-13 Elimination supplies.
© National Association of Emergency Medical Technicians (NAEMT)

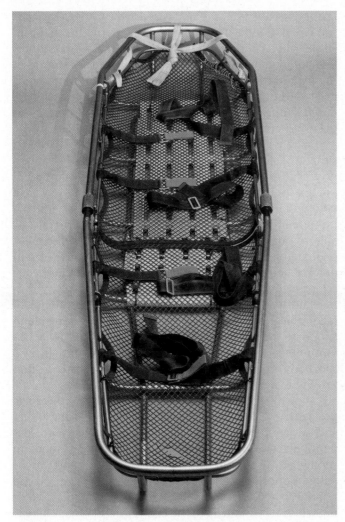

Figure 21-14 Stokes litter. Some models are made of titanium for lightweight transport and split into two sections.
Courtesy of David Bowers.

in feces, the likelihood of decubitus ulcers and resulting sepsis is much greater.

Food and Water Needs

All wilderness patients should be considered to be cold, hungry, and thirsty; that is, they should be considered hypothermic, starved, and dehydrated—or at a slight expense of accuracy, *hypothermic, hypoglycemic,* and *hypovolemic.* Starvation is much more than just hypoglycemia (low blood glucose), and not all starving patients are significantly hypoglycemic. Dehydration is more than just hypovolemia, which refers only to intravascular volume within the blood vascular system. Patients who are dehydrated have also lost water from their cells and the interstitial spaces between the cells.

On the street, water and food are generally not given to patients. There are many reasons not to feed patients during street EMS care. If the patient needs to go to the OR, having food or fluid in the stomach is potentially harmful; it increases the likelihood of vomiting or, more likely, passive regurgitation leading to possible aspiration during induction of anesthesia. Also, a patient will not starve or dehydrate in the time it takes to get to the hospital.

In the wilderness, if a rescued patient needs to go to the OR, it will take time to transport the patient to the hospital, to be evaluated in the ED, and to be prepared for the OR. With wilderness patients, the focus is to ensure that the patient maintains caloric intake and hydration, as transport times are generally delayed. Because the stomach is ideally fasted for several hours before anesthesia, the wilderness medical practitioner may provide food and water to any reasonably alert wilderness patient who can safely swallow.[55,56] Even if a helicopter can quickly expedite an otherwise prolonged rescue, hospitals are capable of taking care of patients with "full" stomachs; for example, people involved in a vehicle crash were not necessarily fasting.

Vomiting and aspiration are always a danger, and careful attention to the patient's airway is always important (e.g., positioning on the side for long transports, even if the patient needs full-body immobilization). Wilderness EMS practitioners may still attempt to provide food and water for their patients, even though they have vomited once or twice. Frequent small sips in many settings can keep a patient hydrated. This concept has transformed many pediatric centers where IV hydration, once the mainstay of treatment for vomiting children, is being replaced with oral hydration. This is good news for wilderness EMS patient care.

When building medical kits, consider adding oral rehydration salts for balanced hydration. Also consider high-calorie, low-volume snacks in the form of gel. Foods high in sugar content can be readily absorbed and provide significant high-yield energy for a patient during evacuation.

Suspension Syndrome

Suspension syndrome has been called by many names, including suspension trauma, harness-induced death, orthostatic intolerance, and harness hang syndrome. *Suspension syndrome* has been established as a better term than these alternatives, as there is little to no direct trauma, and a harness is not needed to cause the condition.[51] The real pathophysiology is a cascade of events that correlates to a syndrome, ultimately culminating as a state of shock caused by blood pooling in dependent lower extremities while the body is held upright without any movement for a prolonged time.[51,57] While uncommon, it remains a real concern for many wilderness-related activities.

Many types of recreationalists (e.g., climbers, cavers) who wear a harness and can have their legs become

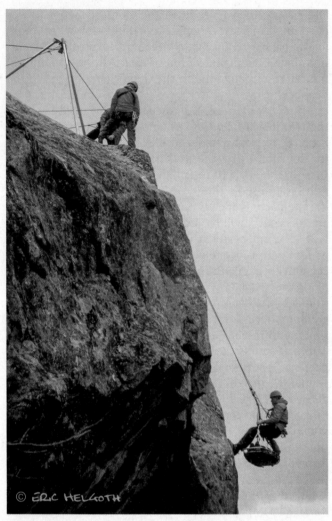

Figure 21-15 Technical proficiency in high-angle terrain is essential for wilderness EMS practitioners. It allows them to take care of patients with potential suspension syndrome as well as prevent it from occurring in rescuers.
Courtesy of Eric Helgoth.

immobile in a dependent position are susceptible to this syndrome. Other cohorts of individuals such as industrial workers, military service members (parachutists), circus performers, and stunt actors who can become suspended vertically as part of their occupation may be exposed to similar pathophysiology. Wilderness EMS practitioners need to be proficient in high-angle terrain to extricate and care for these kinds of patients (**Figure 21-15**).

Suspension syndrome can be worsened by other conditions, such as hypovolemia (e.g., hemorrhage, dehydration), vasodilation (e.g., heat, infection), or any other factors that alter the body's ability to maintain homeostasis (e.g., illicit or prescribed drugs, alcohol). Soldiers standing at attention are trained to make small flexing movements of their calf muscles. This action acts as a pump to accentuate venous return to the heart. By contracting these muscles and the one-way valves in the

lower extremity veins, blood is assisted back into the central circulation. Without this venous pump mechanism, suspension syndrome can develop in a matter of minutes and potentially result in death in as little as 10 minutes if the patient remains suspended upright. Mortimer's landmark 2011 publication in *Wilderness and Environmental Medicine* provides one of the best case report summaries of suspension syndrome.[58]

Whenever a patient experiences a passive hanging situation, blood pools in the lower extremities. Although no blood is lost, a relative hypovolemic state is induced. Some estimate that as much as 60% of the body's blood volume can collect in the lower extremities. This dramatically reduces the preload for the heart, rendering it unable to pump sufficient blood forward with subsequent contractions. Due to this decreased blood flow, the brain quickly becomes affected, and the patient will lose consciousness. This is often called postural syncope, and in most normal and unencumbered settings, the patient will fall to the ground and become horizontal, restoring blood supply to the brain. However, in the technical rescue environment, the patient is often suspended upright and the body's protective mechanisms are thwarted, often leading to death if not quickly reversed.[51]

In addition to venous pooling and decreased cardiac preload, it is thought that additional maladaptive responses contribute to the hemodynamic collapse in suspension syndrome. Hyperkalemia and acidotic blood are thought to contribute to the morbidity and mortality as patients are resuscitated. Pooled blood may have become relatively hypothermic and may cause a systemic cooling when reintroduced to the central circulation. There is some speculation that overlapping problems of asphyxia from certain harnesses causing chest constriction or patient positioning and airway compromise may accelerate the mental status changes and likelihood of death in these patients. While these additional factors may play a role, there are still some pathophysiologic parameters that remain unclear.[59]

Treatment recommendations for suspension syndrome focus on extricating the patient as soon as possible to a supine position. After this critical step, wilderness EMS practitioners can begin traditional BLS and ALS care and rapid transport of the patient to definitive care. Concern has arisen about case studies of "rescue death,"[51,59] where patients experienced cardiac arrest immediately after being extricated from their prolonged suspension. Prior recommendations suggested that a delayed extrication and slow removal of the harness would result in lower morbidity and mortality; however, this is no longer recommended. Mortimer and others have demonstrated that immediate extrication to a supine position provides the best chance for the patient to restore circulation to the heart and brain.[58-60] Standard treatments for crush syndrome and other rhabdomyolysis conditions suggest that IV hydration and possibly even alkalization of the urine with sodium bicarbonate added to IV fluids may be beneficial. These advanced discussions are beyond the scope of this text.

Patients with possible suspension syndrome, even if no clear outward symptoms are present, should be evaluated by a medical professional. Signs and symptoms of delayed rhabdomyolysis (muscle breakdown) and renal failure could develop during rescue or at a later time.

If a patient or rescuer becomes trapped in a suspended vertical position for any period of time, the first step is to immediately call for help and attempt to self-rescue and self-extricate from the situation. If self-rescue is not possible or the victim becomes exhausted, an attempt should be made to support, raise, or move the legs to decrease the dependent pooling of blood. Another preemptive measure would be to engage the body's normal venous pump mechanism by contracting the calf and leg muscles to help return blood to the central circulation. Pushing up against a rock wall or using a set of rope lanyards (e.g., Purcell Prusiks) to provide something to push against may delay the progression of suspension syndrome.

While this life-threatening condition has been reported in the literature, only recently has a better understanding of the pathophysiology and updated treatment recommendations emerged. In summary, the best care for suspension syndrome is to extricate the patient as soon as possible to a supine position and restore blood flow to the vital organs and then continue standard resuscitation protocols.

Eye/Head Protection

During evacuation, pay close attention to ensure you are protecting your patient from iatrogenic injuries, as well as making sure that all the rescuers have the PPE (e.g., helmet, safety glasses) appropriate to the setting. A minor head injury can be made worse by repeated concussion should your patient slip and fall or sustain a secondary impact to the head on a rock during evacuation. Carrying a person through brush and trees, or having unnoticed debris fall onto your patient, can lead to potential eye injuries. As a result, keep your patient in a helmet with goggles or safety glasses for protection. Rescue litters sometimes include a face and head shield.

Sun Protection

Sunlight is essential for the synthesis of vitamin D in the human body, and it also has beneficial effects on mood. However, the ultraviolet (UV) rays of the sun can damage the skin. Acute injury can include superficial, partial-thickness, and full-thickness sunburns seen in some severe cases of exposure. In extreme cases, solar burns may even contribute to shock or death, especially

with other comorbid conditions and trauma. Avoiding exposure to direct sunlight, especially from 1000 to 1500 hours, when UV radiation from the sun is strongest, decreases but does not eliminate the risk of sunburn and long-term damage (photoaging and skin cancers).

Topical sunscreens usually contain combinations of organic chemicals and/or inorganic filters that absorb various wavelengths of UV light. Zinc oxide and titanium dioxide are common examples of inorganic filters. Both types of sunscreens aim to block UV light exposure at two specific frequencies, A and B (UVA and UVB). UVA was once thought to be harmless, but we now know that it works synergistically with UVB to cause sunburn. UVB is responsible for most of the *erythema* (redness) of sunburn. UVA has been implicated in the development of phototoxicity and photoaging.[61] Thus, sun-blocking materials or creams must block both UVA and UVB to be effective. Look for the term *broad-spectrum* sun protection factor (SPF) on the product label to ensure coverage for both UVA and UVB.

The SPF is a numeric measure of how much the clothing or cream increases the minimum dose of UV light to make the skin red (**Figure 21-16**). For example, a sunscreen lotion with a rating of SPF 45 provides protection from sunburn for about 45 times longer than without the sunscreen. An SPF of 10 blocks 90% of UVB radiation, an SPF of 15 blocks 93%, an SPF of 30 blocks 97%, and an SPF of 50 blocks 98%. In 2012, the Food and Drug Administration restricted sunscreen products to an SPF of 50 due to the limited additional protective benefit, but in 2019 proposed a cap of SPF 60+, while allowing for marketing of products with up to SPF 80.[62] The degree of protection against UVA is hard to quantify and is usually much less than protection against UVB.[63,64]

It is advisable to wear protective clothing, such as wide-brimmed hats, pants, and long-sleeved shirts, and to apply sunscreen to exposed skin. Several factors of clothing contribute to the ultraviolet protection factor (UPF), and many outdoor clothing brands now provide a

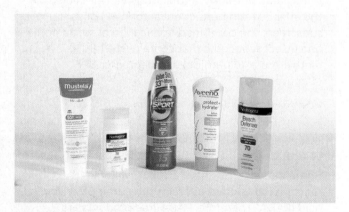

Figure 21-16 Sunscreen.
© Jones & Bartlett Learning. Photographed by Darren Stahlman.

UPF rating. Factors that contribute to the UPF rating of a fabric include the following[65]:

- Composition of the yarns (e.g., cotton, polyester)
- Tightness of the weave or knit (tighter improves the rating; the tightness of the weave probably contributes more than other factors to the UPF of a garment[66])
- Color (darker colors are generally better)
- Stretch (more stretch lowers the rating)
- Moisture (many fabrics have lower ratings when wet)
- Condition (worn and faded garments may have reduced ratings)
- Finishing (some fabrics are treated with UV-absorbing materials)

Protective lotions with a minimum SPF of 15 should be applied to exposed skin to minimize the potential injury from sun exposure. For prolonged evacuations, lotion with an SPF of 30 should be used, but little benefit can be claimed with an SPF 30 alone unless it is reapplied every 90 minutes. Ideally, sunscreens should be applied 15 to 30 minutes before going out into the sun. Most people do not apply a thick enough layer to achieve the claimed SPF. A minimum of 1 ounce (30 milliliters [mL]; about a shot glass full) should be used on all exposed areas for the average adult at the beach. With profuse sweating or water immersion, sunscreen should be reapplied frequently depending on the product label. Generally, water-resistant sunscreen will be effective for up to 40 or 80 minutes, per product description. Further considerations regarding the application of sunscreen are included in **Box 21-3** and **Box 21-4**.

Sunburn is treated as any other burn, and the care is essentially the same in the wilderness as on the street (**Box 21-5**).[63] The only major difference is that in the wilderness, prehospital care practitioners need to be aware

Box 21-3 Factors That Decrease SPF Effectiveness

Wind, heat, humidity, and altitude can all decrease the effective sun protection factor (SPF) of a sunscreen. The combined application of sunscreen and insect repellents that contain DEET (N,N-diethyl-meta-toluamide) also decreases SPF effectiveness.[61]

Data from Prevention and treatment of sunburn. Med Lett Drugs Ther. 2004;46:45.

Box 21-4 Allergic Reactions From Sunscreens

Some patients may have an acute allergic reaction if the lotion contains para-amino benzoic acid (PABA); therefore, PABA-free products are recommended.

© National Association of Emergency Medical Technicians (NAEMT)

Box 21-5 Sunburn Treatment

Prevention
Best prevented with sunscreen SPF > 30, wearing sun-protective clothing.

Pain Relief
Nonsteroidal anti-inflammatory drugs (NSAIDs; e.g., ibuprofen, naproxen, aspirin, indomethacin)
Analgesics: acetaminophen

Immunomodifiers
Corticosteroids: topical or systemic (prednisone)

Skin Care
Cool compresses soaked with water or aluminum acetate solution (Burrow solution)
Aloe vera
Topical anesthetics
Fluid resuscitation (oral or rarely IV) as needed

© National Association of Emergency Medical Technicians (NAEMT)

of and treat the potential delayed infection, fluid loss, dehydration, or sometimes even shock and to recognize that patients with sunburn are at higher risk for hypothermia.

Specifics of Wilderness EMS

This section reviews a few of the most important situations in which proper wilderness trauma care differs from care on the street. Areas covered where operationally specific (expanded scope of practice) protocols could be beneficial include wound management, joint dislocations, cardiopulmonary arrest, and bites and stings.

Wound Management

Wound management encompasses the following:

- *Hemostasis* (stopping bleeding)
- *Antisepsis* (preventing infection)
- Restoration of function (returning the skin to its protective function and restoring a limb or other body part to normal function)
- *Cosmesis* (ensuring pleasant appearance)

In the wilderness, prevention of infection and restoration of function assume great importance.

Hemostasis

Control of bleeding is part of the primary survey. On the street, arterial bleeding can kill. In the wilderness, even venous bleeding can kill if it continues for a sufficient amount of time. Remember, every red blood cell counts. Bleeding control, including standard measures such as

Box 21-6 Updated Hemorrhage Control Principles

In 2015, an international consensus panel, convened by the American Heart Association, published first aid skills, including hemorrhage control principles.[67] These recommended control of severe bleeding by manual direct pressure, gauze and a pressure dressing, hemostatic agents, and a tourniquet. Methods of using pressure points and extremity elevation are of historical note only and not recommended because of the lack of evidence supporting their effectiveness.

Data from Singletary EM, Charlton NP, Epstein JL, et al. Part 15: first aid: 2015 American Heart Association and American Red Cross guidelines update for first aid. *Circulation*. 2015;132(Suppl 2):S574-S589.

Box 21-7 Tourniquet Mistakes to Avoid

- Not using one when the injury indicates it should be used (life-threatening or uncontrolled bleeding)
- Waiting too long to apply the tourniquet (Apply tourniquet first for obvious life-threatening bleeding.)
- Taking it off when the patient is in shock or has a short transport time (less than 1 to 2 hours) to the hospital
- Not taking it off when indicated (i.e., not converting) if applied less than 6 hours
- Not making it tight enough (tourniquet should eliminate distal pulse)
- Not using a second tourniquet if needed (immediately adjacent to the first)
- Periodically loosening the tourniquet to allow blood flow to the injured extremity
- Using a tourniquet for minimal bleeding (when direct pressure/bandaging can be applied successfully)

Modified from Department Defense Lessons Learned from the Committee on Tactical Combat Casualty Care. See Chapter 27 in the 8th edition of *PHTLS: Prehospital Trauma Life Support, Military Edition*.

direct pressure, is as important or more important in the wilderness. Unless medical personnel are part of the actual injured party's group, severe bleeding that is not stopped will probably result in the patient's demise prior to the SAR team's arrival (**Box 21-6**).

Training programs for those venturing into wilderness situations should address these lifesaving skills:

- Tourniquets should be the first option for severe life-threatening bleeding.[21,39,41,51,67] In some situations in the wilderness, multiple patients and limited resources (e.g., at a mass-casualty incident) make it difficult or impossible to apply direct pressure to wounds; a similar challenge exists in a technical situation (e.g., side of a cliff) when extraction is the next critical step and maintaining direct pressure is not feasible. In some situations, a tourniquet that has been in place for less than 6 hours[48] may be converted (i.e., removed and replaced with a different means of bleeding control) to a bandage if there is no longer life-threatening bleeding and hemorrhage can be controlled by other means.[68,69] Specific protocols should be in place for responders to care for patients in these types of settings.
- Well-aimed direct pressure should be applied for 10 to 15 minutes directly on the bleeding site followed by a pressure bandage.
- Hemostatic agents may be useful in wilderness care in the control of severe bleeding. Wilderness medicine practitioners may encounter injured patients who have had hemostatic agents already applied by others in their group. Many of these agents are available for sale to the general public; however, training on how to effectively apply them is still recommended. It is important to remember that even if hemostatic agents are used, direct pressure on the wound remains a critical part of the treatment process.

In the wilderness situation when prolonged application (greater than 2 hours) is anticipated, the tourniquet

should be applied above the wound but as close to the wound as possible (**Box 21-7**). The rationale for this is that the amount of tissue that is ischemic as a result of the tourniquet (and therefore at risk of dying and requiring amputation) is theoretically less than if the tourniquet were applied at the most proximal position possible. (For more about hemostatic agents, tourniquets, and other hemorrhage control principles and preferences, see Chapter 3, *Shock: Pathophysiology of Life and Death*.)

Improvised Tourniquets

In many wilderness situations, responders may have to improvise the tools they use to provide care. Tourniquet improvisation using an available product, such as a belt or clothing article, is a vital skill in the wilderness setting. Although manufactured tourniquets are generally quicker to apply and are likely to achieve hemostasis faster and more reliably,[49] a manufactured tourniquet is not always available in wilderness trauma care.

The U.S. Army Institute of Surgical Research identified key features of a successful tourniquet when evaluating tourniquets for the Iraq and Afghanistan conflicts.[70] These features should be present in the tourniquet supplied in an EMS agency's medical kit and should be the basis for an improvised device[50]:

- At least 1 inch (25 millimeters [mm]) wide (e.g., climbing webbing or belt)
- Windlass or cam to achieve tightening of band
- Ability to capture the tightness

- Easy application (less than 60 seconds to self-apply)
- Adjustable
- Nonslip

Prevention of Infection

After injury in the wilderness, it may be a long time before the wound receives definitive treatment in an ED. Routine wound care in the ED includes appropriate cleaning to prevent infection. Wounds contaminated by dirt or caused by penetration from a dirty object are cleaned with high-pressure irrigation. Uncontaminated wounds are cleaned with low-pressure irrigation.

High-pressure irrigation may cause swelling of wounds, but in the case of contaminated wounds full of dirt and bacteria, the benefit of removing bacteria outweighs the risks from wound swelling.[52,71,72] Infection may set in quickly. After a wound has been open for about 8 hours, bacteria have spread from the skin deep into the wound, and suturing such a wound is associated with a higher chance of leading to a deep wound infection. Deep wound infections develop pressure, which keeps out white blood cells, the body's normal defense mechanism against infection.

Routine wound care in street EMS does not include cleansing the wound because it makes sense to delay wound cleansing for a few minutes until the patient reaches the ED, which is better suited for cleansing and evaluating the patient's wound. Delaying wound care does not make sense in wilderness EMS care. If it will take hours to get to the ED, the wound should be cleaned. In extremely remote areas, the wound could even become infected before the patient arrives at the ED several days later.

Studies have shown that early irrigation is essential to removing bacteria and reducing wound infections.[73-75] It is not necessary or practical to carry sterile solutions for wound irrigation. There is no need to add an antiseptic to the water.[76] Water that is good enough to drink is good enough to irrigate a wound. Water from streams or melted snow can be treated with any standard wilderness drinking water treatment and used to cleanse a wound.[71,77-81]

If the wound is contaminated, it must be irrigated with enough pressure to clean out the bacteria. The original studies showed that a 35-mL syringe with an 18-gauge needle provided an appropriate amount of pressure (5 to 15 pounds per square inch [psi]).[82-84] Squirt the water, at high pressure, throughout the wound. Squirting clean water from a drinking-water bottle or a hydration bladder-backpack system will also work.[85] This procedure, however, causes a major bloodborne pathogen risk to the rescuer; protection from the spray of blood with a gown or a clean trash bag or rain poncho when irrigating is necessary. Eye protection and gloves are essential when caring for these patients.

Sometimes it is necessary to debride the wound of gross dirt and/or foreign material. Wound debridement should be performed with as little trauma to the wound as possible, possibly using a gauze pad or clean cloth, forceps/tweezers, or even gloved fingers. The patient's pain may need to be treated before the wound can be cleaned. Lidocaine applied topically to the wound or injected subcutaneously for local anesthesia can provide relief in most cases. Conversely, narcotic analgesics may impair the patient's ability to ambulate and thus delay the evacuation. Once the irrigation is complete, dress and bandage the wound. Reapply a clean dressing at least daily or more often if the bandage becomes wet or soiled.

If the wound is gaping open, a wet dressing will prevent tissue damage as a result of drying out; change or at least rewet the dressing with clean water several times per day. However, because the wound will be mostly closed by bandaging, a dry dressing can be used in most cases.

Early antibiotic administration is commonly used upon arrival at the ED for patients with significant trauma. Antibiotics are not given in most civilian prehospital emergency medical systems because of the short transport times encountered in the urban environment. Definitive care may be significantly delayed in wilderness settings due to the longer distances to be covered and rescue considerations in rugged terrain, and early antibiotic use may be appropriate in this environment.[52]

Antibiotics administered early after injury are more effective in preventing wound infections. Intramuscular benzylpenicillin begun within 1 hour of injury was found to be effective in preventing streptococcal infections in a swine model of wound infection. If administration was delayed until 6 hours after injury, the medication was not effective.[86]

A military review of antibiotic use on the battlefield recommended that antibiotics be used if arrival at a medical treatment facility was anticipated to be 3 hours or longer.[87] The U.S. Department of Defense's TCCC course advocates the early administration of antibiotics for any open wounds at the point of wounding. TCCC cites multiple case studies where no wound infections developed when service men and women received battlefield antibiotics.[87] TCCC further recommends that oral antibiotics be given to casualties once per day if the casualty has the ability to swallow. Although no comparable studies have been done in the civilian setting, these recommendations make sense for application in the wilderness environment if the physician medical director agrees.

Restoration of Function and Cosmesis: Delayed Closure of Wilderness Wounds

Because of the lack of good lighting, appropriate and clean/sterile supplies, and a warm, dry place to work, in most cases it does not make sense to perform definitive wound closure in the wilderness. It is preferable to simply cleanse and irrigate the wound, dress and bandage, ensure ongoing routine wound care, and then have a **delayed primary closure** performed by the appropriate medical practitioner. As long as the wound is not infected, it is safe to suture the wound several days later as if it had just occurred. Although bacteria move into the wound soon after injury, eventually enough of the body's defenses (e.g., white blood cells) have entered the wound to make it safe to close. If a physician or someone else experienced at wound closure is present, the wound may be closed at the scene. However, it is still reasonable to simply cleanse, dress, and bandage the wound and allow closure to occur later. There is no clear advantage in most situations to closure of the wound in the wilderness environment, and doing so often significantly prolongs evacuation efforts.

Closing a wilderness wound may be important in one situation: when bleeding cannot be controlled in any other way. These situations are uncommon and usually involve a scalp laceration. For this reason, some wilderness medicine practitioners are trained to use disposable surgical staplers to repair scalp wounds. However, wound repair is complex and should not be attempted without sufficient training and experience.[88]

Pain Management

Appropriate pain management in wilderness EMS care can dramatically change the patient's tolerance of the extrication and rescue. The ideal goal is to reduce the pain, and sometimes anxiety along with it, to a tolerable level while ensuring that the patient maintains normal or near normal physiologic function. Alternate pain control strategies are emerging that use ketamine and other shorter acting narcotics such as fentanyl.[89]

Novel delivery strategies are becoming useful and are being adopted for use in the wilderness EMS environment. Transmucosal delivery of fentanyl has had great success in these settings (e.g., military, ski patrol, SAR). Intranasal administration (ketamine, fentanyl, versed) has become a much more frequent route of administration for pain medications during a rescue. NSAIDs, such as ibuprofen, as well as acetaminophen are great non-narcotic options that can provide adequate pain management with few side effects. Some injuries require an expanded pain control regimen, and in those cases narcotics and other pain medications (e.g., ketamine, nitrous oxide, methoxyflurane) can be administered. A hybrid pain control strategy may decrease the total amount of narcotic medication required, as well as decrease dose-related side effects. For example, administering 50 milligrams (mg) of ketamine and 50 micrograms (mcg) of fentanyl intranasally may provide better

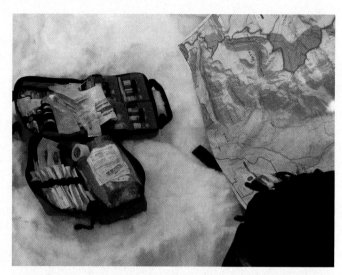

Figure 21-17 Advanced life support medical kit being used on a wilderness rescue of a patient with a femur fracture. Pain management options are crucial for treatment of patients in austere settings.
Courtesy of Will Smith.

analgesia than higher doses of either medication alone. As with any medication, the wilderness EMS practitioner must balance the risk versus benefit of the single agent chosen with the polypharmacy approach. In many rescue settings, the ability to closely monitor a patient can be difficult. A finger pulse oximetry probe may be the only monitoring device that is available, but with appropriate training it may provide sufficient data. **Figure 21-17** shows a wilderness EMS medical kit being used to treat a fractured femur on a backcountry rescue. Choosing an individualized pain control plan for a specific patient, and not using a generic algorithm, is important, as monitoring the patient often can be challenging. Deep procedural sedation, as performed in the hospital, is difficult to perform in the wilderness. Appropriate training, as with other advanced care practices, is essential for administration of many of these advanced medications.

Pain management, however, needs to be approached in a much broader sense and not just in regard to a specific medication that a wilderness EMS practitioner can give. It encompasses much more, including psychological reassurance, physiologic splinting, and medication support. Psychological first aid is an expanding concept and can be a useful tactic in any pain control strategy.[90] A wilderness EMS practitioner must balance all of these options to provide optimal patient care. The Wilderness Medical Society practice guidelines for the treatment of acute pain in remote environments give a good summary of treatment options, that begins with comfort care and PRICE (Protection, Rest, Ice, Compression, Elevation) therapy and builds with more advanced treatments up to intravenous and intraosseous medications.[25,89]

Dislocations

A healthy 20-year-old man was kayaking along a white-water stream when the top of his kayak paddle hit a low-hanging tree branch and caused indirect trauma to his shoulder. Now his right shoulder is deformed and painful. He cannot bring his right arm across his chest or bring his elbow to his side. Distal pulses, capillary refill, sensation, and movement are intact. From the ambulance, the wilderness EMS practitioner hikes a mile through the woods to get to the stream. Should the shoulder be "splinted as it lies," or should the practitioner try to reduce what looks like an anterior shoulder dislocation?

The common practice for fractures and dislocations on the street is to splint them as they lie and transport for definitive treatment. The only exception is the patient whose distal pulse is not palpable, in which case the extremity is realigned anatomically in an effort to restore circulation.

Although "splint it as it lies" is a good general rule for the street, "make it look normal" with physiologic splinting is a better general rule for the wilderness patient. It is certainly appropriate for both fractures and dislocations when transport is delayed, although local scopes of practice must also be considered. In some jurisdictions, front country EMS protocols are beginning to allow reduction techniques for some dislocations.[71]

There are many types of dislocations—finger, toe, shoulder, patella, knee, elbow, hip, ankle, and jaw—and all have been successfully reduced in the wilderness, some more easily than others. It is usually easy to reduce dislocations of the ankle (which are almost always fracture–dislocations), patella, toe, or finger, except the proximal interphalangeal joint of the index finger in some cases. Elbow, knee, and hip dislocations are usually quite difficult. All are much easier with training and practice; in particular, it takes training or experience to know, without a radiograph, when a joint is likely dislocated and to attempt reduction.

Traditional street EMS training courses seldom provide training in dislocation reduction. However, because wilderness dislocations are so common, dislocation reduction of a digit, patella, or shoulder is covered in almost all wilderness EMS training or at orthopedic workshops at wilderness medicine conferences. Those who might provide EMS in the wilderness or who regularly travel in the backcountry are advised to take one of these courses. However, even though the education has been gained, the practitioner must also be certified and credentialed to perform these skills, just like with any other patient care skill.[9,26] In addition, when considering scope of practice, dislocation reduction is one of the circumstances where an EMS physician deployed as part of the field team may be particularly helpful.[39,91,92]

Cardiopulmonary Resuscitation in the Wilderness

Traumatic cardiac arrest on the street has a poor prognosis, even if the scene is within minutes of a level I trauma center. No person survives more than a few minutes of cardiopulmonary resuscitation (CPR) after traumatic arrest.[93-96] This reality is recognized in many street EMS protocols. For traumatic cardiac arrest, consider initiating CPR in the following situations:

- Cardiac arrest occurs in the presence of EMS personnel.
- A victim of penetrating trauma had signs of life within 15 minutes of the arrival of EMS personnel.

Wilderness Traumatic Arrest

The following signs can be uniformly equated with nonsurvivability:

- Decapitation
- Transection of the torso
- Patient is frozen so hard that the patient's chest cannot be compressed
- Patient's rectal temperature is very cold and the same as the environment
- Well-progressed decomposition

The following presumptive signs of death may be of use to wilderness medicine practitioners, although no one sign by itself is reliable:

- **Rigor mortis.** Postmortem rigidity is well known but not always present, and similar rigidity is often observed in hypothermic patients.
- **Dependent lividity.** This finding is common in corpses but can also be found, along with pressure necrosis and frostbite, in some patients exposed to the elements for a long time.
- **Decomposition.** This finding is usually self-evident.
- *Lack of presumptive signs of life.* Hypothermia can mimic death, in that pulses may not be palpable, respirations may be undetectable, and pupils may be dilated and unreactive with no signs of consciousness. However, severely hypothermic patients have occasionally been resuscitated, with full neurologic recovery.

Therefore, in the wilderness context, CPR is inappropriate for most cases of traumatic arrest. It is appropriate for wilderness medicine practitioners and the SAR team members to examine the patient and then gently but firmly tell the companions that the victim is dead and there is no reason to initiate/continue resuscitation. Although it is often difficult to use the word *dead*, euphemisms often lead to misunderstanding and misinterpretation of what is actually being said.

Wilderness Medical Arrest

The term *medical cardiac arrest* applies to a patient who has a contributing underlying medical condition or suffers an acute medical condition (e.g., chest pain, shortness of breath, diabetes) and then sustains a cardiac arrest. Again, in the wilderness context, the chances of survival are poor or nonexistent when the patient is more than a few minutes from CPR or defibrillation.[97-103] It is possible that a SAR team might need to respond to a sudden cardiac arrest—whether sustained by the patient or even a team member. Lightweight defibrillators are now available, and some SAR teams carry them or at least have them at their incident command posts or forward staging locations.[51] As with all medical and other equipment, the weight-to-need-for-use ratio must be examined closely.

There are a variety of other causes of cardiac arrest in the wilderness, such as ventricular fibrillation (VF) cardiac arrest secondary to hypothermia or cardiac arrest secondary to pulmonary embolism. For such cardiac arrests, survival is even less likely than with a cardiac arrest secondary to a myocardial infarction. However, nontraumatic wilderness cardiac arrest might be survivable in the following situations:

- Hypothermia[103,104]
- Cold-water submersion[105-108]
- Lightning strike[109,110]
- Electrocution
- Drug overdose
- Avalanche burial[111,112]

In all of these cases, a patient may appear to be in cardiac arrest but still might be resuscitated by basic CPR. For hypothermia in particular, there is a saying that "Patients are not dead until they are warm and dead." (See Chapter 19, *Environmental Trauma I: Heat and Cold.*) A significant minority of those who appear dead from these mechanisms can be resuscitated. There are special considerations for each of these situations—for example, scene safety for those who have been electrocuted and are still attached to a power line, or the fact that external cardiac compression can actually induce a VF cardiac arrest in a hypothermic patient whose heart is beating just enough to keep the patient alive.[113-116] Although appropriate in a wilderness EMS course, detailed discussion of these topics is beyond the scope of this chapter. (See Chapter 19, *Environmental Trauma I: Heat and Cold*, and Chapter 20, *Environmental Trauma II: Lightning, Drowning, Diving, and Altitude.*)

Two simple and standard wilderness CPR recommendations are as follows[11,31,117]:

- If the patient appears to be in cardiac arrest from causes other than trauma, attempt CPR for 15 to 30 minutes; if, at the end of this time, the patient has not been resuscitated, stop CPR and consider the patient dead.
- Do not start CPR if it will put rescuers at risk and decrease their chances of retreating from the scene safely, given concerns about daylight, terrain, weather, and available nearby shelter.

The NAEMSP's position statement, "Termination of Resuscitation of Nontraumatic Cardiopulmonary Arrest," available on the NAEMSP website, can provide guidance on when to consider termination of a cardiac arrest resuscitation effort.[102]

Bites and Stings

Bites and stings are common wilderness problems. The exact type of bite or sting likely in a wilderness area depends on the specific locale. Local knowledge and resources are important to help guide the care of these patients, but routine patient care guidelines are still necessary.

Insect Bite and Stings

Many insects may become a nuisance in the wilderness settings in North America (e.g., biting flies, mosquitoes) but do not transmit disease. Most people who are bitten or stung by an insect develop only a minor local reaction. While painful, and generally associated with significant anxiety, there are generally no life-threatening issues. However, mosquito-borne diseases, such as West Nile virus and the Zika virus, have prompted high-profile concerns recently. In addition, people traveling to tropical areas must be aware of a host of other vector-transmitted diseases (e.g., malaria, dengue).

Allergic reactions occur on a spectrum from localized signs and symptoms to life-threatening anaphylaxis. The time from the sting to onset of maximal symptoms can be variable, but most severe symptoms usually occur within an hour of the sting. More significant systemic reactions can peak at 48 or more hours, and in some delayed-type hypersensitivities, it may be even longer. Anaphylaxis is reported in 0.3% to 8% of stings.[118-122] At least 40 identified deaths are reported annually in the United States.[121,123,124]

A wilderness EMS practitioner must be able to identify the severity of the reaction from the anxiety often associated with the event. Not all patients who have had a severe allergic reaction before will develop an equally severe reaction upon a second exposure, but they may, or it could be worse. For this reason, it can be extremely difficult to predict who will have a less severe overall reaction, and the practitioner should err on the side of treatment and/or early evacuation.

Some individuals who are stung will progress within a few minutes to a generalized allergic reaction. This

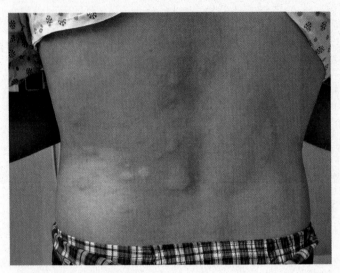

Figure 21-18 Allergic urticaria.

© Chuck Stewart, MD, EMDM, MPH

reaction may range from *urticaria* (hives) to a full-blown anaphylactic reaction. Although the exact spectrum of generalized allergic reaction depends on the contents of the injected toxin (which varies among the many species of bees and wasps) and the allergic history of the patient, one or more of the following are usually seen:

- Urticaria (hives) (**Figure 21-18**)
- Lip and/or facial swelling
- Hoarseness or stridor
- Wheezing and/or shortness of breath
- Abdominal cramping, vomiting, or diarrhea
- Tachycardia or bradycardia
- Hypotension
- Syncope and/or altered mental status

A patient with mild localized or sometimes even diffuse urticaria after a sting will probably do well. If a patient with hives after a bite or sting progresses to real anaphylaxis, however, the most telling early sign is hoarseness and hypotension. The major cause of death after bee sting allergic reaction is airway obstruction from swelling in the airway, and hoarseness is usually the first sign of airway swelling. Any patient with a generalized reaction to an insect bite or sting needs treatment immediately.

Honeybee stingers usually remain in the skin when the insect leaves because the stinger is barbed. Venom from the stinger and venom sac will continue to enter the skin for 45 to 60 seconds if the stinger is not removed; thus it is important to remove the stinger quickly. There has been a great deal of discussion about the proper way to remove a bee stinger, but recent information indicates it really does not matter how it gets out as long as it is removed as soon as possible. Fingernails, a knife blade edge, or a credit card edge are all effective tools for removing an embedded stinger. If a stinger is removed

within 15 seconds of the sting, the severity of the sting is reduced. Other insects such as wasps can cause an allergic reaction, and they can sting a patient multiple times without embedding a stinger.

BLS interventions generally involve keeping the patient sitting in a position of comfort, performing standard airway management, and providing oxygen.

The main medications used to treat allergic reactions to insect bites or stings include the following:

1. *Epinephrine (adrenalin).* Although epinephrine acts for only a few minutes, it can be lifesaving. Repeated dosing may be required in severe cases.
2. *Antihistamines.* Both histamine-1 (e.g., diphenhydramine) and histamine-2 (e.g., famotidine) blockers are used. Anyone who requires epinephrine for a bee sting allergy should also receive an antihistamine.
3. *Steroids* (e.g., prednisone, dexamethasone). Most people who require epinephrine should also receive a steroid to suppress the longer term allergic response.

The most important drug is epinephrine, which acts rapidly to reverse the acute reaction. Epinephrine is available as a pen-sized autoinjector, which is often prescribed to any patient who has had a generalized allergy to bee stings (**Box 21-8**). These autoinjectors are found in many wilderness first aid kits. The Wilderness Medical Society has published a practice guideline on the use of epinephrine in the wilderness.[125] This guideline recommends the administration of epinephrine by wilderness EMS practitioners who are trained to recognize acute anaphylaxis and to give epinephrine.

Some wilderness SAR teams carry drugs for allergic reactions in their medical kits, and the wilderness EMS practitioners have special training in their use. Often, people with a history of severe allergy will carry these medications in their personal first aid kits.

While this chapter focuses on wilderness trauma care, which can involve insect bites and stings, responders

---

Box 21-8 Autoinjectors

Warning: There is another autoinjector medication on the market that has the appearance of an EpiPen autoinjector. The drug is Alsuma, a sumatriptan autoinjector prescribed to treat migraines. This autoinjector could be used by mistake on an anaphylactic patient because there is no warning that it is not epinephrine and has the identical size, color, and cap appearance as the EpiPen released in 2010.[126]

Data from Hawkins S, Weil C, Fitzpatrick D. Letter to the editor: epinephrine autoinjector warning. *Wilderness Environ Med.* 2012;23:371-378.

must keep in mind that a patient may develop a severe allergy from other exposures and foods, and the same patient evaluation and treatment would apply.

Snakebite

There are approximately 3,000 species of snakes, of which some 600 are venomous, but only 200 are considered to be medically significant venomous types.[127,128] Few are found in northern latitudes. Most reside naturally in tropical areas, and many are deadly. Although many snakes have venom glands, there are only two types of native snakes in North America with venom strong enough to cause more than minor irritation to humans. All snakebites have the potential to cause infection and other local tissue damage and should be managed like other puncture wounds.

Coral snakes are small snakes found in the southern parts of North America (**Figure 21-19**). They have venom that is neurotoxic and causes paralysis. These snakes are small, have small front fangs, cannot open their mouths

very far compared to larger snakes, and are rather timid compared to certain crotalids; therefore, serious envenomations are not common. Of the North American coral snakes, the Eastern, or Floridian, has the most toxic venom. The popular rhyme used to identify coral snakes based on colored bands only works for certain North American species and should not be relied on to identify the snake. Signs of envenomation may be delayed up to 15 hours, come on rapidly, and begin with central paralysis (ptosis, double vision, disconjugate gaze, trouble managing oral secretions).[129]

Pit vipers, often called crotalids, are found throughout large portions of North America and include *rattlesnakes* of various types (**Figure 21-20**), *copperheads* (**Figure 21-21**), and *water moccasins*, or *cottonmouths* (**Figure 21-22**). The majority of pit viper bites do not occur in the wilderness but rather in rural, suburban, or even urban areas. A classic example is the intoxicated man who was kissing his pet rattlesnake when he was bitten on the lips or tongue. Bites to other areas of the bodies, especially extremities, are also common (**Figure 21-23**).

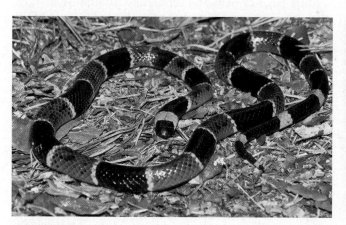

Figure 21-19 Coral snake.
© JasonOndreicka/iStock/Getty Images

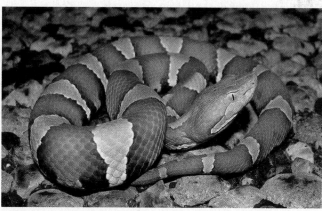

Figure 21-21 Copperhead snake.
© Matt Jeppson/Shutterstock

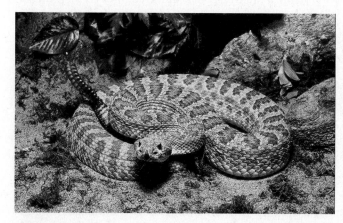

Figure 21-20 Rattlesnake.
© Jason Ondreicka/Thinkstock

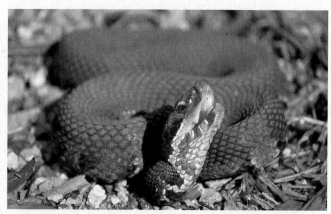

Figure 21-22 Water moccasin (cottonmouth) snake.
© James DeBoer/Shutterstock

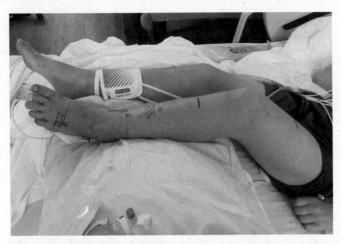

Figure 21-23 Lower left extremity bite from a water moccasin (cottonmouth) snake. Note progressive swelling and ecchymosis.

Courtesy of Ben Abo.

Snakebites are not as rare as one might think. In the United States, almost 10,000 patients are treated each year for snakebites, and approximately 5 die.[130] It is estimated that worldwide there are approximately 421,000 envenomations annually, resulting in 20,000 deaths, although this number may actually be much higher because of poor death records in many countries.[128]

Historically, a variety of prehospital treatments have been attempted by patients, bystanders, or sometimes EMS personnel. The only treatment shown to be effective for envenomated pit viper bites is antivenin (antivenom), which is extremely expensive (thousands of U.S. dollars for a single treatment) and thus not routinely carried in first aid kits. The only street EMS care proven to be helpful is supportive care and transport to the hospital.[131]

The first step in treating snakebite is to *watch for signs of envenomation* (i.e., determine that venom was injected). Only a fraction of bites by pit vipers actually result in envenomation (20% to 25% are dry bites), and the signs of envenomation are fairly distinct. Although signs and symptoms of envenomation usually develop in a few minutes, it is not uncommon for them to be delayed by 6 to 8 hours or perhaps even longer, so transporting to the hospital after a suspected poisonous snakebite is appropriate.[129] Signs of envenomation include the following:

- Severe local redness, swelling, bruising, and pain
- Severe pain and/or tenderness away from bite site (e.g., a bite on the foot with pain or tenderness up in the groin or knee)
- Continued nonsignificant bleeding from the bite
- Paresthesias in the fingers and toes (Paresthesia is unusual sensation, usually caused by damage to nerves or biochemical abnormalities; a feeling of "pins and needles" is a common paresthesia.)

- Metallic taste in the mouth
- Feeling of severe anxiety
- Nausea, vomiting, and abdominal pain

Prehospital Treatment of Suspected Pit Viper Envenomation

When managing a patient with a suspected envenomation, the initial care is similar to any other seriously ill or injured patient[129-134]: Support the ABCs (Airway, Breathing, Circulation), provide oxygen to maintain an adequate oxygen saturation, apply a cardiac monitor, start intravenous therapy (to keep vein open), and monitor the patient's vital signs.

Assess the bite site for signs of envenomation, including erythema, swelling, ecchymosis, tenderness, and the development of blisters or soft-tissue necrosis, and how far pain and/or tenderness travels. Any jewelry or tight clothing should be removed anywhere on the body.

The leading edge of the swelling should be marked with a black pen every 15 minutes to determine the severity of the swelling and rate of progression. Similarly, the leading edge of pain and tenderness should be marked. The involved extremity should be immobilized and positioned at approximately heart level (not elevated or held dependent). Major joints such as the elbow should be maintained in relative extension (less than 45 degrees of flexion). As swelling occurs, constant consideration should be made to ensure any splinting or clothing is not causing circulatory compromise.

If the patient requires pain relief, opiates are preferred for pain relief over NSAIDs because of the risk of bleeding associated with some envenomations and platelet effects with NSAID use.

Do not attempt to kill the snake. A killed or decapitated snake still offers a risk of envenomation to EMS personnel. If circumstances permit, take a photo of the snake from a safe distance. Safety in this scenario cannot be stressed enough.[129]

While a litter rescue is preferred, if necessary, the patient can be slowly walked for evacuation, with frequent rest stops and reassurance to help keep the patient calm. Transport the patient rapidly to an appropriate destination. Notify the receiving facility of the situation while en route so that they can make preparations to receive and treat the patient.

Extremity Immobilization

Pressure immobilization has been used effectively in Australia for field management of *elapid* (cobra, mamba, North American coral) snakebites (**Figure 21-24**).[132] This technique involves immediately wrapping the entire bitten extremity with an elastic wrap or bandage as tightly as would be done for a sprain and then splinting and immobilizing the extremity.

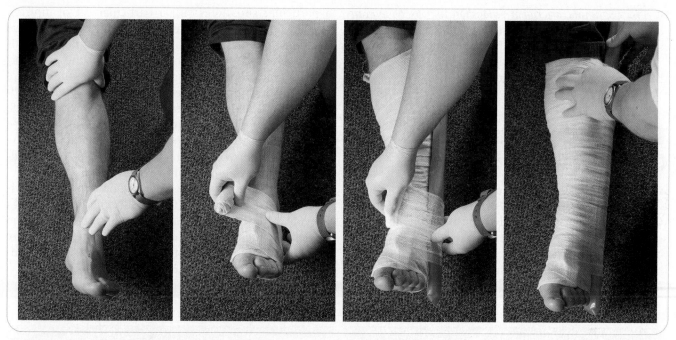

Figure 21-24 Pressure immobilization technique.
© Jones & Bartlett Learning. Photographed by Darren Stahlman.

If the patient is more than 2 hours from medical attention in an area outside of North America, and the bite is on an arm or leg, it might be reasonable to use the pressure immobilization technique. Place a 2- by 2-inch (5- by 5-centimeter [cm]) cloth pad over the bite site. Next, apply an elastic wrap firmly around the involved limb directly over the padded bite site with a margin of at least 4 to 6 inches (10 to 15 cm) on either side of the wound. Take care to check for adequate circulation in the fingers and toes (normal pulses, feeling, and color). An alternative method is to simply wrap the entire limb as tightly as for a sprain with an elastic bandage. The wrap is meant to impede absorption of venom into the general circulation by containing it within the compressed tissue and microscopic blood and lymphatic vessels near the limb surface. Finally, splint the limb to prevent motion. If the bite is on a hand or arm, also apply a sling. It should be noted that this recommendation is controversial, in that some experts believe that localizing venom in a single area might lead to an increased chance for local tissue damage.

Historically, the following treatments have been recommended; however, they are not supported by the literature:

1. *Rest.* Some recommendations insist that those who have been bitten should always avoid exertion. Deaths from North American snakebite are very rare,[129,135] and it is very unlikely that the exertion of hiking out from a wilderness area will make a victim of a snakebite significantly more ill. If the victim can be carried out, that is ideal. However, if waiting for a carryout will delay the victim's arrival at a hospital, the victim should walk out with whatever assistance can be given.

2. *Catching the snake and bringing it to the hospital.* There are numerous reports of bystanders who tried to catch a suspected poisonous snake and were bitten during the attempt. A single antivenin is used for all pit viper venoms in the United States, and treatment is based on clinical degree of envenomation, relying on the previous signs and symptoms. Therefore, identifying a domestic snake is of minor importance compared with the dangers of attempting to catch the snake. A digital photograph of the snake might be useful, but identification is not worth risking an additional bite.

3. *Suction or incision.* Suction, with or without cutting, has been shown to be useless for venomous snakebite. Snakebite kits consisting of suction devices should be left out of all first aid kits and should not be used.[136,137]

4. *Electric shock.* Electric shock applied to the snakebite has been shown to be totally ineffective and should never be used.[138,139]

5. *Cold packs.* Cold packs have been shown to increase tissue damage from North American pit viper bites and should not be used.[140]

6. *Splinting, arterial or venous tourniquets, lymph constrictors, or elastic bandages.* Although widely recommended, none of these treatments has been shown to be effective and may worsen local damage to the bite area.[141]

The Wilderness EMS Context Revisited

At the beginning of this chapter, we asked: "When should we think about wilderness EMS; that is, when should we think and work differently from what we do on the street?" The short answer: "It depends."

Time, distance, weather, and terrain all enter into the decision. The decision that a particular patient, in a particular situation, with a particular set of injuries, needs wilderness care rather than street care is a medical decision—one best made by the prehospital care practitioner directly attending to the patient. If the prehospital care practitioner at the scene can contact the medical oversight practitioner, especially in an area where medical control is likely to be familiar with wilderness EMS, the advice is definitely worth seeking. Ultimately, the decision is up to the prehospital care practitioner at the scene based on scope of practice, local protocols regarding autonomy, and medical oversight.

PHTLS believes that, given a good fund of knowledge, key principles, and training by medical oversight providers in autonomous medical decision making and wilderness medicine, prehospital care practitioners are capable of making the most appropriate decisions regarding patient care in wilderness settings.

SUMMARY

- While many of the principles of *wilderness* EMS are the same as *street* EMS, preferences and practices may change because of the unique circumstances. Balancing these factors becomes the specialty of wilderness EMS practitioners.
- Oversight direction by a knowledgeable physician and specialized training for practitioners who are likely to encounter wilderness EMS situations are integral components of wilderness EMS.
- The acronym LATE—Locate, Access, Treat, Extricate—represents simplified principles in SAR and other wilderness EMS operations.
- Wilderness EMS presents a wide variety of environments and situations requiring unique patient packaging and transport considerations, specialized equipment, modification of standard procedures and protocols, and context-specific safety considerations for both the patient and the responders.
- Initial patient assessment is the same regardless of the environment. The priority of attention is based on the major life threats that can be mitigated immediately at the point of injury.

- In many wilderness situations, responders may have to improvise the tools and methods they use to provide care. They must be skilled in tourniquet use, including improvisational methods, and they must understand how best to adapt standard care practices, such as antibiotic administration, pain management, and cardiopulmonary resuscitation and defibrillation, to the wilderness environment.
- When managing patients in the wilderness, wilderness EMS practitioners must also consider food and water requirements and elimination needs.
- A basic principle of wilderness care is that all patients are hypothermic, hypoglycemic, and hypovolemic until proven otherwise.
- Bites and stings are common wilderness problems. Local knowledge and resources are important to help guide the care of these patients, but routine patient care guidelines are still necessary.

SCENARIO RECAP

You are the medical and team leader for the local SAR team and have been dispatched to a popular canyoneering site in your jurisdiction. The only information you have is a GPS location from a distress signal broadcast via an emergency satellite beacon. The time is about 1800 hours, and current temperature is 74°F (23°C). The weather forecast shows some building thunderstorms throughout the evening and an overnight low of 36°F (2°C). The team begins to plan the response using the LATE acronym: Locate, Access, Treat, Extricate.

Your team assembles the necessary gear, including the still-/swift-water and high-angle rescue kits, their own personal protective equipment, and the standard medical kit, and begins responding to the location. As the team leader, you interface with the incident commander and develop a communication plan with a staged team member to enable a communication relay from the top of the canyon back to the incident command post.

- What are the essential items for a team and individual medical kit to handle the most severe and most likely injuries for this type of rescue scenario?
- What operationally specific (expanded scope of practice) protocols would you want in place to care for patients in remote and/or prolonged care settings? Do you have standing orders, as you are expecting limited communication options?
- What safety concerns should you be considering for your rescue team? How do situational factors such as time of day, location of patient, and experience and training of your team affect safety?

You *locate* the GPS position and find a slot canyon with three known separate 100-ft (30-m) rappels. You attempt to yell and try to make contact but are unable to get any response. When you blow your whistle, you are able to hear a faint whistle blast in return. You and your team safely make your way toward the location. At the top of the second rappel, you find the two members of the party that set off the emergency beacon. They tell you one of their team members sustained an approximately 50-ft (15-m) fall deeper in the canyon at 1300 hours. They had to climb back up from the location to get a signal out on their emergency beacon. Another friend rappelled down to assess the victim and stated the injuries appear to be an angulated open femur fracture, with a lot of pooled blood. He also stated that the patient appeared confused. The patient did not lose consciousness or show any other signs of head trauma. He was wearing a helmet. The friend has been holding pressure on a "pumper" with some continued bleeding.

You continue down the next rappel and establish verbal communication with the friend who is attending to the patient. You direct him to place an improvised tourniquet with 1-inch tubular webbing proximal to the wound that is continuing to bleed. You direct the friend to tighten the webbing by twisting a spare carabiner until the bleeding is stopped and to then secure it in place with another carabiner. The friend reports that the bleeding has been controlled.

Once your additional equipment reaches your location, you begin your final rappel to *access* the patient. Upon reaching the patient, you find a 25-year-old otherwise healthy male awake and now more alert with an obvious open deformed right femur fracture. The friend has tried to get extra clothing around the patient, but the patient is in a shallow pool of cold water and has wet clothing and is shivering. You begin planning and implementing the *treat* portion of your mission, but because it is getting dark, your team will have to wait until morning to *extricate* the patient.

- How can you direct others to provide care in a wilderness setting? Are you familiar with how dispatchers use emergency medical dispatch to assist with prearrival instructions during a 9-1-1 call, and can you remotely direct someone to provide initial care? What else would you direct the friend to perform if you have an additional delay in reaching the patient?
- What are your priorities of care in assessment and intervention? What are the prolonged patient care considerations?
- What is your plan to get this patient packaged and extricated?

As first on the scene, you turn on your headlamp and rapidly assess the area and ensure the safety of yourself, the casualty, and his companions. Your communication relay at the top of the canyon relays the progress of the rescue back to the incident commander. The weather seems to be holding with minimal clouds and no thunderstorms developing, and you decide that you will have to remain at this location through the night. No helicopters are available in the area to perform night operations, and you are not able to safely and efficiently move the patient out of this position tonight. You request the rescue helicopter that had been placed on standby to return at first light to hoist the patient from an opening in the canyon about 328 ft (100 m) from your current location.

There is limited room at the patient's location, but you are able to move him off to the side, so you are no longer under the direct path of other rescuers as they descend to your location, and you are able to carefully move the patient to a dry spot and onto an insulating pad.

Your assessment proceeds along the MARCH PAWS algorithm. You have already remotely identified and controlled the *massive hemorrhage* and now evaluate the tourniquet placed by the friend using tubular webbing. It appears to be moderately effective, so you apply a second tourniquet from your kit adjacent to the first and mark the time it was placed. The second tourniquet completely stopped further bleeding, and you confirm that there is no longer a distal pulse. You perform a blood sweep and detect no other signs of massive hemorrhage. However, when you assess his pelvis, it feels unstable and there is significant pain; therefore you apply a pelvic binder from your medical kit.

He is awake and talking to you with no signs of *airway* compromise. You place your hands on his chest wall and note equal and symmetric chest rise and fall with no signs of *respiratory* distress or chest wall trauma. You check *circulation* by assessing distal pulses and note his heart rate to be rapid with bounding radial pulse of 120 beats per minute. His skin is cool and slightly diaphoretic. You treat the patient's *hypothermia* by removing him from the cold water, exposing his skin, and putting dry warm clothes on him. You direct a teammate to prepare a sleeping pad and bag for a hypothermia wrap with additional heating pads. You assess his *head* and see no overt signs of head or back injury; however, he has had a significant fall and possibly a distracting injury, so you consider the possibility of spinal injury and stabilize his spine using a whole-body vacuum splint. The patient is conscious and alert with an otherwise normal gross neurologic examination. He has some mild nausea but has not vomited, and you administer a 4-mg dose of ondansetron with an orally disintegrating tablet. You treat his *pain* with a 1-gram dose of oral acetaminophen and give a 100-mg subdissociative dose of intranasal ketamine. This brings his pain from 10 out of 10 down to 2 out of 10 and facilitates the completion of your examination and splinting/treatment.

Based on your standing *antibiotic* order protocol for open fractures, you establish an IV now that all other life threats are addressed and administer 2 grams of IV cefazolin after confirming no allergies. You reassess the patient's body (head to toe) for any other *wounds* or injuries and find the only location requiring attention is the open femur fracture. You grossly irrigate the open fracture site with potable water and bandage. Now you know that you have a prolonged extrication and attempt to convert the tourniquet to another form of bleeding control. You are safely able to transition from a tourniquet to a pressure dressing to control the bleeding. You reassess it frequently and confirm that it maintains control. Distal pulses and sensation are regained.

Last, you complete your patient packaging with appropriate *splints*. For the open femur fracture, you use manual traction and bring the leg to anatomic position and provide *physiologic* splinting, with padding and the vacuum mattress to maintain position. The vacuum mattress now is able to splint the entire body, including neck/back, pelvis, and femur fracture without undue pressure spots. You attend to the suspected right wrist fracture, which was not the most significant injury, once higher priority injuries have been addressed. You allow the patient to sip on fluids through the night and to urinate using an adult diaper that you exchange when needed.

The team spends the night out with the patient and his companions, and with the preplanning you are well prepared. Your medical training, along with the prolonged field care guidelines, helps you manage the patient through the night. With your stabilization and treatment, the patient does well overnight, and vital signs

SCENARIO SOLUTION (CONTINUED)

remain stable. Once immobilized, he has very little pain. As morning arrives, the helicopter is able to hoist the patient out of the canyon. A waiting ambulance assumes care of the patient and transports him to the closest appropriate trauma center 45 minutes away. Because the patient has been stable overnight, it was determined that a medical helicopter transport was not needed after conferring with medical control. Your field documentation is passed on with the patient to ensure a continuity of patient care. Once out of the field, you complete a final patient care report. You follow up with the hospital and find that the patient is expected to make a full recovery.

References

1. Wilderness. In: *Merriam-Webster's Collegiate Dictionary*. 11th ed. Merriam-Webster; 2014:1432.

2. McGinnis KK. *Rural and Frontier Emergency Medical Services*. National Rural Health Association; 2004.

3. Liffrig JR, Tarter SL, Schimelpfenig T, et al. Wilderness medicine education. In: Auerbach PS, ed. *Auerbach's Wilderness Medicine*. 7th ed. Elsevier; 2017:2440-2471.

4. Winstead C, Hawkins SC. Wilderness EMS education. In: Hawkins SC, ed. *Wilderness EMS*. Wolters Kluwer; 2018:61-81.

5. Bennett BL. A time has come for wilderness emergency medical service: a new direction. *Wilderness Environ Med*. 2012;23(1):5-6.

6. Warden CR, Millin MG, Hawkins SC, et al. Medical direction of wilderness and other operational emergency services programs. *Wilderness Environ Med*. 2012;23(1):37-43.

7. Millin M. Wilderness EMS medical oversight. In: Hawkins SC, ed. *Wilderness EMS*. Wolters Kluwer; 2018:101-110.

8. Russell K, Weber D, Scheele B, et al. Search and rescue in the intermountain west states. *Wilderness Environ Med*. 2013;24:429-433.

9. National Highway Traffic Safety Administration. *The National EMS Scope of Practice Model*. Department of Transportation/National Highway Traffic Safety Administration; 2005.

10. Millin MG, Johnson DE, Schimelpfenig T, et al. Medical oversight, educational core content, and proposed scopes of practice of wilderness EMS providers: a joint project developed by wilderness EMS educators, medical directors, and regulators using a Delphi approach. *Prehosp Emerg Care*. 2017;21(6):673-681.

11. Smith W. Medical professionals role in search and rescue. In: Rodway G, Weber DC, McIntosh SE, eds. *Mountain Medicine and Technical Rescue*. Carreg; 2016:207-223.

12. Hawkins SC, Millin MC, Smith W. Wilderness emergency medical services and response systems. In: Auerbach P, ed. *Auerbach's Wilderness Medicine*. 7th ed. Elsevier; 2017:1200-1213.

13. Johnson DE, Schimelpfenig T, Hubbel F. Minimum guidelines and scope of practice for wilderness first aid. *Wilderness Environ Med*. 2013;24(4):456-462.

14. Tilton B. *Wilderness First Responder*. Falcon Guides (Globe Pequot Press); 2010.

15. American Society for Testing and Materials. *Standard Guide for Training First Responders Who Practice in Wilderness, Delayed, or Prolonged Transport Settings*. American Society for Testing and Materials; 1995:F1616-F1695.

16. Wilderness Medical Society Curriculum Committee. Wilderness first responder: recommended minimum course topics. *Wilderness Environ Med*. 1999;10:13-19.

17. McNamara EC, Johe DH, Endly DA, eds. *Outdoor Emergency Care*. 5th ed. National Ski Patrol. Brady (Pearson); 2012.

18. Hawkins SC. The relationship between ski patrols and emergency medical services systems. *Wilderness Environ Med*. 2012;23:106-111.

19. Constance BB, Auerbach PS, Johe DH. Prehospital medical care and the National Ski Patrol: how does outdoor emergency care compare to traditional EMS training? *Wilderness Environ Med*. 2012;23:177-189.

20. Spano SJ. National Park Service medicine. In: Auerbach P, ed. *Auerbach's Wilderness Medicine*. 7th ed. Elsevier; 2017: 2487-2497.

21. Smith WR. Integration of tactical EMS in the National Park Service. *Wilderness Environ Med*. 2017;28(2S):S146-S153.

22. Lipman GS, Weichenthal L, Harris NS, et al. Core content for Wilderness Medicine fellowship training of emergency medicine graduates. *Acad Emerg Med*. 2014; 21(2):204-207.

23. Hawkins S, Millin M, Smith W. Care in the wilderness. In: Cone D, Brice JH, Delbridge TR, Myers JB, eds. *Emergency Medical Services: Clinical Practice and System Oversight*. 2nd ed. Vol 2: Medical Oversight of EMS. John Wiley & Sons; 2015:377-391.

24. Vines T, Hudson S. Medical considerations in technical rescue. In: *High-Angle Rope Rescue Techniques: Levels I and II*. 4th ed. Jones & Bartlett Learning; 2016:224-245.

25. Smith WR. Principles of basic technical rescue, packaging, and patient care integration. In: Hawkins SC, ed. *Wilderness EMS*. Wolters Kluwer; 2018:101-110.

26. Hawkins SC. WEMS systems. In: Hawkins SC, ed. *Wilderness EMS*. Wolters Kluwer; 2018:21-59.

27. Zafren K, McCurley L, Shimanski C, et al. Technical rescue. In: Auerbach PS, ed. *Auerbach's Wilderness Medicine*. 7th ed. Elsevier; 2017:1242-1280.

28. Goodman T, Iserson KV, Strich H. Wilderness mortalities: a 13-year experience. *Ann Emerg Med*. 2001;37:279-283.

29. Gentile DA, Morris JA, Schimelpfenig T, Bass SM, Auerbach PS. Wilderness injuries and illnesses. *Ann Emerg Med*. 1992;21:853-861.

30. Singletary EM, Markenson DS. Injury prevention: decision making, safety, and accident avoidance. In: Auerbach PS, ed. *Auerbach's Wilderness Medicine*. 7th ed. Elsevier; 2017:593-616.

31. Isaac JE, Johnson DE. *Wilderness and Rescue Medicine*. 6th ed. Jones & Bartlett Learning; 2013.

32. Hawkins SC. Setting the record straight to reduce fatalities in sinking vehicles. *Emerg Med News*. 2015;37(8):28-29.

33. Butler FK, Blackbourne LH. Battlefield trauma care then and now: a decade of tactical combat casualty care. *J Trauma Acute Care Surg*. 2012;73:S395-S402.

34. Holcomb JB, Stansbury LG, Champion HR, Wade C, Bellamy RF. Understanding combat casualty care statistics. *J Trauma Acute Care Surg*. 2006;60:397-401.

35. Kelly J, Ritenour AE, McLaughlin DF, et al. Injury severity and causes of death from Operation Iraqi Freedom and Operation Enduring Freedom: 2003–2004 versus 2006. *J Trauma*. 2008;6:S21-S27.

36. Eastridge BJ, Mabry RL, Seguin P, et al. Death on the battlefield (2001–2011): implications for the future of combat casualty care. *J Trauma Acute Care Surg*. 2012;73: S431-S437.

37. Kotwal RS, Montgomery HR, Mabry RL, et al. Eliminating preventable death on the battlefield. *Arch Surg*. 2011;146:1350-1358.

38. Bennett BL, Butler FK, Wedmore I, eds. Tactical combat casualty care: transitioning battlefield lessons learned to other austere environments. *Wilderness Environ Med*. 2017;28(2S):S1-S154.

39. Smith B, Bledsoe BE, Nicolazzo P. General management of trauma in the wilderness. In: Hawkins SC, ed. *Wilderness EMS*. Wolters Kluwer; 2018:371-392.

40. Smith W. Episode 3: medical direction with Will Smith, MD [podcast]. RAW Medicine website. Published February 1, 2018. Accessed March 1, 2022. https://rawmedicine.libsyn.com/episode-3-medical-direction-with-will-smith-md

41. What is C-TECC? Committee for Tactical Emergency Casualty Care website. Accessed March 1, 2022. https://www.c-tecc.org/about-us/what-is-ctecc

42. Smith W, Grange K. Mission success: how a rural EMS agency implemented a tactical EMS program. *JEMS*. 2018;43(1):24-30.

43. Chan D, Goldberg R, Tascone A, et al. The effect of spinal immobilization on healthy volunteers. *Ann Emerg Med*. 1994;23(1):48-51.

44. Kwan I, Bunn F, Roberts IG. Spinal immobilisation for trauma patients. *Cochrane Database Syst Rev*. 2001(2): CD002803.

45. Ben-Galim P, Dreiangel N, Mattox KL, et al. Extrication collars can result in abnormal separation between vertebrae in the presence of dissociative injury. *J Trauma*. 2010;69:447-450.

46. Hauswald M, Ong G, Tandeberg D, et al. Out-of-hospital spinal immobilization: its effect on neurologic injury. *Acad Emerg Med*. 1998;5:214-219.

47. Oto B, Corey DJ II, Oswald J, Sifford D, Walsh B. Early secondary neurological deterioration after blunt spinal trauma: a review of the literature. *Acad Emerg Med*. 2015;22:1200-1212.

48. Senz K. New Hampshire rescue squad denies fault in woman's drowning. EMS World website. Published September 10, 2007. Accessed March 1, 2022. https://www.hmpgloballearningnetwork.com/site/emsworld/news/10408685/new-hampshire-rescue-squad-denies-fault-womans-drowning

49. Scheele BM. Technical rescue interface: off-road vehicle and helicopter WEMS response. In: Hawkins SC, ed. *Wilderness EMS*. Wolters Kluwer; 2018:503-518.

50. Kosequat J, Rush SC, Simonsen I, et al. Efficacy of the mnemonic device "MARCH PAWS" as a checklist for pararescuemen during tactical field care and tactical evacuation. *J Spec Operations Med*. 2017;4:80-84.

51. Hawkins SC, Simon RB, Beissinger JP, Simon D. *Vertical Aid: Essential Wilderness Medicine for Climbers, Trekkers, and Mountaineers*. The Countryman Press; 2017.

52. Davis C. Part 2: management of infectious diseases: general infectious diseases in the wilderness environment. In: Hawkins SC, ed. *Wilderness EMS*. Wolters Kluwer; 2018:355-370.

53. Keenan S, Riesberg JC. Prolonged field care: beyond the "Golden Hour." *Wilderness Environ Med*. 2017;28(2S): S135-S139.

54. Gomi T. *Everyone Poops*. Kane/Miller Book Publishers; 1993.

55. Wing-Gaia SL, Askew W. Nutrition, malnutrition and starvation. In: Auerbach PS, ed. *Auerbach's Wilderness Medicine*. 7th ed. Elsevier; 2017:1964-1985.

56. Kenefick RW, Cheuvront SN, Leon LR, Obrien K. Dehydration and rehydration. In: Auerbach PS, ed. *Wilderness Medicine*. 7th ed. Elsevier; 2017:2031-2044.

57. Madsen P, Svendsen LB, Jorgenesen LG, et al. Tolerance to head-up tilt and suspension with elevated legs. *Aviat Space Environ Med*. 1998;69:781-784.

58. Mortimer RB. Risks and management of prolonged suspension in an Alpine harness. *Wilderness Environ Med*. 2011;22:77-86.

59. Seddon P. *Harness Suspension: Review and Evaluation on Existing Information*. Health Safety Executive Books; 2002:CRR 451/2002.

60. Kolb JJ, Smith EL. Redefining the diagnosis and treatment of suspension trauma. *JEMS*. Published June 9, 2015. Accessed March 1, 2022. https://www.jems.com/operations/rescue-vehicle-extrication/redefining-the-diagnosis-and-treatment-of-suspension-trauma/

61. Prevention and treatment of sunburn. *Med Lett Drugs Ther*. 2004;46:45.

62. Department of Health and Human Services. Food and Drug Administration. 21 CFR Parts 201, 310, 347, and 352. Sunscreen drug products for over-the-counter human use. *Federal Register*. Vol 84. No 38. February 26, 2019/Proposed Rules. Accessed April 20, 2022. https://www.govinfo.gov/content/pkg/FR-2019-02-26/pdf/2019-03019.pdf

63. Krakowski AC, Goldenberg A. Exposure to radiation from the sun. In: Auerbach PS, ed. *Auerbach's Wilderness Medicine*. 7th ed. Elsevier; 2017:335-353.

64. Stern RS. Clinical practice: treatment of photoaging. *N Engl J Med*. 2004;350:1526-1534.

65. Richardson SD. Environmental mass spectrometry: emerging contaminants and current issues. *Anal Chem*. 2012;84:747-778.

66. Gies P. Photoprotection by clothing. *Photodermal Photimmunol Photomed*. 2007;23:264-274.

67. Singletary EM, Charlton NP, Epstein JL, et al. Part 15: first aid: 2015 American Heart Association and American Red Cross guidelines update for first aid. *Circulation*. 2015;132(Suppl 2): S574-S589.

68. Kragh JF, Walters TJ, Baer DG, et al. Practical use of emergency tourniquets to stop bleeding in major limb trauma. *J Trauma*. 2008;64(Suppl 2):38-50.

69. Drew B, Bird D, Matteucci M, Keenan S. Tourniquet conversion: a recommended approach in the prolonged field care setting. *J Spec Operations Med*. 2015;15(3):81-85.

70. Kragh JF, Dubick MA. Bleeding control with limb tourniquet use in the wilderness setting: review of science. *Wilderness Environ Med*. 2017;28(Suppl 2):S25-S32.

71. Edlich RF, Rodeheaver GT, Morgan RF, et al. Principles of emergency wound management. *Ann Emerg Med*. 1988;17(12):1284-1302.

72. Edlich RF, Thacker JG, Buchanan L, Rodeheaver GT. Modern concepts of treatment of traumatic wounds. *Adv Surg*. 1979;13:169-197.

73. Bhandari M, Thompson K, Adili A, Shaughnessy SG. High and low pressure irrigation in contaminated wounds with exposed bone. *Int J Surg Invest*. 2000;2(3):179-182.

74. Bhandari M, Adili A, Lachowski RJ. High pressure pulsatile lavage of contaminated human tibiae: an in vitro study. *J Orthop Trauma*. 1998;12(7):479-484.

75. Bhandari M, Schemitsch EH, Adili A, et al. High and low pressure pulsatile lavage of contaminated tibial fractures: an in vitro study of bacterial adherence and bone damage. *J Orthop Trauma*. 1999;13(8):526-533.

76. Anglen JO. Wound irrigation in musculoskeletal injury. *J Am Acad Orthop Surg*. 2001;9(4):219-226.

77. Valente JH, Forti RJ, Freundlich LF, et al. Wound irrigation in children: saline solution or tap water? *Ann Emerg Med*. 2003;41(5):609-616.

78. Backer HD. Field water disinfection. In: Auerbach PS, ed. *Auerbach's Wilderness Medicine*. 7th ed. Elsevier; 2017: 1985-2030.

79. Griffiths RD, Fernandez RS, Ussia CA. Is tap water a safe alternative to normal saline for wound irrigation in the community setting? *J Wound Care*. 2001;10(10):407-411.

80. Moscati R, Mayrose J, Fincher L, Jehle D. Comparison of normal saline with tap water for wound irrigation. *Am J Emerg Med*. 1998;16(4):379-381.

81. Moscati RM, Reardon RF, Lerner EB, Mayrose J. Wound irrigation with tap water. *Acad Emerg Med*. 1998;5(11):1076-1080.

82. Rodeheaver GT, Pettry D, Thacker JG, et al. Wound cleansing by high pressure irrigation. *Surg Gynecol Obstet*. 1975;141(3):357-362.

83. Edlich RF, Reddy VR. Revolutionary advances in wound repair in emergency medicine during the last three decades:

a view toward the new millennium. 5th Annual David R. Boyd, MD, Lecture. *J Emerg Med*. 2001;20(2):167-193.

84. Singer AJ, Hollander JE, Subramanian S, et al. Pressure dynamics of various irrigation techniques commonly used in the emergency department. *Ann Emerg Med*. 1994;24(1):36-40.

85. Luck JB, Campagne D, Falcon Bachs R, et al. Pressures of wilderness improvised wound irrigation techniques: how do they compare? *Wilderness Environ Med*. 2016;27(4):476-481.

86. Mellor SG, Cooper GJ, Bowyer GW. Efficacy of delayed administration of benzylpenicillin in the control of infection in penetrating soft tissue injuries in war. *J Trauma*. 1996;40(Suppl 3):S128-S134.

87. Hospenthal DR, Murray CK, Andersen RC, et al. Guidelines for the prevention of infection after combat-related injuries. *J Trauma*. 2008;64(Suppl 3):S211-S220.

88. Jamshidi R. Wound management. In: Auerbach PS, ed. *Wilderness Medicine*. 7th ed. Elsevier; 2017: 440-450.

89. Russell KW, Scaife CL, Weber DC, et al. Wilderness Medical Society practice guidelines for the treatment of acute pain in remote environments: 2014 update. *Wilderness Environ Med*. 2014;25:S96-S104.

90. McGladrey L. Psychological first aid and stress injuries. In: Hawkins SC, ed. *Wilderness EMS*. Wolters Kluwer; 2018:189-202.

91. Switzer JA, Bovard RS, Quinn RH. Wilderness orthopedics. In: Auerbach PS, ed. *Auerbach's Wilderness Medicine*. 7th ed. Elsevier; 2017:450-492.

92. Kranc DA, Jones AW, Nackenson J, et al. Use of ultrasound for joint dislocation reduction in an austere wilderness setting: a case report. *Prehosp Emerg Care*. 2018;23(2):1-14.

93. Fulton RL, Voigt WJ, Hilakos AS. Confusion surrounding the treatment of traumatic cardiac arrest. *J Am Coll Surg*. 1995;181:209-214.

94. Pasquale MD, Rhodes M, Cipolle MD, et al. Defining "dead on arrival": impact on a level I trauma center. *J Trauma*. 1996;41:726-730.

95. Mattox KL, Feliciano DV. Role of external cardiac compression in truncal trauma. *J Trauma*. 1982;22:934-936.

96. Shimazu S, Shatney CH. Outcomes of trauma patients with no vital signs on admission. *J Trauma*. 1983;23(3):213-216.

97. Forgey WW, Wilderness Medical Society. *Practice Guidelines for Wilderness Emergency Care*. 5th ed. Globe Pequot Press; 2006.

98. Goth P, Garnett G, Rural Affairs Committee, National Association of EMS Physicians. Clinical guidelines for delayed/prolonged transport. I. Cardiorespiratory arrest. *Prehosp Disaster Med*. 1991;6(3):335.

99. Eisenberg MS, Bergner L, Hallstrom AP. Cardiac resuscitation in the community: importance of rapid provision and implications of program planning. *JAMA*. 1979;241:1905-1907.

100. Kellermann AL, Hackman BB, Somes G. Predicting the outcome of unsuccessful prehospital advanced cardiac life support. *JAMA*. 1993;270(12):1433-1436.

101. Bonnin MJ, Pepe PE, Kimball KT, Clark PS. Distinct criteria for termination of resuscitation in the out-of-hospital setting. *JAMA*. 1993;270(12):1457-1462.

102. Millin MG, Khandker SR, Malki A. Termination of resuscitation of nontraumatic cardiopulmonary arrest: resource document for the National Association of EMS Physicians position statement. *Prehosp Emerg Care.* 2011;15(4):547-554.

103. Leavitt M, Podgorny G. Prehospital CPR and the pulseless hypothermic patient. *Ann Emerg Med.* 1984;13:492.

104. Zafren K, Giesbrecht G, Danzl D, et al. Wilderness Medical Society practice guidelines for the out-of-hospital evaluation and treatment of accidental hypothermia: 2014 update. *Wilderness Environ Med.* 2014;25:S66-S85.

105. Keatinge WR. Accidental immersion hypothermia and drowning. *Practitioner.* 1977;219:183-187.

106. Olshaker JS. Near drowning. *Emerg Med Clin North Am.* 1992;10(2):339-350.

107. Bolte RG, Black PG, Bowers RS, et al. The use of extracorporeal rewarming in a child submerged for 66 minutes. *JAMA.* 1988;260(3):377-379.

108. Orlowski JP. Drowning, near-drowning, and ice-water drowning. *JAMA.* 1988;260(3):390-391.

109. Cooper MA, Andrews CJ, Holle RL, et al. Lightning-related injuries and safety. In: Auerbach PS, ed. *Auerbach's Wilderness Medicine.* 7th ed. Elsevier; 2017:71-117.

110. Davis C, Engeln A, Johnson E, McIntosh S, et al. Wilderness Medical Society practice guidelines for the prevention and treatment of lightning injuries: 2014 update. *Wilderness Environ Med.* 2014;25:S86-S95.

111. Durrer B, Brugger H. Recent advances in avalanche survival. Presented at the Second World Congress on Wilderness Medicine. Aspen, CO; 1995.

112. Van Tilburg C, Grissom CK, Zafren K, et al. Wilderness Medical Society practice guidelines for prevention and management of avalanche and nonavalanche snow burial accidents. *Wilderness Environ Med.* 2017;25(28):23-42.

113. Steinman AM. Cardiopulmonary resuscitation and hypothermia. *Circulation.* 1986;74(6, pt 2):29-32.

114. Zell SC. Epidemiology of wilderness-acquired diarrhea: implications for prevention and treatment. *J Wild Med.* 1992;3(3):241-249.

115. Lloyd EL. *Hypothermia and Cold Stress.* Aspen Systems; 1986.

116. Maningas PA, DeGuzman LR, Hollenbach SJ, et al. Regional blood flow during hypothermic arrest. *Ann Emerg Med.* 1986;15(4):390-396.

117. Groves LJ, Cushing TA. General management of medical conditions in the wilderness. In: Hawkins SC, ed. *Wilderness EMS.* Wolters Kluwer; 2018:393-412.

118. Sampson HA, Muñoz-Furlong A, Campbell RL, et al. Second symposium on the definition and management of anaphylaxis: summary report—Second National Institute of Allergy and Infectious Disease/Food Allergy and Anaphylaxis Network symposium. *J Allergy Clin Immunol.* 2006;117:391-397.

119. Graif Y, Romano-Zelekha O, Livne I, et al. Allergic reactions to insect stings: results from a national survey of 10,000 junior high school children in Israel. *J Allergy Clin Immunol.* 2006;117:1435-1439.

120. Golden DB. Insect sting anaphylaxis. *Immunol Allergy Clin North Am.* 2007;27:261-272.

121. Bilò BM, Bonifazi F. Epidemiology of insect-venom anaphylaxis. *Curr Opin Allergy Clin Immunol.* 2008;8:330-337.

122. Graft DF. Insect sting allergy. *Med Clin North Am.* 2006;90: 211-232.

123. Valentine MD, Schuberth KC, Kagey-Sobotka A, et al. The value of immunotherapy with venom in children with allergy to insect stings. *N Engl J Med.* 1990;323:1601-1603.

124. Barnard JH. Studies of 400 *Hymenoptera* sting deaths in the United States. *J Allergy Clin Immunol.* 1973;52:259-264.

125. Gaudio F, Lemery J, Johnson D. Wilderness Medical Society practice guidelines for the use of epinephrine in outdoor education and wilderness settings: 2014 update. *Wilderness Environ Med.* 2014;25:S15-S18.

126. Hawkins S, Weil C, Fitzpatrick D. Letter to the editor: epinephrine autoinjector warning. *Wilderness Environ Med.* 2012;23:371-378.

127. Snakes. *National Geographic.* Accessed March 1, 2022. https://www.nationalgeographic.com/animals/reptiles /facts/snakes-1

128. Kasturiratne A, Wickremasinghe AR, de Silva N, et al. The global burden of snakebite: a literature analysis and modelling based on regional estimates of envenoming and deaths. *PLoS Med.* 2008;5(11):e218. doi: 10.1371/journal .pmed.0050218

129. Abo B. Management of animal bites and envenomation. Hawkins SC, ed. *Wilderness EMS.* Wolters Kluwer; 2018:333-346.

130. O'Neil ME, Mack KA, Gilchrist J, Wozniak EJ. Snakebite injuries treated in United States emergency departments, 2001–2004. *Wilderness Environ Med.* 2007;18(4):281-287.

131. Lavonas EJ, Ruha AM, Banner W, et al. Unified treatment algorithm for the management of crotaline snakebite in the United States: results of an evidence-informed consensus workshop. *BMC Emerg Med.* 2011;11:2. doi: 10.1186/1471-227X-11-2

132. Norris RL, Bush SP, Cardwell MD. Bites by venomous reptiles in Canada, the United States, and Mexico. In: Auerbach PS, ed. *Auerbach's Wilderness Medicine.* 7th ed. Elsevier; 2017:729-760.

133. Warrell DA. Bites by venomous and nonvenomous reptiles worldwide. In: Auerbach PS, ed. *Auerbach's Wilderness Medicine.* 7th ed. Elsevier; 2017:760-828.

134. Kanaan NC, Ray J, Stewart M, et al. Wilderness Medical Society practice guidelines for the treatment of pit viper envenomations in the United States and Canada. *Wilderness Environ Med.* 2015;26:472-487.

135. Curry SC, Kunkel DB. Death from a rattlesnake bite. *Am J Emerg Med.* 1985;3(3):227-235.

136. Bush SP. Snakebite suction devices don't remove venom: they just suck. *Ann Emerg Med.* 2004;43(2):187-188.

137. Alberts MB, Shalit M, LoGalbo F. Suction for venomous snakebite: a study of "mock venom" extraction in a human model. *Ann Emerg Med.* 2004;43(2):181-186.

138. Davis D, Branch K, Egen NB, et al. The effect of an electrical current on snake venom toxicity. *J Wild Med.* 1992; 3(1):48-53.

139. Howe NR, Meisenheimer JL Jr. Electric shock does not save snakebitten rats. *Ann Emerg Med.* 1988;17(3):254-256.

140. Gill KA Jr. The evaluation of cryotherapy in the treatment of snake envenomation. *South Med J.* 1968;63:552-556.

141. Norris RL. A call for snakebite research. *Wilderness Environ Med.* 2000;11(3):149-151.

Suggested Reading

Auerbach PS, ed. *Auerbach's Wilderness Medicine*. 7th ed. Elsevier; 2017.

Hawkins SC, ed. *Wilderness EMS*. Wolters Kluwer; 2018.

Rodway G, McIntosh S, Weber D, eds. *Mountain Medicine and Technical Rescue: A Manual of the Diploma in Mountain Medicine*. Carreg; 2016.

Civilian Tactical Emergency Medical Support (TEMS)

Lead Editors
Faroukh Mehkri, DO
Alexander L. Eastman, MD, MPH, FACS, FAEMS

CHAPTER OBJECTIVES

At the completion of this chapter, you will be able to do the following:

- Describe the components of tactical emergency medical support (TEMS).
- Understand the operational and support functions of TEMS.
- Explain the benefits of a TEMS program.
- Examine how emergency medical care differs in each of the three phases of care in TEMS.
- Relate how remote assessment methodology may be used on a tactical mission.
- Describe the role of medical support for counterterrorism operations.

SCENARIO

Your emergency medical services (EMS) agency provides coverage for the local special weapons and tactics (SWAT) team and has a rigorous, integrated training program with local law enforcement. Your tactical emergency medical support (TEMS) team is called out just after sunset for a barricaded gunman holed up in an old mobile home. As you are preparing for entry, two SWAT officers cross the suspect's yard and approach the house to prepare for a door pull. Shots ring out from the front window, wounding the SWAT officers. One SWAT officer falls in the doorway of the suspect's home. The second falls near an old pickup truck. A patrol officer standing near you yells, "Come on! We need to go get them." You grab the patrol officer by the arm and look to the SWAT commander.

- What should your actions be?
- How will you assess and treat the fallen SWAT officers given the danger of the scene?

INTRODUCTION

Tactical emergency medical support (TEMS) is an out-of-hospital system of care dedicated to enhancing the success of special operations law enforcement missions, reducing mission medical liability and risk, and promoting public safety.[1] TEMS builds on the principles of military medicine, wilderness medicine, disaster response, urban search and rescue, and conventional EMS to create a system of care that supports law enforcement missions and maximizes the clinical outcome for casualties in what is often a resource-poor, prolonged-transport environment, while minimizing the threat to the prehospital care practitioner.

This chapter provides an overview of TEMS. Participation in TEMS and the provision of **tactical casualty care (TCC)** requires specific training and expertise, just as for any other special operations situation. For a detailed overview of TEMS, the National Association of Emergency Medical Technicians offers a 16-hour course devoted to TEMS concepts: Tactical Emergency Casualty Care (TECC).

History and Evolution of Tactical Emergency Medical Support

The first SWAT team was developed in Los Angeles in 1968. Shortly thereafter, the concept of having a "medic" attached to the SWAT team was advanced, similar to the military model of having a combat medic assigned to the squad. Today, TEMS encompasses a broad spectrum of medical services modified in structure and function to operate within the high-risk, high-speed tactical environment. Broad support for TEMS now exists within both the law enforcement and the medical communities.

Over 30 years ago, the Counter Narcotics and Terrorism Operational Medical Support (CONTOMS) course was developed. This program was developed as an evidence-based TEMS curriculum that selected seasoned emergency medical practitioners and immersed them in providing medical care in the tactical environment over the course of 56 hours. Through CONTOMS, an injury database was developed to provide the research data needed to support the efficacy of tactical medicine.

Since then, many courses similar to CONTOMS have been developed. The Tactical Combat Casualty Care (TCCC) courses were developed by the Committee on Tactical Combat Casualty Care, part of the Defense Health Board of the U.S. Department of Defense (DoD). These courses teach the essential medical interventions needed in the tactical environment, which vary depending on the specific tactical situation. The original TCCC project was conducted from 1993 to 1996 as a joint effort of Special Operations medical personnel and the Uniformed Services University. This 4-year research effort culminated with the publication of the original TCCC paper in 1996.[2]

The TCCC Guidelines are now maintained by the Committee on TCCC (CoTCCC), which was established in 2001 by the U.S. Special Operations Command and is now a component of the DoD's Joint Trauma System (JTS). The TCCC Guidelines are updated based on: (1) an ongoing review of the published civilian and military prehospital trauma literature; (2) ongoing interaction with military combat casualty care research laboratories; (3) direct input from experienced combat corpsmen, medics, and pararescue jumpers (PJs); (4) input from the service medical Lessons Learned Centers; (5) case reports discussed at the weekly Joint Theater Trauma System (JTTS) process improvement video-teleconferences; (6) observations on the causes of death in combat fatalities gleaned from JTS-Armed Forces Medical Examiner System (AFMES) conferences; and (7) expert opinion from both military and civilian trauma experts.

There are now three distinct TCCC courses available for different categories of combat personnel including medical and nonmedical. TCCC All Service Members (TCCC-ASM) is a 7-hour course for all service members. TCCC Combat Lifesaver (TCCC-CLS) is a 40-hour course for nonmedical military personnel deploying in support of combat operations. TCCC for Medical Personnel (TCCC-MP) is a 16-hour course for military medical personnel, including medics, corpsmen, and pararescue personnel, deploying in support of combat operations. None of the TCCC courses teaches the operational components of a tactical incident. Knowledge of tactical movement and planning are needed for a complete, well-developed TEMS program. The TCCC-MP program and its medical objectives should be included within any TEMS educational program to address emergency medical care issues in the tactical environment.

In 2013, 27 law enforcement officers died from injuries incurred in the line of duty during felonious incidents.[3] In 2020 that number climbed to 46, which represents an increase of 70%. This increase, in conjunction with an ever-increasing incidence of active shooter/hostile event (ASHE) incidents nationwide, has reinforced the need for TEMS.[4] The National Tactical Officers Association (NTOA) has endorsed TEMS, beginning with its original position statement in 1994, and continues to assert it as standard operating procedures and "an important element of tactical law enforcement" for tactical medics.[5] After the September 11, 2001, attacks, both the National Association of EMS Physicians (NAEMSP) and the American College of Emergency Physicians (ACEP) formally endorsed integrating EMS capabilities into law enforcement special operations.[6,7]

The CoTCCC has established guidelines recognized as the global standard of care for military prehospital medicine. Both the American College of Surgeons Committee on Trauma (ACS-COT) and the National Association of Emergency Medical Technicians (NAEMT) have endorsed the TCCC guidelines. NAEMT offers TCCC courses as specified by the Defense Health Agency Joint Trauma System (DHA-JTS) through its global network of training centers.[8] Though military and law enforcement special operations are unique, similarities exist in the tactical medical care aspects. The NTOA-endorsed TCCC guidelines have provided a strong foundation for the standardization of TEMS protocols.

With the growing recognition that tactical medical care has become an important issue and the work of the CoTCCC to develop the military TCCC educational programs, efforts have been underway to adapt the military information to a civilian setting. A civilian CoTCCC counterpart, the Committee on Tactical Emergency Casualty Care (C-TECC), has developed a set of TECC guidelines that are tailored to address the prehospital high-threat needs of civilian law enforcement.[9] The TECC guidelines have since been incorporated into the National Joint Counterterrorism Awareness Workshop used by the FBI, the Federal Emergency Management Agency, and the National Counterterrorism Center. NAEMT has developed a TECC course for civilian prehospital care practitioners.

While TCCC educational programs and TECC courses are based on similar principles, TCCC and TECC do not always make the same recommendations. Each group includes its own subject matter experts and its own processes for evaluating proposed guideline changes. The differences between the courses reflect the very relevant differences between the military combat and the civilian tactical environments and the subject matter expertise of members of the CoTCCC and C-TECC, respectively.

TEMS Practice Components

Tactical emergency medical support has several distinctions from conventional EMS. Unlike conventional EMS, comprehensive TEMS programs include health maintenance, preventive medicine (e.g., immunizations, proper sleep practices, and physical fitness), medical threat assessments, and coordination of care with a variety of local medical assets. From an operational perspective, TEMS practitioners are frequently faced with treat-and-release decisions. These situations can vary from a TEMS team member who has become dehydrated to an angry prisoner who may have been injured in the tactical operation. Both situations have their unique challenges.

Some states include specific addendums to their EMS protocols that address TEMS practice. TEMS practitioners and their medical directors must be familiar with their local protocols when operating in the tactical environment and when credentialing potential advanced skills.

The TEMS medical skill set is consistent with, and often expanded from, conventional EMS. Although skill sets may be similar, in TEMS, the application of these skills is often heavily influenced by the tactical situation and mission profile. For example, the use of a laryngeal mask airway (LMA) may be clinically indicated for a casualty under normal operational conditions, but, if the casualty will need to be dragged across a linear danger zone or carried over rough terrain, the LMA is not a secure airway and, therefore, may not be appropriate.

Barriers to Traditional EMS Access

The scene of a law enforcement special operation presents various barriers to traditional EMS access. A geographic perimeter is usually established. Within that perimeter, it is rarely obvious which, if any, areas are safe for EMS passage or for performance of medical activities. It is imperative that the medical components not become a liability to the SWAT team's mission. Already scarce law enforcement resources should not need to be diverted to the medical support mission.

The time interval from EMS arrival on scene to patient contact can be a significant source of delay in the initiation of prehospital care in conventional EMS operations.[10] This type of delay can be much longer during tactical missions. Integrated TEMS programs minimize delays because the TEMS practitioners routinely function inside the perimeter as a vital part of the tactical team and can begin treatment of wounds within the first moments of an officer being injured.[11,12]

Some fire and rescue chiefs and EMS administrators may object to their personnel practicing tactical medicine because they perceive it to be too dangerous. When asked why firefighters under their command enter burning buildings—a clearly dangerous situation—they often respond that firefighting is different from law enforcement operations because firefighting personnel are well trained and appropriately equipped against the fire threat. The same argument is true for TEMS (**Box 22-1**).

Box 22-1 Prehospital Care Practitioner Safety

Just as an emergency medical technician (EMT) or paramedic should not enter the hot zone of a hazardous materials incident or a fire scene without appropriate personal protective equipment and training, the EMT or paramedic must apply proper equipment and training when entering the tactical setting.

© National Association of Emergency Medical Technicians (NAEMT)

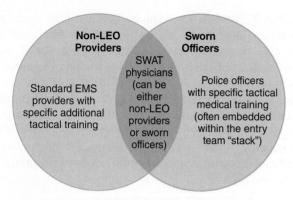

Figure 22-1 TEMS models (operating within secured operational perimeter).

© National Association of Emergency Medical Technicians (NAEMT)

Table 22-1 Phases of Care		
Tactical Situation	**TCCC**	**TECC**
Immediate or active threat (HOT ZONE)	Care under fire/threat	Direct threat care
Threat contained but could resume (WARM ZONE)	Tactical field care	Indirect threat care
No threat (COLD ZONE)	Tactical evacuation care	Evacuation care

© National Association of Emergency Medical Technicians (NAEMT)

It is a violation of basic scene safety principles to utilize EMS personnel who are inadequately trained or equipped for the assignment to enter a secure police perimeter that has not been made safe. Nevertheless, we know that simply waiting for the patient to be delivered outside the perimeter is not an effective option. Delays due to unavailability of TEMS practitioners will result in the unnecessary loss of life or function, whereas far-forward (as close to the point of wounding as possible) medical care in the military has been shown to reduce both mortality and morbidity.[13,14] The duration of the Golden Period is different for each injury and each person, some can wait hours, some only seconds, and as such every effort must be made to treat injuries as soon as feasible. The obvious solution is for the medical support of law enforcement special operations to be performed by well-trained and properly equipped TEMS practitioners who can operate safely within the secured operational perimeter. There are many models for forward operating TEMS personnel. Models may comprise civilian volunteers, sworn officers, police officers with tactical medical training, physicians, or a mix of personnel (**Figure 22-1**). Some include TEMS personnel within the "stack" of the entry team. Others place the TEMS practitioners within the secured perimeter but not in the direct line of fire, usually near the transport vehicles.

Zones of Operation

During tactical missions, the tactical law enforcement team concept of operation divides the target area into zones of operation. The teams establish an **inner perimeter** and **outer perimeter** as geographic boundaries that define the *cold zone* (outside the outer perimeter where no threat should exist), the *warm zone* (between the outer and inner perimeter where the danger of

threat could exist), and the **hot zone** (the area that poses an immediate hazard or in which a responder can become a clear target).[15] This concept is analogous to the zones of operation at a hazardous materials incident. As with any uncontained event, these zones are not static, they are inherently dynamic and it is important to recognize that the geographic boundaries of the various zones may change rapidly as the situation evolves. TEMS practitioners must always maintain situational awareness to minimize risks to themselves and their patients.

Phases of Care

The TCC guidelines, whether from TCCC or TECC, divide the delivery of emergency medical care into *phases of care*, based on the tactical situation and the associated threat at the time care is being provided (**Table 22-1**).[9]

Whether using the TCCC or TECC guidelines, the care that is provided in each phase is essentially the same. The phases of care are dynamic, influenced by minute-to-minute threat assessments, and need not be concentric or contiguous; threat levels change rapidly in the tactical environment. Accordingly, the phases of care may not always coincide with the zones of operation. TEMS personnel must understand the relationship of the two paradigms in order to function effectively and with discipline in a tactical environment (**Box 22-2**).

Care Under Fire/Threat (Direct Threat Care)

During **care under fire/threat (CUFT)**, the threat is direct and immediate. Limited protection exists for the casualty and the responder. Operations inside this area are

Box 22-2 Tactical Combat Casualty Care Guidelines (Tactical Emergency Casualty Care)

Care Under Fire/Threat (Direct Threat Care)

1. Maintain tactical supremacy: Neutralize the threat as soon as possible (e.g., directed fire, smoke, threatening posture, fire suppression, hazardous material mitigation).
2. Ensure cover and/or concealment: Prevent further injury to casualty or additional injury to rescuer.
3. Use tourniquet(s) for life-threatening extremity hemorrhage.
4. *Do not:*
   a. Perform invasive airway management.
   b. Perform cardiopulmonary resuscitation.
   c. Employ strict spinal precautions.

Tactical Field Care (Indirect Threat Care)

1. Initial care of the patient should follow MARCH criteria:
   a. **M**assive bleeding: Control bleeding (tourniquet, hemostatic dressing, conventional pressure dressing) for life-threatening hemorrhage.
   b. **A**irway: Assess for obstruction and secure airway with body positioning, nasopharyngeal airway, advanced airways, or surgical airway. (This decision will be based on unit training and standard medical protocols.)
   c. **R**espirations: Assess and treat for penetrating chest wounds, sucking chest wounds, and tension pneumothoraces.
   d. **C**irculation: Assess for shock. Establish intravenous or intraosseous access, and initiate fluid resuscitation if medically indicated. (This decision will be based on unit training and protocols.)
   e. **H**ead/**H**ypothermia: Protect the casualty from hypothermia. Heat, chemical, or toxic exposures may also be risk factors. Splint any major fracture, and consider spinal motion restriction in the context of a high-risk mechanism of injury.

Tactical Evacuation Care (Evacuation Care)

1. Provide conventional EMS care if appropriate, and use appropriate transport based on given injury and distance to definitive care.
2. Ensure clear routes of egress for prehospital care practitioners and ambulance.
3. Attend to staging considerations.
4. Stay alert for secondary devices and unconventional threats (e.g., flood, crowds, fire).

© National Association of Emergency Medical Technicians (NAEMT)

extremely dangerous and should be limited to reconnaissance and tactical team operators. Safe operation within the hot zone during CUFT requires the use of appropriate personal protective equipment (e.g., ballistic helmets, ballistic vests identical in threat protection level to operators, goggles, shields, boots) and tactical movements (e.g., light/noise discipline, use of cover/concealment, and minimal radio use). An officer down in the front yard of a home with a barricaded concealed gunman shooting from a window exemplifies a typical CUFT scenario.

Casualty care during this phase entails enormous risk and deviates significantly from the principles of conventional EMS. Immediate actions include threat suppression and evacuation of the casualty to cover/concealment. The sooner the threat can be neutralized, the sooner full medical care resources can be brought to bear to treat the casualty. Until that occurs, getting the casualty to cover is imperative. Casualties who are responsive and able to move should be directed to move to cover. If the casualty cannot move, a plan for possible rescue may be considered. Medical care in this phase of the operation is directed toward reducing further injury to the casualty, avoiding responder injury, subduing the threat, and controlling life-threatening extremity hemorrhage. Time is not spent on cervical spine immobilization for penetrating neck trauma, airway management, or "heroic" but likely futile measures such as cardiopulmonary resuscitation (CPR).

Self-aid/buddy aid (SA/BA) are critical components of CUFT. Most nonlethal penetrating injuries sustained by officers are usually not fully incapacitating and will not necessarily remove the officer from the operation entirely.[16] Data from military operations in Vietnam, Iraq, and Afghanistan indicate that training soldiers in SA/BA significantly decreased mortality. In fact, a 67% decrease in fatalities from extremity hemorrhage was appreciated after the initiation of early tourniquet use.[14,17] For example, self-application of a tourniquet to a life-threatening penetrating injury to an extremity could save the victim, minimize further injury, and prevent TEMS practitioners from unnecessarily exposing themselves to hostile fire.

Application of direct pressure and pressure dressings is unrealistic in many CUFT tactical settings and may result in unnecessary blood loss and delay in the evacuation of the casualty to cover. *Tourniquet use for control of extremity hemorrhage is the gold standard during the CUFT phase*, with the benefits of stopping the bleeding clearly outweighing any low risk that may be associated with tourniquet use.[18] The tourniquet should be placed as "high and tight" on the extremity as possible. As opposed to less threatening scenarios, in the CUFT situation the tourniquet should be placed over the clothing. It is vital to ensure that arterial blood flow has been stopped. Non-extremity and junctional wounds are difficult to treat in this phase. An attempt should be made to provide direct pressure to these wounds as the casualty is rapidly moved to a covered position and treatment transitions into the tactical field care phase.

Tactical Field Care (Indirect Threat Care)

During the **tactical field care** phase, threats may continue to exist but are not direct or immediate. For example, in the case of the tactical officer down in the front yard, tactical field care principles would apply once the casualty has been moved behind adequate cover or concealment, or the threat has been suppressed (**Figure 22-2**). It is important to understand the distinction between cover and concealment, as they are key elements of both offensive and defensive tactics.[19] Cover refers to a barrier that offers protection from an incoming projectile (e.g., a bullet) by stopping or deflecting it. Examples of cover include bricks, rocks, steel, or a vehicle engine block; however, the type of cover needed is dependent on the weapon and ammunition used by the assailant. Concealment does not provide protection from a projectile, but rather offers an area or object that is out of the assailant's line of sight.

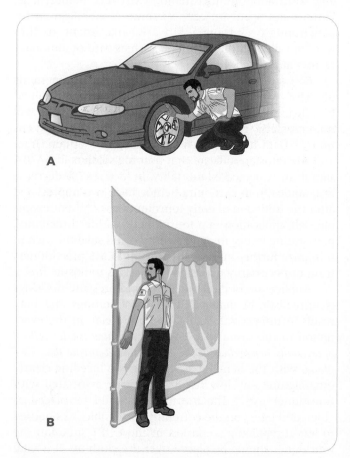

Figure 22-2 **A.** An example of cover. **B.** An example of concealment.

Concealment might be found in bushes, shadows, behind closed blinds or drywall, or even in smoke. Natural terrain offers the potential for either cover (dirt berm, mature tree) or concealment (brush, tall grass).

Threat levels vary significantly in this phase of the operation, mandating a flexible and fluid medical response. The TEMS practitioner must be capable of analyzing dynamic factors, rapidly acquiring data, and quickly weighing all medical decisions in terms of the risks to self and the casualty. In a TEMS scenario, the relatively secure environment may return to a CUFT situation at any point. The adage "just because you *can* do something, does not mean that you should" certainly applies. TEMS practitioners must be disciplined in their medical decision making and interventions on scene.

During tactical field care, if tactically appropriate, care should include a rapid trauma assessment by exposing and assessing all injuries. Interventions should focus on quickly stabilizing the major causes of preventable traumatic death in the tactical environment: compressible hemorrhage, tension pneumothorax, simple airway compromise, and hypothermia.[16,17] The MARCH algorithm should be applied rapidly and initially during tactical field care to address immediate TEMS concerns and stratify the casualty's injuries in order of importance.

Hemorrhage Control

Control of compressible external hemorrhage during tactical field care is critical. Compressible severe external hemorrhage can usually be quickly controlled and should be the first priority. Tourniquets are the first-line treatment of choice for potentially life-threatening extremity hemorrhage when and where application is possible. If the bleeding is life threatening, a tourniquet should be placed "high and tight" in the groin or armpit above the injury, directly on the skin and free of any clothing. It should be placed as snugly as possible, with as much slack removed from the tail as possible before the windlass is tightened. No more than three revolutions (540 degrees) of the windlass should be performed to avoid deforming the chassis of the device.[20] In the event that one tourniquet does not stop the bleeding, it is acceptable and highly recommended to use additional tourniquets side by side until bleeding is controlled, as this provides compression of the artery over a wider area.[17,20] Any tourniquet placed on an extremity during the CUFT phase should be reevaluated to determine the need for its continued use. If bleeding from the injury is determined to not be life threatening, transitioning from a tourniquet to an appropriate pressure dressing may be performed. When there is doubt it is better to err on the side of caution and keep a tourniquet applied, especially if the situation dictates further movement or the conflict has not completely ended.

The current TCCC guidelines recommend the hemostatic dressing Combat Gauze as the dressing of choice, with Celox Gauze, ChitoGauze, XSTAT, and iTClamp as alternatives for hemorrhage in areas not amenable to tourniquet use. After application of any of these dressings, 3 minutes of direct, firm pressure should be applied.[21-27] Practitioners should not use older powder- or granule-type agents, as they have been shown to cause thermal burns, foreign body emboli, and *endothelial* (internal lining of blood vessels) toxicity.[28] Instead, use a packable hemostatic-impregnated gauze for wounds to transition zones (i.e., neck, axilla, and groin). The lack of hemostatic gauze does not hinder a practitioner from utilization of nonimpregnated simplex gauze wound packing. The use of all hemostatic agents and other novel means of wound packing must be approved in advance by the unit's medical director.

Airway Management

Airway management during this phase of care is appropriate if the casualty shows signs of impending airway obstruction or cardiovascular collapse. In conscious casualties with an intact gag reflex, by far the easiest means of airway management is to allow the casualty to sit in a position of comfort, preferably sitting up and leaning forward, to preserve the airway. In unconscious casualties, with or without signs of airway compromise, a trauma jaw thrust followed shortly after by a nasopharyngeal airway (NPA) is recommended as a first-line option. After inserting the NPA, place the casualty into the recovery position to maintain the open airway and prevent aspiration of secretions (**Figure 22-3**). If airway obstruction develops or persists despite the use of an NPA, a properly trained TEMS practitioner may consider inserting an endotracheal tube or supraglottic airway device as the tactical situation allows. These devices are not well tolerated unless the casualty is **obtunded**.

In some cases, a surgical cricothyroidotomy may be indicated. Casualties with airway compromise due to maxillofacial trauma or inhalation burns may warrant a cricothyroidotomy as the first-line airway procedure of choice.[6,17,29] The CricKey device is the preferred option for emergency cricothyrotomy per TCCC Guidelines, and data have shown 100% success rates in cadaver models with combat medics trained to perform this procedure.[30-32] Instructional videos can be found online for this unique device. A cricothyroidotomy is a highly advanced and rarely performed procedure, and training is absolutely crucial to its success. It is up to the TEMS medical director to perform, train, and authorize this intervention, and only a select group of practitioners—often only physicians or critical care paramedics with increased training—will perform this procedure.

Breathing Management

The management of blunt and penetrating chest trauma is especially important for TEMS practitioners. In particular, the TEMS practitioner must be comfortable treating penetrating chest wounds and tension pneumothoraces. Cover all open or sucking penetrating wounds on the torso from the lower neck to the umbilicus with an occlusive dressing directly on skin; numerous different materials are available for improvised use as well as commercially fabricated chest seals, many with excellent adhesive properties. Vented chest seals are preferred and are the recommended option to minimize the risk of developing tension pneumothoraces in sucking chest wounds. It is important to teach TEMS practitioners to quickly wipe the surface of the skin to improve adherence of the material just prior to application.

In a casualty with a penetrating chest wound and progressive respiratory distress, it is reasonable to presume the presence of a tension pneumothorax and perform a needle decompression (NDC) on the side of the penetrating injury to stabilize the patient.[33] Do not rely on findings such as tracheal shift or jugular vein distension, as these signs are late findings and not always present in an early tension pneumothorax; furthermore, they may be difficult to detect in a tactical setting. Even determining absent breath sounds may not be possible in many tactical environments; increasing respiratory distress or evidence of hemodynamic collapse in the presence of penetrating thoracic trauma is enough to justify performing NDC (**Box 22-3**).

Treat a tension pneumothorax by inserting a 14-gauge (or larger), 3.25-inch (8-centimeter [cm])-long needle with catheter into the casualty's fifth intercostal space at the anterior axillary line; alternatively, the

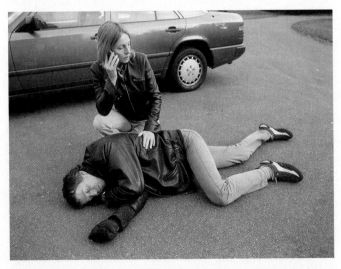

Figure 22-3 A patient who has been placed in the recovery position.
© Cordelia Molloy/Science Photo Library/Science Source

second intercostal space at the midclavicular line lateral to the nipple may be used.[34,35] A casualty with penetrating chest trauma, even if a tension pneumothorax is not present, will generally have some degree of hemothorax or pneumothorax as a result of the primary wound. The additional trauma caused by an NDC will not worsen the casualty's condition in the absence of a tension pneumothorax. Successful NDC is confirmed by improvement in the casualty's respiratory status and, if conditions allow, by hearing a rush of air through the decompression needle as the pressure within the chest is relieved.

It is the TCCC recommendation to use a 14-gauge, 3.25-inch (8-cm) needle and leave the catheter buried to the hub in the casualty.[34-36] The TEMS practitioner must monitor the casualty after the procedure to ensure the catheter has not become dislodged or clotted with blood and that respiratory distress symptoms have not returned. If respiratory distress symptoms return or the catheter becomes obstructed or dislodged, flush the catheter or perform a second NDC adjacent to the first.[17] After an NDC is performed, proper documentation of the indications for the procedure is important, because the casualty will require a subsequent chest tube or further interventions. One last recommendation is that bilateral NDC should be performed prior to discontinuing resuscitation when a casualty with torso trauma or polytrauma suffers prehospital cardiopulmonary arrest.[21] In the case of physician TEMS practitioners or higher level practitioners with medical direction authorization, finger thoracostomy can be substituted for NDC if unavailable or if initial attempts at NDC are unsuccessful.

Vascular Access and Prehospital Fluid Management

Many studies show the benefit of hypotensive ("balanced") resuscitation in trauma patients (see Chapter 3, *Shock: Pathophysiology of Life and Death*, for a detailed discussion).[37,38] Accordingly, delayed intravenous (IV) access is acceptable in certain tactical scenarios. Obtain IV access during the tactical field care phase only if specifically medically indicated. Although traditional trauma training teaches starting IV lines, the use of a single 18-gauge catheter is adequate in

the tactical setting; practitioners must first strive to do no harm and to minimize delays, especially in the tactical setting. The 18-gauge catheter is adequate for rapid delivery of resuscitation fluids and medication, is easier to insert, and limits the number of supplies that need to be carried in the medic aid bag. An IV should not be attempted on an extremity that may have a significant wound proximal to the IV insertion site. The use of a "ruggedized" IV securing system is advisable if the casualty has to be transported a distance before the hand-off to conventional EMS.

If the casualty requires fluid resuscitation or IV medications and IV access cannot be obtained, intraosseous (IO) access is an effective and efficient alternative. IO devices are available for use on the sternum and extremities in the absence of a significant injury to the selected site. As with most advanced medical interventions, this procedure requires a strict training program to instill confidence and competence in the TEMS practitioner. Civilian TEMS injury patterns allow for IO access in both upper and lower extremities with more frequency than military injury patterns. Therefore, it may be appropriate to use the tibial approach for the establishment of the IO line.[39,40] Although the proximal humerus can be used, it has been noted that during movement of the casualty in the tactical environment, the location of the IO device at the widest part of the body (i.e., the shoulders) can easily lead to inadvertent dislodgment.[39-41]

Based on currently accepted hypotensive resuscitation protocols and damage control resuscitation, fluid administration should be reserved for casualties experiencing hemorrhagic shock, as indicated by altered mental status in the absence of a head injury and a weak or absent radial pulse (**Box 22-4**). These findings are indicative of significant blood loss and advanced stages of shock and, coupled with the absence of blood product availability, warrant the administration of fluid.[17,29]

Tactical field care and TEMS have seen much change in the past several years in the realm of fluid management. The choice of resuscitation fluid depends in large part on local protocol and preference. In the context of evidence of improved outcomes with limited crystalloid resuscitation and permissive hypotension, previous recommendations to provide extensive crystalloid fluid administration have been removed.[42,43]

When possible, whole blood is the recommended transfusion strategy in hemorrhage management of TCCC.[44-47] Cold-stored low titer type O whole blood (CS-LTOWB) is the preferred resuscitation fluid for casualties in hemorrhagic shock. Fresh LTOWB from a pre-screened donor pool is the next best option. TCCC then recommends reassessing the casualty after each unit and continuing resuscitation until a palpable radial pulse or improved mental status or systolic blood pressure of 100 millimeters of mercury (mm Hg) is present. If blood products are transfused, TCCC Guidelines now recommend administration of 1 gram of calcium IV/IO after the first transfused product. If a casualty with an altered mental status due to suspected traumatic brain injury has a weak or absent radial pulse, the Guidelines recommend resuscitating as necessary to restore and maintain a normal radial pulse. If blood pressure monitoring is available for these patients, a target systolic pressure between 100 and 110 mm Hg should be established.[48] Specifically, TCCC no longer recommends use of crystalloid solutions for resuscitation in military combat environments. Given the dramatically more limited availability of blood products in civilian tactical scenarios, the complete transition to use of whole blood and away from crystalloid and other nonblood volume expanders has not yet reached most civilian tactical protocols.

Hypothermia

Hypothermia in trauma patients is an independent predictor of mortality.[49] Trauma patients are at high risk for hypothermia, which can occur regardless of the ambient temperature. The longer a patient is exposed to the environment during treatment and evacuation, especially in wet conditions, the more likely they are to develop hypothermia.[50,51] The TEMS practitioner must minimize the casualty's exposure to the elements. Whenever possible, replace or remove any wet or bloody clothing. Use any methods available to keep the casualty warm, such as dry blankets, jackets, sleeping bags, and rescue litters with hypothermic lining. If practical, keep all protective gear on the casualty after ensuring that all injuries have been treated, as this gear will afford protection to the casualty should hostile fire erupt again. For military combat scenarios where prolonged prehospital scenarios are likely in very cold environments, TCCC guidelines recommend placing an active heating blanket on the casualty's anterior torso and under the arms in the axillae. To prevent burns, a heating source should never be placed directly on the skin or wrapped around the torso completely. As soon as possible, the hypothermia enclosure system should be upgraded to a well-insulated enclosure system using a hooded sleeping bag or other readily available insulation inside the enclosure bag and an external vapor barrier shell. In these combat environments, use of a battery-powered warming device to deliver IV resuscitation fluids may also help address hypothermia.[48]

Extraction and Evacuation of Casualties

Extraction is the removal of the casualty from the hot to the warm zone (from within the inner perimeter), whereas evacuation is removal of the casualty from the area within the outer perimeter (warm zone) to the cold zone. Casualty extraction is a physically demanding process that interrupts mission flow and potentially places the tactical team in jeopardy from exposure to hostile fire during the extraction process while in a vulnerable situation dealing with a casualty.

Prior to extracting any casualty, the TEMS practitioner should analyze the transit risk and likelihood of casualty survival. This is a joint decision made with the team leader and, ultimately, it is the decision of the team leader in charge of the overall mission and is influenced by location of injury, weapon of injury, and time of injury.[52] The time required to move a casualty to the cold zone is influenced by the ability of the casualty to assist, the distance involved, the casualty's gear load, relative threat levels of the area, and physical fitness of the team. In some situations, the perpetrator may have a commanding field of fire, creating large unsafe areas, as is the case in the opening scenario. In many civilian tactical operations, the target of the mission may only be one or two perpetrators in a relatively confined location. Missions of these types include high-threat warrant service, narcotics interdiction, and dignitary protection details. These missions tend to be accomplished quickly, with the perpetrator(s) taken into custody or subdued. In these cases, once the area is secured, quick advancement to tactical field care and then to "normal, everyday" EMS care takes place.

The second component of transit risk is the route of travel. Zones of fire are irregularly shaped, noncontiguous geographic areas with dynamic risk levels. Extraction may require crossing linear danger zones, in which case the value of treating in place must be weighed against the need for immediate advanced lifesaving interventions. Commanders must consider their resources prior to initiating a rescue mission. Multiple factors play a role in these high-threat rescues and have historically involved ineffective and unrealistic methods that ultimately increase the risk of unnecessary injury and death. Asymmetric rescues require multiple personnel, potentially specialized equipment (e.g., poleless litter, harnesses, drag straps), and aggressive protective posture prior to implementing egress options (**Figure 22-4**).[53]

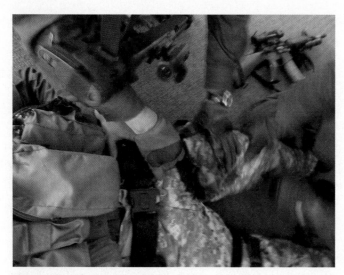

Figure 22-4 Care under fire/threat and extraction.
Courtesy of Commander Al Davis, Ventura Police Department.

Finally, TEMS practitioners must consider their ability to deliver care during transit; for example, during rapid litter movements across a substantial zone of fire, TEMS practitioners may not be able to maintain a manual trauma jaw thrust. In this case, inserting an airway adjunct prior to movement may be prudent. The transit risk, or risk of moving a casualty through a potential zone of fire, is related to the time it takes to traverse the zone and the risks associated with both the route of travel and those risks incurred from providing essential care during transit. As with most decisions in the tactical environment, experience and judgment are critical.

Rapid and Remote Assessment Methodology

The **Rapid and Remote Assessment Methodology (RAM)** was developed by the CONTOMS Program at the Uniformed Services University of the Health Sciences, the U.S. Department of Defense's medical school.[53] The principal purpose of this assessment algorithm is to maximize the opportunity to extract and treat a salvageable casualty while minimizing risk to TEMS practitioners from attempting an unnecessary rescue. This algorithm is most applicable during the CUFT phase of TCC (**Figure 22-5**). Unnecessary rescues fall into two categories: those in which the casualty can self-extract and those in which the casualty is already dead (more appropriately termed a "body recovery"). The RAM provides an organized approach to evaluate the totality of circumstances from a protected position before recommending a rescue attempt to the commander.

The first step in conducting a RAM is to determine if the area is secure. If it is, standard EMS care is appropriate after ensuring that the casualty cannot harm TEMS practitioners. If the area is not secure, use available intelligence to determine whether the casualty is a perpetrator

or otherwise represents a threat. Under such circumstances, *no further medical intervention is indicated until the threat has been controlled*. To do otherwise might jeopardize the safety of tactical officers, TEMS practitioners, and innocent parties. If the casualty is not deemed a perpetrator, a **remote assessment** should be initiated to attempt to evaluate the nature of the injury and the stability of the casualty's condition.

Remote observation is the first technique to be employed during the remote assessment because it allows TEMS practitioners to gather information without revealing their position or intent to the hostile force. Technology available to SWAT teams can improve the reliability of this assessment. For example, a good pair of binoculars or night-vision goggles can often help to ascertain if the casualty is breathing, the rate and quality of respiration, the presence of life-threatening hemorrhage, and the presence of obvious wounds incompatible with life. Unmanned aerial systems (UAS) and aerial drones are becoming more common among tactical teams and can help with RAM observation without compromise of the TEMS practitioners. In cold weather, a respiratory condensation plume can often be seen from the casualty's mouth if the casualty is breathing. Acoustic surveillance equipment, if available, can be deployed to detect speech, moans, groans, and even respiratory sounds. Thermal imaging technology has improved in recent years and may be considered for application in the RAM.

If the casualty appears stable, self-care instructions and reassurance should be communicated to the casualty, if possible, and medical extraction should await an improvement in the tactical situation. A tactical extraction of the casualty may be determined to be optimal by the commander at any time, but the situation and not the casualty's medical stability should primarily inform this decision. If the casualty is unstable, the risk of extraction must be weighed against the benefits of immediate access to medical care. Although this is a command decision, the commander will rely heavily on the TEMS practitioner's assessment of the patient's condition and the need for immediate extraction. If the benefit–risk ratio is sufficiently high, the extraction may proceed.

Although the algorithm seems logical, it is crucial to have a decision structure that fosters good assessment before emotion overtakes reason and a needless rescue is risked. The military experience is filled with examples of casualties incurred to recover a body and of attempts to rescue a casualty who eventually stood up and ran to cover without assistance.[54]

Additional Considerations

Some common conventional EMS interventions may be inappropriate in the tactical situation. CPR, for example, provides little benefit in traumatic arrest and increases

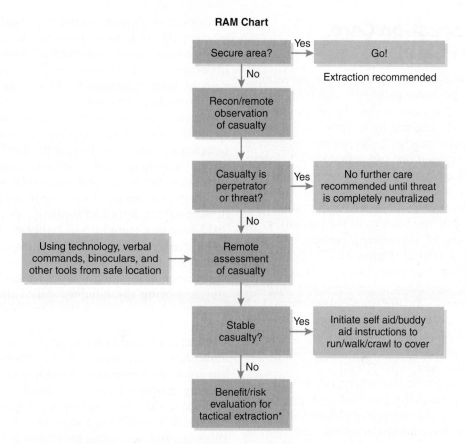

RAM Chart

*The benefit/risk evaluation of tactical extraction will depend on the likelihood of survival of casualty. The decision will ultimately be made by the SWAT commander with significant medical input from the TEMS practitioner.

Figure 22-5 Rapid and Remote Assessment Methodology (RAM) flow chart.
© National Association of Emergency Medical Technicians (NAEMT)

responder exposure.[55] Accordingly, CPR has a very limited role in tactical medical response, and its consideration should be reserved for victims of drowning, electrocution, hypothermia, and some toxic exposures.

The diminished emphasis on CPR, IV access, and fluid management in both phases of CUFT and tactical field care illustrates some of the distinctions between TEMS and conventional EMS. These examples are not meant to substitute for the clinical judgment of the TEMS practitioner.

Analgesia Considerations

One area of brief consideration is that of TEMS pain management. Early TEMS practitioners initially used morphine and titrated, as needed, the frequency and dosage during prehospital missions. However, after discovering the potential use for oral transmucosal fentanyl, this medication was added to the TCCC guidelines for mild to moderate pain in casualties with no compromise in airway or mental status.[56,57] Ketamine is another exceptional

medication with a wide scope of use and limited contraindications, and it was added to TCCC Guidelines in 2012. Ketamine preserves hemodynamics, respiratory rate, and airway reflexes and is not contraindicated in unconscious or obtunded individuals.[56,58] Most casualties requiring analgesia, dissociative amnesia, and procedural sedation can benefit greatly from ketamine use with appropriate monitoring and medical direction approval.

In 2014, TCCC developed a triple option analgesia approach that can be recommended in the civilian realm as well.[58] Initially, oral medications (e.g., nonsteroidal anti-inflammataory drugs [NSAIDs], acetaminophen) are recommended for mild pain with a continually functional member of the team. With moderate pain but without risk of shock or deterioration, oral transmucosal fentanyl (or sublingual sufentanil) is recommended. Finally, if the casualty is in severe pain and at risk for or is experiencing shock or pulmonary compromise, ketamine is the agent of choice with IV fentanyl as an additional option.[50,55-57] Recommendations are dependent on local area availability, preference, and the discretion of the TEMS medical director.

Tactical Evacuation Care (Evacuation Care)

Tactical evacuation care takes place in the operational cold zone, beyond the outer perimeter, and is an area of relatively low risk. The outer perimeter isolates the incident and is typically covered by conventional law enforcement patrol personnel with the primary mission of scene control, event isolation, and general public safety. During the tactical evacuation care phase, medical care continues during transport to the appropriate receiving center. Akin to conventional EMS care of the trauma patient, this may include the transfer of the casualty to an ambulance or the use of alternative emergency vehicles such as an armored vehicle (**Figure 22-6**). Care during this phase is situation- and injury-dependent and based on team standard operating procedures and incident commander decisions. At the incident commander's discretion, and as necessary, medical control may be established beyond reach of the weapons being used by the perpetrator(s), and additional EMS medical resources may also stage in this area.

In the event that alternative emergency vehicles are used in transporting a casualty, standard operating procedures should be rehearsed in depth to include the roles of team members who have limited or no medical training. Additional medical equipment should be staged in these

vehicles, and all team members should be cross-trained in treating the four preventable causes of death (hemorrhage, airway obstruction, pneumothoraces, and hypothermia) by administering lifesaving interventions such as using tourniquets, NPAs, and chest seals and preventing hypothermia.

Even in an area deemed secure, all emergency responders must remain vigilant. Tactical operations are complex and dynamic. During the 1999 Columbine High School shootings, the assailants targeted emergency responders by placing pipe bombs and improvised explosive devices. Fortunately, due to technical failures, these devices did not detonate. Similarly, the perpetrator of the 2012 Aurora, Colorado, movie theater shooting prepared and placed explosives in his apartment. These devices included trip wires and booby traps with flammable material capable of killing officers responding to the scene and destroying the building. All of these devices were handled by astute law enforcement personnel without injury.

The FBI has reported several incidents of intentional ambushes of law enforcement personnel, and the frequency of these events is increasing. In addition, terrorist training manuals have been found that explicitly detail operations that use a barricaded suspect to lure law enforcement personnel to a scene in order to ambush them. Diligence and situational awareness are the cornerstones to safe operations by responding law enforcement officers and TEMS practitioners. In recent years we have seen attacks on civilians and law enforcement utilizing everything from fire to vehicles to organophospate solutions. Astute TEMS practitioners must account for the unexpected injury pattern in an operation.

Mass-Casualty Incidents

Mass-casualty incidents (MCIs) involving active shooters are increasingly common and dangerous, and they present a complex interagency collaboration challenge. The Pulse nightclub shooting in Orlando, Florida, and the Las Vegas Route 91 Harvest country music festival shooting represent tragic examples. TEMS practitioners have a unique role to play in MCI events. First, TEMS teams tend to bridge law enforcement with fire departments and/or EMS systems. Second, TEMS practitioners are trained to work in chaotic, dangerous, and resource-poor environments. Third, TEMS practitioners have broad experience in utilization of various communication modes, immediate action drills, and mission planning. TEMS practitioners are often valuable resources to be considered when undertaking the process of planning and executing a well-coordinated MCI response.[35]

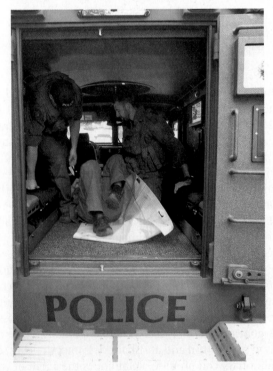

Figure 22-6 Nonstandard tactical evacuation care vehicle.
Courtesy of Commander Al Davis, Ventura Police Department.

Medical Intelligence and Medical Direction

One aspect of the role of the TEMS practitioner is pre-planning, gathering, and maintaining medical intelligence. On local and regional teams, the TEMS practitioner should have an in-depth knowledge of the local EMS and trauma systems, addresses, and contact information. This knowledge will allow the TEMS practitioner to make appropriate decisions regarding evacuation care and patient destination if a casualty should occur on the mission. TEMS teams that function remotely in unknown areas, such as wilderness locations, will have to conduct much more in-depth medical planning to develop an operable evacuation plan and extended care plan.

The role of aeromedical evacuation platforms in TEMS may be of great use; however, the TEMS practitioner must constantly monitor the availability of dedicated aeromedical assets. In addition, the response of an aeromedical evacuation platform to a tactical situation must include appropriate safety precautions to prevent the aeromedical unit from coming under hostile fire.

Finally, given the proliferation of civilian TEMS it is imperative that teams begin to identify and include physician medical directors as part of their leadership teams. Tactical EMS is, at its core, a subspecialty of EMS and should be treated as such. EMS physicians with an interest in tactical medicine must be sought out and retained to help improve officer safety and team performance. EMS physicians adhere to scientific principles of data collection, evidence-based medicine, and good quality management and clinical education programs. These same principles should be brought to the police department and SWAT team in order to produce the highest quality functioning system possible.

SUMMARY

- In general, the principles of medical care in the tactical environment are the same as those to which prehospital care practitioners are accustomed.
- The austerity and danger of the operational environment require that the benefit of every medical intervention be weighed against the risks inherent in delivering that intervention. This determination requires a unique set of decision-making skills.
- The TEMS practitioner constantly needs to balance the benefit of a particular intervention against the special risks inherent in performing the intervention in this environment.
- The tactical situation comprises three phases of care:

  - Care under fire/threat (direct threat care)—the medical care that is provided while under hostile fire or in an actively hazardous situation (hot zone)
  - Tactical field care (indirect threat care)—the medical care that is provided once the immediate hazard has been suppressed or controlled, knowing that the situation could revert to care under fire (warm zone)
  - Tactical evacuation care (evacuation care)—the medical care that is provided once the situation has been deemed safe, which is similar to a standard civilian EMS call (cold zone)
- Medical intelligence gathering allows the TEMS practitioner to know the environment, geography, and available resources of the area in which the tactical operation will be undertaken.

SCENARIO RECAP

Your emergency medical services (EMS) agency provides coverage for the local special weapons and tactics (SWAT) team and has a rigorous, integrated training program with local law enforcement. Your tactical emergency medical support (TEMS) team is called out just after sunset for a barricaded gunman holed up in an old mobile home. As you are preparing for entry, two SWAT officers cross the suspect's yard and approach the house to prepare for a door pull. Shots ring out from the front window, wounding the SWAT officers. One SWAT officer falls in the doorway of the suspect's home. The second falls near an old pickup truck. A patrol officer standing near you yells, "We need to go get them. Come on!" You grab the patrol officer by the arm and look to the SWAT commander.

- What should your actions be?
- How will you assess and treat the fallen SWAT officers given the danger of the scene?

SCENARIO SOLUTION

The SWAT commander orders you to use your Rapid and Remote Assessment Methodology (RAM) to determine the utility of a rescue effort. You use your binoculars and the SWAT team acoustic device to examine the two fallen officers. The first officer, lying in the doorway of the gunman's mobile home, shows no chest wall movement or signs of respiration around his mouth. Despite calls from his fellow officers, you are unable to detect any audible response on the acoustic device.

The second officer has moved behind the engine block of the old pickup truck. You can visualize bleeding from his lower thigh. Fortunately, you have conducted extensive tactical medical training for your officers. You communicate with him via the secure team radio and instruct him to apply a tourniquet high and tight around his groin region. He secures the device and communicates that he has no further injuries.

Based on your recommendation and the threat assessment, the SWAT commander chooses not to undertake a high-risk rescue of the officer showing no signs of life. You remain in contact with the second injured officer while the negotiators work to convince the suspect to surrender. You contact the local trauma center and inform them of a potential incoming casualty. Thirty minutes later, the suspect surrenders and is taken into custody. Your team evacuates the casualty to the local hospital where he undergoes a vascular repair, saving both his leg and his life.

References

1. Rinnert KJ, Hall WL. Tactical emergency medical support. *Emerg Med Clin N Am.* 2002;20:929-952.

2. Butler FK, Hagmann J, Butler EG. Tactical combat casualty care in Special Operations. *Milit Med.* 1996;161(Suppl):1–16.

3. Federal Bureau of Investigation. Crime data explorer. Accessed January 17, 2022. https://crime-data-explorer.app.cloud.gov/pages/home

4. Federal Bureau of Investigation. Uniform crime reports. Accessed October 6, 2021. https://ucr.fbi.gov/leoka

5. National Tactical Officers Association. Position statement on the inclusion of physicians in tactical law enforcement operations. Accessed January 17, 2022. https://www.ntoa.org/sections/tems/tems-position-statement/

6. Heck JJ, Pierluisi G. Law enforcement special operations and medical support. *Prehosp Emerg Care.* 2001;5:403-406.

7. American College of Emergency Physicians. Policy statement on tactical emergency medical support. *Ann Emerg Med.* 2005;45:108.

8. National Association of Emergency Medical Technicians. Pollak AN, ed. *Prehospital Trauma Life Support.* 9th ed. Jones & Bartlett Learning; 2018.

9. Callaway DW, Reed S, Shapiro G, et al. The Committee for Tactical Emergency Care (C-TECC): evolution and application of TCCC guidelines to civilian high threat medicine. *J Special Operations Med.* 2011;11:2.

10. Smith ER, Shapiro G, Sarani B. Fatal wounding pattern and causes of potentially preventable death following the Pulse Night Club shooting event. *Prehosp Emerg Care.* 2018;22(6):662-668.

11. Kanable R. Peak performance: well-trained tactical medics can help the team perform at its best. *Law Enforcement Tech.* August 1999.

12. Cooke, MC. How much to do at the accident scene? *BMJ.* 1999;319:1105-1106. doi: 10.1136/bmj.320.7240.1005/

13. Jagoda A, Pietrzek M, Hazen S, Vayer J. Prehospital care and the military. *Mil Med.* 1992;157(1):11-15. doi: 10.1093/milmed/157.1.11

14. Bellamy RF. The causes of death in conventional land warfare: implications for combat casualty care research. *Mil Med.* 1984;149:55-62.

15. Callaway DW. Tactical emergency services. In: Hogan DE, Burstein JL, eds. *Disaster Medicine.* 2nd ed. Lippincott, Williams and Wilkins; 2007.

16. Gerold KB, Gibbons M, McKay S. The relevance of Tactical Combat Casualty Care (TCCC) guidelines to civilian law enforcement operations. National Tactical Officers TEMS Overview. Updated November 1, 2009. Accessed March 18, 2022. https://www.east.org/content/documents/Military Resources/TCCC/TCCC.pdf

17. Parsons, DL, Mott JC. *Tactical Combat Casualty Care Handbook: Observations, Insights, and Lessons.* Center for Army Lessons Learned; 2012.

18. Kragh JF, Walters TJ, Baer DG, et al. Survival with emergency tourniquet use to stop bleeding in major limb trauma. *Ann Surg.* 2009;249(1):1-7.

19. Thunholm P, Henåker L. A tentative model on effective army combat tactics. *Comparative Strategy.* 2020;39(5):490-504. doi: 10.1080/01495933.2020.1803713

20. Kragh JF, O'Neill ML, Walters TJ, et al. The military emergency tourniquet program's lessons learned with devices and designs. *Mil Med.* 2011;176:10, 1144.

21. Butler FK, Giebner SD, McSwain N, et al., eds. *Prehospital Trauma Life Support.* Military 8th ed. Jones & Bartlett Learning; 2014.

22. Bennett BL, Littlejohn LF, Kheirabadi BS, et al. Management of external hemorrhage in Tactical Combat Casualty Care: chitosan-based hemostatic gauze dressings. *J Spec Oper Med.* 2014;14:12-29.

23. Bennett BL, Littlejohn L. Review of new topical hemostatic dressings for combat casualty care. *Mil Med.* 2014;179:497-514.

24. Littlejohn L, Bennett B, Drew B. Application of current hemorrhage control techniques for backcountry care: part 2: hemostatic dressings and other adjuncts. *Wilderness Environ Med.* 2015;26:246-254.

25. Drew B, Bennett B, Littlejohn L. Application of current hemorrhage control techniques for backcountry care. Part 1: tourniquets and hemorrhage control adjuncts. *Wilderness Environ Med.* 2015;26:236-245.

26. Kheirabadi BS, Edens JW, Terrazas IB, et al. Comparison of new hemostatic granules/powders with currently deployed hemostatic products in a lethal model of extremity arterial hemorrhage in swine. *J Trauma.* 2009;66:316-326.

27. Kheirabadi BS, Mace JE, Terrazas IB, et al. Safety evaluation of new hemostatic agents, smectite granules, and kaolin-coated gauze in a vascular injury wound model in swine. *J Trauma.* 2010;68:269-278.

28. Kheirabadi BS, Edens JW, Terrazas IB, et al. Comparison of new hemostatic granules/powders with currently deployed hemostatic products in a lethal model of extremity arterial hemorrhage in swine. *J Trauma.* 2009;66(2):316-326; discussion 327-328.

29. Butler FK Jr, Hagmann J, Butler EG. Tactical combat casualty care in special operations. *Mil Med.* 1996;161(suppl):3-16.

30. Mabry R, Frankfurt A, Kharod C, et al. Emergency cricothyroidotomy in Tactical Combat Casualty Care. *J Spec Oper Med.* 2015;15:11-19.

31. Hessert MJ, Bennett BL. Optimizing emergent surgical cricothyrotomy for use in austere environments. *Wilderness Environ Med.* 2013;24:53-66.

32. Mabry R, Nichols M, Shiner D, et al. A comparison of two open surgical cricothyroidotomy techniques by military medics using a cadaver model. *Ann Emerg Med.* 2014;63:1-5.

33. Tien HC, Jung V, Riool SB, et al. An evaluation of tactical combat casualty care interventions in a combat environment. *J Am Coll Surg.* 2008;207(2):174-178.

34. Hacked HT, Parse LA, Levy AD, et al. Chest wall thickness in military personnel: implications for needle thoracentesis in tension pneumothorax. *Mil Med.* 2008;172:1260-1263.

35. Zengerink I, Brink PR, Laupland KB, et al. Needle thoracostomy in the treatment of tension pneumothorax in trauma patients: what size needle? *J Trauma.* 2008;64:111-114.

36. Givens ML, Ayotte K, Manifold C. Needle thoracostomy: implications of computed tomography chest wall thickness. *Acad Emerg Med.* 2004;11:211-213.

37. Revell M, Greaves I, Porter K. Endpoints for fluid resuscitation in hemorrhagic shock. *J Trauma.* 2003;54(suppl 5):S63-S67.

38. Morrison CA, Carrick MM, Norman MA, et al. Hypotensive resuscitation strategy reduces transfusion requirements and severe postoperative coagulopathy in trauma patients with hemorrhagic shock: preliminary results of a randomized controlled trial. *J Trauma.* 2011;70(3):652-663.

39. Benson G. Intraosseous access to the circulatory system: an under-appreciated option for rapid access. *J Perioper Pract.* 2015;25:140-143.

40. Byars DV, Tsuchitani SN, Erwin E, et al. Evaluation of success rate and access time for an adult sternal intraosseous device deployed in the prehospital setting. *Prehosp Disaster Med.* 2011;26:127-129.

41. Lewis P, Wright C. Saving the critically injured trauma patient: a retrospective analysis of 1000 uses of intraosseous access. *Emerg Med J.* 2015;32:463-467.

42. Ley E, Clond M, Srour M, et al. Emergency department crystalloid resuscitation of 1.5 L or more is associated with increased mortality in elderly and non-elderly trauma patients. *J Trauma.* 2011;70:398-400.

43. Duke MD, Guidry C, Guice J, et al. Restrictive fluid resuscitation in combination with damage control resuscitation: time for adaptation. *J Trauma.* 2012;73:674-678.

44. Spinella P, Pidcoke H, Strandenes G, et al. Whole blood transfusion for hemostatic resuscitation of major bleeding. *Transfusion.* 2016;56:S190-S202.

45. Cap A, Pidcoke H, DePasquale M, et al. Blood far forward: time to get moving! *J Trauma.* 2015;78:S2-S6.

46. Stubbs J, Zielinski M, Jenkins D. The state of the science of whole blood: lessons learned at Mayo Clinic. *Transfusion.* 2016;56:S173-S881.

47. Spinella PC, Perkins JG, Grathwohl KW, et al. Warm fresh whole blood is independently associated with improved survival for patients with combat-related traumatic injuries. *J Trauma.* 2009;66:S69-S76.

48. Montgomery HR, Drew BG, Torrisi J, et al. TCCC Guidelines Comprehensive Review and Edits 2020: TCCC Guidelines Change 20-05 01 November 2020. *J Spec Oper Med.* 2021;21(2):122-127.

49. Zafren K, Giesbrecht GG, Danzl DF, et al. Wilderness Medical Society practice guidelines for the out-of-hospital evaluation and treatment of accidental hypothermia: 2014 update. *Wilderness Environ Med.* 2014;25(suppl):S66-S85.

50. McKeague AL. Evaluation of patient active warming systems. Military Health System Research Symposium, Tactical Combat Casualty Care breakout session. Ft. Lauderdale, FL. August 2012.

51. Allen PB, Salyer SW, Dubick MA, et al. Preventing hypothermia: comparison of current devices used by the U.S. Army in an in vitro warmed fluid model. *J Trauma.* 2010;69(suppl 1):S154-S161.

52. McKay S, Hoyne S. High threat immediate extraction: the Immediate Reaction Team (IRT) model. *Tactical Edge.* Spring 2007:50-54.

53. Callaway DW. Emergency medical services in disasters. Hogan DE, Burstein JL, eds. *Disaster Medicine.* 2nd ed. Philadelphia, PA: Lippincott, Williams and Wilkins; 2007:127-139.

54. Cloonan C. *Proceedings of the Third International Conference on Tactical Emergency Medical Support.* Bethesda, MD: Uniformed Services University of the Health Sciences; 1999.

55. Rosemary AS, Norris PA, Olson SM, et al. Prehospital traumatic cardiac arrest: the cost of futility. *J Trauma.* 1998;38:468-474.

56. Butler FK, Kotwal RS, Buckenmaier CC III, et al. A triple-option analgesia plan for Tactical Combat Casualty Care. *J Spec Oper Med*. 2014;14:13-25.

57. Kotwal R, O'Connor K, Johnson T, et al. A novel pain management strategy for combat casualty care. *Ann Emerg Med*. 2004;44:121-127.

58. Dickey N, Jenkins D, Butler F. Prehospital use of ketamine in battlefield analgesia. Defense Health Board Memorandum. Published March 8, 2012. Accessed January 17, 2022. https://health.mil/Reference-Center/Reports/2012/03/08/Prehospital-Use-of-Ketamine-in-Battlefield-Analgesia

Suggested Reading

National Association of Emergency Medical Technicians. *PHTLS: Prehospital Trauma Life Support*. Military 9th ed. Jones & Bartlett Learning; 2019.

SPECIFIC SKILLS

Ruggedized Intravenous Line

Principle: To insert and secure an intravenous (IV) line when a trauma patient has to be moved, carried, or transported manually over a distance.

When a trauma patient has to be moved, carried, or manually transported over a distance, IV lines placed in the patient often become dislodged in the effort. The U.S. military has developed a method for initiating and securing IV lines that allows for this kind of movement without loss of the IV access. The skill demonstrated here has been modified from the military for civilian application.

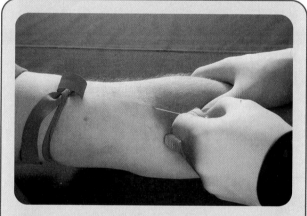

1 The TEMS practitioner obtains IV access according to the usual procedure, using an 18- or 16-gauge IV catheter.

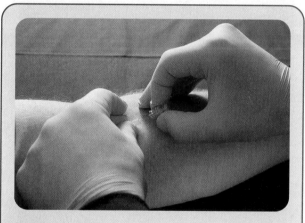

2 The TEMS practitioner attaches a saline lock to the IV catheter.

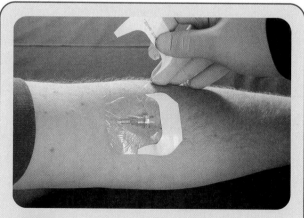

3 The TEMS practitioner covers the IV catheter and saline lock completely with a transparent wound dressing film (e.g., Tegaderm).

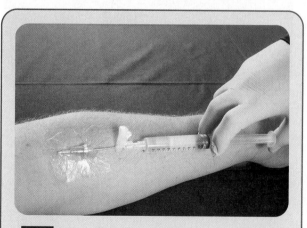

4 The TEMS practitioner flushes the saline lock with 5 milliliters (mL) of normal saline by puncturing directly through the dressing film and rubber stopper of the saline lock.

(continues)

Ruggedized Intravenous Line (continued)

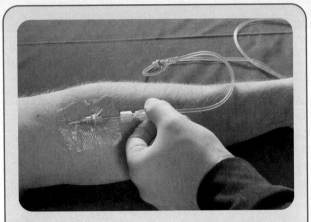

5 The TEMS practitioner inserts a second IV catheter (18 gauge) directly through the dressing film and rubber stopper of the saline lock and administers fluids and medications through this catheter.

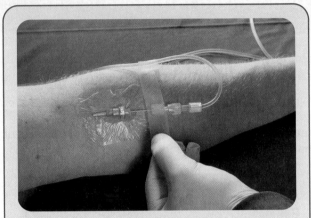

6 The TEMS practitioner secures the second catheter and attaches the IV line to the arm with circumferential application of a Velcro securing device or tape.

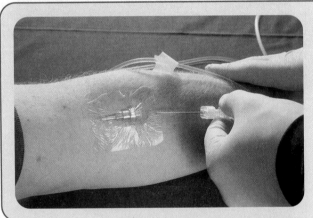

7 If and when the trauma patient must be moved, the securing device or tape, IV line, and second catheter are removed. The primary catheter and saline lock remain in place, thus ensuring rapid IV access once the patient move has been accomplished.

Glossary

Abbreviated Injury Scale (AIS) An injury categorization system that assigns injuries a value between 1 and 6, with (1) being minor, (2) being moderate, (3) being serious, (4) being severe, (5) being critical, and (6) being unsurvivable.

acetylcholine A chemical that functions as a neurotransmitter, released at the end of nerve cells to transmit a nervous system impulse.

acid A chemical substance that has a pH less than 7 and that will neutralize an alkali.

acidosis An accumulation of acids and decreased pH of the blood.

active strategies When referring to injury prevention, prevention steps that require the active participation of the individual; e.g., wearing a helmet.

acute mountain sickness (AMS) A constellation of symptoms that results from travel to high altitude (usually above 8,000 feet [2,400 meters]).

acute respiratory distress syndrome (ARDS) Respiratory insufficiency as a result of damage to the lining of the capillaries and alveoli in the lung, leading to the leakage of fluid into the interstitial spaces and alveoli.

acute tubular necrosis (ATN) Acute damage to the renal tubules, usually due to ischemia associated with shock.

aerosol Solid particles and liquid particles that are suspended in air.

afterload The pressure against which the left ventricle must pump out (eject) blood with each beat.

air density As used in this text, the property of organs having approximately the same weight and density as air, for example, lung tissue.

air-purifying respirator (APR) A device that uses a filter, canister, or cartridge to remove contaminants from ambient air that passes through the air-purifying component and makes the air safe to breathe.

alpha particle A particle emitted during the decay of a radioactive material; consists of two protons and two neutrons, thus giving the particle a positive charge.

alveoli The terminal air sacs of the respiratory tract where the respiratory system meets the circulatory system and gas exchange occurs.

anastomoses A connection between two structures such as two blood vessels or adjacent bowel.

anhidrosis The absence of sweating.

anisocoria Inequality of pupil size.

anterior cord syndrome Damage to the anterior portion of the spinal cord, usually as a result of bony fragments or pressure on spinal arteries.

apneic The absence of breathing.

appendicular skeleton Portion of the skeleton that includes the shoulders and arms as well as the pelvis and legs.

arachnoid mater Spiderweb-like transparent membrane between the dura mater and the pia mater; the middle of the three meningeal membranes surrounding the brain.

aspiration pneumonitis Inflammation and pneumonia caused by inhaling gastric contents or vomitus.

assist control (A/C) ventilation A form of mechanical ventilation; breaths may be assisted by the ventilator if the patient triggers the device by adequately attempting to breathe in or will automatically occur if the patient does not breathe.

ataxic breathing An irregular and uncoordinated breathing pattern with variable tidal volumes and random periods of apnea.

atelectasis Collapse of alveoli or part of the lung.

atherosclerosis A narrowing of the blood vessels; a condition in which the inner layer of the artery wall thickens while fatty deposits build up within the artery.

atlas The first cervical vertebra (C1); the skull perches upon it.

atropine A chemical that competitively inhibits the effect of acetylcholine at parasympathetic nerve endings; anticholinergic medication; used to treat victims of nerve agent poisoning.

austere environment A setting in which resources, supplies, equipment, personnel, transportation, and other aspects of the physical, political, social, and economic environments are extremely limited.

autonomic nervous system The part of the central nervous system that directs and controls the involuntary functions of the body.

autonomy A competent adult patient's right to direct his or her own health care free from interference or undue influence.

autoregulation The biologic process of detecting change within the system and adjusting for that change; in the circulatory system, the process of maintaining a constant blood flow as blood pressure changes.

axial loading The force acting on or applied to the long axis of an object; typically refers to force applied to the spine from the head downward; may also result from the weight of the body being applied to the lower part of the spine, as would occur in a fall from a height landing on the feet.

axis The second cervical vertebra (C2); its shape allows for the wide possible range of rotation of the head. Also, an imaginary line that passes through the center of the body.

baroreceptor A sensory nerve ending that is stimulated by changes in blood pressure. Baroreceptors are found in the walls of the atria of the heart, vena cava, aortic arch, and carotid sinus.

barotrauma Injury to air-containing organs that results from a change in air pressure.

basal level Baseline or minimal level.

basal metabolic rate The number of calories the body burns while at rest, resulting in heat production as a by-product of metabolism.

bases Chemicals with a pH greater than 7; dissolves in water and release hydroxide ions or accept hydrogen ions; cause liquefaction necrosis of tissue.

basilar skull fractures Fractures of the floor of the cranium.

behavioral regulation An individual's conscious response to environmental thermal change and the physical actions taken to keep warm or cool.

beneficence An ethical term that means "to do good"; requires prehospital care providers to act in a manner that maximizes the benefits and minimizes the risks to the patient.

beta particle A high-speed or high-energy electron emitted from radioactive decay.

biologic agent A bacterium, virus, or toxin that can be used as a weapon of mass destruction.

blast lung injury (BLI) Results from exposure to high-order explosive blast overpressure wave; lung damage varies from scattered petechiae to contusions and pulmonary hemorrhage.

blast overpressure Pressure exceeding normal atmospheric pressure that results from a high-order explosive detonation.

blast wave A sharply defined wave front of increased pressure that propagates outward from the center of an explosion.

blast wind The result of the sudden displacement of air from an explosion.

blind nasotracheal intubation (BNTI) A technique of inserting an endotracheal tube through the nares into the trachea without visualizing the larynx and vocal cords.

blister agents A chemical that creates burnlike injuries; used as a weapon of mass destruction.

blunt trauma Nonpenetrating trauma caused by a rapidly moving object that impacts the body.

bradypnea Abnormally slow breathing rate; usually less than 12 breaths per minute.

brain stem The stemlike part of the brain that connects the cerebral hemispheres with the spinal cord.

bronchioles The small divisions of the bronchial tubes through which air passes to the alveoli.

Brown-Séquard syndrome A condition caused by penetrating injury that involves hemitransection of the spinal cord; only one side of the cord is involved.

capillary The smallest type of blood vessel. These minute blood vessels are only one cell wide, allowing for diffusion and osmosis of oxygen and nutrients through the capillary walls.

capnography The method of measuring and monitoring the partial pressure of carbon dioxide in a sample of gas. It can correlate to the arterial.

capnometry The measurement of carbon dioxide in respiratory gas (analysis alone), without a continuous written record or waveform.

cardiac output The volume of blood pumped by the heart (reported in liters per minute).

cardiac tamponade Compression of the heart from an accumulation of fluid in the pericardium surrounding the heart; in the case of trauma, the fluid is usually blood; the accumulation of fluid prevents normal blood return to the heart by compressing the heart, thus impairing circulation.

care under fire/threat (CUFT) Medical attention provided by the first responder or combatant to arrive at the scene of injury while still under active enemy fire or threat.

casualty collection point A location used for the collection, triage, treatment, and evacuation of casualties from a multiple-casualty incident.

cataract A condition of the eye in which the lens becomes progressively more opaque and blocks and distorts light entering the eye and blurs vision.

catecholamines A group of chemicals produced by the body that work as important nerve transmitters. The main catecholamines made by the body are dopamine, epinephrine (also called adrenalin), and norepinephrine.

They are part of the body's sympathetic defense mechanism used in preparing the body to act.

caudad Toward the tail (coccyx).

cavitation The act of forcing tissues of the body out of their normal position; to cause a temporary or permanent cavity (e.g., when the body is struck by a bullet, the acceleration of particles of tissue away from the missile produces an area of injury in which a large temporary cavity occurs).

cellular respiration The use of oxygen by the cells to produce energy.

central chemoreceptors Are cells that are sensitive to changes in brain partial pressure of CO_2 or pH and contribute to the stimulation of breathing elicited by buildup of carbon dioxide in the bloodstream or metabolic acidosis.

central cord syndrome Damage to the central portion of the spinal cord that usually occurs with hyperextension of the cervical area; characterized by weakness or paralysis of the upper extremities but not the lower extremities.

central neurogenic hyperventilation Pathologic rapid and shallow ventilatory pattern associated with head injury and increased intracranial pressure.

cerebellum A portion of the brain that lies beneath the cerebrum and behind the medulla oblongata and is concerned with coordination of movement.

cerebral perfusion pressure (CPP) The amount of pressure needed to maintain cerebral blood flow; calculated as the difference between the mean arterial pressure (MAP) and the intracranial pressure (ICP).

cerebrospinal fluid (CSF) A fluid found in the subarachnoid space and dural sheath; acts as a shock absorber, protecting the brain and spinal cord from jarring impact.

cerebrum The largest part of the brain; responsible for the control of specific intellectual, sensory, and motor functions.

chemosis A watery swelling of the covering (conjunctiva) of the eye.

Cheyne-Stokes ventilation Periodic breathing, wherein the patient's ventilation oscillates between apnea and hyperpnea (i.e., lungs and chemoreceptors are not coordinated well).

chilblains Red or purple skin lesions on the skin that are itchy and painful and appear after cold exposure, particularly in patients with poor underlying circulation.

choke A constriction in the barrel of a shotgun to decrease the amount of pellet spread after firing.

cilia Hairlike vibrating structure of cells that propel foreign particles and mucus from the bronchi.

circumferential burn A burn that encompasses an entire body part such as the arm, leg, or chest. classic heatstroke disorder that results from exposure to high humidity and high temperature, characterized by elevated body temperature above 104°F (40°C) and neurologic abnormalities (altered mental status).

closed fracture A fracture of a bone in which the overlying skin is not interrupted.

coagulative necrosis The type of tissue damage that results from acid exposure; the damaged tissue forms a barrier that prevents deeper penetration of the acid

coagulopathy Impairment in the normal blood-clotting capabilities.

cold-induced diuresis Increased urine production as a result of peripheral vasoconstriction from exposure to cold.

cold-induced vasodilation (CIVD) Physiologic response that occurs once an extremity has been cooled to 50°F (10°C) in an effort to provide some protection from the cold.

command The first component of the incident command system, responsible for all incident oversight and management. It is the only position in the incident command system that must always be staffed.

command staff The public information officer, safety officer, and liaison officer; they report directly to the incident commander.

commission A purposeful act.

commotio cordis Sudden cardiac dysrhythmia, often fatal, that results from a blow to the anterior chest or sternum.

compartment syndrome The clinical findings noted from ischemia and compromised circulation that can occur from vascular injury, causing hypoxia of muscles in an extremity compartment. The cellular edema produces increased pressure in a closed fascial or bony compartment.

competence (1) A legal term referring to a person's general ability to make good decisions for himself or herself; (2) the ability, skill, knowledge, and qualification to do something successfully.

complete cord transection Complete damage and severing of the spinal cord; all spinal tracts are interrupted, and all normal neurologic functions distal to the site are lost.

comprehensive emergency management The steps needed to manage an incident, consisting of four components: mitigation, preparation, response, and recovery.

compressibility The ability to be deformed by the transfer of energy.

compression The type of force involved in impacts resulting in a tissue, organ, or other body part being squeezed between two or more objects or body parts.

compression injury An injury caused by severe crushing and squeezing forces; may occur to the external structure of the body or to the internal organs.

conduction The transfer of heat between two objects in direct contact with each other.

confidentiality The obligation of health care providers to not share patient information that is disclosed to them within the patient–provider relationship to anyone other than those the patient has authorized,

other medical professionals involved in the patient's care, and agencies responsible for processing state and/or federally mandated reporting.

conjunctiva The clear (usually) mucous membrane that covers the sclera (white part of the eye) and lines the eyelids.

contact wound The type of wound that occurs when the muzzle of a gun touches the patient at the time of discharge, resulting in a circular entrance wound, often associated with visible burns, soot, or the imprint of the muzzle.

convection The transfer of heat from the movement or circulation of a gas or liquid, such as the heating of water or air in contact with a body, removing that air (such as by wind) or water, and then having to heat the new air or water that replaces what left.

cord compression Pressure on the spinal cord caused by swelling, bone fragments, or hematoma, which may result in tissue ischemia and, in some cases, may require decompression to prevent a permanent loss of function.

cord concussion The temporary disruption of the spinal cord functions distal to the site of a spinal cord injury.

cord contusion Bruising or bleeding into the tissue of the spinal cord, which may also result in a temporary loss of cord functions distal to the injury.

cord laceration An injury that occurs when spinal cord tissue is torn or cut.

core temperature (1) The temperature at which vital organs are maintained and function best; (2) the measured temperature of the deep structures and organs of the body.

cornea The dome-shaped transparent outer portion of the eye that covers the pupil and colored iris.

corneal abrasion common type of eye injury characterized by a minor cut or scratch on the cornea (the clear, front portion of the eye).

coup-contrecoup injury An injury to the brain that occurs when the head strikes a fixed object, causing an injury at the site of impact (coup) and an injury on the opposite side (contrecoup), where the brain collides with the opposite side of the skull.

cranial vault The space within the skull or cranium.

crepitus A crackling sound made by bone ends grating together.

critical incident stress management (CISM) A group of intervention strategies used to help prevent and manage stress after an incident.

Cushing reflex Characterized by an intracranial hypertension.

cyanosis Blue coloring of skin, mucous membranes, or nail beds indicating unoxygenated hemoglobin and a lack of adequate oxygen levels in the blood; usually secondary to inadequate ventilation or decreased perfusion.

dead space The volume of ventilated air that does not participate in gas exchange, as It either remains in the conducting airways or reaches alveoli that are not perfused or poorly perfused.

debridement The removal, usually surgically, of dead or damaged tissue.

decerebrate posturing Characteristic posture that occurs when a painful stimulus is introduced; the extremities are stiff and extended and the head is retracted. One of the forms of pathologic posturing (response) commonly associated with increased intracranial pressure.

decomposition A state of decay or rotting.

decompression sickness (DCS) A group of disorders that result from the effects of increased pressure on gases in a diver's body.

decontamination Reduction or removal of hazardous chemical, biologic, or radiologic agents.

decorticate posturing A characteristic pathologic posture of a patient with increased intracranial pressure; when a painful stimulus is introduced, the patient is rigidly still with the back and lower extremities extended while the arms are flexed and fists clenched.

deep frostbite Freezing of tissue that affects skin, muscle, and bone.

delayed primary closure Delayed suturing of a wound for 48 to 72 hours to allow any swelling to go down and to ensure that there are no signs of infection.

delayed-sequence intubation (DSI) A technique of medication-assisted intubation that emphasizes preoxygenation with CPAP and apneic oxygenation during intubation.

delirium An abrupt change in mental status secondary to an acute medical condition; generally reversible once the underlying acute process is corrected.

dementia The general term for a decrease in cognitive capabilities that causes interference with daily life.

denuded Having the covering or surface layer removed.

dependent lividity The settling or pooling of blood in the lowest lying portions of a deceased body.

dermatome The sensory area on the body for which a nerve root is responsible. Collectively, they allow the body areas to be mapped out for each spinal level and to help locate a spinal cord injury.

dermis The layer of skin just under the epidermis made up of a framework of connective tissues containing blood vessels, nerve endings, sebaceous glands, and sweat glands.

designated incident facilities An assigned location where specific incident command system functions are performed; for example, incident command is located at the incident command post.

devitalized Lifeless or dead.

diaphragm The dome-shaped muscle that divides the chest and abdomen and that functions as part of the breathing process.

diastole Ventricular relaxation (ventricular filling).

distraction The pulling apart of two structures; e.g., pulling apart the fractured components of a bone or part of the spine.

diverter A device on a shotgun to spread the pellets into a wider, horizontal path when fired.

dorsal root The spinal nerve root responsible for sensory impulses.

DUMBELS A mnemonic that represents the constellation of symptoms associated with the muscarinic effects of nerve agent toxicity (diarrhea, urination, miosis, bradycardia, bronchorrhea, bronchospasm, emesis, lacrimation, salivation, sweating).

dura mater The outer tough membrane covering the spinal cord and brain; the outer of the three meningeal layers. Literally means "tough mother."

dynamic pressure The component of an explosion that is directional and felt as a blast wind.

dysarthria Difficulty speaking.

dysbarism The changes that result physiologically as a result of changes in ambient environmental pressure.

ecchymosis A bluish or purple irregularly formed spot or area resulting from a hemorrhagic area below the skin.

eclampsia A syndrome in pregnant women that includes hypertension, peripheral edema, and seizures; also called toxemia of pregnancy.

edema A local or generalized condition in which some of the body tissues contain an excessive amount of fluid; generally includes swelling of the tissue.

edentulism The absence of teeth.

effective ventilation Total minute ventilation minus dead space ventilation.

elasticity The ability to stretch.

endotracheal (ET) tube A plastic tube that is inserted into the trachea to ensure an open airway and used to assist a patient to breathe.

environmental temperature The thermal temperature of the air surrounding an individual.

epidermis The outermost layer of the skin, which is made up entirely of dead epithelial cells with no blood vessels.

epidural hematoma Arterial bleeding that collects between the skull and dura mater.

epidural space Potential space between the dura mater surrounding the brain and the cranium. Contains the meningeal arteries.

epiglottis A leaf-shaped structure that acts as a gate or flapper valve and directs air into the trachea and solids and liquids into the esophagus.

epinephrine A chemical released from the adrenal glands that stimulates the heart to increase cardiac output by increasing the strength and rate of contractions.

eschar Thick scab of dead tissue, often resulting from a burn.

escharotomy An incision made into an eschar to allow the tissues underlying the tough, leathery damaged skin created by severe burns to expand as they swell.

esophagus The muscular tube that connects the mouth to the stomach.

eucapnic state A condition in which the blood carbon dioxide level is within a normal range.

evaporation Change from liquid to vapor.

event phase The trauma care phase relating to the moment of the actual trauma.

evisceration A condition in which a portion of the intestine or other abdominal organ is displaced through an open wound and protrudes externally outside the abdominal cavity.

exercise-associated hyponatremia (EAH) A life-threatening condition associated with excessive consumption of water (1.5 quarts [1.4 liters] or greater per hour) during prolonged activities leading to marked lowering of the sodium concentration in blood.

exercise-associated hyponatremic encephalopathy (EAHE) A life-threatening condition of cerebral edema resulting from lowered sodium concentration in blood from excessive consumption of water (1.5 quarts [1.4 liters] or greater per hour) during prolonged activities.

exertional heatstroke (EHS) A condition of elevated body temperature, usually in males working or exercising in the heat and humidity, characterized by pale, sweaty skin, elevated body temperature, and altered mentation.

exsanguination Total loss of blood volume, producing death.

extracellular fluid All body fluid that is not contained within cells.

extramural (extraluminal) pressure Pressure in the tissue surrounding the vessel.

extreme altitude An elevation higher than 18,045 feet (5,500 meters).

eyelid lacerations Cuts to the eyelid and constitute a significant subset of facial trauma and are often accompanied by other ocular injuries, including orbital fractures, disruption of the lacrimal drainage system, foreign bodies, corneal abrasions, or open globe.

face-to-face intubation A technique for endotracheal intubation in which the endotracheal tube is inserted orally while the intubator is facing the patient instead of being located at the usual location above the head of the patient.

fascia A flat band of tissue that separates different layers; a fibrous band of tissue that encloses muscle.

field exercise A training event that involves the actual execution and performance of the community disaster-response plan.

finance/administration section The section responsible for all costs and financial actions of the incident.

first-degree frostbite Epidermal injury limited to skin that had brief contact with cold air or metal; involved skin appears white or as yellowish plaque; there is no blister or tissue loss; skin thaws quickly, feels numb, and appears red with surrounding edema; healing occurs in 7 to 10 days.

first phase of death Deaths from traumatic injury that occur within seconds to minutes after the injury.

flail chest A chest with an unstable segment produced by multiple ribs fractured in two or more places or including a fractured sternum.

flail sternum A variation of flail chest that involves fracture of the ribs on both sides of the sternum, allowing the sternum to float freely.

fontanelle The soft, membranous space between the unfused bones of an infant's skull; often referred to as the "soft spot."

foramen magnum The opening at the base of the skull through which the medulla oblongata passes.

foramina A small opening; singular is *foramen*.

fourth-degree frostbite A freezing injury that involves the skin, underlying tissue, muscle, and bone.

fragmentation The breaking up of an object to produce multiple parts or shrapnel.

frostbite The freezing of body tissue as a result of exposure to freezing or below-freezing temperatures.

full thickness burns Burns that involve complete epidermis and dermis.

galea aponeurotica A tough, thick layer of tissue underneath the scalp that covers the cranium.

gamma ray A ray of high-energy electromagnetic radiation released as a result of radioactive material decay.

group training Disaster response training directed at specific response groups.

Haddon Matrix A table that shows the interaction of host, agent, and environmental factors in an incident.

heat stress index The combination of ambient temperature and relative humidity.

heat syncope Fainting or light-headedness after standing for prolonged periods in a hot environment; results from vasodilation and venous blood pooling in the legs, causing low blood pressure.

hemiparesis Weakness limited to one side of the body.

hemiplegia Paralysis on one side of the body.

hemothorax Blood in the pleural space.

high altitude An elevation above 5,000 to 11,480 feet (1,500 to 3,500 meters).

high-altitude cerebral edema (HACE) A life-threatening complication of brain swelling that results from travel to high altitude (usually above 8,000 feet [2,400 meters]).

high-altitude pulmonary edema (HAPE) A life-threatening complication of fluid accumulating in the lungs that results from travel to high altitude (usually above 8,000 feet [2,400 meters]).

high explosives A type of explosive designed to detonate and release its energy very quickly; capable of producing a shock wave, or overpressure phenomenon, that can result in primary blast injury.

homeostasis A constant, stable internal environment; the balance necessary to maintain healthy life processes.

homeotherm A warm-blooded animal.

hot zone An area where the hazardous materials are located, or refers to an area that is considered to be dangerous.

hydrofluoric acid A type of acid; exposure to even small amounts can lead to life-threatening lowering of the serum calcium levels and cardiac dysrhythmias.

hypercarbia An increased level of carbon dioxide in the body.

hyperchloremic acidosis A type of metabolic acidosis (decrease in blood pH) associated with an increase in the amount of chloride ion in the blood; may result from the administration of large amounts of normal saline.

hyperextension Extreme or abnormal extension of a joint; a position of maximum extension. Hyperextension of the neck is produced when the head is extended posterior to a neutral position and can result in a fracture or dislocation of the vertebrae or in spinal cord damage in a patient with an unstable spine.

hyperflexion Extreme or abnormal flexion of a joint. A position of maximum flexion. Increased flexion of the neck can result in a fracture or dislocation of the vertebrae or in spinal cord damage in a patient with an unstable spine.

hyperkalemia A medical term that indicates elevated level of potassium (K+) in the blood.

hyper-rotation Excessive rotation.

hypertension A blood pressure greater than the upper limits of the normal range; generally considered to exist if the patient's systolic pressure is greater than 140 mm Hg.

hypertonic saline Any solution of sodium chloride in water with a concentration of sodium chloride greater than physiologic saline, which is 0.9% sodium chloride, the same as body fluid.

hyphema A collection of blood in the anterior chamber of the eye, between the clear cornea and the colored iris.

hypobaric hypoxia Hypoxia caused by the decrease in atmospheric pressure and the partial pressure of oxygen at increasingly higher altitudes.

hypochlorite An anion composed of chlorine and oxygen with the chemical formula ClO−.

hypopharynx The lower portion of the pharynx that opens into the larynx anteriorly and the esophagus posteriorly.

hypothalamus The area of the brain that functions as the thermoregulatory center and the body's thermostat to control neurologic and hormonal regulation of body temperature.

hypothermia A condition characterized by core body temperature below normal range, usually between 78°F and 90°F (26–32°C).

hypoxemia A condition characterized by below-normal level of oxygen in the blood.

hypoxia A condition in which the body or a region of the body is deprived of adequate oxygen supply at the tissue level.

ICS general staff The chiefs of each of the four major sections of the incident command system (ICS): operations, planning, logistics, and finance/administration.

immersion foot A nonfreezing cold exposure injury caused by prolonged immersion of extremities in wet and moisture that is cool to cold; also referred to as trench foot.

impact phase The phase of the disaster cycle that involves the actual incident or disaster.

Incident action plan (IAP) A continuously updated outline of the overall strategy, tactics, and risk management plans developed by the incident commander or the incident command system staff.

incident commander (IC) The individual responsible for all aspects of a response to an incident, including developing incident objectives, managing all incident operations, setting priorities, and defining the incident command system organization for the particular response; the IC position will always be filled.

incident command post The location at which incident command functions are performed.

incident command system (ICS) A system that defines the chain of command and organization of the various resources that respond during a disaster.

incomplete cord transection Partial transection of the spinal cord in which some tracts and motor/sensory functions remain intact.

independent learning Studying on one's own.

inferior vena cava A major vein that carries deoxygenated blood from the lower half of the body back to the heart.

inhalation The process of drawing air into the lungs.

injury A harmful event that arises from the release of specific forms of physical energy or barriers to normal flow of energy.

injury process Similar to disease, a process involving a host, an agent (in the case of injury the agent is energy), and an environment or situation that allows the host and agent to interact.

Injury Severity Score (ISS) An injury categorization system that categorizes injuries into six anatomically distinct body regions, with (1) being the head and neck, (2) being the face, (3) being the chest, (4) being the abdomen,

inner perimeter A geographic boundary at a hazardous incident surrounding the area of highest danger and potential lethality.

insensible loss The unmeasured loss of water and heat from exhaled air, skin, and mucous membranes.

integrated communications A communications system that allows all responders at an incident to communicate with supervisors and subordinates.

intentional injury Injury associated with an act of interpersonal or selfdirected violence.

intercostal muscles The muscles located between the ribs that connect the ribs to one another and assist with breathing.

interdisaster period The time in between disasters or masscasualty incidents during which risk assessment and mitigation activities are undertaken and when plans for the response to likely events are developed, tested, and implemented.

intermediate-range wound A penetrating gunshot wound that occurs at a distance of approximately 6 to 18 feet (1.8 to 5.5 meters).

intermittent mandatory ventilation (IMV) A form of mechanical ventilation that delivers a set rate and tidal volume to patients.

interstitial fluid The extracellular fluid located between the cell wall and the capillary wall.

intervertebral foramen A notch through which nerves pass in the inferior lateral side of the vertebra.

intracellular fluid Fluid within the cells.

intracranial pressure (ICP) The pressure exerted against the inside of the skull by brain tissue, blood, and cerebrospinal fluid; usually less than 15 mm Hg in adults and 3 to 7 mm Hg in children.

intramural (intraluminal) pressure The pressure exerted against the inside of the walls of blood vessels by the intravascular fluids and blood pressure cycle.

involuntary guarding Rigidity or spasm of the abdominal wall muscles in response to peritonitis.

ionization The process by which a molecule becomes charged by gaining or losing an electron.

iris The colored portion of the eye that contains the adjustable opening of the pupil.

justice That which is fair or just; in medicine, usually refers to how medical resources are distributed with regard to health care.

kinetic energy Energy available from movement. Function of the weight of an item and its speed: KE = 1/2 of the mass × the velocity squared.

kyphosis A forward, humplike curvature of the spine commonly associated with the aging process. Kyphosis may be caused by aging, rickets, or tuberculosis of the spine.

lactated Ringer's solution An intravenous crystalloid solution that is isotonic with blood and used to replenish circulating volume and electrolytes; contains water, sodium, chloride, calcium, potassium, and lactate.

laryngeal mask airway (LMA) An airway management device; the distal end that is inserted into the patient's mouth is shaped like an oval mask to cover the supraglottic structures and isolate the trachea to allow for air passage.

laryngeal tube airway (LTA) Used for mechanical ventilation of the lungs and is an alternative to airway management techniques such as laryngeal mask airway, mask ventilation, and tracheal intubation.

larynx The structure located just above the trachea that contains the vocal cords and the muscles that make them work.

lewisite An oily liquid used as a chemical weapon to produce burnlike blisters; it is a blister agent (vesicant).

liaison officer A command staff member who assists or coordinates with multiple agencies; serves as an intermediary between the incident commander and outside agencies.

Lichtenberg figures A branching or fernlike reddish skin marking that is painless and results from being struck by lightning.

ligament The fibrous connective tissue that connect bones to each other, providing stability and strength to the joint.

liquefaction necrosis The type of tissue injury that occurs when an alkali damages human tissue; the base liquefies the tissue, which allows for deeper penetration of the chemical.

logistics section The section responsible for providing all services, equipment, and facilities for the incident.

logistics section chief The position responsible for directing the logistics function for the incident commander.

long-range wound A penetrating gunshot wound that occurs at a distance greater than 18 feet (5.5 meters).

low explosive A type of explosive that changes relatively slowly from a solid or liquid to a gaseous state (in an action more characteristic of burning than of detonation); because they release their energy much more slowly, low explosives do not produce blast overpressure.

lung sliding sign The movement between the two pleural layers that occurs during respiration (two pleural layers are in apposition to each other, and sliding with respiration).

maceration Softening of the skin as a result of exposure to constant moisture; the skin turns white and breaks down and can easily become infected.

maculopapular rash A skin rash characterized by areas of reddish discoloration (macules) in association with small, raised bumps (papules).

magnesium A highly flammable chemical element used to make incendiary weapons; also an essential electrolyte in human physiology.

mammalian diving reflex A reflex that occurs with submersion in cold water (less than 70°F [21°C]) resulting in rapid slowing of the body's metabolism, spasm of the larynx, shunting of blood from the periphery to the heart and brain, and a marked decrease in heart and respiratory rate.

mass-casualty incident (MCI) An incident (such as a plane crash, building collapse, or fire) that produces a large number of victims from one mechanism, at one place, and at the same time; also referred to as multiple-casualty incident.

mass-casualty incident (MCI) response The postevent actions taken to minimize damage, morbidity, and mortality resulting from the incident.

mean arterial pressure (MAP) The average pressure in the vascular system, estimated by adding one-third of the pulse pressure to the diastolic pressure.

mediastinum The middle of the thoracic cavity containing the heart, great vessels, trachea, main bronchi, and esophagus.

meninges Three membranes that cover the brain tissue and the spinal cord: the dura mater, arachnoid, and pia mater.

minute ventilation (V°) The amount of air exchanged each minute; calculated by multiplying the volume of each breath (tidal volume) by the number of breaths per minute (rate).

minute volume The amount of air exchanged each minute; calculated by multiplying the volume of each breath (tidal volume) by the number of breaths per minute (rate).

mitigation In emergency medicine, a reduction in the loss of life and property by lessening the impact of disasters.

Monro-Kellie doctrine The sum of the volume of brain tissue, blood, and cerebrospinal fluid must remain constant within an intact skull.

MTWHF A mnemonic that represents the constellation of symptoms associated with stimulation of nicotinic receptors, usually after nerve agent exposure; MTWHF

stands for mydriasis (rarely seen), tachycardia, weakness, hypertension, hyperglycemia, fasciculations.

mucocutaneous Made up of or pertaining to both skin and mucous membranes.

multisystem trauma patient A patient with injury to more than one body system.

muscarinic sites An acetylcholine receptor found primarily in smooth muscle and glands.

myocardial hypertrophy An increase in the heart's muscle mass and size.

myoglobin A protein found in muscle that is responsible for giving muscle its characteristic red color.

nasopharyngeal airway (NPA) An airway that is placed in the nostril and follows the floor of the nasal cavity directly posterior to the nasopharynx in order to lift the tongue off of the back of the pharynx and open the airway. This airway is commonly tolerated by patients with a gag reflex.

nasopharynx The upper portion of the airway, situated above the soft palate.

neural arches Two curved sides of the vertebrae.

neutral position The position of a joint that allows for maximal movement; neither flexed nor extended.

Newton's first law of motion A fundamental law of physics stating that a body at rest will remain at rest, and a body in motion will remain in motion unless acted on by an outside force.

Newton's second law of motion A fundamental law of physics stating that the acceleration of an object is directly proportional to the magnitude of the force applied, in the same direction as the force applied, and inversely proportional to the mass of the object.

Newton's third law of motion A fundamental law of physics stating that for every action, there is an equal and opposite reaction.

nicotinic sites An acetylcholine receptor found primarily in skeletal muscle.

nitrogen mustard An oily chemical used as a chemical weapon to produce

burnlike blisters; can also damage the respiratory tract, gastrointestinal tract, and bone marrow; blister agent; vesicant; also used as an anticancer medication.

nonfreezing cold injury (NFCI) A syndrome resulting from damage to peripheral tissues, caused by prolonged (hours to days) exposure to wet/cold; also called immersion foot or trench foot.

nonmaleficence An ethical principle that obligates the medical provider to not take actions that may harm the patient or place the patient in harm's way.

norepinephrine A chemical released by the sympathetic nervous system that triggers constriction of the blood vessels to reduce the size of the vascular container and bring it more closely into proportion with the volume of the remaining fluid.

normal saline An intravenous crystalloid solution comprising water and sodium chloride in a concentration of 0.9%.

obtunded A condition in which the patient's mental capacity is dulled or diminished; mild to moderate decreased level of consciousness with impaired sensory perception.

oculomotor nerve The third cranial nerve; controls pupillary constriction and certain eye movements.

omentum A fold of peritoneum that covers and connects the stomach to other intra-abdominal organs.

omission The failure to act.

oncotic pressure Pressure that determines the amount of fluid within the vascular space.

open fracture A fracture of a bone in which the skin is broken.

open globe A penetrating injury to the eye; injury that involves the full thickness of the cornea or the sclera of the eye.

open pneumothorax A penetrating wound to the chest that causes the chest wall to be opened, producing a preferential pathway for air moving from the outside environment into the thorax.

operations section The section responsible for all tactical operations at the incident.

operations section chief The position responsible for managing all operations activities in the incident command system.

oropharyngeal airway (OPA) An airway that, when placed in the oropharynx superior to the tongue, holds the tongue forward to assist in maintaining an open airway; used only in patients with no gag reflex.

oropharynx The central portion of the pharynx lying between the soft palate and the upper portion of the epiglottis.

orotracheal intubation A method of securing an open and patent airway that involves insertion of a plastic tube through the mouth into the trachea.

osmosis The movement of water (or other solvent) across a membrane from an area that is hypotonic to an area that is hypertonic.

osteoarthritis (OA) A degenerative condition that affects joints, leading to damage of the cartilage in joints that normally provide smooth surfaces for joint movement.

osteophytosis The development of bony outgrowths, usually along joints, particularly of the spine; also referred to as bone spurs.

osteoporosis A loss of normal bone density with thinning of bone tissue and the growth of small holes in the bone. The disorder may cause pain (especially in the lower back), frequent broken bones, loss of body height, and various poorly formed parts of the body. Commonly a part of the normal aging process.

outer perimeter The geographic boundary that defines the "safe zone" where no threat should exist at a hazardous incident.

overpressure phenomenon The sudden increase in atmospheric pressure or shock wave that occurs in proximity to the detonation of a high explosive.

oxygenation The process of providing, treating, or enriching with oxygen.

paradoxical pulse A condition in which the patient's systolic blood pressure drops more than 10 to 15 mm Hg during each inspiration, usually due to the effect of increased intrathoracic pressure such as would occur with tension pneumothorax or from pericardial tamponade.

parasympathetic nervous system The division of the nervous system that maintains normal body functions.

parietal pleura A thin membrane that lines the inner side of the thoracic cavity.

partial thickness burns Burns that involve the epidermis and part of the dermis layer of skin.

passive strategy In injury prevention, a prevention method that requires no action on the part of the individual; e.g., vehicle air bags.

patent Open and clear.

patient care report (PCR) The written report documenting the prehospital care provided to a patient; includes the history, assessment, prehospital interventions, reassessment, and patient response to treatment.

peak overpressure value The maximum value of pressure experienced at a given location at the moment a blast wave from a high explosive reaches the location.

Pediatric Assessment Triangle (PAT) A rapid assessment tool of pediatric patients utilized at the first point of contact; prehospital care providers assess the patient's appearance, work of breathing, and circulation to the skin.

pelvic ring The round shape that comprises the pelvis; made up of the ilium, ischium, pubis, sacrum, and coccyx; also referred to as the pelvic girdle.

penetrating trauma Trauma that results when an object penetrates the skin and injures underlying structures. Generally produces both permanent and temporary cavities.

percutaneous Occurring through the skin; e.g., a needlestick.

pericardial effusion An abnormal build-up of excess fluid between the heart and the sac surrounding the heart, known as the pericardium.

pericardiocentesis A procedure that involves insertion of a needle into the pericardial space to remove accumulated blood or fluid.

peripheral chemoreceptors Carotid and aortic bodies that detect any changes in arterial blood oxygen and initiate reflexes that are important for maintaining homeostasis during hypoxemia.

peritoneal cavity The space in the anterior abdominal cavity that contains the bowel, spleen, liver, stomach, and gallbladder. The peritoneal space is covered by the peritoneum.

peritonitis Inflammation of the peritoneum.

pharynx The throat; a tubelike structure that is a passage for both the breathing and digestive tracts. Oropharynx—area of the pharynx posterior to the mouth; nasopharynx—area of the pharynx beyond the posterior nares of the nose.

physiologic reserve The excess functional capacity of an organ or organ system.

physiologic thermoregulation The process by which the body's temperature is controlled; involves dilation and constriction of blood vessels to help remove or conserve body heat.

pia mater A thin vascular membrane closely adhering to the brain and spinal cord and proximal portions of the nerves; the innermost of the three meningeal membranes that cover the brain.

planning section The ICS section responsible for the collection and evaluation of information related to the incident.

planning section chief The ICS position responsible for collecting and evaluating information and assisting in planning with the incident commander.

pneumothorax An injury that results in air in the pleural space; commonly producing a collapsed lung. A pneumothorax can be open, with an opening through the chest wall to the outside, or closed, resulting from blunt trauma or a spontaneous collapse.

polypharmacy A term used to describe patients taking more than five medications.

positive end-expiratory pressure (PEEP) The pressure in the lungs above atmospheric pressure at the end of expiration; also refers to a ventilatory technique to assist breathing in which an increased amount of pressure is applied to the lungs at the end of expiration to increase the amount of air remaining in the lungs and enhance gas exchange.

post-event phase The trauma care phase relating to the outcome of the traumatic event.

posttraumatic endophthalmitis Infection of the intraocular contents, usually as a result of penetrating trauma to the eye.

posttraumatic stress disorder (PTSD) A mental health condition that results from exposure to a horrific or terrifying event and leads to flashbacks to the incident, nightmares, anxiety, and uncontrollable thoughts about the incident.

powered air-purifying respirator (PAPR) A protective respiratory device that draws ambient air through a filter canister and delivers it under positive pressure to a face mask or hood.

preference The manner in which the principle of care is achieved in the time given and by the prehospital care provider available.

pre-event phase The trauma care phase relating to the circumstances leading up to an injury.

preload The volume and pressure of the blood coming into the heart from the systemic circulatory system (venous return).

preparedness A step of comprehensive emergency management that involves identifying, in advance of an incident, the specific supplies, equipment, and personnel that would be needed to manage an incident, as well as the specific action plan that would be taken if an incident were to occur.

presbycusis A condition characterized by a gradual decline in hearing.

primary contamination Exposure to a hazardous substance at its point of release.

primary hypothermia A decrease in body temperature that occurs when healthy individuals are unprepared for overwhelming acute or chronic cold exposure.

principle An element that must be present, accomplished, or ensured by the health care provider in order to optimize patient survival and outcome; also refers to the four ethical concepts of autonomy, nonmaleficence, beneficence, and justice.

principlism The use of the four ethical principles of autonomy, nonmaleficence, beneficence, and justice, which provide a framework for one to weigh and balance the benefits and burdens of treating a specific patient in order to do what is in the patient's best interest.

privacy The right of patients to control who has access to their personal health information.

prodrome (predisaster) phase The phase in the disaster cycle in which a specific event has been identified as inevitably going to occur and in which specific steps can be taken to mitigate the effects of the ensuing events.

profile A penetrating object's initial size and the degree of change in size that occurs at the time of impact.

public information officer (PIO) The incident command structure (ICS) command staff officer responsible for interacting with the public and media and distributing information.

pulmonary contusion A bruising of the lungs; can be secondary to blunt or penetrating trauma.

pulseless electrical activity A condition characterized by organized electrical activity on cardiac monitoring without an associated palpable pulse.

pulse oximeter A device that measures arterial oxyhemoglobin saturation. The value is determined by measuring the absorption ratio of red and infrared light passed through the tissue.

pulse pressure (1) The increase in pressure (surge) that is created as each new bolus of blood leaves the left ventricle with each contraction; (2) the difference between the systolic and diastolic blood pressures (systolic pressure minus diastolic pressure equals pulse pressure).

quiescent period A state or period of inactivity or dormancy.

radiation The direct transfer of energy from a warm object to a cooler one by infrared radiation.

radiological dispersal device (RDD) This device uses a conventional explosion to disperse radioactive material without a nuclear detonation.

Rapid and Remote Assessment Methodology (RAM) An assessment algorithm utilized to maximize the opportunity to extract and treat a salvageable casualty while minimizing risk to tactical emergency medical service providers.

rapid-sequence intubation (RSI) A technique of medication-assisted intubation that utilizes sedative medications and a fast-acting paralytic agent to render the patient unconscious and unresponsive to minimize the period of risk of aspiration.

rebound tenderness A physical examination finding that occurs by pressing deeply on the abdomen and then quickly releasing the pressure, causing more severe pain when the abdominal pressure is suddenly released.

recovery or reconstruction phase The period during the disaster cycle that addresses the community's resources to endure, emerge, and rebuild from the effects of the disaster through the coordinated efforts of the medical, public health, and community infrastructure (physical and political); this period is usually the longest, lasting months, and perhaps years, before a community fully recovers.

remote assessment A process by which tactical operators and providers gather information without revealing their position or intent to the hostile force; includes remote observation with binoculars, remote acoustic surveillance, and thermal imaging.

rescue, emergency, or relief phase The period during the disaster cycle immediately following the impact, during which response occurs and appropriate management and intervention can save lives.

resource management Agreements and procedures that enable local, state, and federal agencies to work together under one command during a large-scale incident.

respiration The total ventilatory and circulatory processes involved in the exchange of oxygen and carbon dioxide between the outside atmosphere and the cells of the body. Sometimes in medicine limited to meaning breathing and the steps in ventilation.

reticular activating system The central nervous system control center responsible for maintaining the level of consciousness and alertness.

retroperitoneal space The space in the posterior abdominal cavity that contains the kidneys, ureters, bladder, reproductive organs, inferior vena cava, abdominal aorta, pancreas, a portion of the duodenum, colon, and rectum.

rhabdomyolysis The breakdown of muscle tissue with the release of intracellular muscle components into the circulation.

rheumatoid arthritis (RA) An inflammatory disorder caused by an autoimmune response; can lead to joint swelling and deformity.

rifling Grooves on the inside of the barrel that spin a single missile (bullet) in a stable flight pattern toward the target.

rigor mortis The temporary stiffening and rigidity of muscles and joints that occurs after death; typically begins within 2 to 4 hours of death and lasts approximately 36 to 48 hours.

riot control agents A chemical agent used to rapidly and briefly disable those exposed to it by causing irritation to the skin, mucous membranes, lungs, and eyes.

sacrum Part of the spinal column below the lumbar spine containing the five sacral vertebrae (S1–S5), which are connected by immovable joints to form the sacrum. The sacrum is the weight-bearing base of the spinal column and is also a part of the pelvic girdle.

safety officer The incident command structure (ICS) command staff officer who is responsible for monitoring, assessing, and ensuring the safety of emergency personnel.

SAMPLER history A mnemonic to remember the components of the history; stands for symptoms, allergies, medication, past medical and surgical history, last meal, and events leading up to the injury.

sclera The dense, fibrous, white outer layer of the eyeball.

secondary contamination Exposure to a hazardous substance after it has been carried away from the point of origin by a victim, a responder, or a piece of equipment.

secondary hypothermia A decrease in body temperature as a consequence of a patient's systemic disorder, including hypothyroidism, hypoadrenalism, trauma, carcinoma, and sepsis.

second-degree frostbite A freezing injury due to cold exposure that involves the epidermis and superficial dermis; initially appears similar to first-degree injury, but frozen tissues are deeper; after thawing, results in superficial skin blisters surrounded by erythema and edema; there is no permanent loss of tissue; healing occurs in 3 to 4 weeks.

second phase of death Deaths from traumatic injury that occur within minutes to a few hours after the injury.

self-aid/buddy aid (SA/BA) A first-aid procedure employed to help save oneself or save other service personnel's lives. For example, self-application of a tourniquet to a life-threatening injury.

self-contained breathing apparatus (SCBA) A personal protective device consisting of a mask and portable supply of air, used in environments that are oxygen-deficient or pose a risk of toxic inhalation.

self-contained underwater breathing apparatus (SCUBA) A portable breathing device for underwater use, consisting of a mask with tubes connecting to a tank of compressed air.

senescence The process of aging.

sepsis Infection that has spread to involve the entire body.

sequelae Aftereffects or complications of a disease or injury.

shear Change-of-speed force resulting in a cutting or tearing of body parts.

shear force Energy applied to the body that tends to move an organ or part of the body in one direction while the adjacent part moves in a different direction or remains fixed in place.

shear wave See *shear force*.

shock front The boundary between the blast overpressure wave created by a high explosive detonation and normal atmospheric pressure.

shock index (SI) The ratio between heart rate and systolic blood pressure.

shock wave See *shock front*.

simple pneumothorax The presence of air within the pleural space.

simulations A form of training that involves the imitation, enactment, or representation, verbally or with models, of the management of an incident or patient.

single command A command structure in which a single individual is responsible for all of the strategic objectives of the incident. Typically used when an incident is within a single jurisdiction and is managed by a single discipline.

single-system trauma patient A patient who has experienced trauma that involves injury to only one body system.

sniffing position A slightly superior anterior position of the head and neck to optimize ventilation as well as the view during endotracheal intubation.

solar keratitis Burns to the cornea of the eye that result from exposure to ultraviolet light, commonly as a result of reflection off of snow; also referred to as snow blindness.

solid density Tissue density consistent with bone.

span of control In an incident command system, the number of subordinates who report to one supervisor at any level within the response organization; in most situations, one person can effectively supervise only three to seven people or resources.

spinal shock An injury to the spinal cord that results in a temporary loss of sensory and motor function.

spinal stenosis Narrowing of the spinal canal.

spinous process The tail-like structure on the posterior region of the vertebrae.

sprain An acute soft tissue injury of the ligaments within a joint caused by an injury that stresses a joint and overstretches or even ruptures supporting ligaments.

spray The dispersal pattern of pellets fired from a shotgun.

spread See *spray*.

staging area A predetermined area where resources, equipment, and personnel can be located safely and at the ready for assignment.

START triage algorithm A method of evaluating patients and assigning priority for treatment and transport during a mass-casualty incident; involves evaluating the respiratory status, perfusion status, and mental status of the patient.

status epilepticus A life-threatening condition in which a seizure persists for greater than 5 minutes or in which two or more seizures occur without a period of wakening in between.

stellate (starburst) wound A star-shaped wound.

stipple Multiple small dots resulting from gunpowder from point-blank gunshot wounds.

stopping distance The distance over which a moving object comes to a stop; a measure of how quickly energy is dissipated or transferred.

stress wave A supersonic, longitudinal pressure wave that (1) creates high local forces with small, rapid distortions; (2) produces microvascular injury; and (3) is reinforced and reflected at tissue interfaces, thereby enhancing injury potential, especially in gas-filled organs such as the lungs, ears, and intestines.

stroke volume The volume of blood pumped out by each contraction (stroke) of the left ventricle.

subarachnoid hematoma A collection of blood in the cerebrospinal fluid-filled space beneath the arachnoid membrane.

subarachnoid hemorrhage (SAH) Bleeding into the cerebrospinal fluid-filled space beneath the arachnoid membrane.

subconjunctival hemorrhage Bleeding found between the clear conjunctiva covering the eye and the white sclera.

subcutaneous emphysema Accumulation of air in the soft tissues of the body.

subdermal burn A burn injury that involves all layers of the skin, as well as the underlying fat, muscles, bone, or internal organs.

subdural hematoma A collection of blood between the dura mater and the arachnoid membrane.

sublimation A process in which solids emit vapors, bypassing the liquid state.

subluxation A partial or incomplete dislocation.

sulfur mustard An oily, clear to yellow-brown liquid that can be aerosolized by a bomb blast or a sprayer; a vesicant or blister agent used as a weapon of mass destruction.

superficial burn A burn to the epidermis only; red, inflamed, and painful skin.

superficial frostbite A freezing injury due to cold exposure that affects the skin and subcutaneous tissues, resulting in clear blisters when rewarmed.

superior vena cava A major vein that carries deoxygenated blood from the upper portion of the body back to the heart.

supplied air respirator (SAR) A personal protective device consisting of a mask and source of air that is not carried by the responder; used in environments that are oxygen-deficient or pose a risk of toxic inhalation.

supraglottic airway (SGA) An airway device inserted blindly into the mouth and pharynx; designed to isolate the trachea from the esophagus; none of these devices provides a complete seal of the trachea, so the risk of aspiration is lowered but not completely prevented.

surgical cricothyrotomy A procedure to open a patient's airway that is accomplished by making an incision into the cricothyroid membrane in the neck to open the airway into the trachea.

surveillance The process of collecting data within a community, usually for infectious diseases.

suspension syndrome A cascade of events that ultimately culminates as a state of shock caused by blood pooling in dependent lower extremities while the body is held upright without any movement for a prolonged time.

sympathetic nervous system division of the nervous system that produces the fight-or-flight response.

systemic vascular resistance The amount of resistance to the flow of blood through the vessels. It increases as the vessel constricts. Any change in lumen diameter or vessel elasticity can influence the amount of resistance.

systole A rhythmically recurrent contraction of the heart, during which some chambers of the heart muscle contract after refilling with blood.

tachypnea An increased breathing rate.

tactical casualty care (TCC) The emergency medical care provided in a hazardous or tactical situation.

tactical emergency medical support (TEMS) An out-of-hospital system of care dedicated to enhancing the probability of special operations law enforcement mission success, reducing mission medical liability and risk, and promoting public safety.

tactical evacuation care The phase of care in tactical casualty care in which medical care is provided once the threat or hazard has been completely addressed, similar to a conventional emergency medical services (EMS) situation; also referred to as evacuation care.

tactical field care The phase of care in tactical casualty care in which medical care is provided when the threat or hazard has been contained but could resume; also referred to as indirect threat care.

tamponade The closure or blockage of a wound or blood vessel; also, the compression of the heart by the accumulation of blood or fluid in the pericardium.

tendon A band of tough, inelastic, fibrous tissue that connects a muscle to bone.

tension pneumothorax A condition in which the air pressure in the pleural space exceeds the outside atmospheric pressure and cannot escape, the affected side becomes hyperinflated, compressing the lung on the involved side and shifting the mediastinum to the opposite side to partially collapse the other lung; usually progressive and is an imminently life-threatening condition.

tentorium cerebelli An infolding of the dura that forms a covering over the cerebellum. The tentorium is a part of the floor of the upper skull just below the brain (cerebrum).

thermal equilibrium The transfer of heat from a warmer object to a colder object in an effort to create the same temperature between them.

thermal gradient The difference in temperature (high vs. low temperature) between two objects.

thermite An incendiary compound that consists of powdered aluminum and iron oxide that burns furiously at 3,600°F (1,982°C) and scatters molten iron.

thermoregulatory center The area of the brain (hypothalamus) that controls body temperature.

third-degree frostbite A freezing injury due to cold exposure that involves the epidermis and dermis layers; skin is frozen with restricted mobility; after tissue thaws, skin swells and develops blood-filled blisters (hemorrhagic bullae), indicating vascular trauma to deep tissues; skin loss occurs slowly, leading to mummification and sloughing; healing is slow.

third phase of death Deaths from traumatic injury that occur several days or weeks after the initial injury; most often caused by sepsis and organ failure.

tidal volume (V_t) The normal volume of air exchanged with each ventilation. About 500 ml of air is exchanged between the lungs and the atmosphere with each breath in a healthy adult at rest.

total lung capacity (TLC) The total volume of air in the lungs after a forced inhalation.

toxidrome A collection of clinical signs and symptoms that suggest exposure to a certain class of chemical or toxin.

tracheal deviation A clinical sign that indicates change in the position of the trachea away from its normal position in the midline to one side resulting from unequal intrathoracic pressure within the chest cavity.

transesophageal echocardiography A technique of performing ultrasound of the heart using an ultrasound probe inserted into the esophagus.

transmission-based PPE The personal protective equipment used, in addition to standard precautions, to prevent transmission of disease; includes aerosol, contact, and droplet precautions.

transmural pressure The pressure gradient across the vessel wall and is affected by intralymphatic as well as extralymphatic forces.

transverse processes A protuberance at each side of a vertebra near the lateral margins.

trauma chin lift A maneuver used to relieve a variety of anatomic airway obstructions in patients who are breathing spontaneously; accomplished by grasping the chin and lower incisors and then lifting to pull the mandible forward.

trauma jaw thrust A maneuver that allows opening of the airway with little or no movement of the head and cervical spine; the mandible is thrust forward by placing the thumbs on each zygomatic arch and placing the index and long fingers under the mandible and at the same angle, thrusting the mandible forward.

traumatic asphyxia Blunt and crushing injuries to the chest and abdomen with marked increase of intravascular pressure, producing rupture of the capillaries; characterized by a purplish discoloration of the skin of the upper torso and face along with petechiae of the skin.

trench foot A nonfreezing cold exposure injury caused by prolonged immersion of extremities in wet and moisture that is cool to cold; also referred to as immersion foot.

triage French word meaning "to sort"; a process in which a group of patients is sorted according to their priority of need for care. When only several patients are involved, triage involves assessing each patient, meeting all of the patients' highest priority needs first, and then moving to lower priority items. In a mass-casualty incident with a large number of patients involved, triage is done by determining both urgency and potential for survival.

triage officer An individual trained to oversee the process of assigning injury severity categories and prioritization of treatment and transport.

tumble An end-over-end motion. Bullets commonly tumble when resistance is met by the leading edge of the missile.

unified command An ICS command structure in which the incident commanders of all the various agencies responding to an event work together to manage the incident.

unintentional injury An injury that was unplanned and did not involve intent to harm.

units An individual thing or person regarded as single and complete but is also part of a whole or group.

unity of command An incident command system management concept in which each responder has only one direct supervisor.

vapor A solid or liquid in a gaseous state, usually visible as a fine cloud or mist.

vertebral foramen Hole or opening in the bony structure of the vertebrae through which blood vessels and nerves pass.

very high altitude Elevation levels between 11,480 and 18,045 feet (3,500 and 5,500 meters).

vesicant A chemical agent such as sulfur mustard and lewisite used as a weapon of mass destruction; also referred to as blister agent because these agents create an injury that is visually similar to a burn.

vestibular folds The false vocal cords that direct airflow through the vocal cords.

vestibular nuclei The areas of the brain from which the vestibular nerves responsible for balance arise.

viral hemorrhagic fever (VHF) A clinical syndrome caused by several different viruses; typified by the clinical presentation of fever, malaise, and hemorrhagic symptoms.

viscera The internal organs of the body.

visceral pleura A thin membrane that covers the outer surface of each lung.

volatility The likelihood that solids or liquids will vaporize into a gaseous form at room temperature.

voluntary guarding An assessment finding in which the patient tenses the abdominal muscles when the practitioner palpates a tender area of the abdomen.

warning phase The last instructions, notices, and reminders that are communicated to people before the chaos and confusion of a disaster or emergency springs forth.

water density Organs that have a tissue density similar to that of water; e.g., liver, spleen, muscle.

weapons of mass destruction (WMD) A chemical, biologic, radiologic, or explosive agent designed to create significant damage and large numbers of casualties.

white blood cells (WBCs) Nearly colorless blood cells in the circulation responsible for responding to invading microorganisms.

white phosphorus An incendiary agent used in the production of munitions.

work of breathing The physical work or effort performed in moving the chest wall and diaphragm to breathe.

years of potential life lost (YPLL) An estimate of the impact of an injury calculated by subtracting age at death from a fixed age of the group under examination, usually 65 or 70 years, or the life expectancy of the group.

zone of coagulation The region of greatest tissue destruction in a full-thickness burn; the tissue in this zone is necrotic (dead) and is not capable of tissue repair.

zone of hyperemia The outermost zone in a full-thickness burn; it has minimal cellular injury and is characterized by increased blood flow secondary to an inflammatory reaction initiated by the burn injury.

zone of stasis The region next to the zone of coagulation; blood flow to this region is stagnant, and the cells in this zone are injured, but not irreversibly. If they are subsequently deprived of the delivery of oxygen or blood flow, these viable cells will die and become necrotic. Timely and appropriate burn care will preserve blood flow and oxygen delivery to these injured cells.

Index

anhidrosis, 616
anisocoria, 290
antecubital fossa, 478
anterior cord syndrome, 312
anthrax, 586–588
antihistamines, 722
apneic, 178
apneic oxygenation during
    intubation, 231*b*
appendicular skeleton, 406
APR. *See* air-purifying respirator
APRN. *See* Advanced Practice
    Registered Nurse
arachnoid mater, 271
ARDS. *See* acute respiratory distress
    syndrome
arginine vasopressin (AVP), 618
arterial gas embolism, 674
  arterial gas embolism, assessment of, 676
arteriography, 482
ascending nerve tracts, 309
asphyxiant toxidrome, 579
aspiration pneumonitis, 496
assist control (A/C) ventilation, 240
ataxic breathing, 280
atelectasis, 359
atherosclerosis, 497
athletes, heart rate, 70–71
atlas, 308
ATLS. *See* Advanced Trauma Life Support
ATN. *See* acute tubular necrosis
atropine, 581
austere environment, 544
automated external defibrillator
    (AED), 641
autonomic nervous system, 58
autonomy, 32
autoregulation, 273–274
AVP. *See* arginine vasopressin
AVPU scale (Alert, responds to Verbal
    stimulus, responds to Painful
    stimulus, Unresponsive),
    182*b*, 473
axial loading, 311
axis, 308

B
back, secondary survey, 191
backboard debate, 323–324
bag-mask ventilation, 239, 253–254
baroreceptors, 356
barotrauma, 672–675
  of ascent, 673–674
    alternobaric vertigo, 673
    gastrointestinal squeeze, 673
    pulmonary overinflation
      barotrauma, 673–674

decompression sickness,
    674–675, 675*b*
  cardiopulmonary, 675
  cutaneous/lymphatic, 675
  limb pain, 675
  spinal cord, 675
of descent, 672–673
  inner-ear barotraumal, 673
  mask squeeze, 672
  middle-ear squeeze, 672
  reverse squeeze, 672–673
  sinus squeeze, 672
  tooth squeeze, 672
basal level, heat and cold transfer, 608
basal metabolic rate, 607
bases, 453
basic patient packaging, principles
    of, 706, 706*f*
basic *vs.* advanced prehospital care
    practitioner levels, 187
basilar skull fractures, 292
behavioral regulation, 607
beneficence, 32
benzodiazepine therapy, 581
beta particles, 593
biologic agents, 583–592, 583*b*
  concentrated biohazard agent *vs.*
    infected patient, 584–586,
    584–586*b*
  selected agents, 586–592, 587*t*,
    589–590*f*, 589*b*
bites/stings, 721–726, 722–725*f*, 722*b*
blast injuries, 141–144, 391–392
  explosion-related injuries, 141, 142,
    143*t*, 144*f*
  injury from fragments, 142–143
  interaction with body, 142
  multi-etiology injury, 143–144
  physics of, 141–142, 142*f*
blast lung injury (BLI), 575*b*
blast overpressure, 141
blast wave, 141, 572, 573*b*
blast wind, 142, 573*b*, 574
bleeding, 177*b*, 179–181
BLI. *See* blast lung injury
blind nasotracheal intubation
    (BNTI), 228
blocking/decorporation therapy, 597
blood, 54, 57–58, 57*f*
  volume resuscitation, 80
blood pressure, 69–70
blood vessels, 56–57, 56*f*
bloodborne pathogens, 163–167
  hand washing, 166
  hepatitis, 164, 164*b*
  human immunodeficiency virus,
    164–165, 165*b*

occupational exposure management,
    166–167
physical barriers, 165–166
  eye protection, 165
  face shields, 165
  gloves, 165, 166*f*
  gowns, 166
  masks, 165
  resuscitation equipment, 166
  sharp injury prevention, 166, 167*b*
  standard precautions, 165
Blue Star of Life, 6
blunt cardiac injury, 368–369, 368*f*
blunt force injury, 357, 357*f*
blunt trauma, 111–131, 315,
    390–391, 391*b*
  defined, 109
  falls, 125–126
  motor vehicle crashes, 113–122
    frontal impact, 113–116
    lateral-impact, 117–118, 117–118*f*
    occupant protective and restraining
      systems, 120–122
    rear-impact, 116–117, 116*f*
    rollover, 118, 119*f*
    rotational-impact, 118, 119*f*
    types of, 113
    vehicle incompatibility, 118–119
  motorcycle crashes, 122–123
    angular impact, 122, 123*f*
    ejection impact, 122
    head-on impact, 122, 122*f*
    injury prevention, 122–123, 123*f*
  pedestrian injuries, 124–125, 124–125*f*
  regional effects of, 127–131
    abdomen, 130–131, 130–131*f*
    head, 127–128, 127–128*f*
    neck, 128, 128*f*
    thorax, 128–130, 129*f*
  sports injuries, 126–127
BNTI. *See* blind nasotracheal intubation
board device, immobilization of torso to,
    322–323, 322–323*f*
botulinum toxin, 591–592
Boyle's law, 671, 671*f*, 681
bradycardia, 231
bradypnea, 178
brain
  injury, 70. *See also* traumatic brain
    injury (TBI)
  regions of, 272, 273*t*
brain stem, 271
breathing, 469–471, 470*t*, 477, 506
  shock management, 76–77
breathing management, 741–742, 742*b*
British Sleep Society, 531
bronchioles, 208

Combat Application Tourniquet (C-A-T), 95–98
Combat Gauze, 75
Combat Ready Clamp (CRoC), 177b
command structure, 160–163
  incident command system, 160–161
  incident commander, 161–163, 162f
  National Incident Management System, 161
  unified command system, 161
commission, 200
Committee on Tactical Combat Casualty Care (CoTCCC), 28, 177b
common terminology, 547
commotio cordis, 370–371
compartment syndrome, 409, 419
competence, 32
complete cord transection, 312
completing stabilization, 327–328
comprehensive emergency management, 541
compressibility, 126
compression, 112
compression injuries, 389
concentrated biohazard agent vs. infected patient, 584–585, 584–585b
  aerosol precautions, 585, 586b
  contact precautions, 585
  droplet precautions, 585
conduction, heat and cold transfer, 608
confidentiality, 33
conjunctiva, 293
consolidated incident action plans, 547–548
contact burns, 451–452
contact freeze injury, 627, 628b
contact wounds, 140
CONTOMS course. See Counter Narcotics and Terrorism Operational Medical Support course
control zones, 570
convection, heat and cold transfer, 608
COPD. See chronic obstructive pulmonary disease
coral snakes, 723, 723f
cord compression, 312
cord concussion, 312
cord contusion, 312
cord laceration, 312
core temperature, 607
cornea, 293
corneal abrasion, 293
CoTCCC. See Committee on Tactical Combat Casualty Care

Counter Narcotics and Terrorism Operational Medical Support (CONTOMS) course, 736
coup-contrecoup injury, 278
COVID-19 pandemic, 500, 550, 566, 583
Cowley, R. Adams, 33
CPP. See cerebral perfusion pressure
cranial vault, 271
crepitus, 290
crime scenes, 155–156, 155f
critical incident stress management (CISM), 557
critical multisystem trauma patient, 418
critical thinking, 29–31
  assessment steps, 30b
  components of, 29b
  for controling biases, 29–30
  in data analysis, 31
  in patient care, 31
  in rapid decision making, 30
critical trauma patient, 186b
CRoC. See Combat Ready Clamp
crush syndrome, 421–423, 422
CSF. See cerebrospinal fluid
CUFT. See care under fire/threat
Cullen sign, 393
Curry, George J., 5
cushing reflex, 280–281
cyanosis, 357

D

DAN. See Divers Alert Network
data analysis, 31
dead space, 355
debridement, 416, 435
decerebrate posturing, 280
decomposition, 720
decompression sickness, assessment of, 676
decontamination, 158
decontamination, principles of, 571
decorticate posturing, 280
decubitus, 507
deep frostbite, 631
delayed primary closure, 719
delayed-sequence intubation (DSI), 229
delirium, 498
dementia, 498
denuded, 435
dependent lividity, 720
dermatome, 310
dermis, 433
descending nerve tracts, 309
designated incident facilities, 548
detailed physical examination, definition of, 704
devastating neurologic injury, 661

diaphragm, 211
diaphragmatic rupture, 375–376, 376f
diaphyseal, 482
diastole, 54
dilutional hyponatremia, 615
direct threat care, 738–740
disability, 181–183, 473, 474t
  and shock, 77
disaster cycle, 540–544, 541f
  comprehensive emergency management, 541–542
  personal preparedness, 542–544, 542–544b
disaster education/training, 557–558, 558b
disaster management
  cycle, 540–544, 541f
    comprehensive emergency management, 541–542
    personal preparedness, 542–544, 542–544b
  education and training, 557–558, 558b
  mass-casualty incident management, 544–550
    incident command system, 545–548, 545f
    national incident management system, 545
    organization of the incident command system, 548–550, 548f
  medical response, 550–556, 550b
    decontamination, 555–556, 555f
    initial response, 550–551, 551f
    mass destruction, threat of terrorism and weapons of, 544, 555f
    medical assistance teams, 554, 554f
    search and rescue, 551
    transport, 553–554
    treatment, 553
    treatment area, 556
    triage, 551–553, 553f
  psychological response, 556–557
    disasters that affect mental health, characteristics of, 556
    emergency responder stress, 556–557, 557f
    factors impacting psychological response, 556
    interventions, 556
    psychological sequelae of disasters, 556
  response, common pitfalls of, 558–560
    communications, 559
    failure to notify hospitals, 560
    media, 560
    preparedness, 558–559
    scene security, 559

environmental trauma (*continued*)
environment, 623–624, 624*t*
fitness, 624–625
heat acclimatization, 625–626,
626–627*b*
hydration, 624, 625*b*
high-altitude illness, 681–688
acute mountain sickness, 684
epidemiology, 681–682
factors related to, 682–684, 683*t*
high-altitude cerebral edema,
684–686, 685–686*t*
high-altitude pulmonary edema,
686–687
hypobaric hypoxia, 682, 682*t*
prevention, 687–688, 687*b*
lightning-related injuries,
654–660, 654*f*
assessment, 657–658, 658*f*
epidemiology, 654
lightning, injuries from,
655–657, 655*t*
management, 658
mechanism of injury, 654–655
prevention, 658–660, 659–660*b*
physiology, 607–609
homeostasis, 609
thermoregulation/temperature
balance, 607–609, 608*f*
prevention of, 643–644, 644*f*
prolonged transport, 644–646
cold-related illness, 646
heat-related illness, 645
prolonged transport, 688–689
drowning, 688
high-altitude illness, 689
lightning injury, 688
recreational scuba-related diving
injuries, 689
recreational scuba-related injuries,
669–681
AGE and DCS, assessment of,
675–676
barotrauma, 672–675, 675*b*
epidemiology, 670
management, 676–677, 676–677*b*,
678–679*t*
mechanical effects of pressure,
670–671, 671*t*, 671*f*
scuba-related diving injuries,
prevention of, 677–681,
680–681*b*
epidemiological triad, 517, 517*f*
epidermis, 433
epidural hematoma, 271, 276, 276*f*
epidural space, 271
epiglottis, 208

epinephrine, 59, 722
epiphyseal, 482
equity, 528
erythema, 715
eschar, 435
escharotomy, 439
esophagus, 208
ET tube. *See* endotracheal tube
ethics
principles, 31–33
confidentiality, 33
informed consent, 32–33
privacy, 33
truth telling, 33
eucapnic state, 77
euhydration, 610
evacuation care, 746, 746*f*
evaporation, heat and cold
transfer, 608
event phase, in trauma care, 12–13
everyday applicability, 547
Everyone Poops, 710
evisceration, 398, 398*f*
exercise-associated collapse, 614
exercise-associated hyponatremia
(EAH), 617–619, 619*b*,
620*f*, 645
exercise-associated hyponatremic
encephalopathy (EAHE), 618
exercise-associated muscle (heat)
cramps, 611, 613
exertional heatstroke (EHS), 161*b*, 616
expanding bullets, 132*b*
explosion-related injuries, 142,
143*t*, 144*f*
explosions, explosives/incendiary agents,
572–577
categories of, 572–573, 573*b*
evaluation and management, 576
incendiary agents, 577
injury from, 141
injury patterns, 574–576, 576*b*
mechanisms of injury, 573–574, 575*b*
transport considerations, 576–577
explosives, categories of, 572–573
high explosives, 572, 573*b*
low explosives, 573
expose/environment, 183–184, 473
exsanguinating hemorrhage, 176, 291,
291*f*, 506
assessment, 65–66
management, 72–76, 72*f*
direct pressure, 72–73
elevation and pressure points, 76
hemostatic agents, 75–76, 75*f*
junctional hemorrhage, 76, 76*f*
tourniquets, 73–75, 74*f*

extended focused assessment with
sonography in trauma
(eFAST), 358
extracellular fluid, 57
extracranial causes, of secondary brain
injury, 282–285
anemia, 283
coagulopathy, 283–284, 284*t*
hypercapnia, 284
hyperglycemia, 284–285
hyperoxia, 283
hypocapnia, 284
hypoglycemia, 284–285
hypotension, 282–283
hypoxia, 283
seizures, 285
extramural (extraluminal) pressure, 73
extreme altitude, 682
extremities
penetrating trauma, regional effects of,
138, 139*f*
secondary survey, 191
trauma, 482–483
eye protection, 165, 715
eyelid lacerations, 292–293

F

face shields, 165
face-to-face intubation, 228
face-to-face orotracheal intubation,
262–263
facial injuries, 292–295
mandibular fractures, 294–295
midface fractures, 294, 294*f*
nasal fractures, 294
orbit and eye, 292–294, 293*f*
falls, 125–126
Farrington, J. D., 5
fascia, 419
fasciotomy, 419
Federal Emergency Management
Agency (FEMA), 544
FEMA. *See* Federal Emergency
Management Agency
femur fractures, traction splint for,
427–429
Fick principle, 52–53, 53*f*
field exercises, 558
first-degree frostbite, 630–631
first phase of death, 702
flail chest, 359–360, 360*f*
flail sternum, 369
"flash-to-bang" rule, 659–660
fluid administration, 433
fluid resuscitation, 444–446, 444*b*
fluid therapy, 186, 479
fontanelles, 270

food and water needs, 713
FOP. *See* Fraternal Order of Police
foramen magnum, 270
foramina, 270
fourth-degree frostbite, 631
fracture, internal hemorrhage, 77
fragmentation, 132–133, 133*f*
Fraternal Order of Police (FOP), 161
freezing cold injury, 630–632, 631*f*
frontal impact, motor vehicle crashes, 113–116
  down-and-under path, 114–116, 115–116*f*
  up-and-over path, 114, 114*f*
frostbite, 627, 646
frostnip, 627–628
full thickness, 434–435
function and cosmesis, restoration of, 718–719

G

galea aponeurotica, 270
Gallagher, Susan Scavo, 517
gamma rays, 593–594
gastrointestinal anthrax, 586
gastrointestinal tract, penetrating trauma, 138
GCS. *See* Glasgow Coma Scale
genitalia, secondary survey, 191
genitourinary injuries, 401–402
geriatric trauma
  aging, anatomy and physiology of, 494–500, 494*f*
    cardiovascular system, 497
    chronic medical problems, influence of, 495, 495–496*t*, 495*b*
    ears, nose, and throat, 495–496
    musculoskeletal system, 499–500, 499*f*
    nervous system, 497–498
    nutrition/immune system, 500
    renal system, 498–499
    respiratory system, 496–497, 496*f*
    sensory changes, 498, 498*b*
    skin, 500
  assessment, 500–505
    physics of trauma, 500–501, 501*b*
    primary survey, 501–502
    secondary survey, 502–505, 505*f*
  disposition, 509
  elder maltreatment, 508–509
    elder abuse, COVID-19 impact on, 508
    important points, 509, 509*b*
    maltreatment, categories of, 508, 508*f*
  legal considerations, 507–508
    reporting elder abuse, 507–508

management, 506–507
  airway, 506
  breathing, 506
  circulation, 506
  exsanguinating hemorrhage, 506
  immobilization, 506–507, 507*f*
  temperature control, 507
prevention, 510
prolonged transport, 509
GFR. *See* glomerular filtration rate
Glasgow Coma Scale (GCS), 5, 182–183, 182*f*, 466, 473, 487
global positioning system (GPS), 25
glomerular filtration rate (GFR), 498
gloves, 165, 166*f*
Golden Hour, 174
golden principles, 33–34
  of prehospital trauma care, 35–41, 36–37*t*
    accurate communication, 41
    airway management, 38
    bleeding control, 37
    fluid replacement, 40–41
    initiate transport, 40, 40*f*
    pain relief, 41
    physics of trauma, 37–38
    primary survey, 37
    scene safety, 35, 38*f*
    scene situation assessment, 35
    secondary survey, 41
    shock therapy, 39–40
    spinal motion restriction principles, 40
    ventilation and oxygen delivery, 39
gowns, 166
GPS. *See* global positioning system
Grey-Turner sign, 393
group training, 558

H

HACE. *See* high-altitude cerebral edema
Haddon Matrix, 517–518, 519*t*
Haddon, William J., Jr., Dr., 517
hand washing, 166
HAPE. *See* high-altitude pulmonary edema
hazardous materials, 156–157, 156*f*
HBOCs. *See* hemoglobin-based oxygen carriers
head, 127–128
  compression injuries, 127, 127*f*
  maintenance of neutral in-line position of, 324–326, 325*f*, 326*b*
  manual in-line stabilization of, 321
  penetrating trauma, regional effects of, 137, 137–138*f*
  secondary survey, 188–189, 189*f*
  shear injuries, 127–128, 128*f*

head-on impact, motorcycle crashes, 122, 122*f*
head/neck injuries
  cervical vessel injuries, 295–297
    history, 295
    serial examinations, 295
    transport, 295–297, 297*f*
  facial injuries, 292–295
    mandibular fractures, 294–295
    midface fractures, 294, 294*f*
    nasal fractures, 294
    orbit and eye, 292–294, 293*f*
  laryngeal injuries, 295
  scalp injuries, 291–292, 291*f*
  skull fractures, 292, 292*f*
headrests, 117*b*
heart, 54–56, 54–55*f*
heat edema, 611
heat escape lessening posture (HELP), 635
heat exhaustion, 614–615
heat illness, risk factors in, 609–611, 609*b*
  age, 610
  dehydration, 610–611
  medical conditions, 610
  medications, 610
  obesity, fitness/body mass index, 609–610
heat, injuries caused by, 611–619, 612–613*t*
  major heat-related disorders, 614–619, 616*t*, 616*b*, 619*b*, 620*f*
  minor heat-related disorders, 611–614, 613*f*
heat-related illness, 606, 645
  exercise-associated hyponatremia, 645
  heatstroke, 645
  prevention of, 619–627, 621–623*b*
    emergency incident rehabilitation, 627
    environment, 623–624, 624*t*
    fitness, 624–625
    heat acclimatization, 625–626, 626–627*b*
    hydration, 624, 625*b*
heat stress index, 621*f*, 623
heat syncope, 613–614
heatstroke, 615–617, 616*t*, 616*b*, 645
HEAVEN (Hypoxemia, Extremes of size, Anatomic challenge, Vomit/blood/fluid, Exsanguination, Neck) criteria, 227*b*
Heimlich maneuver, 668
HELP. *See* heat escape lessening posture
hematologic failure, 87
hematuria, 401